BURNLEY MACKENZIE
HEALTHCARE LIBRARY
TU05992

Critical Care Obstetrics

Critical Care Obstetrics

EDITED BY

MICHAEL A. BELFORT MBBCH, MD, PhD
Professor of Obstetrics and Gynecology, Department of Obstetrics and Gynecology, University of Utah School of Medicine, Salt Lake City, UT; Director of Perinatal Research, Director of Fetal Therapy, HCA Healthcare, Nashville, TN, USA

GEORGE SAADE MD
Professor of Obstetrics and Gynecology, University of Texas Medical Branch, Galveston, TX, USA

MICHAEL R. FOLEY MD
Chief Medical Officer, Scotsdale Healthcare, Scottsdale, Arizona; Clinical Professor, Department of Obstetrics and Gynecology, University of Arizona College of Medicine, Tucson, AR, USA

JEFFREY P. PHELAN MD, JD
Director of Quality Assurance, Department of Obstetrics and Gynecology, Citrus Valley Medical Center, West Covina; President and Director, Clinical Research, Childbirth Injury Prevention Foundation, City of Industry, Pasadena, CA, USA

GARY A. DILDY, III MD
Director, Maternal-Fetal Medicine, Mountain Star Division, Hospital Corporation of America, Salt Lake City, UT; Clinical Professor, Department of Obstetrics and Gynecology, LSU Health Sciences Center, School of Medicine in New Orleans, New Orleans, LA, USA

FIFTH EDITION

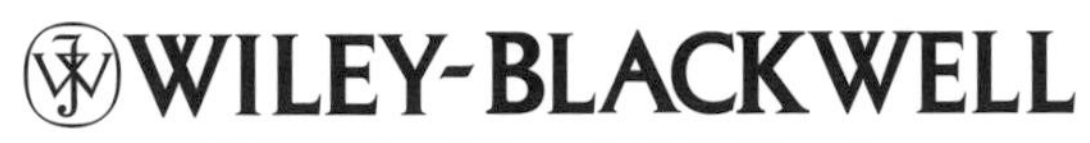

A John Wiley & Sons, Ltd., Publication

Blackwell Publishing was acquired by John Wiley & Sons in February 2007. Blackwell's publishing program has been merged with Wiley's global Scientific, Technical and Medical business to form Wiley-Blackwell.

Registered office: John Wiley & Sons Ltd, The Atrium, Southern Gate, Chichester, West Sussex, PO19 8SQ, UK

Editorial offices: 9600 Garsington Road, Oxford, OX4 2DQ, UK
The Atrium, Southern Gate, Chichester, West Sussex, PO19 8SQ, UK
111 River Street, Hoboken, NJ 07030-5774, USA

For details of our global editorial offices, for customer services and for information about how to apply for permission to reuse the copyright material in this book please see our website at www.wiley.com/wiley-blackwell

Library of Congress Cataloging-in-Publication Data

Evidence-based gastroenterology and hepatology / edited by John W.D. McDonald ... [et al.]. – 3rd ed.
p. ; cm.
Includes bibliographical references and index.
ISBN 978-1-4051-5273-0 (alk. paper)
1. Gastroenterology–Textbooks. 2. Hepatology–Textbooks. 3. Gastrointestinal system–Diseases–Textbooks. 4. Liver–Diseases–Textbooks. 5. Evidence-based medicine–Textbooks. I. McDonald, John W. D.
[DNLM: 1. Gastrointestinal Diseases–diagnosis. 2. Gastrointestinal Diseases–therapy. 3. Evidence-Based Medicine–methods. 4. Liver Diseases–diagnosis. 5. Liver Diseases–therapy. WI 140 E928 2010]
RC801.E95 2010
616.3′3–dc22

2010011010

ISBN: 978-1-4051-5273-0

A catalogue record for this title is available from the British Library

Set in 9.25/12 pt Minion by Toppan Best-set Premedia Limited
Printed and bound in Singapore by Fabulous Printers Pte Ltd

1 2010

Contents

List of Contributors

C. David Adair
Professor and Vice-Chair
Division of Maternal-Fetal Medicine
Department of Obstetrics and Gynecology
University of Tennessee College of Medicine
Chattanooga, TN, USA

Cande V. Ananth
Division of Epidemiology and Biostatistics
Department of Obstetrics, Gynecology and Reproductive Sciences
UMDNJ – Robert Wood Johnson Medical School
New Brunswick, NJ, USA

Katherine W. Arendt
Assistant Professor of Anesthesiology
Mayo Clinic
Rochester, MN, USA

Kelty R. Baker
Department of Internal Medicine
Hematology-Oncology Section and Baylor College of Medicine
Houston, TX, USA

Robert H. Ball
HCA Fetal Therapy Initiative
St Mark's Hospital
Salt Lake City *and*
Division of Perinatal Medicine and Genetics
Departments of Obstetrics
Gynecology and Reproductive Sciences
UCSF Fetal Treatment Center
University of California
San Francisco, CA, USA

Michael A. Belfort
Professor of Obstetrics and Gynecology
Department of Obstetrics and Gynecology
Division of Maternal-Fetal Medicine
University of Utah School of Medicine
Salt Lake City, UT *and*
Director of Perinatal Research
Director of Fetal Therapy
HCA Healthcare
Nashville, TN, USA

Ron Bloom
Professor of Pediatrics
Department of Neonatology
University of Utah Health Sciences
Salt Lake City, UT, USA

Renee A. Bobrowski
Director of Maternal-Fetal Medicine and Women and Children's Services
Department of Obstetrics and Gynecology
Saint Alphonsus Regional Medical Center
Boise, ID, USA

D. Ware Branch
Professor
Department of Obstetrics and Gynecology
University of Utah Health Sciences Center *and*
Medical Director
Women and Newborns Services
Intermountain Healthcare
Salt Lake City, UT, USA

Michael Cackovic
Division of Maternal-Fetal Medicine
Department of Obstetrics, Gynecology and Reproductive Sciences
Yale University School of Medicine
New Haven, CT, USA

Shobana Chandrasekhar
Associate Professor
Department of Anesthesiology
Baylor College of Medicine
Houston, TX, USA

Steven L. Clark
Medical Director
Women's and Children's Clinical Services
Hospital Corporation of America
Nashville, TN, USA

Fred Coleman
Medical Director
Legacy Health Systems
Maternal-Fetal Medicine
Portland, OR, USA

Christian Con Yost
Assistant Professor of Pediatrics
Department of Neonatology
University of Utah Health Sciences
Salt Lake City, UT, USA

Shad H. Deering
Adjunct Assistant Professor
Department of Obstetrics and Gynecology
Uniformed Services University of the Health Sciences
Old Madigan Army Medical Center
Tacoma, WA, USA

Gary A. Dildy III
Director
Maternal-Fetal Medicine
Mountain Star Division
Hospital Corporation of America
Salt Lake City, UT *and*
Clinical Professor
Department of Obstetrics and Gynecology
LSU Health Sciences Center
School of Medicine in New Orleans
New Orleans, LA, USA

Donna Dizon-Townson
Associate Professor
Department of Obstetrics and Gynecology
University of Utah Health Sciences Center
Salt Lake City, UT *and*
Medical Director Clinical Programs Urban South Region
Intermountain Healthcare
Department of Maternal-Fetal Medicine
Provo, UT, USA

M. Bardett Fausett
Consultant to the AF Surgeon General for Obstetrics and Maternal-Fetal Medicine *and*
Chief, Obstetrics and Maternal-Fetal Medicine
San Antonio Military Medical Center *and*
Vice-Chairman, Department of Obstetrics and Gynecology, Wilford Hall Medical Center
Lackland Airforce Base, TX, USA

Ellen Flynn
Clinical Assistant Professor of Psychiatry and Human Behavior
Alpert Medical School of Brown University
Women and Infants Hospital
Providence, RI, USA

Michael R. Foley
Chief Medical Officer
Scotsdale Healthcare
Scottsdale, Arizona *and*
Clinical Professor
Department of Obstetrics and Gynecology
University of Arizona College of Medicine
Tucson, AZ, USA

Jeffrey M. Fowler
Director
Division of Gynecologic Oncology
John G. Boutselis Professor
Department of Obstetrics and Gynecology
James Cancer Hospital and Solove Research Institute
The Ohio State University
Columbus, OH, USA

Alfredo F. Gei
Department of Obstetrics and Gynecology
Methodist Hospital in Houston, Houston, TX USA

Labib Ghulmiyyah
Fellow
Maternal-Fetal Medicine
Department of Obstetrics and Gynecology
University of Texas Medical Branch
Galveston, TX, USA

Cornelia R. Graves
Medical Director
Tennessee Maternal-Fetal Medicine PLC *and*
Director of Perinatal Service
Baptist Hospital *and*
Clinical Professor
Vanderbilt University
Nashville, TN, USA

Kalpalatha K. Guntupalli
Section of Pulmonary Critical Care and Sleep Medicine
Baylor College of Medicine
Houston, TX, USA

Nicola A. Hanania
Section of Pulmonary Critical Care, and Sleep Medicine
Baylor College of Medicine
Houston, TX, USA

Melissa Herbst
Maternal-Fetal Services of Utah
St. Mark's Hospital
Salt Lake City, UT, USA

Calla Holmgren
Department of Obstetrics and Gynecology
University of Utah Medical Center
Salt Lake City, UT, USA

Nazli Hossain
Associate Professor and Consultant Obstetrician and Gynaecologist
Department of Obstetrics and Gynaecology Unit III
Dow University of Health Sciences,
Civil Hospital,
Karachi, Pakistan

Kenneth H. Kim
Clinical Instructor
Division of Gynecological Oncology
Department of Obstetrics and Gynecology
James Cancer Hospital and
Solove Research Institute
The Ohio State University
Columbus, OH, USA

Chad Kendall Klauser
Assistant Clinical Professor
Mount Sinai School of Medicine
New York, NY, USA

Aristides P. Koutrouvelis
Department of Anesthesiology
University of Texas Medical Branch
Galveston, TX, USA

Hee Joong Lee
Department of Obstetrics and Gynecology
The Catholic University of Korea
Seoul, Korea

William C. Mabie
Professor of Clinical Obstetrics and Gynecology
University of South Carolina
Greenville, SC, USA

Antara Mallampalli
Section of Pulmonary, Critical Care, and Sleep Medicine
Baylor College of Medicine
Houston, TX, USA

James N. Martin, Jr
Professor and Director
Department of Obstetrics and Gynecology
Division of Maternal-Fetal Medicine
University of Mississippi Medical Center
Jackson, MS, USA

Kent A. Martyn
Director of Pharmaceutical Services
Citrus Valley Medical Center
West Covina, CA, USA

Suzanne McMurtry Baird
Assistant Professor
Vanderbilt University School of Nursing
Nashville, TN, USA

Joel Moake
Rice University
Houston, TX, USA

Martin N. Montoro
Departments of Medicine and Obstetrics and Gynecology
Keck School of Medicine
University of Southern California
Los Angeles, CA, USA

Carmen Monzon
Clinical Assistant Professor of Psychiatry and Human Behavior
Alpert Medical School of Brown University
Women and Infants Hospital
Providence, RI, USA

Errol R. Norwitz
Louis E. Phaneuf Professor and Chair
Department of Obstetrics and Gynecology
Tufts University School of Medicine
and Tufts Medical Center
Boston, MA, USA

David M. O'Malley
Assistant Professor
Division of Gynecologic Oncology
Department of Obstetrics and Gynecology
James Cancer Hospital and Solove Research Institute
The Ohio State University
Columbus, OH, USA

Gayle Olson
Department of Obstetrics and Gynecology
Division of Maternal-Fetal Medicine
University of Texas Medical Branch
Galveston, TX, USA

Michelle Y. Owens
Department of Obstetrics and Gynecology
Division of Maternal-Fetal Medicine
University of Mississippi Medical Center
Jackson, MS, USA

Luis D. Pacheco
Assistant Professor
Departments of Obstetrics, Gynecology and Anesthesiology
Maternal-Fetal Medicine - Surgical Critical Care
University of Texas Medical Branch
Galveston, TX, USA

Michael J. Paidas
Yale Women & Children's Center for Blood Disorders
Department of Obstetrics, Gynecology and Reproductive Sciences
Yale School of Medicine,
New Haven, CT, USA

Teri Pearlstein
Associate Professor of Psychiatry and Human Behavior and Medicine
Alpert Medical School of Brown University
Women and Infants Hospital
Providence, RI, USA

Jeffrey P. Phelan
Director of Quality Assurance
Department of Obstetrics and Gynecology
Citrus Valley Medical Center
West Covina *and*
President and Director
Clinical Research
Childbirth Injury Prevention Foundation
City of Industry
Pasadena, CA, USA

T. Flint Porter
Associate Professor
Department of Obstetrics and Gynecology
University of Utah Health Science, UT *and*
Medical Director
Maternal-Fetal Medicine
Urban Central Region
Intermountain Healthcare
Salt Lake City, UT, USA

Raymond Powrie
Department of Medicine, Obstetrics and Gynecology
Warren Alpert School of Medicine at Brown University
RI, USA

Fidelma B. Rigby
Department of Obstetrics and Gynecology
MFM Division
MCV Campus of Virginia Commonwealth University
Richmond, VA, USA

Scott Roberts
Department of Obstetrics and Gynecology
The University of Texas Southwestern Medical Center (UTSMC) at Dallas
TX, USA

Julian N. Robinson
Associate Clinical Professor
Harvard Medical School
Division of Maternal-Fetal Medicine
Department of Obstetrics, Gynecology and Reproductive Biology
Brigham and Women's Hospital
Boston, MA, USA

Sheryl Rodts-Palenik
Acadiana Maternal-Fetal Medicine
Lafayette, LA, USA

Roxann Rokey
Director
Department of Cardiology
Marshfield Clinic
Marshfield, WI, USA

David A. Sacks
Department of Research
Southern California Permanente Medical Group
Pasadena, CA, USA

Mark Santillan
Department of Obstetrics and Gynecology
University of Iowa College of Medicine
Iowa City, IA, USA

Anthony Scardella
Professor of Medicine
Division of Pulmonary and Critical Care Medicine
Department of Medicine
University of Medicine and Dentistry of New Jersey-Robert Wood Johnson Medical School
New Brunswick, NJ, USA

William E. Scorza
Chief of Obstetrics
Division of Maternal–Fetal Medicine
Department of Obstetrics
Lehigh Valley Hospital
Allentown, PA, USA

James Scott
Department of Obstetrics and Gynecology
University of Utah, Medical Center
Salt Lake City, UT, USA

Julie Scott
Assistant Professor
Department of Obstetrics and Gynecology
Division of Maternal-Fetal Medicine
University of Colorado Health Sciences Center
Denver, CO, USA

Gail L Seiken
Washington Nephrology Associates
Bethesda, MD, USA

Shailen S. Shah
Director of Operations
Maternal-Fetal Medicine
Virtua Health
Voorhees, NJ *and*
Assistant Professor
Thomas Jefferson University Hospital,
Philadelphia, PA, USA

Howard T. Sharp
Department of Obstetrics and Gynecology
University of Utah School of Medicine
Salt Lake City, UT, USA

Andrea Shields
Director
Antenatal Diagnostic Center
San Antonio Military Medical Center
Lackland Airforce Base, TX, USA

John C. Smulian
Division of Maternal-Fetal Medicine
Department of Obstetrics and Gynecology
Lehigh Valley Health Network
Allentown, PA, USA

Irene Stafford
Maternal-Fetal Medicine
University of Texas Southwestern Medical Center
Dallas, TX, USA

Shawn P. Stallings
Division of Maternal-Fetal Medicine
Department of Obstetrics and Gynecology
University of Tennessee College of Medicine
Chattanooga, TN, USA

Victor R. Suarez
Maternal-Fetal Medicine Attending
Advocate Christ Medical Center
Chicago, IL, USA

Maya S. Suresh
Professor and Interim Chairman
Department of Anesthesiology
Baylor College of Medicine
Houston, TX, USA

Nan H. Troiano
Clinical Nurse Specialist
Women's Services
Labor & Delivery and High Risk Perinatal Unit
Inova Fairfax Hospital Women's Center
Falls Church, Virginia *and*
Columbia University; New-York Presbyterian Hospital
Department of Obstetrics and Gynecology
Division of Maternal-Fetal Medicine *and*
Consultant, Critical Care Obstetrics
New York, USA

James W. Van Hook
Professor and Director
Department of Obstetrics and Gynecology
Division of Maternal-Fetal Medicine
University of Cincinnati College of Medicine
Cincinnati, OH, USA

Michael W. Varner
Department of Obstetrics and Gynecology
University of Utah Health Sciences Center
Salt Lake City, UT, USA

Edward W. Veillon, Jr
Fellow
Maternal-Fetal Medicine
University of Mississippi Medical Center
Jackson, MS, USA

Carey Winkler
MFM Physician
Legacy Health Systems
Maternal-Fetal Medicine Department
Portland, OR, USA

Jerome Yankowitz
Department of Obstetrics and Gynecology
University of Iowa College of Medicine
Iowa City, IA, USA

1 Epidemiology of Critical Illness in Pregnancy

Cande V. Ananth[1] & John C. Smulian[2]

[1]Division of Epidemiology and Biostatistics, Department of Obstetrics, Gynecology and Reproductive Sciences, UMDNJ – Robert Wood Johnson Medical School, New Brunswick, NJ, USA
[2]Division of Maternal-Fetal Medicine, Department of Obstetrics and Gynecology, Lehigh Valley Health Network, Allentown, PA, USA

Introduction

The successful epidemiologic evaluation of any particular disease or condition has several prerequisites. Two of the most important prerequisites are that the condition should be accurately defined and that there should be measurable outcomes of interest. Another requirement is that there must be some systematic way of data collection or surveillance that will allow the measurement of the outcomes of interest and associated risk factors. The epidemiologic evaluation of critical illness associated with pregnancy has met with mixed success on all of these counts.

Historically, surveillance of pregnancy-related critical illness has focused on the well-defined outcome of maternal mortality in order to identify illnesses or conditions that might have led to maternal death. Identification of various conditions associated with maternal mortality initially came from observations by astute clinicians. One of the best examples is the link described by Semmelweiss between hand-washing habits and puerperal fever. In most industrial and many developing countries, there are now population-based surveillance mechanisms in place to track maternal mortality. These often are mandated by law. In fact, the World Health Organization uses maternal mortality as one of the measures of the health of a population [1].

Fortunately, in most industrialized nations the maternal mortality rates have fallen to very low levels. Recent statistics for the United States suggest that overall maternal mortality was 11.5 maternal deaths per 100 000 live births during 1991–97 [2]. Despite this impressively low rate of maternal mortality, tracking maternal deaths may not be the best way to assess pregnancy-related critical illnesses since the majority of such illnesses do not result in maternal death. As stated by Harmer [3], "death represents the tip of the morbidity iceberg, the size of which is unknown." Unlike mortality, which is an unequivocal endpoint, critical illness in pregnancy as a morbidity outcome is difficult to define and, therefore, difficult to measure and study precisely.

There are many common conditions in pregnancy such as the hypertensive diseases, intrapartum hemorrhage, diabetes, thyroid disease, asthma, seizure disorders, and infection that occur frequently and require special medical care, but do not actually become critical illnesses. Most women with these complications have relatively uneventful pregnancies that result in good outcomes for both mother and infant. Nevertheless, each of these conditions can be associated with significant complications that have the potential for serious morbidity, disability and mortality. The stage at which any condition becomes severe enough to be classified as a critical illness has not been clearly defined. However, it may be helpful to consider critical illness as impending, developing, or established significant organ dysfunction, which may lead to long-term morbidity or death. This allows some flexibility in the characterization of disease severity since it recognizes conditions that can deteriorate rather quickly in pregnancy.

Maternal mortality data collection is well established in many places, but specific surveillance systems that track severe complications of pregnancy not associated with maternal mortality are rare. It has been suggested that most women suffering a critical illness in pregnancy are likely to spend some time in an intensive care unit [3–5]. These cases have been described by some as "near-miss" mortality cases [6,7]. Therefore, examination of cases admitted to intensive care units can provide insight into the nature of pregnancy-related critical illnesses and can compliment maternal mortality surveillance. However, it should be noted that nearly two-thirds of maternal deaths might occur in women who never reach an intensive care unit [5].

The following sections review much of what is currently known about the epidemiology of critical illness in pregnancy. Some of the information is based on published studies; however, much of the data are derived from publicly available data that are collected as part of nationwide surveillance systems in the US.

Critical Care Obstetrics, 5th edition. Edited by M. Belfort, G. Saade, M. Foley, J. Phelan and G. Dildy.

Pregnancy-related hospitalizations

Pregnancy complications contribute significantly to maternal, fetal, and infant morbidity, as well as mortality [8]. Many women with complicating conditions are hospitalized without being delivered. Although maternal complications of pregnancy are the fifth leading cause of infant mortality in the US, little is known about the epidemiology of maternal complications associated with hospitalizations. Examination of complicating conditions associated with maternal hospitalizations can provide information on the types of conditions requiring hospitalized care. In the US during the years 1991–92, it was estimated that 18.0% of pregnancies were associated with non-delivery hospitalization with disproportionate rates between black (28.1%) and white (17.2%) women [9]. This 18.0% hospitalization rate comprised 12.3% for obstetric conditions (18.3% among black women and 11.9% among white women), 4.4% for pregnancy losses (8.1% among black women and 3.9% among white women), and 1.3% for non-obstetric (medical or surgical) conditions (1.5% among black women and 1.3% among white women). The likelihood of pregnancy-associated hospitalizations in the US declined between 1986–87 and 1991–92 [9,10].

More recent information about pregnancy-related hospitalization diagnoses can be found in the aggregated National Hospital Discharge Summary (NHDS) data for 1998–99. These data are assembled by the National Center for Health Statistics (NCHS) of the US Centers for Disease Control and Prevention. The NHDS data is a survey of medical records from short-stay, non-federal hospitals in the US, conducted annually since 1965. A detailed description of the survey and the database can be found elsewhere [11]. Briefly, for each hospital admission, the NHDS data include a primary and up to six secondary diagnoses, as well as up to four procedures performed for each hospitalization. These diagnoses and procedures are all coded based on the International Classification of Diseases, ninth revision, clinical modification. We examined the rates (per 100 hospitalizations) of hospitalizations by indications (discharge diagnoses) during 1998–99 in the US, separately for delivery (n = 7965173) and non-delivery (n = 960023) hospitalizations. We also examined the mean hospital lengths of stay (with 95% confidence intervals, CIs). Antepartum and postpartum hospitalizations were grouped as non-delivery hospitalizations.

During 1998–99, nearly 7.4% of all hospitalizations were for hypertensive diseases with delivery, and 6.6% were for hypertensive diseases not delivered (Table 1.1). Mean hospital length of stay (LOS) is an indirect measure of acuity for some illnesses. LOS was higher for delivery-related than for non-delivery-related hospitalizations for hypertensive diseases. Hemorrhage, as the underlying reason for hospitalization (either as primary or secondary diagnosis), occurred much more frequently for delivery- than non-delivery-related hospitalizations. Non-delivery hospitalizations for genitourinary infections occurred three times more frequently (10.45%) than for delivery-related hospitalizations (3.19%), although the average LOS was shorter for non-delivery hospitalizations.

Hospitalizations for preterm labor occurred twice as frequently for non-delivery hospitalizations (21.21%) than for delivery-related hospitalizations (10.28%). This is expected since many preterm labor patients are successfully treated and some of these hospitalizations are for "false labor." Liver disorders were uncommonly associated with hospitalization. However, the mean hospital LOS for liver disorders that occurred with non-delivery hospitalizations was over 31 days, compared with a mean LOS of 3 days if the liver condition was delivery related. Coagulation-related defects required 14.9 days of hospitalization if not related to delivery compared with a mean LOS of 4.9 days if the condition was delivery related. Hospitalizations for embolism-related complications were infrequent, but generally required extended hospital stays.

The top 10 conditions associated with hospital admissions, separately for delivery- and non-delivery-related events, are presented in Figure 1.1. The chief cause for hospitalization (either delivery or non-delivery related) was preterm labor. The second most frequent condition was hypertensive disease (7.37% for delivery related and 6.61% for non-delivery related) followed by anemia (7.13% vs 5.05%). Hospitalizations for infection-related conditions occurred twice more frequently for non-delivery periods (11.65%) than during delivery (5.75%). In contrast, hospitalization for hemorrhage was more frequent during delivery (4.43%) than non-delivery (3.26%). These data provide important insights into the most common complications and conditions associated with pregnancy hospitalization. The LOS data also give some indication of resource allocation needs. While this is important in understanding the epidemiology of illness in pregnancy, it does not allow a detailed examination of illness severity.

Maternal mortality

The national health promotion and disease prevention objectives of the *Healthy People 2010* indicators specify a goal of no more than 3.3 maternal deaths per 100000 live births in the US [12]. The goal for maternal deaths among black women was set at no more than 5.0 per 100000 live births. As of 1997 (the latest available statistics on maternal deaths in the US) this objective remains elusive. The pregnancy-related maternal mortality ratio (PRMR) per 100000 live births for the US was 11.5 for 1991–97 [13], with the ratio over threefold greater among black compared with white women [14]. Several studies that have examined trends in maternal mortality statistics have concluded that a majority of pregnancy-related deaths (including those resulting from ectopic pregnancies, and some cases of infection and hemorrhage) are preventable [1,15,16]. However, maternal deaths due to other complications such as pregnancy-induced hypertension, placenta previa, retained placenta, and thromboembolism, are considered by some as difficult to prevent [17,18].

Table 1.1 Rate (per 100 hospitalizations) of delivery and non-delivery hospitalizations, and associated hospital lengths of stay (LOS) by diagnoses: USA, 1998–99.

Hospital admission diagnosis*	Delivery hospitalization (n = 7,965,173)		Non-delivery hospitalization (n = 960,023)	
	Rate (%)	Mean LOS (95% CI)	Rate (%)	Mean LOS (95% CI)
Hypertensive diseases				
Chronic hypertension	3.05	3.0 (2.9, 3.2)	3.08	2.3 (1.9, 2.7)
Pre-eclampsia/eclampsia	4.08	3.7 (3.6, 3.9)	3.23	2.7 (1.8, 3.6)
Chronic hypertension + pre-eclampsia	0.24	6.3 (4.7, 7.8)	0.30	2.4 (1.8, 2.9)
Hemorrhage				
Placental abruption	1.02	3.9 (3.5, 4.3)	0.72	3.4 (2.2, 4.7)
Placenta previa	0.44	5.5 (4.6, 6.5)	0.13	3.2 (2.0, 4.4)
Hemorrhage (unassigned etiology)	0.24	4.0 (3.2, 4.9)	1.58	1.7 (1.3, 2.2)
Vasa previa	0.17	2.6 (2.0, 3.2)	–	–
Postpartum hemorrhage	2.56	2.6 (2.5, 2.7)	0.83	2.3 (1.3, 2.9)
Infection-related				
Viral infections (not malaria/rubella)	0.93	2.8 (2.6, 3.1)	1.04	2.6 (2.0, 3.2)
Genitourinary infections	3.19	3.4 (2.8, 3.9)	10.45	3.2 (2.5, 3.8)
Infection of the amniotic cavity	1.63	4.2 (3.7, 4.6)	0.16	4.2 (1.7, 6.7)
Anesthesia-related complications	0.02	4.7 (3.5, 5.9)	<0.01	–
Diabetes				
Pre-existing diabetes	0.60	4.6 (3.7, 5.4)	2.40	3.2 (2.7, 3.7)
Gestational diabetes	3.15	2.9 (2.8, 3.1)	2.50	3.5 (3.0, 4.1)
Preterm labor	10.28	3.4 (3.3, 3.6)	21.21	2.5 (2.3, 2.7)
Maternal anemia	7.13	2.9 (2.8, 3.0)	5.05	3.9 (3.2, 4.5)
Drug dependency	0.19	3.0 (2.3, 3.7)	0.53	3.6 (2.3, 4.8)
Renal disorders	0.13	3.4 (2.6, 4.3)	0.86	2.7 (2.1, 3.2)
Liver disorders	0.06	3.0 (2.2, 3.8)	0.08	31.2 (2.7, 59.6)
Congenital cardiovascular disease	0.94	3.0 (2.7, 3.4)	0.98	3.1 (2.3, 3.8)
Thyroid disorders	0.17	2.3 (1.6, 3.0)	0.53	3.0 (1.7, 4.4)
Uterine tumors	0.54	3.8 (3.4, 4.2)	0.63	2.6 (1.5, 3.6)
Uterine rupture	0.11	4.8 (3.3, 6.2)	–	–
Postpartum coagulation defects	0.11	4.9 (3.7, 6.1)	0.07	14.9 (0.2, 47.8)
Shock/hypotension	0.09	3.3 (2.6, 4.0)	0.15	2.2 (0.4, 4.1)
Acute renal failure	0.02	6.9 (4.1, 9.7)	0.02	–
Embolism-related				
Amniotic fluid embolism	0.02	6.8 (1.8, 11.7)	–	–
Blood-clot embolism	<0.01	11.1 (2.7, 19.3)	0.19	5.2 (3.2, 7.5)
Other pulmonary embolism	<0.01	–	–	–

*The diagnoses associated with hospital admissions include both primary and secondary reasons for hospitalizations. Each admission may have had up to six associated diagnoses.

From the 1960s to the mid-1980s, the maternal mortality ratio in the US declined from approximately 27 per 100 000 live births to about 7 per 100 000 live births (Figure 1.2). Subsequently, the mortality ratio increased between 1987 (7.2 per 100 000 live births) and 1990 (10.0 per 100 000 live births). During the period 1991–97, the mortality ratio further increased to 11.5 per 100 000 live births–an overall relative increase of 60% between 1987 and 1997. The reasons for the recent increases are not clear.

Several maternal risk factors have been examined in relation to maternal deaths. Women aged 35–39 years carry a 2.6-fold (95%

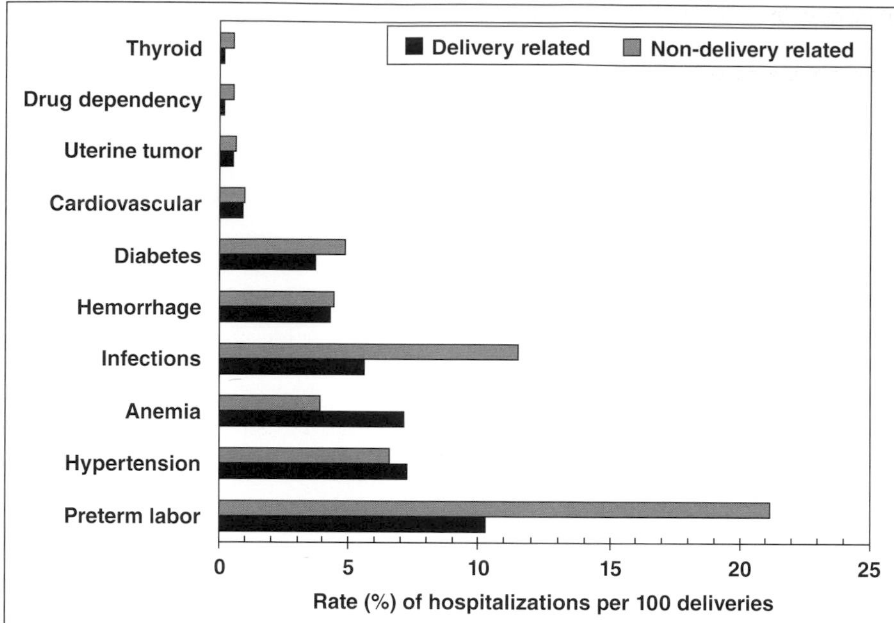

Figure 1.1 Ten leading causes of delivery- and non-delivery-related maternal hospitalizations in the US, 1998–99.

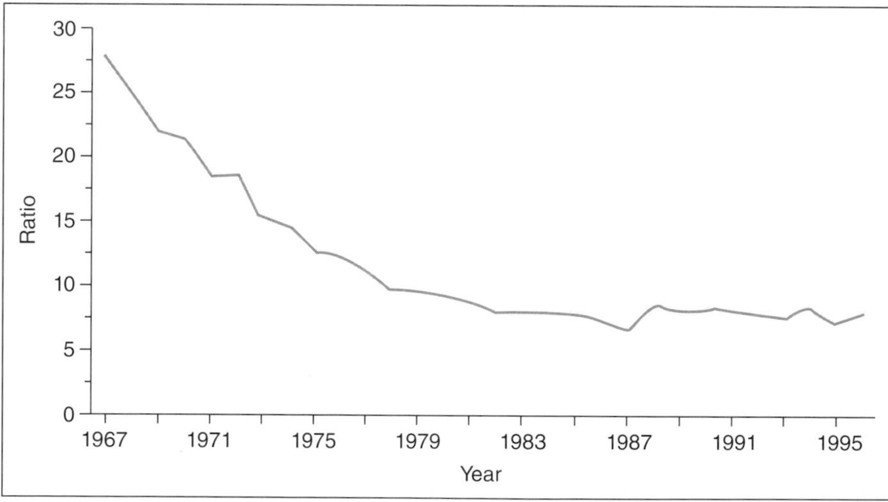

Figure 1.2 Trends in maternal mortality ratio (number of maternal deaths per 100 000 live births) in the US, 1967–96. The term "ratio" is used instead of "rate" because the numerator includes some maternal deaths that were not related to live births and thus were not included in the denominator.

CI 2.2, 3.1) increased risk of maternal death and those over 40 years are at a 5.9-fold (95% CI 4.6, 7.7) increased risk. Black maternal race confers a relative risk of 3.7 (95% CI 3.3, 4.1) for maternal death compared with white women. Similarly, women without any prenatal care during pregnancy had an almost twofold increased risk of death relative to those who received prenatal care [19].

The chief cause for a pregnancy-related maternal death depends on whether the pregnancy results in a live born, stillbirth, ectopic pregnancy, abortion, or molar gestation (Table 1.2). For the period 1987–90, hemorrhage was recorded in 28.8% of all deaths, leading to an overall pregnancy-related mortality ratio (PRMR) for hemorrhage of 2.6 per 100 000 live births, followed by embolism-related deaths (PRMR 1.8), and hypertensive diseases (PRMR 1.6). Among all live births, hypertensive diseases (23.8%) were the most frequent cause of death. Among stillbirths (27.2%) and ectopic (94.9%) pregnancies, the chief cause of death was hemorrhage, while infections (49.4%) were the leading cause of abortion-related maternal deaths.

Understanding the epidemiology of pregnancy-related deaths is essential in order to target specific interventions. Improved population-based surveillance through targeted reviews of all pregnancy-related deaths, as well as additional research to understand the causes of maternal deaths by indication will help in achieving the *Healthy People 2010* goals.

Table 1.2 Pregnancy-related maternal deaths by underlying cause: USA, 1987–90. From Koonin et al. [53].

Cause of death	All outcomes		Outcome of pregnancy (% distribution)						
	%	PRMR*	Live birth	Stillbirth	Ectopic	Abortions†	Molar	Undelivered	Unknown
Hemorrhage	28.8	2.6	21.1	27.2	94.9	18.5	16.7	15.7	20.1
Embolism	19.9	1.8	23.4	10.7	1.3	11.1	0.0	35.2	21.1
Hypertension	17.6	1.6	23.8	26.2	0.0	1.2	0.0	4.6	16.3
Infection	13.1	1.2	12.1	19.4	1.3	49.4	0.0	13.0	9.0
Cardiomyopathy	5.7	0.5	6.1	2.9	0.0	0.0	0.0	2.8	13.9
Anesthesia	2.5	0.2	2.7	0.0	1.9	8.6	0.0	1.8	1.0
Others/unknown	12.8	1.2	11.1	13.6	0.6	11.1	83.3	27.5	19.3
Total	100.0	–	100.0	100.0	100.0	100.0	100.0	100.0	100.0

* Pregnancy-related mortality ratio per 100 000 live births.
† Includes both spontaneous and induced abortions.

Table 1.3 Perinatal mortality rates among singleton and multiple gestations by gestational age and high-risk conditions: USA, 1995–98.

High-risk conditions	20–27 weeks		28–32 weeks		33–36 weeks		≥37 weeks	
	PMR	Relative risk (95% CI)	PMR	Relative risk (95% CI)	PMR	Relative risk (95% CI)	PMR	Relative risk (95% CI)
Singletons								
Number of births	n = 103 755		n = 352 291		n = 1 072 784		n = 13 440 671	
Hypertension	200.4	0.6 (0.5, 0.7)	53.1	0.6 (0.5, 0.6)	13.5	0.6 (0.5, 0.7)	3.6	1.3 (0.5, 0.7)
Hemorrhage	308.9	1.1 (1.0, 1.2)	73.1	1.4 (1.3, 1.5)	19.9	1.6 (1.5, 1.7)	3.6	1.6 (1.5, 1.7)
Diabetes	287.0	1.0 (0.9, 1.1)	60.8	1.2 (1.1, 1.3)	19.5	1.8 (1.7, 1.9)	5.0	2.3 (2.1, 2.4)
SGA	467.4	2.3 (2.1, 2.5)	196.3	6.2 (6.0, 6.4)	56.3	7.8 (7.5, 8.1)	9.1	5.5 (5.4, 5.7)
No complications	297.6	1.0 (Referent)	38.8	1.0 (Referent)	7.0	1.0 (Referent)	1.5	1.0 (Referent)
Multiples								
Number of births	n = 23 055		n = 76 329		n = 147 627		n = 187 109	
Hypertension	183.5	0.7 (0.6, 0.8)	21.4	0.5 (0.4, 0.6)	5.3	0.6 (0.5, 0.7)	4.9	0.8 (0.6, 1.1)
Hemorrhage	251.6	1.0 (0.9, 1.1)	36.6	1.1 (1.0, 1.3)	9.6	1.2 (1.0, 1.4)	6.7	1.3 (1.1, 1.5)
Diabetes	214.9	0.8 (0.7, 1.1)	28.7	0.9 (0.7, 1.2)	9.7	1.3 (1.0, 1.7)	5.9	1.2 (0.9, 1.7)
SGA	394.5	2.0 (1.6, 2.4)	133.4	6.8 (6.3, 7.4)	36.8	7.5 (6.6, 8.4)	24.9	8.6 (7.6, 9.7)
No complications	251.1	1.0 (Referent)	23.4	1.0 (Referent)	5.2	1.0 (Referent)	2.8	1.0 (Referent)

CI, confidence interval; PMR, perinatal mortality rate per 1000 births; SGA, small for gestational age births.
Hypertension includes chronic hypertension, pregnancy-induced hypertension, and eclampsia.
Hemorrhage includes placental abruption, placenta previa, uterine bleeding of undermined etiology.
No complications include those that did not have any complications listed in the table.
Relative risk for each high-risk condition was adjusted for all other high-risk conditions shown in the table.

Perinatal mortality

Perinatal mortality, defined by the World Health Organization as fetal deaths plus deaths of live-born infants within the first 28 days, is an important indicator of population health. Examination of the maternal conditions related to perinatal mortality can provide further information on the association and impact of these conditions on pregnancy outcomes. Table 1.3 shows the results of our examination of perinatal mortality rates among singleton and multiple births (twins, triplets and quadruplets) by gestational age and high-risk conditions. The study population comprises all births in the US that occurred in 1995–98. Data were derived from the national linked birth/infant death files, assembled by the National Center for Health Statistics of the Centers for Disease Control and Prevention [20]. Gestational age was predominantly based on the date of last menstrual period [21], and was grouped as 20–27, 28–32, 33–36, and ≥37 weeks. Perinatal mortality rates were assessed for hypertension (chronic hypertension, pregnancy-induced hypertension, and eclampsia), hemorrhage (placental abruption, placenta previa, and uterine bleeding of undetermined etiology), diabetes (pre-existing and gestational diabetes), and small for gestational age (SGA) births (defined as birth weight below 10th centile for gestational age). We derived norms for the 10th centile birth weight for singleton and multiple births from the corresponding singleton and multiple births that occurred in 1995–98 in the US. Finally, relative risks (with 95% CIs) for perinatal death by each high-risk condition were derived from multivariable logistic regression models after adjusting for all other high-risk conditions.

Perinatal mortality rates progressively decline, among both singleton and multiple births, for each high-risk condition with increasing gestational age (Table 1.3). Among singleton and multiple gestations, with the exception of SGA births, mortality rates were generally higher for each high-risk condition, relative to the no complications group. Infants delivered small for their gestational age carried the highest risk of dying during the perinatal period compared with those born to mothers without complications. Among singleton births, the relative risks for perinatal death for SGA infants were 2.3, 6.2, 7.8, and 5.5 for those delivered at 20–27 weeks, 28–32 weeks, 33–36 weeks, and term, respectively. Among multiple births, these relative risks were similar at 2.0, 6.8, 7.5, and 8.6, respectively, for each of the four gestational age categories.

Pregnancy-related intensive care unit admissions

Evaluation of obstetric admissions to intensive care units (ICUs) may be one of the best ways to approach surveillance of critical illnesses in pregnancy. Unfortunately, there are no publicly available population-based databases for obstetric admissions to ICU that provide sufficiently detailed information to allow in-depth study of these conditions. Therefore, it is reasonable to examine descriptive case series to provide information on these conditions. We reviewed 33 studies published between 1990 and 2006 involving 1 955 111 deliveries and found an overall obstetric-related admission rate to ICU of 0.07–0.89% (Table 1.4). Some of the variation in the rates may be explained by the nature of the populations studied. Hospitals that are tertiary referral centers for large catchment areas typically receive a more concentrated high-risk population. These facilities would be expected to have higher rates of obstetric admissions to an ICU. However, these studies provided sufficient data to allow the exclusion of patients transported from outside facilities. Community-oriented facilities are probably less likely to care for critically ill obstetric patients unless the illnesses develop so acutely that they would preclude transport to a higher-level facility. The largest study of pregnancy-related ICU admissions involved 37 maternity hospitals in Maryland and included hospitals at all care levels [22]. This study found a nearly 30% lower admission rate to ICUs for obstetric patients from community hospitals compared with major teaching hospitals. Another source of variation is the different criteria for admission to the ICU used at different institutions. Finally, there are major differences in the inclusion criteria used for these studies that further contributes to the variability in reported ICU utilization rates.

Reported maternal mortality for critically ill obstetric patients admitted to an ICU is approximately 8.4% (Table 1.4). This reflects the true seriousness of the illnesses of these women. The wide range of mortality from 0% to 33% is due to many factors. Most of the studies were small and just a few deaths may affect rates significantly. The populations studied also differ in underlying health status. Reports from less developed countries had much higher mortality rates. The time period of the study can have an impact. In general, earlier studies had higher maternal mortality rates. These earlier studies represent the early stages of development of care mechanisms for critically ill obstetric patients. They probably reflect part of the "learning curve" of critical care obstetrics, as well as differences in available technology [52]. Regardless, the mortality rate from these ICU admissions is several orders of magnitude higher than the general US population maternal mortality rate of 11.5 per 100 000 live births. Therefore, these cases are a good representation of an obstetric population with critical illnesses.

Illnesses responsible for obstetric intensive care unit admissions

Examination of obstetric ICU admissions provides some insight into the nature of obstetric illnesses requiring critical care. Data were pooled from 26 published studies that provided sufficient details about the primary indication for the ICU admission (Table 1.5). It is no surprise that hypertensive diseases and obstetric hemorrhage were responsible for over 50% of the primary admitting diagnoses. Specific organ system dysfunction was responsible for the majority of the remaining admissions. Of those, pulmonary, cardiac, and infectious complications had the greatest frequency. From these reports, it is apparent that both obstetric and medical complications of pregnancy are responsible for the ICU admissions in similar proportions. There were 16 studies that provided information on 1980 patients as to whether the primary admitting diagnosis was related to an obstetric complication or a medical complication [4,22,23,25,26,36–38,40,42,43,46,49–51,54]. The pooled data indicate that approximately 69.3% (n = 1373) were classified as obstetric related and 30.7% (n = 607) were due to medical complications. These data clearly highlight the complex nature of obstetric critical care illnesses and provide support for a multidisciplinary approach to management since these patients are quite ill with a variety of diseases.

Table 1.4 Obstetric admission rates to an intensive care unit (ICU) and corresponding maternal mortality rates from 33 studies.

Reference	Year(s)	Location	Inclusion criteria	Total deliveries	Obstetric ICU Admissions (rate)	Obstetric ICU deaths (rate)	Fetal/neonatal deaths per ICU admissions
Mabie & Sibai 1990 [22]	1986–89	US	–	22 651	200 (0.88%)	7 (3.5%)	–
Kilpatrick & Matthay 1992 [23]	1985–90	US	Up to 6 weeks PP	8000*	32 (0.4%)	4 (12.0%)	6 (18.8%)
Collop & Sahn 1993 [24]	1988–91	US	<42 weeks	–	20 (–)	4 (20.0%)	7 (35.0%)
El-Solh & Grant 1996 [25]	1989–95	US	Up to 10d PP	–	96 (–)	10/93 (10.8%)	10 (10.4%)
Monoco et al. 1993 [26]	1983–90	US	16 weeks to 2 weeks PP	15 323	38 (0.25%)	7 (18.4%)	4 (10.5%)
Panchal et al. 2000 [27]	1984–97	US	Delivering admission	822 591	1023 (0.12%)	34 (3.3%)	–
Afessa et al. 2001 [28]	1991–98	US	–	–	78 (–)	2 (2.7%)	13 (16.7%)
Gilbert et al. 2000 [29]	1991–98	US	Up to 6 weeks PP	49 349	233 (0.47%)	8 (3.4%)	–
Hogg et al. 2000 [30]	1989–97	US	15 weeks to 6 weeks PP	30 405	172 (0.57%)	23 (13.4%)	2 (1.2%)
Munnur et al. 2005 [31]	1992–2001	US	–	58 000	174(0.3%)	4 (2.3%)	23 (13.2%)
Mahutte et al. 1999 [4]	1991–97	Canada	14 weeks to 6 weeks PP	44 340	131 (0.30%)	3 (2.3%)	
Lapinsky et al. 1997 [32]	1997	Canada	–	25 000*	65 (0.26%)	0	7 (10.8%)
Baskett & Sternadel 1998 [6]	1980–93	Canada	>20 weeks and PP	76 119	55 (0.07%)	2 (3.6%)	–
Hazelgrove et al. 2001 [5]	1994–96	England	Up to 6 weeks PP	122 850	210 (0.17%)	7 (3.3%)	40/200 (20.0%)
DeMello & Restall 1990 [33]	1985–89	England	20–42 weeks	9425	13 (0.14%)	0	–
Selo-Ojeme et al. 2005 [34]	1993–2003	England	14 weeks to 6 weeks PP	31 097	22 (0.11%)	1 (4.5%)	1 (4.5%)
Stephens 1991 [35]	1979–89	Australia	Up to 4 weeks PP	61 435	126 (0.21%)	1 (0.8%)	–
Tang et al. 1997 [36]	1988–95	China	Up to 6 weeks PP	39 350	49 (0.12%)	2 (4.1%)	4 (8.2%)
Ng et al. 1992 [37]	1985–90	China	Delivery related	16 264	37 (0.22%)	2 (5.4%)	–
Cheng & Raman 2003 [38]	1994–1999	Singapore	Up to 1 week PP	13 438	39 (0.28%)	2 (5.1%)	–
Heinonen et al. 2002 [39]	1993–2000	Finland	18 weeks to 4 weeks PP	23 404	22 (0.14%)	1 (4.5%)	–
Keizer et al. 2006 [40]	1990–2001	Netherlands	Obstetrics admissions with illness	18 581	142 (0.76%)	7 (4.9%)	35 (24.6%)
Bouvier-Colle et al. 1996 [41]	1991	France	Up to 6 weeks PP	140 000*	435 (0.31%)	22 (5.1%)	58 (13.3%)
Koeberle et al. 2000 [42]	1986–96	France	Up to 6 weeks PP	27 059*	46 (0.17%)	2 (4.3%)	–
Munnur et al. 2005 [31]	1992–2001	India	–	157 694	754 (0.48%)	189 (25%)	368 (48.81%)
Ryan et al. 2000 [43]	1996–98	Ireland	–	26 164	17 (0.07%)	0	–
Cohen et al. 2000 [44]	1994–98	Israel	20 weeks to 2 weeks PP	19 474	46 (0.24%)	1 (2.3%)	10 (21.7%)
Lewinsohn et al. 1994 [45]	8 yrs	Israel	–	–	58 (–)	4 (6.9%)	–
Loverro et al. 2001 [46]	1987–1998	Italy	–	23 694	41 (0.17%)	2 (4.9%)	5 (12.2%)
Okafor & Aniebue 2004 [47]	1997–2002	Nigeria	–	6544	18 (0.28%)	6 (33%)	–
Platteau et al. 1997 [48]	1992	South Africa	–	–	80 (–)	17 (21.3%)	39 (48.6%)
Demirkiran et al. 2003 [49]	1995–2000	Turkey	–	14 045*	125 (0.89%)	13 (9.6%)	–
Mirghani et al. 2004 [50]	1997–2002	UAE	–	23 383	60 (0.26%)	2 (3.3%)	–
Suleiman et al. 2006 [51]	1992–2004	Saudi Arabia	Up to 6 weeks PP	29 432	64 (0.22%)	6 (9.4%)	8/55 (14.5%)
Summary (pooled data)				1 955 111	4389 (0.22%)	395/4718 (8.4%)	640/2499 (25.6%)

PP, postpartum; (–) indicates data not provided or unable to be calculated (these values excluded from summaries of columns).
* Estimate calculated based on data in paper.

Causes of mortality in obstetric intensive care unit admissions

When specific causes of mortality for the obstetric ICU admissions were reviewed, 26 studies gave sufficient data to assign a primary etiology for maternal death (Table 1.6). Of a total of 138 maternal deaths, over 57% were related to complications of hypertensive diseases, pulmonary illnesses, and cardiac diseases. Other deaths were commonly related to complications of hemorrhage, bleeding into the central nervous system, malignancy, and infection. More importantly, despite an identified primary

Table 1.5 Complications primarily responsible for admission to the intensive care unit for obstetric patients: data summarized from 26 published studies [4–6,22–26,28,31,32,35–37,39,40,42–51].

Category	Category examples	n	Percentage
Hypertensive diseases	Eclampsia, pre-eclampsia, HELLP syndrome, hypertensive crisis	1176	37.4
Hemorrhage	Shock, abruption, previa, postpartum hemorrhage, accreta, uterine rupture	647	20.6
Pulmonary	Pulmonary edema, pneumonia, adult respiratory distress syndrome, asthma, thromboembolic diseases, amniotic fluid embolus	287	9.1
Cardiac	Valvular disease, arrhythmia, cardiomyopathy, infarction	187	5.9
Sepsis/infection	Chorioamnionitis, pyelonephritis, malaria, hepatitis, meningitis, miscellaneous	288	9.2
Central nervous system	Intracranial hemorrhage, seizure (non-eclamptic), arteriovenous malformation	92	2.9
Anesthesia complication	Allergic reaction, failed intubation, high spinal	47	1.5
Gastrointestinal	Pancreatitis, acute fatty liver of pregnancy, inflammatory bowel disease, gallbladder disease	64	2.0
Renal	Renal failure	30	1.0
Hematologic	Thrombotic thrombocytopenic purpura, sickle cell disease, disseminated intravascular coagulation, aspiration	32	1.0
Endocrine	Diabetic ketoacidosis, thyroid storm	52	1.7
Malignancy	Various	17	0.5
Other	Insufficient information to assign to specific organ system but included anaphylaxis, trauma, drug and overdose/ poisoning	227	7.2
Total		3146	100%

etiology for the maternal deaths, nearly all cases were associated with multiorgan dysfunction, which again emphasizes the complex condition of these critically ill women.

As noted earlier, obstetric and medical complications of pregnancy are equally represented in all admissions to the ICU (Table 1.5). However, nearly 40% of all maternal deaths in the ICU were directly related to obstetric conditions (mainly hypertensive diseases, hemorrhage, amniotic fluid embolism and acute fatty liver of pregnancy) with the remaining deaths due to medical conditions (Table 1.6).

Perinatal loss 101th obstetric intensive care unit admissions

When considering the implications of critical illness for obstetric patients, the focus is usually on the mother. However, it is important to re-emphasize that many of these conditions also may have a significant impact on fetal and neonatal outcomes. There is surprisingly little detailed information available on these perinatal outcomes in pregnancies complicated by critical illnesses. However, there are data on perinatal outcomes based on specific disease conditions. Maternal high-risk conditions associated with perinatal mortality in the US are presented in Table 1.3. However, these data do not separate outcomes by severity of maternal illness. We were able to identify 18 studies that provided information on fetal or neonatal mortality rates for obstetric admissions to the ICU (Table 1.4). Fetal and/or neonatal deaths were identified in 640 of the pooled 2499 cases, resulting in an overall mortality rate of 25.6%. Reported rates ranged from 1.2–48.8%. If the large report from India is removed [31], there were 272 of these deaths among 1 745 cases, with a mortality rate of 15.6%. These proportions may not reflect a true perinatal mortality rate since some of the losses may have occurred before 20 weeks gestation. In addition, the denominator includes a number of postpartum admissions for conditions not expected to impact fetal or neonatal mortality. Nevertheless, the high loss rate highlights the importance of considering the fetus when managing critical illnesses in pregnancy.

Summary

In summary, understanding the nature of critical illness in pregnancy is an important and evolving process. We have clearly grown beyond simple mortality reviews for assessment of pregnancy-related critical illness. However, our currently available tools and databases for examining these patients still need improvement. Reports of critically ill women admitted to the ICU have further refined our understanding of these diseases. However, targeted surveillance of obstetric ICU admissions is needed to identify variations in care and disease that may affect management. As our understanding of these conditions continues to mature, we will hopefully gain greater insight into the specific nature of these conditions that will lead to improved prevention strategies and better therapies for the diseases when they occur. In our view, these data will improve our ability to plan and allocate the necessary resources to adequately care for these often complex and severe illnesses.

Table 1.6 Identified primary causes of mortality in obstetric admissions to ICUs reported in 26 studies [4–6,22–26,28,31,32,35–37,39,40,42–51].

Identified etiology	Number	Percentage
Hypertensive diseases	36	26.1
Hypertensive crisis with renal failure		
HELLP syndrome complications		
Eclampsia complications		
Other hypertensive disease complications		
Pulmonary	27	19.6
Pneumonia complications		
Amniotic fluid embolus		
Adult respiratory distress syndrome		
Pulmonary embolus		
Cardiac	16	11.6
Eisenmenger's complex		
Myocardial infarction		
Arrhythmia cardiomyopathy		
Unspecified		
Hemorrhage	14	10.1
Central nervous system hemorrhage	10	7.2
Arteriovenous malformation		
Brain stem hemorrhage		
Intracranial hemorrhage		
Infection	11	8.0
Sepsis		
Tuberculosis meningitis		
Malignancy	8	5.8
Hematologic	2	1.5
Thrombotic thrombocytopenic purpura		
Gastrointestinal	1	0.7
Acute fatty liver of pregnancy		
Poisoning/overdose	2	1.5
Anesthesia complication	1	0.7
Trauma	1	0.7
Unspecified	9	6.5
Total	138	100%

Acknowledgments

We would like to express our sincere appreciation to Anthony Vintzileos, MD, from the Department of Obstetrics and Gynecology, Winthrop-University Hospital, Mineola, NY, for critically reviewing the manuscript and offering several comments that improved its contents. We also appreciate the efficient and excellent assistance of Susan Fosbre during the preparation of this manuscript and thank Laura Smulian for critically proofreading the chapter.

References

1 World Health Organization. *Maternal Mortality: A Global Factbook.* Geneva: World Health Organization, 1991.

2 Morbidity and Mortality Weekly Report – MMWR. Maternal mortality – United States, 1982–1996. US Department of Health and Human Services 1998; 47: 705–707.

3 Harmer M. Maternal mortality – is it still relevant? *Anaesthesia* 1997; 52: 99–100.

4 Mahutte NG, Murphy-Kaulbeck L, Le Q, Solomon J, Benjamin A, Boyd ME. Obstetrics admissions to the intensive care unit. *Obstet Gynecol* 1999; 94: 263–266.

5 Hazelgrove JF, Price C, Pappachan GD. Multicenter study of obstetric admissions to 14 intensive care units in southern England. *Crit Care Med* 2001; 29: 770–775.

6 Baskett TF, Sternadel J. Maternal intensive care and near-miss mortality in obstetrics. *Br J Obstet Gynaecol* 1998; 105: 981–984.

7 Mantel GD, Buchmann E, Rees H, Pattinson RC. Severe acute maternal morbidity: A pilot study of a definition for a near-miss. *Br J Obstet Gynaecol* 1998; 105: 985–990.

8 Scott CL, Chavez GF, Atrash HK, Taylor DJ, Shah RS, Rowley D. Hospitalizations for severe complications of pregnancy, 1987–1992. *Obstet Gynecol* 1997; 90: 225–229.

9 Bennett TA, Kotelchuck M, Cox CE, Tucker MJ, Nadeau DA. Pregnancy-associated hospitalizations in the United States in 1991 and 1992: A comprehensive review of maternal morbidity. *Am J Obstet Gynecol* 1998; 178: 346–354.

10 Franks AL, Kendrick JS, Olson DR, Atrash HK, Saftlas AF, Moien M. Hospitalization for pregnancy complications, United States, 1986 and 1987. *Am J Obstet Gynecol* 1992; 166: 1339–1344.

11 National Center for Health Statistics. Design and operation of the National Hospital Discharge Survey: 1988 redesign. Series I. Programs and collection procedures. US Department of Health and Human Services, CDC 2000; DHHS Publication 2001–1315 (number 39).

12 National Center for Health Statistics. Healthy people 2000 review, 1992. Hyattsville, MD: US Department of Health and Human Services, Public Health Service, CDC, 1993.

13 Morbidity and Mortality Weekly Report – MMWR. Pregnancy-related deaths among Hispanic, Asian/Pacific Islander, and American Indian/Alaska Native women – United States, 1991–1997. US Department of Health and Human Services 2001; 50: 361–364.

14 Morbidity and Mortality Weekly Report – MMWR. Maternal mortality – United States, 1982–1996. US Department of Health and Human Services 1998; 47: 705–707.

15 Sachs BP, Brown DA, Driscoll SG et al. Maternal mortality in Massachusetts: trends and prevention. *N Engl J Med* 1987; 316: 667–672.

16 Syverson CJ, Chavkin W, Atrash HK, Rochat RW, Sharp ES, King GE. Pregnancy-related mortality in New York City, 1980 to1984: Causes of death and associated factors. *Am J Obstet Gynecol* 1991; 164: 603–608.

17 Mertz KJ, Parker AL, Halpin GJ. Pregnancy-related mortality in New Jersey, 1975–1989. *Am J Public Health* 1992; 82: 1085–1088.

18 Berg CJ, Atrash HK, Koonin LM, Tucker M. Pregnancy-related mortality in the United States, 1987–1990. *Obstet Gynecol* 1996; 88: 161–167.

19 Atrash HK, Rowley D, Hogue CJ. Maternal and perinatal mortality. *Curr Opin Obstet Gynecol* 1992; 4: 61–71.

20 MacDorman MF, Atkinson JO. Infant mortality statistics from the linked birth/infant death data set – 1995 period data. *Mon Vital Stat Rep* 1998 Feb 26; 46(6 Suppl 2): 1–22.

21 Taffel S, Johnson D, Heuser R. A method of imputing length of gestation on birth certificates. *Vital Health Stat 2*, 1982 May; 93: 1–11.

22 Mabie WC, Sibai BM. Treatment in an obstetric intensive care unit. *Am J Obstet Gynecol* 1990; 162: 1–4.

23 Kilpatrick SJ, Matthay MA. Obstetric patients requiring critical care. A five-year review. *Chest* 1992; 101: 1407–1412.

24 Collop NA, Sahn SA. Critical illness in pregnancy. An analysis of 20 patients admitted to a medical intensive care unit. *Chest* 1993; 103: 1548–1552.

25 El-Solh AA, Grant BJ. A comparison of severity of illness scoring systems for critically ill obstetrics patients. *Chest* 1996; 110: 1299–1304.

26 Monoco TJ, Spielman FJ, Katz VL. Pregnant patients in the intensive care unit: a descriptive analysis. *South Med J* 1993; 86: 414–417.

27 Panchal S, Arria AM, Harris AP. Intensive care utilization during hospital admission for delivery: Prevalence, risk factors, and outcomes in a statewide population. *Anesthesiology* 2000; 92: 1537–1544.

28 Afessa B, Green B, Delke I, Koch K. Systemic inflammatory response syndrome, organ failure, and outcome in critically ill obstetric patients treated in an ICU. *Chest* 2001; 120: 1271–1277.

29 Gilbert TT, Hardie R, Martin A et al. (Abstract). Obstetric admissions to the intensive care unit: demographic and severity of illness analysis. *Am J Respir Crit Care Med* 2000; 161: A236.

30 Hogg B, Hauth JC, Kimberlin D, Brumfield C, Cliver S. Intensive care unit utilization during pregnancy. *Obstet Gynecol* 2000; 95(Suppl): 62S.

31 Munnur U, Karnad DR, Bandi VDP, Lapsia V, Suresh MS, Ramshesh P, Gardner MA, Longmire S, Guntupalli KK. Critically ill obstetric patients in an American and an Indian public hospital: comparison of case-mix, organ dysfunction, intensive care requirements, and outcomes. *Intensive Care Med* 2005; 31: 1087–1094.

32 Lapinsky SE, Kruczynski K, Seaward GR, Farine D, Grossman RF. Critical care management of the obstetric patient. *Can J Anaesth* 1997; 44: 325–329.

33 DeMello WF, Restall J. The requirement of intensive care support for the pregnant population. *Anesthesia* 1990; 45: 888.

34 Selo-Ojeme DO, Omosaiye M, Battacherjee P, Kadir RA. Risk factors for obstetric admissions to the intensive care unit in a tertiary hospital: a case control study. *Arch Gynecol Obstet* 2005; 272: 207.

35 Stephens ID. ICU admissions from an obstetrical hospital. *Can J Anaesth* 1991; 38: 677–681.

36 Tang LC, Kwok AC, Wong AY, Lee YY, Sun KO, So AP. Critical care in obstetrical patients: An eight-year review. *Chinese Med J* (English) 1997; 110: 936–941.

37 Ng Tl, Lim E, Tweed WA, Arulkumaran S. Obstetric admissions to the intensive care unit – a retrospective review. *Ann Acad Med Singapore* 1992; 21: 804–806.

38 Cheng C, Raman S. Intensive care use by critically ill obstetric patients: a five-year review. *Int J Obstet Anesthesia* 2003; 12: 89–92.

39 Heinonen S, Tyrväinen E, Saarikoski S, Ruokonen E. Need for maternal critical care in obstetrics: a population-based analysis. *Int J Obstet Anesthesia* 2002; 11: 260–264.

40 Keizer JL, Zwart JJ, Meerman RH, Harinck BIJ, Feuth HDM, van Roosmalen . Obstetric intensive care admissions: a 12-year review in a tertiary care centre. *Eur J Obstet Gynecol Reprod Biol* 2006; 128: 152–156.

41 Bouvier-Colle MH, Salanave B, Ancel PY et al. Obstetric patients treated in intensive care units and maternal mortality. Regional teams for the survey. *Eur J Obstet Gynecol Reprod Biol* 1996; 65: 121–125.

42 Koeberle P, Levy A, Surcin S, Bartholin F, Clément G, Bachour K, Boillot A, Capellier G, Riethmuller D. Complications obstétricales graves nécessitant une hospitalization en reanimation: étude retrospective sur 10 ans au CHU de Basançon. *Ann Fr Anesth Réanim* 2000; 19: 445–451.

43 Ryan M, Hamilton V, Bowen M, McKenna P. The role of a high-dependency unit in a regional obstetric hospital. *Anaesthesia* 2000; 55: 1155–1158.

44 Cohen J, Singer P, Kogan A, Hod M, Bar J. Course and outcome of obstetric patients in a general intensive care unit. *Acta Obstet Gynecol Scand* 2000; 79: 846–850.

45 Lewinsohn G, Herman A, Lenov Y, Klinowski E. Critically ill obstetrical patients: Outcome and predictability. *Crit Care Med* 1994; 22: 1412–1414.

46 Loverro G, Pansini V, Greco P, Vimercati A, Parisi AM, Selvaggi L. Indications and outcome for intensive care unit admission during puerperium. *Arch Gynecol Obstet* 2001; 265: 195–198.

47 Okafor UV, Aniebue U. Admission pattern and outcome in critical care obstetric patients. *Int J Obstet Anesthesia* 2004; 13: 164–166.

48 Platteau P, Engelhardt T, Moodley J, Muckart DJ. Obstetric and gynaecological patients in an intensive care unit: A 1 year review. *Trop Doctor* 1997; 27: 202–206.

49 Demirkiran O, Dikmen Y, Utku T, Urkmez S. Critically ill obstetric patients in the intensive care unit. *Int J Obstet Anesthesia* 2003; 12: 266–270.

50 Mirghani HM, Hamed M, Ezimokhai M, Weerasinghe DSL. Pregnancy-related admissions to the intensive care unit. *Int J Obstet Anesthesia* 2004; 13: 82–85.

51 Al-Suleiman SA, Qutub HO, Rahman J, Rahman MS. Obstetric admissions to the intensive care unit: A 12-year review. *Arch Gynecol Obstet* 2006; 274: 4–8.

52 Knaus WA, Draper EA, Wagner DP, Zimmerman JE. An evaluation of outcome from intensive care in major medical centers. *Ann Intern Med* 1986; 104: 410–418.

53 Koonin LM, MacKay AP, Berg CJ, Atrash HK, Smith JC. Pregnancy-related mortality surveillance – United States, 1987–1990. MMWR, Morbidity and Mortality Weekly Report 1997; 46: 17–36.

54 Stevens TA, Carroll MA, Promecene PA, Seibel M, Monga M. Utility of Acute Physiology, Age, and Chronic Health Evaluation (APACHE III) score in maternal admissions to the intensive care unit. *Am J Obstet Gynecol* 2006; 194: 13–15.

2 Organizing an Obstetric Critical Care Unit

Julie Scott[1] & Michael R. Foley[2]

[1]Department of Obstetrics and Gynecology, Division of Maternal-Fetal Medicine, University of Colorado Health Sciences Center, Denver, CO, USA

[2]Scotsdale Healthcare, Scottsdale, Arizona *and* Department of Obstetrics and Gynecology, University of Arizona College of Medicine, Tucson, AZ, USA

Introduction

Critical care unit organization has evolved from the times of Florence Nightingale, who wrote about postoperative recovery areas near the operating suites with attendants at the bedside, to the technologically and medically advanced intensive care units we utilize today [1]. Yet the modern critical care unit is truly only in its infancy stages in that the first National Institutes of Health Consensus Conference pertaining to critical care was convened less than 30 years ago to establish guidelines for protocols of care, design and staffing of these units [2]. Currently there are more than 6000 critical care units in the United States [3]. The medical needs of these critically ill patients are quite complex with not only medical or surgical issues that need to be addressed but also the psychosocial parameters of illness that affect the patient. As a result of these complexities, the critical care team has expanded to include many disciplines with varying levels of organizational management.

An expansion of these critical care models has been applied to obstetric medicine which has a unique population of critically ill women. Pregnancy alters maternal physiology with respect to many organ systems with notable changes pertaining to critical care in the hematologic, cardiopulmonary, renal, endocrine and gastrointestinal systems. In addition to providing care to the mother, we have to consider the needs of the unborn child, which most likely has also been affected by the mother's current health status. Addressing the needs of this population of patients requires specific expertise not only on the part of the obstetric physician, but also nursing and additional ancillary staff who may be providing respiratory support or pharmaceutical interventions. Clearly, these patients require a multiteam approach to provide optimal care.

Critical Care Obstetrics, 5th edition. Edited by M. Belfort, G. Saade, M. Foley, J. Phelan and G. Dildy.

Relevance

Numerous reports in the literature detail the beneficial impact on clinical outcomes when patients are grouped based on severity of illness with physical organization of their care in the same area of the hospital. The rationale driving this model is that the sickest patients are cared for by medical specialists, the brightest nursing staff and ancillary service providers with all the appropriate technology to support their centrally located care. Hence, the reason for organization of cardiac care units, dialysis units, burn units, surgical intensive care units and medical intensive care units. Modernization of medicine with parcelation of expertise care has also occurred in our own specialty, with maternal fetal medicine specialists, for the most part, managing the care of the critically ill obstetric patient. Current literature from tertiary care centers accepting referred patients reports that approximately 0.5–1% of their obstetric population have required care in an intensive care unit [1,2,4].

Patient population

Most obstetricians will concede that pregnancy, with its potential hazards, has the opportunity to produce life-threatening complications. The prior existence of medical disease such as hypertension, diabetes, and autoimmune diseases, to name a few, further complicates the care of mother and child. These and other comorbid medical conditions are becoming more and more prevalent in our obstetric population. The health of our obstetric population reflects that of our nation as a whole, which is changing rapidly secondary to the complications of obesity. The age of our gravidas has also increased, thereby increasing the likelihood of comorbid disease. Further affected are the gravidas, both young and old, with pregnancies that resulted from infertility treatments, with the potential for high-order multiple gestations contributing to pregnancy risks.

Reviews in the literature suggest that obstetric ICU utilization is near 1% in the obstetric population [1,2,4]. The majority of these intensive care admissions were secondary to obstetric complications including hypertensive disorders (pre-eclampsia and eclampsia), respiratory failure as a result of obstetric infection or sepsis, hemorrhage and hemodynamic instability warranting a higher level of care [1,2,4,5]. Antenatally, the majority of ICU admissions were for respiratory support and in the postpartum period for hemodynamic instability with the potential for invasive hemodynamic monitoring. It is important to recognize that the parturient with deteriorating health status secondary to comorbid medical conditions or the healthy parturient who is unstable from an obstetric complication can equally benefit from care in the environment of the intensive care unit (Table 2.1).

Table 2.1 Admission criteria.

Obstetric patients with established medical disease complicating pregnancy
Cardiac
Pulmonary
Renal
Endocrine
Neurologic
Hematologic
Hepatic
Immune
Obstetric patients with obstetric complications
Pre-eclampsia/eclampsia
Hemorrhage and DIC
Pregnancy-related sepsis
Amniotic fluid embolism
Trauma of the obstetric patient requiring intensive monitoring
Pregnant patients requiring invasive hemodynamic monitoring
Pregnant patients with toxicologic insult/poisoning/overdose

Aggressive management of this patient population, combined with the overall better health status, yields lower mortality rates (compared to patients admitted to a standard medical/surgical ICU who are generally older and more infirm) [6].

Members of the team

Critical care management of the obstetric patient requires a multidisciplinary team. The physiologic changes that occur during pregnancy, with their impact on fetal well-being, clearly need to be addressed in order to provide appropriate care. Members of this highly trained team include physicians, nurses, respiratory therapists, clinical pharmacists, and other ancillary healthcare team members. Patient-centered care incorporates all members of the team with the common goal of providing quality, evidence-based care in an efficient, systems-driven model (Figure 2.1). Multidisciplinary teams with protocol-driven care to assist with the critical care decision-making process have been demonstrated to provide improved patient outcomes [7].

Physician staffing

Maternal fetal medicine specialists are among the obstetric providers with the highest level of training to provide critical care to the parturient. Their involvement in the care plan helps facilitate the understanding of the physiologic changes in pregnancy affecting health status, including cardiopulmonary, hemodynamic and gastrointestinal organ systems, among others. Further, their understanding of these processes helps to identify potential *in utero* compromise and complications that jeopardize fetal well-being.

Intensivists whose day-to-day work is in the management of the critically ill patient are vital to the multiprofessional team caring for the obstetric patient. A systematic review in 2002 detailed the importance of intensivist physician staffing in the ICU with data demonstrating reduced ICU and hospital mortal-

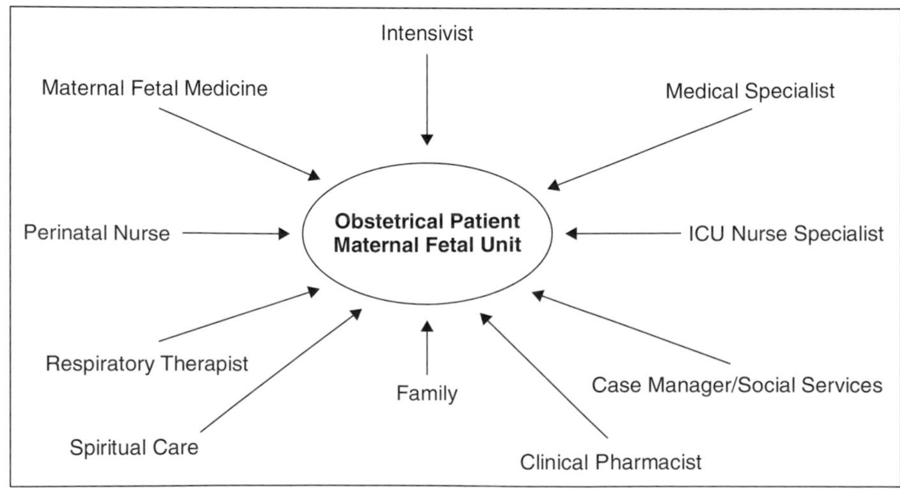

Figure 2.1 Patient-centered approach.

ity and length of stay when there was a greater use of intensivists in the intensive care unit [3]. The intensivists' direct impact on mortality rates has also been demonstrated by Pollack et al. who also showed a decline in mortality-related events, improved efficiency and organization of the ICU in their population [8]. Several different models have been proposed for the involvement of the intensivist and maternal fetal medicine specialist including designation of one or the other as the primary care provider with the other as a consultant or as coproviders with collaborative efforts providing superior patient care. The unique area of expertise that each can provide allows for effective and efficient use of resources [9].

Physician collaborators from other subspecialties may also be helpful. Neonatologists are important team members in the care of the obstetric patient. They help define the fetal and neonatal complications that arise with premature delivery and issues of viability. They are a particularly important resource for families faced with decisions regarding intervention on behalf of the mother and fetus. Other providers include cardiologists and cardiothoracic surgeons for cardiac care and surgical repairs, infectious disease specialists for complicating infectious comorbidities, and neurologists and neurosurgeons to assist with the management of complications relating to hypertensive disorders, including cerebral hemorrhages and infarctions. Working together in an interdisciplinary manner with one physician designated as the primary provider will expand the potential therapeutic options available and provide better care overall.

Nursing staffing

Obstetric nursing has changed drastically over the past 50 years into a complex science with nurses providing highly skilled care for the mother and her fetus with physiologic monitoring of both patients. High-risk obstetric nursing requires a confident and compassionate nurse willing to undertake the complexities and challenges of higher acuity care. In general, the staffing patterns dictated by critical care will demand a 1 : 1 nurse-to-patient ratio in order to meet the needs of the patient and her fetus. With an unstable parturient, this may even require 2 : 1 nurse-to-patient staffing, with a critical care nurse also at the bedside to manage cardiopulmonary monitoring, blood draws, and medication administrations while the obstetric nurse continues to provide fetal monitoring, optimizing maternal positioning and continued surveillance for symptoms significant for preterm labor.

Protocols for staffing, education and core competencies have been described for nurses who care for the critically ill obstetric patient [10]. As these patients are usually a small percentage of the obstetric population, the labor and delivery nurse with a special interest in perinatal nursing care will most often manage the standard obstetric patient. This nurse will need to have mastery of not only the normal physiologic changes of pregnancy, but also the pathophysiologic conditions associated with pregnancy and their impact on the fetus. Additionally, this nurse will be familiar with critical care monitoring techniques and fetal monitoring, with the ability to interpret overall changes that affect fetal well-being. It is recommended that these nurses have at least 1 year of labor and delivery experience with formal instruction in obstetric intensive care [11] (Table 2.2).

Bedside nursing is only one of the many roles that these nurses must master. In addition, the obstetric critical care nurse helps to foster communication between the physician professionals who visit the bedside, provides anticipatory guidance for the patient and her family members who are anxious and concerned, and tends to the psychosocial needs of the patient who may now encounter barriers to mother–child bonding secondary to the ICU environment [10]. These critical care obstetric nurses are highly motivated, enjoy the interactions with team members, and have the ability to facilitate patient care with all the professionals involved. Overall, the collaborative efforts between nurses and physicians in this multidisciplinary team yield better patient outcomes, shorter lengths of stay, decreased overall costs and a heightened sense of professionalism among nursing team members [9,10].

Table 2.2 Obstetric ICU nursing education.

Registered Nurse with at least 1 year of nursing experience in a tertiary care center
Medical surgical nursing
ICU nursing
Labor and delivery unit nursing
Core curriculum
Normal physiologic changes of pregnancy – organ system based
Pathophysiologic alterations of pregnancy
Pregnancy-induced hypertension, pre-eclampsia, eclampsia, HELLP syndrome
Preterm labor management and actions/side effects of tocolytic agents
Cardiac
Respiratory
Renal
Endocrine-specific attention on thyroid disorders, diabetes (pre-existing and gestational)
Hematologic
Sepsis/chorioamnionitis/vascular instability
Monitoring basics
Cardiotocography and contraction monitoring
Basics of telemetry
Invasive hemodynamic monitoring
Principles of mechanical ventilation
Clinical training
ACLS (Advanced Cardiac Life Support)
NRP (Neonatal Resuscitation Program)
Simulated case series
Continuing education
Case review

Other staffing

In order for appropriate clinical services to be provided for patient care, an ICU must have personnel whose main focus is on the administrative details of the unit. Based on the guidelines developed by the Task Force of the American College of Critical Care Medicine and the Society of Critical Care Medicine, units must have designated medical and nursing directors who are responsible for assuring appropriate patient triage through enforcement of patient admission and discharge criteria [12]. These personnel will also promote the continuing education of the staff and directly interface with other unit directors to ensure the quality of care and the appropriateness of services rendered [13]. Implementing technologic advancements, maintaining care protocols and facilitating efforts to improve patient safety and infectious disease control are also important directive responsibilities.

Ancillary staff members also have vital roles in the multidisciplinary team. Nutritional services may be required for patients needing enteral or parenteral feeding, with special consideration of the increased caloric demands of pregnancy. The respiratory therapist is continually updating the team with regard to the pulmonary status of the patient, which may vary from full ventilatory support to supplemental oxygenation as status declines or improves. Case managers and social workers are also integral members who interface with family members and outside services for the transition to either step-down units in the hospital, outpatient facilities or home with various health-related services. Chaplain and spiritual service providers also offer additional support to the patient and her family and assist with the emotional stresses of the ICU environment, disease process, and even potential end-of-life issues.

Unit design: a virtual space

Intensive care unit health costs are exorbitant, approximating 1% of the United States Gross Domestic Product [3]. The management, staffing and organizational models of the intensive care unit have come under scrutiny recently with economic pressure to contain costs [14]. Part of the problem is inappropriate utilization of ICU resources for patients who do not necessarily meet the admission criteria for the unit and its services, thereby increasing the potential costs of care [15]. To that end, the architectural design of an intensive care unit as a finite space with a maximum occupancy will have its own limits. If this space is incorrectly utilized with lower acuity patients then its availability for those who truly need the care will not be available. Many community hospitals do not have the resources to establish a separate designated space for the care of the critically ill obstetric patient. Therefore, the care of this patient is absorbed into the available ICU model which may not have staffing who can properly meet the needs of this specialized patient.

Intensive care unit designs in current use in the United States generally follow two basic models of organization: open and closed. In open ICUs, the organization is such that the attending physician of the patient may admit to the unit without prior approval or with only minimal screening as long as they have appropriate privileges to treat. In this setting, the admission and discharge criteria tend to be less strict. Intensivists are not necessarily the primary provider but are available as consultants with the attending physician of record making the management and treatment plans. An advantage of this model is maintenance of the physician–patient relationship with continuity of care. Familiarity of the patient with the treating doctor fosters trust in the medical management and aids in promoting a positive psychosocial environment, important in healing. Unfortunately, in an open ICU when a patient is admitted by their primary physician (who may not be based in the hospital and likely has a community based private practice) there is a compromise in the care as these physicians are juggling their day to day private practice duties and attempting to manage the patient they admitted to the hospital. At times, this may lead to delays in care and ineffective communication regarding treatment plans with the hospital-based staff caring for the patient because of inconsistent physician availability.

A more structured, intensivist-managed, closed unit model provides advantages that cannot be matched by an open ICU model. Lower morbidity and mortality and decreased length of critical care unit and hospital stay have all been demonstrated with this organizational model [3,8,13]. In this model, a board-certified intensive care specialist directs the care of the critically ill patient with adherence to well-defined admission and discharge criteria. This physician typically has no other competing clinical duties and is dedicated to the care of these patients. This allows a better utilization of healthcare resources with reduction in healthcare expenditure.

Approximately one-quarter of ICUs in the US are closed units [3]. Most intensive care units are organized as a hybrid model with a focus on centralized decision making and management. Collaboration of the intensivist with the attending of record (admitting physician) maximizes the level of care delivered while maintaining continuity of care for the patient. Cordial communication and professional collegiality are important factors for success in this dynamic environment.

Hybridization of the open and closed unit designs usually provides the best care. The obstetric specialist will play a key role in the management of the critically ill parturient. As previously described, a multidisciplinary team is paramount. There are, however, several important questions that need to be addressed. Where in your hospital design should the unit be located? Are there enough resources available for a separate obstetric intensive care unit? Do you have a large enough population of critically ill parturients to make this unit practical and fiscally responsible? For many hospital settings, a separate obstetric intensive care unit is not possible or a practical use of resources.

Therefore, innovative approaches must be considered including the concept of a "virtual obstetric intensive care unit"™ (Michael R. Foley MD). With this practical concept, the ICU is situated and organized not necessarily by location, but by the multispecialty team providing the care to meet the specific needs of the patient. Ideally, this can be accomplished on the labor and delivery unit with obstetric operating suites available for emergencies. Obstetric cardiac patients can have mobile telemetry, dialysis machines can be brought to the bedside for the patient with renal failure, hemodynamic and ventilator support all can be mobilized if no beds are available in the unit. Fetal surveillance by cardiotocography is also not a locale-specific task. The emphasis is on the team providing care to the patient with the organizational leaders being the combined maternal fetal medicine specialist and the medical subspecialist comanaging the illness. For one critically ill obstetric patient, this may mean having the nephrologists and dialysis nurse, in the renal unit, providing their expertise for the patient with renal failure; for another, it may be the cardiologist and telemetry nurse, in the cardiac care unit, treating the hemodynamically unstable arrhythmia, or the intensivist and obstetric specialist, in the labor and delivery unit, administering care to the patient with life-threatening hemorrhage, hypertensive crises and other sequelae from pre-eclampsia and eclampsia.

Importantly, the key features that have been shown to improve outcomes-directed care by an intensivist (including the maternal fetal specialist) with continued care for the patient on the labor and delivery unit have been met. The only modification is the direct locale and potential members of the team, depending on the nature of the critical illness. Proximity to the obstetric operating suite with anesthesia services will allow for immediate surgery for maternal or fetal indications with the potential to limit further morbidities. A "virtual" obstetric critical care unit optimizes the care being delivered by providing a team of specialists who treat the patient where she is located, utilizing the perinatal nurse and other staff as necessary and mobilizing all technical equipment required.

Conclusion

Caring for the critically ill obstetric patient is complex. There are two patients to consider along with alterations of maternal physiology, and the potential pharmacologic considerations to account for. Fortunately, this is a small subset of the entire obstetric population. Efforts to reduce perinatal morbidities and mortality for the critically ill patient have lead practitioners toward models of care similar to those in use in intensive care units. Board-certified intensive care specialists and obstetric specialists, as a part of a multidisciplinary team with ongoing medical education, optimize the care being delivered while utilizing current technologies to support function. Polishing these positive attributes of a "unit" and facilitating care in the best locale for the patient may improve resource utilization and allow for the family-centered environment that a traditional labor and delivery ward provides. The virtual obstetric unit is uniquely situated based on the specific medical needs of the critically ill obstetric patient, thereby eliminating the need to maintain a separate unit in the hospital. Team members are assembled based on the direct clinical application necessary, with centralization through the intensivist or maternal fetal medicine specialist as appropriate.

References

1 Mable WC, Baha MS. Treatment in an obstetric intensive care unit. *Am J Obstet Gynecol* 1990; 162(1): 1–4.
2 Zeeman G, Wendel GD, Cunningham FG. A blueprint for obstetric critical care. *Am J Obstet Gynecol* 2003; 188: 532–536.
3 Pronovost PJ, Angus DC, Dorman T, et al. Physician staffing patterns and clinical outcomes in critically ill patients a systematic review. *JAMA* 2002; 288: 2151–2162.
4 Lapinsky SE, Kruzynski K, Seaward GR, Farine D, Grossman RF. Critical care management of the obstetric patient. *Can J Anaesth* 1997; 44(3): 325–329.
5 Graham SG, Luxton MC. The requirement for intensive care support for the pregnant population. *Anaesthesia* 1989; 44: 581–584.
6 Kilpatrick SJ, Matthay MA. Obstetric patients requiring critical care a five year review. *Chest* 1992; 101: 1407–1412.
7 Wall RJ, Dittus RS, Ely EW. Protocol-driven care in the intensive care unit: a tool for quality. *Critical Care* 2001; 5(6): 283–285.
8 Pollack MM, Katz RW, Ruttimann UE, Getson PR. Improving the outcome and efficiency of intensive care: the impact of an intensivist. *Crit Care Med* 1988; 16: 11–17.
9 Strosberg MA. Intensive care units in the triage mode. An organizational perspective. *Crit Care Clin* 1993; 9(3): 415–424.
10 Brubaker JJ, Teplick FB, McAndrew L. Developing a maternal-fetal intensive care unit. *J Obstet Gynecol Neonat Nurs* 1988; 17(5): 321–326.
11 Graves C. Organizing a critical care obstetric unit. In: Dildy GA III, ed. *Critical Care Obstetrics*, 4th edn. Malden, MA: Blackwell Science, 2004: 13–18.
12 Task Force of the American College of Critical Care Medicine. Guidelines for intensive care unit admission, discharge, and triage. *Crit Care Med* 1999; 27(3): 633–638.
13 Hass BD. Critical care unit organization and patient outcomes. *Crit Care Nurs Quart* 2005; 28(4): 336–340.
14 Marini JJ. Streamlining critical care: responsibilities and cost effectiveness in intensive care unit organization. *Mayo Clin Proc* 1997; 72: 483–485.
15 Iapichino G, Radrizzani D, Ferla L, et al. Description of trends in the course of illness of critically ill patients. Markers of intensive care organization and performance. *Intens Care Med* 2002; 28: 985–989.

3 Critical Care Obstetric Nursing

Suzanne McMurtry Baird[1] & Nan H. Troiano[2]

[1]Vanderbilt University School of Nursing, Nashville, TN, USA
[2]Women's Services, Labor & Delivery and High Risk Perinatal Unit, Inova Fairfax Hospital Women's Center, Falls Church, Virginia *and* Columbia University; New-York Presbyterian Hospital, Department of Obstetrics and Gynecology, Division of Maternal-Fetal Medicine *and* Consultant, Critical Care Obstetrics, New York, USA

Introduction

The essence of critical care nursing lies not in special environments nor amid special equipment, but in the nurse's decision-making process and a willingness to act on those decisions (Tables 3.1 & 3.2). The critically ill obstetric patient requires specialized care directed not only at her identified pathophysiological problems, but also at psychosocial and family issues that become intimately intertwined.

This chapter provides an overview of essential concepts related to critical care obstetric nursing. Standards of nursing care are presented which provide the framework for all professional nursing practice. The inherent need for professional collaboration, communication and teamwork in a critical care setting is reinforced. Case examples are presented which illustrate application of critical care concepts to clinical nursing practice. Finally, strategies are described to adequately prepare nurses to provide quality care to critically ill pregnant women.

Standards of nursing care: framework for critical care obstetric nursing

Standards are the basis for nursing practice. They are an important benchmark against which registered nurses assess their professional practice and by which the quality of practice may be judged. In the USA a variety of sources establish and define standards including local and state statutes (nurse practice acts), the American Nurses Association (ANA), national professional nursing organizations, documentary evidence, established references, and expert witness testimony [3]. In other countries similar bodies take on these responsibilities.

Nursing is a dynamic profession that has undergone significant change over time. Thus, regardless of their source, standards should be dynamic to reflect the current state of knowledge applicable to nursing practice.

Critical Care Obstetrics, 5th edition. Edited by M. Belfort, G. Saade, M. Foley, J. Phelan and G. Dildy. © 2010 Blackwell Publishing Ltd.

Critical care technology: critical concepts and application to clinical practice

Technological adjuncts are an integral part of providing care to selected critically ill obstetric patients. Examples of such critical care technology include invasive hemodynamic monitoring and mechanical ventilation. Thus, critical concepts related to use of invasive hemodynamic monitoring and mechanical ventilation during pregnancy are presented. Case examples are provided to illustrate application of these concepts to bedside clinical nursing practice.

Invasive hemodynamic monitoring: concepts for intrapartum nursing practice

The ability to obtain continuous hemodynamic and oxygen transport data has led to a better understanding of pathophysiological processes in disease states during pregnancy and to an improved ability to use data to guide therapeutic decision-making. In general, invasive hemodynamic monitoring is indicated during pregnancy for patients with complications that are refractory to conventional therapy or who have conditions that place her at significant risk for cardiopulmonary compromise or end-organ dysfunction. One such condition is coronary artery disease.

Pulmonary artery catheterization during pregnancy is discussed in detail in Chapter 16 of this text. Cardiac disease during pregnancy including specific principles related to the medical care of patients with coronary artery disease is thoroughly addressed in Chapter 20.

Caring for the pregnant woman with significant cardiac disease during the intrapartum period presents unique challenges for the critical care team. Comprehensive discussion of specific critical care nursing issues related to this patient population is beyond

Table 3.1 Standards of clinical nursing practice: standards of care.

Standard	Statement
I Assessment	The nurse collects patient health data
II Diagnosis	The nurse analyzes the assessment data in determining diagnoses
III Outcome identification	The nurse identifies expected outcomes individualized to the patient
IV Planning	The nurse develops a plan of care that prescribes interventions to attain expected outcomes
V Implementation	The nurse implements the interventions identified in the plan of care
VI Evaluation	The nurse evaluates the patient's progress toward attainment of outcomes

Table 3.2 Standards of clinical nursing practice: standards of professional performance.

Standard	Statement
I Quality of care	The nurse systematically evaluates the quality and effectiveness of nursing practice
II Performance appraisal	The nurse evaluates his/her own nursing practice in relation to professional practice standards and relevant statutes and regulations
III Education	The nurse acquires and maintains current knowledge in nursing practice
IV Collegiality	The nurse contributes to the professional development of peers, colleagues, and others
V Ethics	The nurse's decisions and actions on behalf of patient are determined in an ethical manner
VI Collaboration	The nurse collaborates with the patient, significant others, and healthcare providers in providing patient care
VII Research	The nurse uses research findings in practice
VIII Resource utilization	The nurse considers factors related to safety, effectiveness, and cost in planning and delivering patient care

the scope of this chapter. Additional resources are available that address topics including classification of cardiac disorders during pregnancy, general principles of nursing care, nursing diagnoses, interventions to promote maternal and fetal stabilization, and specific nursing care issues related to coronary artery disease [9–12].

Certain technical issues related to invasive hemodynamic monitoring require attention when caring for the critically ill obstetric patient. Historically, these issues have often been considered the domain of either the physician or the nurse. However, such compartmentalization of responsibility is in direct conflict to the concept of collaboration and team centric approach. More importantly, it promotes a great disservice to the quality of patient care. Nurses and physicians with extensive clinical experience in obstetric practice cannot imagine a professional environment in which nursing responsibilities related to electronic monitoring of fetal and maternal status are limited to application of monitoring devices, operation of the equipment, and the ability to change the monitoring paper, with interpretation of data and initiation of all necessary interventions the sole responsibility of a physician. In fact, physicians depend on nurses to assess and interpret patient data, communicate significant findings in a timely manner, initiate appropriate nursing interventions and evaluate the patient's response to interventions. In other words, physicians expect nurses to utilize the nursing process as a framework for patient care. The same concept applies to the practice of critical care, especially when technological adjuncts such as invasive hemodynamic monitoring or mechanical ventilation are utilized in the care of a unique patient population.

Central venous access

Several critical care obstetric nursing issues relate to establishment of central venous access. Because of pulmonary physiologic changes associated with pregnancy and the increased risk of pneumothorax, the preferred site for central venous access during pregnancy is the internal jugular vein. Advantages include the ease by which this vessel can be compressed in the case of hemorrhage, decreased risk of pneumothorax, and, when the right internal jugular vein is cannulated, the thoracic duct is avoided. The nurse should assist with proper positioning of the patient to facilitate successful performance of the procedure. It is also imperative that the uterus be displaced laterally during establishment of central venous access and catheter placement to prevent reduction in venous return, cardiac output, supine hypotension, and a concomitant decrease in uterine perfusion. Displacement may be accomplished manually or by placing a wedge under the patient's hip. Depending on the gestational age, assessment of fetal status may be accomplished via continuous electronic fetal monitoring (EFM).

The potential for central line-associated bloodstream infection (CLA-BSI) is of considerable concern in any critical care setting. Research over the last decade has focused on a number of care activities that have been shown to reduce the incidence of catheter-related infections. Four major risk factors are associated with increased catheter-related infection rates: cutaneous colonization of the insertion site, moisture under the dressing, length of time the catheter remains in place, and the technique of care and placement of the central line [13]. Appropriate hand hygiene is the cornerstone of any infection prevention program. Use of maximal sterile barriers (MSBs) has also been shown to reduce infection by improving sterile technique during catheter insertion. The Centers for Disease Control (CDC) guidelines on central line management rate MSBs as the highest-level evidence available for reducing central venous catheter (CVC) infections and recommends adopting this procedure. Research studies have not evaluated what the assisting personnel should wear. Existing guidelines recommend that minimal practice for assisting personnel should be universal precautions, unless the nurse comes into contact with or crosses over the sterile field [15]. Providone iodine has been the most widely used antiseptic for cleansing skin before central catheter line insertion in the United States. Recent data demonstrated that use of chlorhexidine gluconate (CHG) rather than providone iodine reduced the risk of CLA-BSI by approximately 50% in hospitalized patients who required short-term catheterization [16]. The CDC also recommends that application of antibiotic ointment at the insertion site be avoided, as it promotes fungal infections and antibiotic resistance. Replacement of intravenous administration sets and add-on devices is recommended no more frequently than at 72-hour intervals, unless catheter-related infection is suspected or has been documented. In addition, strategies for implementing a comprehensive CLA-BSI prevention program and a tool and process for defect analysis as part of a statewide collaborative effort in Michigan have recently been described [17].

Heparin flush

The addition of heparin to flush solutions used in continuous hemodynamic pressure monitoring lines is another issue that requires special consideration during pregnancy. According to the American Association of Critical Care Nurses' Thunder Project, the risk of non-patency of pressure monitoring lines is greatest in women with short non-femoral lines who do not receive other anticoagulants or thrombolytics and have non-heparinized flush solutions [18]. Since pregnancy is a hypercoagulable state, most procoagulant factors including factors V, VII, VIII, IX, X, XII, and prothrombin are increased during pregnancy. Fibrinolysis is prolonged during pregnancy because of reduction in the levels of antithrombin III and plasminogen activator. Collectively, these provide evidence to support heparinization of hemodynamic pressure monitoring lines when caring for the critically ill pregnant woman. Flush solutions for this patient population usually contain a concentration of between 3 and 5 units of heparin per mL of flush solution.

Cardiac output evaluation

Cardiac output is most often assessed at the bedside by the critical care nurse using the thermodilution method. Temperature of the injectate solution is an issue when caring for the critically ill pregnant woman. Numerous studies report favorable correlation between room temperature and iced injectate solutions for thermodilution cardiac output assessment in the absence of either low or high cardiac output states. The normal range described in these studies has most often been defined as an expected cardiac output greater than 4.0 L/min but less than 8.0 L/min. However, correlation is poor in patients with low or high cardiac output states [19]. Based on these data, iced injectate is recommended if cardiac output is expected to be less than 3.5 L/min or greater than 8.0 L/min. Pregnant women most often are expected to have cardiac outputs greater than 8.0 L/min during an acute or critical illness. Such high cardiac outputs are also expected during labor, birth, and immediately postpartum. It is also imperative that cardiac output assessment be performed between uterine contractions. A number of physiologic events occur during uterine contractions, including autotransfusion of blood from the uterus into the maternal central circulation, which in turn produces significant alteration in cardiac output. Thus, careful assessment for the presence of uterine contractions and proper timing of cardiac output measurements are crucial. This concept is of special concern when pulmonary artery catheters with capability for continuous cardiac output are considered for use during pregnancy. This capability utilizes another thermal-based approach whereby small quantities of heat are emitted via the catheter at the right atrial/right ventricular level using a resistance element. Blood temperature is monitored near the catheter tip a short distance downstream. Assessments are made and averaged at extremely frequent intervals and the averages continuously displayed on the monitor. Thus, near-continuous measurement of cardiac output is available. Though data from these instruments appear to correlate well with those from conventional thermodilution techniques, the inability to eliminate measurements during uterine contractions increases the risk of erroneous data collection as well as inappropriate comparison of fluctuations in data over time. Cardiac output factors into the formula for calculation of significant hemodynamic parameters including systemic vascular resistance, pulmonary vascular resistance, and left ventricular stroke work index. In addition, formulas used for calculation of significant oxygen transport parameters also include cardiac output. These include oxygen delivery, oxygen consumption, and the oxygen extraction ratio. Utilization of this clinical data reduces the likelihood of clinical errors.

Case example: Coronary artery disease and intrapartum nursing care

The following case example illustrates critical clinical practice concepts related to intrapartum nursing care of a pregnant woman with significant cardiac disease who required invasive hemodynamic monitoring. The case involved a 32-year-old pregnant woman admitted at 39 weeks gestation to the critical care obstetric (CCOB) service in the labor and delivery unit of a local tertiary care hospital for planned induction of labor.

Her medical history was significant for development of shortness of breath and dyspnea on exertion less than 2 years before her current pregnancy. A stress electrocardiogram was performed and interpreted as abnormal, as were results of a subsequent nuclear stress test. Coronary angiography was performed which indicated total occlusion of the right coronary artery, 80% occlusion of the midsegment and total occlusion of the distal segment of the left anterior descending coronary artery. A four-vessel coronary artery bypass graft (CABG) was performed which was complicated by a postoperative myocardial infarction (MI). Subsequent care included cardiac rehabilitation with exercise and medications to optimize cardiac function. Echocardiograms performed during the period of cardiac rehabilitation revealed the presence of persistent decreased left ventricular dysfunction and mild pulmonary hypertension.

Her obstetric history was significant for an unplanned pregnancy which occurred approximately 1 year following her CABG and MI. She decided to undergo termination of the pregnancy after consultation with a cardiologist and perinatologist. Less than a year later, she presented at 9 weeks estimated fetal gestational age (EGA) for consultation with a perinatologist. She was subsequently referred to a perinatologist at a local tertiary care center. Initial evaluation included an echocardiogram which indicated persistent moderate to severe left ventricular dysfunction, an ejection fraction between 25 and 30%, and elevated pulmonary artery pressures. The consultation included a thorough discussion with the patient and her husband of the potential risk of morbidity and mortality associated with continuation of the pregnancy, as well as components of a multidisciplinary plan of care should continuation of the pregnancy be desired. Both the patient and her husband verbalized a strong desire to continue the pregnancy. Thus, prenatal care continued, without development of additional maternal or fetal complications.

She was admitted to the CCOB service at 39 weeks gestation for planned induction of labor and vaginal delivery. Any decision to perform a cesarean section would be based on development of obstetric indications. Maternal and fetal assessment findings at the time of admission were all reassuring. Occasional uterine contractions were noted and her cervix was approximately 1 cm dilated and long. On the evening of admission, the induction process was started with the insertion of a Foley catheter into the cervix and the bulb inflated. A neonatologist met with the patient, her husband, and other family members to answer questions and reinforce the plan of care for the baby. Maternal and fetal assessment findings throughout the night remained reassuring.

The following morning, an intravenous infusion of oxytocin was initiated. Regional anesthesia via epidural block was initiated, after administration of an intravenous crystalloid bolus. Monitoring techniques included continuous maternal electrocardiogram (ECG) with the ability to monitor two leads (II and V_5) simultaneously, to detect myocardial ischemia or dysrhythmias. An arterial catheter was utilized for continuous blood pressure assessment and access for obtaining blood samples. Hourly assessment of both intake and output, continuous arterial oxygen saturation monitoring, and auscultation of breath sounds were part of the nursing plan of care. Continuous electronic monitoring of the FHR and uterine activity was also utilized. Equipment for invasive hemodynamic and oxygen transport monitoring had been assembled, prepared, and available at the bedside. In addition, necessary equipment and resources for delivery and immediate care of the baby were made available in the patient's room. The charge nurse in labor and delivery kept neonatal nursing and medical personnel updated on the patient's progress on a regular basis.

Approximately 5 hours after initiation of the oxytocin infusion, nursing assessment of maternal status revealed diminished urinary output for 2 consecutive hours. In addition, the patient complained of new-onset shortness of breath and a cough. Auscultation of the lungs revealed the presence of crackles bilaterally. Vital signs included a blood pressure of 100/61, a normal sinus rhythm of 82, and arterial oxygen saturation (S_aO_2) of 94% on room air. Regular uterine contractions were noted every 2–4 min, moderate to palpation, and uterine resting tone was not consistently relaxed to palpation. Assessment of fetal status revealed a normal baseline rate, no FHR accelerations, and the onset of repetitive FHR decelerations. The CCOB nurse interpreted these findings as indicative of an adverse change in maternal and fetal status. Nursing interventions were initiated including administration of supplemental oxygen by mask, elevation of the head of the patient's bed, lateral displacement of the uterus, discontinuation of the oxytocin infusion and prompt notification of the CCOB physician. The physician ordered that the oxytocin infusion remain off until the hemodynamic and oxygenation status of the patient could be further assessed. A fiberoptic pulmonary artery catheter with capability of continuous mixed venous oxygen saturation (SvO_2) monitoring was inserted via the right internal jugular vein without complications. Initial maternal hemodynamic and oxygen transport assessment data are presented in Table 3.3. Fetal heart rate and uterine activity noted on the EFM tracing at the time the decision was made to initiate invasive hemodynamic monitoring, and after initial maternal hemodynamic and oxygen transport data were obtained are presented in Figures 3.1 and 3.2 respectively.

Interpretation by the nurse of initial hemodynamic data indicated the patient had a significantly low cardiac output (CO). Analysis of the determinants of cardiac output revealed a high left preload, high right afterload, and significantly impaired left ventricular contractility. Assessment by the nurse of the pulmonary artery waveform revealed the presence of large V waves. The exact reason for all V-wave abnormalities is not always clear. Under most circumstances, the regurgitation of blood into the atrium during ventricular systole or a non-compliant atrium accounts for most large V waves. However, if the V waves appear to increase in a patient with severe left ventricular dysfunction, an acute episode of failure may be imminent. Interpretation of oxygen transport data indicated the patient also had a significantly low oxygen delivery (DO_2). Analysis of determinants of oxygen delivery indicated the primary cause of the patient's critically low DO_2 was her low cardiac output. The mixed venous oxygen saturation (SvO_2), indicative of oxygen saturation of hemoglobin returned to the heart via the venous system, was significantly low for an obstetric patient. Most likely this was related to the critically low cardiac output state. The oxygen extraction ratio, an expression of the balance between oxygen supply and demand, was significantly elevated, thus indicative of diminished oxygen reserve. Interpretation of FHR data included a normal baseline rate,

Table 3.3 Case example. Initial maternal hemodynamic and oxygen transport data following initiation of invasive hemodynamic monitoring.

Maternal assessment findings	
Vital signs	
Blood pressure	71/31 mmHg
Heart rate	75
Respiratory rate	26
S_aO_2	97%
SvO_2	55%
Hemodynamic values	
CVP	2 mmHg
PAP	71/27 mmHg
PCWP	24 mmHg
CO	3.2 L/min
CI	2.0 L/min/m^2
SVR	1037 dyne/s/cm^5
PVR	518 dyne/s/cm^5
LVSWI	7 g/m^2
Oxygen transport values	
C_aO_2	15 mL/dL
CvO_2	9 mL/dL
DO_2	480 mL/min
VO_2	192 mL/min
O_2ER	40%

CVP, central venous pressure; PAP, pulmonary artery pressure; PCWP, pulmonary capillary wedge pressure; CO, cardiac output; CI, cardiac index; SVR, systemic vascular resistance; PVR, pulmonary vascular resistance; LVSWI, left ventricular stroke work index.

C_aO_2, arterial oxygen content; CvO_2, venous oxygen content; DO_2, oxygen delivery; VO_2, oxygen consumption; O_2ER, oxygen extraction ratio.

absence of FHR accelerations, and the presence of persistent FHR decelerations with each uterine contraction, despite discontinuation of oxytocin.

Nursing diagnoses, based upon interpretation of these assessment findings, included decreased cardiac output, impaired gas exchange, impaired maternal and fetal oxygen transport, activity intolerance related to inadequate oxygen reserve, and anxiety. Desired outcomes included optimization of cardiac output, maternal and fetal oxygen transport and gas exchange, optimization of oxygen reserve, and reduction in the level of patient anxiety.

To develop a plan of care, the CCOB physician was contacted and the assessment findings and nursing diagnoses were discussed. Collaboration resulted in a plan of care intended to achieve the desired outcomes. Interventions to optimize cardiac output focused on improvement of left ventricular contractility and correction of the patient's high left preload. Dobutamine was administered by intravenous infusion for inotropic support. The method of action is stimulation of beta receptors in the heart muscles which increases contractility, thereby increasing stroke volume and cardiac output. The initial dosage was 2.5 μg/kg/min. In the absence of an appreciable increase in SvO_2, the dosage was increased to 5.0 μg/kg/min. Assessment of the ECG tracing revealed no tachydysrhythmias or ventricular ectopy. Within 5 minutes following the change in the dobutamine dosage, the continuous SvO_2 monitor indicated a significant improvement. Thus, hemodynamic and oxygen transport data were obtained and are presented in Table 3.4.

Evaluation of the patient's response to interventions ensued. Interpretation of these data indicates significant improvement in left ventricular contractility, normalization of left preload, and improvement in cardiac output. In addition, oxygen delivery increased significantly which in turn increased the patient's

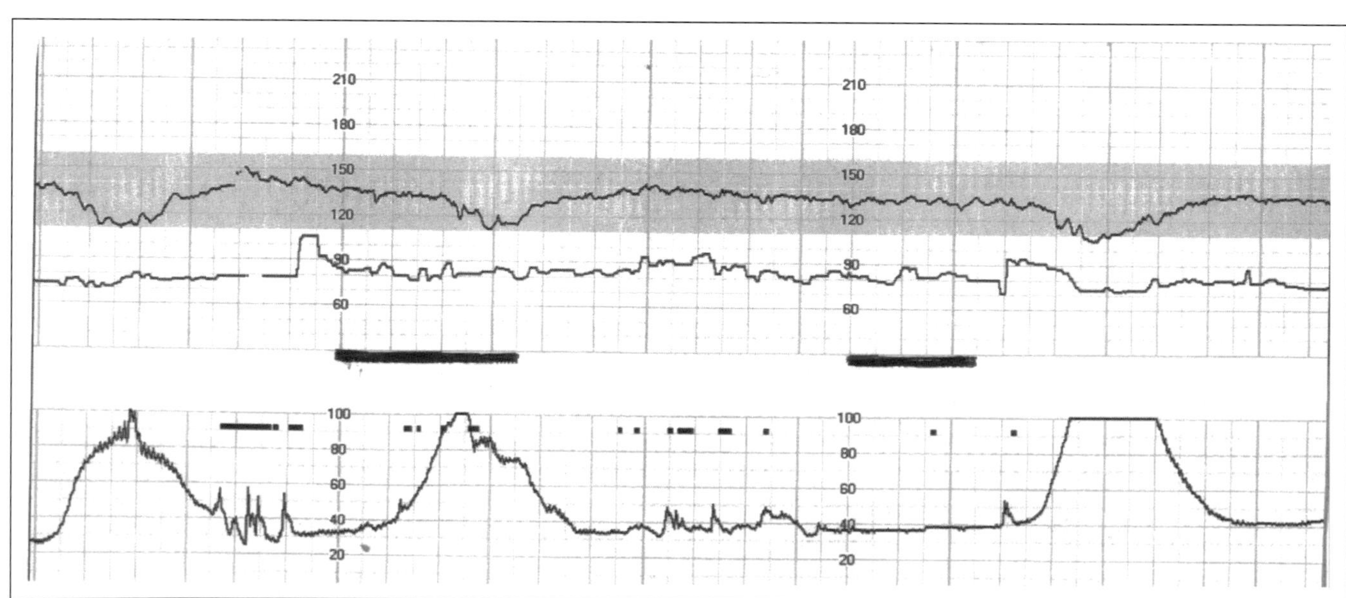

Figure 3.1 Case example. Fetal heart rate and uterine activity at the time the decision was made to initiate invasive hemodynamic monitoring.

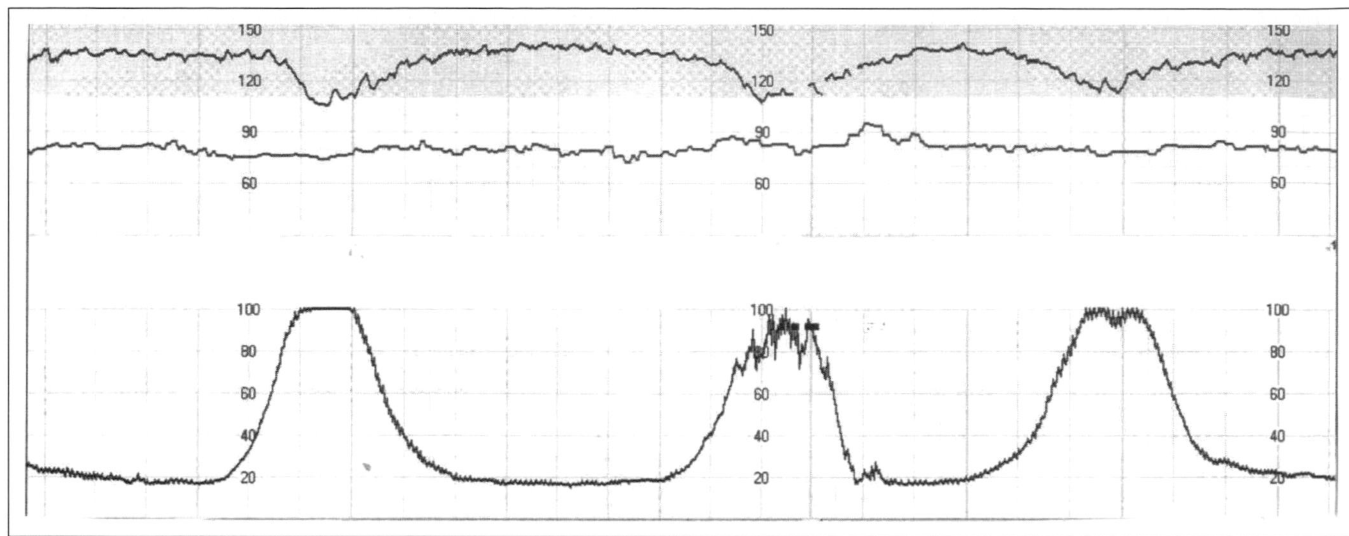

Figure 3.2 Case example. Fetal heart rate and uterine activity at the time initial maternal hemodynamic and oxygen transport data were obtained.

Table 3.4 Case example. Maternal hemodynamic and oxygen transport data following interventions.

Maternal assessment findings	
Vital signs	
Blood pressure	127/75 mmHg
Heart rate	84
Respiratory rate	21
S_aO_2	99%
SvO_2	75%
Hemodynamic values	
CVP	3 mmHg
PAP	52/14 mmHg
PCWP	11 mmHg
CO	5.6 L/min
CI	3.6 L/min/m^2
SVR	1271 dyne/s/cm^5
PVR	228 dyne/s/cm^5
LVSWI	54 g/m^2
Oxygen transport values	
C_aO_2	16 mL/dL
CvO_2	129 mL/dL
DO_2	896 mL/min
VO_2	224 mL/min
O_2ER	25%

CVP, central venous pressure; PAP, pulmonary artery pressure; PCWP, pulmonary capillary wedge pressure; CO, cardiac output; CI, cardiac index; SVR, systemic vascular resistance; PVR, pulmonary vascular resistance; LVSWI, left ventricular stroke work index.

C_aO_2, arterial oxygen content; CvO_2, venous oxygen content; DO_2, oxygen delivery; VO_2, oxygen consumption; O_2ER, oxygen extraction ratio.

oxygen reserve. Arterial oxygen saturation improved to 99% and remained at that level following discontinuation of supplemental oxygen by mask. Resolution of adventitious lung sounds as well as oliguria was also noted. Subsequent fetal assessment findings are presented in Figure 3.3. Interpretation of these data indicates a normal baseline FHR, presence of accelerations and absence of FHR decelerations. The frequency of uterine contractions was every 2½ to 4½ minutes and mild to moderate upon palpation. Uterine resting tone was also noted to be consistently relaxed upon palpation. Collectively, these subsequent maternal and fetal assessment findings were considered reassuring.

The attending CCOB physician performed a digital vaginal examination which revealed the cervix to be 3 cm dilated and soft. An amniotomy was subsequently performed with clear fluid noted. An internal fetal ECG electrode was applied and an intrauterine pressure catheter inserted. The decision was made to resume the oxytocin infusion, continue the dobutamine infusion, and reassess maternal and fetal status in accordance with unit guidelines. The plan of care was discussed with the patient, her husband and family members. They remained with the patient in accordance with the visitation policy within the labor and delivery unit. Their presence and support facilitated reduction in the patient's anxiety level.

As labor continued, both maternal and fetal status remained reassuring, until the nurse noted an abrupt change in the FHR tracing. Changes in the FHR tracing are presented in Figures 3.4 and 3.5. Assessment of the tracing revealed the onset of variable decelerations, caused by umbilical cord compression, which were followed by a prolonged deceleration. Assessment of uterine activity revealed no evidence of over stimulation. Findings included the presence of contractions every 2½ to 3 minutes, 65–80 mmHg in intensity, lasting between 50 and 60 seconds, with a normal uterine resting tone of approximately 20 mmHg.

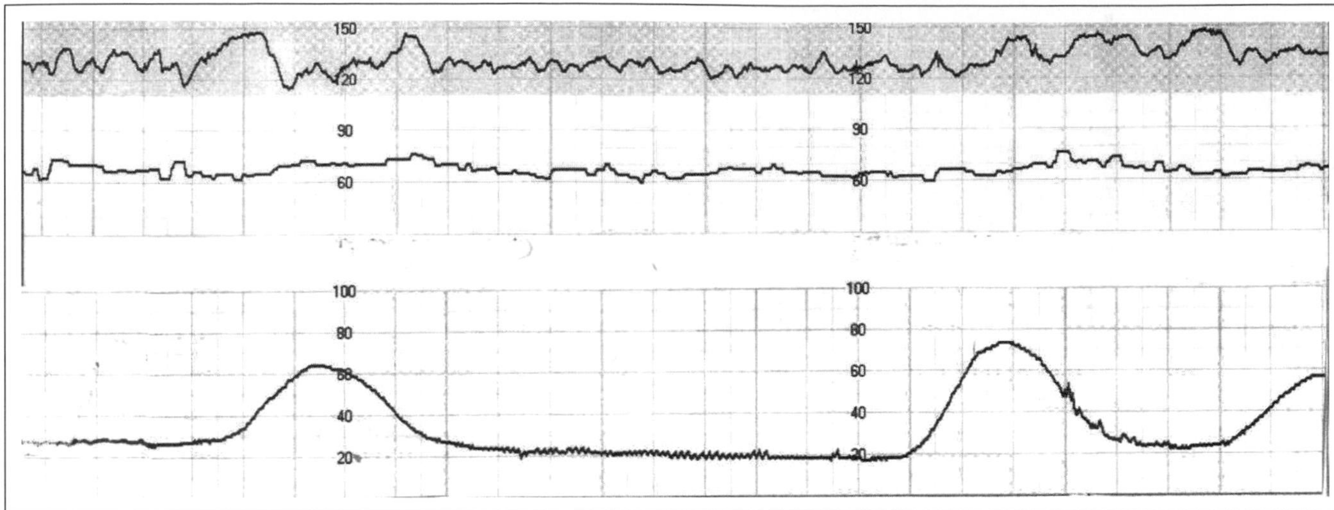

Figure 3.3 Case example. Fetal heart rate and uterine activity following interventions.

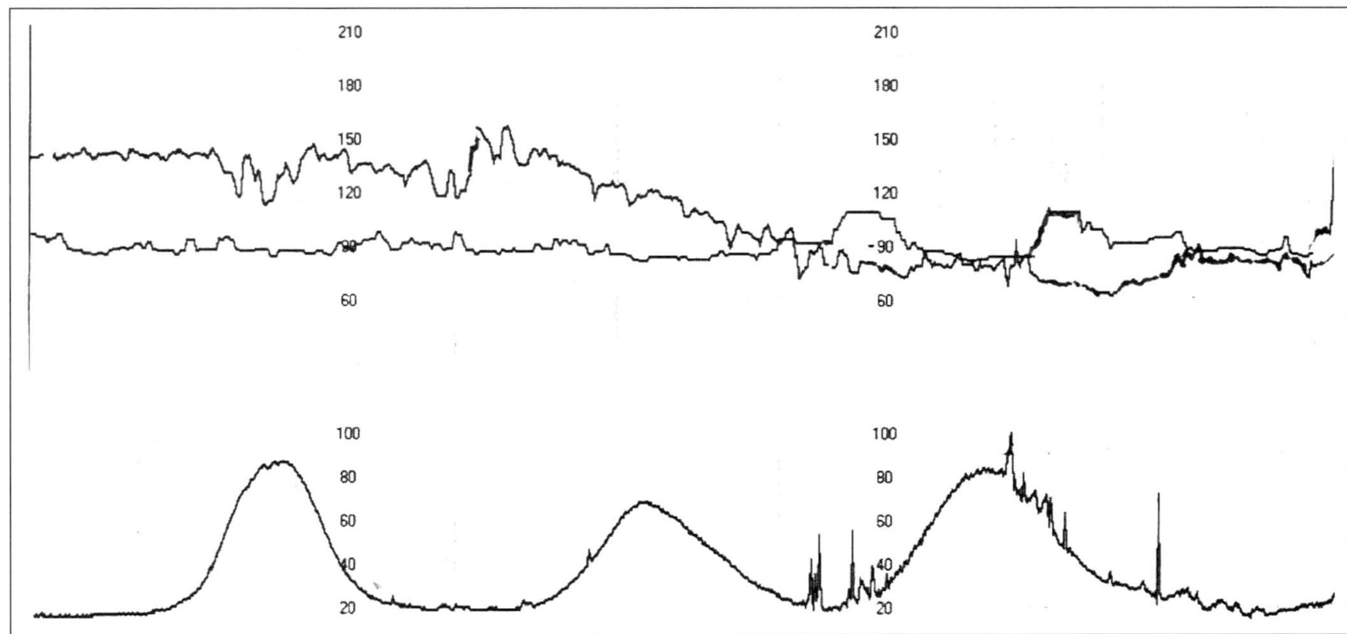

Figure 3.4 Case example. Adverse fetal heart rate changes during labor.

The nurse interpreted the prolonged deceleration as non-reassuring and immediately initiated appropriate interventions. The charge nurse was notified of the need for immediate assistance and was asked to notify the CCOB physician of the adverse change in fetal status. The nurse performed a digital vaginal exam which ruled out the presence of an umbilical cord prolapse. The cervix was noted to be 4 cm dilated and 90% effaced. A second nurse arrived and immediately began respositioning the patient in order to decrease umbilical cord compression. The first prolonged deceleration lasted 5 minutes and resolved following maternal repositioning. To determine if the change in fetal status might be related to a change in maternal hemodynamic status, the CCOB nurse assessed the pulmonary capillary wedge pressure, cardiac output and other routine vital signs. Assessment of these findings revealed no adverse change in maternal hemodynamic status. Collaboration with the physician resulted in a plan of care directed toward alleviating the cord compression. An amnioinfusion was subsequently initiated during which a second prolonged deceleration lasting 4 minutes was noted. The patient was again repositioned and the amnioinfusion continued. Fetal responses following these interventions are depicted in Figure 3.6. The FHR baseline remained normal, FHR variability was present, variable decelerations continued but no further prolonged decelerations developed. Approximately 2 hours later, the patient's

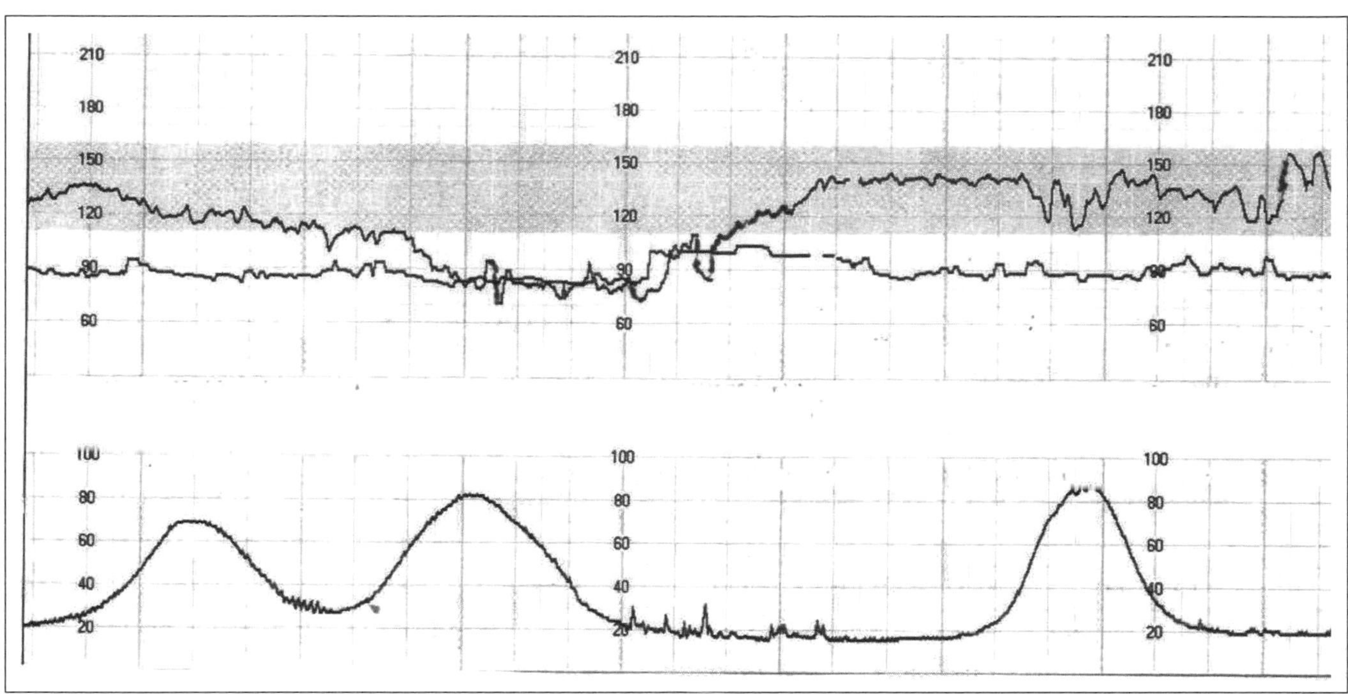

Figure 3.5 Case example. Adverse fetal heart rate changes during labor (continued).

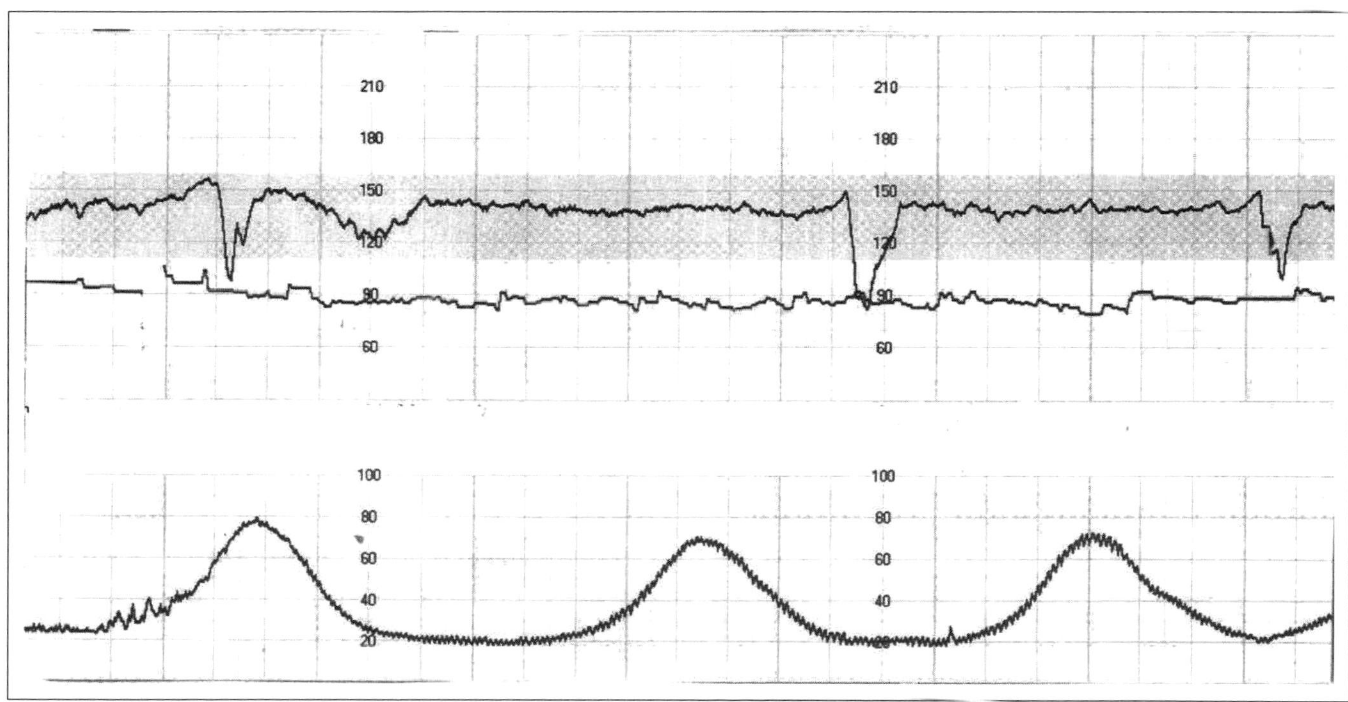

Figure 3.6 Case example. Fetal heart rate following amnioinfusion.

cervix was reassessed and found to be 8–9 cm dilated with the fetal vertex at 0 station. Maternal and fetal status remained reassuring until a significant decrease in SvO_2 was noted during the second stage of labor. Following evaluation by the physician, the decision was made to provide assistance to expedite delivery. She subsequently had a forceps-assisted vaginal delivery of a baby girl. Neonatal personnel were present to assess the baby and provide necessary care. Apgar scores and cord blood gases were normal. The baby was transferred to the transitional nursery for further assessment, but a short time later was considered sufficiently stable to be returned to labor and delivery to stay in the room with the patient and her family.

Mechanical ventilation during pregnancy: critical concepts for nursing practice

General indications for the initiation of mechanical ventilation include inadequate arterial oxygenation, inadequate alveolar ventilation, and excessive respiratory workload. Complications during pregnancy may cause respiratory or ventilatory failure that necessitates mechanical ventilatory support. Such complications include severe pre-eclampsia or eclampsia, pulmonary edema, pneumonia, sepsis, pulmonary embolism, neurological insult, drug overdose, trauma, or aspiration. A thorough and specific discussion of airway management in critical illness is presented in Chapter 9 of this text. Guidelines for the medical diagnosis of respiratory and ventilatory failure, criteria upon which these diagnoses are based, modes of mechanical ventilation, settings and goals, complications, and weaning techniques are included in that chapter. Detailed discussions of disease processes during pregnancy that may lead to respiratory failure are presented elsewhere in this text.

Caring for the obstetric patient requiring mechanical ventilation presents unique challenges to the healthcare team. Comprehensive discussion of specific nursing care issues related to care of such patients is beyond the scope of this chapter. Additional resources are available that address topics including nursing diagnoses associated with care of the obstetric patient requiring mechanical ventilation, assessment of ventilation and oxygenation, airway care, strategies for prevention of nosocomial infection, and psychosocial support [20,21].

The following physiologic concepts are significant and should be incorporated in the framework for clinical nursing care of the obstetric patient requiring mechanical ventilation. The nurse should first recall that numerous changes in the maternal respiratory system occur during pregnancy. These result from endocrine, physical and mechanical influences throughout pregnancy. The net physiologic result is a decrease in maternal P_aCO_2 to a level less than half that of the fetus. This leads in turn to increased bicarbonate excretion by the maternal kidneys. This compensatory mechanism serves to maintain the maternal arterial pH between 7.40 and 7.45. Thus, normal arterial blood gases during pregnancy reflect a state of compensated respiratory alkalemia. Additional cardiovascular changes significantly increase cardiac output throughout pregnancy, with further increases noted during labor, birth, and the immediate postpartum period. Collectively, these alterations significantly increase the rate of oxygen delivery. Because of the high oxygen diffusion gradient during pregnancy, oxygen diffuses from the maternal alveoli into the maternal circulation, binding to red blood cells at a more rapid rate. Oxygen is subsequently transported via the placenta to fetal tissues. In addition, a right shift in the maternal oxyhemoglobin dissociation curve occurs during pregnancy. Thus, the affinity of oxygen to hemoglobin is decreased, in turn facilitating oxygen diffusion and transport. The left shift in the fetal oxyhemoglobin dissociation curve increases the affinity of oxygen to fetal hemoglobin. Thus, an optimum environment is created for maternal–fetal gas exchange.

Based on the theory of venous equilibration, it is apparent that the uterine venous PO_2 is the major determinant of umbilical venous PO_2. The oxygen saturation of uterine venous blood is affected by three variables: oxygen saturation of maternal arterial blood, oxygen content of maternal blood, and uterine blood flow. Any reduction in maternal P_aO_2 thus decreases uterine venous PO_2 and umbilical venous PO_2.

Uterine contractions cause a reduction in uterine blood flow secondary to a significant increase in uterine vascular resistance. In addition to the effect of uterine contractions, a number of maternal conditions may impair oxygen delivery. In essence, any condition that causes maternal uterine venous PO_2 to be reduced will also result in decreased oxygen transport to the fetus.

For these reasons, it is especially important for the nurse to frequently assess the hemodynamic and oxygen transport status of the obstetric patient requiring mechanical ventilation. Appropriate interpretation by the nurse of assessment findings is critical. If a pregnant woman has diminished arterial oxygen content because of anemia, decreased arterial oxygen saturation (S_aO_2), or a low P_aO_2, or decreased cardiac output, catecholamines subsequently redistribute blood flow in favor of vital maternal organ systems. Thus, alterations in uterine activity or the fetal heart rate may be indicative of decreased oxygen transport or perfusion. It is common to find this dynamic process illustrated at the bedside when assessment by the nurse of the electronic fetal monitor (EFM) tracing reveals adverse changes in maternal–fetal status. Initiation of appropriate nursing interventions, including notification of the physician of significant assessment findings, is imperative. In the event that adverse changes in maternal or fetal status persist, despite initiation of appropriate interventions, or acute deterioration in maternal or fetal status occurs, decisions regarding delivery of the fetus may be necessary. Thus, the plan of care should provide for the capability to perform emergent delivery via cesarean section should it become necessary. In addition, the potential urgent need for appropriate personnel and resources to resuscitate and stabilize the newborn should be anticipated and addressed in the plan of care.

In addition to physiologic concepts which provide a framework for critical care obstetric nursing care, significant psychosocial principles should be incorporated in any plan of patient care. Obstetric critical care can benefit from data in the critical care literature that address family and patient needs in a critical care setting. Obstetric literature and extensive experience in implementation of a family-centered approach to care of the pregnant woman can also be used to identify the need for humane care in an obstetric critical care setting [22,23]. Use of mechanical ventilation subjects the obstetric patient to physical and psychosocial stress. It is also a difficult time for the patient's family and support system. Concern for the condition of the pregnant woman as well as the well-being of the fetus produces stress and anxiety for the patient and her family. Numerous reports have shown that hospital admission for a critical illness may cause a crisis within a family. Historically, visitation restrictions were imposed in intensive care units (ICUs) to provide patients time for rest. Visiting hours became so restrictive that many family members felt they had lost their loved one with the admission to the ICU. A result was conflict between the duties of the critical care nurse and the rights of the patient and family members.

The unique challenges inherent in providing care to this patient population were presented in a study by Jenkins et al. which described the characteristics and outcomes of obstetric patients who required mechanical ventilation [24]. Data that were collected included maternal demographics, medical condition that necessitated mechanical ventilatory support, delivery status, duration of ventilation, onset of parturition while receiving ventilation, mode of delivery, and maternal and early neonatal morbidity or death. A summary of results from the study is presented in Table 3.5. The three most frequent diagnoses that produced complications which led to the need for mechanical ventilation were pre-eclampsia or eclampsia (43%), labor or preterm labor (14%), and pneumonia (12%). Overall, 43 of the 51 patients (84%) included in the study were cared for in labor and delivery, with care directed by a critical care perinatologist, a critical care obstetric nurse, with consultations provided by other intensivists, depending on the clinical picture.

Table 3.5 Demographics and delivery characteristics of 51 obstetric patients requiring mechanical ventilation.

Characteristic	Value
Age (years)*	28.2 ± 7.4
Gravidity (number)*	3.0 ± 2.1
Parity (number)*	1.3 ± 1.9
Race (%)	
White	56
Black	38
Asian, other	6
Estimated gestational age on admission (weeks)*	31.6 ± 5.1
Length of stay (days)*	10.9 ± 3.6
Days on ventilator*	3.4 ± 3.6
Pulmonary artery catheter used (number)	33 (65%)
Undelivered on admission (number)	43
Delivered during admission (number)	37 (86%)
Vaginal delivery (number)	13 (35%)
Cesarean delivery (number)	24 (65%)
Labor during ventilation (number)	11 (30%)
EGA at delivery (weeks)*	32.6 ± 4.9
Birth weight (g)*	2131 ± 1906
Neonatal intensive care nursery admission (number)	28 (76%)
Fetal/neonatal death (number)	4 (11%)
Maternal deaths (number)	7 (14%)

* Data are given as mean ± standard deviation.

Case example: Mechanical ventilation during pregnancy

The following case excerpts illustrate significant clinical practice concepts related to nursing care of a pregnant woman who required mechanical ventilation. The case involved a 25-year-old primigravida at 33 weeks estimated fetal gestational age (EGA). Her prenatal course had been uncomplicated until she developed an upper respiratory infection. Despite outpatient treatment her symptoms worsened and she was subsequently admitted to a local community hospital where she was diagnosed with pneumonia. She was refractory to the prescribed medical treatment regimen, her condition worsened and a pulmonary consult was obtained. The decision was made to transfer her to the medical intensive care unit (MICU) for further care. Endotracheal intubation was performed and a 7.0 Fr endotracheal tube was inserted without complications. A volume-cycled ventilator was utilized for mechanical ventilatory support. Central venous access was also accomplished via the right internal jugular vein and a central venous pressure (CVP) catheter was inserted. Following stabilization, the decision was made to transport the patient to a tertiary care center that had an established the CCOB service within the labor and delivery unit. Following initial assessment by the CCOB physician and CCOB nurse, the decision was made to replace the CVP catheter with a fiberoptic pulmonary artery (PA) catheter with the capability to continuously monitor mixed venous oxygen saturation (SvO_2). Initial maternal assessment findings and ventilator settings obtained and documented upon admission to the tertiary care center are presented in Table 3.6. Initial assessment findings pertaining to the fetal heart rate (FHR) and uterine activity are presented in Figure 3.7.

Interpretation by the nurse of initial hemodynamic data indicated the patient had a significantly low cardiac output (CO). Analysis of the four determinants of cardiac output revealed a low preload, high afterload, decreased left ventricular contractility, and sinus tachycardia. Vasoconstriction and tachycardia most likely represented compensatory mechanisms but were not sufficient to produce an adequate cardiac output. In addition, decreased contractility of the left ventricle could be indicative of impending heart failure. Interpretation of oxygen transport data indicated the patient had a significantly low oxygen delivery (DO_2). Analysis of determinants of oxygen delivery, in addition to cardiac output, previously interpreted to be significantly low, revealed low arterial oxygen content (CaO_2). In addition, oxygen consumption (VO_2) was low, possibly an indication of altered organ system perfusion or impaired ability of organ systems to extract oxygen, a condition referred to as delivery-dependent oxygen consumption. During assessment of the patient's respiratory status, the nurse noted the presence of tachypnea as well as an apparent increased work of breathing. Lungs were clear bilaterally to auscultation. Interpretation of arterial blood gases revealed an elevated pH, low P_aCO_2, and low P_aO_2, indicating respiratory alkalemia. The presence of alkalemia produces a left shift of the oxyhemoglobin dissociation curve. Such a shift increases the affinity or binding of oxygen to hemoglobin which subsequently impairs the release of oxygen from hemoglobin for

Table 3.6 Case example. Initial maternal assessment findings and ventilator settings upon admission to the CCOB service.

Maternal assessment findings		Maternal assessment findings	
Vital signs		*Oxygen transport values*	
Blood pressure	100/52	C_aO_2	12 mL/dL
Heart rate	132	CvO_2	7 mL/dL
Respiratory rate		DO_2	504 mL/min
Set	14	VO_2	210 mL/min
Total	36	O_2ER	42%
S_aO_2	100%		
		Ventilator settings upon arrival	
Arterial blood gases		Mode	Assist control
pH	7.52	Tidal volume (Vt)	600 mL
P_aO_2	92 mmHg	Rate (set)	14
P_aCO_2	18 mmHg	F_iO_2	0.60
Base excess	+3.8	PEEP	5 cmH_2O
		PSV	5 cmH_2O
Hemodynamic values			
CVP	4 mmHg		
PAP	16/4 mmHg		
PCWP	3 mmHg		
CO	4.2 L/min		
CI	2.3 L/min/m^2		
SVR	1219 dyne/s/cm^5		
PVR	95 dyne/s/cm^5		
LVSWI	34 gM/m^2		

CVP, central venous pressure; PAP, pulmonary artery pressure; PCWP, pulmonary capillary wedge pressure; CO, cardiac output; CI, cardiac index; SVR, systemic vascular resistance; PVR, pulmonary vascular resistance; LVSWI, left ventricular stroke work index.
C_aO_2, arterial oxygen content; CvO_2, venous oxygen content; DO_2, oxygen delivery; VO_2, oxygen consumption; O_2ER, oxygen extraction ratio.
F_iO_2, fraction of inspired oxygen; PEEP, positive end-expiratory pressure; PSV, pressure support ventilation.

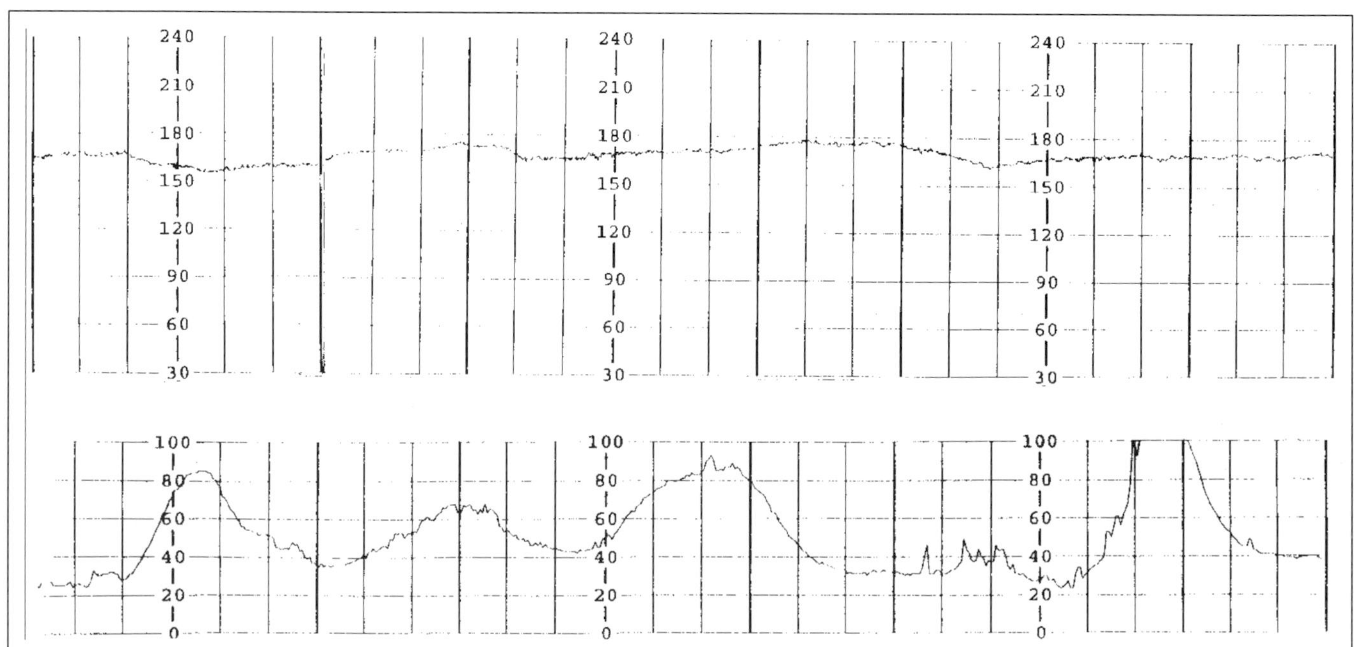

Figure 3.7 Case example. Initial fetal heart rate and uterine activity upon admission to the CCOB service.

transport to tissues. Interpretation of FHR data included the presence of a baseline fetal tachycardia, a relatively smooth FHR baseline via external or indirect monitoring, absence of FHR accelerations, and the presence of repetitive late decelerations of the FHR. Regular uterine contractions were evident on the EFM tracing. Manual palpation by the nurse revealed the contractions to be mild to moderate in intensity and the uterine resting tone was also noted to be inadequate.

Nursing diagnoses, based upon interpretation of assessment findings, included decreased cardiac output, impaired gas exchange, ineffective breathing pattern, impaired maternal and fetal oxygen transport, and anxiety [25]. Desired outcomes included optimization of cardiac output, maternal and fetal oxygen transport and gas exchange, as well as establishment of an effective breathing pattern and reduction in the level of patient anxiety.

In order to develop a plan of care, the CCOB physician was contacted and the assessment findings and nursing diagnoses were discussed. Collaboration resulted in a plan of care intended to achieve the desired outcomes. Interventions to optimize cardiac output began with correction of the patient's low preload. As demonstrated by the Starling curve, within certain physiologic limits, the higher the filling pressure in the ventricles during diastole, the greater the quantity of blood that will be ejected during systole. In addition, increased filling pressures may improve ventricular contractility, also known as the inotropic state of the heart, thus further increasing cardiac output. Rapid intravenous administration of crystalloid fluid was initiated in order to increase left preload and improve left ventricular contractility. This process is both delicate and dynamic. The goal is to determine and maintain the optimal pulmonary capillary wedge pressure (PCWP) that, in turn, optimizes left ventricular contractility and cardiac output. Frequent assessment by the nurse of critical data is imperative, since an excessively high PCWP may further diminish the function of the left ventricle, decrease cardiac output, and lead to congestive failure and pulmonary edema. In addition to administration of intravenous fluid, the nurse repositioned the patient to optimize preload and displaced the uterus laterally to facilitate venous return to the heart. In order to further facilitate oxygen transport, the CCOB physician ordered administration of 2 units of packed red blood cells (PRBCs). Since 98–99% of oxygen is chemically bound to hemoglobin, in contrast to the 1–2% of oxygen which is dissolved under pressure in the plasma, though the patient was not anemic, it was thought that even a modest increase in hemoglobin would significantly improve arterial oxygen content and, thus, oxygen delivery.

Interventions to optimize maternal–fetal gas exchange and oxygen transport also included changes in mechanical ventilator settings. The mode of mechanical ventilation was changed to synchronized intermittent mandatory ventilation (SIMV). This was based on the rationale that, when the mode of assist control is utilized, the "triggering" of breaths above the set number of breaths to be delivered by the machine may result in excessive elimination of carbon dioxide. Since a compensated respiratory alkalemia exists during normal pregnancy, further reduction in levels of carbon dioxide increase the risk of development of respiratory alkalemia. Assessment findings that supported this concept included the arterial blood gas results. The arterial oxygen saturation of 100% could be the result of a left shift of the oxyhemoglobin dissociation curve. In addition, tachypnea significantly increased the total number of breaths delivered by the machine at the preset tidal volume. Initiation of SIMV allowed both spontaneous patient breaths at her own tidal volume, and a set number of mechanical cycles timed to coincide with spontaneous effort. The level of positive end-expiratory pressure (PEEP) was increased in order to recruit additional alveoli for participation in gas exchange. In addition, the level of pressure support was increased in order to decrease the patient's workload during spontaneous breaths. The fraction of inspired oxygen (F_iO_2) was decreased to 0.40.

A number of interventions were initiated to reduce patient anxiety. First, an open policy of visitation, which allows visiting 24 hours a day, commensurate with the standard visitation policy within the labor and delivery unit, was initiated. This facilitated involvement of the patient's husband and other family members in the overall plan of care. Opportunities for more frequent discussions between the family and members of the healthcare team facilitated a better understanding of prescribed interventions, goals of therapy, and patient progress. In addition, the family had more opportunities to ask questions and express concerns. A method was identified which allowed the patient to communicate with the CCOB nurse, family members, and other members of the healthcare team. An arterial catheter was utilized for repetitive collection of blood for arterial blood gas assessment. The endotracheal tube was secured and care was taken to minimize movement of the tube which has been well documented as a source of discomfort, irritation and anxiety in patients receiving mechanical ventilatory support. A closed, or "in line", system was utilized for endotracheal suctioning. This system eliminates the need to disconnect ventilator tubing from the endotracheal tube when suctioning is indicated. Finally, every attempt was made to minimize extraneous stimulation such as bright lights, alarms, and general noise originating from outside the patient's room.

A consultation with a neonatologist was obtained who provided multiple opportunities for the patient and family to verbalize questions. Equipment, supplies and other resources were made available in the patient's room, in the event delivery occurred and immediate neonatal care was needed.

Evaluation of the patient's response to these interventions ensued. Subsequent maternal assessment findings are presented in Table 3.7. Interpretation of these data indicates significant improvement in cardiac output, optimization of preload, and improved left ventricular contractility. In addition, oxygen delivery increased significantly, as did arterial oxygen content. Oxygen consumption increased indicative of improved oxygen delivery and oxygen extraction capability. Arterial blood gases indicated a compensated respiratory alkalemia, the normal acid–base state expected during pregnancy. Resolution of the patient's tachypnea also occurred and her work of breathing was decreased. Subsequent fetal assessment findings are presented in Figure 3.8.

Table 3.7 Case example. Maternal assessment findings and ventilator settings following interventions.

Maternal assessment findings		Maternal assessment findings	
Vital signs		*Oxygen transport variables*	
Blood pressure	97/50	C_aO_2	16 mL/dL
Heart rate	96	CvO_2	12 mL/dL
Respiratory rate		DO_2	1632 mL/min
Set	12	VO_2	408 mL/min
Total	21	O_2ER	25%
S_aO_2	97%		
		Ventilator settings	
Arterial blood gases		Mode	SIMV
pH	7.41	Tidal volume (Vt)	600 mL
P_aCO_2	30 mmHg	Rate (Set)	12
P_aO_2	164 mmHg	F_iO_2	0.40
Base excess	+2.6	PEEP	8 cmH_2O
		PSV	10 cmH_2O
Hemodynamic values			
CVP	4 mmHg		
PAP	28/14 mmHg		
PCWP	12 mmHg		
CO	10.2 L/min		
CI	5.6 L/min/m^2		
SVR	486 dyne/s/cm^5		
PVR	56 dyne/s/cm^5		
LVSWI	95 gM/m^2		

CVP, central venous pressure; PAP, pulmonary artery pressure; PCWP, pulmonary capillary wedge pressure; CO, cardiac output; CI, cardiac index; SVR, systemic vascular resistance; PVR, pulmonary vascular resistance; LVSWI, left ventricular stroke work index.

C_aO_2, arterial oxygen content; C_vO_2, venous oxygen content; DO_2, oxygen delivery; VO_2, oxygen consumption; O_2ER, oxygen extraction ratio.

F_iO_2, fraction of inspired oxygen; PEEP, positive end-expiratory pressure; PSV, pressure support ventilation.

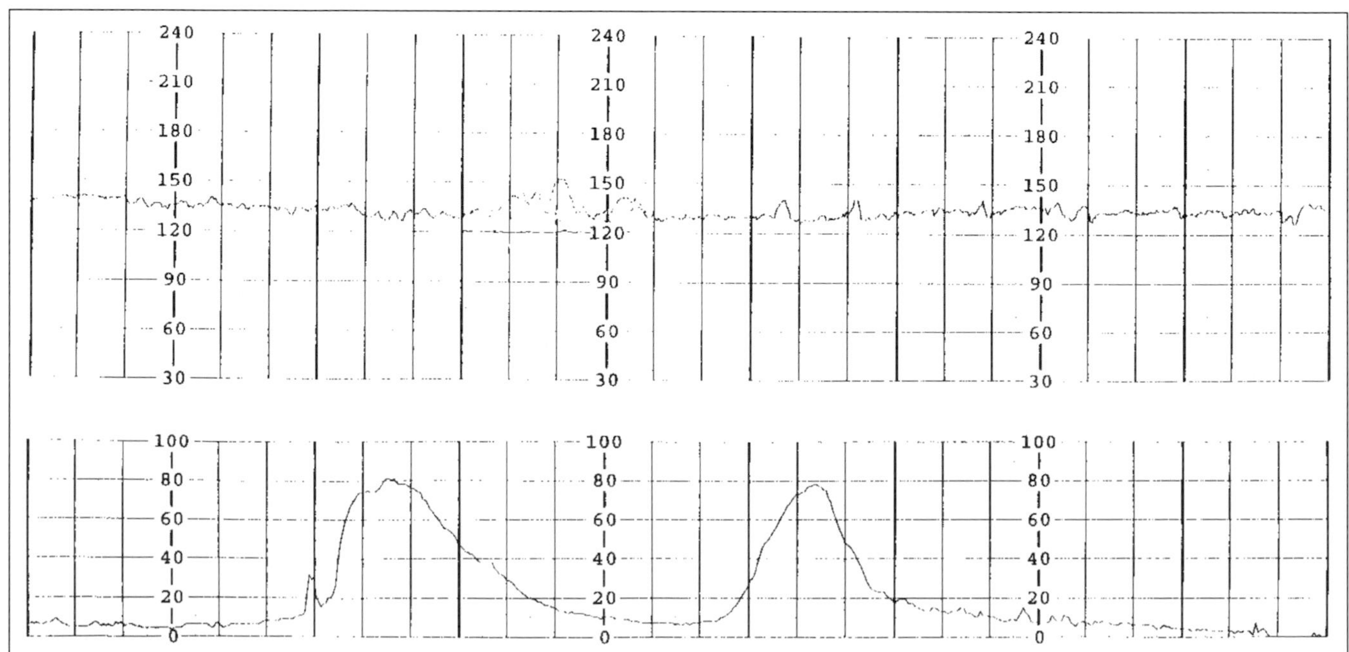

Figure 3.8 Case example. Subsequent fetal heart rate and uterine activity following interventions.

Interpretation of these data indicates a normal baseline FHR, presence of accelerations and absence of FHR decelerations. In addition, decreased uterine contraction frequency was noted and uterine resting tone by palpation was normal. Collectively, these subsequent maternal and fetal assessment findings were considered reassuring.

Strategies to prepare nurses to care for critically ill obstetric patients

When creating a program to care for critically ill obstetric women, careful attention should be paid to the identification of nursing competencies necessary to create a safe practice environment. The theoretical basis for this enhanced level of practice should be presented in a consistent and organized fashion. Thorough discussion of content to be included would cover maternal physiology and common pathophysiology of pregnancy complications that are common in the critically ill obstetric population. However, didactic material should be accompanied by the opportunity for nurses to gain clinical practice in a mentored, supervised setting to verify competency of skills. The subject of critical care obstetric staff is addressed in Chapter 2 of this text. Additional resources are available in the literature to address this subject.

References

1 Clark SL, Phelan JP, Cotton DB, eds. Critical Care Obstetrics. Medical Economics Books, Oradell, New Jersey, 1987.

2 Hankins GDV. Foreword. In: Harvey CJ, ed. *Critical Care Obstetrical Nursing*. Gaithersburg, Maryland: Aspen Publishers, Inc., 1991.

3 Fedorka P. Defining the standard of care. In *AWHONN's Liability Issues in Perinatal Nursing*. Philadelphia: Lippincott, 1997.

4 American Nurses Association. Standards of Clinical Nursing Practice. Washington, DC, 1991.

5 Association of Women's Health, Obstetric and Neonatal Nurses. Standards for Professional Nursing Practice in the Care of Women and Newborns, 6th edn. Washington, DC, 2003.

6 Joint Commission for Accreditation of Healthcare Organizations. Comprehensive Accreditation Manual for Hospitals: The Official Handbook (CAMH), 2007.

7 Page A. *Keeping Patients Safe: Transforming the Work Environment of Nurses*. Washington, DC: The National Academy Press, 2003.

8 Baggs JG, Schmitt MH, Mushlin AI, Mitchell PH, Eldredge DH, Hutson AD. Association between nurse-physician collaboration and patient outcomes in three intensive care units. *Crit Care Med* 200; 31, 956–959.

9 Baird SM, Kennedy B. Myocardial infarction in pregnancy. *J Perinat Neonat Nurs* 2006; 220(4): 311–321.

10 Witcher PM. Promoting fetal stabilization during maternal hemodynamic instability or respiratory insufficiency. *Crit Care Nurs Q* 2006; 29(1): 70–76.

11 Drummond SB, Troiano NH. Cardiac disorders during pregnancy. In: Mandeville LK, Troiano NH, eds. *AWHONN'S High-Risk and Critical Care Intrapartum Nursing*, 2nd edn. Philadelphia: Lippincott, 1999: 173–184.

12 Sala DJ. Myocardial infarction. In: *NAACOG's Clinical Issues in Perinatal and Women's Health Nursing: Critical Care Obstetrics*. Philadelphia: Lippincott, 1992: 443–453.

13 Centers for Disease Control and Prevention. Guidelines for the prevention of intravascular catheter-related infections. *MMWR Morbidity Mortality Weekly* 2002; 51(RR-10): 3–36.

14 American Association of Critical Care Nurses. *Practice Alert: Preventing Catheter Related Bloodstream Infections*. Washington, DC, 2005.

15 Preuss T, Wiegand DLM. Pulmonary artery catheter insertion (assist) and pressure monitoring. In: Wiegand DLM, Carlson KK, eds. *AACN Procedure Manual for Critical Care, 5th edn*. St. Louis: Elsevier Saunders, Inc., 2005: 549–569.

16 Chaiyakunapruk N, Veenstra DL, Lipsky BA, Saint S. Chlorhexidine compared with providone-iodine solution for vascular catheter-site care: A meta-analysis. *Ann Intern Med* 2002; 136: 792–801.

17 Posa PJ, Harrison, D, Vollman KM. Elimination of central line-associated bloodstream infections: Application of the evidence. *AACN Advanced Critical Care* 2006; 17(4): 446–454.

18 American Association of Critical Care Nurses. Evaluation of the effects of heparinized and nonheparinized flush solutions on the patency of arterial pressure monitoring lines: the AACN "Thunder Project". *Am J Crit Care* 1993; 2: 3–13.

19 Wallace DC, Winslow EH. Effects of iced and room temperature injectate on cardiac output measurements in critically ill patients with decreased and increased cardiac outputs. *Heart Lung* 1993; 22: 55–63.

20 Troiano NH, Dorman K. Mechanical ventilation during pregnancy. In: Mandeville LK, Troiano NH, eds. *AWHONN'S High-Risk and Critical Care Intrapartum Nursing*, 2nd edn. Philadelphia: Lippincott, 1999: 84–99.

21 Troiano NH, Baird SM. Critical care of the obstetrical patient. In: Kinney MR, Dunbar SB, Brooks-Brunn JA, Molter N, Vitello-Cicciu JM, eds. *AACN's Clinical Reference for Critical Care Nursing*, 4th edn. St Louis: Mosby, 1998: 1219–1239.

22 Martin-Arafeh J, Watson CL, Baird SM. Promoting family centered care in high risk pregnancy. *J Perinat Neonat Nurs* 1999; 13(1).

23 Harvey MG. Humanizing the intensive care unit experience. *NAACOG's Clinical Issues in Perinatal and Women's Health Nursing: Critical Care Obstetrics*. 1992; 3(3): 369–376.

24 Jenkins TM, Troiano NH, Graves CR, Baird SM, Boehm FH. Mechanical ventilation in an obstetric population: characteristics and delivery rates. *Am J Obstet Gynecol* 2003; 188(2): 549–552.

25 North American Nursing Diagnosis Association. *NANDA Nursing Diagnoses: Definitions and Classification*. Philadelphia: Lippincott, 2003–2004.

4 Pregnancy-Induced Physiologic Alterations

Errol R. Norwitz[1] & Julian N. Robinson[2]

[1]Department of Obstetrics and Gynecology, Tufts University School of Medicine and Tufts Medical Center, Boston, MA, USA
[2]Harvard Medical School, Division of Maternal-Fetal Medicine, Department of Obstetrics, Gynecology and Reproductive Biology, Brigham and Women's Hospital, Boston, MA, USA

Physiologic adaptations occur in the mother in response to the demands of pregnancy. These demands include support of the fetus (volume support, nutritional and oxygen supply, and clearance of fetal waste), protection of the fetus (from starvation, drugs, toxins), preparation of the uterus for labor, and protection of the mother from potential cardiovascular injury at delivery. Variables such as maternal age, multiple gestation, ethnicity, and genetic factors affect the ability of the mother to adapt to the demands of pregnancy. All maternal systems are required to adapt; however, the quality, degree, and timing of the adaptation vary from one individual to another and from one organ system to another. This chapter reviews in detail the normal physiologic adaptations that occur within each of the major maternal organ systems. A detailed discussion of fetal physiology is beyond the scope of this review. A better understanding of the normal physiologic adaptations of pregnancy will improve the ability of clinicians to anticipate the effects of pregnancy on underlying medical conditions and to manage pregnancy-associated complications.

Cardiovascular system

Critical illnesses that compromise the cardiovascular system are among the most challenging problems affecting pregnant women. When evaluating patients for cardiovascular compromise, it is important to be aware of the pregnancy-associated changes and how these changes influence the various maternal hemodynamic variables, including blood volume, blood pressure (BP), heart rate, stroke volume, cardiac output, and systemic vascular resistance (SVR). Factors such as maternal age, multiple pregnancy, gestational age, body habitus, positioning, labor, regional anesthesia, and blood loss may further complicate the management of such patients. This section reviews in detail the effects of pregnancy on the maternal cardiovascular system, and the relevance of this information in the management of the critically ill obstetric patient.

Blood volume

Maternal plasma volume increases by 10% as early as the 7th week of pregnancy. As summarized in Figure 4.1, this increase reaches a plateau of around 45–50% at 32 weeks, remaining stable thereafter until delivery [1–6]. Although the magnitude of the hypervolemia varies considerably between women, there is a tendency for the same plasma volume expansion pattern to be repeated during successive pregnancies in the same woman [4,7]. Moreover, the magnitude of the hypervolemia varies with the number of fetuses [7,8]. In a longitudinal study comparing blood volume estimations during term pregnancy with that in the same patient after pregnancy, Pritchard [7] demonstrated that blood volume in a singleton pregnancy increased by an average of 1570 mL (+48%) as compared with 1960 mL in a twin pregnancy (Table 4.1). There is a similar but less pronounced increase in red cell mass during pregnancy (see Figure 4.1), likely due to the stimulatory effect of placental hormones (chorionic somatomammotropin, progesterone, and possibly prolactin) on maternal erythropoiesis [9,10]. These changes account for the maternal dilutional anemia that develops in pregnancy despite seemingly adequate iron stores [11]. Hemodilution is maximal at around 30–32 weeks of gestation.

The physiologic advantage of maternal hemodilution of pregnancy remains unclear. It may have a beneficial effect on the uteroplacental circulation by decreasing blood viscosity, thereby improving uteroplacental perfusion and possibly preventing stasis and resultant placental thrombosis [12]. Blood volume changes are closely related to maternal morbidity, and hypervolemia likely serves as a protective mechanism against excessive blood loss at delivery. Pre-eclamptic women, for example, are less tolerant of peripartum blood loss because, although total body fluid overloaded, they have a markedly reduced intravascular volume as compared with normotensive parturients, due primarily to an increase in capillary permeability (Table 4.2) [13]. The precise etiology for this increased capillary permeability in the

Critical Care Obstetrics, 5th edition. Edited by M. Belfort, G. Saade, M. Foley, J. Phelan and G. Dildy.

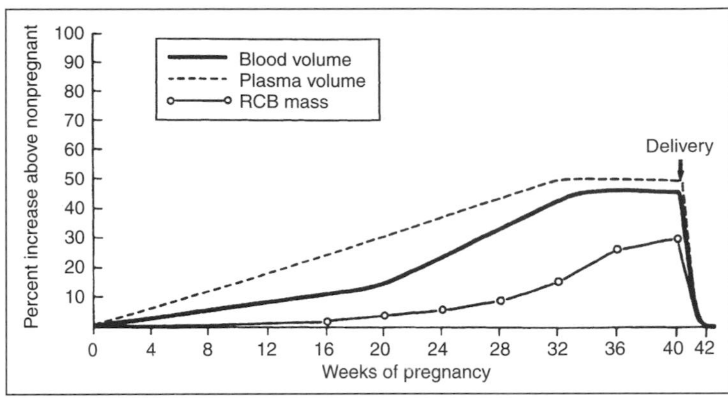

Figure 4.1 Blood volume changes during pregnancy. (Reproduced with permission McLennon and Thouin [1].)

Table 4.1 Blood and red cell volumes in normal women late in pregnancy and again when not pregnant.

	Late pregnancy	Non-pregnant	Increase (mL)	Increase (%)
Single fetus (n = 50)				
Blood volume	4820	3250	1570	48
RBC volume	1790	1355	430	32
Hematocrit	37.0	41.7	–	–
Twins (n = 30)				
Blood volume	5820	3865	1960	51
RBC volume	2065	1580	485	31
Hematocrit	35.5	41.0	–	–

Reproduced by permission from Pritchard JA. Changes in the blood volume during pregnancy and delivery. *Anesthesiology* 1965; 26: 393.

Table 4.2 Blood volume changes in five women.

	Non-pregnant	Normal pregnancy	Eclampsia
Blood volume (mL)	3035	4425	3530
Change (%)*	–	+47	+16
Hematocrit (%)	38.2	34.7	40.5

Blood volume estimation (chromium 51) during antepartum eclampsia, again when non-pregnant, and finally at a comparable time in a second pregnancy uncomplicated by hypertension.

* Change in blood volume (%) as compared with non-pregnant women.

Adapted by permission from Pritchard JA, Cunningham FG, Pritchard SA. The Parkland Memorial Hospital protocol for treatment of eclampsia: evaluation of 245 cases. *Am J Obstet Gynecol* 1984; 148: 951.

setting of pre-eclampsia is not clear, but it appears to involve excessive levels of circulating antiangiogenic factors [14–16].

Normal maternal blood volume expansion also appears to be important for fetal growth. Salas et al. [17] compared maternal plasma volume as measured by Evans blue dye dilution in term pregnancies with normal and growth-restricted fetuses. Pregnancies complicated by fetal intrauterine growth restriction (IUGR) had significantly lower mean maternal plasma volumes as compared with pregnancies with well-grown fetuses (2976 ± 76 mL vs 3594 ± 103 mL, respectively). Moreover, recent studies have found that low pre-pregnancy plasma volumes in formerly pre-eclamptic women predispose to a recurrence of pre-eclampsia and adverse pregnancy outcome in a subsequent pregnancy [18]. The physiologic mechanisms responsible for these pregnancy-associated changes in blood volume are not fully understood. Pregnancy may best be regarded as a state of volume overload resulting primarily from renal sodium and water retention, with a shift of fluid from the intravascular to the extravascular space. Indeed, in addition to fetal growth, a substantial part of maternal weight gain during pregnancy results from fluid accumulation. Unlike other arterial vasodilatory states, pregnancy is associated with an increase in renal glomerular filtration and filtered sodium load [19], leading to an increase in urinary sodium and water excretion [20]. To prevent excessive fluid loss and resultant compromise to uteroplacental perfusion, mineralocorticoid activity increases to promote sodium and water retention by the distal renal tubules. The increased mineralocorticoid activity results primarily from extra-adrenal conversion of progesterone to deoxycorticosterone [21]. It is also possible that another as yet unidentified vasodilator(s) may be responsible for the volume expansion, since studies in pregnant baboons have demonstrated that systemic vasodilation precedes the measured increase in maternal blood volume [22]. The net result of these two opposing mechanisms is an accumulation during pregnancy of approximately 500–900 mEq of sodium and 6–8 L of total body water [23,24].

There is also evidence to suggest that the fetus may contribute to the increase in maternal plasma volume. Placental estrogens are known to promote aldosterone production by directly activating the renin–angiotensin system, and the capacity of the placenta to synthesize estrogens is dependent in large part on the availability of estrogen precursor (dehydroepiandrosterone) from the fetal adrenal. As such, the fetus may regulate maternal plasma

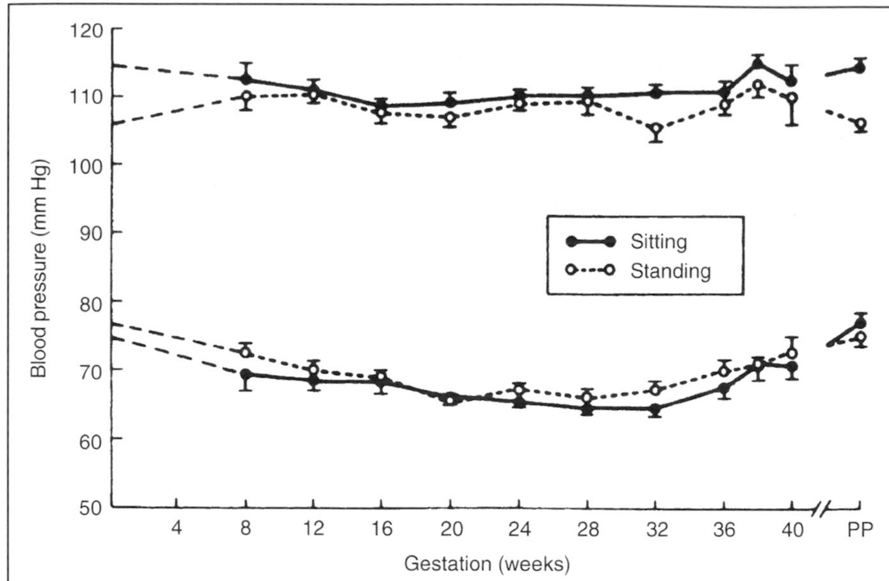

Figure 4.2 Sequential changes in systolic and diastolic BP throughout pregnancy with subjects sitting and standing (n = 69; values are mean ± SEM). Postpartum (PP) values drawn on the ordinate are used as a baseline, and dashed lines represent the presumed changes during the first 8 weeks. (Reprinted by permission of the publisher from Wilson M, Morganti AA, Zervodakis I, et al. Blood pressure, the renin-aldosterone system, and sex steroids throughout normal pregnancy. *Am J Med* 68: 97. Copyright 1980 by Excerpta Medica Inc.)

volume through its effect on the placental renin–angiotensin system [25]. In support of this mechanism, pregnancies complicated by IUGR have lower circulating levels of aldosterone and other vasodilator substances (prostacyclin, kallikrein) as compared with pregnancies with well-grown fetuses [17]. However, the fetus is not essential for the development of gestational hypervolemia, because it develops also in complete molar pregnancies [26].

Blood pressure

Blood pressure (BP) is the product of cardiac output and SVR, and reflects the ability of the cardiovascular system to maintain perfusion to the various organ systems, including the fetoplacental unit. Maternal BP is influenced by several factors, including gestational age, measurement technique, and positioning.

Gestational age is an important factor when evaluating BP in pregnancy. For example, a maternal sitting BP of 130/84 mmHg would be considered normal at term but concerningly high at 20 weeks of gestation. A sustained elevation in BP of ≥140/90 should be regarded as abnormal at any stage of pregnancy. Earlier reports suggested that an increase in BP of ≥30 mmHg systolic or ≥15 mmHg diastolic over first- or early second-trimester BP should be used to define hypertension; however, this concept is no longer valid since many women exhibit such changes in normal pregnancy [27,28].

Blood pressure normally decreases approximately 10% by the 7th week of pregnancy [6]. This is likely due to systemic vasodilation resulting from hormonal (progesterone) changes in early pregnancy. Indeed, studies in baboons have shown that the fall in arterial BP that occurs very early in pregnancy is due entirely to the decrease in SVR [22]. The resultant increase in cardiac output does not fully compensate for the diminished afterload, thereby providing a reasonable explanation for a lower mean arterial BP during the first trimester.

Systolic and diastolic BP continue to decrease until midpregnancy and then gradually recover to non-pregnant values by term. A longitudinal study of 69 women during normal pregnancy demonstrated that the lowest arterial BP occurs at around 28 weeks of gestation (Figure 4.2) [29]. BP measurements can be affected by maternal positioning. In this same series, BP was lowest when measured with the patient in the left lateral decubitus position, and increased by approximately 14 mmHg when patients were rotated into the supine position [29] (Figure 4.3). Despite the difference in absolute measurements, the pattern of BP change throughout pregnancy was unaffected (see Figure 4.3) For the sake of consistency and standardization, all BP measurements in pregnancy should be taken with the patient in the sitting position.

Blood pressure measurements are also subject to change depending on the technique used to attain the measurements. In a series of 70 pregnant women, Ginsberg and Duncan [30] demonstrated that mean systolic and diastolic BP were lower (by −6 mmHg and −15 mmHg, respectively) when measurements were taken directly using a radial intra-arterial line as compared with indirect measurements using a standard sphygmomanometer. Conversely, Kirshon and colleagues [31] found a significantly lower systolic (but not diastolic) BP when using an automated sphygmomanometer as compared with direct radial intra-arterial measurements in a series of 12 postpartum patients.

Heart rate

Maternal heart rate increases as early as the 7th week of pregnancy and by late pregnancy is increased approximately 20% as compared with postpartum values [29] (Figure 4.4). It is likely that

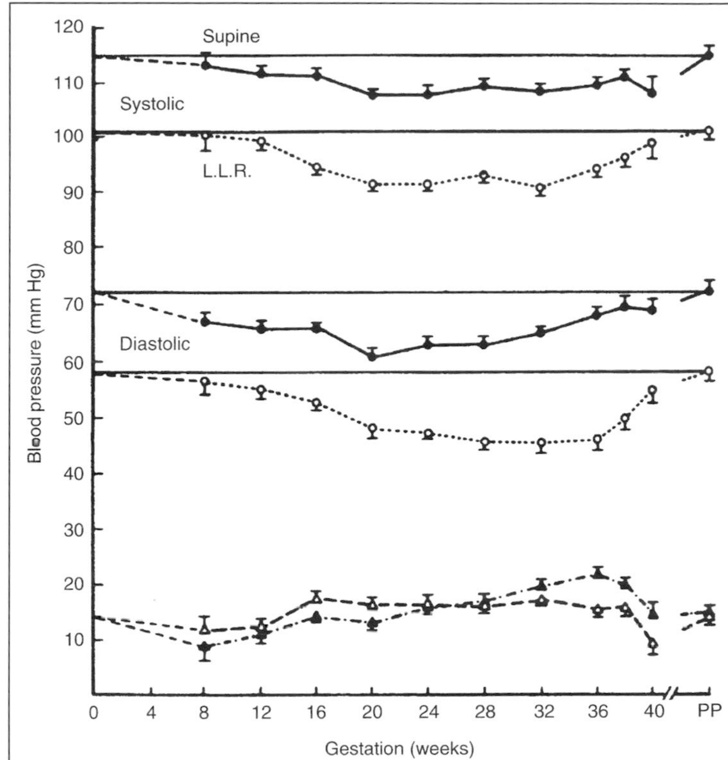

Figure 4.3 Sequential changes in BP throughout pregnancy with subjects in the supine and left lateral decubitus positions (n = 69; values are mean ± SEM). The calculated change in systolic (open triangles) and diastolic (closed triangles) BP produced by repositioning from the left lateral decubitus to the supine position is illustrated. LLR, left lateral recumbent; PP, postpartum. (Reprinted by permission of the publisher from Wilson M, Morganti AA, Zervodakis I, et al. Blood pressure, the renin-aldosterone system, and sex steroids throughout normal pregnancy. *Am J Med* 68: 97. Copyright 1980 by Excerpta Medica Inc.)

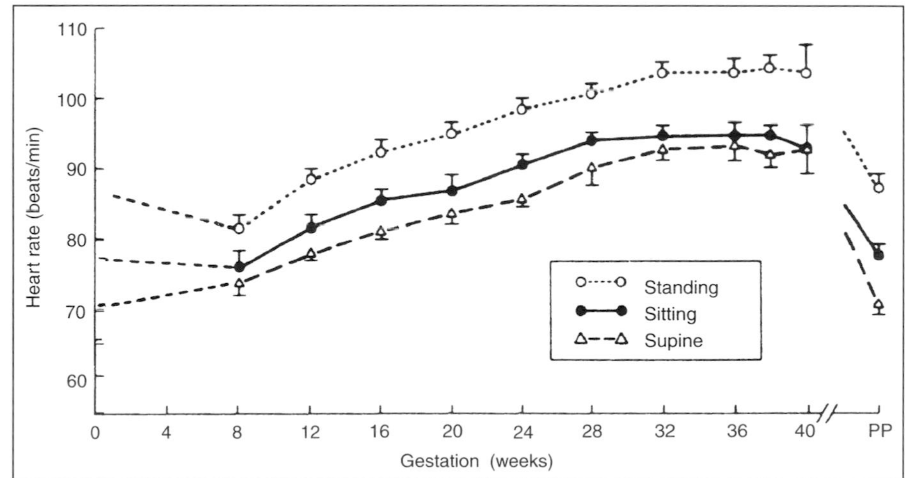

Figure 4.4 Sequential changes in mean heart rate in three positions throughout pregnancy (n = 69; values are mean ± SEM). PP, postpartum. (Reprinted by permission of the publisher from Wilson M, Morganti AA, Zervodakis I, et al. Blood pressure, the renin-aldosterone system, and sex steroids throughout normal pregnancy. *Am J Med* 68: 97. Copyright 1980 by Excerpta Medica Inc.)

the increase in heart rate is a secondary (compensatory) effect resulting from the decline in SVR during pregnancy [32]. However, a direct effect of hormonal factors cannot be entirely excluded. Although human chorionic gonadotropin (hCG) is an unlikely candidate [33], free thyroxine levels increase by 10 weeks and remain elevated throughout pregnancy [33,34]. The possibility that thyroid hormones may be responsible for the maternal tachycardia warrants further investigation.

In addition to pregnancy-associated changes, maternal tachycardia can also result from other causes (such as fever, pain, blood loss, hyperthyroidism, respiratory insufficiency, and cardiac disease) which may have important clinical implications for critically ill parturients. For example, women with severe mitral stenosis must rely on diastolic ventricular filling to achieve satisfactory cardiac output. Because left ventricular diastolic filling is heart rate dependent, maternal tachycardia can severely limit the capacity of such women to maintain an adequate BP, and can lead to cardiovascular shock and "fetal distress". As such, the management of patients with severe mitral stenosis should include, among other parameters, careful control of maternal heart rate and cardiac preload.

Cardiac output and stroke volume

Cardiac output is the product of heart rate and stroke volume, and reflects the overall capacity of the left ventricle to maintain systemic BP and thereby organ perfusion. Cardiac index is calculated by dividing cardiac output by body surface area (Table 4.3). Although useful in non-pregnant women, cardiac index is less useful in pregnant women because the normal correlation between cardiac output and body surface area is lost in pregnancy [35]. This may be explained, in part, by the observation that the du Bois and du Bois [36] body surface area nomogram widely used to calculate cardiac index is based on nine non-gravid subjects and, as such may not apply to pregnant women.

Linhard [37] was the first to report a 50% increase in cardiac output during pregnancy using the indirect Fick method. Others have studied maternal cardiac output by invasive catheterization [38–41], dye dilution [42–46], impedance cardiography [47,48], and echocardiography or Doppler ultrasound [49–53]. Despite controversy about the relative contributions of stroke volume and heart rate, maternal cardiac output increases as early as 10 weeks' gestation and peaks at 30–50% over non-pregnant values by the latter part of the second trimester. This rise, from 4.5 to 6.0 L/min, is sustained for the remainder of the pregnancy. Nulliparous women have a higher mean cardiac output than multiparous women [53].

Beginning in the late 1940s, right heart catheterization provided a more refined although invasive method for studying cardiac output. Hamilton [38] measured cardiac output in 24 non-gravid and 68 normal pregnant women by this technique. Cardiac output averaged 4.51 ± 0.38 L/min in non-pregnant women. In pregnancy, cardiac output began to increase at approximately 10–13 weeks' gestation, reached a maximum of 5.73 L/min at 26–29 weeks, and returned to non-pregnant levels by term. These observations have been confirmed by subsequent cross-sectional right heart catheterization studies in pregnant women [39,40].

Longitudinal studies using Doppler and M-mode echocardiography to interrogate maternal cardiac output throughout pregnancy report conflicting results about the relative contributions of heart rate and stroke volume. Katz and colleagues [49] attributed the elevation in cardiac output (+59% by the third trimester; n = 19) to increases in both heart rate and stroke volume, whereas the study by Mashini et al. [51] showed that the increase (+32% in the third trimester; n = 16) was due almost exclusively to maternal tachycardia. Laird-Meeter et al. [50] have suggested that the initial increase in cardiac output prior to 20 weeks' gestation is due to maternal tachycardia, whereas that observed after 20 weeks results from an increase in stroke volume due primarily to reversible myocardial hypertrophy. Mabie and colleagues [54], on the other hand, attributed the increase in cardiac output (from 6.7 ± 0.9 L/min at 8–11 weeks to 8.7 ± 1.4 L/min at 36–39 weeks; n = 18) to augmentation of both heart rate (+29%) and stroke

Table 4.3 Cardiovascular parameters.

Parameter	Units	Comment/derivation
	Measured directly using minimally invasive techniques	
Systolic blood pressure (SBP)	mmHg	
Diastolic blood pressure (DBP)	mmHg	
Heart rate	beats/min (bpm)	
	Measured directly using invasive techniques	
Central venous pressure (CVP)	mmHg	Reflects right ventricular preload
Pulmonary artery SBP	mmHg	
Pulmonary artery DBP	mmHg	
Pulmonary capillary wedge pressure (PCWP)	mmHg	Reflects left ventricular preload
	Derived from measured values	
Pulse pressure	mmHg	= SBP – DBP
Mean arterial pressure (MAP)	mmHg	= DBP + (pulse pressure/3)
Systemic vascular resistance (SVR)	dynes/sec/cm^{-5}	= (MAP – CVP) (80)/CO
Peripheral vascular resistance (PVR)	dynes/sec/cm^{-5}	= (MPAP – PCWP) (80)/CO
Cardiac output (CO)	L/min	= MAP/SVR = HR (beats/min) × SV (mL/beat)
Stroke volume (SV)	mL/beat	= CO (L/min)/HR (beats/min)
Cardiac index (CI)	L/min/m^2	= CO (L/min)/body surface area (m^2)
Stroke volume index (SVI)	mL/beat/m^2	= SV (mL/beat)/body surface area (m^2)

volume (+18%) (Figure 4.5). The conflicting nature of these studies can be attributed, in part, to the positioning of the patient during examination (lateral recumbent versus supine position). It must also be emphasized that although M-mode echocardiographic estimation of stroke volume correlates well with angiographic studies in non-gravid subjects, similar validation studies have not been carried out during pregnancy [55,56]. For this reason, ultrasound measurements of maternal volume flow in pregnancy have been validated only against similar measurements attained by thermodilution techniques [57–61].

One criticism of the above studies is that the maternal hemodynamic measurements in pregnancy are usually compared with those from postpartum control subjects. This comparison may not be valid, however, because cardiac output remains elevated for many weeks after delivery [60,62]. To address this issue, Robson et al. [63] measured cardiac output by Doppler echocardiography in 13 women before conception and again at monthly intervals throughout pregnancy. Maternal heart rate was significantly elevated by 5 weeks' gestation, and continued to increase thereafter, reaching a plateau at around 32 weeks (+17% above midpregnancy values). Stroke volume was increased by 8 weeks, with maximal values (+32% over midpregnancy levels) attained at 16–20 weeks. Overall, maternal cardiac output increased from 4.88 L/min at 5 weeks to 7.21 L/min (+48%) at 32 weeks. The mechanisms responsible for the increase in maternal cardiac output during pregnancy remain unclear. An increase in circulating blood volume is unlikely to contribute significantly to this effect, because hemodynamic studies in pregnant baboons have shown that the increase in cardiac output develops much earlier than does the gestational hypervolemia [22]. Burwell et al. [64] noted that the increase in plasma volume, cardiac output, and heart rate during pregnancy was similar to that seen in patients with arteriovenous shunting, and proposed that these hemodynamic changes are the result of the low-pressure, high-volume arteriovenous shunting that characterizes the uteroplacental circulation. A third hypothesis is that hormonal factors (possibly steroid hormones) may act directly on the cardiac musculature to increase stroke volume and hence cardiac output, analogous to the mechanisms responsible for the decrease in venous tone seen in normal pregnancy [65] or after oral contraceptive administration [66]. In support of this hypothesis, high-dose estrogen administration has been shown to increase stroke volume and cardiac output in male transsexuals [67]. To further investigate this hypothesis, Duvekot and colleagues [32] studied serial echocardiographic, hormonal, and renal electrolyte measurements in 10 pregnant women. The authors propose that the inciting event may be the fall in SVR that leads, in turn, to a compensatory tachycardia with activation of volume-restoring mechanisms. In this manner, the increased stroke volume may be a direct result of "normalized" vascular filling in the setting of systemic afterload reduction. These data support the conclusion of Morton and co-workers [68] that early stroke volume increases are caused by a "shift to the right" of the left ventricular pressure–volume curve (Frank–Starling mechanism).

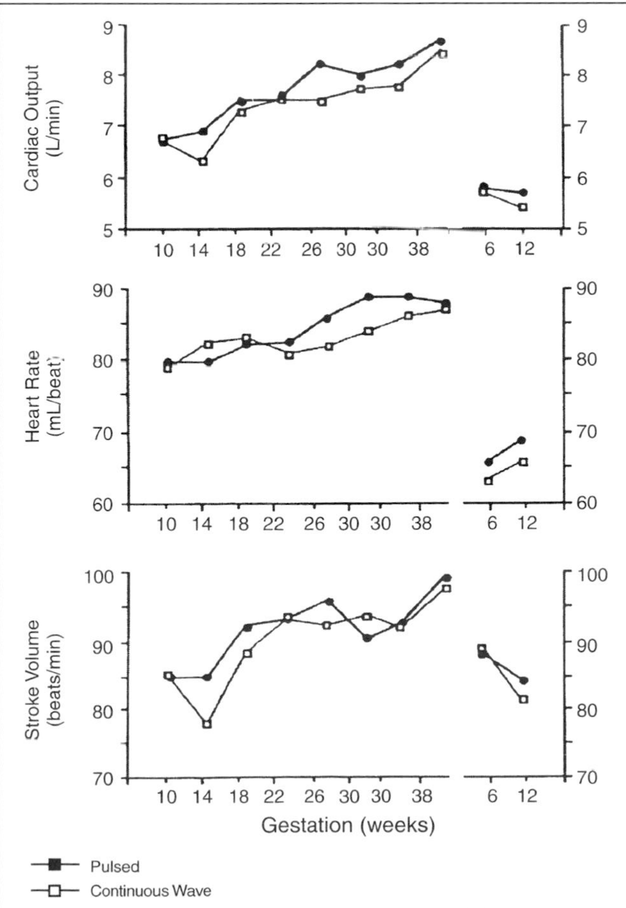

Figure 4.5 Hemodynamic changes during pregnancy and postpartum. (Reproduced by permission from Mabie W, DiSessa TG, Crocker LG, et al. A longitudinal study of cardiac output in normal human pregnancy. *Am J Obstet Gynecol* 1994; 170: 849.)

The cardiovascular changes in women carrying multiple pregnancies are greater than those described for singleton pregnancies. Two-dimensional and M-mode echocardiography of 119 women with twins showed that cardiac output was 20% higher than in women carrying singletons, and peaked at 30 weeks of gestation [69]. This increase was due to a 15% increase in stroke volume and 4.5% increase in heart rate.

Systemic vascular resistance

Systemic vascular resistance (SVR) is a measure of the impedance to the ejection of blood into the maternal circulation (i.e. afterload). Bader et al. [40] used cardiac catheterization to investigate the effect of pregnancy on SVR. They demonstrated that SVR decreases in early pregnancy, reaching a nadir at around 980 dynes/sec/cm^{-5} at 14–24 weeks. Thereafter, SVR rises progressively for the remainder of pregnancy, approaching a pre-pregnancy value of around 1240 dynes/sec/cm^{-5} at term. These findings are consistent with subsequent studies [41] which found a mean SVR of 1210 ± 266 dynes/sec/cm^{-5} during late pregnancy.

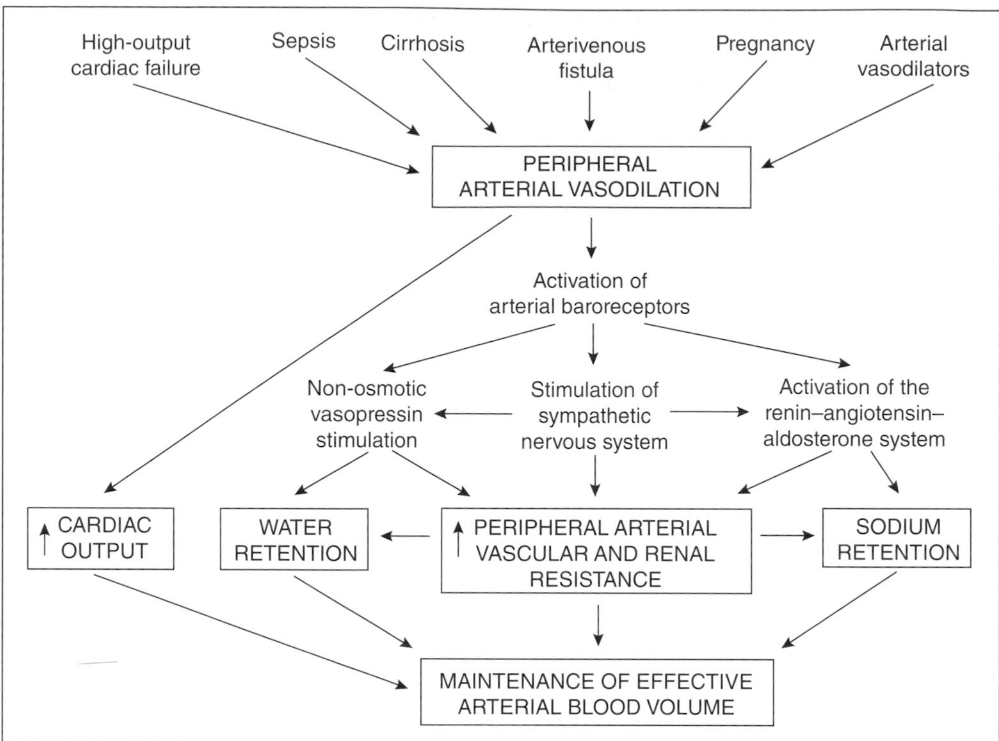

Figure 4.6 Unifying hypothesis of renal sodium and water retention initiated by peripheral arterial vasodilation. (Reprinted by permission from the American College of Obstetricians and Gynecologists. *Obstet Gynecol* 1991; 77: 632.)

When describing the physiologic relationship between pressure and flow, it is customary to report vascular impedance as a ratio of pressure to flow (see Table 4.3). The observed decrease in SVR during pregnancy results primarily from a decrease in mean arterial pressure coupled with an increase in cardiac output. It is important to recognize the inverse relationship between cardiac output and SVR.

Peripheral arterial vasodilation with relative underfilling of the arterial circulation is likely the primary event responsible for the decrease in SVR seen in early pregnancy [70,71]. The factors responsible for this vasodilation are not clear but likely include hormonal factors (progesterone) and peripheral vasodilators such as nitric oxide [72]. The existence of a pregnancy-specific vasodilatory substance has been postulated but it has yet to be characterized. Cardiac afterload is further reduced by the progressive development of the low-resistance uteroplacental circulation. The decrease in SVR in early pregnancy leads to activation of compensatory homeostatic mechanisms designed to maintain arterial blood volume by increasing cardiac output and promoting sodium and water retention (summarized in Figure 4.6). This is accomplished through activation of arterial baroreceptors, upregulation of vasopressin, stimulation of the sympathetic nervous system, and increased mineralocorticoid activity. In addition to vasodilation, creation of a high-flow, low-resistance circuit in the uteroplacental circulation also contributes significantly to the decline in peripheral vascular resistance [63].

Whether atrial natriuretic peptide (ANP) has a role to play in the regulation of SVR in pregnancy is still unclear. ANP is a peptide hormone produced by atrial cardiocytes, which promotes renal sodium excretion and diuresis in non-pregnant subjects [73]. *In vitro*, ANP has been shown to promote vasodilation in vascular smooth muscle pretreated with angiotensin II. Circulating ANP levels increase in pregnancy, suggesting that ANP may play a role in decreasing maternal SVR [74,75]. Earlier cross-sectional studies did not correlate ANP levels with blood volume and hemodynamic measurements. In a prospective longitudinal study, Thomsen et al. [76] demonstrated that plasma ANP levels were positively correlated with Doppler ultrasound estimates of peripheral vascular resistance. Although their results substantiate the physiologic importance of ANP in the regulation of blood volume, the authors conclude that ANP does not function as a significant vasodilator during pregnancy.

Regional blood flow

Significant regional blood flow changes have been documented during pregnancy. For example, renal blood flow increases by 30% over non-pregnant values by midpregnancy and remains elevated for the remainder of pregnancy [77,78]. As a result, glomerular filtration rate increases 30–50% [70]. Similarly, skin perfusion increases slowly to 18–20 weeks' gestation but rises rapidly thereafter, reaching a plateau at 20–30 weeks that persists until approximately 1 week postpartum [79]. This is likely due to vasodilation of dermal capillaries [80,81] and may serve as a mechanism by which the excess heat of fetal metabolism is allowed to dissipate from the maternal circulation. Pulmonary blood flow increases during pregnancy from 4.88 L/min in early pregnancy to 7.19 L/min at 38 weeks, an increase of around 32% [82,83]. A small decrease in pulmonary vascular resistance was noted at 8 weeks without any subsequent significant change thereafter. However, both non-invasive [82] and invasive studies [40,41,84] have shown that mean pulmonary artery pressure remains stable at around 14 mmHg, which is not significantly different from the non-gravid state.

The most dramatic change in regional blood flow in pregnancy occurs in the uterus. Uterine blood flow increases from approximately 50 mL/min at 10 weeks to 500 mL/min at term [85,86]. At term, therefore, uterine blood flow accounts for over 10% of maternal cardiac output. This increase in blood flow is likely related to hormonal factors, because animal studies have shown a significant decrease in uterine vascular resistance in response to exogenous administration of estrogen and progesterone [87,88].

Effect of posture on maternal hemodynamics

Prior to the 1960s, clinical investigators did not fully appreciate the effects of postural change on maternal hemodynamics and patients were often studied in the supine position. The unique angiographic studies of Bieniarz et al. [89,90] demonstrate that the gravid uterus can significantly impair vena caval blood flow in >90% of women studied in the supine position, thereby predisposing pregnant women to dependent edema and varicosities of the lower extremities. Moreover, impairment of central venous return in the supine position can result in decreased cardiac output, a sudden drop in BP, bradycardia, and syncope [91]. These clinical features were initially described by Howard et al. [92] and are now commonly referred to as the "supine hypotensive syndrome." Symptomatic supine hypotension occurs in 8% [93] to 14% [94] of women during late pregnancy. It is likely that women with poor collateral circulation through the paravertebral vessels may be predisposed to symptomatic supine hypotension, because these vessels usually serve as an alternative route for venous return from the pelvic organs and lower extremities [95]. In addition to impairing venous return, compression by the gravid uterus in the supine position can also result in partial obstruction of blood flow through the aorta and its ancillary branches, leading, for example, to diminished renal blood flow [77,96].

The clinical significance of supine hypotension is not clear. Vorys et al. [97] demonstrated an immediate 16% reduction in cardiac output when women in the latter half of pregnancy were moved from the supine to the dorsal lithotomy position, likely due to the compressive effect of the gravid uterus on the vena cava (Table 4.4). To investigate the effect of gestational age on the maternal cardiovascular response to posture, Ueland and Hansen [44] measured changes in resting heart rate, stroke volume, and cardiac output for 11 normal gravid women in various positions (sitting, supine, and left lateral decubitus) throughout their pregnancies (Figure 4.7). Maternal heart rate was maximal (range, +13% to +20% compared with postpartum values) at 28–32 weeks of pregnancy, and was further elevated in the sitting position. Stroke volume increased early in pregnancy, with maximal values by 20–24 weeks (range, +21% to +33%), followed by a progressive decline towards term that was most

Table 4.4 Changes in cardiac output with maternal position.

Late-trimester women (n = 31)	Change from supine (%)
Horizontal left side	+14
Trendelenburg left side	+13
Lithotomy	−16
Supine Trendelenburg	−18

Reproduced by permission from Vorys N, Ullery JC, Hanusek GE. The cardiac output changes in various positions in pregnancy. *Am J Obstet Gynecol* 1961; 82: 1312.)

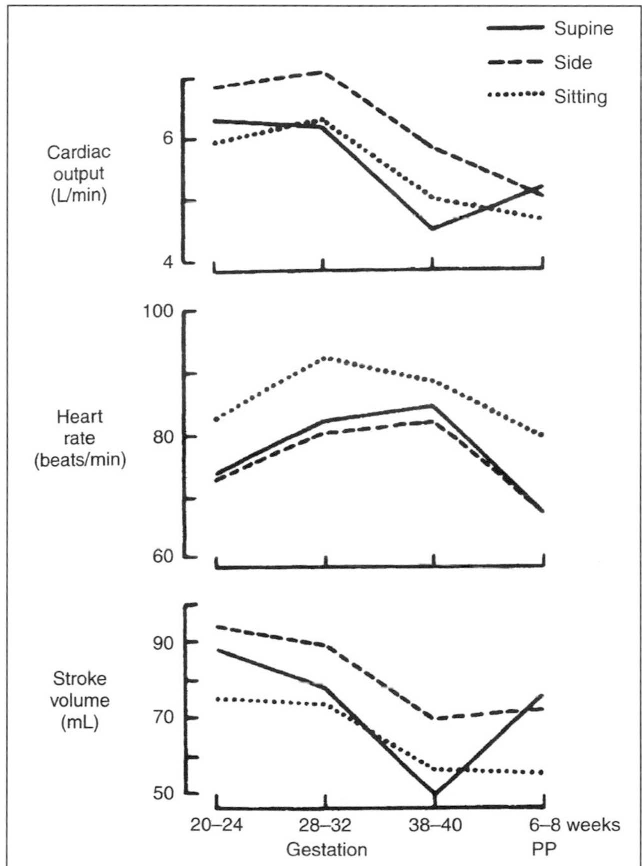

Figure 4.7 Effect of posture on maternal hemodynamics. PP, postpartum. (Reproduced by permission from Ueland K, Metcalfe J. Circulatory changes in pregnancy. *Clin Obstet Gynecol* 1975; 18: 41; modified from Ueland K, Novy MJ, Peterson EN, et al. Maternal cardiovascular dynamics. IV. The influence of gestational age on the maternal cardiovascular response to posture and exercise. *Am J Obstet Gynecol* 1969; 104: 856.)

striking in the supine position. Indeed, measurements of stroke volume and cardiac output in the supine position at term were even lower than the corresponding values in the postpartum period (see Figure 4.7). On an optimistic note, Calvin and associates [94] were able to demonstrate that supine hypotension does not normally result in significant oxygen desaturation.

To investigate the effect of standing on the maternal hemodynamic profile, Easterling et al. [98] measured cardiac output and SVR in the recumbent, sitting, and standing positions in women during early (11.1 ± 1.4 weeks) and late (36.7 ± 1.6 weeks) pregnancy. A change from the recumbent to standing position resulted in a decrease in cardiac output of around 1.7 L/min at any stage of gestation with a compensatory SVR augmentation (Table 4.5). Of note, the compensatory increase in SVR was significantly blunted in late pregnancy as compared with non-pregnant subjects, which may be related to the altered response to norepinephrine observed during pregnancy [99,100]. In addition to confirming these findings, Clark et al. [101] were able to demonstrate that maternal BP was essentially unaffected by standing in the third trimester of pregnancy, despite varying effects on cardiac output (Table 4.6). The observed decrease in left ventricular stroke work index on standing (−22%) was attributed to the subject's inability to compensate for the decrease in stroke volume by heart rate alone as a result of Starling forces. Intrapulmonary shunting is not affected by maternal position [102]. Whether such postural changes have any clinical significance in terms of placental perfusion, birthweight, and/or preterm delivery is unclear at this time [103,104].

Conventional wisdom teaches us that low blood pressure in pregnancy is reassuring, but recent studies suggest that sustained low blood pressure in the third trimester (defined as a maximum diastolic blood pressure <65 mmHg) is a risk factor for stillbirth and growth restriction [105–108]. The rise in blood pressure in the third trimester of pregnancy likely represents a healthy physiologic response of the maternal cardiovascular system to the relative inability of the placenta to keep pace with fetal growth, and

Table 4.5 Net change in hemodynamic parameters from recumbent to standing positions.

	Non-pregnant	Early pregnancy	Late pregnancy	*P**
MAP (mmHg)	78 ± 8.3	4.7 ± 7.7	5.0 ± 11.3	NS
Heart rate (bpm)	15.5 ± 9.2	25.7 ± 11.8	16.7 ± 11.2	NS
CO (L/min)	−1.8 ± 0.84	−1.8 ± 0.79	−1.7 ± 1.2	NS
Stroke volume (mL/beat)	−41.1 ± 15.8	−38.7 ± 14.5	−30.8 ± 17.5	NS
SVR (dynes/sec/cm^{-5})	732 ± 363	588 ± 246	379 ± 214	0.005

Data are presented as mean ± SD.
* Determined by analysis of variance.
CO, cardiac output; MAP, mean arterial pressure; NS, not significant; SVR, systemic vascular resistance.
Reproduced with permission from the American College of Obstetricians and Gynecologists. *Obstet Gynecol* 1988; 72: 550.

Table 4.6 Hemodynamic alterations in response to position change late in third trimester of pregnancy.

Hemodynamic parameter	Position			
	Left lateral	Supine	Sitting	Standing
MAP (mmHg)	90 ± 6	90 ± 8	90 ± 8	91 ± 14
CO (L/min)	6.6 ± 1.4	6.0 ± 1.4*	6.2 ± 2.0	5.4 ± 2.0*
Heart rate (bpm)	82 ± 10	84 ± 10	91 ± 11	107 ± 17*
SVR (dynes/sec/cm^{-5})	1210 ± 266	1437 ± 338	1217 ± 254	1319 ± 394
PVR (dynes/sec/cm^{-5})	76 ± 16	101 ± 45	102 ± 35	117 ± 35*
PCWP (mmHg)	8 ± 2	6 ± 3	4 ± 4	4 ± 2
CVP (mmHg)	4 ± 3	3 ± 2	1 ± 1	1 ± 2
LVSWI (g/min/m^{-2})	43 ± 9	40 ± 9	44 ± 5	34 ± 7*

* $p < 0.05$, compared with left lateral position.
CO, cardiac output; CVP, central venous pressure; LVSWI, left ventricular stroke work index; MAP, mean arterial pressure; PCWP, pulmonary capillary wedge pressure; PVR, pulmonary vascular resistance; SVR, systemic vascular resistance.
Reproduced with permission from Clark SL, Cotton DB, Pivarnik JM, et al. Position change and central hemodynamic profile during normal third-trimester pregnancy and postpartum. *Am J Obstet Gynecol* 1991; 164: 884.)

may be necessary to achieve optimal birthweight. Indeed, interventions designed to interfere with this increase in blood pressure in the latter half of pregnancy (such as antihypertensive medications) have repeatedly been shown to be associated with low birthweight [109,110]. The mechanism by which low blood pressure leads to stillbirth is not well understood. One possible explanation is that, in women with a low baseline blood pressure, a further drop in systemic pressure, such as may occur when a woman rolls over onto her back during sleep with resultant supine hypotension, may result in a drop in placental perfusion below a critical threshold, resulting in fetal demise.

Central hemodynamic changes associated with pregnancy

To establish normal values for central hemodynamics, Clark and colleagues [41] interrogated the maternal circulation by invasive hemodynamic monitoring. Ten primiparous women underwent right heart catheterization during late pregnancy (35–38 weeks) and again at 11–13 weeks postpartum (Table 4.7). When compared with postpartum values, late pregnancy was associated with a significant increase in heart rate (+17%), stroke volume (+23%), and cardiac output (+43%) as measured in the left lateral recumbent position. Significant decreases were noted in SVR (−21%), pulmonary vascular resistance (−34%), serum colloid osmotic pressure (−14%), and the colloid osmotic pressure to pulmonary capillary wedge pressure gradient (−28%). No significant changes were found in the pulmonary capillary wedge or central venous pressures, which confirmed previous studies [40].

Table 4.7 Central hemodynamic changes associated with late pregnancy.

	Non-pregnant	Pregnant	Change (%)
MAP (mmHg)	86 ± 8	90 ± 6	NS
PCWP (mmHg)	6 ± 2	8 ± 2	NS
CVP (mmHg)	4 ± 3	4 ± 3	NS
Heart rate (bpm)	71 ± 10	83 ± 10	+17
CO (L/min)	4.3 ± 0.9	6.2 ± 1.0	+43
SVR (dynes/sec/cm^{-5})	1530 ± 520	1210 ± 266	−21
PVR (dynes/sec/cm^{-5})	119 ± 47	78 ± 22	−34
Serum COP (mmHg)	20.8 ± 1.0	18.0 ± 1.5	−14
COP–PCWP gradient (mmHg)	14.5 ± 2.5	10.5 ± 2.7	−28
LVSWI (g/min/m^{-2})	41 ± 8	48 ± 6	NS

Measurements from the left lateral decubitus position are expressed as mean ± SD (n = 10). Significant changes are noted at the *P* p<0.05 level, paired two-tailed t-test.

CO, cardiac output; COP, colloid osmotic pressure; CVP, central venous pressure; LVSWI, left ventricular stroke index; MAP, mean arterial pressure; NS, non-significant; PCWP, pulmonary capillary wedge pressure; PVR, pulmonary vascular resistance; SVR, systemic vascular resistance.

Adapted with permission from Clark SL, Cotton DB, Lee W, et al. Central hemodynamic assessment of normal term pregnancy. *Am J Obstet Gynecol* 1989; 161: 1439.

Hemodynamic changes during labor

Repetitive and forceful uterine contractions (but not Braxton-Hicks contractions) have a significant effect on the cardiovascular system during labor. Each uterine contraction in labor expresses 300–500 mL of blood back into the systemic circulation [111,112]. Moreover, angiographic studies have shown that the change in shape of the uterus during contractions leads to improved blood flow from the pelvic organs and lower extremities back to the heart. The resultant increase in venous return during uterine contractions leads to a transient maternal bradycardia followed by an increase in cardiac output and compensatory bradycardia. Indeed, using a modified pulse pressure method for estimating cardiac output, Hendricks and Quilligan [112] showed a 31% increase in cardiac output with contractions as compared with the resting state.

Other factors that may be responsible for the observed increase in maternal cardiac output during labor included pain, anxiety, Valsalva, and maternal positioning [44,45,113,114]. Using the dye-dilution technique to measure hemodynamic parameters in 23 pregnant women in early labor with central catheters inserted into their brachial artery and superior vena cava, Ueland and Hansen [44,45] demonstrated that change in position from the supine to the lateral decubitus position was associated with an increase in both cardiac output (+21.7%) and stroke volume (+26.5%), and a decrease in heart rate (−5.6%). Figure 4.8 summarizes the effect of postural changes and uterine contractions on maternal hemodynamics during the first stage of labor. Under these conditions, uterine contractions resulted in a 15.3% rise in cardiac output, a 7.6% heart rate decrease, and a 21.5% increase in stroke volume. These hemodynamic changes were of less

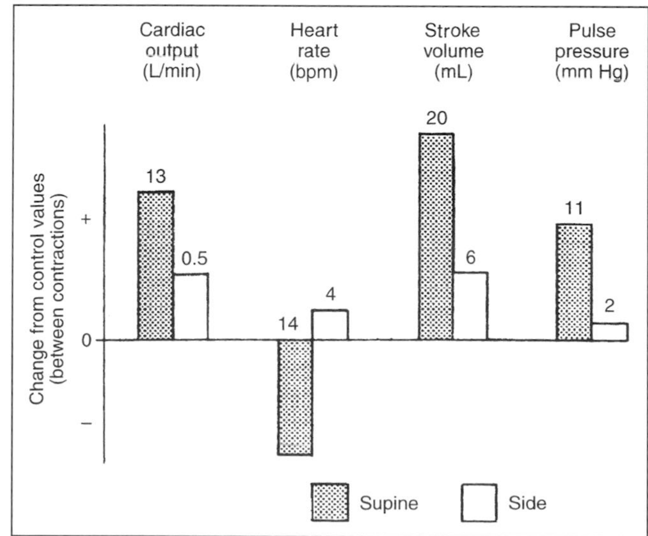

Figure 4.8 Effect of posture on the maternal hemodynamic response to uterine contractions in early labor. (Reproduced by permission from Ueland K, Metcalfe J. Circulatory changes in pregnancy. *Clin Obstet Gynecol* 1975; 18: 41; modified from Ueland K, Hansen JM. Maternal cardiovascular dynamics. II. Posture and uterine contractions. *Am J Obstet Gynecol* 1969; 103: 8.)

magnitude in the lateral decubitus position, although cardiac output measurements between contractions were actually higher when patients were on their side.

The first stage of labor is associated with a progressive increase in cardiac output. Kjeldsen [115] found that cardiac output increased by 1.10 L/min in the latent phase, 2.46 L/min in the accelerating phase, and 2.17 L/min in the decelerating phase as compared with antepartum values. Ueland and Hansen [45] described a similar increase in cardiac output between early and late first stages of labor. In a more detailed analysis, Robson and colleagues [58] used Doppler ultrasound to measure cardiac output serially throughout labor in 15 women in the left lateral position under meperidine labor analgesia. Cardiac output measured between contractions increased from 6.99 L/min to 7.88 L/min (+13%) by 8 cm cervical dilation, primarily as a result of increased stroke volume. A further increase in cardiac output was evident during contractions, due to augmentation of both heart rate and stroke volume. Of interest, the magnitude of the contraction-associated augmentation in cardiac output increased as labor progressed: ≤3 cm (+17%), 4–7 cm (+23%), and ≥8 cm (+34%). Similar results were reported by Lee et al. [116] using Doppler and M-mode echocardiography to study the effects of contractions on cardiac output in women with epidural analgesia. Under epidural analgesia, however, the effect of contractions on heart rate was minimal.

Although a detailed discussion of the effect of labor analgesia on maternal hemodynamics is beyond the scope of this chapter and is dealt with in detail elsewhere in this book, the increase in cardiac output during the labor was not as pronounced in women with regional anesthesia as compared with women receiving local anesthesia (paracervical or pudendal). These data suggest that the relative lack of pain and anxiety in women with regional analgesia may limit the absolute increase in cardiac output encountered at delivery. Alternatively, the fluid bolus required for regional anesthesia may itself affect cardiac output. Indeed, Robson and coworkers [117] found that infusion of 800 mL of Ringer's lactate prior to epidural anesthesia resulted in a 12% increase in stroke volume and an overall augmentation of cardiac output from 7.01 to 7.70 L/min. It is likely that this change is responsible, at least in part, for the altered response of the maternal cardiovascular system to labor in the setting of regional anesthesia.

Hemodynamic changes during the postpartum period

The postpartum period is associated with significant hemodynamic fluctuations, due largely to the effect of blood loss at delivery. Using chromium-labeled erythrocytes to quantify blood loss, Pritchard and colleagues [118] found that the average blood loss associated with cesarean delivery was 1028 mL, approximately twice that of vaginal delivery (505 mL). They also demonstrated that healthy pregnant women can lose up to 30% of their antepartum blood volume at delivery with little or no change in their postpartum hematocrit. These findings were similar to those of other investigators [119,120].

Ueland [114] compared blood volume and hematocrit changes in women delivered vaginally (n = 6) with those delivered by elective cesarean (n = 34) (Figure 4.9). The average blood loss at vaginal delivery was 610 mL, compared with 1030 mL at cesarean. In women delivered vaginally, blood volume decreased steadily for the first 3 days postpartum. In women delivered by cesarean, however, blood volume dropped off precipitously within the first hour of delivery, but remained fairly stable thereafter. As a result, both groups had a similar drop-off in blood volume (−16.2%) at the third postpartum day (see Figure 4.9). The differences in postpartum hematocrit between women delivered vaginally (+5.2% on day 3) and those delivered by cesarean (−5.8% on day 5) suggest that most of the volume loss following vaginal delivery was due to postpartum diuresis. This diuresis normally occurs between day 2 and day 5 postpartum, and allows for loss of the excess extracellular fluid accumulated during pregnancy [121], with a resultant 3 kg weight loss [122]. Failure to adequately

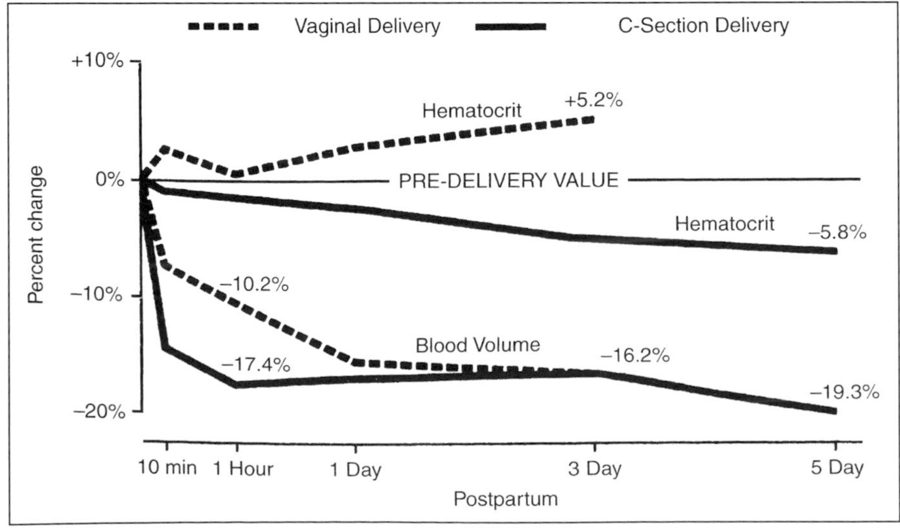

Figure 4.9 Percentage change in blood volume and venous hematocrit following vaginal or cesarean delivery. (Reproduced by permission from Metcalfe J, Ueland K. Heart disease and pregnancy. In: Fowler NO, ed. *Cardiac Diagnosis and Treatment*, 3rd edn. Hagerstown, MD: Harper and Row, 1980: 1153–1170.)

diurese in the first postpartum week may lead to excessive accumulation of intravascular fluid, elevated pulmonary capillary wedge pressure, and pulmonary edema [123].

Significant changes in cardiac output, stroke volume, and heart rate also occur after delivery [115]. Ueland and Hansen [45] demonstrated a dramatic increase in cardiac output (+59%) and stroke volume (+71%) within the first 10 minutes after delivery in 13 women who delivered vaginally under regional anesthesia. At 1 hour, cardiac output (+49%) and stroke volume (+67%) in these women were still elevated, with a 15% decrease in heart rate and no significant change in BP. The increase in cardiac output following delivery likely results from increased cardiac preload due to the autotransfusion of blood from the uterus back into the intravascular space, the release of vena caval compression from the gravid uterus, and the mobilization of extravascular fluid into the intravascular compartment.

These changes in maternal cardiovascular physiology resolve slowly after delivery. Using M-mode and Doppler echocardiography, Robson et al. [60] measured cardiac output and stroke volume in 15 healthy parturients at 38 weeks (not in labor) and then again at 2, 6, 12, and 24 weeks postpartum. Their results show a decrease in cardiac output from 7.42 L/min at 38 weeks to 4.96 L/min at 24 weeks postpartum, which was attributed to a reduction in both heart rate (−20%) and stroke volume (−18%). By 2 weeks postpartum, there was a substantial decrease in left ventricular size and contractility as compared with term pregnancy. By 24 weeks postpartum, however, echocardiographic studies demonstrated mild left ventricular hypertrophy that correlated with a slight diminution in left ventricular contractility as compared with age-matched non-gravid controls. Because the echocardiographic parameters in the control subjects were similar to those in previously published reports, it is likely that this small diminution in myocardial function 6 months after delivery is a real observation. This is an interesting finding, because patients with peripartum cardiomyopathy usually develop their disease within 5–6 months of delivery [124].

Respiratory system

There are numerous changes in the maternal respiratory system during pregnancy. These changes result initially from the endocrine changes of pregnancy and, later, from the physical and mechanical changes brought about by the enlarging uterus. The net physiologic result of these changes is a lowering of the maternal PCO_2 to less than that of the fetus, thereby facilitating effective exchange of CO_2 from the fetus to the mother.

Changes in the upper airways

The elevated estrogen levels and increases in blood volume associated with pregnancy may contribute to mucosal edema and hypervascularity in the upper airways of the respiratory system. Although one study failed to demonstrate an increased prevalence or severity of upper airway symptomatology in pregnancy, this study was of modest numbers (33 pregnant patients) and confined only to the first trimester [125]. The weight of evidence in the literature suggests that such changes do lead to an increased prevalence of nasal stuffiness, rhinitis, and epistaxis during pregnancy. Epistaxis can be severe and recurrent. Indeed, there are several case reports of epistaxis severe enough to cause "fetal distress" [125] and to be life-threatening to the mother [127]. The peculiar condition of "rhinitis of pregnancy" was recognized as far back as 1898 [128]. It has been reported to complicate up to 30% of pregnancies [129] although since, in some cases, the condition likely predated the pregnancy, the incidence of rhinitis attributable to pregnancy is somewhat lower at around 18% [129]. Symptoms of eustachian tube dysfunction are also frequently reported in pregnancy [130].

The factors responsible for the changes in the upper airways are not clearly understood. Animal studies have reported nasal mucosa swelling and edema in response to exogenous estrogen administration [131,132] and in pregnancy [132]. Increased cholinergic activity has been demonstrated in the nasal mucosa of pregnant women [133] and following estrogen administration to animals [134]. Although an estrogen-mediated cholinergic effect may explain the maternal rhinitis seen in pregnancy, other factors such as allergy, infection, stress, and/or medications may also be responsible [129]. As such, the occurrence of rhinitis in pregnancy should not be attributed simply to a normal physiologic process until other pathologic mechanisms have been excluded.

Changes in the mechanics of respiration

The mechanics of respiration change throughout pregnancy. In early pregnancy, these changes result primarily from hormonally-mediated relaxation of the ligamentous attachments of the chest. In later pregnancy, the enlarging uterus leads to changes in the shape of the chest. The lower ribs flare outwards, resulting in a 50% increase in the subcostal angle from around 70° in early pregnancy [135]. Although this angle decreases after delivery, it is still significantly greater (by approximately 20%) at 24 weeks postpartum than that measured at the beginning of pregnancy [135]. The thoracic circumference increases by around 8% during pregnancy and returns to normal shortly after delivery [135]. Both the anteroposterior and transverse diameters of the chest increase by around 2 cm in pregnancy [136,137]. The end result of these anatomic changes is elevation of the diaphragm by approximately 5 cm [137] and increase in excursion [138]. On the other hand, both respiratory muscle function and ribcage compliance are unaffected by pregnancy [135]. The relative contribution of the diaphragm and intercostal muscles to tidal volume is also similar in late pregnancy and after delivery [139]. As such, there is no significant difference in maximum respiratory pressures before and after delivery [135,138].

In later pregnancy, abdominal distension and loss of abdominal muscle tone may necessitate greater use of the accessory muscles of respiration during exertion. The perception of increased inspiratory muscle effort may contribute to a subjective experience of dyspnea [140]. Indeed, 15% of pregnant women report an increase in dyspnea in the first trimester as compared with almost 50% by 19 weeks and 76% by 31 weeks' gestation [141]. Labor is a condition requiring considerable physical exertion with extensive use of the accessory muscles. Acute diaphragmatic fatigue has been reported in labor [140].

Physiologic changes in pregnancy

Static lung volumes change significantly throughout pregnancy (Table 4.8; Figure 4.10). There is a modest reduction in the total lung capacity (TLC) [137]. The functional reserve capacity (FRC) also decreases because of a progressive reduction in expiratory reserve volume (ERV) and residual volume (RV) [135,137,142–146]. The inspiratory capacity (IC) increases as the FRC decreases. It is important to note that these changes are relatively small and vary considerably between individual parturients as well as between reported studies. In one report, for example, the only parameter that consistently changed in all women studied was the FRC [143]. Data from a review [146] of three large studies [143,148,149] comparing static lung volumes in pregnant and non-pregnant women are summarized in Table 4.8.

Table 4.8 Changes in static lung volumes in pregnant women at term.

Static lung volumes	Change from non-pregnant state
Total lung capacity (TLC)	↓ 200–400 mL (–4%)
Functional residual capacity (FRC)	↓ 300–500 mL (–17% to –20%)
Expiratory reserve volume (ERV)	↓ 100–300 mL (–5% to –15%)
Reserve volume (RV)	↓ 200–300 mL (–20% to –25%)
Inspiratory capacity (IC)	↑ 100–300 mL (+5% to +10%)
Vital capacity (VC)	Unchanged

Data from Baldwin GR, Moorthi DS, Whelton JA, MacDonnell KH. New lung functions in pregnancy. *Am J Obstet Gynecol* 1977; 127: 235.

It is commonly accepted that the decrease in ERV and FRC results primarily from the upward displacement of the diaphragm in pregnancy. It has also been suggested that this displacement further reduces the negative pleural pressure, leading to earlier closure of the small airways, an effect that is especially pronounced at the lung bases [146]. The modest change in TLC and lack of change in vital capacity (VC) suggests that this upward displacement of the diaphragm in pregnancy is compensated for by such factors as the increase in transverse thoracic diameter, thoracic circumference, and subcostal angle [135].

Respiratory rate and mean inspiratory flow are unchanged in pregnancy [135]. On the other hand, ventilatory drive (measured as mouth occlusion pressure) is increased during pregnancy, leading to a state of hyperventilation as evidenced by an increase in minute ventilation, alveolar ventilation, and tidal volume [135,147]. Moreover, these changes are evident very early in pregnancy. Minute ventilation, for example, is already increased by around 30% in the first trimester of pregnancy as compared with postpartum values [135,148,150,151]. Overall, pregnancy is associated with a 30–50% (approximately 3 L/min) increase in minute ventilation, a 50–70% increase in alveolar ventilation, and a 30–50% increase in tidal volume [147]. Although ventilatory dead space may increase by approximately 50% in pregnancy, the net effect on ventilation may be so small (approximately 60 mL) that it may not even be detectable [147]. Another reported change in ventilation during pregnancy is a decrease in airway resistance

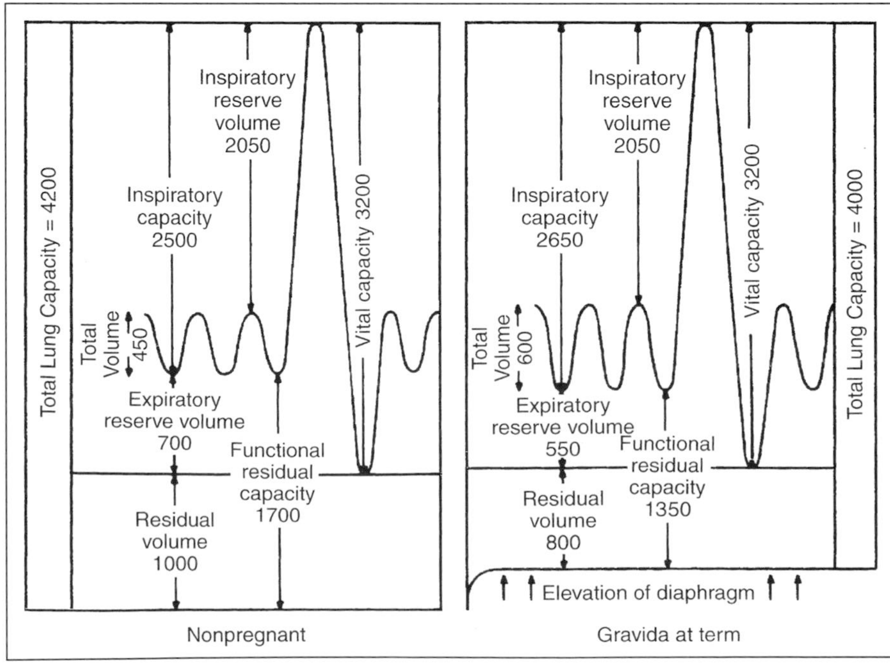

Figure 4.10 Respiratory changes during pregnancy (Note: all volumes are given in mL.) (Reproduced by permission from Bonica JJ. *Principles and Practice of Obstetrical Analgesia and Anesthesia*. Philadelphia: FA Davis, 1962.)

[144], while pulmonary compliance is thought to remain unchanged [135,145]. The hyperventilation of pregnancy has been attributed primarily to a progesterone effect. Indeed, minute ventilation had been shown to increase in men following exogenous progesterone administration [152]. However, other factors, such as the increased metabolic rate associated with pregnancy, may also have a role to play [153].

Changes in maternal acid–base status

Pregnancy represents a state of compensated respiratory alkalosis. CO_2 diffuses across membranes far faster than oxygen. As such, it is rapidly removed from the maternal circulation by the increased alveolar ventilation, with a concomitant reduction in the P_aCO_2 from a normal level of 35–45 mmHg to a lower level of 27–34 mmHg [137,147]. This leads in turn to increased bicarbonate excretion by the maternal kidneys, which serves to maintain the arterial blood pH between 7.40 and 7.45 (as compared with 7.35–7.45 in the non-pregnant state) [136,137,147]. As a result, serum bicarbonate levels decrease to 18–21 mEq/L in pregnancy [137,147]. The increased minute ventilation in pregnancy leads to an increase in P_aO_2 to 101–104 mmHg as compared with 80–100 mmHg in the non-pregnant state [136,137,147] and a small increase in the mean alveolar–arterial (A–a) O_2 gradient to 14.3 mmHg [154]. It should be noted, however, that a change from the sitting to supine position in pregnant women can decrease the capillary PO_2 by 13 mmHg [155] and increase the mean (A–a) O_2 gradient to 20 mmHg [154].

Genitourinary system

Alterations in renal tract anatomy

Because of the increased blood volume, the kidneys increase in length by approximately 1 cm during pregnancy [156]. The urinary collecting system also undergoes marked changes during pregnancy, with dilation of the renal calyces, renal pelvices, and ureters [157]. This dilation is likely secondary to the smooth muscle relaxant effects of progesterone, which may explain how it is that dilation of the collecting system can be visualized as early as the first trimester. However, an obstructive component to the dilation of the collecting system is also possible, due to the enlarging uterus compressing the ureters at the level of the pelvic brim [158]. Indeed, the right-sided collecting system tends to undergo more marked dilation than the left side, likely due to dextrorotation of the uterus [159]. These anatomic alterations may persist for up to 4 months postpartum [160].

The end result of these anatomic changes is physiologic obstruction and urinary stasis during pregnancy, leading to an increased risk of pyelonephritis in the setting of asymptomatic bacteriuria. Moreover, interpretation of renal tract imaging studies needs to take into account the fact that mild hydronephrosis and bilateral hydroureter are normal features of pregnancy, and do not necessarily imply pathologic obstruction.

Alterations in renal physiology

The glomerular filtration rate (GFR), as measured by creatinine clearance, increases by approximately 50% by the end of the first trimester to a peak of around 180 mL/min [161]. Effective renal plasma flow also increases by around 50% during early pregnancy and remains at this level until the final weeks of pregnancy, at which time it declines by 15–25% [162]. These physiologic changes result in a decrease in serum blood urea nitrogen (BUN) and creatinine levels during pregnancy, such that a serum creatinine value of greater than 0.8 mg/dL may be an indicator of abnormal renal function. An additional effect of the increased GFR is an increase in urinary protein excretion. Indeed, urinary protein loss of up to 260 mg/day can be considered normal during pregnancy [163].

Renal tubular function is also significantly changed during pregnancy. The filtered load of sodium increases significantly due to the increased GFR and the action of progesterone as a competitive inhibitor of aldosterone. Despite this increased filtered load of sodium, the increase in tubular reabsorption of sodium results in a net retention of up to 1 g of sodium per day. The increase in tubular reabsorption of sodium is likely a result of increased circulating levels of aldosterone and deoxycorticosterone [164]. Renin production increases early in pregnancy in response to rising estrogen levels, resulting in increased conversion of angiotensinogen to angiotensin I and II and culminating in increased levels of aldosterone. Aldosterone acts directly to promote renal tubular sodium retention.

Loss of glucose in the urine (glycosuria) is a normal finding during pregnancy, resulting from increased glomerular filtration and decreased distal tubular reabsorption [161]. This observation makes urinalysis an unreliable screening tool for gestational diabetes mellitus. Moreover, glycosuria may be a further predisposing factor to urinary tract infection during pregnancy.

Pregnancy is a period of marked water retention. During pregnancy, intravascular volume expands by around 1–2 L and extravascular volume by approximately 4–7 L [161]. This water retention results in a decrease in plasma sodium concentration from 140 to 136 mmol/L [165] and in plasma osmolality from 290 to 280 mosmol/kg [165]. Plasma osmolality is maintained at this level throughout pregnancy due to a resetting of the central osmoregulatory system.

Gastrointestinal system

Alterations in gastrointestinal anatomy

Gingival hyperemia and swelling are common in pregnancy, and the resultant gingivitis often presents as an increased tendency for bleeding gums during pregnancy. The principal anatomic alterations of the gastrointestinal tract result from displacement or pressure from the enlarging uterus. Intragastric pressure rises in pregnancy, likely contributing to heartburn and an increased incidence of hiatal hernia in pregnancy. The appendix is displaced progressively superiorly and laterally as pregnancy advances, such that the pain associated with appendicitis may be localized to the right upper quadrant at term [166]. Another anatomic alteration commonly seen in pregnancy is an increased incidence of hemorrhoids, which likely results from the progesterone-mediated relaxation of the hemorrhoidal vasculature, pressure from the enlarging uterus, and the increased constipation associated with pregnancy.

Alterations in gastrointestinal physiology

Many of the physiologic changes affecting gastrointestinal physiology during pregnancy are the result of a progesterone-mediated smooth muscle relaxant effect. Lower esophageal sphincter tone is decreased, resulting in increased gastroesophageal reflux and symptomatic heartburn [167]. Gastric and small bowel motility may also be decreased, leading to delayed gastric emptying and prolonged intestinal transit times [168]. Such effects may contributed to pregnancy-related constipation by facilitating increased large intestine water reabsorption and may explain, at least in part, the increased risk of regurgitation and aspiration with induction of general anesthesia in pregnancy. Of interest, more recent studies have suggested that delayed gastric emptying is only significant around the time of delivery and, rather than being a pregnancy-related phenomenon, may result primarily from anesthetic medications given during labor [169].

Early studies suggested that the progesterone-dominant milieu of pregnancy resulted in a decrease in gastric acid secretion and an increase in gastric mucin production [170], and that these changes accounted for the apparent rarity of symptomatic peptic ulcer disease during pregnancy. However, more recent studies have shown no significant change in gastric acid production during pregnancy [171]. It is possible that the apparent protective effect of pregnancy on peptic ulcer disease may be a result of under-reporting, since dyspeptic symptoms may be attributed to pregnancy-related heartburn without a complete evaluation.

Hepatobiliary changes in pregnancy

Although the liver does not change in size during pregnancy, its position is shifted upwards and posteriorly, especially during the third trimester. Other physical signs commonly attributed to liver disease in non-pregnant women (such as spider nevi and palmar erythema) can be normal features of pregnancy, and are likely due to increased circulating estrogen levels. Pregnancy is associated with dilation of the gallbladder and biliary duct system, which most likely represents a progesterone-mediated smooth muscle relaxant effect [172].

Liver function tests change during pregnancy. Circulating levels of transaminases, including aspartate transaminase (AST) and alanine transaminase (ALT), as well as γ-glutamyl transferase (γGT) and bilirubin, are normal or slightly diminished in pregnancy [173]. Knowledge of the normal range for liver function tests in pregnancy as compared with non-pregnant patients is important, for example, when evaluating patients with pre-eclampsia. Prothrombin time (PT) and lactic acid dehydrogenase (LDH) levels are unchanged in pregnancy. Serum albumin and protein levels are decreased in pregnancy, most likely as a result of hemodilution from the increased plasma volume. Serum alkaline phosphatase (ALP) levels are markedly increased, especially during the third trimester of pregnancy, and this is almost exclusively as a result of the placental isoenzyme fraction.

Gallbladder function is considerably altered during pregnancy. This is due primarily to progesterone-mediated inhibition of cholecystokinin, which results in decreased gallbladder motility and stasis of bile within the gallbladder [172]. In addition, pregnancy is associated with an increase in biliary cholesterol concentration and a decrease in the concentration of select bile acids (especially chenodeoxycholic acid), both of which contribute to the increased lithogenicity of bile. Such changes serve to explain why cholelithiasis is more common during pregnancy.

Hematologic system

The functions of the hematologic system include supplying tissues and organ systems with oxygen and nutrients, removal of CO_2 and other metabolic waste products, regulation of temperature, protection against infection, and humoral communication. In pregnancy, the developing fetus and placenta impose further demands and the maternal hematologic system must adapt in order to meet these demands. Such adaptations included changes in plasma volume as well as the numbers of constituent cells and coagulation factors. All these changes are designed to benefit the mother and/or fetus. However, some changes may also bring with them potential risks. It is important for the obstetric care provider to have a comprehensive understanding of both the positive and negative effects of the pregnancy-associated changes to the maternal hematologic system.

Changes in red blood cell mass

Red blood cell mass increases throughout pregnancy. In a landmark study using chromium (^{51}Cr)-labeled red blood cells, Pritchard [7] reported an average increase in red blood cell mass of around 30% (450 mL) in both singleton and twin pregnancies. Of note, the increase in red blood cell mass lags significantly behind the change in plasma volume and, as such, occurs later in pregnancy and continues until delivery [4,174,175]. The difference in timing between the increase in red blood cell mass and plasma volume expansion results in a physiologic fall of the hematocrit in the first trimester (so-called physiologic anemia of pregnancy), which persists until the end of the second trimester. Erythropoiesis is stimulated by erythropoietin (which increases in pregnancy) as well as by human placental lactogen, a hormone produced by the placenta which is more abundant in later pregnancy [176]. There are different opinions as to what ought to be regarded as the definition of anemia in pregnancy, but an historical and widely accepted value is that of a hemoglobin concentration <10.0 g/dL [7]. The increase in red blood cell mass serves to optimize oxygen transport to the fetus, while the decrease in blood viscosity resulting from the physiologic anemia of pregnancy will improve placental perfusion and offer the mother some protection from obstetric hemorrhage.

Iron stores in healthy reproductive-age women are marginal, with two-thirds of such women having suboptimal iron stores [177]. The major reason for low iron stores is thought to be menstrual blood loss. The total iron requirement for pregnancy has been estimated at around 980 mg. This amount of iron is not provided by a normal diet. As such, iron supplementation is recommended for all reproductive-age and pregnant women.

Changes in white blood cell count

Serum white blood cell count increases in pregnancy due to a selective bone marrow granulopoiesis [175]. This results in a "left shift" of the white cell count, with a granulocytosis and increased numbers of immature white blood cells. The white blood cell count is increased in pregnancy and peaks at around 30 weeks' gestation [175,178] (Table 4.9). Although a white blood cell count of 5000–12 000/mm^3 is considered normal in pregnancy, only around 20% of women will have a white blood cell count of greater than 10 000/mm^3 in the third trimester [175].

Changes in platelet count

Most studies suggest that platelet counts decrease in pregnancy [179,180], although some studies show no change [181]. Since pregnancy does not appear to change the lifespan of platelets [182], it is likely that the decrease in platelet count with pregnancy is primarily a dilutional effect. Whether there is increased consumption of platelets in pregnancy is controversial. Fay et al. [183] reported a decrease in platelet count due to both hemodilution and increased consumption that reached a nadir at around 30 weeks' gestation. This study, along with the observation that the mean platelet volume increase in pregnancy is indicative of a younger platelet population [184], suggests that there may indeed be some increased platelet consumption in pregnancy.

The lower limit of normal for platelet counts in pregnancy is commonly accepted as the same as that for non-pregnant women (i.e. 150 000/mm^3). A maternal platelet count less than 150 000/mm^3 should be regarded as abnormal, although the majority of cases of mild thrombocytopenia (i.e. 100 000–150 000/mm^3) will have no identifiable cause. Such cases are thought to result primarily from hemodilution. This condition has been termed "gestational thrombocytopenia." It is evident in around 8% of pregnancies [185] and poses no apparent risk to either mother or fetus.

Table 4.9 White blood cell count in pregnancy.

	White blood cell count (cells/mm^3)	
	Mean	Normal range
First trimester	8000	5110–9900
Second trimester	8500	5600–12 200
Third trimester	8500	5600–12 200
Labor	25 000	20 000–30 000

Data from Pitkin R, Witte D. Platelet and leukocyte counts in pregnancy. *JAMA* 1979; 242: 2696.)

Changes in coagulation factors

Pregnancy is associated with changes in the coagulation and fibrinolytic cascades that favor thrombus formation. These changes include an increase in circulating levels of factors XII, X, IX, VII, VIII, von Willebrand factor, and fibrinogen [186]. Factor XIII, high molecular weight kininogen, prekallikrein, and fibrinopeptide A (FPA) levels are also increased, although reports are conflicting [186]. Factor XI decreases and levels of prothrombin and factor V are unchanged [186]. In contrast, antithrombin III and protein C levels are either unchanged or increased, and protein S levels are generally seen to decrease in pregnancy [186]. The observed decrease in fibrinolytic activity in pregnancy is likely due to the marked increase in the plasminogen activator inhibitors, PAI-I and PAI-2 [187]. The net result of these changes is an increased predisposition to thrombosis during pregnancy and the puerperium. Genetic risk factors for coagulopathy may also be present. Such factors include, among others, hyperhomocysteinemia, deletions or mutations of genes encoding for factor V Leiden or prothrombin 20210A, and altered circulating levels of protein C, protein S or antithrombin III.

The hypercoagulable state of pregnancy helps to minimize blood loss at delivery. However, these same physiologic changes also put the mother at increased risk of thromboembolic events, both in pregnancy and in the puerperium. In one large epidemiologic study, the incidence of pregnancy-related thromboembolic complications was 1.3 per 1000 deliveries [188].

Endocrine system

The pituitary gland

The pituitary gland enlarges by as much as 135% during normal pregnancy [189]. This enlargement is generally not sufficient to cause visual disturbance from compression of the optic chiasma, and pregnancy is not associated with an increased incidence of pituitary adenoma.

Pituitary hormone function can vary considerably during normal pregnancy. Plasma growth hormone levels begin to increase at around 10 weeks' gestation, plateau at around 28 weeks, and can remain elevated until several months postpartum [190]. Prolactin levels increase progressively throughout pregnancy, reaching a peak at term. The role of prolactin in pregnancy is not clear, but it appears to be important in preparing breast tissue for lactation by stimulating glandular epithelial cell mitosis and increasing production of lactose, lipids, and certain proteins [191].

The thyroid gland

A relative deficiency of iodide is common during pregnancy, due often to a relative dietary deficiency and increased urinary excretion of iodide. There are also increased demands on the thyroid gland to increase its uptake of available iodide from the circulation during pregnancy, leading to glandular hypertrophy. The thyroid gland also enlarges as a result of increased vascularity and cellular hyperplasia [33]. However, evidence of frank goiter is not a feature of normal pregnancy, and its presence always warrants appropriate investigation.

Thyroid-binding globulin increases significantly during pregnancy under the influence of estrogen, and this leads to an increase in the total and bound fraction of thyroxine (T_4) and tri-iodothyronine (T_3). This increase begins as early as 6 weeks' gestation and reaches a plateau at around 18 weeks [33]. However, the free fractions of T_4 and T_3 remain relatively stable throughout pregnancy and are similar to non-pregnant values. Thyroid-stimulating hormone (TSH) levels fall slightly in early pregnancy as a result of the high circulating hCG levels, which have a mild thyrotropic effect [192]. TSH levels generally return to normal later in pregnancy. These physiologic changes in thyroid hormone levels have important clinical implications when selecting appropriate laboratory tests for evaluating thyroid status during pregnancy. As a general rule, total T_4 and T_3 levels are unhelpful in pregnancy. The most appropriate test for detecting thyroid dysfunction is the high-sensitivity TSH assay. If this is abnormal, free T_4 and free T_3 levels should be measured.

The adrenal glands

Although the adrenal glands do not change in size during pregnancy, there are significant changes in adrenal hormone levels. Serum cortisol levels increase significantly in pregnancy, although the vast majority of this cortisol is bound to cortisol-binding globulin, which increases in the circulation in response to estrogen stimulation. However, free cortisol levels also increase in pregnancy by around 30% [193].

Serum aldosterone levels increase throughout pregnancy, reaching a peak during the third trimester [194]. This increase likely reflects an increase in renin substrate production, which results in increased levels of angiotensin II that, in turn, stimulates the adrenal glands to secrete aldosterone. Aldosterone functions to retain sodium at the level of the renal tubules, and likely balances the natriuretic effects of progesterone.

Circulating levels of adrenal androgens are also increased in pregnancy. This is due in part to increased levels of sex hormone-binding globulin, which retards their clearance from the maternal circulation. The conversion of adrenal androgens (primarily androstenedione and testosterone) to estriol by the placenta effectively protects the fetus from androgenic side effects.

The endocrine pancreas

β-cells in the islets of Langerhans within the pancreas are responsible for insulin production. β-cells undergo hyperplasia during pregnancy, resulting in increased insulin secretion. This insulin hypersecretion is likely responsible for the fasting hypoglycemia seen in early pregnancy. Peripheral resistance to circulating insulin increases as pregnancy progresses, due primarily to the increased production of insulin antagonists such as human placental lactogen. Such placental insulin antagonists result in the normal postprandial hyperglycemia seen in pregnancy [195].

Immune system

One of the more interesting issues is not why some pregnancies fail, but how is it that any pregnancies succeed? Immunologists would argue that the fetus acquires its genetic information equally from both parents and, as such, represents a foreign tissue graft (hemiallograft). It should therefore be identified as "foreign" by the maternal immune system and destroyed. This is the basis of transplant rejection. Successful pregnancy, on the other hand, is dependent on maternal tolerance (immunononreactivity) to paternal antigen. How is it that the hemiallogeneic fetus is able to evade the maternal immune system? In 1953, Medawar proposed that mammalian viviparous reproduction represents a unique example of successful transplantation (known colloquially as *nature's transplant*) [196]. Several hypotheses have been put forward to explain this apparent discordance.

1 The conceptus is not immunogenic and, as such, does not evoke an immunologic response.

2 Pregnancy alters the systemic maternal immune response to prevent immune rejection.

3 The uterus is an immunologically privileged site.

4 The placenta is an effective immunologic barrier between mother and fetus.

The answer to this intriguing question likely incorporates a little of each of these hypotheses [197].

Pregnancy is not a state of non-specific systemic immunosuppression. In experimental animals, for example, mismatched tissue allografts (including paternal skin grafts and ectopic fetal tissue grafts) are not more likely to be accepted in pregnant as compared with non-pregnant animals. However, there is evidence to suggest that the intrauterine environment is a site of partial immunologic privilege. For example, foreign tissue allograft placed within the uterus will ultimately be rejected, even in hormonally-primed animals, but this rejection is often slower and more protracted than tissue grafts at other sites [198].

Trophoblast (placental) cells are presumed to be essential to this phenomenon of immune tolerance, because they lie at the maternal–fetal interface where they are in direct contact with cells of the maternal immune system. It has been established that chorionic villous trophoblasts do not express classic major histocompatibility complex (MHC) class II molecules [199]. Surprisingly, cytotrophoblasts upregulate a MHC class Ib molecule, HLA-G, as they invade the uterus [200]. This observation, and the fact that HLA-G exhibits limited polymorphism [201], suggests functional importance. The exact mechanisms involved are not known but may include upregulation of the inhibitory immunoglobulin-like transcript 4, an HLA-G receptor that is expressed on macrophages and a subset of natural killer (NK) lymphocytes [202]. Cytotrophoblasts that express HLA-G come in direct contact with maternal lymphocytes that are abundant in the uterus during early pregnancy. Although estimates vary, a minimum of 10–15% of all cells found in the decidua are leukocytes [203,204]. Like invasive cytotrophoblasts, these maternal lymphocytes have unusual properties. Most are CD56+ NK cells. However, compared with peripheral blood lymphocytes, decidual leukocytes have low cytotoxic activity [205]. Trophoblast cells likely help to recruit these unusual maternal immune cells through the release of specific chemokines [206].

Cytotoxicity against trophoblast cells must be selectively inhibited to prevent immune rejection and pregnancy loss. The factors responsible for this localized immunosuppression are unclear but likely include cytotrophoblast-derived interleukin-10, a cytokine that inhibits alloresponses in mixed lymphocyte reactions [207]. Steroid hormones, including progesterone, have similar effects [208]. The complement system may also be involved, since deletion of the complement regulator, Crry, in mice leads to fetal loss secondary to placental inflammation [209]. Finally, pharmacologic data, also from studies in mice, suggest that trophoblasts express an enzyme, indoleamine 2,3-dioxygenase, that rapidly degrades tryptophan, which is essential for T-cell activation [210]. Whether this mechanism occurs in humans is not known, although human syncytiotrophoblasts express indoleamine 2,3-dioxygenase [211] and maternal serum tryptophan concentrations fall during pregnancy [212].

Although pregnancy does not represent a state of generalized maternal immunosuppression, there is evidence of altered immune function [198]. The major change in the maternal immune system during pregnancy is a move away from cell-mediated immune responses toward humoral or antibody-mediated immunity. Absolute numbers and activity of T-helper 1 cells and NK cells decline, whereas those of T-helper 2 cells increase. Clinically, the decrease in cellular immunity during pregnancy leads to an increased susceptibility to intracellular pathogens (including cytomegalovirus, varicella, and malaria). The decrease in cellular immunity may also explain why cell-mediated immunopathologic diseases (such as rheumatoid arthritis) frequently improve during pregnancy [198]. Although pregnancy is characterized by enhanced antibody-mediated immunity, the levels of immunoglobulins A (IgA), IgG, and IgM all decrease in pregnancy. This decrease in titers is due primarily to the hemodilutional effect of pregnancy and has few, if any, clinical implications [213]. The peripheral white blood cell (leukocyte) count rises progressively during pregnancy [178] (see Table 4.9), primarily because of increased numbers of circulating segmented neutrophils and granulocytes. The reason for this leukocytosis is not clear, but it is likely secondary to elevated estrogen and cortisol levels. It probably represents the reappearance in the circulation of leukocytes previously shunted out of the circulation.

Although maternal IgM and IgA are effectively excluded from the fetus, maternal IgG does cross the placenta [214,215]. Fc receptors are present on trophoblast cells and the transport of IgG across the placenta is accomplished by way of these receptors through a process known as endocytosis. IgG transport from mother to fetus begins at around 16 weeks' gestation and increases as gestation proceeds. However, the vast majority of IgG acquired by the fetus from the mother occurs during the last 4 weeks of pregnancy [214,216]. The human fetus begins to produce IgG shortly after birth, but adult values are not attained until approximately 3 years of age [215].

Conclusion

Physiologic adaptations occur in all maternal organ systems during pregnancy; however, the quality, degree, and timing of the adaptation vary from one organ system to another and from one individual to another. Moreover, maternal adaptations to pregnancy occur before they appear to be necessary. Such physiologic modifications may be prerequisites for implantation and normal placental and fetal growth. It is important that obstetric care providers have a clear understanding of such physiologic adaptations, and how pre-existing variables (such as maternal age, multiple gestation, ethnicity, and genetic factors) and pregnancy-associated factors (including gestational age, labor, and intrapartum blood loss) interact to affect the ability of the mother to adapt to the demands of pregnancy. A better understanding of the normal physiologic adaptations of pregnancy will improve the ability of clinicians to anticipate the effects of pregnancy on underlying medical conditions and to better manage pregnancy-associated complications, such as pre-eclampsia, pulmonary edema, and pulmonary embolism.

References

1 McLennon CE, Thouin LG. Blood volume in pregnancy. *Am J Obstet Gynecol* 1948; 55: 1189.

2 Caton WL, Roby CC, Reid DE, et al. The circulating red cell volume and body hematocrit in normal pregnancy and the puerperium. *Am J Obstet Gynecol* 1951; 61: 1207.

3 Hytten FE, Paintin DB. Increase in plasma volume during normal pregnancy. *J Obstet Gynaecol Br Commonw* 1963; 70: 402.

4 Lund CJ, Donovan JC. Blood volume during pregnancy. Significance of plasma and red cell volumes. *Am J Obstet Gynecol* 1967; 98: 394–404.

5 Scott DE. Anemia during pregnancy. *Obstet Gynecol Annu* 1972; 1: 219–244.

6 Clapp JF, Seaward BL, Sleamaker RH, et al. Maternal physiologic adaptations to early human pregnancy. *Am J Obstet Gynecol* 1988; 159: 1456–1460.

7 Pritchard JA. Changes in the blood volume during pregnancy and delivery. *Anesthesiology* 1965; 26: 394.

8 Rovinsky JJ, Jaffin H. Cardiovascular hemodynamics in pregnancy. I. Blood and plasma volumes in multiple pregnancy. *Am J Obstet Gynecol* 1965; 93: 1.

9 Jepson JH. Endocrine control of maternal and fetal erythropoiesis. *Can Med Assoc J* 1968; 98: 844–847.

10 Letsky EA. Erythropoiesis in pregnancy. *J Perinat Med* 1995; 23: 39–45.

11 Cavill I. Iron and erythropoiesis in normal subjects and in pregnancy. *J Perinat Med* 1995; 23: 47–50.
12 Koller O. The clinical significance of hemodilution during pregnancy. *Obstet Gynecol Surv* 1982; 37: 649–652.
13 Pritchard JA, Cunningham FG, Pritchard SA. The Parkland Memorial Hospital protocol for treatment of eclampsia: evaluation of 245 cases. *Am J Obstet Gynecol* 1984; 148: 951.
14 Maynard SE, Min JY, Merchan J, et al. Excess placental soluble fms-like tyrosine kinase 1 (sFlt1) may contribute to endothelial dysfunction, hypertension, and proteinuria in preeclampsia. *J Clin Invest* 2003; 111: 649–658.
15 Levine RJ, Maynard SE, Qian C, et al. Circulating angiogenic factors and the risk of preeclampsia. *N Engl J Med* 2004; 350: 672–684.
16 Buhimschi CS, Magloire L, Funai E, et al. Fractional excretion of angiogenic factors in women with severe preeclampsia. *Obstet Gynecol* 2006; 107: 1103–1114.
17 Salas SP, Rosso P, Espinoza R, et al. Maternal plasma volume expansion and hormonal changes in women with idiopathic fetal growth retardation. *Obstet Gynecol* 1993; 81: 1029–1034.
18 Aardenburg R, Spaanderman ME, van Eijndhoven HW, de Leeuw PW, Peeters LL. A low plasma volume in formerly preeclamptic women predisposes to the recurrence of hypertensive complications in the next pregnancy. *J Soc Gynecol Investig* 2006; 13: 598–604.
19 Schrier RW, Briner VA. Peripheral arterial vasodilation hypothesis of sodium and water retention in pregnancy: implications for pathogenesis of preeclampsia-eclampsia. *Obstet Gynecol* 1991; 77: 632–639.
20 Oparil S, Ehrlich EN, Lindheimer MD. Effect of progesterone on renal sodium handling in man: relation to aldosterone excretion and plasma renin activity. *Clin Sci Mol Med* 1975; 49: 139–147.
21 Winkel CA, Milewich L, Parker CR Jr, et al. Conversion of plasma progesterone to desoxycorticosterone in men, nonpregnant, and pregnant women, and adrenalectomized subjects. *J Clin Invest* 1980; 66: 803–812.
22 Phippard AF, Horvath JS, Glynn EM. Circulatory adaptation to pregnancy – serial studies of hemodynamics, blood volume, renin and aldosterone in the baboon (*Papio hamadryas*). *J Hypertens* 1986; 4: 773–779.
23 Seitchik J. Total body water and total body density of pregnant women. *Obstet Gynecol* 1967; 29: 155–166.
24 Lindheimer MD, Katz AI. Sodium and diuretics in pregnancy. *N Engl J Med* 1973; 288: 891–894.
25 Longo LD, Hardesty JS. Maternal blood volume: measurement, hypothesis of control, and clinical considerations. *Rev Perinatal Med* 1984; 5: 35.
26 Pritchard JA. Blood volume changes in pregnancy and the puerperium. IV. Anemia associated with hydatidiform mole. *Am J Obstet Gynecol* 1965; 91: 621.
27 Villar MA, Sibai BM. Clinical significance of elevated mean arterial pressure in second trimester and threshold increase in systolic and diastolic blood pressure during third trimester. *Am J Obstet Gynecol* 1989; 160: 419–424.
28 American College of Obstetricians and Gynecologists. *Hypertension in pregnancy. Technical Bulletin No. 219.* Washington, DC: American College of Obstetricians and Gynecologists, 1996.
29 Wilson M, Morganti AA, Zervodakis I, et al. Blood pressure, the renin-aldosterone system, and sex steroids throughout normal pregnancy. *Am J Med* 1980; 68: 97–107.
30 Ginsberg J, Duncan SL. Direct and indirect blood pressure measurement in pregnancy. *J Obstet Gynaecol Br Commonw* 1969; 76: 705.
31 Kirshon B, Lee W, Cotton DB, Giebel R. Indirect blood pressure monitoring in the postpartum patient. *Obstet Gynecol* 1987; 70: 799–801.
32 Duvekot JJ, Cheriex EC, Pieters FA, et al. Early pregnancy changes in hemodynamics and volume homeostasis are consecutive adjustments triggered by a primary fall in systemic vascular tone. *Am J Obstet Gynecol* 1993; 169: 1382–1392.
33 Glinoer D, de Nayer P, Bourdoux P, et al. Regulation of maternal thyroid during pregnancy. *J Clin Endocrinol Metab* 1990; 71: 276–287.
34 Harada A, Hershman JM, Reed AW, et al. Comparison of thyroid stimulators and thyroid hormone concentrations in the sera of pregnant women. *J Clin Endocrinol Metab* 1979; 48: 793–797.
35 Van Oppen AC, van der Tweel I, Duvekot JJ, Bruinse HW. Use of cardiac output in pregnancy: is it justified? *Am J Obstet Gynecol* 1995; 173: 923–928.
36 Du Bois D, du Bois EF. A formula to estimate the approximate area if height and weight be known. *Arch Intern Med* 1916; 17: 864.
37 Linhard J. Uber das minutevolumens des herzens bei ruhe und bei muskelarbeit. *Pflugers Arch* 1915; 1612: 234.
38 Hamilton HGH. The cardiac output in normal pregnancy as determined by the Cournard right heart catheterization technique. *J Obstet Gynaecol Br Emp* 1949; 56: 548.
39 Palmer AJ, Walker AHC. The maternal circulation in normal pregnancy. *J Obstet Gynaecol Br Emp* 1949; 56: 537.
40 Bader RA, Bader MG, Rose DJ, et al. Hemodynamics at rest and during exercise in normal pregnancy as studied by cardiac catheterization. *J Clin Invest* 1955; 34: 1524.
41 Clark SL, Cotton DB, Lee W, et al. Central hemodynamic assessment of normal term pregnancy. *Am J Obstet Gynecol* 1989; 161: 1439–1442.
42 Walters WAW, MacGregor WG, Hills M. Cardiac output at rest during pregnancy and the puerperium. *Clin Sci* 1966; 30: 1–11.
43 Lees MM, Taylor SH, Scott DB, et al. A study of cardiac output at rest throughout pregnancy. *J Obstet Gynaecol Br Commonw* 1967; 74: 319–328.
44 Ueland K, Hansen JM. Maternal cardiovascular dynamics. II. Posture and uterine contractions. *Am J Obstet Gynecol* 1969; 103: 1–7.
45 Ueland K, Hansen JM. Maternal cardiovascular hemodynamics. III. Labor and delivery under local and caudal anesthesia. *Am J Obstet Gynecol* 1969; 103: 8–18.
46 Ueland K, Novy MJ, Peterson EN, et al. Maternal cardiovascular dynamics. IV. The influence of gestational age on the maternal cardiovascular response to posture and exercise. *Am J Obstet Gynecol* 1969; 104: 856–864.
47 Atkins AF, Watt JM, Milan P. A longitudinal study of cardiovascular dynamic changes throughout pregnancy. *Eur J Obstet Gynecol Reprod Biol* 1981; 12(4): 215–224.
48 Atkins AFJ, Watt JM, Milan P, et al. The influence of posture upon cardiovascular dynamics throughout pregnancy. *Eur J Obstet Gynecol Reprod Biol* 1981; 12(6): 357–372.
49 Katz R, Karliner JS, Resnik R. Effects of a natural volume overload state (pregnancy) on left ventricular performance in normal human subjects. *Circulation* 1978; 58: 434–441.

50 Laird-Meeter K, van de Ley G, Bom TH, et al. Cardiocirculatory adjustments during pregnancy – an echocardiographic study. *Clin Cardiol* 1979; 2: 328–332.
51 Mashini IS, Albazzaz SJ, Fadel HE, et al. Serial noninvasive evaluation of cardiovascular hemodynamics during pregnancy. *Am J Obstet Gynecol* 1987; 156: 1208–1214.
52 Easterling TR, Benedetti TJ, Schmucker BC, Millard SP. Maternal hemodynamics in normal and preeclamptic pregnancies: a longitudinal study. *Obstet Gynecol* 1990; 76: 1061–1069.
53 Van Oppen ACC, van der Tweel I, Alsbach GPJ, et al. A longitudinal study of maternal hemodynamics during normal pregnancy. *Obstet Gynecol* 1996; 88: 40–46.
54 Mabie WC, DiSessa TG, Crocker LG, et al. A longitudinal study of cardiac output in normal human pregnancy. *Am J Obstet Gynecol* 1994; 170: 849–856.
55 Pombo JF, Troy BL, Russell RO. Left ventricular volumes and ejection fraction by echocardiography. *Circulation* 1971; 43: 480–490.
56 Murray JA, Johnston W, Reid JM. Echocardiographic determination of left ventricular dimensions, volumes, and performance. *Am J Cardiol* 1972; 30: 252–257.
57 Easterling TR, Watts DH, Schmucker BC, Benedetti TJ. Measurement of cardiac output during pregnancy: validation of Doppler technique and clinical observations in preeclampsia. *Obstet Gynecol* 1987; 69: 845–850.
58 Robson SC, Dunlop W, Boys RJ, Hunter S. Cardiac output during labor. *BMJ* 1987; 295: 1169–1172.
59 Robson SC, Dunlop W, Moore M, Hunter S. Combined Doppler and echocardiographic measurement of cardiac output: theory and application in pregnancy. *Br J Obstet Gynaecol* 1987; 94: 1014–1027.
60 Robson SC, Hunter S, Moore M, Dunlop W. Haemodynamic changes during the puerperium: a Doppler and M-mode echocardiographic study. *Br J Obstet Gynaecol* 1987; 94: 1028–1039.
61 Lee W, Rokey R, Cotton DB. Noninvasive maternal stroke volume and cardiac output determinations by pulsed Doppler echocardiography. *Am J Obstet Gynecol* 1988; 158: 505–510.
62 Capeless EL, Clapp JF. When do cardiovascular parameters return to their preconception values? *Am J Obstet Gynecol* 1991; 165: 883–886.
63 Robson SC, Hunter S, Boys RJ, Dunlop W. Serial study of factors influencing changes in cardiac output during human pregnancy. *Am J Physiol* 1989; 256: H1060–1065.
64 Burwell CS, Strayhorn WD, Flickinger D, et al. Circulation during pregnancy. *Arch Intern Med* 1938; 62: 979.
65 McCalden RA. The inhibitory action of oestradiol-17b and progesterone on venous smooth muscle. *Br J Pharmacol* 1975; 53: 183–192.
66 Wook JE, Goodrich SM. Dilation of the veins with pregnancy or with oral contraceptive therapy. *Trans Am Clin Climatol Assoc* 1964; 76: 174.
67 Slater AJ, Gude N, Clarke IJ, Walters WA. Haemodynamic changes and left ventricular performance during high-dose oestrogen administration to male transsexuals. *Br J Obstet Gynaecol* 1986; 93: 532–538.
68 Morton M, Tsang H, Hohimer R, et al. Left ventricular size, output, and structure during guinea pig pregnancy. *Am J Physiol* 1984; 246: R40–48.
69 Kametas NA, McAuliffe F, Krampl E, Chambers J, Nicolaides KH. Maternal cardiac function in twin pregnancy. *Obstet Gynecol* 2003; 102: 806–815.
70 Schrier RW. Pathogenesis of sodium and water retention in high-output and low-output cardiac failure, nephrotic syndrome, cirrhosis, and pregnancy. *N Engl J Med* 1988; 319: 1127–1134.
71 Schrier RW. Body fluid volume regulation in health and disease: a unifying hypothesis. *Ann Intern Med* 1990; 113: 155–159.
72 Seligman SP, Kadner SS, Finlay TH. Relationship between preeclampsia, hypoxia, and production of nitric oxide by the placenta. *Am J Obstet Gynecol* 1996; 174: abstract.
73 Brenner BM, Ballermann BJ, Gunning ME, Zeidel ML. Diverse biological actions of atrial natriuretic peptide. *Physiol Rev* 1990; 70: 665–669.
74 Cusson JR, Gutkowska, J, Rey E, et al. Plasma concentration of atrial natriuretic factor in normal pregnancy. *N Engl J Med* 1985; 313: 1230–1231.
75 Thomsen JK, Storm TL, Thamsborg G, et al. Increased concentration of circulating atrial natriuretic peptide during normal pregnancy. *Eur J Obstet Gynecol Reprod Biol* 1988; 27: 197–201.
76 Thomsen JK, Fogh-Anderson N, Jaszczak P, Giese J. Atrial natriuretic peptide (ANP) decrease during normal pregnancy as related to hemodynamic changes and volume regulation. *Acta Obstet Gynecol Scand* 1993; 72: 103–110.
77 Chesley LC. Renal functional changes in normal pregnancy. *Clin Obstet Gynecol* 1960; 3: 349.
78 Gabert HA, Miller JM. Renal disease during pregnancy. *Obstet Gynecol Surv* 1985; 40: 449–461.
79 Katz M, Sokal MM. Skin perfusion in pregnancy. *Am J Obstet Gynecol* 1980; 137: 30–34.
80 Burt CC. Peripheral skin temperature in normal pregnancy. *Lancet* 1949; 2: 787.
81 Herbert CM, Banner EA, Wakim KG. Variations in the peripheral circulation during pregnancy. *Am J Obstet Gynecol* 1958; 76: 742.
82 Kitabatake A, Inoue M, Asao M, et al. Noninvasive evaluation of pulmonary hypertension by a pulsed Doppler technique. *Circulation* 1983; 68: 302–309.
83 Robson SC, Hunter S, Boys J, Dunlop W. Serial changes in pulmonary haemodynamics during human pregnancy: a non-invasive study using Doppler echocardiography. *Clin Sci* 1991; 80: 113–117.
84 Werko L. Pregnancy and heart disease. *Acta Obstet Gynecol Scand* 1954; 33: 162.
85 Metcalfe J, Romney SL, Ramsy LH, et al. Estimation of uterine blood flow in normal human pregnancy at term. *J Clin Invest* 1955; 34: 1632.
86 Assali NS, Rauramo L, Peltonen T. Measurement of uterine blood flow and uterine metabolism. VIII. Uterine and fetal blood flow and oxygen consumption in early human pregnancy. *Am J Obstet Gynecol* 1960; 79: 86–98.
87 Ueland K, Parer JT. Effects of estrogens on the cardiovascular system of the ewe. *Am J Obstet Gynecol* 1966; 96: 400–406.
88 Caton D, Abrams RM, Clapp JF, et al. The effect of exogenous progesterone on the rate of blood flow of the uterus of ovariectomized sheep. *Q J Exp Physiol Cogn Med Sci* 1974; 59: 225–231.
89 Bieniarz J, Maqueda E, Caldeyro-Barcia R. Compression of aorta by the uterus in late human pregnancy. I. Variations between femoral and brachial artery pressure with changes from hypertension to hypotension. *Am J Obstet Gynecol* 1966; 95: 795–808.
90 Bieniarz J, Crottogini JJ, Curuchet E, et al. Aortocaval compression by the uterus in late human pregnancy. II. An arteriographic study. *Am J Obstet Gynecol* 1968; 100: 204.

91 Kerr MG. Cardiovascular dynamics in pregnancy and labour. *Br Med Bull* 1968; 24: 19.
92 Howard BK, Goodson JH, Mengert WF. Supine hypotensive syndrome in late pregnancy. *Obstet Gynecol* 1953; 1: 371.
93 Holmes F. Incidence of the supine hypotensive syndrome in late pregnancy. *J Obstet Gynaecol Br Emp* 1960; 67: 254.
94 Calvin S, Jones OW, Knieriem K, Weinstein L. Oxygen saturation in the supine hypotensive syndrome. *Obstet Gynecol* 1988; 71: 872–877.
95 Kinsella SM, Lohmann G. Supine hypotensive syndrome. *Obstet Gynecol* 1994; 83 (5 Pt 1): 774–788.
96 Lindheimer MD, Katz AI. Renal function in pregnancy. *Obstet Gynecol Annu* 1972; 1: 139–176.
97 Vorys N, Ullery JC, Hanusek GE. The cardiac output changes in various positions in pregnancy. *Am J Obstet Gynecol* 1961; 82: 1312.
98 Easterling TR, Schmucker BC, Benedetti TJ. The hemodynamic effects of orthostatic stress during pregnancy. *Obstet Gynecol* 1988; 72: 550–552.
99 Barron WM, Mujais SK, Zinaman M, et al. Plasma catecholamine responses to physiologic stimuli in normal human pregnancy. *Am J Obstet Gynecol* 1986; 154: 80–84.
100 Nisell H, Lunell N, Linde B. Maternal hemodynamics and impaired fetal growth in pregnancy-induced hypertension. *Obstet Gynecol* 1988; 71: 163–166.
101 Clark SL, Cotton DB, Pivarnik JM, et al. Position change and central hemodynamic profile during normal third-trimester pregnancy and postpartum. *Am J Obstet Gynecol* 1991; 164: 883–887.
102 Hankins GDV, Harvey CJ, Clark SL, et al. The effects of maternal position and cardiac output on intrapulmonary shunt in normal third-trimester pregnancy. *Obstet Gynecol* 1996; 88: 327–330.
103 Naeye RL, Peters EC. Working during pregnancy: effects on the fetus. *Pediatrics* 1982; 69: 724–727.
104 Henriksen TB, Hedegaard M, Secher NJ, Wilcox AJ. Standing at work and preterm delivery. *Br J Obstet Gynaecol* 1995; 102: 198–206.
105 Friedman EA, Neff RK. Hypertension-hypotension in pregnancy. Correlation with fetal outcome. *JAMA* 1978; 239: 2249–2251.
106 Grunberger W, Leodolter S, Parschalk O. Maternal hypotension: fetal outcome in treated and untreated cases. *Gynecol Obstet Invest* 1979; 10: 32–38.
107 Ng PH, Walters WA. The effects of chronic maternal hypotension during pregnancy. *Aust NZ J Obstet Gynaecol* 1992; 32: 14–16.
108 Steer PJ, Little MP, Kold-Jensen T, Chapple J, Elliott P. Maternal blood pressure in pregnancy, birth weight, and perinatal mortality in first births: prospective study. *BMJ* 2004; 329: 1312–1317.
109 Easterling TR, Brateng D, Schmucker B, Brown Z, Millard SP. Prevention of preeclampsia: a randomized trial of atenolol in hyperdynamic patients before onset of hypertension. *Obstet Gynecol* 1999; 93: 725–734.
110 Von Dadelszen P, Ornstein MP, Bull SB, Logan AG, Koren G, Magee LA. Fall in mean arterial pressure and fetal growth restriction in pregnancy hypertension: a meta-analysis. *Lancet* 2000; 355: 87–92.
111 Adams JQ, Alexander AM. Alterations in cardiovascular physiology during labor. *Obstet Gynecol* 1958; 12: 542.
112 Hendricks ECH, Quilligan EJ. Cardiac output during labor. *Am J Obstet Gynecol* 1958; 76: 969.
113 Winner W, Romney SL. Cardiovascular responses to labor and delivery. *Am J Obstet Gynecol* 1966; 96: 1004.
114 Ueland K. Maternal cardiovascular dynamics. VII. Intrapartum blood volume changes. *Am J Obstet Gynecol* 1976; 126: 671–677.
115 Kjeldsen J. Hemodynamic investigations during labor and delivery. *Acta Obstet Gynecol Scand* 1979; 89(Suppl): 1–252.
116 Lee W, Rokey R, Cotton DB, Miller JF. Maternal hemodynamic effects of uterine contractions by M-mode and pulsed-Doppler echocardiography. *Am J Obstet Gynecol* 1989; 161: 974–977.
117 Robson SC, Hunter R, Boys W, et al. Changes in cardiac output during epidural anaesthesia for caesarean section. *Anaesthesia* 1989; 44: 475–479.
118 Pritchard JA, Baldwin RM, Dickey JC, Wiggins KM. Blood volume changes in pregnancy and the puerperium. II. Red blood cell loss and changes in apparent blood volume during and following vaginal delivery, cesarean section, and cesarean section plus total hysterectomy. *Am J Obstet Gynecol* 1962; 84: 1271.
119 Wilcox CF, Hunt AR, Owen FA. The measurement of blood lost during cesarean section. *Am J Obstet Gynecol* 1959; 77: 772.
120 Newton M, Mosey LM, Egli GE, et al. Blood loss during and immediately after delivery. *Obstet Gynecol* 1961; 17: 9.
121 Cunningham FG, MacDonald PC, Gant NF, Leveno KJ, Gilstrap LC III. The puerperium. In: Cunningham FG, MacDonald PC, Gant NF, Leveno KJ, Gilstrap LC III, eds. *Williams' Obstetrics*, 19th edn. Norwalk, CT: Appleton and Lange, 1993: 467.
122 Chesley LC, Valenti C, Uichano L. Alterations in body fluid compartments and exchangeable sodium in early puerperium. *Am J Obstet Gynecol* 1959; 77: 1054.
123 Hankins GD, Wendel GD, Cunningham FG, et al. Longitudinal evaluation of hemodynamic changes in eclampsia. *Am J Obstet Gynecol* 1984; 150: 506–512.
124 Lee W, Cotton DB. Peripartum cardiomyopathy: current concepts and clinical management. *Clin Obstet Gynecol* 1989; 32: 54–67.
125 Sobol SE, Frenkiel S, Nachtigal D, Wiener D, Teblum C. Clinical manifestations of sinonasal pathology during pregnancy. *J Otolaryngol* 2001; 30: 24–28.
126 Braithwaite JM, Economides DL. Severe recurrent epistaxis causing antepartum fetal distress. *Int J Gynaecol Obstet* 1995; 50: 197–198.
127 Howard DJ. Life-threatening epistaxis in pregnancy. *J Laryngol Otol* 1985; 99: 95–96.
128 MacKenzie JN. The physiological and pathological relations between the nose and the sexual apparatus of man. *Alienist Neurol* 1898; 19: 219.
129 Mabry RL. Rhinitis of pregnancy. *South Med J* 1986; 79: 965.
130 Schatz M, Zieger RS. Diagnosis and management of rhinitis during pregnancy. *Allergy Proc* 1988; 9: 545–554.
131 Mortimer H, Wright RP, Collip JB. The effect of the administration of oestrogenic hormones on the nasal mucosa of the monkey (*Macata mulatta*). *Can Med Assoc J* 1936; 35: 504.
132 Taylor M. An experimental study of the influence of the endocrine system on the nasal respiratory mucosa. *J Laryngol Otol* 1961; 75: 972.
133 Toppozada H, Michaels L, Toppozada M, et al. The human respiratory mucosa in pregnancy. *J Laryngol Otol* 1982; 96: 613–626.
134 Reynolds SRM, Foster FI. Acetylcholine-equivalent content of the nasal mucosa in rabbits and cats, before and after administration of estrogen. *Am J Physiol* 1940; 131: 422.
135 Contreras G, Guitierrez M, Beroiza T, et al. Ventilatory drive and respiratory muscle function in pregnancy. *Am Rev Respir Dis* 1991; 144: 837–841.

136 Weinberger SE, Weiss ST, Cohen WR, Weiss JW, Johnson TS. Pregnancy and the lung: state of the art. *Am Rev Respir Dis* 1980; 121: 559–581.

137 Elkus R, Popovich J. Respiratory physiology in pregnancy. *Clin Chest Med* 1992; 13: 555–565.

138 Gilroy RJ, Mangura BT, Lavietes MH. Rib cage and abdominal volume displacements during breathing in pregnancy. *Am Rev Respir Dis* 1988; 137: 668–672.

139 Macklem PT, Gross D, Grassino GA, Roussos C. Partitioning of inspiratory pressure swings between diaphragm and intercostals/accessory muscles. *J Appl Physiol* 1978; 44: 200–208.

140 Nava S, Zanotti E, Ambrosino N, Fracchia C, Scarabelli C, Rampulla C. Evidence of acute diaphragmatic fatigue in a "natural" condition. The diaphragm during labor. *Am Rev Respir Dis* 1992; 146: 1226–1230.

141 Milne JA, Howie AD, Pack AI. Dyspnoea during normal pregnancy. *Br J Obstet Gynaecol* 1978; 85: 260–264.

142 Thomson JK, Cohen ME. Studies on the circulation in pregnancy. II. Vital capacity observations in normal pregnant women. *Surg Gynecol Obstet* 1938; 66: 591.

143 Cugell DW, Frank NR, Gaensler EA, Badger TL. Pulmonary function in pregnancy. I. Serial observations in normal women. *Am Rev Tuberc* 1953; 67: 598.

144 Rubin A, Russo N, Goucher D. The effect of pregnancy upon pulmonary function in normal women. *Am J Obstet Gynecol* 1956; 72: 964.

145 Gee JB, Packer BS, Millen JE, Robin ED. Pulmonary mechanics during pregnancy. *J Clin Invest* 1967; 46: 945–952.

146 Baldwin GR, Moorthi DS, Whelton JA, MacDonnell KF. New lung functions in pregnancy. *Am J Obstet Gynecol* 1977; 127: 235–239.

147 Crapo RO. Normal cardiopulmonary physiology during pregnancy. *Clin Obstet Gynecol* 1996; 39: 3–16.

148 Alaily AB, Carrol KB. Pulmonary ventilation in pregnancy. *Br J Obstet Gynaecol* 1978; 85: 518–524.

149 Norregard O, Shultz P, Ostergaard A, Dahl R. Lung function and postural changes during pregnancy. *Respir Med* 1989; 83: 467.

150 Pernoll ML, Metcalfe J, Kovach PA, Wachtel R, Dunham MJ. Ventilation during rest and exercise in pregnancy and postpartum. *Respir Physiol* 1975; 25: 295–310.

151 Milne JA. The respiratory response to pregnancy. *Postgrad Med J* 1979; 55: 318–324.

152 Zwillich CW, Natalino MR, Sutton FD, Weil JV. Effects of progesterone on chemosensitivity in normal men. *J Lab Clin Med* 1978; 92: 262–269.

153 Bayliss DA, Millhorn DE. Central neural mechanisms of progesterone action: application to the respiratory system. *J Appl Physiol* 1992; 73: 393–404.

154 Awe RJ, Nicotra MB, Newsom TD, et al. Arterial oxygenation and alveolar–arterial gradients in term pregnancy. *Obstet Gynecol* 1979; 53: 182–186.

155 Ang CK, Tan TH, Walters WA, et al. Postural influence on maternal capillary oxygen and carbon dioxide tension. *BMJ* 1969; 4: 201–204.

156 Cietak KA, Newton JR. Serial quantitative maternal nephrosonography in pregnancy. *Br J Radiol* 1985; 58: 405–414.

157 Shulman A, Herlinger H. Urinary tract dilatation in pregnancy. *Br J Radiol* 1975; 48: 638–645.

158 Dure-Smith P. Pregnancy dilatation of the urinary tract: the iliac sign and its significance. *Radiology* 1970; 96: 545–550.

159 Hertzberg BS, Carroll BA, Bowie JD, et al. Doppler US assessment of maternal kidneys: analysis of intrarenal resistivity indexes in normal pregnancy and physiologic pelvicaliectasis. *Radiology* 1993; 186: 689–692.

160 Fried A, Woodring JH, Thompson TJ. Hydronephrosis of pregnancy. *J Ultrasound Med* 1983; 2: 255–259.

161 Davison JM, Hytten FE. The effect of pregnancy on the renal handling of glucose. *Br J Obstet Gynaecol* 1975; 82: 374–381.

162 Lindheimer MD, Barron WM. Renal function and volume homeostasis. In: Gleicher N, Buttino L, Elkayam U, et al, eds. *Principles and Practice of Medical Therapy in Pregnancy*, 3rd edn. Stanford, CT: Appleton and Lange, 1998: 1043–1052.

163 Higby K, Suiter CR, Phelps JY, Siler-Khodr T, Langer O. Normal values of urinary albumin and fetal protein excretions during pregnancy. *Am J Obstet Gynecol* 1994; 171: 984–989.

164 Barron WM, Lindheimer MD. Renal sodium and water handling in pregnancy. *Obstet Gynecol Annu* 1984; 13: 35–69.

165 Davison JM, Vallotton MB, Lindheimer MD. Plasma osmolality and urinary concentration and dilution during and after pregnancy. *Br J Obstet Gynaecol* 1981; 88: 472–479.

166 Baer JL, Reis RA, Artens RA. Appendicitis in pregnancy with changes in position and axis of the normal appendix in pregnancy. *JAMA* 1932; 98: 1359.

167 Van Thiel DH, Gavaler JS, Joshi SN, Sara RK, Stremple J. Heartburn of pregnancy. *Gastroenterology* 1977; 72: 666–668.

168 Parry E, Shields R, Turnbull AC. Transit time in the small intestine in pregnancy. *J Obstet Gynaecol Br Commonw* 1970; 77: 900–901.

169 Radberg G, Asztely M, Cantor P, Rehfeld JF, Jarnfeldt-Samsioe A, Svanvik J. Gastric and gall bladder emptying in relation to the secretion of cholecystokinin after a meal in late pregnancy. *Digestion* 1989; 42: 174–180.

170 Vasicka A, Lin TJ, Bright RH. Peptic ulcer and pregnancy: review of hormonal relationships and a report of one case of massive hemorrhage. *Obstet Gynecol Surv* 1957; 12: 1.

171 Waldum HL, Straume BK, Lundgren R. Serum group I pepsinogens during pregnancy. *Scand J Gastroenterol* 1980; 15: 61–64.

172 Braverman DZ, Johnson ML, Kern F. Effects of pregnancy and contraceptive steroids on gallbladder function. *N Engl J Med* 1980; 302: 262–264.

173 Girling JC, Dow E, Smith JH. Liver function tests in preeclampsia: importance of comparison with a reference range derived for normal pregnancy. *Br J Obstet Gynaecol* 1997; 104: 246–250.

174 Pirani BBK, Campbell DM, MacGillivray I. Plasma volume in normal first pregnancy. *J Obstet Gynaecol Br Commonw* 1973; 80: 884–887.

175 Peck TM, Arias F. Hematologic changes associated with pregnancy. *Clin Obstet Gynecol* 1979; 22: 785–798.

176 Jepson JH, Lowenstein L. Role of erythropoietin and placental lactogen in the control of erythropoiesis during pregnancy. *Can J Physiol Pharmacol* 1968; 46: 573–576.

177 Scott DE, Pritchard JA. Iron deficiency in healthy young college women. *JAMA* 1967; 199: 897–900.

178 Pitkin R, Witte D. Platelet and leukocyte counts in pregnancy. *JAMA* 1979; 242: 2696–2698.

179 Sejeny SA, Eastham RD, Baker SR. Platelet counts during normal pregnancy. *J Clin Pathol* 1975; 28: 812–814.

180 O'Brien JR. Platelet counts in normal pregnancy. *J Clin Pathol* 1976; 29: 174.

181 Fenton V, Saunders K, Cavill I. The platelet count in pregnancy. *J Clin Pathol* 1977; 30: 68–69.
182 Wallenburg HC, van Kessel PH. Platelet lifespan in normal pregnancy as determined by a nonradioisotopic technique. *Br J Obstet Gynaecol* 1978; 85: 33–36.
183 Fay RA, Bromham DR, Brooks JA, et al. Platelets and uric acid in the prediction of pre-eclampsia. *Am J Obstet Gynecol* 1985; 152: 1038–1039.
184 Rakoczi I, Tallian F, Bagdany S, Gati I. Platelet lifespan in normal pregnancy and pre-eclampsia as determined by a non-radioisotope technique. *Thromb Res* 1979; 15: 553–556.
185 Burrows RF, Kelton JG. Thrombocytopenia at delivery: a prospective survey of 6,715 deliveries. *Am J Obstet Gynecol* 1990; 162: 731–734.
186 Hellgren M. Hemostasis during pregnancy and puerperium. *Hemostasis* 1996; 26(Suppl 4): 244–247.
187 Davis GL. Hemostatic changes associated with normal and abnormal pregnancies. *Clin Lab Sci* 2000; 13: 223–228.
188 Lindqvist P, Dahlback B, Marsal K. Thrombotic risk during pregnancy: a population study. *Obstet Gynecol* 1999; 94: 595–599.
189 Gonzalez JG, Elizondo G, Saldivar D, Nanez H, Todd LE, Villarreal JZ. Pituitary gland growth during normal pregnancy: an in vivo study using magnetic resonance imaging. *Am J Med* 1988; 85: 217–220.
190 Kletzky OA, Rossman F, Bertolli SI, Platt LD, Mischel DR Jr. Dynamics of human chorionic gonadotropin, prolactin, and growth hormone in serum and amniotic fluid throughout normal human pregnancy. *Am J Obstet Gynecol* 1985; 151: 878–884.
191 Anderson JR. Prolactin in amniotic fluid and maternal serum during uncomplicated human pregnancy. *Dan Med Bull* 1982; 29: 266.
192 Ballabio M, Poshyachinda M, Ekins RP. Pregnancy-induced changes in thyroid function: role of human chorionic gonadotropin as putative regulator of maternal thyroid. *J Clin Endocrinol Metab* 1991; 73: 824–831.
193 Nolten WE, Rueckert PA. Elevated free cortisol index in pregnancy: possible regulatory mechanisms. *Am J Obstet Gynecol* 1981; 139: 492–498.
194 Watanabe M, Meeker CI, Gray MJ, Sims EA, Solomon S. Secretion rate of aldosterone in normal pregnancy. *J Clin Invest* 1963; 42: 1619.
195 Phelps RL, Metzger BE, Freinkel N. Carbohydrate metabolism in pregnancy. XVII. Diurnal profiles of plasma glucose, insulin, free fatty acids, triglycerides, cholesterol, and individual amino acids in late normal pregnancy. *Am J Obstet Gynecol* 1981; 140: 730–736.
196 Medawar PB. Some immunological and endocrinological problems raised by the evolution of viviparity in vertebrates. *Symp Soc Exper Biol* 1953; 7: 320.
197 Norwitz ER, Schust DJ, Fisher SJ. Implantation and the survival of early pregnancy. *N Engl J Med* 2001; 345: 1400–1408.
198 Wilder R. Hormones, pregnancy, and autoimmune diseases. *Ann NY Acad Sci* 1998; 840: 45–50.
199 Redman CW. HLA-DR antigen on human trophoblast: a review. *Am J Reprod Immunol* 1983; 3: 175–177.
200 Kovats S, Main EK, Librach C, Stubblebine M, Fisher SJ, DeMars R. A class I antigen, HLA-G, expressed in human trophoblasts. *Science* 1990; 248: 220–224.
201 Bainbridge DR, Ellis SA, Sargent IL. Little evidence of HLA-G mRNA polymorphism in Caucasian or Afro-Caribbean populations. *J Immunol* 1999; 163: 2023–2027.
202 Allan DS, Colonna M, Lanier LL, et al. Tetrameric complexes of human histocompatibility leukocyte antigen (HLA)-G bind to peripheral blood myelomonocytic cells. *J Exp Med* 1999; 189: 1149–1156.
203 Starkey PM, Sargent IL, Redman CW. Cell populations in human early pregnancy decidua: characterization and isolation of large granular lymphocytes by flow cytometry. *Immunology* 1988; 65: 129–134.
204 King A, Burrows T, Verma S, Hiby S, Loke YW. Human uterine lymphocytes. *Hum Reprod Update* 1998; 4: 480–485.
205 Deniz G, Christmas SE, Brew R, Johnson PM. Phenotypic and functional cellular differences between human CD3-decidual and peripheral blood leukocytes. *J Immunol* 1994; 152: 4255–4261.
206 Drake PM, Gunn MD, Charo IF, et al. Human placental cytotrophoblasts attract monocytes and CD56 (bright) natural killer cells via the actions of monocyte inflammatory protein 1-alpha. *J Exp Med* 2001; 193: 1199–1212.
207 Roth I, Corry DB, Locksley RM, Abrams JS, Litton MJ, Fisher SJ. Human placental cytotrophoblasts produce the immunosuppressive cytokine interleukin 10. *J Exp Med* 1996; 184: 539–548.
208 Pavia C, Siiteri PK, Perlman JD, Stites DP. Suppression of murine allogeneic cell interactions by sex hormones. *J Reprod Immunol* 1979; 1: 33–38.
209 Xu C, Mao D, Holers VM, Palanca B, Cheng AM, Molina H. A critical role for murine complement regulator crry in fetomaternal tolerance. *Science* 2000; 287: 498–501.
210 Munn DH, Zhou M, Attwood JT, et al. Prevention of allogeneic fetal rejection by tryptophan catabolism. *Science* 1998; 281: 1191–1194.
211 Kamimura S, Eguchi K, Yonezawa M, Sekiba K. Localization and developmental change of indoleamine 2,3-dioxygenase activity in the human placenta. *Acta Med Okayama* 1991; 45: 135–139.
212 Schrocksnadel H, Baier-Bitterlich G, Dapunt O, Wachter H, Fuchs D. Decreased plasma tryptophan in pregnancy. *Obstet Gynecol* 1996; 88: 47–50.
213 Baboonian C, Griffiths P. Is pregnancy immunosuppressive? Humoral immunity against viruses. *Br J Obstet Gynaecol* 1983; 90: 1168–1175.
214 Gitlin D, Kumate J, Morales C, Noriega C, Arevalo N. The turnover of amniotic fluid protein in the human conceptus. *Am J Obstet Gynecol* 1972; 113: 632–645.
215 Cunningham FG, MacDonald PC, Gant NF, Leveno KJ, Gilstrap LC III. The morphological and functional development of the fetus. In: Cunningham FG, MacDonald PC, Gant NF, Leveno KJ, Gilstrap LC III, eds. *Williams' Obstetrics*, 19th edn. Norwalk, CT: Appleton and Lange, 1993: 165–207.
216 Gitlin D. Development and metabolism of the immune globulins. In: Kagan BM, Stiehm ER, eds. *Immunologic Incompetence*. Chicago: Year Book, 1971.

5 Maternal–Fetal Blood Gas Physiology

Renee A. Bobrowski
Department of Obstetrics and Gynecology, Saint Alphonsus Regional Medical Center, Boise, ID, USA

Introduction

Abnormalities in acid–base and respiratory homeostasis are common among patients requiring intensive medical support, but many clinicians find the physiology cumbersome. As a result of both their illness and our therapeutic interventions, critically ill patients frequently require assessment of metabolic and respiratory status. An understanding and clinical application of basic physiologic principles is therefore essential to the care of these patients. It is also important that clinicians involved in the care of critically ill gravidas be familiar with the metabolic and respiratory changes of pregnancy as well as their effect on arterial blood gas interpretation.

The arterial blood gas provides information regarding acid–base balance, oxygenation, and ventilation. A blood gas should be considered when a patient has significant respiratory symptoms or experiences oxygen desaturation, or as a baseline in the evaluation of pre-existing cardiopulmonary disease. In this chapter we focus on fundamental physiology, analytic considerations, effective interpretation of an arterial blood gas, and acid–base disturbances.

Essential physiology

Acid–base homeostasis

Normal acid–base balance depends on production, buffering, and excretion of acid. The delicate balance that is crucial for survival is maintained by buffer systems, the lungs and kidneys. Each day, approximately 15 000 mEq of volatile acids (e.g. carbonic acid) are produced by the metabolism of carbohydrates and fats. These acids are transported to and removed via the lungs as carbon dioxide (CO_2) gas. Breakdown of proteins and other substances results in 1–1.5 mEq/kg/day of non-volatile or fixed acids (predominantly phosphoric and sulfuric acids), which are removed by the kidneys.

Buffers are substances that can absorb or donate protons and thereby resist or reduce changes in H^+ ion concentration. Acids produced by cellular metabolism move out of cells and into the extracellular space where buffers absorb the protons. These protons are then transported to the kidney and excreted in urine. The intra- and extracellular buffer systems that maintain homeostasis in the human include the carbonic acid–bicarbonate system, plasma proteins, hemoglobin, and bone.

The carbonic acid–bicarbonate system is the principal extracellular buffer. Its effectiveness is predominantly due to the ability of the lungs to excrete carbon dioxide. In this system, bicarbonate, carbonic acid and carbon dioxide are related by the equation:

$$\underset{\substack{\text{Gaseous}\\\text{phase}\\\downarrow\\\textit{Lung}}}{CO_2} \leftrightarrow \underset{\text{Dissolved}}{H_2O + CO_2} \leftrightarrow \underset{\substack{\text{Carbonic}\\\text{acid}}}{H_2CO_3} \underset{\substack{\textit{Carbonic}\\\textit{anhydrase}}}{\leftrightarrow} \underset{\substack{\text{Bicarbonate}\\\downarrow\\\textit{Kidney}}}{H^+ + HCO_3^-}$$

Carbon dioxide is produced as an end-product of aerobic metabolism and physically dissolves in body fluids. A portion of dissolved CO_2 reacts with water to form carbonic acid, which dissociates into bicarbonate and hydrogen ions. The concentration of carbonic acid is normally very low relative to that of dissolved CO_2 and HCO_3^-. If the H^+ ion concentration increases, however, the acid load is buffered by bicarbonate, and additional carbonic acid is formed. The equilibrium of the equation is then driven to the left, and excess acid can be excreted as carbon dioxide gas.

The Henderson–Hasselbalch equation expresses the relationship between the reactants of the carbonic acid–bicarbonate system under conditions of equilibrium:

Critical Care Obstetrics, 5th edition. Edited by M. Belfort, G. Saade, M. Foley, J. Phelan and G. Dildy.

$$\text{pH} = \text{pK} + \log\frac{[\text{HCO}_3^-]}{(s)\text{P}_{\text{CO}_2}} = \frac{\text{metabolic}}{\text{respiratory}}$$

As the equation demonstrates, the ratio of $[HCO_3^-]$ to PCO_2 determines pH (H^+ ion concentration) and not individual or absolute concentrations. This ratio is influenced to a large extent by the function of the kidneys (HCO_3^-) and lungs (PCO_2). The constant *s* represents the solubility coefficient of CO_2 gas in plasma and relates PCO_2 to the concentration of dissolved CO_2 and HCO_3^-. The value of *s* is 0.03 mmol/L/mmHg at 37°C. The dissociation constant (pK) of blood carbonic acid is equivalent to 6.1 at 37°C.

The lungs are the second component of acid–base regulation. Alveolar ventilation controls PCO_2 independent of bicarbonate excretion. When the bicarbonate concentration is altered, respiratory changes attempt to return the ratio of $[HCO_3^-]/PCO_2$ toward the normal 20/1. Thus, in the presence of metabolic acidosis (decreased HCO_3^-), ventilation increases, PCO_2 is lowered, and the ratio normalizes. In metabolic alkalosis, the opposite occurs as PCO_2 rises in response to the primary increase in HCO_3^-.

The kidney is the final element of acid–base regulation. The main functions of the renal system are excretion of fixed acids and regulation of plasma bicarbonate levels. Carbonic acid that has been transported to the kidney dissociates into H^+ and HCO_3^- in renal tubular cells. Each H^+ ion secreted into the tubular lumen is exchanged for sodium, and HCO_3^- is passively reabsorbed into the blood. Essentially all bicarbonate must be reabsorbed by the kidney before acid can be excreted, because the loss of one HCO_3^- is equivalent to the addition of one H^+ ion. Mono- and diphasic phosphates and ammonia are urinary buffers that combine with H^+ ions in the renal tubules and are excreted. Under normal conditions, the amount of H^+ excreted approximates the amount of non-volatile acids produced.

The buffer systems, the lungs and kidneys interact to maintain very tight control of the body's acid–base balance. The sequence of responses to a H^+ ion load and the time required for each may be summarized:

Extracellular buffering → Respiratory buffering → Renal excretion
by HCO_3^- (immediate) — $PCO_2 \downarrow$ s (minutes to hours) — of $H^+ \uparrow$ s (hours to days)

In contrast, when PCO_2 changes:

Intracellular buffering → Renal excretion of H^+
(minutes) — (hours to days)

Unlike the response to an acid load, no extracellular buffering occurs with a change in PCO_2. Since HCO_3^- is not an effective buffer against H_2CO_3, the only protection against respiratory acidosis or alkalosis is intracellular buffering (i.e. by hemoglobin) and renal H^+ ion excretion.

Acid–base disturbances

Disturbances in acid–base balance are classified according to whether the underlying process results in an abnormal rise or fall in arterial pH. The suffix *-osis* refers to a pathologic process that causes a gain or loss of acid or base. Thus, *acidosis* describes any condition that leads to a fall in blood pH if the process continues uncorrected. Conversely, *alkalosis* characterizes any process that will cause a rise in pH if unopposed. The terms acidosis and alkalosis do not require the pH to be abnormal. The suffix *-emia* refers to the state of the blood, and *acidemia* and *alkalemia* are appropriately used when blood pH is abnormally low (<7.36) or high (>7.44), respectively [1].

In addition, alterations in acid–base homeostasis are classified based upon whether the underlying mechanism is metabolic or respiratory. If the primary abnormality is a net gain or loss of CO_2, this is respiratory acidosis or alkalosis, respectively. Alternatively, a net gain or loss of bicarbonate results in metabolic alkalosis or acidosis, respectively. If only one primary process is present, then the acid–base disturbance is simple, and bicarbonate and PCO_2 always deviate in the same direction. A mixed disturbance develops when two or more primary processes are present, and the changes in HCO_3^- and PCO_2 are in opposite directions.

The compensatory response attempts to normalize the $[HCO_3^-]/PCO_2$ ratio and maintain pH. Renal and pulmonary function must be adequate for these responses to be effective and adequate time must be allowed for the complete response. The compensatory response for a primary respiratory abnormality is via the bicarbonate system or acid excretion by the kidney and requires several days for a complete response. Compensation for a metabolic aberration is through ventilation changes and occurs quite rapidly.

Compensatory responses cannot, however, completely return the pH to normal, with the exception of chronic respiratory alkalosis. The more severe the primary disorder, the more difficult it is for the pH to return to normal. When the pH is normal but PCO_2 and HCO_3^- are abnormal or the expected compensatory responses do not occur, then a second primary disorder exists. The four types of acid–base abnormalities and the compensatory response associated with each are listed in Table 5.1.

Respiratory and acid–base changes during pregnancy

A variety of physiologic changes occur during pregnancy, affecting maternal respiratory function and gas exchange. As a result, an arterial blood gas obtained during pregnancy must be interpreted with an understanding of these alterations. Since these changes begin early in gestation and persist into the puerperium, they must be taken into consideration regardless of the stage of pregnancy [2]. In addition, the altitude at which a patient lives will affect arterial blood gas values, and normative data for each individual population should be established [3].

Minute ventilation increases by 30–50% during pregnancy [4,5] and alveolar and arterial PCO_2 decrease. Normal maternal arterial PCO_2 levels range from 26 to 32 mmHg [6–8]. Since the

Table 5.1 Summary of acid–base disorders: the primary disturbance, compensatory response, and expected degree of compensation.

	Primary disturbance	Compensatory response	Expected degree of compensation
Metabolic acidosis	Decreased HCO_3^-	Decreased P_{CO_2}	P_aCO_2 = [1.5 × (serum bicarbonate)] + 8 P_aCO_2 = last two digits of pH
Metabolic alkalosis	Increased HCO_3^-	Increased P_{CO_2}	P_aCO_2 = [0.7 × (serum bicarbonate)] + 20
Respiratory acidosis	Increased P_{CO_2}	Increased HCO_3^-	Acute: pH Δ = 0.08 × (measured P_aCO_2 − 40)/10 Chronic: pH Δ = 0.03 × (measured P_aCO_2 − 40)/10
Respiratory alkalosis	Decreased P_{CO_2}	Decreased HCO_3^-	Acute: pH Δ = 0.08 × (40 − measured P_aCO_2)/10 Chronic: pH Δ = 0.03 × (40 − measured P_aCO_2)/10

Table 5.2 Arterial blood gas values during pregnancy at sea level. Normative data should be established for individual populations residing at high altitude.

Parameter	Normal range
pH	7.40–7.46
P_{CO_2}	26–32 mmHg
P_{O_2}	101–106 mmHg
HCO_3^-	18–21 mEq/L

fetus depends upon the maternal respiratory system for carbon dioxide excretion, the decreased maternal PCO_2 creates a gradient that allows the fetus to offload carbon dioxide. Thus, fetal PCO_2 is approximately 10 mmHg higher than the maternal level when uteroplacental perfusion is normal.

Maternal alveolar oxygen tension increases as alveolar carbon dioxide tension decreases, and arterial PO_2 levels rise as high as 106 mmHg during the first trimester [7,9]. Airway closing pressures increase with advancing gestation, causing a slight fall in arterial PO_2 in the third trimester (101–104 mmHg) [7,9,10]. The arterial PO_2 level, however, is dependent upon the altitude at which the patient resides. The mean arterial PO_2 for gravidas at sea level ranges from 95 to 102 mmHg [9,11], while the average values reported for those living at 1388 m are 87 mmHg [12] and 61 mmHg at 4200 m [13]. As with carbon dioxide transfer, the fetus depends upon the oxygen gradient for continued diffusion across the placenta. Maternal arterial oxygen content, uterine artery perfusion and maternal hematocrit contribute to fetal oxygenation and compromise of any of these factors can cause fetal hypoxemia and eventually acidemia [14].

Despite the increased ventilation, maternal arterial pH remains essentially unchanged during pregnancy [7,15]. A slightly higher pH value has been noted in women living at a moderate altitude, with a reported mean of 7.46 at 1388 m above sea level [3]. Bicarbonate excretion by the kidney is increased during normal pregnancy to compensate for the lowered PCO_2, and serum bicarbonate levels are normally 18–21 mEq/L [2,7,8,16]. Thus, the metabolic state of pregnancy is a chronic respiratory alkalosis with a compensatory metabolic acidosis (Table 5.2).

Oxygen delivery and consumption

All tissues require oxygen for the combustion of organic compounds to fuel cellular metabolism. The cardiopulmonary system serves to deliver a continuous supply of oxygen and other essential substrates to tissues. Oxygen delivery is dependent on oxygenation of blood in the lungs, oxygen-carrying capacity of the blood and cardiac output. Under normal conditions, oxygen delivery (DO_2) exceeds oxygen consumption (VO_2) by about 75% [17]. The amount of oxygen delivered is determined by the cardiac output (CO, L/min) times the arterial oxygen content (CaO_2 mL/O_2/dL):

$$DO_2 = CO \times C_aO_2 \times 10\ dL/L$$

Arterial oxygen content (CaO_2) is determined by the amount of oxygen that is bound to hemoglobin (S_aO_2) and by the amount of oxygen that is dissolved in plasma ($P_aO_2 \times 0.003$):

$$C_aO_2 = (1.39 \times Hb \times S_aO_2) + (P_aO_2 \times 0.003)$$

It is clear from this formula that the amount of oxygen dissolved in plasma is negligible and, therefore, that arterial oxygen is dependent largely on hemoglobin concentration and arterial oxygen saturation. Oxygen delivery can be impaired by conditions that affect either cardiac output (flow), arterial oxygen content, or both (Table 5.3). Anemia leads to low arterial oxygen content because of a lack of hemoglobin binding sites for oxygen [18]. The patient with hypoxemic respiratory failure will not have sufficient oxygen available to saturate the hemoglobin molecule. Furthermore, it has been demonstrated that desaturated hemoglobin is altered structurally in such a fashion as to have a diminished affinity for oxygen [19]. It must be kept in mind that the amount of oxygen actually available to tissues also is affected by the affinity of the hemoglobin molecule for oxygen. Thus, the oxyhemoglobin dissociation curve (Figure 5.1) and those conditions that influence the binding of oxygen either negatively or positively must be considered when attempts are made to maximize oxygen delivery [20]. An increase in the plasma pH level or a decrease in temperature or 2,3 diphosphoglycerate (2,3-DPG) will increase hemoglobin affinity for oxygen, shifting the curve to the left and resulting in diminished tissue oxygenation. If the

Table 5.3 Commonly used formulas for assessment of oxygenation.

	Formula	Normal value
Est. alveolar oxygen tension	$P_AO_2 = 145 - P_aCO_2$	
Pulmonary capillary oxygen content	$C_{c'}O_2 = [Hb](1.39) + (P_AO_2)(0.003)$	
Arterial oxygen content	$C_aO_2 = (1.39 \times Hb \times S_aO_2) + (P_aO_2 \times 0.003)$	18–21 mL/dL
Mixed venous oxygen content	$C\bar{v}O_2 = (1.39 \times Hb \times S\bar{v}O_2) + (P\bar{v}O_2)(0.003)$	
Oxygen delivery	$DO_2 = C_aO_2 \times Q_T \times 10$	640–1,200 mLO$_2$/min
Oxygen consumption	$\dot{V}O_2 = Q_T\,(C_aO_2 - C_vO_2) = 13.8\,(Hb)\,(Q_T)\,(S_aO_2 - S_vO_2)/100$	180–280 mLO$_2$/min
Shunt equation	$\dfrac{Q_{sp} = Cc'O_2 - C_aO_2}{Q_tCc'O_2 - C\bar{v}O_2}$	3–8%
Estimated shunt	$\text{Est. Qsp/Qt} = \dfrac{Cc'O_2 - CaO_2}{[Cc'O_2 - CaO_2] + [CaO_2 - CvO_2]}$	

P_aCO_2, partial pressure of arterial carbon dioxide; P_aO_2, partial pressure of arterial oxygen; $P\bar{v}O_2$, partial pressure of venous oxygen; Hb, hemoglobin; S_aO_2, arterial oxygen saturation; $S\bar{v}O_2$, venous oxygen saturation; Q_T, cardiac output.

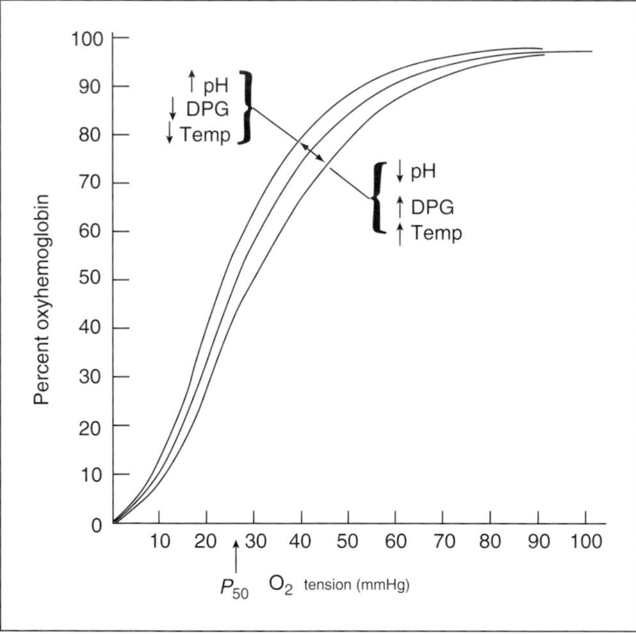

Figure 5.1 The oxygen binding curve for human hemoglobin A under physiologic conditions (middle curve). The affinity is shifted by changes in pH, diphosphoglycerate (DPG) concentration, and temperature, as indicated. P_{50} represents the oxygen tension at half saturation. (Reproduced by permission from Bunn HF, Forget BG. Hemoglobin: molecular, genetic, and clinical aspects. Philadelphia: WB Saunders, 1986.)

plasma pH level or temperature falls, or if 2,3-DPG increases, hemoglobin affinity for oxygen will decrease and more oxygen will be available to tissues [20].

In certain clinical conditions, such as septic shock and adult respiratory distress syndrome, there is maldistribution of flow relative to oxygen demand, leading to diminished delivery and loss of vascular autoregulation, producing regional and microcirculatory imbalances in blood flow [21]. This mismatching of blood flow with metabolic demand causes excessive blood flow to some areas, with relative hypoperfusion of other areas, limiting optimal systemic utilization of oxygen [21].

The patient with diminished cardiac output secondary to hypovolemia or pump failure is unable to distribute oxygenated blood to tissues. Therapy directed at increasing volume with normal saline, or with blood if the hemoglobin level is less than 10 g/dL, increases oxygen delivery in the hypovolemic patient. The patient with pump failure may benefit from inotropic support and afterload reduction in addition to supplementation of intravscular volume.

Relationship of oxygen delivery to consumption

Oxygen consumption (VO_2) is the product of the arteriovenous oxygen content difference ($C_{(a-v)}O_2$) and cardiac output. Under normal conditions, oxygen consumption is a direct function of the metabolic rate [22].

$$VO_2 = C_{(a-v)}O_2 \times CO \times 10 \text{ dL/L}$$

The oxygen extraction ratio (OER) is the fraction of delivered oxygen that is actually consumed:

$$OER = VO_2/DO_2$$

The normal OER is about 0.25. A rise in the OER is a compensatory mechanism employed when oxygen delivery is inadequate for the level of metabolic activity. An OER of less than 0.25 suggests flow maldistribution, peripheral diffusion defects, or fractional shunting [22]. As the supply of oxygen is reduced, the fraction extracted from blood increases and oxygen consumption is maintained. If a severe reduction in oxygen delivery occurs, the limits of oxygen extraction are reached, tissues are unable to sustain aerobic energy production, and consumption decreases. The level of oxygen delivery at which oxygen consumption begins to decrease has been termed the "critical DO_2" [23]. At the critical DO_2, tissues begin to use anerobic glycolysis, with resultant lactate production and metabolic acidosis [23]. If this oxygen deprivation continues, irreversible tissue damage and death ensue.

Oxygen delivery and consumption in pregnancy

The physiologic anemia of pregnancy results in a reduction in the hemoglobin concentration and arterial oxygen content. Oxygen delivery is maintained at or above normal despite this because cardiac output increases 50%. It is important to remember, therefore, that the pregnant woman is more dependent on cardiac output for maintenance of oxygen delivery than the non-pregnant patient [24]. Oxygen consumption increases steadily throughout pregnancy and is greatest at term, reaching an average of 331 mL/min at rest and 1167 mL/min with exercise [10]. During labor, oxygen consumption increases by 40–60%, and cardiac output increases by about 22% [25,26]. Because oxygen delivery normally far exceeds consumption, the normal pregnant patient usually is able to maintain adequate delivery of oxygen to herself and her fetus, even during labor. When a pregnant patient's oxygen delivery decreases, however, she can very quickly reach the critical DO_2, especially during labor, compromising both herself and her fetus. The obstetrician, therefore, must make every effort to optimize oxygen delivery before allowing labor to begin in the compromised patient.

Blood gas analysis

The accuracy of a blood gas determination relies upon many factors, including blood collection techniques, specimen transport, and laboratory equipment. Up to 16% of specimens may be improperly handled, diminishing diagnostic utility in a number of cases [27]. Factors that can influence blood gas results include excessive heparin in the collection syringe, catheter dead space, air bubbles in the blood sample, time delays to laboratory analysis as well as other less common causes. This section highlights considerations for obtaining a blood sample and potential sources of error, and briefly describes laboratory methods.

Sample collection

The collection syringe typically contains heparin to prevent clotting of the specimen. Excessive heparin in the syringe before blood collection, however, can significantly decrease the PCO_2 and bicarbonate of the sample. The spurious PCO_2 level results in a falsely lowered bicarbonate concentration when calculated using the Henderson–Hasselbalch equation. Although sodium heparin is an acid, pH is minimally affected because whole blood is an adequate buffer. Expelling all heparin except that in the dead space of the syringe and needle will ensure adequate dilution by obtaining a minimum of 3 mL of blood and reduce or avoid anticoagulant-related errors [28].

In the intensive care setting, an arterial catheter is often placed when frequent blood sampling is anticipated. Dilutional errors occur when a blood sample is contaminated with fluids in the catheter [29]. An adequate volume of maintenance fluid or flush solution must be withdrawn from the catheter and discarded before obtaining the sample for analysis. But the difficulty is estimating the appropriate amount to withdraw. Although a 2.5-mL discard volume has been suggested, it has also been recommended that each intensive care unit establish its own policy based upon individual catheter and connection systems [1,30,31].

Air bubbles in the collection syringe cause time-dependent changes in the arterial blood gas. Air trapped as froth accelerates these changes because of the increased surface area [32]. The degree of change in PO_2 depends upon the initial PO_2 of the sample. Since an air bubble has a PO_2 of 150 mmHg (room air), the bubble will cause a falsely elevated PO_2 if the sample PO_2 is <150 mmHg. The opposite occurs if the sample has an initial PO_2 >150 mmHg. [1,33]. Oxygen saturation is most significantly affected when the sample PO_2 is <60 mmHg since saturation changes rapidly with changes in PO_2, as predicted by the oxyhemoglobin dissociation curve. PCO_2 in the sample decreases within several minutes of exposure to ambient air [32,34].

When a blood sample remains at room temperature following collection, PO_2 and pH may decrease while PCO_2 increases. Specimens analyzed within 10–20 minutes of collection give accurate results even when transported at room temperature [35,36]. In most clinical settings, however, the time between sampling and laboratory analysis of the specimen exceeds this limit. Therefore, the syringe should be placed into an ice bath immediately after sample collection. The combination of ice and water provides better cooling of the syringe than ice alone, and a sample may be stored for up to 1 hour without adversely affecting blood gas results [34].

Several additional factors can influence blood gas results. Insufficient time between an adjustment in fractional inspired oxygen or mechanical ventilator settings and blood gas analysis may not accurately reflect the change. Equilibration is quite rapid, however, and has been reported to occur as soon as 10 minutes after changing ventilator settings of postoperative cardiac patients [37]. General anesthesia with halothane will falsely elevate PO_2 determination as it mimics oxygen during sample analysis [38–41]. Finally, severe leukocytosis causes a false lowering of PO_2 due to consumption by the cells in the collection syringe [42]. The effect of the white blood cells may be minimized, but not necessarily eliminated, by cooling the sample immediately after it is obtained.

The blood gas analyzer

The blood gas analyzer is designed to simultaneously measure the pH, PO_2, and PCO_2 of blood. An aliquot of heparinized blood is injected into a chamber containing one reference and three measuring electrodes. Each measuring electrode is connected to the reference electrode by a Ag/AgCl wire. The electrodes and injected sample are kept at a constant 37°C by a warm water bath or heat exchanger. The accuracy of the measurements depends upon routine calibration of equipment, proper sample collection, and constant electrode temperature.

Blood pH and PCO_2 are potentiometric determinations, with the potential difference between each electrode and the reference electrode quantitated. The pH electrode detects hydrogen ions, and the electrical potential developed by the electrode varies with the H^+ ion activity of the sample. The potential difference between the pH and reference electrode is measured by a voltmeter and converted to the pH. The PCO_2 electrode is actually a modified pH electrode. A glass electrode is surrounded with a weak bicarbonate solution and enclosed in a silicone membrane. Carbon dioxide in the sample diffuses through this membrane which is permeable to CO_2 but not water and H^+ ions. As CO_2 diffuses through the membrane, the pH of the bicarbonate solution changes. Thus, the pH measured by the electrode is related to CO_2 tension.

The measurement of PO_2 is amperometric, as the current generated between an anode and cathode estimates the partial pressure of oxygen. The PO_2 electrode surrounds a membrane permeable to oxygen but not other blood constituents. The electrode consists of an anode and a cathode, and constant voltage is maintained between them. An electrolytic process that occurs in the presence of oxygen produces current, and the magnitude of the current is proportional to the partial pressure of oxygen in the sample. As oxygen tension increases, the electrical current generated between the anode and cathode increases.

Bicarbonate concentration as reported on a blood gas result is not directly measured in the blood gas laboratory. Once pH and PCO_2 are determined, bicarbonate concentration is calculated using the Henderson–Hasselbalch equation or determined from a nomogram. In contrast, the total serum CO_2 (tCO_2) content is measured by automated methods and reported with routine serum electrolyte measurements.

Oxygen saturation (SO_2) is the ratio of oxygenated hemoglobin to total hemoglobin. It can be plotted graphically once PO_2 is determined, calculated using an equation that estimates the oxyhemoglobin dissociation curve, or determined spectrophotometrically by a co-oximeter. The latter is the most accurate method since saturation is determined by a direct reading.

Pulse oximetry

The oximetry system determines arterial oxygen saturation by measuring the absorption of selected wavelengths of light in pulsatile blood flow [43]. Oxyhemoglobin absorbs much less red and slightly more infrared light than reduced hemoglobin. Oxygen saturation is therefore the ratio of red to infrared absorption.

Red and infrared light from light-emitting diodes are projected across a pulsatile tissue bed and analyzed by a photodetector. The absorption of each wavelength of light varies cyclically with pulse. The patient's heart rate, therefore, is also determined. When assessing the accuracy of the arterial saturation measured by the pulse oximeter, correlation of the oximeter determined heart rate and the patient's actual pulse rate indicates proper electrode placement. The oximetry probe is usually placed on a nail bed or ear lobe. Under ideal circumstances, most oximeters measure saturation (S_pO_2) to within 2% of S_aO_2 [43].

Pulse oximetry is ideal for non-invasive arterial oxygen saturation monitoring near the steep portion of the oxyhemoglobin dissociation curve, namely at a P_aO_2 less than or equal to 70 mmHg [44]. P_aO_2 levels greater than or equal to 80 mmHg result in very small changes in oxygen saturation, namely 97–99%. Large changes in the P_aO_2 from 90 mmHg to 60 mmHg can occur without significant change in arterial oxygen saturation. This technique, therefore, is useful as a continuous monitor of the adequacy of blood oxygenation and not as a method to quantitate the level of impaired gas exchange [45].

Poor tissue perfusion, hyperbilirubinemia, and severe anemia may cause inaccurate oximetry readings [44]. Carbon monoxide poisoning leads to an overestimation of the P_aO_2. When methemoglobin levels exceed 5%, the pulse oximeter cannot reliably predict oxygen saturation. Methylene blue, the treatment for methemoglobinemia, will also lead to inaccurate oximetry readings. Normal values for maternal pulse oximetry readings (S_pO_2) are dependent upon gestational age, position, and altitude of residence [46–48].

Mixed venous oxygenation

The mixed venous oxygen tension (P_VO_2) and mixed venous oxygen saturation (S_VO_2) are parameters of tissue oxygenation [22]. P_VO_2 is 40 mmHg with a saturation of 73%. Saturations less than 60% are abnormally low. These parameters can be measured directly by obtaining a blood sample from the distal port of the pulmonary artery catheter. The S_VO_2 also can be measured continuously with a fiberoptic pulmonary artery catheter. Mixed venous oxygenation is a reliable parameter in the patient with hypoxemia or low cardiac output, but findings must be interpreted with caution. When the S_VO_2 is low, oxygen delivery can be assumed to be low. However, normal or high does not guarantee that tissues are well oxygenated. In conditions such as septic shock and adult respiratory distress syndrome, the maldistribution of systemic flow may lead to abnormally high S_VO_2 in the face of severe tissue hypoxia [21]. The oxyhemoglobin dissociation curve must be considered when interpreting the S_VO_2 as an indicator of tissue oxygenation [19]. Conditions that result in a left shift of the curve cause the venous oxygen saturation to be normal or high, even when the mixed venous oxygen content is low. The S_VO_2 is useful for monitoring trends in a particular patient, because a significant decrease will occur when oxygen delivery has decreased secondary to hypoxemia or a fall in cardiac output.

Blood gas interpretation

The processes leading to acid–base disturbances are well described, and blood gas analysis may facilitate identification of the cause of a serious illness. Since many critically ill patients have metabolic and respiratory derangements, correct interpretation of a blood gas is fundamental to their care. Misinterpretation, however, can result in treatment delays and inappropriate therapy. Several methods of acid–base interpretation have been devised, including graphic nomograms and step-by-step analysis. Each method is detailed in this section to aid in rapid and correct diagnosis of disturbances in acid–base balance.

Blood gas results are not a substitute for clinical evaluation of a patient, and laboratory values do not necessarily correlate with the degree of clinical compromise. A typical example is the patient with an acute exacerbation of asthma who experiences severe dyspnea and respiratory compromise before developing hypercapnea and hypoxemia. Thus, a blood gas is an adjunct to clinical judgment, and decision-making should not be based on a single test.

Graphic nomogram

Nomograms are a graphic display of an equation and have been designed to facilitate identification of simple acid–base disturbances [49–52]. Figure 5.2 is an example of a nomogram with arterial blood pH represented on the *x*-axis, HCO_3^- concentration on the *y*-axis, and arterial PCO_2 on the regression lines. Nomograms are accurate for simple acid–base disturbances, and a single disorder can be identified by plotting measured blood gas values. When blood gas values fall between labelled areas, a mixed disorder is present and the nomogram does not apply. These complex disorders must then be characterized by quantitative assessment of the expected compensatory changes (Table 5.1).

A systematic approach to an acid–base abnormality

Several different approaches for blood gas interpretation have been devised [53–55]. A six-step approach modified from Narins and Emmitt provides a simple and reliable method to analyze a blood gas, particularly when a complicated mixed disorder is present [33,56,57]. This method, adjusted for pregnancy, is as follows (Figure 5.3).

1 *Is the patient acidemic or alkalemic?* If the arterial blood pH is <7.36, the patient is acidemic, while a pH >7.44 defines alkalemia.

2 *Is the primary disturbance respiratory or metabolic?* The primary alteration associated with each of the four primary disorders is shown in Table 5.1.

3 *If a **respiratory disturbance** is present, is it acute or chronic?* The equations listed in Table 5.1 are used to determine the acuteness of the disturbance. The expected change in the pH is calculated and the measured pH is compared to the pH that would be expected based on the patient's PCO_2.

4 *If a **metabolic acidosis** is present, is the anion gap increased?* Metabolic acidosis is classified according to the presence or absence of an anion gap.

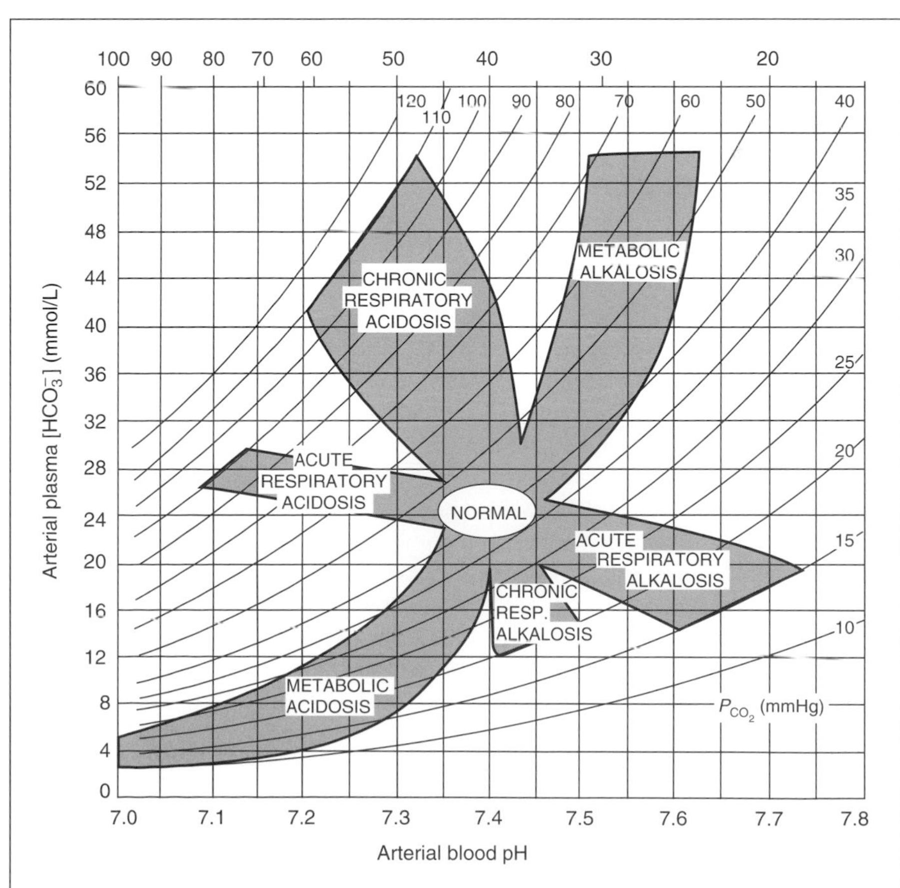

Figure 5.2 Nomogram for interpretation of simple acid–base disorders. (Reproduced by permission from Cogan MJ. In: Brenner BM, Rector FC Jr, eds. The Kidney. Philadelphia: WB Saunders, 1986: 473.)

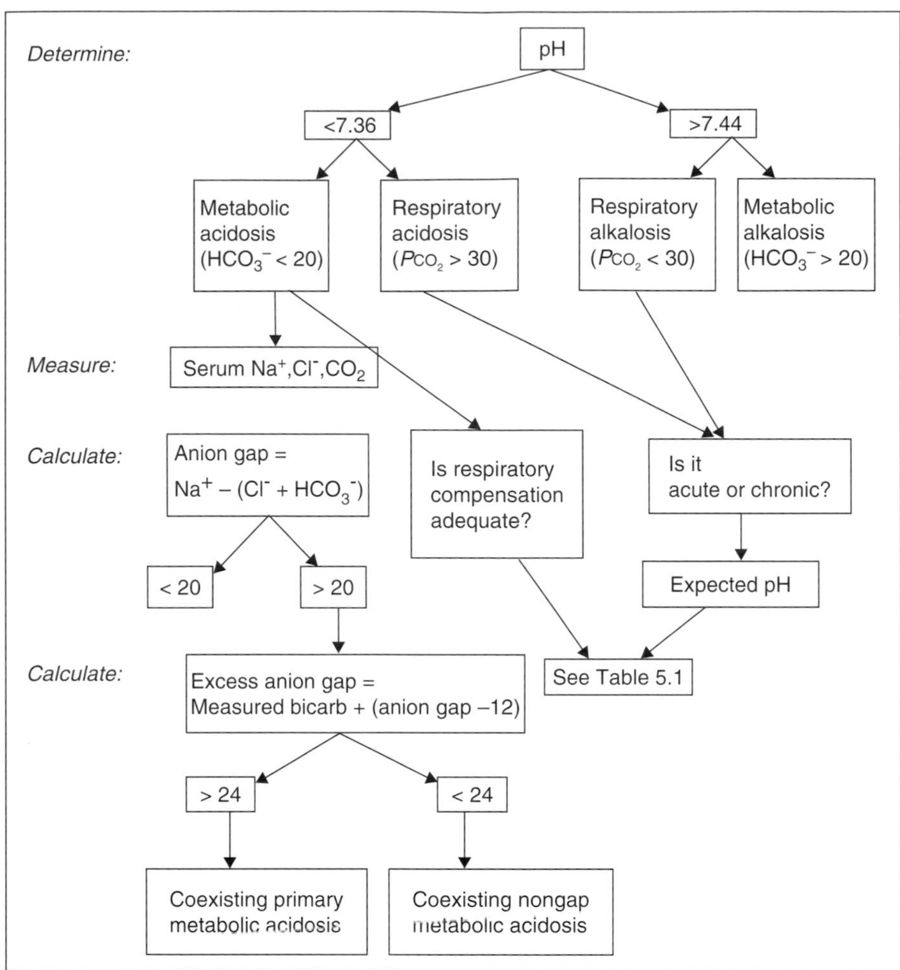

Figure 5.3 A systematic approach to the interpretation of an arterial blood gas during pregnancy.

5 *If a* ***metabolic disturbance*** *is present, is the respiratory compensation adequate?* The expected PCO_2 for a given degree of metabolic acidosis can be predicted by Winter's formula (Table 5.1), since the relationship between PCO_2 and HCO_3^- is linear. Predicting respiratory compensation for metabolic alkalosis, however, is not nearly as consistent as with acidosis.

6 *If the patient has an anion gap metabolic acidosis, are additional metabolic disturbances present?* The excess anion gap represents bicarbonate concentration before the anion gap acidosis developed. By calculating the excess gap, an otherwise undetected non-anion gap acidosis or metabolic alkalosis may be detected.

Respiratory components of the arterial blood gas

Partial pressure of arterial oxygen: P_aO_2

The P_aO_2 reflects the lung's ability to provide adequate arterial oxygen. Normal arterial oxygen tension during pregnancy ranges from 87 to 106 mmHg, depending upon the altitude at which a patient lives. Although P_aO_2 has been reported to decrease by 25% when samples are obtained from gravidas in the supine position [11], arterial blood gas values have been shown to be unaffected by a change in maternal position [3]. Abnormal gas exchange, inadequate ventilation or both can lead to a fall in P_aO_2. Hypoxemia is defined as a P_aO_2 below 60 mmHg or a saturation less than 90%. At this level, the oxygen content of blood is near its maximum for a given hemoglobin concentration and any additional increase in arterial oxygen tension will increase oxygen content only a small amount.

The amount of oxygen combined with hemoglobin is related to the P_aO_2 by the oxyhemoglobin dissociation curve and influenced by a variety of factors (Figure 5.4). The shape of the oxyhemoglobin dissociation curve allows P_aO_2 to decrease faster than oxygen saturation until the P_aO_2 is approximately 60 mmHg. A left shift of the curve increases hemoglobin's affinity for oxygen and oxygen content, but decreases release of O_2 in peripheral tissues. The fetal or neonatal oxyhemoglobin dissociation curve is shifted to the left as a result of fetal hemoglobin and lower levels of 2,3-DPG. (Figure 5.4) The increased affinity of hemoglobin for oxygen allows the fetus to extract maximal oxygen from maternal blood. A shift to the right has the opposite effect, with decreased oxygen affinity and content but increased release in the periphery.

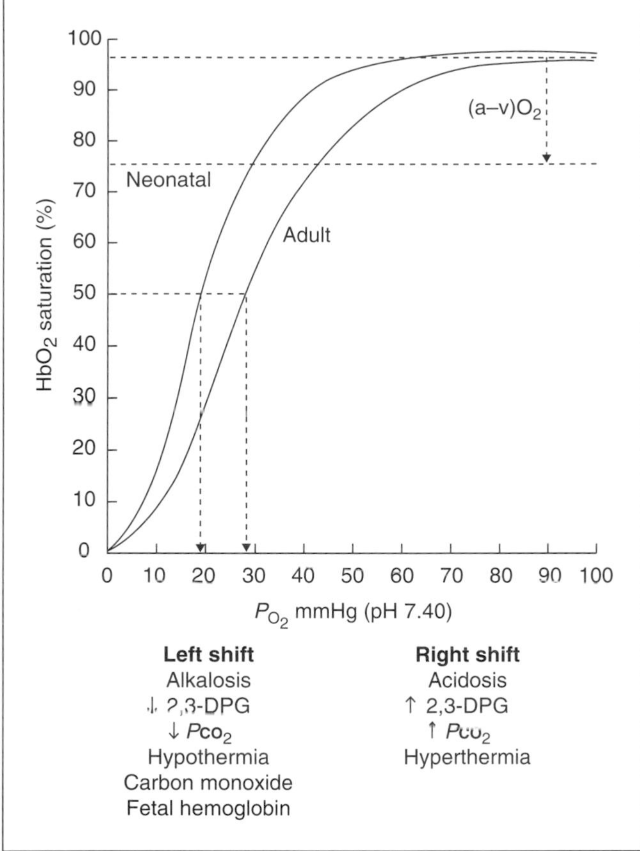

Figure 5.4 Maternal and fetal oxyhemoglobin dissociation curves. 2,3-DPG, 2,3-diphosphoglycerate. (Reproduced by permission from Semin Perinatol. WB Saunders, 1984; 8:168.)

Assessment of lung function

Impairment of lung function can be estimated using an oxygen tension- or oxygen content-based index. Oxygen tension-based indices include: (i) expected P_aO_2 for a given fraction of inspired oxygen (F_iO_2); (ii) P_aO_2/F_iO_2 ratio; and (iii) alveolar–arterial oxygen gradient ($P_{(A-a)}O_2$). These methods are quick and easy to use but have limitations in the critically ill patient [58]. The shunt calculation (Qsp/Qt) is an oxygen content-based index and is the most reliable method of determining the extent to which pulmonary disease is contributing to arterial hypoxemia. The need for a pulmonary artery blood sample is a disadvantage, however, as not all patients require invasive monitoring. The estimated shunt calculation (est. Qsp/Qt) is derived from the shunt equation and is the optimal method to estimate lung compromise when a pulmonary artery catheter is not in place.

The expected P_aO_2 is an oxygen tension-based calculation and can be quickly estimated by multiplying the actual percentage of inspired oxygen by 6 [59]. Thus, a patient receiving 50% oxygen has an expected PO_2 of (50×6) or 300 mmHg. Alternatively, the F_iO_2 (e.g. 0.50 in a patient receiving 50% oxygen) may be multiplied by 500 to estimate the minimum PO_2 [60]. The P_aO_2/F_iO_2 ratio has been used to estimate the amount of shunt. The normal ratio is 500–600 and correlates with a shunt of 3–5% while a shunt of 20% or more is present when the ratio is less than 200.

Calculation of the alveolar–arterial oxygen gradient is also an oxygen tension calculation. The A–a gradient is most reliable when breathing room air and is normally less than 20. An increased gradient indicates pulmonary dysfunction. A–a gradient values, however, can change unpredictably with changes in F_iO_2 and vary with alterations in oxygen saturation and consumption. Thus, the utility of this measurement in critically ill patients has been questioned since these patients often require a high F_iO_2 and have unstable oxygenation [61]. Additionally, the A–a gradient appears to be unreliable in the assessment of lung impairment during pregnancy [11].

Oxygen content-based indices include the shunt equation and estimated shunt as derived from the shunt equation (Table 5.3). The estimated shunt has been shown to be superior to the oxygen tension-based indices described above [58]. The patient is given 100% oxygen for at least 20 minutes before determining arterial and venous blood gases and hemoglobin. Since the estimated shunt equation does not require a pulmonary artery blood sample, the $C_{(a-v)}O_2$ difference is assumed to be 3.5 mL/dL. A normal shunt in non-pregnant patients is less than 10%, while a 20–29% shunt may be life-threatening in a patient with compromised cardiovascular or neurologic function, and a shunt of 30% and greater usually requires significant cardiopulmonary support.

Intrapulmonary shunt values during normal pregnancy, however, have been reported to be nearly three times above the mean for non-pregnant individuals [12]. The mean Qs/Qt in normotensive primiparous women at 36–38 weeks gestation ranges from 10% in the knee–chest position to 13% in the standing position and 15% in the lateral position. The increased Qs/Qt can be explained by the physiologic changes of pregnancy as follows. Lung volumes decrease during gestation and the amount of shunt increases. In addition, pulmonary blood flow increases secondary to increased cardiac output. The combined effect of decreased lung volumes and increased pulmonary flow results in a higher intrapulmonary shunt during pregnancy.

Oxygenation of peripheral tissues

An adequate P_aO_2 is only the initial step in oxygen transport, however, and it does not guarantee well-oxygenated tissues. The degree of intrapulmonary shunt, oxygen delivery, and oxygen consumption all contribute to adequate tissue oxygenation. Accurate assessment of peripheral oxygenation requires measurement of arterial and venous partial pressures of oxygen, arterial and venous oxygen saturation, hemoglobin, and cardiac output (Table 5.3).

The amount of O_2 (mL) contained in 100 mL of blood defines oxygen content. Oxygen delivery (DO_2) is the volume of O_2 brought to peripheral tissues in 1 minute and consumption (VO_2) is the volume used by the tissues in 1 minute. Under normal conditions, delivery of oxygen is 3–4 times greater than consumption. Oxygen extraction measures the amount of O_2 transferred to tissues from 100 mL of blood and can be thought of as $CaO_2 - CvO_2$. Thus, an O_2 extraction of 3–4 mL/dL suggests adequate cardiac reserve to supply additional oxygen if demand increases. Inadequate cardiac reserve is indicated by an O_2 extraction of 5 mL/dL or greater, and tissue extraction must be increased to meet changing metabolic needs [62].

Mixed venous oxygen tension (P_vO_2) and saturation (S_vO_2) are measured from pulmonary artery blood. These measurements are better indicators of tissue oxygenation than arterial values since venous blood reflects peripheral tissue extraction. Normal arterial oxygen saturation is 100% and venous saturation is 75%, yielding a normal arteriovenous difference ($S_aO_2 - S_vO_2$) of 25%. An increased S_vO_2 (>80%) can occur when oxygen delivery increases, oxygen consumption decreases, (or some combination of the two), cardiac output increases, or the pulmonary artery catheter tip is in a pulmonary capillary instead of the artery. A decrease in S_vO_2 (<50–60%) may be due to increased oxygen consumption, decreased cardiac output or compromised pulmonary function. The venous oxygen saturation may not change at all, however, even with significant cardiovascular changes.

Partial pressure of arterial carbon dioxide: P_aCO_2

The metabolic rate determines the amount of carbon dioxide that enters the blood. Carbon dioxide is then transported to the lung as dissolved CO_2, bicarbonate, and carbamates. It diffuses from blood into alveoli and is removed from the body by ventilation, or the movement of gas into and out of the pulmonary system. Measurement of the arterial partial pressure of carbon dioxide allows assessment of alveolar ventilation in relation to the metabolic rate.

Ventilation (V_E) is the amount of gas exhaled in 1 minute and is the sum of alveolar and dead space ventilation ($V_E = V_A + V_{DS}$). Alveolar ventilation (V_A) is that portion of the lung that removes CO_2 and transfers O_2 to the blood, while dead space (V_{DS}) has no respiratory function. As dead space increases, ventilation must increase to maintain adequate alveolar ventilation. Dead space increases with a high ventilation–perfusion ratio (V/Q) (i.e. an acute decrease in cardiac output, acute pulmonary embolism, acute pulmonary hypertension, or ARDS) and positive-pressure ventilation.

Since P_aCO_2 reflects the balance between production and alveolar excretion of carbon dioxide, accumulation of CO_2 indicates failure of the respiratory system to excrete the products of metabolism. The primary disease process may be respiratory or a process outside the lungs. Extrapulmonary processes that increase metabolism and CO_2 production include fever, shivering, seizures, sepsis, and physiologic stress. Parenteral nutrition with glucose providing more than 50% of non-protein calories can also contribute to high CO_2 production.

Recognizing respiratory acid–base imbalance is important because of the need to assist in CO_2 elimination. As V_E increases, the work of breathing can cause fatigue and respiratory failure. It is important to recognize that the P_aCO_2 may initially be normal, but rises as the work of breathing exceeds a patient's functional reserve. Ventilatory failure occurs when the pulmonary system can no longer provide adequate excretion of CO_2. Clinically, this is recognized as tachypnea, tachycardia, intercostal muscle retraction, accessory muscle use, diaphoresis and paradoxical breathing.

The metabolic component of the arterial blood gas: bicarbonate

Measurement of bicarbonate reflects a patient's acid–base status. The bicarbonate concentration reported with a blood gas is calculated using the Henderson–Hasselbalch equation and represents a single ionic species. Total serum CO_2 (tCO_2) content is measured with serum electrolytes and is the sum of the various forms of CO_2 in serum. Bicarbonate is the major contributor to tCO_2, and additional forms include dissolved CO_2, carbamates, carbonate, and carbonic acid. The calculated bicarbonate concentration does not include carbonic acid, carbonate, and carbamates.

Frequently, arterial and venous blood samples are obtained simultaneously, making arterial blood gas bicarbonate and venous serum tCO_2 measurements available. Venous serum tCO_2 content is 2.5–3 mEq/L higher than arterial blood gas bicarbonate, since CO_2 content is higher in venous than arterial blood and all species of carbon dioxide are included in the determination of tCO_2. If the blood sample is arterial, the tCO_2 content reported on the electrolyte panel should be 1.5–2 mEq/L higher than the calculated bicarbonate. The tCO_2 measured directly with serum electrolytes will be higher because it includes the different forms of CO_2. Since both blood gas bicarbonate and electrolyte tCO_2 determinations are usually available, there is a split of opinion as to the relative clinical utility of each[63]. A recent review, however, concludes that calculated and measured bicarbonate values are close enough in most cases that either is acceptable for clinical use [64].

Disorders of acid–base balance

Metabolic acidosis

Metabolic acidosis is diagnosed on the basis of a decreased serum bicarbonate and arterial pH. The baseline bicarbonate concentration during pregnancy should, of course, be kept in mind when interpreting bicarbonate concentration. Metabolic acidosis develops when fixed acids accumulate or bicarbonate is lost. Accumulation of fixed acid occurs with overproduction as in diabetic ketoacidosis or lactic acidosis, or with decreased acid excretion as in renal failure. Diarrhea, a small bowel fistula, and renal tubular acidosis can all result in loss of extracellular bicarbonate.

Although the clinical signs associated with metabolic acidosis are not specific, multiple organ systems may be affected. Tachycardia develops with the initial fall in pH, but bradycardia usually predominates as the pH drops below 7.10. Acidosis causes venous constriction and impairs cardiac contractility, increasing venous return while cardiac output decreases. Arteriolar dilation

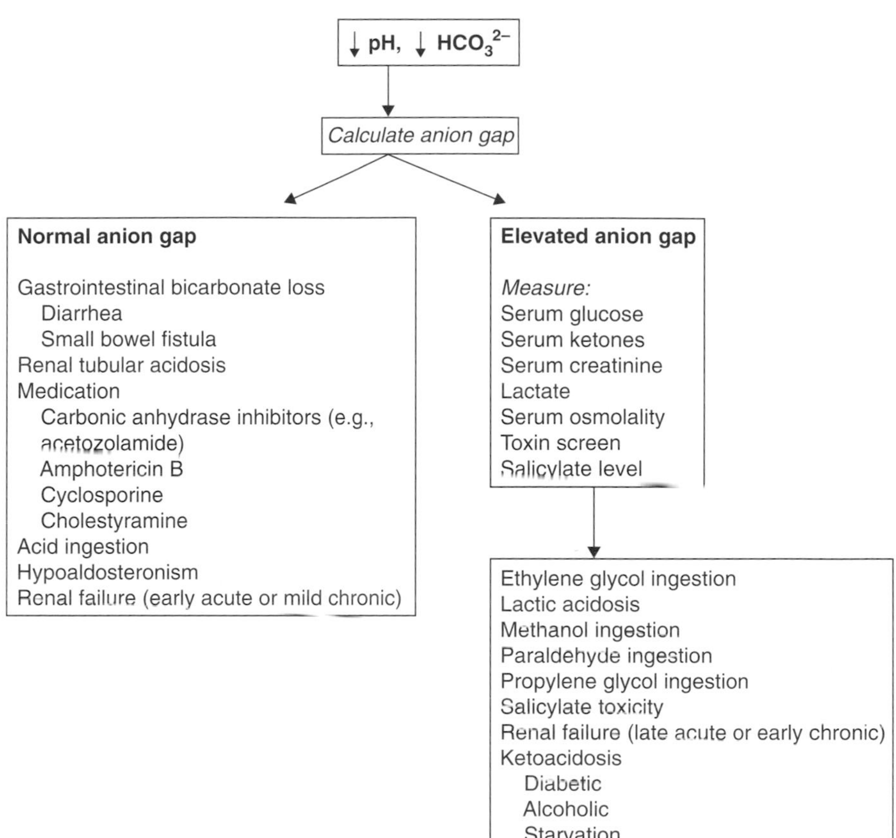

Figure 5.5 Etiology and evaluation of metabolic acidosis.

occurs at pH <7.20. Respiratory rate and tidal volume increase in an attempt to compensate for the acidosis. Maternal acidosis can result in fetal acidosis as H^+ ions equilibrate across the placenta, and fetal pH is generally 0.1 pH units less than the maternal pH.

The compensatory response to metabolic acidosis is an increase in ventilation that is stimulated by the fall in the pH. Hyperventilation lowers PCO_2 as the body attempts to return the $[HCO_3^-]/PCO_2$ ratio toward normal. The respiratory response is proportional to the degree of acidosis and allows calculation of the expected PCO_2 for a given bicarbonate level (Table 5.1). When the measured PCO_2 is higher or lower than expected for the measured serum bicarbonate, a mixed acid–base disorder must be present. This formula is ideally applied once the patient has reached a steady state, when PCO_2 nadirs 12–24 hours after the onset of acidosis [56].

The classification of metabolic acidosis as non-anion gap or anion gap acidosis helps determine the pathologic process. Once a metabolic acidosis is detected, serum electrolytes should be obtained to calculate the anion gap. Frequently the clinical history and a few additional diagnostic studies can identify the underlying abnormality (Figure 5.5) [65].

Electroneutrality in the body is maintained because the sum of all anions equals the sum of all cations. Na^+, K^+, Cl^-, and HCO_3^- are the routinely measured serum ions while Mg^+, Ca^{2+}, proteins (particularly albumin), lactate, HPO_4^- and SO_4^- are the unmeasured ions. Na^+ and K^+ account for 95% of cations while HCO_3^- and Cl^- represent 85% of anions [66]. Thus, unmeasured anions are greater than unmeasured cations. The anion gap is the difference between measured plasma cations (Na^+) minus measured anions (Cl^-, HCO_3^-) and is derived.

$$\text{Total anions} = \text{Total cations}$$

$$\textbf{Measured anions} + \text{unmeasured anions} = \textbf{measured cations} + \text{unmeasured cations}$$

$$\left([\mathbf{Cl^-}]+[\mathbf{tCO_2}]+\text{unmeasured anions}\right)=\left([\mathbf{Na^+}]+\text{unmeasured cations}\right)$$

$$\text{Unmeasured anions} - \text{unmeasured cations} = [\mathbf{Na^+}]-([\mathbf{Cl^-}]+[\mathbf{tCO_2}])$$

$$\textit{Anion gap} = [\boldsymbol{Na^+}]-([\boldsymbol{Cl^-}]+[\boldsymbol{tCO_2}])$$

A normal anion gap is 8–16 mEq/L. Potassium may be included as a measured cation, although it contributes little to the accuracy or utility of the gap. If K^+ is included in the calculation, however, the normal range becomes 12–20 mEq/L [67].

A change in the gap involves a change in unmeasured cations or anions. An elevated gap is most commonly due to an accumulation of unmeasured anions that include organic acids (i.e. keto-acids or lactic acid), or inorganic acids (i.e. sulfate and phosphate) [68]. A decrease in cations (i.e. magnesium and calcium) will also increase the gap, but the serum level is usually life-threatening.

The following example demonstrates use of the anion gap in a patient who had been experiencing dysuria, polyuria, and polydypsia of several days duration. Initial evaluation of this 19-year-old gravida at 24 weeks gestation was notable for a serum glucose level of 460 mg/dL and 4+ urinary ketones. Further investigation revealed: arterial pH of 7.30, HCO_3^- of 14 mEq/L, serum Na^+ of 133 mEq/L, K^+ of 4.1 mEq/L, tCO_2 of 15 mEq/L, and Cl^- of 95 mEq/L. The anion gap was determined:

$$\begin{aligned}\text{Anion gap} &= [Na^+]-([Cl^-]+[tCO_2^-])\\ &= 133\ \text{mEq/L}-(95\ \text{mEq/L}+15\ \text{mEq/L})\\ &= 133\ \text{mEq/L}-110\ \text{mEq/L}\\ \text{Anion gap} &= 23\ \text{mEq/L}\end{aligned}$$

The elevated anion gap is the result of unmeasured organic anions or ketoacids that have accumulated and decreased serum bicarbonate. As this patient with type I diabetes mellitus receives insulin therapy, the anion gap will normalize, reflecting disappearance of the ketoacids from the serum.

The limitations of the anion gap, however, should be recognized. Various factors can lower the anion gap, but its importance is not so much in the etiology of the decrease as in its ability to mask an elevated gap. Since albumin accounts for the majority of unmeasured anions, the gap decreases as albumin levels fall. For each 1 g decrease in albumin, the gap may be lowered by 2.5–3 mEq/L. The most common cause of a lowered gap is decreased serum albumin. Other less common causes include markedly elevated levels of unmeasured cations (K^+, Mg^+, and Ca^{2+}), hyperlipidemia, lithium carbonate intoxication, multiple myeloma, and bromide or iodide intoxication.

Although an elevated anion gap is traditionally associated with metabolic acidosis, it may also occur in the presence of severe metabolic alkalosis. The ionic activity of albumin changes with increasing pH and protons are released. The net negative charge on each molecule increases, thereby increasing unmeasured anions. Volume contraction leads to hyperproteinemia and augments the anion gap.

If an anion gap acidosis is present, the ratio of the change in the anion gap (the delta gap) to the change in HCO_3^- can be helpful in determining the type of disturbances present:

$$\frac{\Delta\text{gap}}{\Delta HCO_3^-}=\frac{\text{Anion gap}-12}{24-[HCO_3^-]}$$

In simple anion gap metabolic acidosis, the ratio approximates 1.0, since the decrease in bicarbonate equals the increase in anions. The delta gap for the patient with diabetes and ketoacidosis previously described is calculated as follows:

$$\begin{aligned}\frac{\Delta\text{gap}}{\Delta HCO_3^-}&=\frac{\text{Anion gap}-12}{24-[HCO_3^-]}\\ &=\frac{23-12}{24-14}\\ &=\frac{11}{10}=1.1\end{aligned}$$

The delta gap is 0 when the acidosis is a pure non-anion gap acidosis. A delta gap of 0.3–0.7 is associated with one of two mixed metabolic disorders: (i) a high anion gap acidosis and respiratory alkalosis and (ii) high anion gap with a pre-existing normal or low anion gap. A ratio greater than 1.2 implies a metabolic alkalosis superimposed on a high anion gap acidosis or a mixed high anion gap acidosis and chronic respiratory acidosis. The use of the delta gap is, however, limited by the wide range of normal values for the anion gap and bicarbonate, and its accuracy has been questioned [69].

When a normal anion gap metabolic acidosis is present, the urinary anion gap may be helpful in distinguishing the cause of the acidosis:

$$\text{urinary anion gap}=[\text{urine } Na^+]+[\text{urine } K^+]-[\text{urine } Cl^-]$$

The urinary anion gap is a clinically useful method to estimate urinary ammonium (NH_4^+) excretion. Since the amount of NH_4^+ excreted in the urine cannot be directly measured, the urinary anion gap helps determine whether the kidney is responding appropriately to a metabolic acidosis [70]. Normally, the urine anion gap is positive or close to zero. A negative gap ($Cl^- > Na^+$ and K^+) occurs with gastrointestinal bicarbonate loss and NH_4^+ excretion by the kidney increases appropriately. In contrast, a positive gap ($Cl^- < Na^+$ and K^+) in a patient with acidosis suggests impaired distal urinary acidification with inappropriately low NH_4^+ excretion.

A variety of processes can lead to metabolic acidosis and therapy will depend on the underlying condition. Adequate oxygenation should be ensured and mechanical ventilation instituted for impending respiratory failure. The use of bicarbonate solutions to correct acidosis has been suggested when arterial pH is less than 7.10 or bicarbonate is lower than 5 mEq/L. Bicarbonate solutions must be administered with caution since an "overshoot" alkalosis can lower seizure threshold, impair oxygen availability to peripheral tissues, and stimulate additional lactate production.

Metabolic alkalosis

Metabolic alkalosis is characterized by a rise in serum bicarbonate concentration and an elevated arterial pH. The most impressive clinical effects of metabolic alkalosis are neurologic and include confusion, obtundation, and tetany. Cardiac arrhythmias, hypotension, hypoventilation and various metabolic aberrations may accompany these neurologic changes.

Metabolic alkalosis results from a loss of acid or the addition of alkali. The development of metabolic alkalosis occurs in two phases, with the initial addition or generation of HCO_3^- followed by the inability of the kidney to excrete the excess HCO_3^-. The two most common causes of metabolic alkalosis are excessive loss of gastric secretions and diuretic administration. Once established, volume contraction, hypercapnea, hypokalemia, glucose loading, and acute hypercalcemia promote HCO_3^- reabsorption by the kidney and sustain the alkalosis.

The degree of respiratory compensation for metabolic alkalosis is more variable than with metabolic acidosis, and formulas to estimate the expected P_aCO_2 have not proven useful [56]. Alkalosis tends to cause hypoventilation but P_aCO_2 rarely exceeds 55 mmHg [56,71]. Tissue and red blood cells attempt to lower HCO_3^- by exchanging intracellular H^+ ions for extracellular Na^+ and K^+.

Once metabolic alkalosis is diagnosed, determination of urinary chloride concentration can be helpful in determining the etiology (Figure 5.6). Urinary chloride is a more reliable indicator of volume status than urinary sodium concentration in this group of patients. Sodium is excreted in the urine with bicarbonate to maintain electroneutrality and occurs independently of volume status. Therefore, low urinary chloride in patients with volume contraction accurately reflects sodium chloride retention by the kidney.

A urinary chloride concentration <10 mEq/L that improves with sodium chloride administration is a chloride-responsive metabolic alkalosis. In contrast, a urine chloride >20 mEq/L indicates that the alkalosis will not improve with saline administration and is a chloride-resistant alkalosis. Urine chloride levels must be interpreted with caution since levels are falsely elevated when obtained within several hours of diuretic administration.

Treatment of metabolic alkalosis is aimed at eliminating excess bicarbonate and reversing factors responsible for maintaining the alkalosis. If the urinary chloride level indicates a responsive disorder, infusion of sodium chloride will correct the abnormality. Conversely, saline administration will not correct a chloride resistant disorder and can be harmful. Treatment of the primary disease will concurrently correct the alkalosis. Although mild alkalemia is generally well tolerated, critically ill surgical patients with a pH ≥ 7.55 have increased mortality [72,73].

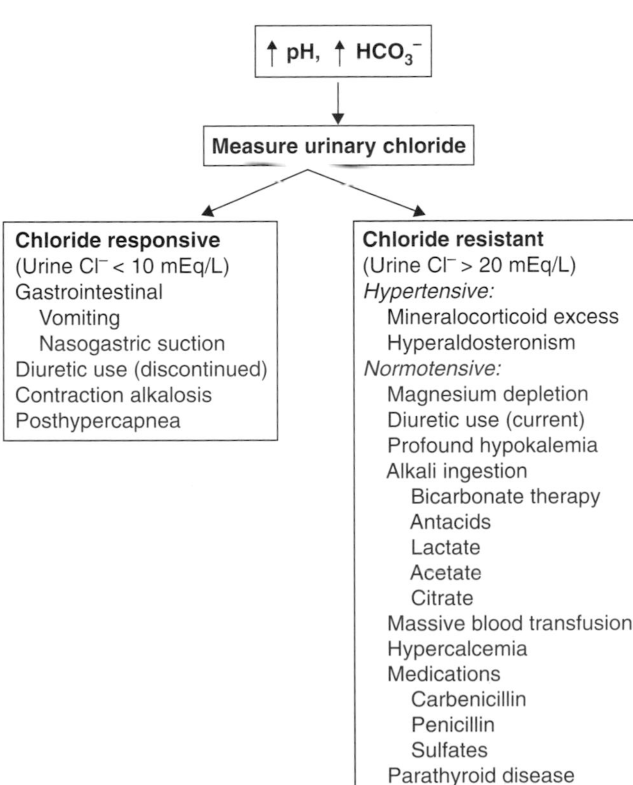

Figure 5.6 Etiology and evaluation of metabolic alkalosis.

Respiratory acidosis

Respiratory acidosis is characterized by hypercapnea (a rise in PCO_2) and a decreased arterial pH. The development of respiratory acidosis indicates the failure of carbon dioxide excretion to match CO_2 production. A variety of disorders can contribute to this acid–base abnormality (Table 5.4). It is important to remember that the normal PCO_2 in pregnancy is 30 mmHg, and normative data for non-pregnant patients do not apply to the gravida.

The clinical manifestations of acute respiratory acidosis are particularly evident in the central nervous system. Since carbon dioxide readily penetrates the blood–brain barrier and cerebrospinal fluid buffering capacity is not as great as blood, PCO_2 elevations quickly decrease the pH of the brain. Thus, neurologic compromise may be more significant with respiratory acidosis than metabolic acidosis [59]. Acute hypercapnia also decreases

Table 5.4 Causes of respiratory acidosis.

Airway obstruction
Aspiration
Laryngospasm
Severe bronchospasm
Impaired ventilation
Pneumothorax
Hemothorax
Severe pneumonia
Pulmonary edema
Adult respiratory distress syndrome
Circulatory collapse
Massive pulmonary embolism
Cardiac arrest
CNS depression
Medication
Sedatives
Narcotics
Cerebral infarct, trauma or encephalopathy
Obesity–hypoventilation syndrome
Neuromuscular disease
Myasthenic crisis
Severe hypokalemia
Guillain–Barré
Medication

cerebral vascular resistance, leading to increased cerebral blood flow and intracranial pressure.

The compensatory response depends on the duration of the respiratory acidosis. In acute respiratory acidosis, the respiratory center is stimulated to increase ventilation. Carbon dioxide is neutralized in erythrocytes by hemoglobin and other buffers, and bicarbonate is generated. An acute disturbance implies that renal compensation is not yet complete. Sustained respiratory acidosis (longer than 6–12 hours) stimulates the kidney to increase acid excretion, but this mechanism usually requires 3–5 days for full compensation [74].

The primary goal in the management of respiratory acidosis is to improve alveolar ventilation and decrease arterial PCO_2. Assessment and support of pulmonary function are paramount when a patient has respiratory acidosis. Carbon dioxide accumulates rapidly, and PCO_2 rises 2–3 mmHg/min in a patient with apnea. The underlying condition should be rapidly corrected and may include relief of an airway obstruction or pneumothorax, administration of bronchodilator therapy, narcotic reversal, or a diuretic.

Adequate oxygenation is crucial because hypoxemia is more life-threatening than hypercapnia. In the pregnant patient, hypoxemia also compromises the fetus. Uterine perfusion should be optimized and maternal oxygenation ensured since the combination of maternal hypoxemia and uterine artery hypoperfusion profoundly affects the fetus. When a patient cannot maintain adequate ventilation despite aggressive support, endotracheal intubation and mechanical ventilation should be performed without delay.

Table 5.5 Causes of respiratory alkalosis.

Pulmonary disease
Pneumonia
Pulmonary embolism
Pulmonary congestion
Asthma
Drugs
Salicylates
Xanthines
Nicotine
CNS disorders
Voluntary hyperventilation
Anxiety
Neurologic disease
Infection
Trauma
Cerebrovascular accident
Tumor
Other causes
Pregnancy
Pain
Sepsis
Hepatic failure
Iatrogenic mechanical hyperventilation

Respiratory alkalosis

Respiratory alkalosis is characterized by hypocapnea (decreased PCO_2) and an increased arterial pH. Acute hypocapnea frequently is accompanied by striking clinical symptoms, including paresthesias, circumoral numbness, and confusion. Tachycardia, chest tightness, and decreased cerebral blood flow are some of the prominent cardiovascular effects. Chronic respiratory alkalosis, however, is usually asymptomatic.

Respiratory alkalosis is the result of increased alveolar ventilation (Table 5.5). Hyperventilation can develop from stimulation of brainstem or peripheral chemoreceptors and nociceptive lung receptors. Higher brain centers can override chemoreceptors and occurs with involuntary hyperventilation. Respiratory alkalosis is commonly encountered in critically ill patients in response to hypoxemia or acidosis, or secondary to central nervous system dysfunction.

The compensatory response is divided into acute and chronic phases. In acute alkalosis, there is an instantaneous decrease in H^+ ion concentration due to tissue and red blood cell buffer release of H^+ ions. If the duration of hypocapnea is greater than a few hours, renal excretion of bicarbonate is increased and acid excretion is decreased. This response requires at least several days to reach a steady state. Chronic respiratory alkalosis is the only acid–base disorder in which the compensatory response can return the pH to normal.

Respiratory alkalosis may be diagnostic of an underlying condition and is usually corrected with treatment of the primary problem. Hypocapnea itself is not life-threatening but the disease causing the alkalosis may be. The presence of respiratory alkalosis should always raise suspicion for hypoxemia, pulmonary embolism, or sepsis. These conditions, however, can be overlooked if the only concern is correction of the alkalosis. Mechanical ventilation may lead to iatrogenic respiratory alkalosis and the PCO_2 can usually be corrected by lowering the machine-set respiratory rate. [75]

References

1 Kruse JA. Acid–base interpretations. *Crit Care* 1993; 14: 275.

2 MacRae DJ, Palavradji. Maternal acid–base changes in pregnancy. *J Obstet Gynaecol Br Cwlth* 1967; 74: 11.

3 Hankins GDV, Harvey CJ, Clark SL, Uckan EM. The effects of maternal position and cardiac output on intrapulmonary shunt in normal third-trimester pregnancy. *Obstet Gynecol* 1996; 88: 327.

4 Cruikshank DP, Hays PM. Maternal physiology in pregnancy. In: Gabbe S, Niebyl J, Simpson JL, eds. *Obstetrics: Normal and Problem Pregnancies*, 2nd edn. New York: Churchill Livingstone, 1991: 129.

5 Artal R, Wiswell R, Romem Y, Dorey F. Pulmonary responses to exercise in pregnancy. *Am J Obstet Gynecol* 1986; 154: 378.

6 Liberatore SM, Pistelli R, Patalano F et al. Respiratory function during pregnancy. *Respiration* 1984; 46: 145.

7 Andersen GJ, James GB, Mathers NP et al. The maternal oxygen tension and acid–base status during pregnancy. *J Obstet Gynaecol Br Cwlth* 1969; 76: 16.

8 Dayal P, Murata Y, Takamura H. Antepartum and postpartum acid–base changes in maternal blood in normal and complicated pregnancies. *J Obstet Gynaecol Br Cwlth* 1972; 79: 612.

9 Templeton A, Kelman GR. Maternal blood-gases, (PA|d2dend-Pa|d2dend (Maternal blood-gases, PaO2–PaO2, physiological shunt and VD/VT in normal pregnancy) physiological shunt and V|dDdend/V|dTdend in normal pregnancy. *Br J Anaesth* 1976; 48: 1001.

10 Pernoll ML, Metcalfe J, Kovach PA et al. Ventilation during rest and exercise in pregnancy and postpartum. *Respir Physiol* 1975; 25: 295.

11 Awe RJ, Nicotra MB, Newsom TD, Viles R. Arterial oxygenation and alveolar-arterial gradients in term pregnancy. *Obstet Gynecol* 1979; 53: 182.

12 Hankins GDV, Clark SL, Uckan EM et al. Third trimester arterial blood gas and acid–base values in normal pregnancy at moderate altitude. *Obstet Gynecol* 1996; 88: 347.

13 Sobrevilla LA, Cassinelli MT, Carcelen A et al. Human fetal and maternal oxygen tension and acid–base status during delivery at high altitude. *Am J Obstet Gynecol* 1971; 111: 1111.

14 Novy MJ, Edwards MJ. Respiratory problems in pregnancy. *Am J Obstet Gynecol* 1967; 99: 1024.

15 Weinberger SE, Weiss ST, Cohen WR et al. Pregnancy and the lung. *Am Rev Respir Dis* 1980; 121: 559.

16 Lucius H, Gahlenbeck H, Kleine HO et al. Respiratory functions, buffer system, and electrolyte concentrations of blood during human pregnancy. *Respir Physiol* 1970; 9: 311.

17 Cain SM. Peripheral uptake and delivery in health and disease. *Clin Chest Med* 1983; 4: 139.

18 Stock MC, Shapiro BA, Cane RD. Reliability of SvO_2 in predicting A-VDO_2 and the effect of anemia. *Crit Care Med* 1986; 14: 402.

19 Bryan-Brown CW, Back SM, Malcabalig et al. Consumable oxygen: oxygen availability in relation to oxyhemoglobin dissociation. *Crit Care Med* 1973; 1: 17.

20 Perutz MF. Hemoglobin structure and respiratory transport. *Sci Ann* 1978; 239: 92.

21 Rackow EC, Astiz M. Pathophysiology and treatment of septic shock. *JAMA* 1991; 266: 548.

22 Shoemaker WC, Ayers S, Grenuik A et al. *Textbook of Critical Care*, 2nd edn. Philadelphia: WB Saunders, 1989.

23 Shibutani K, Komatsu T, Kubal K et al. Critical levels of oxygen delivery in anesthetical man. *Crit Care Med* 1983; 11: 640.

24 Barron W, Lindheimer M. *Medical Disorders During Pregnancy*, 1st edn. Mosby-Year Book, St Louis, 1991: 234.

25 Gemzell CA, Robbe H, Strom G et al. Observations on circulatory changes and muscular work in normal labor. *Acta Obstet Gynecol Scand* 1957; 36: 75.

26 Ueland K, Hansen JM. Maternal cardiovascular hemodynamics: II. Posture and uterine contractions. *Am J Obstet Gynecol* 1969; 103: 1.

27 Walton JR, Shapiro BA, Wine C. Pre-analytic error in arterial blood gas measurement. *Respir Care* 1981; 26: 1136.

28 Bloom SA, Canzanello VJ, Strom JA, Madias NE. Spurious assessment of acid–base status due to dilutional effect of heparin. *Am J Med* 1985; 79: 528.

29 New W. Pulse oximetry. *J Clin Monit* 1985; 1: 126.

30 Al-Ameri MW, Kruse JA, Carlson RW. Blood sampling from arterial catheters: minimum discard volume to achieve accurate laboratory results. *Crit Care Med* 1986; 14: 399.

31 Bhaskaran NC, Lawler PG. How much blood for a blood gas? *Anesthesiology* 1988; 43: 811.

32 Biswas CK, Ramos JM, Agroyannis B, Kerr DNS. Blood gas analysis: effect of air bubbles in syringe and delay in estimation. *Br Med J* 1982; 284: 923.

33 Morganroth ML. Six steps to acid–base analysis: clinical applications. *J Crit Ill* 1990; 5: 460.

34 Harsten A, Berg B, Inerot S, Muth L. Importance of correct handling of samples for the results of blood gas analysis. *Acta Anesthesiol Scand* 1988; 32: 365.

35 Mueller RG, Lang GE. Blood gas analysis: effect of air bubbles in syringe and delay in estimation. *Br Med J* 1982; 285: 1659.

36 Madiedo G, Sciacca R, Hause L. Air bubbles and temperature effect on blood gas analysis. *J Clin Pathol* 1980; 33: 864.

37 Schuch CS, Price JG. Determination of time required for blood gas homeostasis in the intubated, post-open-heart *surgery* adult following a ventilator change. *NTI Res Abs* 1986; 15: 314.

38 McHugh RD, Epstein RM, Longnecker DE. Halothane mimics oxygen in oxygen microelectrodes. *Anesthesiology* 1979; 50: 47.

39 Douglas IHS, McKenzie PJ, Ledingham IM, Smith G. Effect of halothane on PO_2 electrode. *Lancet* 1978; 2: 1370.

40 Maekawa T, Okuda Y, McDowall DG. Effect of low concentrations of halothane on the oxygen electrode. *Br J Anaesth* 1980; 52: 585.

41 Dent JG, Netter KJ. Errors in oxygen tension measurements caused by halothane. *Br J Anaesth* 1976; 48: 195.

42 Hess CE, Nichols AB, Hunt WB. Pseudohypoxemia secondary to leukemia and thrombocytopenia. *N Engl J Med* 1979; 301: 363.

43 Nearman HS, Sampliner JE. Respiratory monitoring. In: Berk JL, Sampliner JE, eds. *Handbook of critical care*, 3rd edn. Boston: Little Brown, 1982: 125–143.

44 Demling BK, Knox JB. Basic concepts of lung function and dysfunction: oxygenation, ventilation and mechanics. *New Horiz* 1993; 1: 362.

45 Huch A, Huch R, Konig V et al. Limitations of pulse oximetry. *Lancet* 1988; 1: 357.

46 Dildy GA, Loucks CA, Porter TF, Sullivan CA, Belfort MA, Clark SL. *Many normal pregnant women residing at moderate altitude have lower arterial oxygen saturations than expected*. Society for Gynecologic Investigation, Atlanta, GA, March 1998.

47 Dildy GA, Sullivan CA, Moore LG, Richlin ST, Loucks CA, Belfort MA, Clark SL. *Altitude reduces and pregnancy increases maternal arterial oxygen saturation*. Society for Maternal-Fetal Medicine, San Francisco, CA, January 1999.

48 Richlin S, Cusick W, Sullivan C, Dildy GA, Belfort MA. *Normative oxygen saturation values for pregnant women at sea level*. The American College of Obstetricians and Gynecologists, New Orleans, LA, May 1998.

49 Goldberg M, Green SB, Moss ML et al. Computer-based instruction and diagnosis of acid–base disorders. *JAMA* 1973; 223: 269.

50 Davenport HW. Normal acid–base paths. In: *The ABC of Acid–Base Chemistry*, 6th edn. Chicago: University of Chicago Press, 1974: 69.

51 Arbus GS. An in vivo acid–base nomogram for clinical use. *Can Med Assoc J* 1973; 109: 291.

52 Cogan MJ. In: Brenner BM, Rector FC Jr, eds. *The Kidney*, 3rd edn. Philadelphia: WB Saunders, 1986: 473.

53 Haber RJ. A practical approach to acid–base disorders. *West J Med* 1991; 155: 146.

54 Ghosh AK. Diagnosing acid-base disorders. *J Assoc Physicians India* 2006;54:720–724.

55 Tremper KK, Barker SJ. Blood-gas analysis. In: Hall JB, Schmidt GA, Wood LDH, eds. *Principles of Critical Care*. New York: McGraw-Hill, 1992: 181–196.

56 Narins RG. Acid–base disorders: definitions and introductory concepts. In: Narins RG, ed. *Clinical Disorders of Fluid and Electrolyte Metabolism*, 5th edn. New York: McGraw-Hill, 1994: 755–767.

57 Morganroth ML. An analytic approach to diagnosing acid–base disorders. *J Crit Ill* 1990; 5: 138.

58 Cane RD, Shapiro BA, Templin R, Walther K. Unreliability of oxygen tension-based indices in reflecting intrapulmonary shunting in critically ill patients. *Crit Care Med* 1988; 16: 1243.

59 Wilson RF. Acid–base problems. *In: Critical Care Manual: Applied Physiology and Principles of Therapy*, 2nd edn. Philadelphia: FA Davis, 1992: 715–756.

60 Shapiro BA, Peruzzi WT. Blood gas analysis. In: Civetta J, Taylor R, Kirby J, eds. *Critical Care*, 2nd edn. Philadelphia: Lippincott, 1992: 325–342.

61 Narins RG, Emmett M. Simple and mixed acid–base disorders: a practical approach. *Medicine* 1980; 59: 161.

62 Shapiro BA, Peruzzi WT. Interpretation of blood gases. In: Ayers SM, Grenvik A, Holbrook PR, Shoemaker WC, eds. *Textbook of Critical Care*, 3rd edn. Philadelphia: WB Saunders, 1995: 278–294.

63 Kruse JA, Hukku P, Carlson RW. Relationship between the apparent dissociation constant of blood carbonic acid and severity of illness. *J Lab Clin Med* 1989; 114: 568.

64 Kruse JA. Calculation of plasma bicarbonate concentration versus measurement of serum CO_2 content. pK` revisited. *Clin Int Care* 1995; 6: 15.

65 Battle DC, Hizon M, Cohen E et al. The use of the urinary anion gap in the diagnosis of hyperchloremic metabolic acidosis. *N Engl J Med* 1988; 318: 594.

66 Preuss HG. Fundamentals of clinical acid–base evaluation. *Clin Lab Med* 1993; 13: 103.

67 Kruse JA. Use of the anion gap in intensive care and emergency medicine. In: Vincent MJ, ed. *Yearbook of intensive care and emergency medicine*. New York: Springer, 1994: 685–696.

68 Oh MS, Carroll HJ. Current concepts: the anion gap. *N Engl J Med* 1977; 297: 814.

69 Salem MM, Mujais SK. Gaps in the anion gap. *Arch Intern Med* 1992; 152: 1625.

70 Halperin ML, Richardson RMA, Bear RA et al. Urine ammonium: the key to the diagnosis of distal renal tubular acidosis. *Nephron* 1988; 50: 1.

71 Wilson RF. Blood gases: pathophysiology and interpretation. In: *Critical Care Manual: Applied Physiology and Principles of Therapy*, 2nd edn. Philadelphia: FA Davis, 1992: 389–421.

72 Wilson RF, Gibson D, Percinel AK et al. Severe alkalosis in critically ill surgical patients. *Arch Surg* 1972; 105: 197.

73 Rimmer JM, Gennari FJ. Metabolic alkalosis. *J Intensive Care Med* 1987; 2: 137.

74 Nanji AA, Whitlow KJ. Is it necessary to transport arterial blood samples on ice for pH and gas analysis? *Can Anaesth Soc J* 1984; 31: 568.

75 Ng RH, Dennis RC, Yeston N et al. Factitious cause of unexpected arterial blood-gas results. *N Engl J Med* 1984; 310: 1189.

6 Fluid and Electrolyte Balance

William E. Scorza[1] & Anthony Scardella[2]

[1]Division of Maternal–Fetal Medicine, Department of Obstetrics, Lehigh Valley Hospital, Allentown, PA, USA
[2]University of Medicine and Dentistry, Robert Wood Johnson Medical School, New Brunswick, NJ, USA

The physiologic effects of pregnancy on normal fluid dynamics and renal function

The infusion of fluid remains a cornerstone of therapy when treating critically ill pregnant women with hypovolemia. An understanding of the distribution and pharmacokinetics of plasma expanders, as well as knowledge of normal renal function and fluid dynamics during pregnancy, is needed to allow for prompt resuscitation of patients in various forms of shock, as well as to provide maintenance therapy for other critically ill patients.

The total body water (TBW) ranges from 45% to 65% of total body weight in the human adult. TBW is distributed between two major compartments, the intracellular fluid (ICF) space and the extracellular fluid (ECF) space. Two-thirds of the TBW resides in the ICF space and one-third in the ECF space. The ECF is further subdivided into the interstitial and intravascular spaces in a ratio of 3 : 1. Regulation of the ICF is mostly achieved by changes in water balance, whereas the changes in plasma volume are related to the regulation of sodium balance. Because water can freely cross most cell membranes, the osmolalities within each compartment are the same. When water is added into one compartment, it distributes evenly throughout the TBW, and the amount of volume added to any given compartment is proportional to its fractional representation of the TBW. Infusions of fluids that are isotonic with plasma are distributed initially within the ECF; however, only one-fourth of the infused volume remains in the intravascular space after 30 minutes. Because most fluids are a combination of free water and isotonic fluids, one can predict the space of distribution and thus the volume transfused into each compartment.

During pregnancy, the ECF accumulates 6–8 L of extra fluid, with the plasma volume increasing by 50% [1]. Both plasma and red cell volumes increase during pregnancy. The plasma volume increases slowly but to a greater extent than the increase in total blood volume during the first 30 weeks of pregnancy and is then maintained at that level until term [2]. The plasma volume to ECF ratio is also increased in pregnancy [3]. Plasma volume is increased by a greater fraction in multiple pregnancies [4,5], with the increase being proportional to the number of fetuses [6]). Reduced plasma volume expansion has been shown to occur in pregnancies complicated by fetal growth restriction [7,8], hypertensive disorders [3,4,9,10,11,12], prematurity [11,13], oligohydramnios [11,14], and maternal smoking [15]. In pregnancy-induced hypertension the total ECF is unchanged [3,16], supporting an altered distribution of ECF between the two compartments, possibly secondary to the rise in capillary permeability. A similar mechanism may occur in other conditions in which the plasma volume is reduced; the clinician needs to be cognizant of this when choosing fluids for resuscitation. Blood volume decreases over the first 24 hours postpartum [17]), with non-pregnant levels reached at 6–9 weeks postpartum [18]. With intrapartum hemorrhage, ICF can be mobilized to restore the plasma volume [17]).

Red cell mass increases about 24% during the course of pregnancy [5]. A physiologic hemodilution and relative anemia of pregnancy occur because the rise in plasma volume exceeds the increase in red cell mass. The decrease in the hematocrit is characterized by a gradual fall until week 30, followed by a gradual rise afterward [19]. This is also associated with a decrease in whole blood viscosity, which may be beneficial for intervillous perfusion [20]. With hemorrhagic shock and mobilization of fluid from the ICF, the hematocrit, and thus oxygen-carrying capacity, would be further reduced, requiring replacement with appropriate fluids.

The glomerular filtration rate (GFR) increases during pregnancy, and peaks approximately 50% above non-pregnant levels by 9–11 weeks gestation. This level is sustained until the 36th week [21]. The cause of this increase in GFR is unknown. Postulated mechanisms include an increased plasma and ECF volume, a fall in intrarenal oncotic pressure due to decreased albumin, and an increased level of a number of hormones including prolactin [22,23,24].

Critical Care Obstetrics, 5th edition. Edited by M. Belfort, G. Saade, M. Foley, J. Phelan and G. Dildy.

Table 6.1 Characteristics of various volume-expanding agents.

Agent	Na^+ (mEq/L)	Cl^- (mEq/L)	Lactate (mEq/L)	Osmolarity (mosmol/L)	Oncotic pressure (mmHg)
Ringer's lactate	130	109	28	275	0
Normal saline	154	154	0	310	0
Albumin (5%)	130–160	130–160	0	310	20
Hetastarch (6%)	154	154	0	310	30

Several aspects of tubular function are affected during pregnancy. Sodium retention occurs throughout pregnancy. The total amount of sodium retained during the course of pregnancy is approximately 950 mEq. A number of factors may contribute to the enhanced sodium reabsorption seen in pregnant patients. Increased levels of aldosterone, deoxycortisone, progesterone, and plactental lactogen as well as decreased plasma albumin have all been implicated [21]. The tendency to retain sodium is offset in part by factors that favor sodium excretion in pregnancy, among which the most important is a higher GFR. Heightened levels of progesterone favor sodium excretion by competitive inhibition of aldosterone [25]. Increased calcium absorption from the small intestine occurs in order to meet the increased needs of the pregnant woman for calcium. Calcium excretion does increase during pregnancy, serum calcium and albumin are both decreased, but total ionized calcium remains unchanged. During the first and second trimester plasma uric acid levels decrease but gradually reach prepregnancy values in the third trimester.

The effects of pregnancy on acid–base balance are well known. There is a partially compensated respiratory alkalosis that begins early in pregnancy and is sustained throughout. The expected reduction in arterial PCO_2 is to about 30 mmHg with a concomitant rise in the arterial pH to approximately 7.44 [26]. The pH is maintained in this range by increased bicarbonate excretion that keeps serum bicarbonate levels between 18 and 21 mEq/L [26]. The chronic hyperventilation seen in pregnancy is thought to be secondary to increased levels of circulating progesterone, which may act directly on brainstem respiratory neurons [27].

Fluid resuscitation

Controversy exists as to the appropriate intravenous (IV) solutions to use in the management of hypovolemic shock. As long as physiologic endpoints are used to guide therapy and adjustments are made based on the individual's needs, side effects associated with inadequate or overaggressive resuscitation can be avoided. In most types of critical illness, intravascular volume is decreased. Hemorrhagic shock has been shown to deplete the ECF compartment with an increase in intracellular water secondary to cell membrane and sodium–potassium pump dysfunction [28–31]. After trauma, surgical patients are found to have an expanded ECF, while the intravascular volume is depleted [32]. Most available studies of fluid balance have been conducted in patients in the non-pregnant state; very little data exist documenting these changes in pregnant women. Whatever the underlying pathology, intravascular volume is decreased in many types of critical illness. Successful resuscitation thus remains dependent on the prompt restoration of intravascular volume.

Crystalloid solutions

The most commonly employed crystalloid products for fluid resuscitation are 0.9% saline and lactated Ringer's solutions. The contents of normal saline and Ringer's lactate solutions are shown in Table 6.1. These are isotonic solutions that distribute evenly throughout the extracellular space but will not promote ICF shifts.

Isotonic crystalloids

Isotonic crystalloid solutions are generally readily available, easily stored, non-toxic, and reaction-free. They are an inexpensive form of volume resuscitation. The infusion of large volumes of 0.9% saline and Ringer's lactate is not a problem clinically; when administered in large volumes to patients with traumatic shock, acidosis does not occur [33]. The excess circulating chloride ion resulting from saline infusion is excreted readily by the kidney. In a similar manner, the lactate load in Ringer's solution does not potentiate the lactacidemia associated with shock [34], nor has it been shown to effect the reliability of blood lactate measurements [33].

Using the Starling–Landis–Staverman equation for fluid flux across a microvascular wall, one can predict that crystalloids will distribute rapidly between the ICF and ECF. Equilibration within the extracellular space occurs within 20–30 minutes after infusion. In healthy non-pregnant adults, approximately 25% of the volume infused remains in the intravascular space after 1 hour. In the critically ill or injured patient, however, only 20% or less of the infusion remains in the circulation after 1–2 hours [35,36]. The volemic effects of various crystalloid solutions compared with albumin and whole blood are shown in Table 6.2. At equivalent volumes, crystalloids are less effective than colloids for expansion of the intravascular volume. Two to 12 times the volume of crystalloids are necessary to achieve similar hemodynamic and volemic endpoints [30,36–40]. The rapid equilibration between the ICF and ECF seen with crystalloid infusion

Table 6.2 Typical volemic effects of various resuscitative fluids after 1-L infusion.

Fluid*	ICV (mL)	ECV (mL)	IV (mL)	PV (mL)
0.5% Dextrose/water	660	340	255	85
Normal saline or lactated Ringer's	−100	1100	825	275
Albumin	0	1000	500	500
Whole blood	0	1000	0	1000

* Based on infusion of 1L volumes.

ECV, extracellular volume; IV, interstitial volume; IVC, intracellular volume; PV, plasma volume.

(From Carlson RW, Rattan S, Haupt M. Fluid resuscitation in conditions of increased permeability. *Anesth Rev* 1990; 17(suppl 3): 14.)

reduces the incidence of pulmonary edema [41,42], whereas exogenous colloid administration promotes the accumulation of interstitial fluid [43,44].

Indications

Shock

Crystalloids–either normal saline or Ringer's lactate–are used to replenish plasma volume deficits and replace fluid and electrolyte losses from the interstitium [32,40,45–48]. Patients in shock from any cause should receive immediate volume replacement with crystalloid solution during the initial clinical evaluation. Aggressive administration of crystalloid may promptly restore blood pressure and peripheral perfusion. Given in a quantity of 3–4 times the amount of blood lost, they can adequately replace an acute loss of up to 20% of the blood volume, although 3–5 L of crystalloid may be required to replace a 1 L blood loss [43,48–51]. After the initial resuscitation with crystalloid, the selection of fluids becomes controversial, especially if microvascular integrity is not preserved (as in sepsis, burns, trauma, and anaphylaxis). Further fluid resuscitation should be guided by continuous bedside observation of urine output, mental status, heart rate, pulse pressure, respiratory rate, blood pressure, and temperature monitoring, together with serial measurements of hematocrit, serum albumin, platelet count, prothrombin, and partial thromboplastin times. More aggressive monitoring is required in patients who remain in shock or fail to respond to the initial resuscitatory efforts and in patients with poor physiologic reserve who are unlikely to tolerate imprecisions in resuscitation efforts.

Diagnosis of oliguria

In critically ill patients, it is often extremely difficult to distinguish volume depletion from congestive heart failure (CHF). Because prerenal hypoperfusion resulting in a urine output of less than 0.5 mL/kg/h can result in renal failure, it is extremely important to separate the two conditions and treat accordingly. An adequate fluid challenge consists of at least 500 mL of Ringer's lactate or normal saline administered over 5–10 minutes. Increasing the patient's IV infusion rate to 200 mL/h or giving the bolus over 30 minutes or longer will not expand the intravascular volume sufficiently to help differentiate the etiology or treat the volume depletion. If there is no response from the initial fluid challenge, one may repeat it. If no increase in urine output occurs, one is probably not dealing with intravascular depletion, and further fluid management should be guided by invasive monitoring with a pulmonary artery catheter or repetitive echocardiograms. Patients with CHF do not experience a prolonged increase in vascular volume because crystalloid fluids distribute out of the intravascular space rapidly with only a transient increase in intravascular volume.

Side effects

Crystalloid solutions are generally non-toxic and free of side effects. However, fluid overload may result in pulmonary, cerebral, myocardial, mesenteric, and skin edema; hypoproteinemia; and altered tissue oxygen tension.

Pulmonary edema

Isotonic crystalloid resuscitation lowers the colloid oncotic pressure (COP) [52,53], although it is uncertain whether such alterations in COP actually worsen lung function [28,36,41,42]. The lung has a variety of mechanisms that act to prevent the development of pulmonary edema. These include increased lymphatic flow, diminished pulmonary interstitial oncotic pressure, and increased interstitial hydrostatic pressure. Together they limit the effect of the lowered COP [52]. In patients with intact microvascular integrity, studies have failed to demonstrate an increase in extravascular lung water after appropriate crystalloid loading [54]. Irrespective of the amount of fluid administered, strict attention to physiologic endpoints, and oxygenation are essential in order to prevent pulmonary edema.

Peripheral edema

Peripheral edema is a frequent side effect of fluid resuscitation but can be limited by appropriate monitoring of the resuscitatory effort. Excess peripheral edema may result in decreased oxygen tension in the soft tissue, promoting complications such as poor wound healing, skin breakdown, and infection [55–57]. Despite this, burn patients have shown improvement in survival after massive crystalloid resuscitation [58].

Bowel edema

Edema of the gastrointestinal system seen with aggressive crystalloid resuscitation may result in ileus and diarrhea, probably secondary to hypoalbuminemia [59]. This may be limited by monitoring of the COP and correction of hypo-oncotic states.

Central nervous system

Under normal circumstances, the brain is protected from volume-related injury by the blood–brain barrier and cerebral autoregulation. However, a patient in shock may have a primary or coincidental CNS injury, which may damage either or both of these protective mechanisms. In this situation, the COP and osmotic gradients should be monitored closely to prevent edema.

Colloid solutions

Colloids are large-molecular-weight substances to which cell membranes are relatively impermeable. They increase COP, resulting in the movement of fluid from the interstitial compartment to the intravascular compartment. Their ability to remain in the intravascular space prolongs their duration of action. The net result is a lower volume of infusate necessary to expand the intravascular space when compared with crystalloid solutions.

Albumin

Albumin is the colloidal agent against which all others are judged [60]. Albumin is produced in the liver and represents 50% of hepatic protein production [61]. It contributes to 70–80% of the serum COP [52,62]. A 50% reduction in the serum albumin concentration will lower the COP to one-third of normal [62]).

Albumin is a highly water-soluble polypeptide with a molecular weight ranging from 66300 to 69000 daltons [62] and is distributed unevenly between the intravascular (40%) and interstitial (60%) compartments [62]. The normal serum albumin concentration is maintained between 3.5 and 5 g/dL and is affected by albumin secretion, volume of distribution, rate of loss from the intravascular space, and degradation. The albumin level also is well correlated with nutritional status [63]. Hypoalbuminemia secondary to diminished production (starvation) or excess loss (hemorrhage) results in a decrease in its degradation and a compensatory increase in its distribution in the interstitial space [61,64]. In acute injury or stress with depletion of the intravascular compartment, interstitial albumin is mobilized and transported to the intravascular department by lymphatic channels or transcapillary refill [65]. Albumin synthesis is stimulated by thyroid hormone [66] and cortisol [67] and decreased by an elevated COP [68].

The capacity of albumin to bind water is related to the amount of albumin given as well as to the plasma volume deficit [67,69]. One gram of albumin increases the plasma volume by approximately 18 mL ([52,70,71]. Albumin is available as a 5% or 25% solution in isotonic saline. Thus, 100 mL of 25% albumin solution increases the intravascular volume by approximately 450 mL over 30–60 minutes [36]. With depletion of the ECF, this equilibration is not sufficiently brisk or complete unless supplementation with isotonic fluids is provided as part of the resuscitation regimen [52]. A 500-mL solution of 5% albumin containing 25 g of albumin will increase the intravascular space by 450 mL. In this instance, however, the albumin is administered in conjunction with the fluid to be retained.

Infused albumin has an initial plasma half-life of 16 hours, with 90% of the albumin dose remaining in the plasma 2 hours after administration [52,72]. The albumin equilibrates between the intravascular and interstitial compartments over a 7–10-day period [73], with 75% of the albumin being absent from the plasma in 2 days. In patients with shock, the administration of plasma albumin has been shown to significantly increase the COP for at least 2 days after resuscitation [53].

Indications

Albumin is used primarily for the resuscitation of patients with hypovolemic shock. In the United States, 26% of all albumin administered to patients is given to treat acute hypovolemia (surgical blood loss, trauma, hemorrhage) while an additional 12% is given to treat hypovolemia due to other causes, such as infection [74]. A major goal in the resuscitation of a patient in acute shock is to replace the intravascular volume in order to restore tissue perfusion. In patients with acute blood loss of greater than 30% of blood volume, it probably should be used early in conjunction with a crystalloid infusion to maintain peripheral perfusion. Treatment goals are to maintain a serum albumin of greater than 2.5 g/dL in the acute period of resuscitation. With non-edematous patients, 5% albumin and crystalloid can be used, but with edematous patients, 25% albumin may assist the patient in mobilizing her own interstitial volume. In patients with suspected loss of capillary wall integrity (especially in the lung in patients at risk for the subsequent development of acute respiratory distress syndrome), the use of albumin should be limited, because it crosses the capillary wall and exerts an oncotic influence in the interstitial space, worsening pulmonary edema. Albumin may be used in patients with burns [61] once capillary integrity is restored, approximately 24 hours after the initial event.

The use of albumin in patients with volume depletion regardless of the cause is not without controversy. In one meta-analysis of 30 relatively small randomized clinical trials comparing the use of albumin or plasma protein fraction with no administration or the administration of crystalloids in critically ill patients with hypovolemia or burns, the authors found no evidence that albumin decreased mortality [75]. A later meta-analysis of randomized clinical trials of albumin use found that in many trials included for analysis, problems with randomization were present. In addition there was significant heterogeneity among the various studies [76]. The authors of this study concluded that there was no hard evidence that albumin was beneficial. They surmised that albumin and large volume crystalloid infusions were equivalent in terms of mortality in critically ill patients. Finally, given the lack of data supporting a beneficial effect of albumin on mortality in critically ill patients, the cost of this therapy also becomes a factor. One study projected that compared to albumin, the use of the least expensive, fully approved colloid would save nearly $300 million per year in the United States [74].

Side effects

A number of potential adverse effects of albumin have been reported. This agent may accentuate respiratory failure and contribute to the development of pulmonary edema. However, the presence or absence of infection, together with the method of resuscitation and volumes used, affect respiratory function far more than the type of fluid infused [42,48,77–79]. Albumin may lower the serum ionized calcium concentration, resulting in a negative inotropic effect on the myocardium [44,80–82], and it may impair immune responsiveness. Infusion of albumin results in moderate to transient abnormalities in prothrombin time, partial thromboplastin time, and platelet counts [83]. However, the clinical implications of these defects, if any, are unknown. Albumin-induced anaphylaxis is reported in 0.47–1.53% of recipients [61]. These reactions are short-lived and include urticaria, chills, fever and rarely, hypertension. Although albumin is derived from pooled human plasma, there is no known risk of hepatitis or acquired immune deficiency syndrome. This is because it is heated and sterilized by ultrafiltration.

Hetastarch

Hetastarch is a synthetic colloid molecule that closely resembles glycogen. It is prepared by incorporating hydroxyethyl ether into the glucose residues of amylopectin [84]. Hetastarch is available clinically as a 6% solution in normal saline. The molecular weight of the particles is 480 000 daltons, with 80% of the molecules in the range of 30 000–2 400 000 daltons. Hetastarch is metabolized rapidly in the blood by alpha-amylase [85–87], with the rate of degradation dependent on the dose and the degree of glucose hydroxyethylation or substitution [87–89].

There is an almost immediate appearance of smaller-molecular-weight particles (molecular weight, 50 000 daltons or less) in the urine after IV infusion of hetastarch [90]. Forty per cent of this compound is excreted in the urine after 24 hours, with 46% excreted by 2 days and 64% by 8 days [86,91]. Bilirubin excretion accounts for less than 1% of total elimination in humans [92]. The larger particles are metabolized by the reticuloendothelial system [93–95] and remain in the body for an extended period [89,96]. Blood alpha-amylase also degrades larger particles to smaller starch polymers and free glucose. The smaller particles eventually are cleared through the urine and bowel. The amount of glucose thus produced does not cause significant hyperglycemia in a diabetic animal model [97]. The half-life of hetastarch represents a composite of the half-lives of the various-sized particles. Ninety per cent of a single infusion of hetastarch is removed from the circulation within 42 days, with a terminal half-life of 17 days [86].

Indications

Hetastarch is an effective long-acting plasma volume-expanding agent that can be used in patients suffering from shock secondary to hemorrhage, trauma, sepsis, and burns. It initially expands plasma volume by an amount equal to or greater than the volume infused [69,98,99]. The volume expansion seen after the infusion of hetastarch is equal to or greater than that produced by dextran 70 [94,100,101] or 5% albumin. The plasma volume remains 70% expanded for 3 hours after the infusion and 40% expanded for 12 hours after the infusion [94]. At 24 hours after infusion, the plasma volume expansion is approximately 28%, with 38% of the drug actually remaining intravascular [102]. The increase in intravascular volume has been associated with improvement in hemodynamic parameters in critically ill patients [91,103–105]. Hetastarch also has been shown to increase the COP to the same degree as albumin [53,105]. The maximum recommended daily dose for adults is 1500 mL/70kg of body weight.

Side effects

Starch infusions increase serum amylase levels two- to threefold. Peak levels occur 12–24 hours after infusion, with elevated levels present for 3 days or longer [90,106–108]. No alterations in normal pancreatic function have been noted [107]. Liver dysfunction with ascites secondary to intrahepatic obstruction after hetastarch infusions has been reported [44].

Hetastarch does not seem to promote histamine release [109] or to be immunogenic [110,111]. Anaphylactic reactions occur in less than 0.1% of the population, with shock or cardiopulmonary arrest occurring in 0.01% [92]. When given in doses below 1500 mL/day, hetastarch has not been associated with clinical bleeding, but minor alterations in laboratory measurements may be seen [100,112]. There is a transient decrease in the platelet count, prolonged prothrombin and partial thromboplastin times, acceleration of fibrinolysis, reduced levels of factor VIII, a decrease in the tensile clot strength and platelet adhesion, and an increased bleeding time [113–116]. Hetastarch-induced disseminated intravascular coagulation [117] and intracranial bleeding in patients with subarachnoid hemorrhage have been documented [118,119].

Electrolyte disorders

Although almost any metabolic disorder can occur coincidentally with pregnancy, there are a few electrolyte disturbances of special importance that can specifically complicate pregnancy such as:

- water intoxication (hyponatremia)
- hyperemesis gravidarum
- hypokalemia associated with betamimetic tocolysis
- hypocalcemia with magnesium sulfate treatment for pre-eclampsia
- hypermagnesemia in treatment for pre-eclampsia.

Physiologic control of volume and osmolarity

Under normal physiologic conditions sodium and water are major molecules responsible for determining volume and tonicity of the ECF. These are in turn controlled by the influence of the renin–angiotensin aldosterone system and the action of antidiuretic hormone (ADH) otherwise known as arginine vasopressin (AVP).

A decrease in ECF volume for any reason causes the juxtaglomerular complex in the kidney to sense a decrease in pressure resulting in an release of renin, which through angiotensin I and angiotensin II, stimulates the adrenal cortex to secrete aldosterone. This results in an increase in sodium reabsorption in the renal collecting tubule. Water follows the sodium, restoring the extracellular volume to normal.

When the osmolarity of the ECF increases above a predetermined set point (usually 280–300 mosmol/L), the posterior pituitary is stimulated via the hypothalamus to release AVP which acts at the level of the collecting tubule to maximally stimulate the reabsorption of water into the circulation. Three types of receptors have been identified for AVP. Receptors 1A are located in the smooth muscle of the endothelium and myocardium. Stimulation of these receptors causes vasoconstriction. Type 2 AVP receptors reside in the collecting tubule and stimulation of these receptors results in reabsorbtion of water. Receptors 1B in the anterior pituitary mediate the release of adrenocorticotropin [120]. The reabsorbed water dilutes the plasma solute, restoring normal tonicity. When osmolarity of the ECF decreases, AVP secretion is shut down and water reabsorption is inhibited. Therefore, normal tonicity is once again restored. Although this is the main regulatory mechanism for the control of osmolarity, there are other physiologic stimuli for controlling the secretion of AVP. Decreased blood pressure and decreased blood volume are problems commonly encountered in obstetric hemorrhage. These stimuli result in an increase in AVP. In addition, vomiting is also a potent stimulus for the release of AVP [121]. Pregnancy is associated with a decrease in tonicity and plasma osmolarity beginning in early gestation resulting in a new steady state. It appears that the osmotic threshold for release of AVP and thirst (which stimulates drinking and is another way of increasing ECF water) are decreased. In general, this leads to a decrease of about 10 mosmol/L below non-pregnant levels [122]. The serum osmolarity can be measured in the laboratory but it can also be estimated for clinical purposes. Sodium and the ions associated with it account for almost 95% of the solute in ECF. To estimate the plasma osmolarity the following formula can be used [121]:

$$P_{osm} = 2.1 \times \text{plasma sodium concentration.}$$

Disturbances in sodium metabolism

Hyponatremia

Hyponatremia is defined as plasma sodium concentration of less than 135 mEq/L. Lowering the plasma osmolarity results in water movement into cells, leading to cellular overhydration, which is responsible for most of the symptoms associated with this disorder. Hyponatremia occurs when there is the addition of free water to the body or an increased loss of sodium. After ingestion of the water load there is a fall in plasma osmolarity (P_{osm}) resulting in decreased secretion and synthesis of AVP. This leads to decreased water reabsorption in the collecting tubule, the production of dilute urine and rapid excretion of excess water. When the plasma sodium is less than 135 mEq/L and/or the P_{osm} is below 275 mosmol/kg, AVP secretion generally ceases. A defect in renal water excretion will thus lead to hyponatremia. A reduction in free water excretion is caused by either decreased generation of free water in the loop of Henle and distal tubule or enhanced water permeability of the collecting tubules due to the presence of AVP (see Table 6.3). Hyponatremia may occur with normal renal water excretion in primary polydipsia and in conditions where there is a resetting of the plasma osmostat, such as in psychosis and malnutrition [123]. Levels of atrial natriuretic peptide (ANP) and aldosterone lead to significant alteration in serum sodium excretion in twins as opposed to singleton pregnancy [124]. True hyponatremia may be accompanied by a normal plasma osmolality because of hyperglycemia, azotemia or after the administration of hypertonic mannitol [125].

Table 6.3 Common causes of decreased hyponatremia.

Hypovolemic hyponatremia
Gastrointestinal losses (vomiting, diarrhea)
Renal losses (salt wasting nephropathy, renal tubular acidosis)
Skin losses (burns)
Diuretics
Evolemic hyponatremia
Syndrome of inappropriate ADH secretion
Drugs (e.g. indomethacin, chlorpropanamide, barbiturates)
Tumors
CNS diseases
Physical and emotional distress
Glucocorticoid deficiency
Adrenal insufficiency
Hypothyroidism
Hypervolemic hyponatremia
Edematous states (heart failure, nephrotic syndrome, cirrhosis)

Etiology

Oxytocin is a polypeptide hormone secreted by the posterior pituitary. It differs from the other posterior pituitary polypeptide hormone, AVP, by only two amino acids. Although oxytocin serves an entirely different physiologic function, there is some AVP effect exerted by oxytocin. When oxytocin is infused at a rate of about 45 mU/min the antidiuretic effect is maximal and equal to the maximal effect of AVP. At a rate of 20 mU/min, the antidiuretic effect is about half the maximal effect of AVP [126,127]. When oxytocin is infused in high concentrations or for prolonged periods of time in dextrose 5% water (D5%W) or hypotonic solutions, oxytocin-induced water intoxication can occur. This provides a classic example of the clinical presentation of hyponatremia. The use of a balanced salt solution such as 0.9% normal saline as the vehicle for administration of oxytocin virtually eliminates the problem. Oxytocin infusion for the treatment of stillbirth, and prolonged induction of labor still results in this problem [128–130]. As of 2002, approximately 2% of hospitals in the United States [131] were still using D5%W to dilute oxytocin for infusion [132].

Hyperemesis is another example of a disorder unique to pregnancy that can lead to severe electrolyte disturbance. Hyperemesis gravidarum complicates between 0.3% and 2% of all pregnancies. It can result in depletion of sodium, potassium, chloride, and other electrolytes. Hyponatremia can occur in severe cases causing lethargy, seizures, and rarely Wernicke's encephalopathy. Wernicke's encephalopathy, secondary to thiamin deficiency, is characterized by confusion, ataxia, and abnormal eye movement. Overaggressive treatment of hyponatremia in these patients can lead to central pontine myelinolysis [133,134].

Rarely preeclampsia can present with hyponatremia as a result of SIADH or hypervolemic hyponatremia. The case reports more often involve twins but singleton pregnancys can also be affected. [135]

Postpartum hemorrhage severe enough to cause anterior pituitary necrosis, otherwise known as Sheehan's syndrome, has been associated with hyponatremia. The pituitary necrosis is associated with adrenocorticotropin deficiency and inappropriate antidiuretic hormone secretion. Hypothyroidism, which can also cause hyponatremia, may also play a part in the etiology [136].

Clinical presentation

Patients initially complain of headache, nausea, and vomiting, progressing to disorientation and obtundation, followed by seizure and coma. Hyponatremia may result in cerebral edema, permanent neurologic deficits, and death. The severity of the symptoms correlates with the degree of cerebral edema together with the speed at which this occurs, as well as the degree in reduction in the plasma sodium concentration [137,138] (see Table 6.4).

The diagnosis of hyponatremia is established through a good history and physical examination and appropriate laboratory tests. The history should focus on fluid volume losses such as vomiting and diarrhea and whether replacement fluids were hypotonic or isotonic. Symptoms of renal failure should be sought, as well as diuretic use or other medications including nicotine, tricyclic antidepressants, antipsychotic agents, antineoplastic drugs, narcotics, non-steroidal anti-inflammatory medications, methylxanthines, chlorpropamide, and barbiturates. Psychiatric history and an assessment of physical and emotional status is also important because compulsive water drinking may also cause hyponatremia. Laboratory evaluation should include serum electrolytes, BUN, creatinine, urinalysis with urine electrolytes, and an estimation of the serum osmolarity as described previously.

Pseudohyponatremia is a condition in which the measured serum Na^+ appears to be low but in fact the actual amount of sodium in the serum is unchanged. This happens when high amounts of large molecules which do not contribute to osmolality "dilute" the Na^+. This occurs most frequently with hyperlipidemia. The presence of a low plasma sodium and normal osmolarity suggests pseudohyponatremia but does not confirm it. The cause of pseudohyponatremia is investigated by examining the serum, which may have a milky appearance in patients with hyperlipidemia, and measurement of the serum lipid profile, plasma proteins, plasma sodium, osmolarity, and glucose.

A urine osmolarity below 100 mosmol/kg (specific gravity <1.003) is seen with primary polydipsia or a reset osmostat. A urine osmolarity of greater than 100 mosmol/kg is seen in patients with a syndrome of inappropriate ADH secretion (SIADH). When evaluating hyponatremia associated with hypo-osmolarity, one needs to distinguish between SIADH, effective circulating volume depletion, adrenal insufficiency, and hypothyroidism. Urinary sodium excretion is less than 25 mEq/L in hypovolemic states and greater than 40 mEq/L in SIADH, reset osmostat, renal disease, and adrenal insufficiency. A BUN <10 mg/dL [139], a serum creatinine <1 mg/dL and a serum urate <4.0 mg/dL [140] are all suggestive of normal circulating volume.

Three important considerations should be taken into account when considering the treatment of hyponatremia. First, the duration, referring to whether the condition is less than or greater than 48 hours. Second, whether the patient is hypovolemic, euvolemic or hypervolemic. Third, the severity of symptoms must be considered. Hypovolemic hyponatremia can be treated with normal saline. Euvolemic hyponatremia as in SIADH can be treated with fluid restriction. If neurologic symptoms are present 3% saline may be necessary with or withour furosimide added to increase solute free water excretion. Normal saline will increase the net retention of water and can exacerbate the hyponatremia and therefore it is not recommended in this situation. Hypervolemic hyponatremia associated with congestive heart failure, cirrihosis and edematous states usually is treated with water restriction , furosimide or spironolactone [141].

Vigorous therapy with hypertonic saline is required with acute hyponatremia when symptoms are present or the sodium concentration is <110 mEq/L.

Overly rapid correction of hyponatremia can be harmful, leading to central demyelinating lesions (central pontine myelinolysis). This is characterized by paraparesis or quadraparesis, dysarthria, dysphagia, coma, and less commonly seizures. It is best diagnosed by magnetic resonance imaging, but it may not be detected radiologically for 4 weeks [142]. To minimize this complication chronic hyponatremia should be corrected at a speed of less than 0.5 mEq/L per hour [142]. The degree of correction over the first day (<12 mEq/L), however, seems to be more important than the rate at which it is corrected [143]. In patients with acute, symptomatic hyponatremia the risk of cerebral edema is greater than the risk of central pontine myelinolysis. Rapid correction at a rate of 1.5–2 mEq/L per hour for 3–4 hours should be restricted to only those patients with acute symptomatic hyponatremia. With concomitant hypokalemia, replacement potassium may raise the plasma sodium at close to the maximum rate [144]; therefore, the appropriate treatment is 0.45% sodium chloride

Table 6.4 Neurologic symptoms associated with an acute reduction in plasma sodium.

Plasma sodium level (mEq/L)	Symptoms
120–125	Nausea, malaise
115–120	Headache, lethargy, obtundation
<115	Seizures, coma

containing 40 mEq of potassium in each liter. For rapid replacement of sodium depletion in patients with symptomatic hypo-osmolality, the IV administration of sodium as hypertonic saline will effectively correct the hypo-osmolality. The sodium needed to raise the sodium concentration to a chosen level is approximated to 0.5 × lean body weight (kg) × (Na) where Na is the desired serum sodium minus the actual serum sodium. Sodium may be administered as a 3% sodium chloride solution. With hyponatremia secondary to the excessive water accumulation, the water may be removed rapidly by administration of IV furosemide. Additional treatment with hypertonic saline may be appropriate in some cases. Furosemide results in the loss of water and sodium but the latter is given back as hypertonic saline, with the net result being the loss of water only [145]. In extreme cases peritoneal dialysis or hemodialysis may be required. The usual adult starting dose of furosemide for this purpose is 40 mg, IV. The same dose can be repeated at 2–4-hour intervals while hypertonic saline is being given. Potassium supplements are usually needed with this therapy. Chronic hyponatremia may be treated by water restriction or by an increase in renal water excretion. Water restriction may be difficult to achieve in patients with heart failure. In these and similar patients, administration of a loop diuretic such as furosemide in conjunction with an angiotensin-converting enzyme (ACE) inhibitor [146] is effective. ACE inhibitors should be restricted to postpartum patients, because of documented oligohydramnios and renal anomalies associated with their use. Mannitol has been administered with furosemide as a proposed alternative to 3% hypertonic saline for the treatment of acute hyponatremia (<48 hours' duration). This therapy may be considered in the acute setting when hypertonic saline is not available and significant neurologic symptoms or seizures are present with acute hyponatremia [147,148].

A new class of drugs collectively referred to as "vaptans" have emerged for the treatment of hyponatremia. These medications act as vasopressin receptor antagonists, blocking the action of AVP in the renal tubule, pituitary or smooth muscle depending upon receptor selectivity [120]. Conivaptan (Vaprisol, Astellas) is a combined V1A/V2 receptor and has been approved by the FDA for use in euvolemic patients with hyponatremia. It may be used in hyponatremia associated with SIADH, hypothyroidism and adrenal insufficiency. It has also been found to be effective in treatment of hypervolemic hyponatremia [149,150]. Tolvaptan is a selective V2 receptor which has also undergone trials. There are no reports of conivaptan use in pregnancy yet, nor is there any information regarding its safety or teratogenecity. Relcovaptan (SR 49059), a vasopressin V1a, has been studied for its inhibitory effect on uterine contractions [151].

Hypernatremia

Etiology

Hypernatremia is defined as an increased sodium concentration in plasma water. This is characterized by a serum sodium of >145 mosmol/L and represents a hyperosmolar state. The increased P_{osm} results in water moving extracellularly, with cellular dehydration occurring. However, the extracellular volume in hypernatremia may be normal, decreased, or increased [152]. Hypernatremia results from water loss, sodium retention, or a combination of both (see Table 6.5). Loss of water is due to either increased loss or reduced intake and gain of sodium is due to either increased intake or reduced renal excretion. As shown in Table 6.5, there are numerous disorders responsible for hypernatremia. However, there are two important conditions specific to pregnancy that can result in hypernatremia. The first is iatrogenic and caused by hypertonic saline used for second-trimester induced abortion. Twenty per cent hypertonic saline, which is infused into the amniotic sac as an abortifacient, can gain access to the maternal vascular compartment resulting in acute, profound hypernatremia, hyperosmolar crisis, and disseminated intravascular coagulopathy. Fortunately, this method has mostly been abandoned in the United States, but it is still performed in other countries [153].

Transient diabetes insipidus of pregnancy (TDIP) has become a well recognized, although unusual condition. It is characterized by polyuria, polydipsia, and normal or increased serum sodium. Most importantly, a majority of these patients develop pre-eclampsia or liver abnormalities such as acute fatty liver of pregnancy.

As noted previously, pregnancy is associated with a lower threshold for thirst and a lower osmolarity threshold for ADH release. In addition, the placenta produces vasopressinase, which is a cysteine-aminopeptidase that breaks down the bond between 1-cysteine and 2-tyrosine of vasopressin (ADH), effectively neutralizing the antidiuretic effect of the hormone [154,155]. The liver is believed to be the major site for degradation of vasopressinase and active liver disease can decrease the clearance of vasopressinase.

Women who are symptomatic or mildly symptomatic before pregnancy develop progressively increasing polyuria and polydipsia as the ability of endogenous ADH to effect reabsorption of water in the kidney is overwhelmed. There are probably at least

Table 6.5 Causes of hypernatremia.

Water loss
Insensible loss: burns, respiratory infection, exercise
Gastrointestinal loss: gastroenteritis, malabsorption syndromes, osmotic diarrhea
Renal loss: central diabetes insipidus (transient diabetes insipidus of pregnancy, Sheehan's syndrome, cardiopulmonary arrest), nephrogenic diabetes insipidus (X-linked recessive, sickle-cell disease, renal failure, drugs–lithium, diuresis with mannitol, or glucose)
Decreased water intake
Hypothalamic disorders
Loss of consciousness
Limited access to water or inability to drink
Sodium retention
Increased intake of sodium or administration of hypertonic solutions
Saline-induced abortion

two subsets of women who develop TDIP. In the first group women are minimally symptomatic before pregnancy and have subclinical cranial diabetes insipidus (DI). The inability to produce enough ADH, combined with increased vasopressinase activity, leads to clinically evident DI. In this group pre-eclampsia and liver abnormalities do not seem to develop. In the second subset, abnormal liver function leading to decreased metabolism of vasopressinase causes increased inactivation of ADH in clinical manifestations of DI [156]. It is in the second group that the incidence of pre-eclampsia and abnormal liver function seems to be increased. Interestingly, it appears that there is a higher preponderance of male infants in mothers who develop TDIP. In one report, which reviewed 17 pregnancies with TDIP, 16 had abnormal liver function tests, 12 had diastolic blood pressures ≥90 mmHg and 6 had significant proteinuria [155].

This form of TDIP tends not to recur in subsequent pregnancies [157]. Patients who present with polyuria and polydipsia must be evaluated for previously unrecognized diabetes mellitus, pre-eclampsia, and liver disease. If these are excluded, serum electrolytes, creatinine, liver enzymes, bilirubin, uric acid, complete blood count with differential and peripheral smear, urinalysis for electrolytes, specific gravity, osmolality, protein and 24-hour urine collection for total protein, and creatinine clearance should be ordered. The diagnosis of diabetes insipidus can be made by a water deprivation test. Water is withheld and hourly serum sodium and osmolality are determined as well as urine osmolality and specific gravity. Normally, when water is withheld, sodium and therefore osmolality, should rise as the urine becomes more concentrated, urine osmolality increases and urine volume decreases. In DI the urine osmolality fails to rise and dilute urine continues to be produced. After exogenous ADH is administered (DDAVP should be used in pregnancy), patients with TDIP should respond by concentrating the urine. Failure to concentrate the urine suggests a rarer form of nephrogenic diabetes insipidus. In nephrogenic diabetes insipidus the collecting tubule of the kidney is unable to respond to ADH. Caution is advised if a water deprivation test is performed in pregnancy because as plasma volume decreases, uterine hypoperfusion could be of consequence, especially in a patient who may have surreptitious pre-eclampsia. Electronic fetal monitoring should be performed during the test. Because osmolarity is reduced in pregnancy, lower serum osmolarity criteria for the diagnosis of DI in pregnancy are recommended. Administration of DDAVP will help differentiate nephrogenic DI from cranial DI.

DDAVP (1-desamino-8 D-argenine-vasopressin) is a synthetic analog of ADH and is not subject to breakdown by vasopressinase. Therefore, this is an ideal drug for the treatment of TDIP. It can be administered by a nasal spray (10–20 μg) or subcutaneously (1–4 μg). DDAVP has negligible pressor or oxytoxic effects. Failure to respond to DDAVP suggests nephrogenic DI.

Clinical presentation

The symptoms are primarily neurologic. The earliest findings are lethargy, weakness, and irritability. These may progress to seizures, coma, and death [158,159]. It is often difficult to discern whether the symptoms are secondary to neurologic disease or hypernatremia. Patients may also exhibit signs of volume expansion or volume depletion. With DI the patient may complain of nocturia, polyuria, and polydipsia.

Diagnosis

Hypernatremia usually causes altered mental status; therefore, obtaining a good history is difficult. Physical examination should help to evaluate the volume status of the patient as well as demonstrate any focal neurologic abnormalities. A urine specific gravity of less than 1.010 usually indicates diabetes insipidus. Administration of ADH in this situation will differentiate central diabetes insipidus (ADH response is an increase in specific gravity with a decrease in urine volume) from nephrogenic diabetes insipidus (no change) [160]. A specific gravity greater than 1.023 is often seen with excessive insensible or gastrointestinal water losses, primary hypodipsia, and excessive administration of hypertonic fluids. Urine volume should be recorded, because volumes in excess of 5 L/day are seen with lithium toxicity, primary polydipsia, hypercalcemia, central diabetes insipidus, and congenital nephrogenic diabetes insipidus. A water restriction test may be the only way to differentiate the etiologies of CDI and NDI.

Management

Hypernatremia is treated by either the addition of water or removal of sodium, the choice of which depends on the status of the body's sodium and water content. If water depletion is the cause of hypernatremia, water is added. If sodium excess is the cause, sodium needs to be removed. Rapid correction of hypernatremia can cause cerebral edema, seizures, permanent neurologic damage, and death [137]. The plasma sodium content should be lowered slowly to normal unless the patient has symptomatic hypernatremia. Hypernatremia of TDIP is generally mild because the thirst mechanism is uninhibited. Hypernatremia secondary to other causes tends to be more severe. When hypernatremia is secondary to water loss calculation of the water deficit is essential. The water deficit can be estimated by the following equation:

$$\text{water deficit} = \text{body weight (kg)} \times 0.55 \times \text{Na}/\text{Na}_b$$

where Na_b is the desired sodium level and Na is the difference between the desired and observed serum sodium. This relationship allows calculation of the volume of fluid replacement necessary to reduce the sodium to the desired level. In acute, symptomatic, hypernatremia sodium may be reduced by 6–8 mEq/L in the first 4 hours. But thereafter, the rate of decline should not exceed 0.5 mEq/L/h. As with hyponatremia, chronic hypernatremia usually does not cause CNS symptoms and therefore does not require rapid correction. As with hyponatremia, a safe rate of correction is 0.7 mEq/L/h or 12 mEq/L/day [161]. The type of fluid administered to correct losses depends on the patient's clinical state. Dextrose in water, either orally or IV, can be given to patients with pure water loss. If sodium depletion is also present, such as in vomiting or diarrhea, 0.25 mol/L saline is recommended. In hypotensive patients, normal saline should be used until tissue perfusion has been corrected. Thereafter, a more dilute saline solution should be used.

In patients with excess sodium, the restoration of normal volume usually initiates natriuresis, but if natriuresis does not occur promptly, sodium may be removed with diuretics. Furosemide with a dextrose 5% solution can be used in this situation, but care must be taken not to allow serum sodium concentration to decline too rapidly. Furosemide can be administered at doses of up to 60 mg, IV every 2–4 hours. Patients with renal failure can be treated with dialysis.

Nephrogenic diabetes, which does not respond to ADH or DDAVP, requires treatment with a thiazide diuretic combined with a low-sodium, low-protein diet. Subjects with primary hypodipsia should be educated to drink on schedule. Stimulation of the thirst center with chlorpropamide has met with some success in these patients [162].

Abnormalities in potassium metabolism

Total body potassium (K^+) averages approximately 50 mEq/kg body weight, or about 3500 mEq in a 70-kg non-pregnant individual, but only 2% of it is extracellular [163]. During pregnancy there is an accumulation of 300–320 mEq of potassium [163,164]. Approximately 200 mEq of it is in the products of conception. Serum plasma levels change little from the non-pregnant state, with an average decrease in serum potassium (K^+) of approximately 0.2–0.3 mEq/L. The serum K^+ level is determined by three factors: K^+ consumption, whether taken in by diet or administered by parenteral solutions; K^+ loss through the kidney and GI tract; and the shifting between extracellular and intracellular compartments. Renal excretion of potassium is determined by the reabsorption of potassium and most importantly by the secretion of potassium in the distal and collecting tubule of the kidney. Aldosterone enhances the secretion of potassium in the distal tubules and collecting ducts and also increases the permeability of the luminal cellular membranes of the tubules, further facilitating K^+ excretion [121]. Acute acidosis decreases the kidneys' ability to secrete K^+, while alkalosis enhances the secretion of potassium into the distal tubules. The shifting of K^+ between the extracellular space and the intracellular space is controlled by the sodium–potassium ATPase pump (Na^+–K^+-ATPase pump), which actively transports sodium (Na^+) out of the cell and in turn moves K^+ into the cell. Acid–base balance plays a critical role in the function of the Na^+–K^+-ATPase pump. In simple terms, acidosis inhibits the function of the Na^+–K^+-ATPase pump and alkalosis enhances it. Thus, acidosis will result in flux of K^+ out of the cell and decreased secretion of K^+ into the distal renal tubules and collecting ducts, leading to hyperkalemia. Alkalosis has the opposite effect, resulting in hypokalemia.

Hypokalemia

Etiology

The causes of hypokalemia are listed in Table 6.6. One particular cause of hypokalemia of special interest in obstetrics is the administration of intravenous β_2-adrenergic agonists for the treatment of preterm labor [165]. β_2-receptor stimulation by agents such as terbutaline and has widespread metabolic effects. Stimulation of the β_2-receptors in the liver results in glycogenolysis and gluconeogenesis, and causes an elevation in serum glucose. The increase in glucose as well as direct stimulation of β_2-receptors in the pancreatic islet cells causes secretion of insulin. Most importantly the Na^+–K^+-ATPase pump is directly stimulated by these agents. A significant decrease in serum potassium occurs within minutes of intravenous administration of β_2-agonists, even before glucose and insulin levels increase. As glucose levels rise and insulin secretion increases, K^+ levels fall even further as K^+ is shifted into the cell [166]. Although an intracellular shift of K^+ caused by insulin-induced glucose uptake may contribute to the hypokalemia, it seems that the most important cause is the direct β_2-adrenergic stimulation [167]. Renal excretion does not seem to be a factor in β_2-agonist-induced hypokalemia [166].

Table 6.6 Causes of hypokalemia.

Redistribution within the body
β_2-agonists
Glucose and insulin therapy
Acute alkalosis or correction of acute acidosis
Familial periodic paralysis
Barium poisoning
Reduced intake
Chronic starvation
Pica
Increased loss
Gastrointestinal loss
Prolonged vomiting or nasogastric suction
Diarrhea or intestinal fistula
Villous adenoma
Renal loss
Primary hypoaldosteronism
Secondary hypoaldosteronism (renal artery stenosis, diuretic therapy, malignant hypertension)
Cushing's syndrome and steroid therapy
Bartter's syndrome
Carbenoxolone
Licorice-containing substances
Renal tubular acidosis
Acute myelocytic and monocytic leukemia
Magnesium deficiency

The severity of the hypokalemia is dependent upon the pretreatment concentration of serum K^+. The effect is more pronounced when the pretreatment K^+ concentration is high and the effect is reduced in patients with pre-existing hypokalemia. Nevertheless, patients with pre-existing hypokalemia may be at greater risk of developing the complications of hypokalemia [168]. Since the hypokalemia associated with intravenous administration of β_2-agonists represents an intracellular shift with unchanged total body K^+ and hypokalemic side effects are uncommon, serum K^+ of 2.5 mmol/L generally does not require K^+ replacement. At levels <2.5 mmol/L serious cardiac arrhythmias have been reported with β_2-agonist tocolysis, and replacement of K^+ is recommended [166].

Bartter's syndrome is an autosomal recessive disorder characterized by hypokalemia, hyperaldosteronism, sodium wasting, normal blood pressure, hypochloremic alkalosis, and hyperplasia of the juxtaglomerular apparatus [169]. Increasing numbers of cases are being reported in the literature [170,171]. Hypokalemia is responsible for most of the symptoms of Bartter's syndrome and therapy is directed toward increasing the K^+ concentration with supplements and K^+-sparing diuretics. Over one-third of patients with Bartter's syndrome also suffer magnesium wasting and increased magnesium supplementation may also be required for treatment.

Pica in pregnancy is more common than realized and often goes unrecognized [172]. Geophagia with ingestion of clay during pregnancy is a common practice in some parts of the US and around the world. The clay binds K^+ in the intestine and if enough is ingested it can cause hypokalemic myopathy [173]. Questioning about pica should be included in the history for patients who present with hypokalemia and symptoms as noted below.

Clinical presentation

Muscle weakness, hypotonia and mental status changes may occur when the serum K^+ is below 2.5 mmol/L. ECG changes occur in 50% of patients with hypokalemia [174] and involve a decrease in T-wave amplitude in addition to the development of prominent U-waves. Hypokalemia can potentiate arrhythmias due to digitalis toxicity [174].

Diagnosis

After obtaining a history and physical examination, serum and urine electrolytes plus serum calcium and magnesium should be obtained. The urine potassium will help differentiate renal from extrarenal losses. A urine potassium below 30 mEq/L signifies extrarenal losses, seen commonly in patients with diarrhea or redistribution within the body (see Table 6.6). A urine potassium of greater than 30 mEq/L is seen with renal losses. In this situation, a serum bicarbonate will help separate renal tubular acidosis (<24 mEq/L) from other causes. A urine chloride less than 10 mEq/L is seen with vomiting, nasogastric suctioning, and overventilation. A level greater than 10 mEq/L is seen with diuretic and steroid therapy.

Management

Hypokalemia is treated either by the administration of potassium or by preventing the renal loss of potassium. Once the potassium falls below 3.5 mEq/L, there is already a 200 mEq deficit in potassium; therefore, any additional decrease in potassium is significant regardless of the magnitude [175].

If the serum potassium level is below 2.5 mEq/L, clinical symptoms or ECG changes are generally present, and one should initiate IV therapy. While it is theoretically useful to estimate the potassium deficit before initiating therapy, such calculations are of limited value because they can vary considerably secondary to transcellular shifts. As a rough estimate, a serum potassium of 3.0 mEq/L is associated with a potassium deficit of 350 mEq, and a potassium level of 2.0 mEq/L with a deficit of 700 mEq. Oral replacement is preferred unless the potassium level is critically low, symptoms are present or EKG changes exist. The recommended IV replacement dose is 0.7 mEq/kg lean body weight over 1–2 hours [176]. In obese patients, 30 mEq/m^2 body surface area is administered. The dose should not increase the serum potassium by more than 1.0–1.5 mEq/L unless an acidosis is present. In life-threatening situations, a rate in excess of 100 mEq/h may be used [176]. If aggressive replacement therapy does not correct the serum potassium, magnesium depletion should be considered and the magnesium then replaced.

With an underlying metabolic alkalosis, one should use potassium chloride for replacement of hypokalemia. The chloride salt is necessary to correct the alkalosis, which otherwise would result in the administered potassium being lost in the urine. When rapidly replacing potassium chloride, glucose-containing solutions should not be used because they will stimulate release of insulin, which will drive potassium into the cells. Potassium at concentrations exceeding 40 mEq/L may produce pain at the infusion site and may lead to sclerosis of smaller vessels; thus, it is advisable to split the dosage and administer each portion via a separate peripheral vein. One should avoid central venous infusion of potassium at high concentrations because this can produce life-threatening cardiotoxicity.

Renal loss of potassium is prevented either by treating its cause or by the administration of potassium-sparing diuretics. Spironolactone (25–150 mg twice a day), triamterine (50–100 mg twice a day), or amiloride (5–20 mg/day) is effective in reducing potassium loss. Mild potassium loss can be replaced orally in the form of potassium chloride or KPO_4. Amiloride should be administered with food to avoid gastric irritation.

Hyperkalemia

Hyperkalemia is defined as a serum potassium greater than 5.5 mEq/L. Because of its potential for producing dysrhythmias, hyperkalemia should be managed far more aggressively than hypokalemia. Pseudohyperkalemia is defined as an increase in potassium concentration only in the local blood vessel or in vitro and has no physiologic consequences. Hemolysis during venepuncture, thrombocytosis (greater than 1 million/μL), and severe leukocytosis (over 50000) cause psuedohyperkalemia. Pseudohyperkalemia should always be investigated immediately, with careful attention paid to avoiding cell trauma during blood collection. Both thrombocytosis and leukocytosis release potassium from the platelets and WBCs during blood clotting [177,178]. Suspected pseudohyperkalemia should be investigated by obtaining simultaneous serum potassium specimens from clotted and unclotted specimens. The potassium in the clotted sample should be 0.3 mEq/L higher than in the unclotted specimen.

Etiology

The causes of hyperkalemia can be classified according to three basic mechanisms: redistribution within the body, increased potassium intake, or reduced renal potassium excretion (Table 6.7). Severe tissue injury leads to direct release of potassium due to disruption of cell membranes. Rhabdomyolysis and hemolysis cause hyperkalemia only when causing renal failure. Metabolic acidosis results in increased potassium shift across membranes, with reduced renal excretion of potassium. This can increase the serum potassium by up to 1 mEq/L [176]. Hyperkalemia is less predictable with organic causes of acidosis, such as diabetic and lactic acidosis, when compared with the inorganic causes of acidosis [179]. Respiratory acidosis does not often produce hyperkalemia. Digitalis toxicity leads to disruption of the membrane Na^+–K^+-ATPase pump, which normally keeps potassium intracellular [180].

Diminished renal potassium excretion is due to renal failure, reduced aldosterone or aldosterone responsiveness, or reduced distal delivery of sodium. Renal failure usually does not cause hyperkalemia until the GFR is below 10 mL/min or urine output is less than 1 L [181]. Deficiency of aldosterone may be due to an absence of hormone, such as occurs in Addison's disease, or may be part of a selective process, such as occurs in hyporeninemic hypoaldosteronism, which is the most common cause of chronic hyperkalemia [182]. Unfractionated heparin and low molecular weight heparin, even in a small dose, can reversibly inhibit aldosterone synthesis causing hyperkalemia. Angiotensin-converting enzyme inhibitors, potassium-sparing diuretics, and non-steroidal anti-inflammatory agents limit the supply of renin or angiotensin II, resulting in decreased aldosterone and hyperkalemia. Severe dehydration may result in the delivery of sodium to the distal nephron being markedly reduced with the development of hyperkalemia [245]. Life-threatening arrhythmias and cardiac arrest have been reported in patients who underwent induction of general anesthesia for cesarean section with succinylcholine after they were treated for preterm labor with prolonged bed rest and intravenous magnesium sulfate infusion combined with β_2-adrenergic agonists. Sudden increases in serum potassium concentrations ranging from 5.7 to 7.2 occurred in patients shortly after induction of anesthesia with the muscle-blocking agent succinylcholine. The administration of succinylcholine in immobilized patients may cause a hazardous hyperkalemic response. In addition, patients with burns, infections, or neuromuscular disease are at risk for massive hyperkalemia after succinylcholine injection. It is speculated that extrajunctional acetylcholine receptors develop in these patients so that potassium is released from the entire muscle instead of the neuromuscular junction alone. This increase of potassium release is referred to as upregulation of acetylcholine receptors [183]. Severe hyperkalemia has also been reported in intravenous drug abusers treated with prolonged parenteral magnesium sulfate in the absence of an obvious cause [184].

Table 6.7 Causes of hyperkalemia.

Redistribution within the body
Severe tissue damage (e.g. myonecrosis)
Insulin deficiency
Metabolic acidosis
Digitalis toxicity
Severe acute starvation
Hypoxia
Increased potassium intake
Overly aggressive potassium therapy
Failure to stop therapy when depletion corrected
Reduced renal excretion of potassium
Adrenal insufficiency
Drugs
Angiotensin-converting enzyme inhibitors
Potassium-sparing diuretics
Non-steroidal anti-inflammatory agents
Heparin
Succinylcholine
Renal glomerular failure
Magnesium sulfate

Clinical presentation

Skeletal muscle and cardiac conduction abnormalities are the dominant features of clinical hyperkalemia. Neuromuscular weakness may occur, with severe flaccid quadriplegia being common [185]. ECG changes begin when the serum potassium reaches 6.0 mEq/L and are always abnormal when a serum level of 8.0 mEq/L is reached [181]. The earliest changes are tall, narrow T waves in precordial leads V2–4. The T wave in hyperkalemia has a narrow base, which helps to separate it from other causes of tall T waves. As the serum potassium level increases, the P-wave amplitude decreases with lengthening of the P–R interval until the P waves disappear. The Q–R–S complex may be prolonged, resulting in ventricular asystole. Occasionally, gastrointestinal symptoms occur.

Diagnosis

After obtaining a history and physical examination, serum and urine electrolytes plus serum calcium and magnesium should be obtained. The urine potassium will help differentiate renal from extrarenal losses. A urine potassium above 30 mEq/L suggests a transcellular potassium shift; below this level, reduced renal excretion is suggested.

Management

Therapy always should be initiated when the serum potassium exceeds 6.0 mEq/L, irrespective of ECG findings, because ventricular tachycardia can appear without premonitory ECG signs [176]. Therapy should be monitored by frequent serum potassium level sampling and ECG. The plan is to acutely manage the hyperkalemia and then achieve and maintain a normal serum level (Table 6.8).

The mainstay of therapy for patients with acute and severe hyperkalemia is administration of calcium. This may be a lifesaving medication in an emergency. Calcium directly antagonizes the action of potassium and decreases excitation potential at the membrane. Calcium gluconate is the preferred agent because inadvertent extravasation of calcium chloride into soft tissues can cause a severe inflammation and tissue necrosis. Ten milliliters of a 10% solution of calcium gluconate (approximately 1 g) can be infused over 2–3 minutes. The effect is rapid, occurring over a few minutes, but is short lived, lasting only about 30 minutes. If no effect is noted, characterized by changes in the ECG, the dose can be repeated once. Measures must be taken to achieve a more prolonged effect to lower potassium levels. Another time-honored, proven therapy is to cause a shift of potassium into the cells by infusing glucose and insulin. Ten units of regular insulin can be mixed in 500 mL of 20% dextrose in water (D20%W) and infused over 1 hour. Diluting standard D50%W can make 20% glucose. Alternatively 10–20 units of regular insulin can be infused more rapidly in D50%W. The onset of action should occur over 15–30 minutes and the duration of action is hours. The serum glucose potassium should fall by 1 mEq/L within about an hour. Sodium bicarbonate has been recommended as a tertiary agent to lower the serum potassium; however its efficacy for treatment of patients with renal failure has been called into doubt [186,187]. It may be more efficacious in patients suffering with concomitant metabolic acidosis. In theory raising the pH of blood will increase uptake of potassium by the cells. One to three ampules of $NaHCO_3$, 44–132 mEq, can be mixed with D5%W and infused over 1 hour or 1–2 ampules can be administered over 10 minutes. β_2-adrenergic agents such as salbutamol and albuterol administered parenterally or by nebulizer have been shown to be efficacious in the treatment of hyperkalemia. The mechanism of action has been described previously. β_2-adrenergic agents are familiar to most obstetricians and can be considered in the less acute management of patients with hyperkalemia. A paradoxical initial rise in serum potassium has been reported and caution is advised if considering this in initial treatment [188]. Dialysis may be necessary in patients with acute or chronic renal failure if these measures fail to return potassium to safe levels.

Table 6.8 Management of hyperkalemia.

Acute management
Calcium gluconate
10 mL (10% solution) IV over 3 min; repeat in 5 min if no response
Insulin–glucose infusion
10 units regular insulin in 500 mL of 20% dextrose and infuse over 1 hour
Sodium bicarbonate
1–2 ampules (44–88 mEq) over 5–10 min
Furosemide
40 mm IV
Dialysis
Chronic management
Kayexalate
Oral: 30 g in 50 mL of 20% sorbitol
Rectal: 50 g in 200 mL of 20% sorbitol retention enema

In less acute situations any offending agents contributing to hyperkalemia should be stopped, potassium intake adjusted, and therapy instituted. Removal of potassium may be accomplished by several routes including through the gastrointestinal tract, through the kidneys, or by hemodialysis or peritoneal dialysis. A potassium exchange resin, sodium polystyrene sulfonate (Kayexalate), may be administered either orally or by enema. It is more effective when given with sorbitol or mannitol, which cause osmotic diarrhea. One tablespoon of Kayexalate mixed with 100 mL of 10% sorbitol or mannitol can be given by mouth 2–4 times a day. Premixed preparations are generally available in hospital pharmacies. Complications such as intestinal necrosis and perforation have been reported with this treatment and recently its use has been put into question [189]. Loop diuretics, mineralocorticoids or increased salt intake enhance the urinary excretion of potassium. Finally, in cases of severe refractory or life-threatening hyperkalemia, either hemodialysis or peritoneal dialysis may be necessary.

Abnormalities in calcium metabolism

Calcium circulates in the blood in one of three forms. Between 40 and 50% of calcium is bound to serum protein, mostly albumin, and is non-diffusible. Approximately 10% is bound to other anions such as citrate or phosphate and is diffusible. The remainder is unbound ionized calcium, which is diffusible and the most physiologically active form. The normal serum range for the ionized fraction is between 1.1 and 1.3 mmol/L [190]. The total serum calcium levels may not accurately reflect the ionized calcium level. Alteration of the patient's serum albumin concentration can influence the protein bound fraction, leading to an incorrect assessment of the ionized calcium level. It is the ionized calcium that determines the normalcy of the physiologic state. Therefore, measurement of the ionized calcium is preferred for clinical decision-making. If the ionized calcium cannot be measured by the laboratory the total calcium and serum albumin should be measured simultaneously and a correction factor used to estimate whether hypocalcemia is present. The normal range of serum calcium is 8.6–10.5 mg/dL and the normal range for serum albumin is 3.5–5.5 g/dL. One simply adds 0.8 mg/dL for every 1 g/dL albumin concentration below 4 g/dL. For example, if the total serum calcium is 7.8 mg/dL and the serum albumin is

3.0 g/dL, using the correction factor $1 \times 0.8 + 7.8 = 8.6$. Therefore, this patient would not be in the hypocalcemic range. In pregnancy, serum albumin concentration drops with a compensatory increase in ionized calcium activity. In a condition such as pre-eclampsia albumin levels may drop even further. Calcium levels are also influenced by blood pH. Acidosis leads to decreased binding of calcium to serum proteins and an increase in the ionized calcium level. Alkalosis has the opposite effect. Free fatty acids increase calcium binding to albumin. Serum levels of free fatty acids are often increased during critical illness as a result of illness-induced elevations of plasma concentrations of epinephrine, glucagon, growth hormone, and corticotropin as well as decreases in serum insulin concentrations.

Serum calcium levels are normally maintained within a very narrow range. Calciferol, obtained either in the diet or formed in the skin, is converted to 1α,25-dihydroxycalciferol by reactions in the liver and kidney and is commonly referred to as 1,25-dihydroxyvitamin D. This substance enhances calcium absorption in the gut. Parathyroid hormone (PTH) is secreted in accordance to a feedback relationship with calcium. As calcium levels drift lower, PTH is secreted and as calcium levels increase, PTH secretion is inhibited. Calcitonin stimulates calcium entry into bone due to the action of osteoblasts and its effect is less important in calcium control than PTH. PTH stimulates osteoclastic absorption of bone leading to release of calcium into the extracellular fluid. In addition, PTH stimulates calcium reabsorption in the distal tubules of the kidney.

Hypocalcemia

The most commonly encountered derangement in calcium homeostasis in pregnancy is hypocalcemia associated with magnesium sulfate ($MgSO_4 \cdot 7H_2O$) therapy used to treat pre-eclampsia, eclampsia, and preterm labor. Magnesium sulfate is usually administered as a 3–6 g bolus over 15–30 minutes, followed by a 1–3 g/h continuous infusion [191]. Within 1 hour of initiation of intravenous magnesium sulfate infusion, both total and ionized calcium levels decline rapidly. Serum ionized and total calcium concentrations have been shown to decline 11% and 22% respectively during infusion for the treatment of pre-eclampsia. These levels are 4–6 standard deviations below the mean normal serum calcium concentration [192,193]. Serum albumin is often significantly decreased in pre-eclampsia and can contribute to the lower serum calcium levels; however, other mechanisms are probably responsible for this effect. Urinary calcium excretion increases 4.5-fold during magnesium sulfate infusions at a rate three times greater than observed in normal controls [194]. Some have noted decreased PTH levels in response to magnesium sulfate administration, an effect that would cause decreased calcium reabsorption in the kidney and decreased serum calcium levels [195]. Cruikshank demonstrated not only increased levels of PTH but also increased levels of 1,25-dihydroxyvitamin D during magnesium sulfate infusions. It is hypothesized that magnesium ions compete with calcium ions for common reabsorptive sites or mechanisms in the nephron. The increased delivery of magnesium to the distal tubule and collecting duct results in increased magnesium reabsorption and less availability for resorptive sites for calcium, leading to increased urinary calcium loss [194,196].

Nifedipine, a calcium channel blocker, is used both as a tocolytic agent in the treatment of preterm labor and as an antihypertensive in pregnancy. Magnesium sulfate administered concomitantly with nifedipine may thoretically enhance the effect of hypocalcemia resulting in neuromuscular blockade or myocardial suppression [197].

Others have not found a clinically significant difference in toxicity when magnesium sulfate and nifedipine were used together [198].

Therapy with both magnesium and nifedipine does not increase the risk of serious magnesium-related maternal side effects in women with pre-eclampsia [199].

Etiology

Common non-obstetric causes of hypocalcemia include both metabolic and respiratory alkalosis, sepsis, magnesium depletion, and renal failure (Table 6.9). Magnesium deficiency is common in critically ill patients and also may cause hypocalcemia [200,201]. One cannot correct a calcium deficiency until the magnesium deficit has been corrected.

Sepsis can lead to hypocalcemia, presumably as a result of calcium efflux across a disrupted microcirculation [202]. This effect may be linked to an underlying respiratory alkalosis; this combination confers a poor prognosis. Hypocalcemia commonly is seen in patients with acute pancreatitis and also is associated with a poor prognosis [203]. Renal failure leads to phosphorus retention, which may cause hypocalcemia as a result of calcium precipitation, inhibition of bone resorption, and suppression of renal 1-hydroxylation of vitamin D [204,205]. Thus, the treatment of hypocalcemia in this setting is to lower the serum PO_4 level. Citrated blood (massive blood transfusion), albumin, and radiocontrast dyes are the most common chelators that cause

Table 6.9 Causes of hypocalcemia.

Magnesium sulfate infusion
Massive blood transfusion
Acid–base disorders
Respiratory and metabolic alkalosis
Shock
Renal failure
Malabsorption syndrome
Magnesium depletion
Hypoparathyroidism
Surgically produced
Idiopathic
Pancreatitis
Fat embolism syndrome
Drugs
Heparin, aminogylcosides, cis-platinum, phenytoin, phenobarbital, and loop diuretics

hypocalcemia in critically ill patients. Primary hypoparathyroidism is seen rarely, whereas secondary hypoparathyroidism after neck surgery is a common cause of hypocalcemia [206].

Clinical presentation

Hypocalcemia may present with a variety of clinical signs and symptoms. The most common manifestations are caused by increased neuronal irritability and decreased cardiac contractility [203]. Neuronal symptoms include seizures, weakness, muscle spasm, paresthesias, tetany, and Chvostek's and Trousseau's signs. Neither Chvostek's nor Trousseau's signs are sensitive or specific [207]. Cardiovascular manifestations include hypotension, cardiac insufficiency, bradycardia, arrhythmias, left ventricular failure, and cardiac arrest. ECG findings include Q–T and S–T interval prolongation and T-wave inversion. Other clinical findings include anxiety, irritability, confusion, brittle nails, dry scaly skin, and brittle hair.

Serum calcium levels may drop to very low levels during continuous intravenous administration of magnesium. Although hypocalcemic tetany has been reported during treatment for pre-eclampsia, it is so rare that compensatory protective mechanisms must be acting [208].

Parathyroid hormone levels have been shown to rise 30–50% after infusion of magnesium sulfate and its associated hypocalcemia. 1,25-dihydroxyvitamin D rises by more than 50% and the placenta is a significant source of this vitamin. Such a response leads to increased calcium released from bone and increased gastrointestinal absorption, perhaps limiting the progressive decline in calcium concentration. It is not necessary to replace depleted calcium in pre-eclamptic patients with magnesium-induced hypocalcemia, unless the ionized calcium levels fall dangerously low and obvious clinical signs of hypocalcemia ensue. In the authors' and editors' collective experience it has not been necessary to replace calcium in severely pre-eclamptic or eclamptic patients. The administration of calcium could interfere with the therapeutic effect of magnesium sulfate.

Treatment

All patients with an ionized calcium concentration below 0.8 mmol/L should receive treatment. Life-threatening arrhythmias can develop when the ionized calcium level approaches 0.5–0.65 mmol/L. Acute symptomatic hypocalcemia is a medical emergency that necessitates IV calcium therapy (Table 6.10).

Table 6.10 Calcium preparations.

Parenteral	*Rate*
Calcium gluconate	1.0 mL/min
Calcium chloride	0.5 mL/min
Oral	*Contents*
Calcium carbonate	500 mg calcium
Calcium gluconate	500 mg calcium

With acute symptoms, a calcium bolus can be given at an initial dose of 100–200 mg IV over 10 minutes, followed by a continuous infusion of 1–2 mg/kg/h. This will raise the serum total calcium by 1 mg/dL, with levels returning to baseline by 30 minutes after injection. Intravenous calcium preparations are irritating to veins and should be diluted (10-mL vial in 100 mL of D5%W and warmed to body temperature). If IV access is not available, calcium gluconate may be given intramuscularly (IM) [209].

Anticonvulsant drugs, sedation, and paralysis may help eliminate signs of neuronal irritability. Once the serum calcium is in the low normal range, oral replacement with enteral calcium is recommended.

Hypercalcemia

Etiology

The finding of hypercalcemia is a relatively rare occurrence in women of the reproductive age group. Gastroesophageal reflux is very common in pregnancy and it is treated often with calcium-based antacids. In addition calcium intake is generally supplemented throughout gestation. Hypercalcemia caused by milk alkali syndrome can develop with excessive use of antacids and is reported in pregnancy [210]. The most common cause of hypercalcemia in the general population is hyperparathyroidism secondary to a benign adenoma. Approximately 80% are single, benign adenomas, while multiple adenomas or hyperplasia of the four parathyroid glands also may cause hyperparathyroidism. In patients treated in the intensive care unit hypercalcemia is more likely to be related to malignancy. Ten to 20% of patients with malignancy develop hypercalcemia because of direct tumor osteolysis of bone and secretion of humoral substances that stimulate bone resorption [211,212]. Other causes of hypercalcemia are listed in Table 6.11. There are rare reports cases of parathyroid carcinoma in pregnancy, accounting for a minority of cases [213].

Table 6.11 Causes of hypercalcemia.

Milk alkali syndrome
Malignancy
Hyperparathyroidism
Chronic renal failure
Recovery from acute renal failure
Immobilization
Calcium administration
Hypocalciuric hypercalcemia
Granulomatous disease
Sarcoidosis
Tuberculosis
Hyperthryroidism
AIDS
Drug-induced
Lithium, theophylline, thiazides, and vitamin D or A

Clinical presentation

Although women are twice as likely as men to develop hyperparathyroidism, the peak incidence is in women over the age of 45 years. In non-pregnant individuals the disorder is generally asymptomatic and detected on screening metabolic profiles. This is not the case in pregnancy, where approximately 70% of individuals exhibit symptoms of hypercalcemia [214]. Constipation, anorexia, nausea, and vomiting are common. Severe hypertension and arrhythmias have been reported in patients with hypercalcemia during pregnancy. Other symptoms include fatigue, weakness, depression, cognitive dysfunction, and hyporeflexia. ECG changes include Q–T segment shortening. Nephrolithiasis may occur in a third of these patients and pancreatitis in 13%. This is in contrast to non-pregnant individuals with hyperparathyroidism who have an incidence of 1.5% of pancreatitis [214].

Diagnosis

Calcium derangements in neonates and infants may indicate disorders of maternal calcium metabolism. Hypocalcemic tetany and seizures in infants have been reported in mothers diagnosed with hypercalcemia. Therefore, serum calcium levels should be measured in mothers whose infants are born with metabolic bone disease or abnormal serum calcium levels [215]. After a complete history and physical examination is obtained, serum electrolytes, total and ionized calcium, magnesium, PO_4, and albumin should be obtained. Serum PTH, thyroid-stimulating hormone (TSH), T_3 and T_4 should be obtained and an ECG performed. Renal function should be assessed with a 24-hour urine collection for calcium, creatinine, creatinine clearance, and total volume to help distinguish hypocalciuric from hypercalciuric syndromes.

Treatment

Surgical removal of the abnormal parathyroid gland is the only long-term effective treatment for primary hyperparathyroidism. Surgery is optimally performed in the first and second trimester on symptomatic patients with serum calcium over 11 mg/dL. The major complication from surgical treatment is hypocalcemia, which can be treated with a calcium gluconate infusion. Calcium gluconate can be diluted in 5% dextrose and infused at a rate of 1 mg/kg body weight per hour [214]. Medical therapy (Table 6.12) needs to be initiated when the serum calcium reaches 13 mg/dL or if patients are symptomatic at levels greater than 11. Patients with hypercalcemia are usually dehydrated. Hyperuricemia resulting from hypercalcemia compounds the volume deficit and further elevates the serum calcium level. The first step in management of hypercalcemia is restoration of intravascular volume. Not only will volume expansion dilute the serum calcium, but volume expansion with isotonic saline inhibits sodium reabsorption and increases calcium excretion. After the intravascular volume is restored, furosemide or ethacrynic acid, the loop diuretics, may be administered. Their major effect is in preventing volume overload in patients predisposed to CHF. Although they may increase sodium and calcium excretion, the additional benefit is questionable and their administration necessitates vigilant monitoring and replacement of potassium and magnesium. Thiazide diuretics inhibit renal calcium excretion and are contraindicated in the treatment of hypercalcemia. Bisphosphonates are medications that inhibit osteoclast-mediated bone reabsorption. Pamidronate is most commonly used and should be administered early in the therapy of hypercalcemia after volume restoration with normal saline has been accomplished. A single dose of 30–60 mg, diluted in 500 mL of 0.9% saline or 5% dextrose in D5%W can be infused over 4 hours. However, for severe hypercalcemia 90 mg can be infused over 24 hours. The maximal hypocalcemic effect is observed in 1–2 days and its effect generally lasts for weeks. Pamidronate has been used in pregnancy for the treatment of malignant hypercalcemia with no ill effect reported on the fetus [216]. Animal studies have failed to demonstrate a teratogenic effect of the medication [217]. However, it does bind to fetal bone and limited experience with its use in pregnancy warrants caution. Calcitonin inhibits bone resorption and increases urinary calcium excretion. Its effect is rapid and can lower serum calcium 1–2 mg/dL within several hours. It can be administered subcutaneously or intramuscularly in doses of 4–8 IU/kg every 6–12 hours. Unfortunately, tachyphylaxis develops over days and its effectiveness is decreased. Nevertheless, it is safe, relatively free of side effects and compatible with use in renal failure. Glucocorticoids may be beneficial in hypercalcemia secondary to sarcoidosis, multiple myeloma and vitamin D intoxication. They are generally considered a secondary or tertiary agent and require doses of 50–100 mg of prednisone in divided doses per day. Oral phosphate, which has been a mainstay of therapy in the past, has fallen out of common usage because of more effective medications noted above. It can have a modest effect in decreasing calcium levels by inhibiting calcium absorption and promoting calcium deposition in bone. Mithramycin is another agent whose use has been supplanted by pamidronate. It is associated with serious side effects such as thrombocytopenia, coagulopathy, and renal failure.

Table 6.12 Acute management of hypercalcemia.

Agent	Dose	Comments
0.9% Saline	300–500 mL/h	Adjust infusion to maintain urine output at ≥200 mL/h. Add furosemide if volume overload or CHF
Pamidronate	30–60 mg in 500 mL 0.9% saline or D5%W over 4h	Maximal effect in 2 days; lasts for weeks
Calcitonin	4 IU/kg IM or subcutaneously q 12h	Tachyphylaxis develops
Steroids	Prednisone 20–50 mg b.i.d.	Multiple myeloma, sarcoidosis, vitamin D toxicity
Phosphates	0.5–1 g p.o. t.i.d.	Requires normal renal function
Hemodialysis		Severe hypercalcemia, renal failure, CHF

Hemodialysis can be highly effective in the treatment of severe hypercalcemia or hypercalcemia refractory to other methods of treatment. It is generally reserved as a last line of therapy.

Magnesium imbalances

Hypomagnesemia

Magnesium (Mg^{2+}) is the second most abundant intracellular cation in the body. It is a cofactor for all enzyme reactions involved in the splitting of high-energy adenosine triphosphate (ATP) bonds required for the activity of phosphatases. Such enzymes are essential and provide energy for the Na^+–K^+-ATPase pump, proton pump, calcium ATPase pump, neurochemical transmission, muscle contraction, glucose–fat–protein metabolism, oxidative phosphorylation, and DNA synthesis [218–220]. Magnesium is also required for the activity of adenylate cyclase.

Magnesium is not distributed uniformly within the body. Less than 1% of total body magnesium is found in the serum, with 50–60% found in the skeleton and 20% in muscle [218]. Serum levels, thus, may not reflect true intracellular stores accurately and may be normal in the face of magnesium depletion or excess [219,221]. In the blood, there are three fractions: an ionized fraction (55%), which is physiologically active and homeostatically regulated; a protein-bound fraction (30%); and a chelated fraction (15%).

Magnesium can be viewed as a calcium-channel blocker. Intracellular calcium levels rise as magnesium becomes depleted. Many calcium channels have been shown to be magnesium dependent and higher concentrations of magnesium inhibit the flux of calcium through both intracellular, extracellular channels and from the sarcoplasmatic reticulum. Hypomagnesemia enhances the vasoconstrictive effect of catecholemines and angiotensin II in smooth muscle [222].

It is estimated that at least 65% of critically ill patients develop hypomagnesemia. The normal magnesium concentration is between 1.7 and 2.4 mg/dL (1.4–2.0 mEq/L); however, a normal reading should not deter one from considering hypomagnesemia in the presence of a suggestive clinical presentation [223].

Etiology

Hypomagnesemia results from at least one of three causes: decreased intake, increased losses from the gastrointestinal tract or kidney, and cellular redistribution. Hypomagnesemia is common in patients receiving total parenteral nutrition and increased supplementation may be required to assure adequate magnesium intake. Increased renal losses secondary to the use of diuretics and amnioglycosides constitute the most common cause of magnesium loss in a hospital setting (Table 6.13). Diuretics such as furosemide and ethacrynic acid and amnioglycosides inhibit magnesium reabsorption in the loop of Henle and also block absorption at this site, leading to increased urinary losses [224]. Up to 30–40% of patients receiving aminoglycosides will develop hypomagnesemia [225,226].

Table 6.13 Causes of hypomagnesemia.

Drug-induced
Diuretics (furosemide, thiazides, mannitol)
Aminoglycosides
Neoplastic agents (cis-platinum, carbenicillin, cyclosporine)
Amphotericin B
Digoxin
Thyroid hormone
Insulin
Malabsorption, laxative abuse, fistulas
Malnutrition
Hyperalimentation and prolonged IV therapy
Renal losses
Glomerulonephritis, interstitial nephritis
Tubular disorders
Hyperthyroidsm
Diabetic ketoacidosis
Pregnancy and lactation
Sepsis
Hypothermia
Burns
Blood transfusion (citrate)

Hypomagnesemia can result from internal redistribution of magnesium. Following the administration of glucose or amino acids, magnesium shifts into cells [227,228]. A similar effect is seen with increased catecholemine levels, correction of acidosis, and hungry bone syndromes. Lower gastrointestinal tract secretions are rich in magnesium; thus, severe diarrhea leads to hypomagnesemia.

Clinical presentation

The signs and symptoms of hypomagnesemia are very similar to those of hypocalcemia and hypokalemia, and it is not entirely clear whether hypomagnesemia alone is responsible for these symptoms [229,230]. Most symptomatic patients have levels below 1.0 mg/dL. Cardiovascular symptoms include hypertension, heart failure, arrhythmias, increased risk for digitalis toxicity, and decreased pressor response [227,228,231–234]. The ECG may demonstrate a prolonged P–R and Q–T interval with S–T depression. Tall, peaked T-waves occur early and slowly broaden with decreased amplitude together with the development of a widened Q–R–S interval as the magnesium level falls. As with hypocalcemia, there is increased neuronal irritability with weakness, muscle spasms, tremors, seizures, tetany, confusion, psychosis, and coma. Patients also complain of anorexia, nausea, and abdominal cramps.

Diagnosis

Following a complete history, physical examination, and ECG, serum electrolyte, calcium, magnesium, and PO_4 levels should be obtained. A 24-hour urine magnesium measurement is helpful in separating renal from non-renal causes. An increased urinary magnesium level suggests increased renal loss of magnesium as the etiology of hypomagnesemia.

Treatment

Patients with life-threatening arrhythmias, acute symptomatic hypomagnesemia, or severe hypomagnesemia are best treated with IV magnesium sulfate [235–240]. A 2-g bolus of magnesium sulfate is administered IV over 1–2 minutes, followed by a continuous infusion at a rate of 2 g/h. After a few hours, this can be reduced to a 0.5–1.0 g/h maintenance infusion. Magnesium chloride is used in patients with concurrent hypocalcemia, because sulfate can bind calcium and worsen hypocalcemia. During magnesium replacement, one should monitor the serum levels of magnesium, calcium, potassium, and creatinine. Blood pressure, respiratory status, and neurologic status (mental alertness, deep tendon reflexes) should be assessed periodically. As magnesium sulfate is renally excreted, its dose should be reduced in patients with renal insufficiency.

With moderate magnesium deficiency, 50–100 mEq magnesium sulfate per day (600–1200 mg elemental magnesium) can be administered in patients without renal insufficiency. Mild asymptomatic magnesium deficiency can also be replaced with diet alone. It can take up to 3–5 days to replace intracellular stores.

Magnesium is important for the maintenance of normal potassium metabolism [219,240]. Magnesium deficiency can lead to renal potassium wasting, resulting in a cellular potassium deficiency. Magnesium levels must, therefore, be adequate before successful correction of potassium deficiency.

Hypermagnesemia

Hypermagnesemia, like hypomagnesemia, is difficult to detect because of the unreliability of serum levels in predicting clinical symptoms. New technology has been developed to more accurately measure ionized magnesium levels and this is gaining wider acceptance in practice. However, the clinical utility of measuring serum ionized magnesium levels has not been substantiated. Hypermagnesemia (serum magnesium >3 mg/dL or 2.4 mEq/L or 1.2 mmol/L) occurs in up to 10% of hospitalized patients [231], most commonly secondary to iatrogenic causes [219,236,238,241].

Etiology

The most common cause of hypermagnesemia in the critically ill obstetric population is treatment for pre-eclampsia/eclampsia and preterm labor with magnesium sulfate infusion. Magnesium sulfate remains the mainstay for the treatment of pre-eclampsia and has been shown to be a better agent for the prevention/treatment of eclampsia than phenytoin and other agents. The most common medical illness associated with hypermagnesemia is renal failure usually in combination with excess magnesium ingestion. The usual sources of excess magnesium ingestion are magnesium-containing antacids and cathartics. Other causes include diabetic ketoacidosis, pheochromocytoma, hypothyroidism, Addison's disease, and lithium intoxication.

Clinical presentation

Hypermagnesemia can lead to neuromuscular blockade and depressed skeletal muscle function. Conduction through the cardiac conducting system is slowed, with ECG changes noted at a serum concentration as low as 5 mEq/L and heart block seen at 7.5 mEq/L [221]. In patients not suffering from pre-eclampsia, hypotension may be seen at levels between 3.0 and 5.0 mEq/L [221]. Loss of deep tendon reflexes occurs at a serum concentration of 10 mEq/L (12 mg/dL), with respiratory paralysis occurring at a serum concentration of 15 mEq/L (18 mg/dL). Cardiac arrest occurs at a serum concentration of greater than 25 mEq/L (30 mg/dL).

Diagnosis

A complete history and physical examination should be performed. Special attention should be directed at soliciting a history of concomitant calcium-channel blocker use with magnesium sulfate for treatment of preterm labor. Neuromuscular blockade, profound hypotension, and myocardial depression have been associated with this practice [197,198,242]. ECG, serum electrolyte, calcium, magnesium, and PO_4 levels should be obtained.

Treatment

Intravenous calcium gluconate (10 mL of 10% solution over 3 minutes) is effective in reversing the physiologic effects of hypermagnesemia [243]. Calcium gluconate should not be administered to patients being treated for pre-eclampsia/eclampsia with magnesium levels in the therapeutic range of 4–8 mg/dL because this may counteract the therapeutic effect of magnesium in the prevention of seizures. In patients with other disorders hemodialysis is the recommended therapy. In patients who can tolerate fluid therapy, aggressive infusion of IV saline with furosemide may be effective in increasing renal magnesium losses. All agents containing magnesium should be discontinued. Supralethal levels of hypermagnesemia can be successfully corrected with prompt recognition and treatment [244]. Supplemental oxygen delivery and ventilation support are assessed via continuous monitoring of S_pO_2 by pulse oximetry.

References

1 Gallery EDM, Brown MA. Volume homeostasis in normal and hypertensive human pregnancy. *Baillieres Clin Obstet Gynecol* 1987; 1: 835–851.

2 Wittaker PG, Lind T. The intravascular mass of albumin during human pregnancy: A serial study in normal and diabetic women. *Br J Obstet Gynaecol* 1993; 100: 587–592.

3 Brown MA, Zammitt VC, Mitar DM. Extracellular fluid volumes in pregnancy-induced hypertension. *J Hypertens* 1992; 10: 61–68.

4 MacGillivray I, Campbell D, Duffus GM. Maternal metabolic response to twin pregnancy in primigravidae. *J Obstet Gynaecol Br Cmwlth* 1971; 78: 530–534.

5 Thomsen JK, Fogh-Andersen N, Jaszczak P et al. Atrial natriuretic peptide decrease during normal pregnancy as related to hemodynamic changes and volume regulation. *Acta Obstet Gynecol Scand* 1993; 72: 103–110.

6 Fullerton WT, Hytten FE, Klopper AL et al. A case of quadruplet pregnancy. *J Obstet Gynaecol Br Cmwlth* 1965; 72: 791–796.

7 Hytten FE, Paintin DB. Increase in plasma volume during normal pregnancy. *J Obstet Gynaecol Br Cmwlth* 1973; 70: 402.

8 Salas SP, Rosso P, Espinoza R et al. Maternal plasma volume expansion and hormonal changes in women with idiopathic fetal growth retardation. *Obstet Gynecol* 1993; 81: 1029–1033.

9 Arias F. Expansion of intravascular volume and fetal outcome in patients with chronic hypertension and pregnancy. *Am J Obstet Gynecol* 1965; 123: 610.

10 Gallery ED, Hunyor SN, Gyory AZ. Plasma volume contraction: a significant factor in both pregnancy-associated hypertension (preeclampsia) and chronic hypertension in pregnancy. *Q J Med* 1979; 48: 593–602.

11 Goodlin RC, Quaife MA, Dirksen JW. The significance, diagnosis, and treatment of maternal hypovolemia as associated with fetal/maternal illness. *Semin Perinatol* 1981; 5: 163–174.

12 Sibai BM, Anderson GD, Spinnato JA et al. Plasma volume findings in patients with mild pregnancy-induced hypertension. *Am J Obstet Gynecol* 1983; 147: 16–19.

13 Raiha CE. Prematurity, perinatal mortality, and maternal heart volume. *Guy's Hosp Rep* 1964; 113: 96.

14 Goodlin RC, Anderson JC, Gallagher TF. Relationship between amniotic fluid volume and maternal plasma volume expansion. *Am J Obstet Gynecol* 1983; 146: 505–511.

15 Pirani BBK, MacGillivray I. Smoking during pregnancy. Its effect on maternal metabolism and fetoplacental function. *Obstet Gynecol* 1978; 52: 257–263.

16 Brown MA, Zammit VC, Lowe SA. Capillary permeability and extracellular fluid volumes in pregnancy-induced hypertension. *Clin Sci (Lond)* 1989; 77: 599–604.

17 Ueland K. Maternal cardiovascular dynamics. VII. Intrapartum blood volume changes. *Am J Obstet Gynecol* 1976; 126: 671–677.

18 Lund CJ, Donovan JC. Blood volume during pregnancy. Significance of plasma and red cell volumes. *Am J Obstet Gynecol* 1967; 98: 394–403.

19 Peeters LL, Buchan PC. Blood viscosity in perinatology. *Rev Perinatol Med* 1989; 6: 53.

20 Peeters LL, Verkeste CM, Saxena PR et al. Relationship between maternal hemodynamics and hematocrit and hemodynamic effects of isovolemic hemodilution and hemoconcentration. I. The awake late-pregnancy guinea pig. *Pediatr Res* 1987; 21: 584–589.

21 Dafinis E, Sabatini, S. The effect of pregnancy on renal function: physiology and pathophysiology. *Am J Med Sci* 1992; 303: 184–205.

22 Chesley LC. The kidney. In: Chesley LC, ed. *Hypertensive disorders in pregnancy*. New York: Appleton-Century-Crofts 1978: 154 197.

23 Baylis C. The mechanism of the increase in glomerular filtration rate in the twelve-day pregnant rat. *J Physiol* 1980; 305: 405–414.

24 Walker J, Garland HO. Single nephron function during prolactin-induced pseudopregnancy in the rat. *J Endocrinol* 1985; 107: 127–131.

25 Oparil S, Ehrlich EN, Lindheimer MD. Effect of progesterone on renal sodium handling in man: Relation to aldosterone excretion and plasma renin activity. *Clin Sci Mol Med* 1975; 44: 139–147.

26 Elkus R, Popovich J Jr. Respiratory physiology in pregnancy. *Clin Chest Med* 1992; 13: 555–565.

27 Skatrud J, Dempsey J, Kaiser DG. Ventilatory response to medroxyprogesterone acetate in normal subjects: Time course and mechanism. *J Appl Physiol* 1978; 44: 393–394.

28 Skillman JJ, Awwad HK, Moore FD. Plasma protein kinetics of the early transcapillary refill after hemorrhage in man. *Surg Gynecol Obstet* 1967; 125: 983–996.

29 Skillman JJ, Restall DS, Salzman EW. Randomized trial of albumin vs electrolyte solutions during abdominal aortic operations. *Surgery* 1975; 78: 291–303.

30 Skillman JJ, Rosenoer VM, Smith PC. Improved albumin synthesis in postoperative patients by amino acid infusion. *N Engl J Med* 1976; 295: 1037–1040.

31 Carrico CJ, Canizaro PC, Shires GT. Fluid resuscitation following injury; rational for the use of balanced salt solutions. *Crit Care Med* 1976; 4: 46–54.

32 Shoemaker WC, Bryan Brown CW, Quigley L et al. Body fluid shifts in depletion and post-stress states and their correction with adequate nutrition. *Surg Gynecol Obstet* 1973; 136: 371–374.

33 Lowery BD, Cloutier CT, Carey LC. Electrolyte solutions in resuscitation in human hemorrhagic shock. *Surg Gynecol Obstet* 1971; 133: 273–284.

34 Trudnowski RJ, Goel SB, Lam FT et al. Effect of Ringer's lactate solution and sodium bicarbonate on surgical acidosis. *Surg Gynecol Obstet* 1967; 125: 807–814.

35 Carey JS, Scharschmidt BF, Culliford AT et al. Hemodynamic effectiveness of colloid and electrolyte solutions for replacement of simulated operative blood loss. *Surg Gynecol Obstet* 1970; 131: 679–686.

36 Hauser CJ, Shoemaker WC, Turpin I et al. Oxygen transport responses to colloids and crystalloids in critically ill surgical patients. *Surg Gynecol Obstet* 1980; 150: 811–816.

37 Hanshiro PK, Weil MH. Anaphylactic shock in man. *Arch Intern Med* 1967; 119: 129–140.

38 Dawidson I, Gelin LE, Hedman L et al. Hemodilution and recovery from experimental intestinal shock in rats: a comparison of the efficacy of three colloids and one electrolyte solution. *Crit Care Med* 1981; 9: 42–46.

39 Dawidson I, Eriksson B. Statistical evaluations of plasma substitutes based on 10 variables. *Crit Care Med* 1982; 10: 653–657.

40 Moss GS, Lower RJ, Jilek J et al. Colloid or crystalloid in the resuscitation of hemorrhagic shock. A controlled clinical trial. *Surgery* 1981; 89: 434–438.

41 Virgilio RW. Crystalloid vs colloid resuscitation [reply to letter to editor]. *Surgery* 1979; 86: 515.

42 Virgilio RW, Rice CL, Smith DE. Crystalloid vs colloid resuscitation: is one better? A randomized clinical study. *Surgery* 1979; 85: 129–139.

43 Siegel DC, Moss GS, Cochin A et al. Pulmonary changes following treatment for hemorrhagic shock: saline vs colloid infusion. *Surg Forum* 1970; 921: 17–19.

44 Lucas CE, Denis R, Ledgerwood AM et al. The effects of hespan on serum and lymphatic albumin, globulin and coagulant protein. *Ann Surg* 1988; 207: 416–420.

45 Takaori M, Safer P. Acute severe hemodilution with lactated Ringer's solution. *Arch Surg* 1967; 94: 67–73.

46 Moss GS, Siegel DC, Cochin A et al. Effects of saline and colloid solutions on pulmonary function in hemorrhagic shock. *Surg Gynecol Obstet* 1971; 133: 53–58.

47 Lowe RJ, Moss GS, Jilek J et al. Crystalloid vs colloid in the etiology of pulmonary failure after trauma: a randomized trial in man. *Surgery* 1977; 81: 676–683.

48 Virgilio RW, Smith DE, Zarins CK. Balanced electrolyte solutions: experimental and clinical studies. *Crit Care Med* 1979; 7: 98–106.

49 Baue AE, Tragus ET, Wolfson SK. Hemodynamic and metabolic effects of Ringer's lactate solution in hemorrhagic shock. *Ann Surg* 1967; 166: 29–38.

50 Waxman K, Holness R, Tominaga G et al. Hemodynamic and oxygen transport effects of pentastarch in burn resuscitation. *Ann Surg* 1989; 209: 341–345.

51 Singh G, Chaudry KI, Chaudry IH. Crystalloid is as effective as blood in resuscitation of hemorrhagic shock. *Ann Surg* 1992; 215: 377–382.

52 Lewis RT. Albumin: role and discriminative use in surgery. *Can J Surg* 1980; 23: 322–328.

53 Haupt MT, Rackow EC. Colloid osmotic pressure and fluid resuscitation with hetastarch, albumin and saline solutions. *Crit Care Med* 1982; 10: 159–162.

54 Miller RD, Robbins TO, Tong MJ et al. Coagulation defects associated with massive blood transfusions. *Ann Surg* 1971; 174: 794–801.

55 Myers MB, Cherry G, Heimburger S et al. Effect of edema and external pressure on wound healing. *Arch Surg* 1967; 94: 218–222.

56 Hohn DC, Makay RD, Holliday B et al. Effect of oxygen tension on microbicidal function of leukocytes in wounds and in vitro. *Surg Forum* 1976; 27: 18–20.

57 Kaufman BS, Rackow EC, Falk JL. The relationship between oxygen delivery and consumption during fluid resuscitation of hypovolemic and septic shock. *Chest* 1984; 85: 336–340.

58 Barone JE, Snyder AB. Treatment strategies in shock: use of oxygen transport measurements. *Heart Lung* 1991; 20: 81–85.

59 Granger DW, Udrich M, Parks DA et al. Transcapillary exchange during intestinal fluid absorption. In: Sheppard AP, Granger DW, eds. *Physiology of the Intestinal Circulation*. New York: Raven, 1984: 107.

60 Tullis JL. Albumin. I. Background and use. *JAMA* 1977; 237: 355–360.

61 Rothschild MA, Oratz M, Schreiber SS. Albumin synthesis. *N Engl J Med* 1972; 286: 748–756, 816–820.

62 Thompson WL. Rational use of albumin and plasma substitutes. *Johns Hopkins Med J* 1975; 136: 220–225.

63 Grant JP, Custer PB, Thurlow J. Current techniques of nutritional assessment. *Surg Clin North Am* 1981; 61: 437–463.

64 Rosenoer VM, Skillman JJ, Hastings PR et al. Albumin synthesis and nitrogen balance in postoperative patients. *Surgery* 1980; 87: 305–312.

65 Moss GS, Proctor JH, Homer LD. A comparison of asanguineous fluids and whole blood in the treatment of hemorrhagic shock. *Surg Gynecol Obstet* 1966; 129: 1247–1257.

66 Rothschild MA, Schreiber SS, Oratz M et al. The effects of adrenocortical hormones on albumin metabolism studies with albumin-I131. *J Clin Invest* 1958; 37: 1229–1235.

67 Rothschild MA, Bauman A, Yalow RS et al. The effect of large doses of desiccated thyroid on the distribution and metabolism of albumin-I131 in euthyroid subjects. *J Clin Invest* 1957; 36: 422–428.

68 Liljedahl SO, Rieger A. Blood volume and plasma protein. IV. Importance of thoracic-duct lymph in restitution of plasma volume and plasma proteins after bleeding and immediate substitution in the splenectomized dog. *Acta Chir Scand* 1968; 379(suppl): 39–51.

69 Lamke LO, Liljedahl SO. Plasma volume changes after infusion of various plasma expanders. *Resuscitation* 1976; 5: 93–102.

70 Holcroft JW, Trunkey DD. Extravascular lung water following hemorrhagic shock in the baboon: comparison between resuscitation with Ringer's lactate and plasmanate. *Ann Surg* 1974; 180: 408–417.

71 Granger DN, Gabel JC, Drahe RE et al. Physiologic basis for the clinical use of albumin solutions. *Surg Gynecol Obstet* 1978; 146: 97–104.

72 Berson SA, Yalow RS. Distribution and metabolism of I131 labeled proteins in man. *Fed Proc* 1957; 16: 13S–18S.

73 Sterling K. The turnover rate of serum albumin in man as measured by I-131 tagged albumin. *J Clin Invest* 1951; 30: 1228–1237.

74 Boldt J. The good, the bad and the ugly: Should we completely banish human albumin from our intensive care units? *Anesth Analg* 2000; 91: 887–895.

75 Cochrane Injuries Group. Human albumin administration in critically ill patients: systematic review of randomised controlled trials. *BMJ* 1998; 317: 235–240.

76 Ferguson N, Stewart T, Etchells. Human albumin administration in critically ill patients. *Intensive Care Med* 1999; 25: 323–325.

77 Vito L, Dennis RC, Weisel RD. Sepsis presenting as acute respiratory insufficiency. *Surg Gynecol Obstet* 1974; 138: 896–900.

78 Shoemaker WC, Schluchter M, Hopkins JA et al. Comparison of the relative effectiveness of colloids and crystalloids in emergency resuscitation. *Am J Cardiol* 1981; 142: 73–84.

79 Poole GV, Meredith JW, Pernell T et al. Comparison of colloids and crystalloids in resuscitation from hemorrhagic shock. *Surg Gynecol Obstet* 1982; 154: 577–586.

80 Weaver DW, Ledgerwood AM, Lucas CE et al. Pulmonary effects of albumin resuscitation for severe hypovolemic shock. *Arch Surg* 1978; 113: 387–392.

81 Lucas CE, Ledgerwood AM, Higgins RF et al. Impaired pulmonary function after albumin resuscitation from shock. *J Trauma* 1980; 20: 446–451.

82 Kovalik SG, Ledgerwood AM, Lucas CE et al. The cardiac effect of altered calcium homeostasis after albumin resuscitation. *J Trauma* 1981; 21: 275–279.

83 Cogbill TH, Moore EE, Dunn EI et al. Coagulation changes after albumin resuscitation. *Crit Care Med* 1981; 9: 22–26.

84 Solanke TF, Khwaja MS, Madojemu EI. Plasma volume studies with four different plasma volume expanders. *J Surg Res* 1971; 11: 140–143.

85 Farrow SP, Hall M, Ricketts CR. Changes in the molecular composition of circulating hydroxyethyl starch. *Br J Pharmacol* 1970; 38: 725–730.

86 Yacobi A, Stoll RG, Sum CY et al. Pharmacokinetics on hydroxyethyl starch in normal subjects. *J Clin Pharmacol* 1982; 22: 206–212.

87 Ferber HP, Nitsch E, Forster H. Studies on hydroxyethyl starch. Part II: changes of the molecular weight distribution for hydroxyethyl starch types 450/0.7, 450/0.3, 300/0.4, 200/0.7, 200/0.5, 200/0.3, 200/0.1 after infusion in serum and urine of volunteers. *Arzneimittelforschung* 1985; 35: 615–622.

88 Thompson WL, Britton JJ, Walton RP. Persistence of starch derivatives and dextran when infused after hemorrhage. *Pharmacol Exp Ther* 1962; 136: 125–132.

89 Mishler JM, Ricketts CR, Parkhouse EJ. Post transfusion survival of hydroxyethyl starch 450/0.7 in man: a long term study. *J Clin Pathol* 1980; 33: 155–159.

90 Mishler JM, Borberg H, Emerson PM. Hydroxyethyl starch, an agent for hypovolemic shock treatment. II. Urinary excretion in normal volunteers following three consecutive daily infusions. *Br J Pharmacol* 1977; 4: 591–595.

91 Puri VK, Paidipaty B, White L. Hydroxyethyl starch for resuscitation of patients with hypovolemia in shock. *Crit Care Med* 1981; 9: 833–837.

92 Ring J, Messmer K. Incidence and severity of anaphylactoid reactions to colloid volume substitutes. *Lancet* 1977; 1: 466–469.

93 Bogan RK, Gale GR, Walton RP. Fate of 14C-label hydroxyethyl starch in animals. *Toxicol Appl Pharmacol* 1969; 15: 206–211.

94 Metcalf W, Papadopoulos A, Tufaro R et al. A clinical physiologic study of hydroxyethyl starch. *Surg Gynecol Obstet* 1970; 131: 255–267.

95 Thompson WL, Fukushima T, Rutherford RB et al. Intravascular persistence, tissue storage, and excretion of hydroxyethyl starch. *Surg Gynecol Obstet* 1970; 131: 965–972.

96 Mishler JM, Ricketts CR, Parkhouse EJ. Changes in molecular composition of circulating hydroxyethyl starch following consecutive daily infusions in man. *Br J Clin Pharmacol* 1979; 7: 505–509.

97 Hofer RE, Lanier WL. Effect of hydroxyethyl starch solutions on blood glucose concentrations in diabetic and nondiabetic rats. *Crit Care Med* 1992; 20: 211–215.

98 Ballinger WF. Preliminary report on the use of hydroxyethyl starch solution in man. *J Surg Res* 1966; 6: 180–183.

99 Kilian J, Spilker D, Borst R. Effect of 6% hydroxyethyl starch, 45% dextran 60 and 5.5% oxypolygelatine on blood volume and circulation in human volunteers. *Anaesthesist* 1975; 24: 193–197 (in German).

100 Lee WH, Cooper N, Weidner MG. Clinical evaluation of a new plasma expander: hydroxyethyl starch. *J Trauma* 1968; 8: 381–393.

101 Khosropour R, Lackner F, Steinbereithner K et al. Comparison of the effect of pre- and intraoperative administration of medium molecular weight hydroxyethyl starch (HES 200/0.5) and dextran 40 (60) in vascular surgery. *Anaesthesist* 1980; 29: 616–622 (in German).

102 Laks H, Pilon RN, Anderson W et al. Acute normovolemic hemodilution with crystalloid vs colloid replacement. *Surg Forum* 1974; 25: 21–22.

103 Diehl JT, Lester JL 3rd, Cosgrove DM. Clinical comparison of hetastarch and albumin in postoperative cardiac patients. *Ann Thorac Surg* 1982; 34: 674–679.

104 Shatney CH, Deapiha K, Militello PR et al. Efficacy of hetastarch in the resuscitation of patients with multisystem trauma and shock. *Arch Surg* 1983; 118: 804–809.

105 Kirklin JK, Lell WA, Kouchoukos NT. Hydroxyethyl starch vs albumin for colloid infusion following cardiopulmonary bypass in patients undergoing myocardial revascularization. *Ann Thorac Surg* 1984; 37: 40–46.

106 Boon JC, Jesch F, Ring J et al. Intravascular persistence of hydroxyethyl starch in man. *Eur Surg Res* 1976; 8: 497–503.

107 Kohler H, Kirch W, Horstmann HJ. Hydroxyethyl starch-induced macroamylasemia. *Int J Clin Pharmacol Biopharm* 1977; 15: 428–431.

108 Korttila K, Grohn P, Gordin A et al. Effect of hydroxyethyl starch and dextran on plasma volume and blood hemostasis and coagulation. *J Clin Pharmacol* 1984; 24: 273–282.

109 Lorenz W, Doenicke A, Freund M et al. Plasma histamine levels in man following infusion of hydroxyethyl starch: a contribution to the question of allergic or anaphylactoid reactions following administration of a new plasma substitute. *Anaesthesist* 1975: 24: 228–230.

110 Maurer PH, Berardinelli B. Immunologic studies with hydroxyethyl starch (HES): a proposed plasma expander. *Transfusion* 1968; 8: 265–268.

111 Ring J, Seifert B, Messmer K et al. Anaphylactoid reactions due to hydroxyethyl starch infusion. *Eur Surg Res* 1976; 8: 389–399.

112 Muller N, Popov-Cenic S, Kladetzky RG et al. The effect of hydroxyethyl starch on the intra- and postoperative behavior of haemostasis. *Bibl Anat* 1977; 16: 460–462.

113 Solanke TF. Clinical trial of 6% hydroxyethyl starch (a new plasma expander). *Br Med J* 1968; 3: 783–785.

114 Weatherbee L, Spencer HH, Knopp CT et al. Coagulation studies after the transfusion of hydroxyethyl starch protected frozen blood in primates. *Transfusion* 1974; 14: 109–115.

115 Strauss RG, Stump DC, Henriksen RA. Hydroxyethyl starch accentuates von Willebrand's disease. *Transfusion* 1985; 25: 235–237.

116 Mattox KL, Maningas PA, Moore EE et al. Prehospital hypertonic saline/dextran infusion for post-traumatic hypotension. *Ann Surg* 1991; 213: 482–491.

117 Chang JC, Gross HM, Jang NS. Disseminated intravascular coagulation due to intravenous administration of hetastarch. *Am J Med Sci* 1990; 300: 301–303.

118 Cully MD, Larson CP, Silverberg GD. Hetastarch coagulopathy in a neurosurgical patient. *Anesthesiology* 1987; 66: 706–707.

119 Damon L, Adams M, Striker RB et al. Intracranial bleeding during treatment with hydroxyethyl starch. *N Engl J Med* 1987; 317: 964–965.

120 Ali F, Guglin M, Vaitkevicius P. Theraputic potential of vasopressin receptor antagonists. *Drug* 2007; 67(6): 847–858.

121 Guyton AC, Hall JE. Regulation of extracellular fluid, osmolarity and sodium concentration. In: Guiton AC, Hall JE, eds. *Textbook of Medical Physiology*, 9th edn. Philadelphia, Pennsylvania: WB Saunders Company, 1996: 349–365.

122 Lindheimer MD, Davison JM. Osmoregulation, the secretion of arginine vasopressin and its metabolism during pregnancy. *Eur J Endocrinol* 1995; 132(2): 133–143.

123 Anderson RJ, Chung H-M, Kluge R, Schrier RW. Hyponatremia: a prospective analysis of its epidemiology and pathogenetic role of vasopressin. *Ann Intern Med* 1985; 102: 164–168.

124 Thomsen JK, Fogh-Andersen N, Jaszczak P. Atrial natriuretic peptide, blood volume, aldosterone, and sodium excretion during twin pregnancy. *Acta Obstet Gynecol Scand* 1994; 73: 14–20.

125 Weisberg LS. Pseudohyponatremia: a reappraisal. *Am J Med* 1989; 86: 315–318.

126 Abdul-Karim R, Assali NS. Renal function in human pregnancy, V Effects of oxytocin on renal hemodynamics and water electrolyte excretion. *J Lab Clin Med* 1961; 57: 522–532.

127 Chesley LC. Management of preeclampsia and eclampsia. In: Chesley LC, ed. *Hypertensive Disorders in Pregnancy*. New York: Appleton-Century-Crofts, 1978: 345.

128 Josey WE, Pinto AP, Plante RF. Oxytocin induced water intoxication. *Am J Obstet Gynecol* 1969; 104: 926.

129 Morgan DB, Kirwan NA, Hancock KW et al. Water intoxication and oxytocin infusion. *Br J Obstet Gynaecol* 1977; 84: 6–12.

130 Wang JY, Shih HL, Yuh FL et al. An unforgotten cause of acute hyponatremia: water intoxication due to oxytocin administration in a pregnant woman. *Nephron* 2000; 86: 342–343.
131 Moen V, Brundin L, Rundgren M et al. Hyponatremia complicated labor – rare or unrecognized? A prospective observational study. *BJOG* 2009; 116(4): 552–561.
132 Ruchala PL, Metheny N,Essenpreis H et. al. Current practice in oxytocin dilution and fluid administration for induction of labor. *J Obstet Gynecol Neonatal Nurs* 2002; 31(5): 545–550.
133 Theunissen IM, Parer JT. Fluids and electrolytes in pregnancy. *Clin Obstet Gynecol* 1994; 34(1): 3–15.
134 Burneo J, Vizcarra D, Miranda H, Central pontine myelinolysis and pregnancy. A case report and review of the literature. *Rev Neurol* 2000; 30(11): 1036–1040.
135 Sandhu G, Ramaiyah S, Chan C, et al. Pathophysiology and management of preeclampsia-associated severe hyponatremia. *Am J Kidney Dis* 2010; 55(3): 599–603.
136 Boulanger E, Pagniez D, Roueff S, Sheehan syndrome presenting as early postpartum hyponatremia. *Nephrol Dial Transplant* 1999; 14 (11): 2714–2715.
137 Pollock AS, Arieff AL. Abnormalities of cell volume regulation and their functional consequences. *Am J Physiol* 1980; 239: F195–205.
138 Arieff AI. Hyponatremia, convulsions, respiratory arrest, and permanent brain damage after elective *surgery* in healthy women. *N Engl J Med* 1986; 314: 1529–1535.
139 Decaux G, Genette F, Mockel J. Hypouremia in the syndrome of inappropriate secretion of antidiuretic hormone. *Ann Intern Med* 1980; 93: 716–717.
140 Beck LH. Hypouricemia in the syndrome of inappropriate secretion of antidiuretic hormone. *N Engl J Med* 1979; 301: 528–530.
141 Biwas M, Davies JS. Hyponatremia in clinical practice. *Postgraduate Med J* 2007; 83: 373–378.
142 Sterns RH. The treatment of hyponatremia: first, do no harm. *Am J Med* 1990; 88: 557–560.
143 Soupart A, Penninckx R, Stenuit A et al. Treatment of chronic hyponatremia in rats by intravenous saline: comparison of rate versus magnitude of correction. *Kidney Int* 1992; 41: 1662–1667.
144 Kamel KS, Bear RA. Treatment of hyponatremia: a quantitative analysis. *Am J Kidney Dis* 1993; 21: 439–443.
145 Hantman D, Rossier B, Zohlman R et al. Rapid correction of hyponatremia in the syndrome of appropriate secretion of antidiuretic hormone. *Ann Intern Med* 1973; 78: 870–875.
146 Packer M, Medina N, Yushnak M. Correction of dilutional hyponatremia in severe chronic heart failure by converting-enzyme inhibition. *Ann Intern Med* 1984; 100: 782–789.
147 Berl T. Mannitol a therapeutic alternative in the treatment of acute hyponatremia. *Crit Care Med* 2000; 28(6): 2152–2153.
148 Porzio P, Halberthal M, Bohn D et al. Treatment of acute hyponatremia: Ensuring the excretion of a predictable amount of electrolyte-free water. *Crit Care Med* 2000; 28(6): 1905–1910.
149 Hussar D, New drugs 07, part 1. *Nursing* 2007; 37(2): 51–58.
150 Zeltser D, Rosansky S, Verbalis JG et al. Assessment of the efficacy and safety of intravenous conivaptan in euvolemic and hypervolemic hyponatremia. *Am J Nephrol* 2007; 27(5); 447–457.
151 Steinwall M, BossmarT, BrouardR, The effect of reclovaptan (sR49059) , an orally active vasopressin V1a receptor antagonist, on uterine contractions in preterm labor. *Gynecol Endocrinol* 2005; 20(2): 104–109.
152 Oh MS, Carroll HJ. Hypernatremia. In: Hurst JW, ed. *Medicine for the Practicing Physician*, 3rd edn. Boston: Butterworth-Heinemann, 1992: 1293.
153 Ananthakrishnan S. Diabetes insipidus in pregnancy: etiology, evaluation, and management. *Endocr Pract* 2009; 15(4): 377–382.
154 Sjoholm I, Ymam L. Degradation of oxytocin lysine – vasopressin, angiotensin II, angiotensin II-amide by oxytocinase. *Acta Pharmacol Suecca* 1967; 4: 65–76.
155 Krege J, Katz VL, Bowes WA Jr. Transient diabetes insipidus of pregnancy. *Obstet Gynecol Surv* 1989; 44(11): 789–795.
156 Williams DJ, Metcalf KA, Skingle AI. Pathophysiology of transient cranial diabetes insipidus during pregnancy. *Clin Endocrinol (Oxf)* 1993; 38: 595–600.
157 Tur-Kasm I, Paz I, Gleicher W. Disorders of the pituitary and hypothalamus. In: Gleicher N, Butino L et al., eds. *Principles and Practice of Medical Therapy in Pregnancy*, 3rd edn. Stamford, Connecticut: Appleton & Lange, 1998: 424–430.
158 Ross EJ, Christie SB. Hypernatremia. *Medicine* 1969; 48: 441–473.
159 Arieff AI, Guisado R. Effects on the central nervous system of hypernatremic and hyponatremic states. *Kidney Int* 1976; 10: 104–116.
160 Miller M, Dalakos T, Moses AM et al. Recognition of partial defects in antidiuretic hormone secretion. *Ann Intern Med* 1970; 73: 721–729.
161 Blum D, Brasseur D, Kahn A, Brachet E. Safe oral rehydration of hypertonic dehydration. *J Pediatr Gastroenterol Nutr* 1986; 5: 232–235.
162 Bode HH, Harley BM, Crawford JD. Restoration of normal drinking behavior by chlorpropamide in patients with hypodipsia and diabetes insipidus. *Am J Med* 1971; 51: 304–313.
163 Lindeheimer MD, Richardson DA, Ehrlich EN. Potassium homeostasis in pregnancy. *J Reprod Med* 1987; 32(7): 517–532.
164 Godfrey BE, Wadsworth GR. Total body potassium in pregnant women. *J Obstet Gynaecol Br Cmwlth* 1970; 77: 244–246.
165 Anotayanouth S, Subhedar NV, Garner P et al. Betamimetics for inhibiting preterm labor. *Cochrane Database Syst Rev* 2004; Oct 18(4): CD004325.
166 Braden GL, von Oeyen PT, Germain MJ. Ritodrine and terbutaline-induced hypokalemia in preterm labor: Mechanisms and consequences. *Kidney Int* 1997; 51: 1867–1875.
167 Cano A, Tovar I, Parrilla JJ et al. Metabolic disturbances during intravenous use of ritodrine: Increased insulin levels and hypokalemia. *Obstet Gynecol* 1985; 65: 356–360.
168 Hildebrandt R, Weitzel HK, Gundert-Remy U. Hypokalemia in pregnant women treated with β_2 mimetic drug fenoterol–A concentration and time dependent effect. *J Perinat Med* 1997; 25(2): 173–179.
169 O'Sullivan E, Monga M, Graves W. Bartter's syndrome in pregnancy – a case report and review. *Am J Perinatol* 1997; 14(1): 55–57.
170 Johnson JR, Miller RS, Samuels P. Bartter syndrome in pregnancy. *Obstet Gynecol* 2000; 95(6 Part 2): 1035.
171 Nohira T, Nakada T, Akutagawa O et al. Pregnancy complicated with Bartter's syndrome: A case report. *J Obstet Gynaecol Res* 2001; 27(5): 267–274.
172 Smulian JC, Motiwala S, Sigman RC. Pica in a rural obstetric population. *South Med J* 1995; 88: 1236–1240.
173 Ukaonu C, Hill DA, Christensen F. Hypokalemic myopathy in pregnancy caused by clay ingestion. *Obstet Gynecol* 2003; 102(5 pt 2): 1169–1171.

174 Flakeb G, Villarread D, Chapman D. Is hypokalemia a cause of ventricular arrhythmias? *J Crit Ill* 1986; 1: 66.
175 Marino P. Potassium. In: Marino P, ed. *The ICU Book*. Philadelphia: Lea & Febiger, 1991: 478.
176 Smith JD, Bia MJ, DeFronzo RA. Clinical disorders of potassium metabolism. In: Arieff AI, DeFronzo RA, eds. *Fluid, Electrolyte and Acid–Base Disorders*. New York: Churchill Livingstone, 1985: 413.
177 Hartman RC, Auditore JC, Jackson DP. Studies in thrombocytosis. I. Hyperkalemia due to release of potassium from platelets during coagulation. *J Clin Invest* 1958; 37: 699.
178 Robertson GL. Abnormalities of thirst regulation. *Kidney Int* 1984; 25: 460–469.
179 Oster JR, Perez GO, Vaamonde CA. Relationship between blood pH and phosphorus during acute metabolic acidosis. *Am J Physiol* 1978; 235:F345–351.
180 Bismuth C, Gaultier M, Conso F et al. Hyperkalemia in acute digitalis poisoning: prognostic significance and therapeutic implications. *Clin Toxicol* 1973; 6: 153–162.
181 Williams ME, Rosa RM. Hyperkalemia: disorders of internal and external potassium balance. *J Intensive Care Med* 1988; 3: 52.
182 Phelps KR, Lieberman RL, Oh MS et al. Pathophysiology of the syndrome of hyporeninemic hypoaldosteronism. *Metabolism* 1980; 29: 186–199.
183 Sato K, Nishiwaki K, Kuno N et al. Unexpected hyperkalemia following succinylcholine administration in prolonged immobilized parturients treated with magnesium and ritodrine. *Anesthesiology* 2000; 93(6): 1539–1541.
184 Spital A, Greenwell R. Severe hyperkalemia during magnesium sulfate therapy in two pregnant drug abusers. *South Med J* 1991; 84(7): 919–921.
185 Villabona C, Rodriguez P, Joven J. Potassium disturbances as a cause of metabolic neuromyopathy. *Intensive Care Med* 1987; 13: 208–210.
186 Allon M, Shanklin N. Effect of bicarbonate administration on plasma potassium in dialysis patients: interactions with insulin and albuterol. *Am J Kidney Dis* 1996; 28(4): 508–514.
187 Greenberg A. Hyperkalemia treatment options. *Semin Nephrol* 1998; 18(1): 46–57.
188 Mandelberg A, Krupnik Z, Houri S et al. Salbutamol metered-dose inhaler with spacer for hyperkalemia: how fast? How safe? *Chest* 1999; 115(3): 617–622.
189 Stems Rh, Rojas M, Bernstein P, et al. Ion exchange resinsfor the treatment of hyperkalemia: Are they safe and effective? *J Soc Nephrol* 2010: [Epup ahead of print].
190 Marino P. Calcium and phosphorus. In: Marino P, ed. *The ICU Book*. Philadelphia: Lea & Febiger, 1991: 499.
191 ACOG Technical Bulletin No. 219, January 1996: 518.
192 Cruikshank DP, Pitkin RM, Reynolds WA et al. Effects of magnesium sulfate treatment on perinatal calcium metabolism. I–Maternal and fetal responses. *Am J Obstet Gynecol* 1979; 134: 243–249.
193 Cruikshank DP, Chan GM, Doerrfeld D. Alterations in vitamin D and calcium metabolism with magnesium sulfate treatment of preeclampsia. *Am J Obstet Gynecol* 1993; 168: 1170–1177.
194 Cruikshank DP, Pitkin RM, Donnelly E et al. Urinary magnesium, calcium and phosphate excretion during magnesium sulfate infusion. *Obstet Gynecol* 1981; 58: 430–434.
195 Cholst IN, Steinberg SF, Tropper PJ et al. The influence of hypermagnesemia on serum calcium and parathyroid hormone levels in human subjects. *N Engl J Med* 1984; 310: 1221–1225.
196 Carney SL, Wong NL, Quamme GA et al. Effect of magnesium deficiency on renal magnesium and calcium transport in the rat. *J Clin Invest* 1980; 65: 180–188.
197 Snyder SW, Cardwill MS. Neuromuscular blockade with magnesium sulfate and nifedipine. *Am J Obstet Gynecol* 1989; 161(1): 35–36.
198 Kurtzman JL, Thorp JM Jr, Spielman FJ, Mueller RC, Cerfalo RC. Do nifedipine and verapamil potentiate the cardiac toxicity of magnesium sulfate? *Am J Perinatol* 1993; 10(6): 450–452.
199 Magee LA, Miremadi S, Li J et al. Therapy with both magnesium and nifedipine does not increase the risk of serious magnesium-related maternal side effects in women with preeclampsia. *Am J Obstet Gynecol* 2005; 1: 153–163.
200 Anast CS, Winnacker JL, Forte LR, Burns TW. Impaired release of parathyroid hormone in magnesium deficiency. *J Clin Endocrinol Metab* 1976; 42: 707–717.
201 Zaloga GP, Wilkens R, Tourville J et al. A simple method for determining physiologically active calcium and magnesium concentrations in critically ill patients. *Crit Care Med* 1987; 15: 813–816.
202 Zaloga GP, Chernow B. The multifactorial basis for hypocalcemia during sepsis. Studies of the parathyroid hormone-vitamin D axis. *Ann Intern Med* 1987; 107: 36–41.
203 Zaloga GP, Chernow B. Stress-induced changes in calcium metabolism. *Semin Respir Med* 1985; 7: 56.
204 Chernow B, Rainey TG, Georges LP, O'Brian JT. Iatrogenic hyperphosphatemia: a metabolic consideration in critical care medicine. *Crit Care Med* 1981; 9: 772–774.
205 Zaloga GP. Phosphate disorders. *Probl Crit Care* 1990; 4: 416.
206 Nagant De Deuxchaisnes C, Krane SM. Hypoparathyroidism. In: Avioli LV, Krane SM, eds. *Metabolic Bone Disease*, vol 2. Orlando, FL: Academic, 1978: 217.
207 Zaloga GP, Chernow B. Calcium metabolism. *Clin Crit Care Med* 1985; 5.
208 Monif GR, Savory J. Iatrogenic maternal hypocalcemia following magnesium sulfate therapy. *JAMA* 1972; 219(11): 1469–1470.
209 Haynes RC, Murad F. Agents affecting calcification: calcium, parathyroid hormone, calcitonin, vitamin D, and other compounds. In: Gilman AG, Goodman LS, Rall TW, Murad F, eds. *Goodman and Gilman's The Pharmacological Basis of Therapeutics*. New York: Macmillan, 1985: 1517.
210 Ennen CS, Magann EF. Milk alkali syndrome presenting as acute renal insufficiency during pregnancy. *Obstet Gynecol* 2006; 108(3 pt 2): 785–786.
211 Benabe JE, Martinez-Maldonado R. Disorders of calcium metabolism. In: Maxwell MH, Kleeman CR, Narins RG, eds. *Clinical Disorders of Fluid and Electrolyte Metabolism*, 4th edn. New York: McGraw-Hill, 1987: 758.
212 Mundy GR. *Calcium Homeostasis: Hypercalcemia and Hypocalcemia*. London: Martin Dunitz, 1989: 1.
213 Montoro MN, Paler RJ, Goodwin TM et al. Parathyroid carcinoma during pregnancy. *Obstet Gynecol* 2000; 96(5 Part 2): 841.
214 Mestamen JH. Parathyroid disorders of pregnancy. *Semin Perinatol* 1998; 22(6): 485–496.
215 Thomas AK, McVie R, Levine SN. Disorders of maternal calcium metabolism implicated by abnormal calcium metabolism in the neonate. *Am J Perinatol* 1999; 16(10): 515–520.
216 Illidge TM, Hussey M, Godden CW. Malignant hypercalcaemia in pregnancy and antenatal administration of intravenous pamidronate. *Clin Oncol (R Coll Radiol)* 1996; 8(4): 257–258.

217 Graepel P, Bentley P, Fritz H et al. Reproductive studies with pamidronate. *Arzneimittelforschung* 1992; 42(5): 654–667.

218 Quamme GA, Dirks KJ. Magnesium metabolism. In: Maxwell MH, Kleeman CR, Narins RG, eds. *Clinical Disorders of Fluid and Electrolyte Metabolism*, 4th edn. New York: McGraw-Hill 1987: 297.

219 Zaloga GP, Roberts JE. Magnesium disorders. *Probl Crit Care* 1990; 4: 425.

220 Salem M, Munoz R, Chernow B. Hypomagnesemia in critical illness. A common and clinically important problem. *Crit Care Clin* 1991; 7: 225–252.

221 Reinhart RA. Magnesium metabolism. A review with special reference to the relationship between intracellular content and serum levels. *Arch Intern Med* 1988; 148: 2415–2420.

222 Dacey MJ. Hypomagnesemic disorders. *Crit Care Clin* 2001; 17(1): 155–173.

223 Marino P. Magnesium: the hidden ion. In: Marino P, ed. *The ICU ook*. Philadelphia: Lea & Febiger, 1991: 489.

224 Ryan MP. Diuretics and potassium/magnesium depletion. *Direction Am J Med* 1987; 82: 38A.

225 Zaloga GP, Chernow B, Pock A et al. Hypomagnesemia is a common complication of aminoglycoside therapy. *Surg Gynecol Obstet* 1984; 158: 561–565.

226 Elin RJ. Magnesium metabolism in health and disease. *Dis Mon* 1988; 34: 161–218.

227 Berkelhammer C, Bear RA. A clinical approach to common electrolyte problems: hypomagnesemia. *Can Med Assoc J* 1985; 132: 360–368.

228 Brauthbar N, Massry SG. Hypomagnesemia and hypermagnesemia. In: Maxwell MH, Kleeman CR, Narins RG, eds. *Clinical Disorders of Fluid and Electrolyte Metabolism*, 4th edn. New York: McGraw-Hill, 1987: 831.

229 Kingston ME, Al-Siba'i MB, Skooge WC. Clinical manifestations of hypomagnesemia. *Crit Care Med* 1986; 14: 950–954.

230 Zaloga GP. Interpretation of the serum magnesium level. *Chest* 1989; 95: 257–258.

231 Iseri LT, Freed J, Bures AR. Magnesium deficiency and cardiac disorders. *Am J Med* 1975; 58: 837–846.

232 Burch GE, Giles TD. The importance of magnesium deficiency in cardiovascular disease. *Am Heart J* 1977; 94: 649–651.

233 Rasmussen HS, McNair P, Norregard P et al. Intravenous magnesium in acute myocardial infarction. *Lancet* 1986; 1: 234–236.

234 Abraham AS, Rosenmann D, Kramer M et al. Magnesium in the prevention of lethal arrhythmias in acute myocardial infarction. *Arch Intern Med* 1987; 147: 753–755.

235 Flink EB. Therapy of magnesium deficiency. *Ann NY Acad Sci* 1969; 162: 901–905.

236 Mordes JP, Wacker WE. Excess magnesium. *Pharmacol Rev* 1977; 29: 273–300.

237 Heath DA. The emergency management of disorders of calcium and magnesium. *Clin Endocrinol Metab* 1980; 9: 487–502.

238 Rude RK, Singer FR. Magnesium deficiency and excess. *Annu Rev Med* 1981; 32: 245–259.

239 Cronin RE, Knochel JP. Magnesium deficiency. *Adv Intern Med* 1983; 28: 509–533.

240 Whang R, Flink EB, Dyckner T et al. Magnesium depletion as a cause of refractory potassium repletion. *Arch Intern Med* 1985; 145: 1686–1689.

241 Stewart AF, Horst R, Deftos LJ et al. Biochemical evaluation of patients with cancer-associated hypercalcemia: evidence for humoral and nonhumoral groups. *N Engl J Med* 1980; 303: 1377–1383.

242 Waisman GD, Mayorga LM, Camera MI, Vignolo CA, Martinotti A. Magnesium plus nifedipine: potentiation of hypotensive effect in preeclampsia? *Am J Obstet Gynecol* 1988; 159(2): 308–309.

243 Fassler CA, Rodriguez RM, Badesch DB et al. Magnesium toxicity as a cause of hypotension and hypoventilation. *Arch Intern Med* 1985; 14: 1604–1606.

244 Bohman VR, Cotton DB. Supralethal magnesemia with patient survival. *Obstet Gynecol* 1990; 76: 984–985.

245 Oh MS. Selective hypoaldosteronism. *Resident Staff Phys* 1982; 28: 46S.

7 Cardiopulmonary Resuscitation in Pregnancy

Andrea Shields[1] & M. Bardett Fausett[2]

[1]Antenatal Diagnostic Center, San Antonio Military Medical Center, Lackland Airforce Base, Texas, USA

[2]Obstetrics and Maternal-Fetal Medicine, San Antonio Military Medical Center *and* Department of Obstetrics and Gynecology, Wilford Hall Medical Center, Lackland Airforce Base, Texas, USA

Introduction

Sudden cardiac arrest (SCA) is a leading cause of death in the United States and Canada. An estimated 330 000 people die annually in the United States from SCA in out-of-hospital and emergency department settings [1]. This translates to 0.55 per thousand people in the US, and 1 in 30 000 gravid women who will suffer SCA each year. Overall maternal mortality is significantly higher in developing countries including mortality from SCA. Women of childbearing age are commonly healthy and the overall risk of death is low in developed nations. These facts, along with the additional life involved, make SCA in pregnancy unexpected and particularly devastating.

Women are most likely to survive cardiopulmonary arrest when attended by providers skilled in basic and advanced cardiopulmonary resuscitative techniques. The mechanical and physiologic changes of pregnancy impact every phase of the resuscitation process. In this chapter, we review the most recent American Heart Association (AHA) cardiopulmonary resuscitation (CPR) guidelines and emphasize pregnancy-specific modifications. We do not address infant and child resuscitation in this chapter but the practicing obstetrician should likewise be expert with neonatal resuscitation. In this chapter, we will consider other relevant pregnancy-related issues such as perimortem cesarean section and the ethical dilemma of prolonged maternal life support for fetal maturation.

The initial objective of CPR and emergency cardiac care (ECC) is to maintain adequate oxygenation and vital organ perfusion. CPR restores hemodynamic stability in 40–60% of arrested patients; however, prolonged survival is lower with underlying illness [2]. Overall outcome, particularly full neurologic recovery, is improved by early initiation of CPR and defibrillation. Most victims of SCA demonstrate ventricular fibrillation at some point leading to full arrest. Ventricular fibrillation is best treated by electrical cardioversion performed within the first 5 minutes after collapse [3]. Since the majority of SCA occurs outside of the hospital setting, it is uncommon for emergency medical service personnel to be contacted and arrive at the victim's side within these critical 5 minutes [4]. Thus, achieving a high survival rate depends upon public training in CPR and well-organized public access defibrillation programs. Considering all victims, out-of-hospital survival rates for SCA victims are only 6% but can improve to 75% when victims are given high-quality CPR [4]. Outside of the hospital, SCA is usually associated with catastrophic trauma and is rarely a survivable event for pregnant women even in developed countries.

In the hospital, SCA in pregnancy is usually associated with peripartum events [5]. In such circumstances delivery of high-quality CPR is likely to have a significant impact on survival rates. Thus, hospital personnel involved in the care of pregnant women should be expertly trained and facile in techniques of cardiopulmonary resuscitation. Obstetrical units should have proper resuscitative equipment readily available and staff members be engaged in ongoing programs to train and maintain CPR competency. In one recent evaluation of obstetric training programs, the authors concluded that even basic life support knowledge and skills are inadequate and ongoing training is necessary [6].

Current cardiac care recommendations

In December 2005, the American Heart Association published an update to the guidelines for lay and professional Basic and Advanced Cardiac Life Support (BLS/ACLS). A summary of the ABCDs of lay and provider rescuer BLS is shown in Table 7.1. The primary changes to the 2005 resuscitation guidelines were meant to simplify algorithms and promote their early application to SCA victims. The new guidelines include four major changes relevant to women of reproductive age and are applicable to both lay and provider rescuer CPR [7]. These general changes are summarized in Table 7.2.

Critical Care Obstetrics, 5th edition. Edited by M. Belfort, G. Saade, M. Foley, J. Phelan and G. Dildy.

Airway	Head tilt/chin lift unless trauma then use jaw thrust
Breathing: Initial	2 breaths at 1 second/breath
Rescue breathing without chest compressions	10–12 breaths/min
Rescue breaths with advanced airway	8–10 breaths/min
Foreign body obstruction	Abdominal thrusts
Circulation	
Pulse check (≤10 s)	Carotid
Compression landmarks	Lower half of sternum, between nipples
Compression method	Heel of one hand with the other on top; push hard and fast and allow complete recoil
Compression depth	1½ to 2 inches
Compression rate	100/min
Compression : ventilation ratio	30 : 2 (either one or two rescuers)
Defibrillation	
AED	After 5 cycles of CPR if out of hospital

Table 7.1 Summary of CPR ABCDs (modified from "Summary of BLS ABCD maneuvers for infants, children and adults")[68].

Table 7.2 Summary of key changes in 2005 CPR guidelines [4].

Deliver more effective chest compressions	Early, consistent, fast, hard
Single compression : ventilation ratio for all but neonates	30 : 2
Rescue breaths	Given over 1 second; 500–600 mL for adults
Defibrillation	After first shock go directly to compression : ventilations × 2 min

First, there is significant emphasis on, and recommendations to improve, delivery of effective chest compressions. The key words are early, consistent, fast and hard. This emphasis is made because half of chest compressions (even by healthcare providers) are too shallow. The chest is often not allowed to recoil adequately between compressions and interruptions are too common. Complete chest wall recoil increases cardiac filling by increasing negative pressure, promoting venous return and maximizing cardiac output with the subsequent compression. The first few compressions after interruption are not as effective as those that follow. Thus, inadequate compressions, incomplete chest recoil and frequent interruptions all significantly decrease circulation and oxygen delivery and decrease survival [7].

The second new recommendation is for a single 30 : 2 compression to ventilation ratio for all victims except newborns. The guideline authors note most cases of cardiac arrest in adults are not hypoxia-induced. Consequently, circulation is more critical than ventilation in the first minute of CPR. Since the blood flow to the lungs is diminished (25–33%) during arrest/CPR, victims need less ventilation than normal. In contrast, newborn cardiac arrest is commonly related to hypoxia so more ventilations (5:1) to compressions are indicated and remain part of the new guidelines [7].

The third recommendation is that each rescue breath should be given over 1 second (rather than 1–2 seconds) and produces a visible chest rise. The visible chest rise ensures efficacy and the 1-second breath provides adequate tidal volume (500–600 mL) while avoiding hyperinflation. Rescuers are to take a normal breath before giving the rescue breath. Frequent rescue breathing interrupts and delays chest compressions. Hyperinflation increases intrathoracic pressure leading to decreased blood return to the chest. This results in diminished efficacy of the next several compressions and increases the risk of gastric insufflation.

The final new major recommendation is that during ventricular fibrillation (VF) cardiac arrest, a single shock should be given followed by immediate CPR. CPR is to begin even before the first rhythm check 2 minutes later. Historically, rhythm analysis by automated defibrillators available before 2005 resulted in delays of more than 30 seconds before giving the first post-shock compressions. Current defibrillators eliminate VF more than 85% of the time. Thus, in a case where the first shock fails, CPR is likely to convey greater value than a second shock. Even when a shock eliminates VF, it usually takes several minutes for a normal effective rhythm to return. A brief period of CPR can increase energy and oxygen to the heart, increasing the likelihood that the heart will be able to continue effective blood flow. There is no evidence that postdefibrillation chest compressions provoke recurrent VF. For similar reasons, lay rescuer CPR recommendations now eliminate the initial check for pulse after giving the initial two rescue breaths [7].

Key changes to recommendations for provider-level and hospital-based adult BLS include use of the 30 : 2 ventilation to compression ratio (even with two rescuers) until an advanced airway is in place. As noted in the general guidelines above, before an advanced airway is in place, rescuers should perform 5 cycles of CPR after shock before the next rhythm check. Even once the advanced airway is in place, rescuers should perform 2 minutes of CPR after shock before the next rhythm check. With two or more rescuers and an advanced airway in place, rescuers no longer provide cycles of compressions with pauses for ventilation. One rescuer provides 8–10 breaths per minute (1 every 6–8 seconds) while the other rescuer provides continuous compressions. Where possible, rescuers should rotate the compressor role every 2 minutes, taking no more than 5 seconds to do so. After 2–3 minutes of CPR, rescuers typically perform chest compressions less effectively [7]. The general provider BLS algorithm is shown in Figure 7.1 and the pulseless arrest ACLS algorithm in Figure 7.2. Algorithms for tachycardia and bradycardia are not included here but are usually available on all "code carts".

Patient population and etiologies of SCA in pregnancy

Of women who suffer SCA during pregnancy, most have thromboembolic-, followed by hemorrhage-, related events [8]. The most common causes of SCA during pregnancy are listed in Table 7.3. Victims of SCA in pregnancy are younger and have fewer underlying medical conditions than non-pregnant victims [8]. However, maternal age and underlying medical problems continue to increase in developed countries due to elective delayed childbearing and advanced reproductive technologies.

Pregnancy increases the risk of venous thromboembolic disease (VTE) due to hormonally stimulated increases of virtually all of the procoagulant proteins. The risk of VTE is amplified by conditions necessitating bed rest such as gestational hypertensive disorders and preterm labor. The risk is highest in the immediate postpartum period, [9] probably due to the tissue trauma and decreased physical activity associated with delivery.

Lipo-oxidative injury to the coronary vessels is the most common cause of SCA in non-pregnant individuals but is an uncommon cause of SCA in pregnancy. However, the added physiologic stress of pregnancy can unveil underlying congenital or acquired valve disease. Pregnancy does increase the risk of myocardial infarction 3–4-fold over otherwise comparable non-pregnant women. The pregnancy-related MI risk is significantly greater in women older than 30 years [10]. Additionally, pregnant women have a relatively increased risk of coronary artery and aortic dissections compared to non-pregnant women with otherwise similar demographic characteristics [11]. This may be due to progesterone-mediated relaxation of smooth muscle.

Pregnancy-specific conditions associated with SCA

Turning now to pregnancy-specific conditions associated with SCA, we first highlight the anaphylactoid syndrome of pregnancy also called amniotic fluid embolus (AFE). This disorder is characterized by an anaphylaxis-like syndrome that is associated with cardiac depression, cardiopulmonary collapse and coagulopathy. The disorder is highly lethal with a 50–65% risk of cardiac arrest and maternal death [12–15]. This catastrophic condition is discussed in detail in Chapter 35 but the reader is encouraged to remember that this disorder is associated with profound vascular leak, and over-resuscitation with crystalloid fluids can result in massive pulmonary edema. Therapy targeted to support the cardiovascular system and correct the coagulopathy while avoiding over-resuscitation with crystalloid fluid may be helpful [16].

Gestational hypertensive disorders occur more frequently than thromboembolic disorders and both occur more commonly than anaphylactoid syndrome of pregnancy [14]. Women with hypertensive disorders of pregnancy are at increased risk of SCA for several reasons including the associated underlying endothelial injury and inflammatory response. Hypertension may necessitate medical therapy and magnesium is often used for seizure prophylaxis. Both may be associated with cardiac compromise leading to SCA [17–20]. Profound hypotension and SCA can occur in women with pre-eclampsia treated concurrently with calcium channel antagonists and magnesium sulfate. In cases of cardiopulmonary compromise due to magnesium sulfate toxicity, resuscitation must include calcium rescue. The typical dose is 1 g of intravenous calcium carbonate.

ABCDs in pregnancy

If breathing stops first, then the heart often continues to pump for several minutes usually providing enough oxygen in the lungs and bloodstream to support life for up to 6 minutes [21]. In contrast, when the heart stops first, oxygen in the lungs and bloodstream cannot be circulated to vital organs. The patient whose heart and respirations have stopped for less than 4 minutes has an excellent chance of recovery if CPR is administered immediately and is followed by ACLS within 4 minutes [22]. By 4–6 minutes, brain damage may occur, and after 6 minutes, brain damage will almost always occur. Therefore, the initial goals of CPR are to deliver oxygen to the lungs and provide a means of circulation to the vital organs. Initially circulation is provided via closed-chest compression followed by ACLS, with restoration of the heart as the mechanism of circulation. These goals are achieved by remembering the "ABCDs" of the primary and secondary survey (Table 7.1). The primary survey consists of airway management using non-invasive techniques, breathing with positive-pressure ventilations, and performing CPR until equipment for external defibrillation arrives. Out-of-hospital and BLS tools required include gloved hands, a barrier device for CPR, and an automated external defibrillator (AED) for defibrillation. A secondary survey requires the use of advanced, invasive techniques as the rescuer attempts to resuscitate, stabilize, and transfer the patient to a higher level of care if indicated (i.e. hospital or intensive care setting). Potentially reversible causes of cardiopulmonary arrest should also be considered and addressed at this stage (Table 7.4).

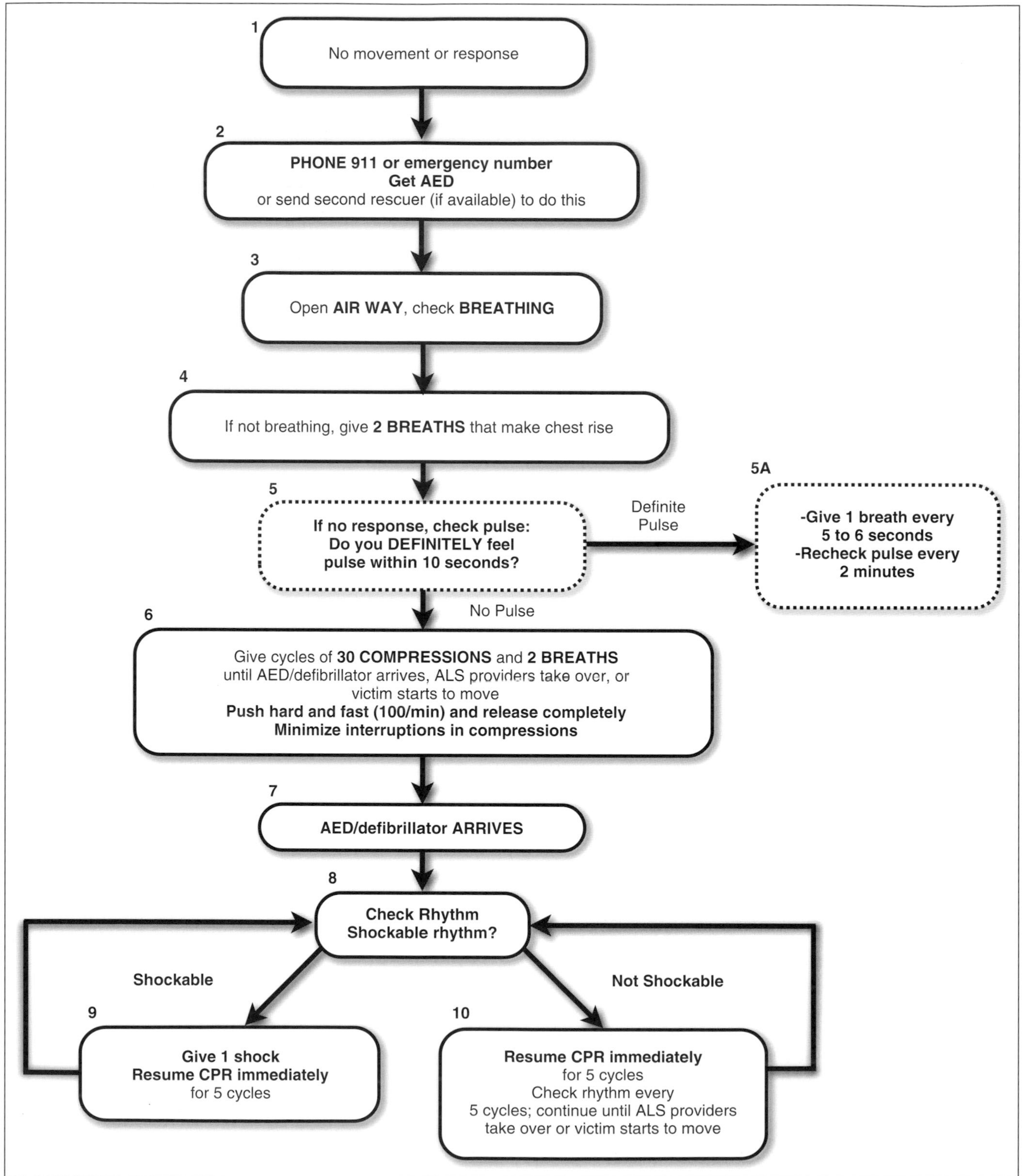

Figure 7.1 ACLS Adult BLS Provider Algorithm. Modified from Circulation 2005; 112: IV-58–IV-66.

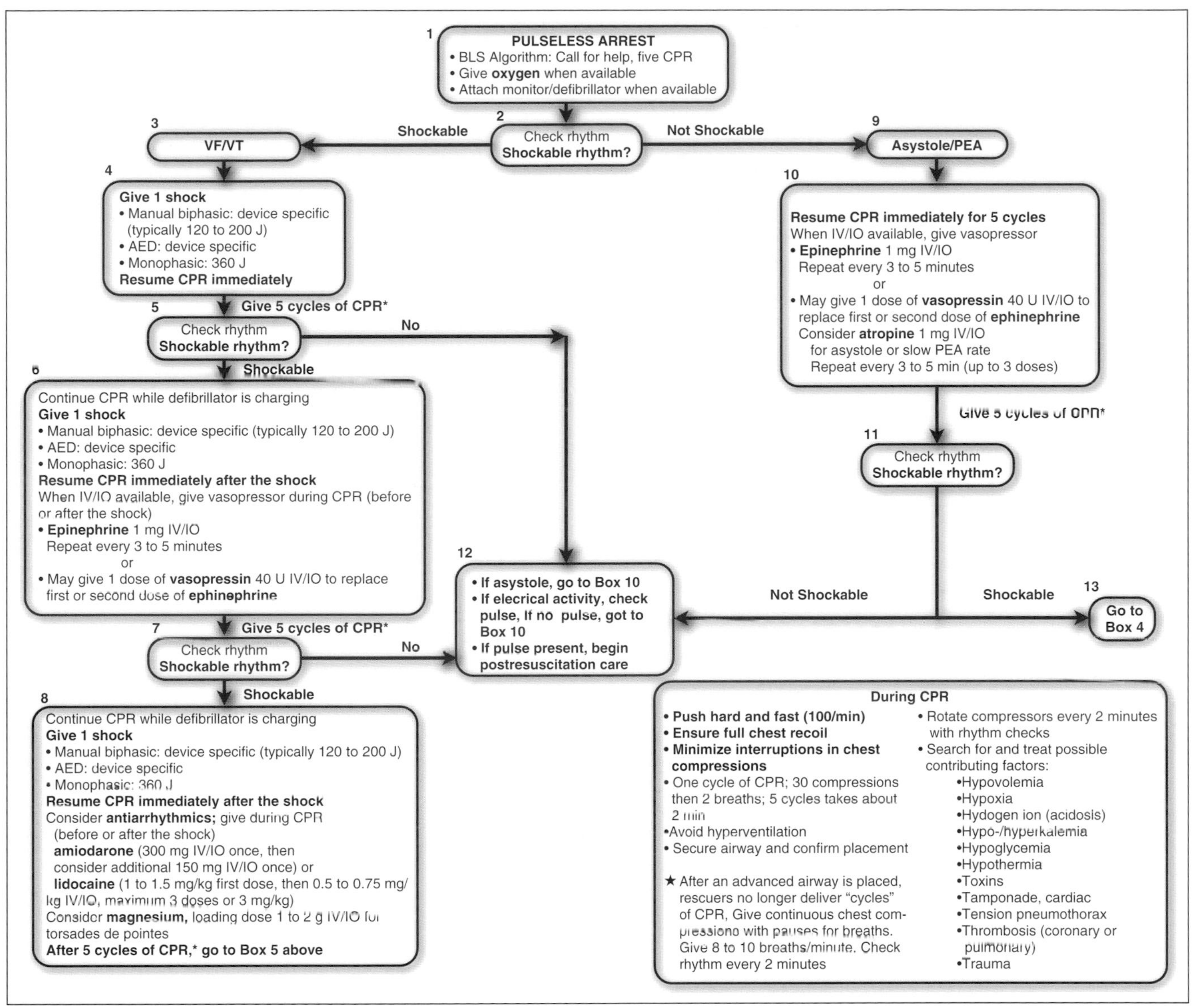

Figure 7.2 ACLS Adult Pulseless Arrest Algorithm. Modified from Circulation 2005; 112: IV-58–IV-66.

Airway

Delivery of oxygen is achieved by positioning the patient, opening the airway, and delivering rescue breaths. In the absence of muscle tone, the tongue and epiglottis frequently obstruct the airway. The head tilt with the chin-lift maneuver (Figure 7.3) or the jaw thrust maneuver (Figure 7.4) facilitates airway access. If foreign material appears in the mouth, it should be removed. If air does not enter the lungs with rescue breathing, reposition the head and repeat the attempt at rescue breathing. Persistent obstruction may require the Heimlich maneuver (subdiaphragmatic abdominal thrusts), chest thrusts, removal of foreign body if now visualized, and rescue breathing. The Heimlich maneuver cannot be used in the late stages of pregnancy or in the obese choking victim. Airway obstruction may occur in a choking victim as well as the patient experiencing a cardiopulmonary arrest. The conscious women with only partial airway obstruction should be allowed to attempt to clear the obstruction herself. Rescuers should avoid the finger sweep in a conscious patient.

In the first half of pregnancy, airway obstruction can be relieved with the Heimlich maneuver or abdominal thrusts. From a standing position the rescuer wraps his arms around the victim's waist, making a fist with one hand and placing the thumb side of the fist against the victim's abdomen in the midline slightly above the umbilicus and well below the top of the xiphoid process. The rescuer grasps the fist with the other hand and presses the fist into the victim's abdomen with quick, distinct, upward thrusts. The thrusts are continued until the object is expelled or the victim is unconscious. The unconscious victim is placed supine, the heel of one hand remains against the victim's abdomen, in the midline slightly above the umbilicus but below the top of the xiphoid. The

Table 7.3 Causes of cardiac arrest during pregnancy [69].

Venous thromboembolism
Pregnancy-induced hypertension
Sepsis
Amniotic fluid embolism
Hemorrhage
Placental abruption
Placenta previa
Uterine atony
Disseminated intravascular coagulation
Trauma
Iatrogenic
Medication errors or allergy
Anesthetic complications
Hypermagnesemia
Pre-existing heart disease
Congenital
Acquired

Table 7.4 Potentially reversible causes of cardiac arrest.

Hypovolemia
Hypoxia
Hydrogen ion acidosis
Hyper- or hypokalemia, other metabolic
Hypothermia
Tablets (drug overdose)
Trauma
Tamponade, cardiac
Tension pneumothorax
Thrombosis, coronary
Thrombosis, pulmonary
Toxins (e.g. amniotic fluid)

second hand lies directly on top of the first, and quick upward thrusts are administered.

In the latter half of pregnancy, the gravid uterus or maternal habitus may necessitate the use of chest thrusts instead of abdominal thrusts. Chest thrusts in a conscious sitting or standing victim require placing the thumb side of the fist on the middle of the sternum, avoiding the xiphoid and the ribs. The rescuer then grabs his or her own fist with the other hand and performs chest thrusts until either the foreign object is dislodged or the patient loses consciousness. The unconscious patient is placed supine. The rescuer's hand closest to the patient's head is placed 2 fingerbreadths above the xiphoid. The long axis of the heel of the provider's hand rests on the long axis of the sternum and the other hand lies over the first, with the fingers either extended or interlaced. The elbows are extended and the chest is compressed 1.5–2 inches. Up to 5 abdominal or chest thrusts are given followed by repetition of the jaw-lift, foreign body visualization, and attempted ventilation. These steps are repeated until effective or until a surgical airway can be obtained by emergency cricothyrotomy or jet-needle insufflation.

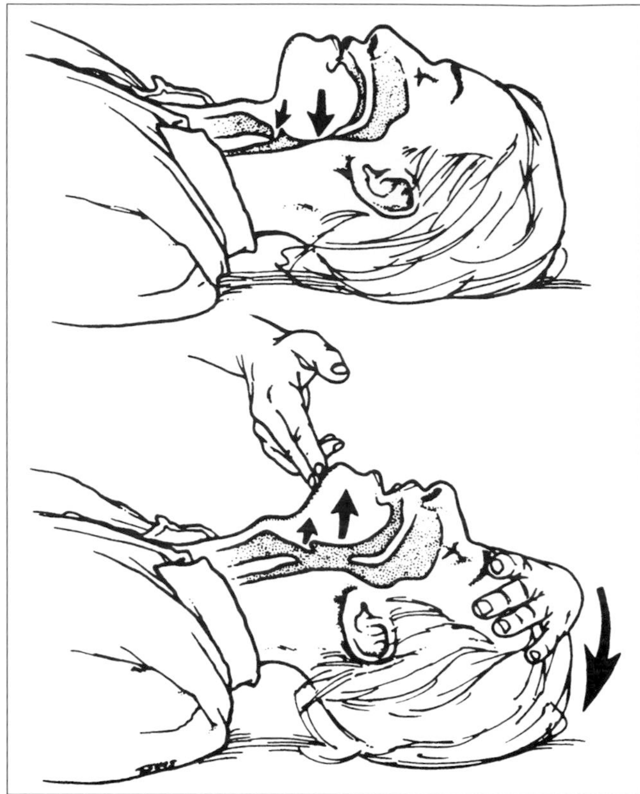

Figure 7.3 Head tilt, chin lift.

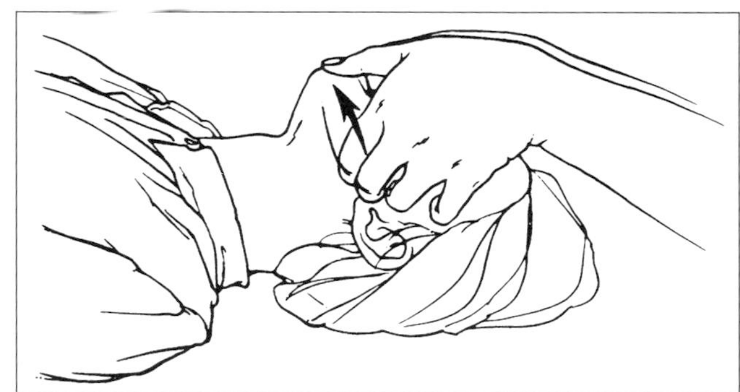

Figure 7.4 Jaw thrust.

If, after clearing any obstruction, the patient is unresponsive but breathing spontaneously, she is placed in the recovery position to keep the airway open. The pregnant victim is placed on her left side. The left arm is placed at a right angle to the victim's torso, while the right arm is placed across her chest with the back of her hand under the lower cheek. The victim's right thigh is flexed at a right angle to the torso, across the left leg, with the right knee resting on the surface. The victim's head is tilted back to maintain the airway, using the right hand to maintain the head tilt. Fetal monitoring should begin as soon as possible and breathing is monitored regularly. If breathing does not resume after clearing the airway or if it stops, the emergency medical system is activated and the BCDs of CPR continued.

In cases of a witnessed respiratory arrest when the airway is known to be clear but the victim is not breathing, the airway must be protected from aspiration and kept patent, and the BLS/ACLS algorithms begun. Endotracheal intubation by direct laryngoscopy is the preferred method for maintaining airway patency for the gravid arrest victim. Alternative techniques for airway management include endotracheal intubation by light stylet, esophageal tracheal combitube, laryngeal mask airway, and transtracheal ventilation. Tracheal intubation offers advantages of securely protecting the airway, facilitating oxygenation and ventilation, and providing a route for drug administration during a cardiac arrest.

In the hospital setting immediate confirmation of the tracheal tube is typically done using non-physical examination techniques, such as end-tidal (ET) carbon dioxide indicators. The presence of ET CO_2 is a reliable measure of pulmonary perfusion and, therefore, can measure the efficacy of CPR. Esophageal detector devices may also be used to confirm tracheal tube placement but false-negative results may be obtained in women in late gestation. False-negative results are due to decreased functional residual capacity (FRC) and tracheal compression in late pregnancy. Consequently, the gold standard for confirmation in the pregnant women remains repeat direct visualization [23].

Even with advanced airway techniques, airway access and maintenance can be difficult in pregnancy due to enlarged breasts and increased pharyngeal edema. Rescuers may find it necessary to use a slightly smaller endotracheal tube than normal [24]. Also, progesterone relaxes the smooth muscle of the lower esophageal sphincter and increases the propensity of the gravida to reflux and aspirate.

Breathing

Rescue breathing may occur mouth-to-mouth, mouth-to-nose, mouth-to-mask, bag valve-to-mask, or ultimately by endotracheal intubation. The current guidelines call for a ratio of 2 ventilations to 30 compressions in one- or two-person CPR, pausing for ventilations in the absence of an advanced airway. With a protected airway, the 2005 guidelines call for continuous chest compression with rescue breaths every 6 seconds [25].

In pregnancy, the expanding breast tissue decreases chest wall compliance, making ventilation more difficult. The enlarging uterus results in upward displacement of the diaphragm leading to a decrease in the functional residual capacity (FRC) of the lungs. Maternal minute ventilation increases, probably due to a central effect of progesterone. The decrease in FRC combined with the increase in oxygen demand predisposes the pregnant woman to rapid decreases in arterial and venous oxygen tension during periods of decreased ventilation. The chronic increase in ventilation in pregnancy leads to a decline in arterial carbon dioxide tension. The maternal kidney compensates for this respiratory alkalosis by reducing serum bicarbonate concentration. The maternal respiratory alkalosis enhances fetal excretion of carbon dioxide. Hence, increases in maternal carbon dioxide levels promote fetal acidosis. During periods of hypoxia there is also decreased uteroplacental blood flow which further promotes fetal acidosis. Thus, the demands of the fetus and normal maternal adaptations to those demands promote rapid maternal hypoxia and acidosis in the presence of hypoventilation. This makes it more difficult to resuscitate the mother and ultimately the fetus.

Circulation

An adequately functioning heart and sufficient quality and quantity of blood are necessary to deliver oxygen to the tissues. In the pulseless patient, external chest compressions provide a means of circulation, as originally described by Kouwenhoven and colleagues in 1960 [26]. The initial belief that the chest compressions cause direct compression of the heart between the sternum and the spine, leading to a rise in ventricular pressure, closure of the mitral and tricuspid valves, forcing blood into the pulmonary artery and aorta, has been disproved. We now understand the primary mechanism of blood movement involves compression-mediated fluctuations in the intrathoracic pressure that create an arteriovenous pressure gradient peripherally [27]. External chest compressions cause a rise in intrathoracic pressure, which is distributed to all the intrathoracic structures. Competent venous valves prevent transmission of this pressure to extrathoracic veins, whereas the arteries transmit the increased pressure to extrathoracic arteries, creating an artificial venous pressure gradient and forward blood flow. Werner et al. [28] used echocardiography to support the notion of the heart as a passive conduit, rather than a pump, by demonstrating that the mitral and tricuspid valves remain open during CPR.

With or without an advanced airway, when chest compressions are required, they should be given at a rate of approximately 100/min. Chest compressions should only be interrupted for brief assessments and application of electrical therapy when indicated by the specific rhythm and cardiac circulatory effectiveness. The BLS algorithms include the use of automated external defibrillators (AEDs). AED availability and rapid deployment has lead to improved survival. ACLS involves additional electrical and pharmacologic therapy, invasive monitoring, and other therapeutic techniques to correct cardiac arrhythmias, metabolic imbalances, and other causes of cardiac arrest. Defibrillators can be used without significant complications to the fetus in pregnant women [29]. The fetus has a relatively high fibrillation threshold and the electrical current density reaching the fetus is small. Nanson and colleagues evaluated women during and after pregnancy and compared transthoracic impedance values. Because there was no significant difference, the authors concluded that no modifications to the recommendations for non-pregnant patients were necessary [30].

Concurrent with establishing cardiac function, resuscitators must assure that arrest victims have adequate quality and quantity of blood remaining in the vascular tree for circulation. Although volume administration, which can lead to decreased cerebral and coronary blood flow, is generally not recommended during treatment of cardiac arrest, it should be strongly considered in cardiopulmonary arrest related to postpartum hemorrhage or circulatory collapse as seen with amniotic fluid embolism. Accordingly, early in the resuscitation, resources should be mobilized to obtain blood products to refill the vascular tree and manage ongoing hemorrhage. Current data suggest that the optimal product for resuscitations involving massive hemorrhage is whole blood or reconstitutes thereof. However, overzealous fluid resuscitation, particularly with crystalloid fluids, before controlling hemorrhage and in the early phases of resuscitation, actually decreases survival [31–35]. Factor VII concentrates, now available in many medical centers in the United States, provide an improved means of correcting coagulopathies also common to obstetric hemorrhage. There are now several reports of using recombinant factor VII concentrates in uncontrolled obstetric hemorrhage [31–35]. The reader is referred to Chapter 22 in this text for more information regarding the management of hemorrhage in pregnancy.

This stage of the primary and secondary survey of BLS/ACLS should include an assessment of the fetal status and whether or not delivery of the fetus would be of benefit to mother and/or fetus. Morris and colleagues [36] evaluated neonatal survival following emergency cesarean section in trauma patients presenting to nine Level I trauma centers. The authors suggest adding Doppler fetal heart tone (FHT) assessment to the primary survey along with assessment of maternal circulation. If FHTs are not present, the authors suggest the fetus should otherwise be ignored and treatment directed toward maternal survival. Nonetheless, delivery of the fetus can be considered in the secondary survey if fetal distress is present. More importantly, delivery may be a means of improving effectiveness of maternal CPR efforts even in cases of antecedent fetal death. This has led to a recommendation by some to avoid using precious time for assessment of fetal status when moving forward with cesarean section for maternal benefit [37].

The effect of pregnancy on cardiopulmonary resuscitation

Pregnancy produces physiologic changes that have profound effects on cardiopulmonary resuscitation. Pregnancy-specific physiologic changes and recommended intervention changes to CPR are summarized in Tables 7.5 and 7.6. There are significant changes in the pulmonary, cardiovascular and renal systems. Some of these changes have been briefly described above. A more comprehensive description of these changes and their impact on CPR follows.

From the circulatory perspective, pregnancy represents a high-flow, low-resistance state characterized by a high cardiac output (CO) and low systemic vascular resistance (SVR). Cardiac output increases by 50% of non-pregnant values. The uterus receives up to 30% of cardiac output compared with 2–3% in the non-gravid patient. The increase in CO satisfies the increase in oxygen demands of the growing fetus, the placenta, and the mother.

In the latter half of pregnancy, aortocaval compression by the gravid uterus renders resuscitation more difficult in the pregnant woman than in her non-pregnant counterpart. The pregnant uterus exerts pressure on the inferior vena cava common iliac vessels, and abdominal aorta. In the supine position, such uterine obstruction may lead to sequestration of up to 30% of circulating blood volume [38], decreasing venous return, causing supine hypotension, and decreasing effectiveness of thoracic compressions. Furthermore, the enlarged uterus poses an obstruction to forward blood flow, particularly when arterial pressure and volume are decreased, as in cardiac arrest.

The use of drugs for resuscitation

Changes in the gravida woman's response to drugs may also hinder effective resuscitation. Vasopressors used in ACLS, especially alpha-adrenergic or combined alpha and beta agents, are capable of producing uteroplacental vasoconstriction, leading to decreased fetal oxygenation and carbon dioxide exchange.

Clinical experience with the pharmacologic agents used in ACLS is limited in pregnancy, particularly when the drugs are used for acute life-threatening situations. In the acute situation, absent or poor maternal cardiac output produces fetal hypoxia and hypercarbia. Thus, despite the potential for uteroplacental vascular vasoconstriction, the benefits of these drugs in restoring maternal circulation outweigh their risks.

Most of the data concerning fetal effects of these drugs come from chronic use rather than limited dosing in the acute arrest setting. Beginning with the 2000 American Heart Association ACLS guidelines, amiodarone became the drug of choice for treatment of wide-complex tachycardia, stable narrow-complex tachycardia, monomorphic and polymorphic VT, and potentially for shock-refractory VF/VT. Placental transfer occurs with amiodarone at approximately a quarter of the maternal dose. Amiodarone has been labeled a category D drug by the manufacturer. With chronic use, fetal effects such as growth restriction, hypothyroid goiter, enlarged fontanels, and transient bradycardia in the newborn have all been reported [39]. The drug has been used to successfully treat resistant fetal tachycardia both transplacentally and by direct insertion into the umbilical cord [39]. As with the vasopressors, the concerns raised about chronic use should not negate using amiodarone for maternal resuscitation.

Vasopressin was added as a first-line pressor agent in the 2000 CPR guidelines. However, in the 2005 guidelines epinephrine remains the drug of choice as the first-dose pressor agent given in various scenarios given the available data. Nonetheless vasopressin may have a lower adverse affect profile than epinephrine and the 2005 guidelines allow its use primarily to use primarily when a second pressor dose is required [40,41]. See Figure 7.2. Some controversy remains about high-dose (>1 mg and usually 4–5 mg) epinephrine in these scenarios [41–44]. At present, the consensus appears to be to use regular-dose epinephrine initially

Table 7.5 Relevant maternal physiologic changes in pregnancy and their effect on CPR [66,70,71].

Measured parameter	Direction of change	Values in normal pregnancy	Effect on CPR
Respiratory			
Pharyngeal edema	Increases	–	May need smaller endotracheal tube, increases difficulty with intubation and airway control
Minute ventilation	Increases 50%	–	Increased development of hypercarbia
Oxygen consumption	Increases 20%	–	More rapid development of hypoxia
FRC	Decreases 20%	–	More rapid development of hypoxia
Arterial PCO_2	Decreases	28–32 torr	
Serum bicarbonate	Decreases	18–21 mEq/L	Decreased acid buffering capability
Chest wall compliance	Decreases	–	More difficult intubation, increased ventilation pressures
Cardiovascular			
Cardiac output	Increases 50%	6.2 ± 1.0 L/min	Increases the circulatory demand during CPR
Blood volume	Increases 30–50%	–	Dilutional anemia with decreased O_2 carrying capacity
Heart rate	Increases 15–20%	83 ± 10 beats/min	
SVR	Decreases 20%	1210 ± 256 dynes/sec/cm^{-5}	
COP	Decreases 15%	18 ± 1.5 mmHg	Propensity to pulmonary edema
PCWP	Decreases	7.5 ± 1.8 mmHg	
Aortocaval compression	Increases	–	Lateral uterine displacement required to maintain venous return and hence cardiac output
Hematologic			
Most clotting factors	Increase	–	Propensity to thrombosis; thromboembolic disease high on differential diagnosis
Gastrointestinal			
Motility	Decreases	–	Increased risk of aspiration, need to protect airway
Lower esophageal sphincter tone	Decreases	–	Increased risk of aspiration, need to protect airway
Renal			
Compensated respiratory alkalosis	Increases	–	Modification of target values and increase ventilation required, avoid bicarbinate in CPR
Glomerular filtration rate	Increases	–	Drug clearance may be modified

but consider high dose for prolonged, resistant cardiac arrest [45]. Spohr et al. recently summarized the current data regarding drug therapy for CPR [45]. Adenosine, lidocaine, procainamide, and beta-blockers, also used in the treatment of tachyarrhythmias, all appear to be safe in pregnancy [46].

Resuscitators should remember that during pregnancy, the volume of distribution and drug metabolism may vary from non-pregnant norms. Page [47] reviewed the multiple factors contributing to altered therapeutic blood levels of drugs in pregnancy. They include increased intravascular volume, reduced drug protein binding, increased clearance of renally excreted drugs, progesterone-activated increased hepatic metabolism, and altered gastrointestinal absorption due to changes and gastric secretion and gut motility. The agents used in ACLS are recommended in standard doses. However, if the victim does not respond to standard doses, higher doses should be considered to account for the expanded plasma volume of pregnancy.

Modifications of basic life support and advanced cardiac life support in pregnancy

The anatomic and physiologic changes of pregnancy require several modifications in ECC (Tables 7.5 & 7.6). Most important, to affect an increase in venous return and reduced supine hypotension, the uterus must be displaced to the left. Left lateral displacement can be achieved by: (i) manual displacement of the uterus by a member of the resuscitation team; (ii) positioning of the patient on an operating room table that can be tilted laterally; (iii) positioning a wedge under the right hip; (iv) using a Cardiff resuscitation wedge or (v) using a human wedge [48]. The human wedge kneels on the floor with the patient's back placed on the thighs of the human wedge. The human wedge uses one arm to stabilize the patient's shoulder and the other arm to stabilize the pelvis. The human wedge maneuver has the advantage that it may

Table 7.6 Primary and secondary ABCD surveys: modifications for pregnant women. Reproduced from [72].

ACLS Approach	Modifications to BLS and ACLS Guidelines
Primary ABCD Survey	
Airway	No modifications.
Breathing	No modifications.
Circulation	Place the woman on her left side with her back angled 15° to 30° back from the left lateral position. Then start chest compressions. *or* Place a wedge under the woman's right side (so that she tilts toward her left side). *or* Have one rescuer kneel next to the woman's left side and pull the gravid uterus laterally. This maneuver will relieve pressure on the inferior vena cava.
Defibrillation	No modifications in dose or pad position. Defibrillation shocks transfer no significant current to the fetus. Remove any fetal or uterine monitors before shock delivery.
Secondary ABCD Survey	
Airway	Insert an advanced airway early in resuscitation to reduce the risk of regurgitation and aspiration. Airway edema and swelling may reduce the diameter of the trachea. Be prepared to use a tracheal tube that is slightly smaller than the one you would use for a non-pregnant woman of similar size. Monitor for excessive bleeding following insertion of any tube into the oropharynx or nasopharynx. No modifications to intubation techniques. A provider experienced in intubation should insert the tracheal tube. Effective preoxygenation is critical because hypoxia can develop quickly. Rapid sequence intubation with continuous cricoid pressure is the preferred technique. Agents for anesthesia or deep sedation should be selected to minimize hypotension.
Breathing	No modifications of confirmation of tube placement. Note that the esophageal detector device may suggest esophageal placement despite correct tracheal tube placement. The gravid uterus elevates the diaphragm: Patients can develop hypoxemia if either oxygen demand or pulmonary function is compromised. They have less reserve because functional residual capacity and functional residual volume are decreased. Minute ventilation and tidal volume are increased. Tailor ventilatory support to produce effective oxygenation and ventilation.
Circulation	Follow standard ACLS recommendations for administration of all resuscitation medications. Do not use the femoral vein or other lower extremity sites for venous access. Drugs administered through these sites may not reach the maternal heart unless or until the fetus is delivered.
Differential diagnosis and decisions	Decide whether to perform emergency hysterotomy. Identify and treat reversible causes of the arrest. Consider causes related to pregnancy and causes considered for all ACLS patients (see the 6 H's and 6 T's, in Part 7.2: "Management of Cardiac Arrest").

be employed without equipment, utilizing an untrained person. Its obvious disadvantage of the wedge is that it must be displaced when defibrillation becomes necessary. The back of an upside down chair may also function as a leaning post to support a woman in a laterally tilted position.

The maternal propensity for hypoxia and hypercapnia (which lead to decreases *in utero*placental perfusion) suggests that the pregnant woman may benefit from sodium bicarbonate in an arrest situation in order to keep maternal pH greater than 7.10. This idea is hazardous and should be discarded. Sodium bicarbonate crosses the placenta very slowly. Accordingly, with rapid correction of maternal metabolic acidosis, her respiratory compensation will cease with normalization of her PCO_2 toward the non-pregnant state. For example, if the maternal PCO_2 increases from 20 to 40 mmHg as a result of bicarbonate administration, fetal PCO_2 will also increase. However, the fetus will not receive the benefit of the bicarbonate. If the fetal pH was 7.0 before maternal bicarbonate administration, the normalization of maternal pH will be achieved at the expense of increasing the fetal PCO_2 by 20 mmHg, resulting in a reduction in fetal pH to approximately 6.84. Even in the non-pregnant state, sodium bicarbonate is considered potentially harmful in patients with hypoxic lactic acidosis, such as commonly occurs in non-intubated patients undergoing prolonged cardiopulmonary arrest. Carbon dioxide generated in tissues is not well cleared by low blood flow [49]. Adequate ventilation and restoration of perfusion are the mainstays of control of acid–base balance during cardiac arrest. The buffering of blood with bicarbonate does not benefit the patient [50].

Thrombolytic therapy

Unfractionated and low molecular weight heparins have been used extensively during pregnancy. In cases of acute cardiopulmonary thrombosis, therapy with these agents has proven helpful in both non-pregnant and pregnant patients. There is much less data regarding the use of other thrombolytic therapies during pregnancy including recombinant tissue plasminogen activators (TPA). Generally, pregnancy is considered a contraindication to TPA therapy but there are several case reports of successful use during pregnancy [51–53]. The use of such agents increases the risk of hemorrhage, particularly in the scenario when operative delivery has or is likely to occur. Nonetheless, the use of these agents should not be completely excluded when alternative therapies have been unsuccessful.

Complications and aftercare of cardiopulmonary resuscitation during pregnancy

Unfortunately, CPR is rarely effective in restoring spontaneous circulation and permitting neurologically intact recovery to hospital discharge. Successful resuscitation is reported in 6–15% of patients suffering in-hospital cardiac arrest [54,55]. In pregnancy, survival may be even less likely given the maternal physiologic changes that predispose her to rapid hypoxia and complicated resuscitative efforts. Fortunately, the paucity of underlying disease may improve the likelihood of success.

For survivors, cardiopulmonary resuscitation may impose secondary complications on both mother and fetus. Ongoing supportive and therapeutic care will be necessary, paying careful attention to common areas of injury and ongoing risk. Care is best accomplished by a multidisciplinary team. Neonatal and maternal care providers should assess for injuries. Maternal injuries may include: (i) fractures of ribs and sternum; (ii) hemothorax and hemopericardium; (iii) rupture of internal organs (especially the spleen and uterus); and (iv) lacerations of organs (most notably the liver). Damaging effects to the fetus consist of central nervous toxicity from medications and reduced uteroplacental perfusion with possible fetal hypoxemia and acidemia. Fetal monitoring may be used to assess ongoing fetal status; however, maternal resuscitation should be the primary goal.

Perimortem cesarean delivery

Historically, perimortem cesarean delivery (PMCD) was a widely accepted practice. In fact, the term *cesarean* developed from the Roman period (715–763 BC) when PMCD was practiced under the law of Caesar (*lex Cesare*), not for maternal or fetal benefit, rather to allow woman and children to be buried separately for religious ritual [56]. In ancient Greek mythology the first cesarean section was performed by Apollo, on his wife Coronois, as she was being burned on a funeral pyre. Their son, Asclepius, is said to be the demigod of medicine and healing. The Staff of Asclepius, a rod entwined with a single serpent, has become the symbol for physicians across the globe.

The first documented case of maternal survival from a PMCD took place in Switzerland, when a farmer named Jacob Nufer performed a cesarean delivery on his own wife [57]. Since then, over 250 reports of maternal survival from PMCD have been described. Recognition that the gravid uterus may prevent proper CPR techniques by restoring adequate cardiac output, has led many to theorize that immediate PMCD may assist in maternal resuscitation. The theory is that the low-resistance, high-volume uteroplacental unit sequesters blood and hinders effective CPR. Delivery leads to a decrease in aortocaval obstruction, and increase in effectiveness of compressions, and an increase in maternal cardiac output. In a recent review by Katz et al., 12 of 22 case reports showed a sudden and often dramatic improvement in pulseless gravidas following uterine evacuation [58].

When considering PMCD, several factors need to be addressed. Clearly, the timing of the operation is critical for infant survival. Survival appears to be inversely proportional to the time between the mother's cardiac arrest and her delivery. In 1986, Katz et al. introduced the idea of the "4-minute rule" for PMCD, basing their recommendations on the idea that maternal neurologic injury would commence 6 minutes after the cessation of cerebral perfusion [59]. If delivery is accomplished within 5 minutes of maternal cardiac arrest, intact neurologic survival is likely [15,59]. Beyond 15 minutes, neonatal death or impaired survival is generally seen. Primate studies confirm brain damage *in utero* with as little as 6 minutes of complete asphyxia and severe cellular damage occurring by 8 minutes [60]. Nonetheless scattered reports describe infant survival at longer intervals following arrest, implying that cesarean delivery should be performed post arrest if signs of fetal life are still present [61,62].

In light of the evolving timing of the limits of fetal viability, one group of authors attempted to develop an algorithm to assist clinicians in determining when and who would benefit from a postmortem cesarean section [36]. The "potentially salvageable" infant was defined as an estimated gestational age of at least 26 weeks with the confirmation of fetal cardiac activity by Doppler ultrasound. In this group, 75% of the infants survived. The authors postulated that 60% of the infant deaths may have been avoided by earlier recognition of fetal distress and earlier cesarean delivery. With evolving technology, determination of what gestational age defines fetal viability will be left to the discretion of the delivering physician and the resources available for neonatal resuscitation. To date, we have not identified any lawsuits brought against physicians for the wrongful performance of a PMCD.

The 4-minute limit to initiate delivery, as advocated by Katz and colleagues [58,59] and the American College of Obstetricians and Gynecologists is derived from the theoretical physiologic advantages for resuscitating the mother, as well as from extrapolation of data on infant survival. While such data suggests an ideal arrest-to-delivery interval, in actual practice these goals are rarely achieved. It must be emphasized that no data exist to prospectively document actual maternal benefits of perimortem cesarean section. There are many anecdotal examples of improved maternal response to resuscitation after perimortem cesarean. However, maternal death remains the most likely outcome regardless of arrest-to-delivery interval. None-the-less, in light of both the anecdotal experiences suggesting benefit to mother and fetus, and the dismal outcomes without intervention, we support the concept of the 4-minute rule based on the currently available evidence. In the setting of perimortem cesarean section performed for the likely salvageable fetus, the staff should be well versed in the techniques of neonatal resuscitation as these infants are likely to suffer from respiratory and circulatory depression at birth. Women with chronic illnesses are less likely to have a normal surviving infant by perimortem cesarean section, compared to previously healthy women who suffer cardiac arrest following an acute obstetric event.

The neurologically impaired patient following resuscitation

On the rare occasion when a patient is successfully resuscitated but left brain dead and a cesarean section has not been performed, several medical, social, ethical and legal dilemmas follow. In most circumstances, advance directives are not available to guide the physician in the decision-making process. A decision must be made, based on gestational age, family wishes (or medical power of attorney), and available resources, on whether to extend the maternal life for fetal benefit.

To arrive at a decision involving the prolongation of pregnancy in a brain-dead pregnant patient, the physician must be guided by basic ethical and legal principles. If an advance directive is available and deemed lawful, it must be interpreted within the context of the situation and with the patient's values in mind. If a durable power of attorney or next of kin are not available, or if there is conflict within the family, then legal counsel is recommended. Keep in mind that the decision to prolong maternal life for the benefit of the fetus must first be consistent with the values of the patient as determined by the next of kin. Historically, gestational age at the timing of the event was often cited as the most important variable, with the assumption that prolongation of a pregnancy was rarely successful beyond 2–4 weeks, and thus should only be considered in the gravid women beyond 24 weeks gestational age [63]. However, more recent cases have demonstrated that pregnancy can be prolonged for as long as 204 days following severe neurologic injury, and as early as 15 weeks gestation in a brain-dead patient [64,65]. Therefore, the more relevant questions for the physician and family are if prolongation of the pregnancy is what the patient would have wanted and if so, when is the appropriate time for delivery to optimize the health of the neonate?

If the decision is made to prolong the pregnancy, a unique set of medical complications must also be addressed in anticipation of expected physiologic changes following brain death. Discussion of the somatic support of a brain dead gravida is beyond the scope of this chapter, but is covered comprehensively in a review by Mallampalli and colleagues [66].

Case presentation

A 22-year-old primigravida was admitted to the hospital for mild pre-eclampsia and preterm contractions at 32 weeks. Her pregnancy was remarkable for a 12-year history of insulin-dependent diabetes. Her blood sugar control was reasonable on an insulin pump. She had no overt consequences of microvascular injury. She was given pneumatic compression stockings for use while in bed. The 2-week admission was remarkable for episodes of shortness of breath associated with ambulation and with pneumatic compression stocking use. She was evaluated clinically. Chest X-ray, pulse oximetry, and an ECG were performed. Thromboembolic disease was entertained but ultimately considered unlikely. Because of the discomfort with the compression stockings they were discontinued and she was started on thromboprophylactic doses of heparin. She labored spontaneously in the 36th week but had arrest of dilatation at 8 cm.

After unsuccessful oxytocin labor stimulation, she was taken for cesarean section on a weekend morning. The delivery occurred using the labor epidural from a recumbent position with a left lateral tilt. Just as the rectus fascia was incised, she suddenly expressed great anxiety, attempted to sit up and then collapsed unresponsive. Cardiac monitoring initially showed bradycardia to the 40s and then became erratic. There was no palpable pulse. Within the first 2 minutes of the event, a hospital "code blue" was initiated, the baby was quickly delivered, endotracheal intubation was attempted and chest compressions begun. The initial intubation was unsuccessful and bag/mask ventilation was performed. Two 1-mg doses of epinephrine followed by 1 mg of atropine were given intravenously without response. Lidocaine and calcium were given and a second attempt at endotracheal intubation was successful within 4 minutes into the resuscitation. The cardiac monitors showed only a flat line tracing.

External cardiac monitors were disconnected. Cardioversions with 200, 360 and 360 J were attempted with intermittent CPR and rhythm monitoring without a positive response. Four mg of epinephrine was given intravenously; there was no response.

Eight minutes into the resuscitation, the potential etiologies of the arrest were reviewed. Given the absence of an apparent coagulopathy, anaphalactoid syndrome of pregnancy was considered unlikely. However, the history of previous events, now more suspicious for possible thromboembolic phenomenon, put a large pulmonary embolism at the top of the differential diagnoses. The pulseless electrical activity (PEA) identified earlier in the resuscitation supported this possibility.

Left lateral thoracotomy and pericardotomy were performed and open cardiac massage was initiated. Within 30 seconds a palpable beat was noted with subsequent beats following in increasingly rapid succession. By 12–15 minutes into the resuscitation the patient had a sustained rhythm and a blood pressure of 70/40. Bilateral chest tubes were placed. She was given 80 mg/kg of heparin. An hour into the resuscitation a portable pulmonary arteriogram demonstrated bilateral distal filling defects in the pulmonary vasculature. Ultimately, to maintain an adequate blood pressure, the patient was given multiple 4-mg doses of epinephrine. She needed levoephedrin, dopamine and neosynephrin drips and required cardiac massage on two subsequent occasions to maintain an adequate cardiac output. She received a total of 10 units of packed red blood cells during the first 4 hours of the resuscitation and 2 units of FFP. Crystalloid fluids were limited to 800 mL during the first 3 hours. Three hours into the resuscitation her pupils were fixed and dilated. There was no response to stimulation despite the fact that no pharmacologic sedation had been given. The patient was warmed, the wounds closed and she was transferred to the ICU. Within 18 hours of the arrest she was appropriately responsive. She was extubated within 72 hours. She was discharged from the hospital on post arrest day 40 with moderate lower extremity spasticity and short-term memory loss but otherwise neurologically intact. Her cardiac output at discharge was 25%. Over the course of 2 years her cardiac and neurologic function completely normalized. The baby has done well.

Summary

Sudden cardiac arrest is uncommon in pregnancy and is usually catastrophic when it occurs. Because SCA arrest in pregnancy is a rare event, medical facilities and personnel must maintain competency by training and practice. While successful resuscitation is uncommon, early aggressive resuscitation by well-trained and skilled attendants improves the likelihood of survival.

The latest guidelines for CPR by the American Heart Association make several recommendations for change from the previous algorithms. Pregnancy necessitates several modifications to standard CPR that include displacement of the uterus off the vena cava to facilitate venous return. Modifications to pharmacologic or electrical therapy are usually not necessary.

Immediate action is critical for both mother and baby. In pregnant and non-pregnant individuals there is a window of opportunity in the first 5 minutes after the arrest. This short window of time includes decisions about and performance of emergency cesarean section if that course is elected. Urgent cesarean delivery in SCA victims may be of benefit to both mother and baby.

Precisely because SCA is an uncommon event on the labor and delivery unit, it is often unexpected. Thus, training and drilling for such events should be a priority in order to maintain a state of alert and readiness by hospital personnel. We concur with Morris and colleagues [67] that the best opportunity for good outcome occurs when inertia can be avoided. We must avoid (i) the inertia of fear that proven procedures and medications in non-pregnant patients will adversely affect the fetus, (ii) the inertia of indecision about emergent surgical delivery, (iii) the inertia of hopelessness for the desperately ill mother, delivered or undelivered, and (iv) the peculiarly American condition of medicolegal dystocia.

References

1 Zheng ZJ et al. Sudden cardiac death in the United States, 1989 to 1998. *Circulation* 2001; 104: 2158–2163.

2 Thel MC, O'Connor CM. Cardiopulmonary resuscitation: historical perspective to recent investigations. *Am Heart J* 1999; 137: 39–48.

3 Cobb LA et al. Changing incidence of out-of-hospital ventricular fibrillation, 1980–2000. *JAMA* 2002; 288: 3008–3013.

4 2005 American Heart Association Guidelines for Cardiopulmonary Resuscitation and Emergency Cardiovascular Care. *Circulation* 2005; 112(24 Suppl): IV1–203.

5 Dildy GA, Clark SL. Cardiac arrest during pregnancy. *Obstet Gynecol Clin North Am* 1995; 22: 303–314.

6 Pandey U, Russell IF, Lindow SW. How competent are obstetric and gynaecology trainees in managing maternal cardiac arrests? *J Obstet Gynaecol* 2006; 26: 507–508.

7 2005 American Heart Association Guidelines for Cardiopulmonary Resuscitation and Emergency Cardiovascular Care. *Circulation* 2005; 112(24 Suppl): 116.

8 Berg CJ et al. Pregnancy-related mortality in the United States, 1991–1997. *Obstet Gynecol* 2003; 101: 289–296.

9 Heit JA et al. Trends in the incidence of venous thromboembolism during pregnancy or postpartum: a 30-year population-based study. *Ann Intern Med* 2005; 143: 697–706.

10 James AH et al. Acute myocardial infarction in pregnancy: a United States population-based study. *Circulation* 2006; 113: 1564–1571.

11 Phillips LM et al. Coronary artery dissection during pregnancy treated with medical therapy. *Cardiol Rev* 2006; 14: 155–157.

12 Martin SR, Foley MR. Intensive care in obstetrics: an evidence-based review. *Am J Obstet Gynecol* 2006; 195: 673–689.

13 Tuffnell DJ. United Kingdom amniotic fluid embolism register. *BJOG* 2005; 112: 1625–1629.

14 Samuelsson E, Hellgren M, Hogberg U. Pregnancy-related deaths due to pulmonary embolism in Sweden. *Acta Obstet Gynecol Scand* 2007; 86: 435–443.

15 Clark SL et al. Amniotic fluid embolism: analysis of the national registry. *Am J Obstet Gynecol* 1995; 172(4 Pt 1): p. 1158–1167; discussion 1167–1169.

16 De Jong MJ, Fausett MB. Anaphylactoid syndrome of pregnancy. A devastating complication requiring intensive care. *Crit Care Nurse* 2003; 23: 42–48.

17 Garner EG, Smith CV, Rayburn WF. Maternal respiratory arrest associated with intravenous fentanyl use during labor. A case report. *J Reprod Med* 1994; 39: 818–820.
18 Swartjes JM, Schutte MF, Bleker OP. Management of eclampsia: cardiopulmonary arrest resulting from magnesium sulfate overdose. *Eur J Obstet Gynecol Reprod Biol* 1992; 47: 73–75.
19 Richards A, Stather-Dunn L, Moodley J. Cardiopulmonary arrest after the administration of magnesium sulphate. A case report. *S Afr Med J* 1985; 67: 145.
20 McCubbin JM et al. Cardiopulmonary arrest due to acute maternal hypermagnesaemia. *Lancet* 1981; 1(8228): p. 1058.
21 American Heart Association. *Textbook of Basic Life Support for Health-Care Providers.* Dallas: American Heart Association, 1994.
22 Eisenberg MS, Bergner L, Hallstrom A. Cardiac resuscitation in the community. Importance of rapid provision and implications for program planning. *JAMA* 1979; 241: 1905–1907.
23 Barnes TA et al. Cardiopulmonary resuscitation and emergency cardiovascular care. Airway devices. *Ann Emerg Med* 2001; 37(4 Suppl): S145–S151.
24 American Heart Association. 2005 American Heart Association Guidelines for Cardiopulmonary Resuscitation and Emergency Cardiovascular Care. *Circulation* 2005; 112(24 Suppl): p. IV150–IV153.
25 American Heart Association. 2005 American Heart Association Guidelines for Cardiopulmonary Resuscitation and Emergency Cardiovascular Care. *Circulation* 2005; 112(24 Suppl): p. IV-19–IV-34.
26 Kouwenhoven WB, Jude JR, Knickerbocker GG. Closed-chest cardiac massage. *JAMA* 1960; 173: 1064–1067.
27 Rudikoff MT et al. Mechanisms of blood flow during cardiopulmonary resuscitation. *Circulation* 1980; 61: 345–352.
28 Werner JA et al. Visualization of cardiac valve motion in man during external chest compression using two-dimensional echocardiography. Implications regarding the mechanism of blood flow. *Circulation* 1981; 63: 1417–1421.
29 Ogburn PL Jr et al. Paroxysmal tachycardia and cardioversion during pregnancy. *J Reprod Med* 1982; 27: 359–362.
30 Nanson J et al. Do physiological changes in pregnancy change defibrillation energy requirements? *Br J Anaesth* 2001; 87: 237–239.
31 Sapsford W et al. Recombinant activated factor VII increases survival time in a model of incompressible arterial hemorrhage in the anesthetized pig. *J Trauma* 2007; 62: 868–879.
32 Franchini M, Lippi G, Franchi M. The use of recombinant activated factor VII in obstetric and gynaecological haemorrhage. *BJOG* 2007; 114: 8–15.
33 Haynes J, Laffan M, Plaat F. Use of recombinant activated factor VII in massive obstetric haemorrhage. *Int J Obstet Anesth* 2007; 16: 40–49.
34 Palomino MA et al. Recombinant activated factor VII in the management of massive obstetric bleeding. *Blood Coagul Fibrinolysis* 2006; 17: 226–227.
35 Ahonen J, Jokela R. Recombinant factor VIIa for life-threatening post-partum haemorrhage. *Br J Anaesth* 2005; 94: 592–595.
36 Morris JA Jr et al. Infant survival after cesarean section for trauma. *Ann Surg* 1996; 223: 481–488; discussion 488–491.
37 Varma R. Caesarean section after cardiac arrest. *BMJ* 2003. See http://www.bmj.com/cgi/eletters/327/7426/1277#41863.
38 Lee RV et al. Cardiopulmonary resuscitation of pregnant women. *Am J Med* 1986; 81: 311–318.
39 Briggs GG, Freeman RK, Yaffe SJ, eds. *Drugs in Pregnancy and Lactation*, 6th edn. Philadelphia: Lippincott Williams and Wilkins, 2002: 1595.
40 Daga MK, Singh KJ, Kumar N. Emerging role of vasopressin. *J Assoc Physicians India* 2006; 54: 376–380.
41 Miano TA, Crouch MA. Evolving role of vasopressin in the treatment of cardiac arrest. *Pharmacotherapy* 2006; 26: 828–839.
42 Choux C et al. Standard doses versus repeated high doses of epinephrine in cardiac arrest outside the hospital. *Resuscitation* 1995; 29: 3–9.
43 Berg RA et al. High-dose epinephrine results in greater early mortality after resuscitation from prolonged cardiac arrest in pigs: a prospective, randomized study. *Crit Care Med* 1994; 22: 282–290.
44 Polin K, Leikin JB. High-dose epinephrine in cardiopulmonary resuscitation. *JAMA* 1993; 269: 1383; author reply 1383–1384.
45 Spohr F, Wenzel V, Bottiger BW. Drug treatment and thrombolytics during cardiopulmonary resuscitation. *Curr Opin Anaesthesiol* 2006; 19: 157–165.
46 Rubin PC. Current concepts: beta-blockers in pregnancy. *N Engl J Med* 1981; 305: 1323–1326.
47 Page RL, Hamdan MH, Joglar JA. Arrhythmias occurring during pregnancy. *Card Electrophysiol Rev* 2002; 6(1–2): p. 136–139.
48 Goodwin AP, Pearce AJ. The human wedge. A manoeuvre to relieve aortocaval compression during resuscitation in late pregnancy. *Anaesthesia* 1992; 47: 433–434.
49 Adrogue HJ et al. Assessing acid-base status in circulatory failure. Differences between arterial and central venous blood. *N Engl J Med* 1989; 320: 1312–1316.
50 American Heart Association, Part 7.4: Monitoring and medications. *Circulation* 2005; 112(24 suppl): p. IV78–IV83.
51 Johnson DM et al. Thrombolytic therapy for acute stroke in late pregnancy with intra-arterial recombinant tissue plasminogen activator. *Stroke* 2005; 36: e53–e55.
52 Murugappan A et al. Thrombolytic therapy of acute ischemic stroke during pregnancy. *Neurology* 2006; 66: 768–770.
53 Ahearn GS et al. Massive pulmonary embolism during pregnancy successfully treated with recombinant tissue plasminogen activator: a case report and review of treatment options. *Arch Intern Med* 2002; 162: 1221–1227.
54 Diem SJ, Lantos JD, Tulsky JA. Cardiopulmonary resuscitation on television. Miracles and misinformation. *N Engl J Med* 1996; 334: 1578–1582.
55 Karetzky M, Zubair M, Parikh J. Cardiopulmonary resuscitation in intensive care unit and non-intensive care unit patients. Immediate and long-term survival. *Arch Intern Med* 1995; 155: 1277–1280.
56 Ritter JW. Postmortem cesarean section. *JAMA* 1961; 175: 715–716.
57 Weber CE. Postmortem cesarean section: review of the literature and case reports. *Am J Obstet Gynecol* 1971; 110: 158–165.
58 Katz V, Balderston K, DeFreest M. Perimortem cesarean delivery: were our assumptions correct? *Am J Obstet Gynecol* 2005; 192: 1916–1920; discussion 1920–1921.
59 Katz VL, Dotters DJ, Droegemueller W. Perimortem cesarean delivery. *Obstet Gynecol* 1986; 68: 571–576.
60 Windle WF. Brain damage at birth. Functional and structural modifications with time. *JAMA* 1968; 206: 1967–1972.
61 Kaiser RT. Air embolism death of a pregnant woman secondary to orogenital sex. *Acad Emerg Med* 1994; 1: 555–558.
62 Selden BS, Burke TJ. Complete maternal and fetal recovery after prolonged cardiac arrest. *Ann Emerg Med* 1988; 17: 346–349.

63 Dillon WP et al. Life support and maternal death during pregnancy. *JAMA* 1982; 248: 1089–1091.
64 Bernstein IM et al. Maternal brain death and prolonged fetal survival. *Obstet Gynecol* 1989; 74(3 part 2): p. 434–437.
65 Sim KB. Maternal persistent vegetative state with successful fetal outcome. *J Korean Med Sci* 2001; 16: 669–672.
66 Mallampalli A, Guy E. Cardiac arrest in pregnancy and somatic support after brain death. *Crit Care Med* 2005; 33(10 Suppl): S325–S331.
67 Morris S, Stacey M. Resuscitation in pregnancy. *BMJ* 2003; 327(7426): 1277–1279.
68 American Heart Association. 2005 American Heart Association Guidelines for Cardiopulmonary Resuscitation and Emergency Cardiovascular Care. *Circulation* 2005; 112(24 Suppl): IV-12–IV-18.
69 Mallampalli A, Powner DJ, Gardner MO. Cardiopulmonary resuscitation and somatic support of the pregnant patient. *Crit Care Clin* 2004; 20: 747–761, x.
70 Clark SL et al. Central hemodynamic assessment of normal term pregnancy. *Am J Obstet Gynecol* 1989; 161(6 Pt 1): 1439–1442.
71 Fujitani S, Baldisseri MR. Hemodynamic assessment in a pregnant and peripartum patient. *Crit Care Med* 2005; 33(10 Suppl): S354–S361.
72 American Heart Association. 2005 American Heart Association Guidelines for Cardiopulmonary Resuscitation and Emergency Cardiovascular Care. *Circulation* 2005; 112(24 Suppl): p. IV152.

8 Neonatal Resuscitation

Christian Con Yost & Ron Bloom
Department of Neonatology, University of Utah Health Sciences, Salt Lake City, UT, USA

Introduction

Under normal circumstances, the transition from womb to world is a series of dramatic and rapid physiologic changes leading to the birth of an infant prepared to continue the processes of growth and development. The goal of delivering a healthy infant intact ready to continue normal development is, unfortunately, not always possible. Pregnancies and/or deliveries complicated by common and uncommon conditions, discussed throughout this text, are at increased risk of failing to successfully make the transition to extrauterine life. Modern diagnostic tools often, but not always, allow for anticipation of infants at risk of not making a successful transition, and, thus, permit the perinatal team to plan for neonatal resuscitation and/or medically necessary interventions. However, more acute and often unanticipated conditions such as a sudden prolapsed cord, an abruption or a previously unrecognized congenital anomaly may result in the need for an unanticipated, but nevertheless, skillful resuscitation.

At birth, neonatal resuscitation may be necessary. However, because it is not possible to predict every infant who may require resuscitation, the ability to conduct an effective resuscitation is an integral part of the considerations and planning for any delivery. Regardless of level of care, a trained and experienced team, readily available, is an integral part of perinatal care. These teams must be provided with appropriate and well functioning equipment needed to resuscitate a newborn [1]. Skilled and experienced personnel with the right equipment can usually intervene successfully on a compromised infant's behalf.

The approach to neonatal resuscitation has continually changed since the late 1980s when the teaching of neonatal resuscitation became commonplace. Over the last 20 years, we have reconsidered our approach to resuscitation and have questioned some of our previous assumptions. We are now considering approaches to assisted ventilation and the use of oxygen from a whole new perspective.

This chapter will not address the details of exactly how to perform a resuscitation. This is very well taught in the Neonatal Resuscitation Program of the American Academy of Pediatrics/American Heart Association [2] and the details exceed the bounds of this chapter. What we will discuss are some of the new ideas, approaches and principles as well as some basic elements of neonatal resuscitation. In this context, we will discuss the role of continuous positive airway pressure versus intermittent mandatory ventilation. We will also discuss the growing dialogue regarding the use of oxygen in the resuscitative process.

Elements of birth depression

Causes of birth depression

While all deliveries involve a complex physiologic transition at birth, infants of those mothers cared for by the high-risk obstetric team, especially if premature, are at a greater risk of birth depression. The newborn infant may be depressed at birth through a variety of mechanisms, some of which are unrelated to asphyxia. Birth depression requiring resuscitation of a neonate cannot always be predicted, but at least among infants born of high-risk pregnancies, it should be expected.

Maternal or placental conditions can result in birth depression. For example, diminished uterine blood flow may result from maternal hypotension, eclampsia, regional anesthesia or uterine contractions. Placental abnormalities such as an abruption, edema, or inflammatory changes may reduce placental gas exchange. Fetoplacental blood flow may also be compromised due to sustained and unrelieved cord compression from a nuchal or prolapsed umbilical cord.

Compromising conditions or events may also be primarily fetal in origin. These include drug-induced central nervous system (CNS) depression, CNS anomalies, spinal cord injury, mechanical airway obstruction, pulmonary immaturity, congenital anomalies and infection. All of these events or conditions, maternal and

Critical Care Obstetrics, 5th edition. Edited by M. Belfort, G. Saade, M. Foley, J. Phelan and G. Dildy.

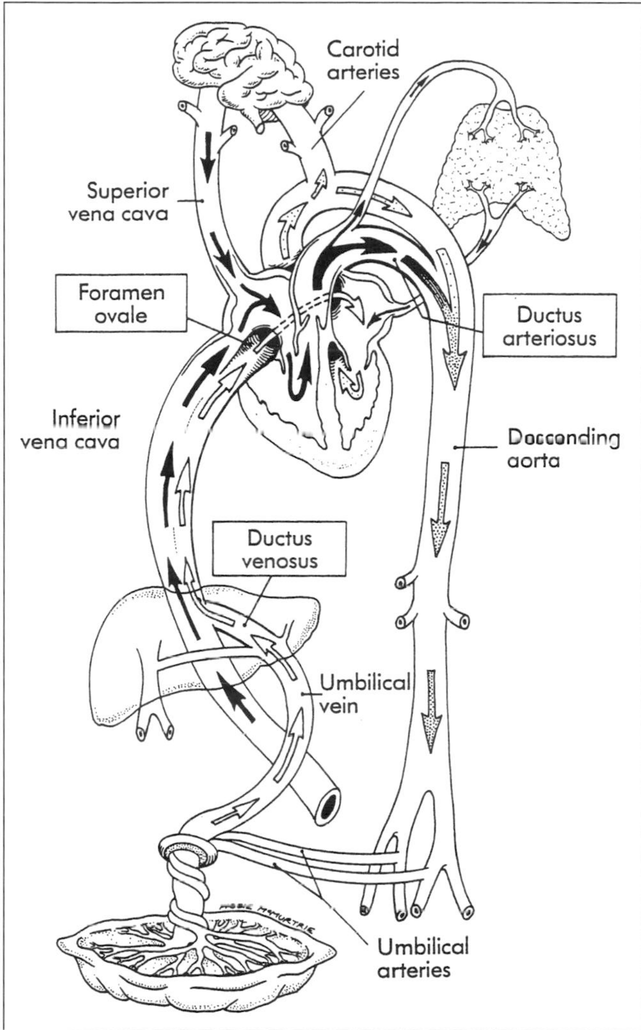

Figure 8.1 Fetal circulation. (Reproduced by permission from Faranoff M, Martin RJ, eds. *Neonatal-Perinatal Medicine: Diseases of the Fetus and Newborn*, 7th edn. St Louis: Mosby, 2002: 417.)

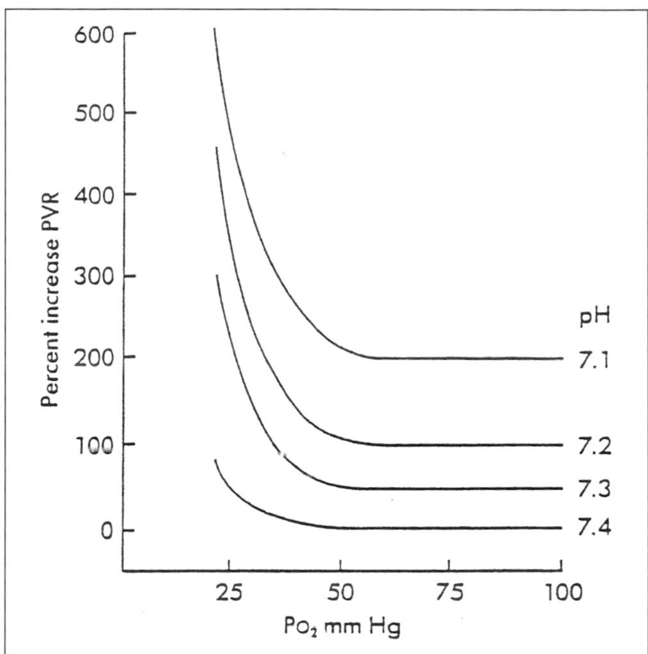

Figure 8.2 Pulmonary vascular resistance (PVR) in the calf. (From [3].)

fetal, may occur at the time of delivery or significantly before the events of parturition. It is important to note that intrauterine ischemic events, even those quite remote from the delivery of the infant, may extend into the newborn period resulting in a compromised infant.

Response to hypoxia

In the normal fetal circulation, blood returning to the heart from the body and placenta is primarily shunted through the foramen ovale to the left side of the heart facilitating oxygenated blood to going to the head and the heart. Blood that reaches the right ventricle is shunted through the ductus arteriosus to the aorta, bypassing the lungs as a result of a high pulmonary vascular resistance [3]. This serves the fetus well as the major organ of gas exchange is the placenta (Figure 8.1).

However, if the fetus or newborn is subjected to "hypoxic" conditions the physiologic response is to exacerbate or maintain an increase in pulmonary vascular resistance. For the neonate, without connection to the placenta after the cord is clamped, maintenance of the fetal circulation shunts blood away from the lungs, the only available organ of gas exchange.

In the circumstances of progressive asphyxia, the fetus or newborn responds with an increase in systemic vascular resistance or vasoconstriction. This decreases blood flow to the musculature and the intestines, while attempting to increase blood flow to the head and heart. Thus, blood flow to the cardiac and cerebral vessels is maximized at the expense of "non-vital" organs. This pattern of blood flow, if prolonged, results in an increasing acidosis [4,5]. The increasing acidosis along with the hypoxia further increases the pulmonary vascular resistance, exacerbating the problem (Figure 8.2). For both fetus and newborn, cardiac output and blood pressure are maintained to the vital organs initially, but will, in the face of increased hypoxia and acidosis fail, as the myocardium fails [6].

Primary and secondary apnea

Superimposed on these circulatory and hemodynamic changes is a characteristic respiratory pattern response to asphyxia. The fetus or neonate will initiate gasping respirations (which may occur *in utero*) and, should the asphyxia persist, enter an apneic phase known as primary apnea. If the asphyxia continues, the primary apnea will be followed by a period of irregular gasping respirations. Continued asphyxia will lead to a period of unremitting apnea known as secondary apnea. Figure 8.3 illustrates the respiratory and cardiovascular effects of asphyxia.

If an infant is in primary apnea and exposed to oxygen when gasping respirations ensue, exposure to oxygen may be sufficient

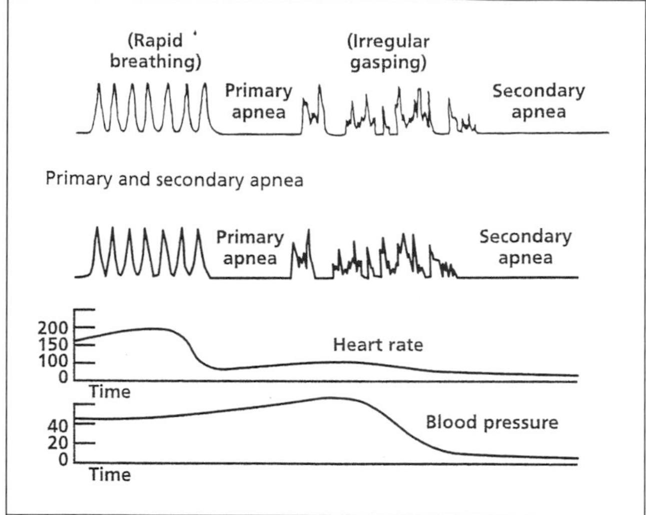

Figure 8.3 Heart rate and blood pressure changes during apnea. (Reproduced by permission from *Textbook of Neonatal Resuscitation*, 4th edn. Elk Grove, IL: American Academy of Pediatrics/American Heart Association, 2000: 1–7.)

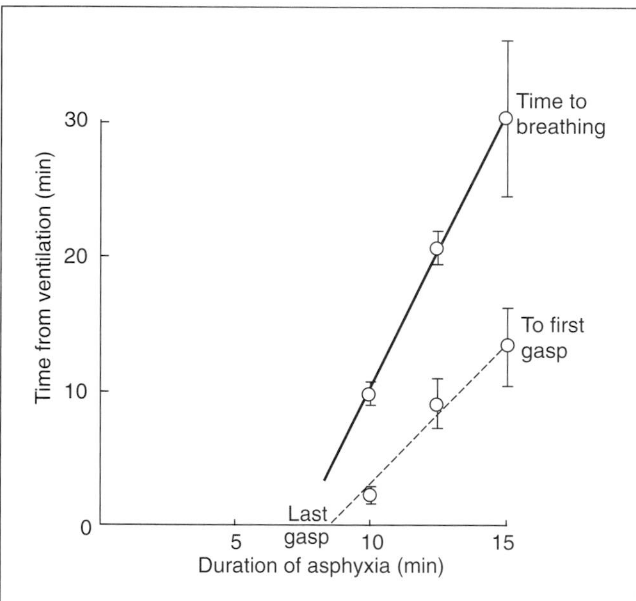

Figure 8.4 Time from ventilation to first gasp and to rhythmic breathing in newborn monkeys asphyxiated for 10, 12.5, and 15 minutes at 30°C. (From Adamsons K et al. Resuscitation by positive-pressure ventilation and tris-hydroxymethyl-aminomethane of rhesus monkeys asphixiated at birth. *J Pediatr* 1964; 65: 807.)

to reverse the process. However, once the infant reaches secondary apnea, positive-pressure ventilation is required to initiate spontaneous ventilation. Furthermore, the longer the duration of secondary apnea, the longer it will take for spontaneous respiratory effort to return following the administration of positive-pressure ventilation (Figure 8.4) [7,8].

It is very important to understand that asphyxia may begin *in utero*. The infant may go through primary apnea *in utero* and be born in secondary apnea. Thus, it is extremely difficult to assess the degree of asphyxia at the time of birth. For this reason, the resuscitative efforts should begin immediately for all infants born with any degree of depression. To wait may only subject the infant to a potentially prolonged resuscitation and an increased risk of neonatal brain damage.

Use of the Apgar score

The Apgar score, which is not routinely given until 1 minute of age, should *not* be used to guide decisions regarding resuscitation interventions. If an infant is born in secondary apnea intervention should be initiated immediately rather than waiting until 1 minute. The Apgar score is intended to provide a "snapshot" look at the condition of the infant at any one moment in time – it is not to be used as a guide for initiating resuscitation.

Elements of a resuscitation

Overview (Figure 8.5)

The ability to provide for a prompt and effective resuscitation should be available for all infants regardless of the relative risk for resuscitation as estimated by prenatal complications, fetal heart tracings or complications of labor. For infants who are known to be at high risk of being born depressed, based upon the clinical circumstances, the need for resuscitation should be anticipated and prepared for before the moment of delivery.

After delivery, a quick assessment allows for appropriate triaging of the infant. If the infant is term, breathing or crying, with good muscle tone and clear amniotic fluid there is no further need for resuscitation and the infant may be handed to an eager mother. The infant who is preterm, and who has any difficulty with breathing, reduced muscle tone or stained amniotic fluid should be placed on a preheated radiant warmer for further evaluation.

If the neonate is placed on a radiant warmer, the initial steps include drying and warming, correct airway positioning, clearing the airway by suctioning of the mouth and nose, and assessment of respiratory effort, heart rate and color. This should occur within the first few seconds of life and is independent of the 1-minute Apgar score. Subsequent efforts are dictated by assessment of respiratory effort, heart rate and color.

Gasping or apnea, or a heart rate below 100, should prompt initiation of assisted ventilation. Most infants will respond to assisted ventilation alone. In an infant with persistent central cyanosis but adequate spontaneous respirations and a heart rate greater than 100 beats per minute, free-flow oxygen may be all that is necessary.

While the long-term effects of asphyxia are sometimes unavoidable, a prompt and effective resuscitation will in most cases, restore spontaneous respiratory effort and reverse the hypoxia,

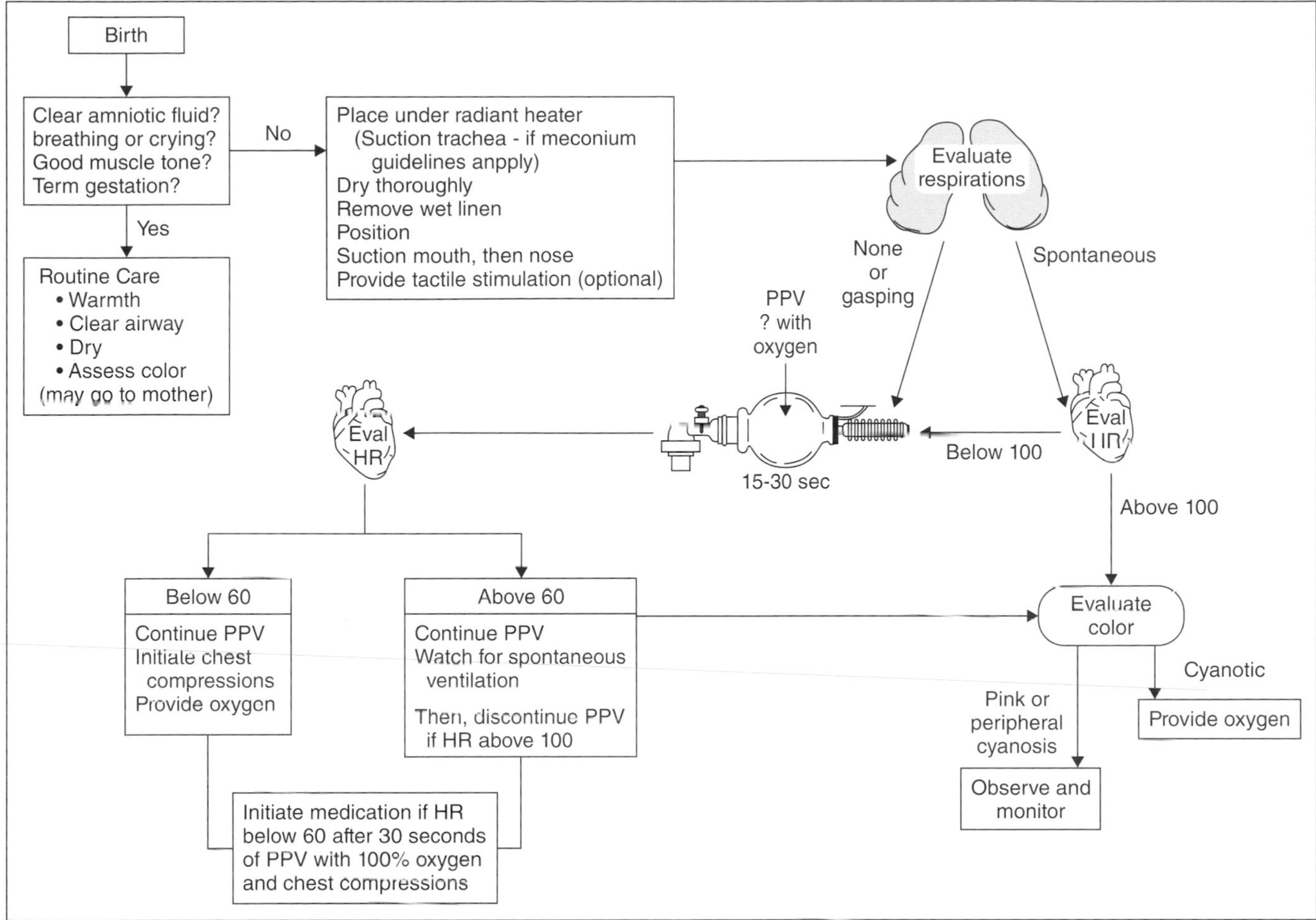

Figure 8.5 Overview of resuscitation in the delivery room. HR, heart rate; PPV, positive-pressure ventilation. (Modified from *Textbook of Neonatal Resuscitation*, 4th edn; Elk Grove, IL; American Academy of Pediatrics/American Heart Association, 2000. Originally published in Faranoff AA, Martin RJ, eds. *Neonatal-Perinatal Medicine: Diseases of the Fetus and Newborn*, 7th edn. St Louis: Mosby, 2002: 434.)

ischemia, hypercapnia and acidosis and minimize the long-term consequences to the child (Box 8.1).

In those very few infants who do not respond to ventilation, chest compressions and, possibly, medications may be needed. However, before chest compressions or medications are given, it must be assured that the infant is being provided with appropriate positive-pressure ventilation.

The resuscitative steps for infants with special circumstances such as thick meconium-stained amniotic fluid, pneumothorax, congenital diaphragmatic hernia or erythroblastosis/hydrops will be discussed later in this chapter.

Importance of establishing ventilation

In the vast majority of resuscitations, the initiation of effective positive-pressure ventilation alone will restore spontaneous respirations and heart rate. In an exceedingly important and often overlooked paper, Pearlman et al. reported on a large series of over 30 000 deliveries [9]. In their experience only 0.12% of infants required chest compressions or medication. Of note is the fact that in those infants with persistent neonatal depression, 75% were believed to be due to ineffective or improper ventilatory support. Thus, if adequate ventilation is established, in less than one-tenth of 1% is there any need to progress onto chest compression or medications.

Preparation for a resuscitation

Anticipation

It must be assumed that the infant delivered of a mother requiring critical care to support and maintain a pregnancy may require resuscitation. Thus, preparation is the first step to assure neonatal resuscitation. A careful review of the antepartum and peripartum maternal history, as well as careful assessment of the infant's response to labor, will frequently identify the potential for the delivery of a depressed infant (Box 8.2). This review will help assure that the resuscitative team is less likely to be caught unprepared or surprised by an infant born in a high-risk situation who requires immediate resuscitation. If the infant is vigorous and

Box 8.1 Consequences of asphyxia

Central nervous system
Cerebral hemorrhage
Cerebral edema
Hypoxic-ischemic encephalopathy
Seizures

Lung
Delayed onset of respiration
Respiratory distress syndrome
Meconium aspiration syndrome

Cardiovascular system
Myocardial failure
Papillary muscle necrosis
Persistent fetal circulation

Renal system
Cortico/tubular/medullary necrosis

Gastrointestinal tract
Necrotizing enterocolitis

Blood
Disseminated intravascular coagulation

(From Faranoff AA, Martin, RJ, eds. *Neonatal-Perinatal Medicine: Diseases of the Fetus and Newborn*, 7th edn. St Louis: Mosby, 2002: 420.)

pink despite its high-risk situation, it will be only a pleasant surprise to those preparing for resuscitation.

Traditionally, a cesarean delivery of any type has been considered high risk. Enough information is now available to state that the uncomplicated repeat cesarean section carries no greater risk for the infant than a vaginal delivery [10].

Anticipation of the potential need for resuscitation has been made easier by technologic advances allowing better prenatal assessment of the fetus. But, not all events compromising an infant's response to labor may be predicted. For this reason, equipment and personnel must be immediately available to intervene on behalf of the infant requiring an unanticipated resuscitation.

Equipment

Whenever an infant is delivered, appropriate equipment must be close at hand and in good working order. Having the correct equipment and skilled individuals to establish adequate ventilation is imperative. It is unacceptable for a team member to have to leave the delivery room in order to retrieve an essential piece of equipment.

Adequate personnel

Individuals vested with the responsibility of resuscitating infants should be adequately trained, readily available and capable of working together as a team. Adequate training involves more than simple completion of a certification course on the resuscitation of the newborn infant. The Neonatal Resuscitation Program of the American Heart Association/American Academy of Pediatrics and similar courses serve simply as starting points. They do not qualify one to assume independent responsibility in the delivery room. Those having completed a course, but still lacking the expertise gained through experience must be adequately supervised and supported by experienced personnel. Ultimately, the ability to resuscitate neonates is not determined by professional designation or course completion, but by experience and expertise.

Finally, those responsible for resuscitating an infant must be capable of working together as a team. If individuals are aware of and able to fulfill their respective responsibilities as well as anticipate the needs of other team members, the tension inherent in a difficult resuscitation will be reduced. In those institutions where resuscitations are uncommon events, frequent mock code drills will help to maintain skills and develop coordination among team members.

Initial steps and evaluation

To its mother or not?

Most infants are vigorous, cry upon birth and breathe easily thereafter. The decision to bypass resuscitative efforts should, however, be based on data collected during a brief triage of the infant. The infant born at term without obvious deformity or the passage of meconium *in utero*, who immediately after birth is vigorous, is breathing easily and who exhibits good tone, may be triaged to its mother if those are the wishes of the parents. A light blanket and some drying of the infant by the mother and delivery room staff will help to establish an appropriate thermal environment but should not hinder frequent and adequate assessments of the neonate's condition.

If, however, the infant is premature, has passed meconium *in utero* or exhibits any degree of respiratory distress, hypotonia, or obvious malformations, the infant should be placed onto a radiant warmer for the initial steps of resuscitation. There a more thorough assessment can be performed and possible further resuscitative interventions begun.

Initial steps

Thermal management

Temperatures in delivery rooms are typically lower than the neutral thermal environment for neonates. This can leave the newly delivered, wet infant at risk for cold stress. Immediately after birth, the infant with any degree of compromise, or for whom there is any concern, should be placed in the microenvironment of a preheated radiant warmer. The infant should be thoroughly dried with all wet blankets removed to reduce evaporative heat loss. These simple measures can minimize the signifi-

Box 8.2 Factors associated with neonatal depression and asphyxia

Antepartum risk factors	*Intrapartum risk factors*
Maternal diabetes	Emergency cesarean section
Pregnancy-induced hypertension	Forceps or vacuum-assisted delivery
Chronic hypertension	Breech or other abnormal presentation
Chronic maternal illness	Premature labor
Cardiovascular	Precipitous labor
Thyroid	Chorioamnionitis
Neurologic	Prolonged rupture of membranes (>18 hours before delivery)
Pulmonary	Prolonged labor (>24 hours)
Renal	Prolonged second stage of labor (>2 hours)
Fetal anemia or isoimmunization	Persistent fetal bradycardia
Previous fetal or neonatal death	Non-reassuring fetal heart rate patterns
Bleeding in second or third trimester	Use of general anesthesia
Maternal infection	Uterine hyperstimulation
Polyhydramnios	Narcotics given to mother within 4 hours of delivery
Oligohydramnios	Meconium-stained amniotic fluid
Premature rupture of membranes	Prolapsed cord
Post-term gestation	Abruptio placentae
Multiple gestation	Placenta previa
Size–dates discrepancy	Significant intrapartum bleeding
Fetal hydrops	
Drug therapy, e.g.	
magnesium	
adrenergic-blocking drugs	
Maternal substance abuse	
Fetal malformation	
Diminished fetal activity	
No prenatal care	
Age <16 or >35 years	

(Modified from *Textbook of Neonatal Resuscitation*, 4th edn; Elk Grove, IL; American Academy of Pediatrics/American Heart Association, 2000. Originally published in Faranoff AA, Martin RJ, eds. *Neonatal-Perinatal Medicine: Diseases of the Fetus and Newborn*, 7th edn. St Louis: Mosby, 2002: 420.)

cant drop in infant core body temperature experienced immediately after birth [11]. This is particularly important for the infant with any degree of compromise. Hypoxia reduces the infant's homeostatic response to cold stress, and without intervention, the hypoxic infant will undergo a greater than normal drop in core body temperature [12]. Hypothermia also reduces the clearance of metabolic acidosis and thus prolongs the recovery from perinatal asphyxia [13].

The premature and/or small infant represents an especially difficult problem from the aspect of temperature control. As a result of the lack of subcutaneous tissue and thin skin they tend to have greater evaporative water loss across the skin than a term infant. In addition, the large surface area to body mass ratio also facilitates heat loss and a decrease in body temperature.

There are three things that can be done to help diminish heat loss in the preterm/small infant. The first two should be done before the anticipated delivery: (i) increase the temperature of the delivery room and (ii) make sure that the radiant warmer is preheated before the birth of the infant. Finally, for infants less than 28 weeks, it is now recommended that consideration be given to placing the infant in a standard, food-quality 1-gallon polyethylene bag that can easily be obtained from a grocery store. A hole is cut in the closed end of the bag and the bag slipped over the baby with his or her head coming out of the hole. The "zipper" end can then be closed (Figure 8.6). This allows a resuscitation to proceed with minimal evaporative heat loss and full visualization of the infant. The infant can be placed in the bag in place of, or after, drying. A preheated transport incubator can be used to help maintain body temperature during transport to the nursery or NICU.

Clearing the airway

The airway is normally cleared with the use of a bulb syringe or suction catheter. The mouth is suctioned first and then the nose.

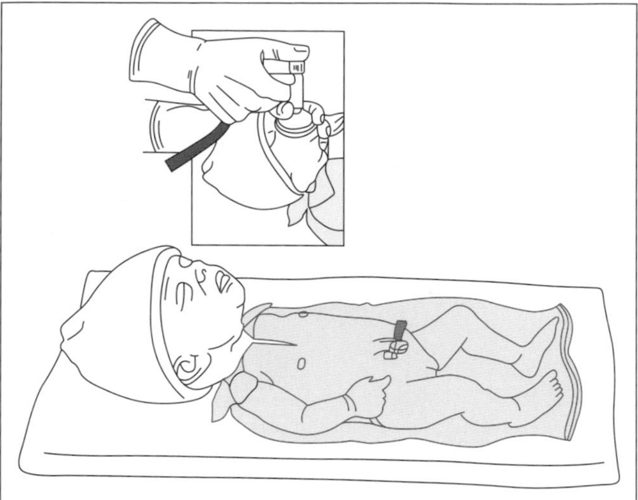

Figure 8.6 Use of plastic bag for reducing evaporative heat loss. (Reproduced from *Textbook of Neonatal Resuscitation*, 5th edn. Elk Grove, IL: American Academy of Pediatrics/American Heart Association, 2006: 8–6.)

This is done to first clear secretions in the mouth and potentially prevent their aspiration should deep breaths occur with nasal suctioning. Gentle suctioning of the mouth will avoid the reflex bradycardia associated with stimulation of the posterior pharynx [14]. The infant exposed to meconium *in utero* represents a special case and will be discussed later.

Tactile stimulation

Drying and suctioning are generally sufficient to stimulate respirations in the newborn infant. Other methods such as flicking the feet or rubbing the back have been traditionally used to stimulate a more vigorous respiratory response. If there is no immediate response to these supplemental methods, positive-pressure ventilation should be promptly initiated. Continued tactile stimulation in an unresponsive infant will not succeed and may prolong the asphyxial process. If, after suctioning and tactile stimulation an infant exhibits apnea or a heart rate of ≥100 beats/min, positive-pressure ventilation should be initiated.

Free-flow oxygen

The use of oxygen has become a topic which has been subject to a great deal of discussion and, in some sense, controversy. This is related to the potentially harmful effects of hyperoxia, especially in an asphyxiated infant. As prolonged hypoxia is to be avoided, it is also necessary to avoid hypoxemia. Most of what has been written involves the role of oxygen in infants who are in need of active resuscitation with ventilatory support, which we will discuss later in this chapter. However, in the infant who is breathing spontaneously with no or minimal significant signs of respiratory distress and whose heart rate is above 100, yet who remains cyanotic, there is general agreement that there is a need for supplemental oxygen. However, when to introduce the oxygen and at what levels to start are not well agreed upon.

It is now clear that at about 1 minute, following an uncomplicated birth, most infants breathing room air will only attain an oxygen saturation of around 60–70%. By 5 minutes, most infants have reached ranges in the mid- to high 80% range and, in many infants, it may take 10 minutes to reach oxygen saturations of 90% or higher [15,16]. This matter may be complicated by individual variation in the clinical assessment of color during the transition of a neonate.

In the breathing infant with a heart rate of above 100 who appears cyanotic, the use of a pulse oximeter may be of some value. Using the newer pulse oximetry models with placement of the oximeter probe on the right hand (preductal), it should be possible to obtain an S_pO_2 reading by a couple of minutes of age in most infants. If the S_pO_2 is less than 85% then blended oxygen can be provided to whatever extent is necessary to raise the S_pO_2 to between 85% to 90%, or until it is quite clear that additional oxygen makes no difference in the oxygen saturations, in which case the infant is likely to have cyanotic congenital heart disease.

Having said this, it is important to understand that we do not know what the optimal oxygen saturation of a transitioning newborn is at any point in time. Thus, the best we can do is to have oxygen blenders and pulse oximeters in delivery units that deal with high-risk infants in order to provide some guidance so that the supplemental oxygen can be provided at the levels which are no higher than necessary. If the infant is in need of supplemental oxygen, it seems prudent to start at about 40% and move up or down as indicated.

Free-flow oxygen in high concentrations can easily be administered by oxygen mask (with escape holes) or by cupping the hand around the end of the oxygen tubing and holding this close to the infant's nose and mouth. A flow-inflating (anesthesia) bag and mask or a mask on the end of a T-tube device (such as the Neopuff®) held lightly over the infant's nose and mouth may also deliver a measured concentration of inspired oxygen. Caution should be used to avoid a seal of the mask to the face so as to avoid providing positive pressure to the lung. A self-inflating bag is not capable of providing free-flow oxygen. Cold, dry oxygen can be given in an emergency; however, a persistent need for free-flow oxygen should prompt humidification and heating of the oxygen.

Assisted ventilation

If an infant is not breathing, is breathing but incapable of sustaining a heart rate of above 100, or is in significant respiratory distress and requiring supplemental oxygen, some form of assisted ventilation may be necessary. This may be simply the provision of a continuous positive end-expiratory pressure to a spontaneously breathing infant or intermittent mandatory positive-pressure ventilation with end-expiratory pressure to infants who are not breathing or are in significant respiratory distress.

When resuscitating a newborn, one must establish a functional residual capacity (FRC) and provide tidal volumes breaths. In the past when positive-pressure ventilation was used the concerns were to provide a peak inspiratory pressure capable of effecting chest movement that resembled an "easy breath". In recent years we have taken into consideration the potential lung damage that can come from over-inflation that may occur if chest movement is the only indicator of adequate ventilation. We have also begun to recognize that there is a potential for damage when the lungs are allowed to deflate to an end-expiratory pressure of zero with the induction of shear stresses upon re-inflation. This has led to the use of a positive end-expiratory pressure, especially when ventilating premature infants, whose immature lungs may well be more susceptible to shear stresses than the term infant [17].

Tidal volume ventilation

In a resuscitation of a newborn, one has to provide tidal volume breaths that are sufficient to promote adequate gas exchange, but which do not over-distend the lung. The parameter most often used for monitoring adequacy of inspiratory flow while bagging is chest wall movement. What is not known is how chest wall movement relates to appropriate expansion of alveoli and true tidal volume in the non-uniformly inflated lung of the neonate, and especially the premature infant with lung disease. It is quite possible, in fact, even likely, that when chest wall movement is used as a guide for positive-pressure ventilation in the delivery room we are overdistending more compliant portions of the lung in our quest for chest rise. This is especially problematic in the immature, surfactant-deficient lung which may be subject to non-uniform expansion. In these circumstances positive-pressure inspiratory gas may be forced into those areas that are more compliant, overdistending those areas of the lung.

These issues become important to consider as we now realize that overdistention of the alveoli can induce lung damage. There is good evidence that overdistention of the lung (volutrauma) is of greater concern than trauma caused by high pressure (barotrauma) [18].

Wada et al. demonstrated that in preterm lambs ventilated for 30 minutes at high tidal volumes, compared to controls, there was a decrease in compliance, lower ventilatory efficiencies and a decreased subsequent response to surfactant [19]. Bjorklund et al. showed that only six large breaths delivered with manual ventilation immediately after birth created enough injury in the lung to result in an attenuated response to surfactant, greater difficulty in ventilating the animal and more widespread lung injury in histologic sections [20].

Overdistention of the lung can induce a series of events that lead to lung injury, e.g. interstitial and alveolar edema, as well as the initiation of an inflammatory response by attraction and activation of neutrophils and macrophages. Simply stretching the lung opens stretch-activated ion channels and increases epithelial and endothelial permeability. It can also result in conformational changes in the membrane molecules. Studies at both a cell level and of whole lung have shown that overdistention can alter cell metabolism leading to a cascade of cytokines and chemokines which are proinflammatory and lead to further lung injury [21].

Thus, there is good evidence that overdistention of the lung promotes lung injury. However, at this point our ability to assure appropriate tidal volume is very limited. We have neither the knowledge nor the tools to assure appropriate tidal volumes in the immediate newborn lung during resuscitation.

How then do we approach a positive-pressure inflation? Where in the past we looked for a "easy rise and fall of the chest" or provided enough positive pressure to reach certain pressure values, now it is recommended that just enough pressure be provided to improve the heart rate, color and muscle tone. These signs are considered the best indicators that inflation pressures are adequate. If these signs are not improving, then one should look for the presence of chest movement and increase the pressure, assuming that one has a good face-mask seal [22].

Keep in mind that in order to establish an FRC, it may be necessary to use higher pressures and longer inspiratory times for the first few breaths than for subsequent breaths.

Positive end-expiratory pressure (PEEP)

We are concerned with not only the degree of inspiration but also the expiratory wing of the breath. In surfactant-deficient animals, ventilation without end-expiratory pressure may result in collapse of the distal units of the lung. Repeated re-expansion of units of the lung that are allowed to become atelectatic at end-expiration leads to shear stresses on the lung that results in similar consequences as those induced by overexpansion of the lung.

When surfactant-deficient rabbit lungs are allowed to attain low end-expiratory volumes they have reduced compliance and greater histologic lung injury than those lungs ventilated at a higher end-expiratory volume maintained with end-expiratory pressures [23]. When rat lungs are ventilated with a low end-expiratory lung volume there is increased cytokine release [24] and increased pulmonary edema [25]. It has also been shown that when saline-lavaged rabbit lungs or preterm lambs are ventilated at low lung volumes there is an impaired response to surfactant. On the other hand, there is also evidence that if preterm lamb lungs are held open at end-expiration with positive end-expiratory pressure, surfactant function is preserved [26,27]. For a very long time we have used end-expiratory pressure with all infants who are on ventilators.

Thus, in addition to avoiding overexpansion of the lung, it also may be important to resuscitate infants, especially the premature infant, using an end-expiratory pressure. This may help avoid the potential damage which can result from repeated re-opening of lung units that are allowed to become atelectatic at end-expiration.

Now, many neonatologists routinely use an end-expiratory pressure when they resuscitate an infant with positive-pressure ventilation to prevent the lung from collapsing at end-expiration with the induction of shear stress upon the subsequent inflation.

Continuous positive airway pressure (CPAP)

End-expiratory pressure, in the form of mask CPAP, is becoming more and more frequently used in the delivery room with infants who are spontaneously breathing yet have some degree of respiratory distress. The goal is the same as discussed above, namely helping to recruit and maintain alveoli open by preventing collapse of alveoli at end-expiration. In breathing preterm lambs when the use of CPAP was compared with intubation and positive-pressure ventilation, it has been shown that at 2 hours of age, those animals resuscitated and treated only with CPAP have higher lung volumes, as well as less evidence of an inflammatory response or acute lung injury [28].

In 1987 the incidence of chronic lung disease was examined at eight institutions throughout the United States. Of note was the fact that Columbia University, had the lowest incidence of chronic lung disease and the most frequent use of CPAP as method of resuscitation and ventilatory support in the nursery [29]. This was confirmed again in 2000 when the incidence of chronic lung disease was examined at two Boston hospitals (22%) and compared to the hospital at Columbia University (4%). The conclusion of the paper was that "… most of the increased risk of CLD among very low birth weight infants hospitalized at 2 Boston NICUs, compared with those at Babies' Hospital, was explained simply by the initiation of mechanical ventilation." [30].

There are a great number of cohort studies indicating that the use of CPAP for ventilatory support in the delivery room reduces the number of infants who need to be ventilated. There are, however, no randomized, controlled clinical trials of sufficient power that compare the use of CPAP with positive-pressure ventilation in neonatal resuscitation. In spite of the lack of "gold standard" trials, the use of CPAP is becoming more and more accepted [31]. The 2006 edition of the American NRP points out that "Some neonatologists recommend administering CPAP to a spontaneously breathing baby …" The Australian Neonatal Resuscitation guidelines point out that there are no randomized controlled trials of CPAP and then go on to say: "However, there is accumulating evidence that it is beneficial and no evidence of harm when used with babies with stiff lungs. Therefore, CPAP or PEEP (at least 5 cmH_2O) should now be considered when resuscitating very premature infants." [32].

Resuscitation devices

It is now recommended that any device used in assisted ventilation be capable of controlling peak inspiratory pressure and end-expiratory pressure as well as inspiratory time. In addition, the device should be able to deliver a variable amount of oxygen ranging from room air to 100%.

There are three devices currently in use that, with various degrees of ease, can meet these requirements. These are the self-inflating bag, the flow-inflating bag and a T-tube device with CPAP and PEEP capability. Regardless of what device is used, those who participate as part of the neonatal resuscitation team should be trained, comfortable and proficient in its use.

If a self-inflating or flow-inflating bag is used, the volume must be appropriate for the newborn infant (200–750 mL total volume) and capable of delivering high concentrations of oxygen. An infant will only require between 5 and 8 cc/kg with each ventilation. A large bag makes it difficult to provide such small volumes. Those who routinely use a flow-inflating bag believe it gives greater responsiveness and greater individual control. Self-inflating bags, however, require less expertise and experience to use effectively than do flow-inflating bags. They will require a special attachment to provide end-expiratory pressure (PEEP); however, they cannot deliver CPAP. Self-inflating bags also require an oxygen reservoir to provide variable concentrations of oxygen.

To guard against the delivery of excessive pressure to the infant's lungs, all resuscitation bags should be equipped with a pressure gauge, a pressure-relief valve (pop-off valve) or both. Pop-off valves ideally vent pressures of greater than 30–40 cmH_2O, but great variability can exist between individual bags [16]. Should pressures greater than 30–40 cmH_2O be needed to establish adequate chest rise, a finger can easily be placed over the pop-off valve. Any bag without a pop-off valve should have a pressure gauge. Pressure gauges with built-in pressure release valves are available.

A T-tube device capable of providing both CPAP and PEEP, controlling the peak-inspiratory pressure as well as the inspiratory time, has been developed (Figure 8.7). The most common one on the market today is called the NeoPuff®.

It is important to check any apparatus for defects before every resuscitation. Reusable bags will develop leaks and cracks over time, and bag reassembly after cleaning may not be correct. It is greatly preferable to discover a faulty bag and mask before it is urgently needed. The apparatus can quickly be checked for function by occluding the air outlet and squeezing the bag or occluding the opening in the T-tube. A pressure should be generated and reflected on the pressure gauge and/or the pop-off valve should vent air above 30–40 cmH_2O.

Use of mask-CPAP

As pointed out previously, in infants who are breathing yet exhibit some degree of respiratory distress and/or an oxygen need, the use of CPAP has become increasingly more common. The easiest way to do this is with the NeoPuff®. After setting the F_iO_2 and the desired degree of continuous positive airway pressure, the attached mask can be sealed to the face, permitting the infant to exhale against a continuous pressure. The same effect can be obtained with a flow-inflating bag by use of the flow-control valve.

Although there are no well-established values at which to start CPAP most neonatologists will begin with at least 5 cmH_2O pressure and move up, if necessary. It is uncommon to go to pressures in excess of 8 cmH_2O. Care must be taken to avoid providing excessive end-expiratory pressure to an infant with good lung compliance.

Use of positive-pressure ventilation

In the infant who is not breathing, has inadequate respirations to keep the heart rate above 100 or who has an excessive work of breathing and a high F_iO_2 requirement on CPAP, there is a need for positive-pressure ventilation. Any of the three devices that

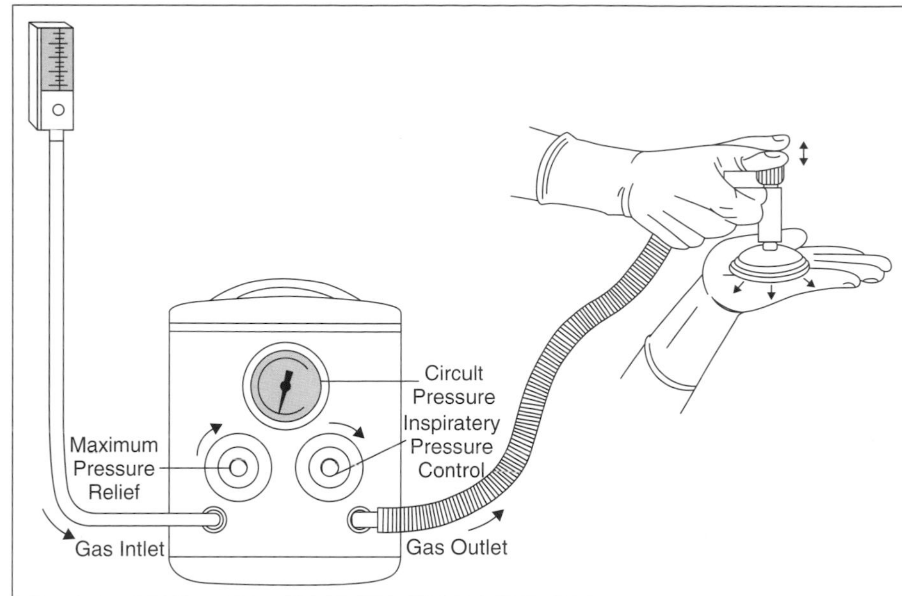

Figure 8.7 T-tube device capable of providing CPAP and PEEP. (Reproduced from *Textbook of Neonatal Resuscitation*, 5th edn. Elk Grove, IL: American Academy of Pediatrics/American Heart Association, 2006: 3–55.)

have been discussed are capable of providing positive-pressure ventilation. However, in order to add end-expiratory pressure to prevent alveolar collapse at end-expiration, one needs to add a device to the self-inflating bag. Initially, positive-pressure ventilation will be provided with a mask.

Positive-pressure ventilation, like the first spontaneous breaths in the healthy infant, must establish FRC and an adequate tidal volume to halt the development or progression of the asphyxial process. To prevent overdistention of the lungs, the goal is to use just enough pressure to effect an improvement in heart rate, oxygen saturation/color, muscle tone and spontaneous breathing. The first breaths may require a greater peak inspiratory pressure and a longer inspiratory time than subsequent breaths. It is recommended that the rate of ventilation should be between 40 and 60 breaths per minute.

If the infant improves, yet continues to need positive-pressure ventilation, be aware of how much tidal volume you are providing. If the chest movement is enough to make the infant appear to be taking deep breaths, you are probably overinflating the lungs. In addition, to increasing the risk of the type of lung damage we previously discussed, you are also at an increased risk for producing a pneumothorax.

If no improvement occurs with the first few breaths, it may be necessary to increase the inspiratory pressure. However, before you do this, check to see if there is any chest movement and have someone listen with a stethoscope to assess breath sounds. If these are poor first check to see if there is an adequate seal between the mask and the face and make sure the airway is not blocked. If these are OK, and there is no improvement, increase the pressure. If there continues to be no improvement, it may be necessary to intubate the infant and provide positive pressure through the endotracheal tube. Table 8.1 describes common problems associated with inadequate chest expansion and potential corrective actions easily performed in the delivery room.

Table 8.1 Problems associated with inadequate chest expansion.

Problem	Correction
Inadequate face mask seal	Reapply mask to face Alter position of hand that holds mask
Blocked airway	
Bag and mask	Check infant's position Suction mouth, oropharynx, and nose Insert oral airway if indicated (Pierre–Robin, macroglossia)
Bag and endotracheal tube	Suction the tube
Misplaced endotracheal tube	Remove endotracheal tube, ventilate with bag and mask, replace tube
Inadequate pressure	Increase pressure, taking care not to overexpand the chest; may require adjusting or overriding the pop-off valve

(Reproduced by permission from Faranoff AA, Martin, RJ, eds. *Neonatal-Perinatal Medicine: Diseases of the Fetus and Newborn*, 7th edn. St Louis: Mosby, 2002: 429.)

Endotracheal intubation

The task of endotracheal intubation is best accomplished by two people. One inserts the tube into the airway, while the other assists and then assesses for correct placement of the tube by listening for equal breath sounds on both sides of the chest. Uncuffed endotracheal tube sizes ranging from 2.0 to 4.0 should be available in the delivery suite. A 2.5 endotracheal tube will be small enough for all but the 500–600-g, extremely low birth weight infants (Table 8.2). If a soft, flexible wire stylet is used to assist with endotracheal tube placement, it should not extend past the tip of the endotracheal tube, thus ensuring that the stylet does not damage the tracheal wall or carina. A tip to lip distance in cm should be used to estimate depth of placement (Table 8.3).

When the tube is placed in the airway, whichever resuscitation device one is using should be attached to the endotracheal tube and a series of breaths initiated. Placement should initially be checked both by auscultation of equal breath sounds on both sides of the chest along with a lack of significant auscultated gastric breath sounds or of significant gastric distension. The placement should be confirmed by the use of a small, portable exhaled CO_2 detector.

Complications of endotracheal intubation include hypoxia, bradycardia, infection and contusions or lacerations to the structures of the upper airway, including the vocal cords themselves. Rarely but tragically, the trachea or esophagus will be perforated. The utmost care must be given to placement of the endotracheal tube to avoid such complications. Even more vigilance must be exercised if an endotracheal tube is placed with the use of a stylet.

Room air versus 100% oxygen

The use of room air as opposed to 100% oxygen in the resuscitation of an infant is a source of much debate. The references for the animal and human work can be gleaned from two recent review articles [33,34]. Multiple animal studies have provided evidence indicating that the generation of oxygen free radicals during the reperfusion phase of ischemic injury is associated with increased damage. After a pilot study demonstrating no difference in outcomes of resuscitation with room air versus 100% oxygen, a seminal and, to date, the only large multicenter controlled study was done [35]. This study enrolled 609 infants to more rigorously test the hypothesis that room air resuscitation of the asphyxiated infant would not increase morbidity and mortality. There were no significant differences in mortality, incidence and severity of hypoxic-ischemic encephalopathy, acid–base status, oxygen saturations or arterial oxygen concentrations.

There are human data to indicate that the initial use of 100% oxygen increases the time to the onset of spontaneous respiration, increases the time of resuscitation, results in a lower 5-minute Apgar score, increases oxidative stress and results in some, at least in the short term, oxidative injury in the kidney and heart. There is also a suggestion that there is an increased neonatal mortality, although this finding is debated. There have been a limited number of randomized controlled human studies, which individually and when looked at in a meta-analysis [36] indicated that starting resuscitation with room air and adding oxygen if needed, does no harm.

The American NRP recommends that 100% oxygen should be used when resuscitating term infants with cyanosis or a need for positive pressure ventilation. When resuscitating the pre-term infant one should use a blender and pulse oximeter and begin somewhere between room air and 100% oxygen; increasing or decreasing the F_iO_2 upon the response of the infant.

On the other hand, the Australian Neonatal Resuscitation Guidelines state that “However, at present, the best available evidence suggests air should be used initially with supplemental oxygen reserved for infants whose condition does not improve after effective ventilatory support.” [32]. The Canadian recommendations indicate that positive-pressure ventilations should be initiated with room air and supplemental oxygen used at 90 seconds of age if the heart rate is below 100 beats per minute or cyanosis persists [37]. Others have suggested starting with an F_iO_2 of 40% and moving up or down as necessary.

Table 8.2 Endotracheal tube sizes.

Tube size (mm ID)	Weight (g)	Gestational age (weeks)
2.0*	500–600 or less	25–26 or less
2.5	<1000	<28
3.0	1000–2000	28–34
3.5	2000–3000	34–38
3.5–4.0	>3000	>38

* May be needed if a size 2.5Fr tube does not fit.
ID, internal diameter.
(Reproduced by permission from Faranoff AA, Martin, RJ, eds. *Neonatal-Perinatal Medicine: Diseases of the Fetus and Newborn*, 7th edn. St Louis: Mosby, 2002: 426.)

Table 8.3 Endotracheal tube placement.

Weight (kg)	Depth of insertion (cm from upper lip)
1	7*
2	8
3	9
4	10

* Infants weighing less than 750 g may require only 6 cm insertion.
(Reproduced by permission from *Textbook of Neonatal Resuscitation*, 4th edn. Elk Grove, IL: American Academy of Pediatrics/American Heart Association, 2000: 5–19.)

Chest compressions

As emphasized above, in all but a fraction of 1% of infants, provision of positive-pressure ventilation will be sufficient to overcome any bradycardia and lead to spontaneous respirations. If, however, after ventilation with 100% oxygen, the newborn remains bradycardic, chest compressions will be needed to maintain systemic blood flow.

The American Heart Association/American Academy of Pediatrics currently recommends beginning chest compression for a heart rate of less than 60 beats/min. This can be done with the two-finger method, or the thumb method may be used to administer adequate chest compressions. However, regardless of the method used, those responsible for chest compressions and for continued ventilation of the infant must position themselves so that they do not interfere with one another. It is helpful for a third team member to monitor for palpable pulses during compressions.

It is currently recommended that chest compressions occur 90 times a minute with ventilation interposed after every third compression. Thus, in a 2-second period, 3 compressions and 1 breath are given. This provides 90 compressions and 30 respirations in each minute. Intermittently, chest compressions should be stopped to check for a spontaneous heart rate. If the spontaneous heart rate is greater than 60 beats/min compressions may be stopped.

If well-coordinated chest compressions and ventilation do not raise the infant's heart rate above 60 beats/min within 30 seconds, support of the cardiovascular system with medications is indicated.

Medications

If the heart rate remains below 60/min, despite ventilation and chest compression, the first action should be to ensure that ventilations and compressions are well coordinated and optimal and 100% oxygen is being used before proceeding with medications. Epinephrine is indicated when, in the rare infant, positive-pressure ventilation and chest compressions fail to correct the neonatal bradycardia. Where the infant appears to be in shock, there is evidence of blood loss and the infant is not responding to resuscitation, volume expanders may be indicated.

Clearly, the best choice for giving epinephrine or volume expanders is via an umbilical venous catheter. If, while preparing for placement of the venous catheter, epinephrine is needed, it can be given via an endotracheal tube. Resuscitative placement of the umbilical vein catheter differs from postresuscitative placement. The umbilical catheter is inserted slightly past the level of the skin – only to the point where blood is first able to be aspirated. This avoids the devastating complication of hepatic necrosis caused by infusion of medications through a catheter inadvertently wedged in a hepatic vein. Any doubt about the position of the umbilical catheter should prompt removal and reinsertion of the catheter to just past the level of the skin.

Epinephrine

Epinephrine should be used as the first-line agent for persistent bradycardia in the face of adequate positive-pressure ventilation with 100% oxygen. It may be given via intravenous catheter or via endotracheal tube while intravenous access is being acquired. It may be re-administered every 3–5 minutes as needed for bradycardia. It remains uncertain as to whether an increase in the standard IV epinephrine dosage should routinely be given when epinephrine is administered via the endotracheal tube. The most current recommendations are that 0.3–1 mL/kg of a 1 : 10 000 solution of epinephrine be used via the endotracheal route. If epinephrine is given via an umbilical venous catheter, the recommended dose is 0.1–0.3 mL/kg of a 1 : 10 000 solution. Given concern about adverse outcomes when high-dose epinephrine has been used for adult resuscitations, routine use of higher epinephrine doses cannot be recommended.

When epinephrine alone is not effective, consideration should be given to the possibility of hypovolemic shock. There is no role for the use of sodium bicarbonate in an acute neonatal resuscitation.

Volume expanders

After administration of epinephrine, if the infant exhibits signs of shock such as poor capillary refill, weak pulses or a pale appearance, or there is evidence or suspicion of acute blood loss a volume expander may be indicated. With a placental abruption or a placental previa, blood loss may be obvious. However, an infant may lose blood into the maternal circulation and this may not be obvious.

The recommended volume expander, and the most easily available is normal saline at a dose of 10 mL/kg via the umbilical vein given over 5–10 minutes. Ringer's lactate can also be used. If severe fetal anemia is documented or expected, type O Rh-negative packed red blood cells should be used, if available.

The drug-depressed infant

Although relatively uncommon, respiratory depression may occur in the infant whose mother received inhalational anesthetic before cesarean section delivery or who was given a narcotic analgesic less than 4 hours before delivery. With the inhalational anesthetics, adequate ventilation will effectively clear them from the infant. If the infant's mother received a narcotic analgesic less than 4 hours before delivery and there is continued respiratory depression after effective positive-pressure ventilation has restored the heart rate and color, naloxone (Narcan) may be useful in antagonizing the narcotic agent's respiratory depression. The standard dose is 0.1 mg/kg of a 1.0 mg/mL solution. The referred route of administration is intravenous. It may be administered intramuscularly, but this route of administration is associated with a delayed onset of action.

It is important to note that the duration of action of the naloxone may be significantly shorter than the duration of action of the narcotic analgesic. Therefore, repeated doses may be necessary. Narcan should never be given to the infant born of a mother with a narcotics addiction. The infant may have acute withdrawal symptoms, including seizures.

If an infant is not breathing, it is important to stress that the first intervention is the administration of positive-pressure ventilation to establish a good heart rate and color, regardless of how sure you are of the fact that narcotics were given to the mother within 4 hours before delivery. Only then, in the face of recent narcotic administration, should a narcotic antagonist be considered.

Immediate care after establishing adequate ventilation and circulation

Once an infant is stabilized after resuscitation, the next steps require deliberate consideration. The future course of the infant's resuscitation is related to the degree of cardiorespiratory compromise. Many infants will quickly improve, and develop good lung compliance, adequate pulmonary blood flow and spontaneous respiratory drive. In these infants, assisted ventilation can be withdrawn in a matter of minutes. Attention must be paid to the amount of assistance they receive as they improve. There is a tendency to overventilate the recovering infant after a successful resuscitation. Furthermore, some degree of inspired oxygen may be all that is necessary to support the recovering infant after an effective resuscitation.

Prolonged assisted ventilation

Prolonged ventilatory assistance is often linked to the time required to resume spontaneous respirations. Some asphyxiated infants, as well as premature infants, may also demonstrate some degree of lung disease and, hence, may require ventilatory assistance even after the resumption of spontaneous respirations. At times, infants with lung disease start out well on their own, but very shortly require ventilatory assistance, in the form of intermittent mechanical ventilation (IMV) or continuous positive airway pressure (CPAP), to maintain adequate ventilation and oxygenation. Whenever an infant requires prolonged ventilatory support, the infant should be managed by physicians and nurses who are comfortable providing assisted ventilation to infants. The use of arterial blood gases taken from an umbilical arterial catheter or peripheral arterial line should be used to guide further ventilatory management.

Dopamine

There are times when the severely asphyxiated infant will have suffered so much compromise despite the previous steps in the resuscitation that poor cardiac output and hypertension remain in spite of the volume boluses which were given. For such infants, dopamine should be used. starting at an intravenous infusion rate of 5 μg/kg/min, increasing, if necessary, to 20 μg/kg/min. If the dose of 20 μg/kg/min is reached without improvement, further increases in the infusion rate are unlikely to make a difference. By the time one is far enough into the resuscitation to reach the point at which dopamine is needed, there should have been some consultation with a neonatologist or pediatrician who is experienced in taking care of sick newborns.

Glucose

As soon as the hypoxia has been corrected, an infusion of glucose at about 5 mg/kg/min should be started (approximately 80 cc/kg/day of 10% glucose). Adjustment of the glucose infusion rate should be made in response to serial, follow-up blood glucose measurements. The asphyxiated infant may have depleted glycogen stores, especially myocardial glycogen stores, and it is important to provide fuel to such an infant. The glucose infusion also prevents the hypoglycemia that is frequently associated with perinatal compromise.

Fluids

The urine output of any infant undergoing an episode of depression should be carefully monitored. Oliguria may occur in asphyxiated infants, and an infant can easily be overloaded with fluid. Fluid should be restricted until there is evidence of adequate urine output. The need to restrict fluid and yet give glucose emphasizes the importance of considering glucose infusion in terms of milligrams per kilogram of body weight per minute, rather than in the amount of 10% glucose to be given. The concentration of glucose will depend on how much fluid can be given to the infant.

Thermal management

Any infant who has undergone an active resuscitation should be carefully observed. This requires that the infant be clothed only in a diaper and kept in either an incubator or a radiant warmer so that thermal neutrality can be maintained. The temperature of the infant should be monitored frequently. As important as it is to prevent hypothermia, it is equally important to avoid hyperthermia.

Feeding

During the asphyxial process, ischemia of the intestine may occur as a result of vasoconstriction of the mesenteric blood vessels. Due to the association between gut ischemia and the development of necrotizing enterocolitis, it may be prudent to withhold enteral feedings from the asphyxiated infant for anywhere up to a few days.

Other problems

Other complications of the post-asphyxial infant include hypocalcemia, disseminated intravascular coagulation, seizures, cerebral edema, and intracerebral hemorrhage.

Special problems during resuscitation

Meconium aspiration

Infants with meconium-stained amniotic fluid are at an increased risk for aspiration of meconium. Although not all infants who pass meconium are depressed or have problems, it is true that if meconium is present in the amniotic fluid, there is a chance that the meconium will enter the mouth of the fetus and be aspirated into the lungs. Aspiration of meconium into the lungs may create ball-valve obstructions throughout the lung, leading to possible air trapping and pneumothorax. Aspirated meconium may further create a reactive inflammation in the lungs that will hinder gas exchange and may be associated with persistent pulmonary hypertension. This perpetuates the fetal circulation pattern and further impairs ventilation and oxygenation of the infant.

The management of infants born through meconium-stained amniotic fluid has represented a controversial area, with varying recommendations over time. Current recommendations [1] take into account recent studies showing no advantages from tracheal suctioning in vigorous, term infants born through meconium-stained amniotic fluid [38]. The current recommendations are based upon two observations: the presence of meconium of any kind and the baby's level of activity. A vigorous infant is defined as an infant with strong respiratory efforts, good muscle tone and a heart rate of >100/min.

Vigorous, term infants born through meconium-stained amniotic fluid, thick or thin, need not be handled in a special way. If an infant is born through meconium-stained amniotic fluid and has depressed respirations, depressed muscle tone and/or a heart rate of less than 100/min then the infant should have the mouth and trachea suctioned.

The best method to remove meconium from the trachea is to insert an endotracheal tube and attach an adapter so that suction can be directly applied, using regulated wall suction at approximately 100 mmHg, as the tube is withdrawn (Figure 8.8). The trachea can then be reintubated and suctioned again, if necessary. One should not try to use a suction catheter inserted through the endotracheal tube to suction meconium.

Because some infants with thick meconium-stained amniotic fluid may be severely asphyxiated, it may not be possible to clear the trachea completely before beginning positive-pressure ventilation. Clinical judgment determines the number of reintubations needed.

Pneumothorax

Whenever positive-pressure ventilation is used a pneumothorax is a potential problem. A pneumothorax should be suspected in all infants who appear to be improving and then suddenly deteriorate. The infant with a pneumothorax may present with unequal breath sounds and distant heart sounds, or the heart sounds may be shifted from the normal position in the left side of the chest. The affected side of the chest may appear to be slightly more distended and less mobile with ventilation than the unaffected side. Acute oxygen desaturation and cyanosis may be noted. If the pleural air generates enough tension, cardiac venous return may be impaired. This may result in hypotension due to a significant drop in cardiac output.

The signs and symptoms of a pneumothorax are usually easily recognized in the otherwise stable infant who suddenly takes a turn for the worse. A high index of suspicion for early pneumothorax must, however, be maintained in the unstable infant requiring resuscitation, for in this circumstance the signs and symptoms are not as obvious.

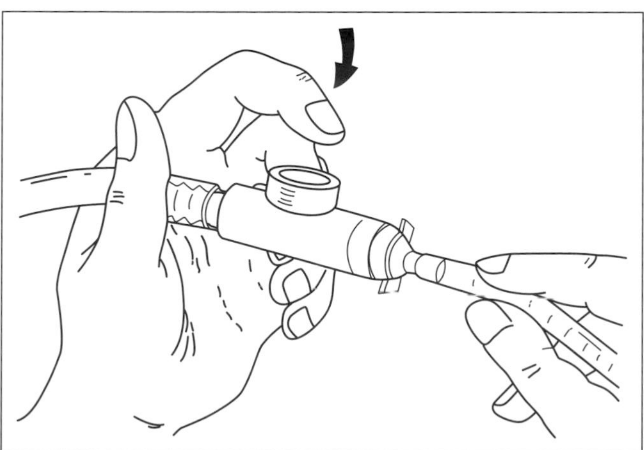

Figure 8.8 Adapter to connect endotracheal tube to mechanical suction. (Reproduced by permission from *Textbook of Neonatal Resuscitation*. Elk Grove, IL; American Academy of Pediatrics/American Heart Association, 1994, rev. 1996: 5–68.)

Diaphragmatic hernia

Congential diaphragmatic hernia undiagnosed before birth is an unusual, but not uncommon, event in the contemporary practice of perinatal medicine. In any infant known or suspected to have a diaphragmatic hernia, one should always use an endotracheal tube for ventilation to prevent gas from entering the intestines. Forcing air into the intestine with bag-and-mask positive-pressure ventilation increases the chances of inflating the intrathoracic bowel and further compromising pulmonary function. An orogastric tube should be placed as soon as possible to remove as much air as possible from the intestines.

Erythroblastosis/hydrops

The hydropic infant is likely not only to be severely anemic, but also to have marked ascites, pleural effusions and pulmonary edema. These infants are also more likely to be asphyxiated *in utero* as well as to be born prematurely, adding respiratory distress syndrome to the list of complications. Thus, successful resuscitation of an infant with hydrops demands preparation of a coordinated team with preassigned responsibilities. The team should be prepared at delivery to perform a thoracentesis, paracentesis, and a complete resuscitation, in addition to an immediate partial exchange transfusion, with O-negative blood cross-matched against the mother, if available.

Establishment of adequate positive-pressure ventilation with immediate tracheal intubation is essential as poor lung compliance and marked pulmonary edema are the rule in this setting. If adequate ventilation cannot be established and significant abdominal distension is noted, paracentesis with removal of significant ascites will often allow improved diaphragmatic excursion and improve ventilation and oxygenation. Consideration should be given to performing a thoracentesis for removal of significant pleural effusions if evidence for significant fluid accumulations exists. Information obtained from prenatal ultrasound examinations can help predict the amount of fluid present. Careful attention must be paid to the maintenance of intravascular volume and the prevention of shock, especially after the removal of large amounts of peritoneal or pleural fluid.

A hematocrit obtained in the delivery room will determine the need for an exchange transfusion (usually partial) in the delivery room. If the infant is extremely anemic and in need of immediate oxygen-carrying capacity, catheters should be inserted into both the umbilical artery and vein to permit a slow, isovolemic exchange with packed red cells. This should result in minimal impact on the hydropic infant's already tenuous hemodynamic status. These lines can also be transduced for central venous and central arterial pressures. Then critical information for managing the hydropic infant's volume can be more easily attained. This information is even more essential if large fluid volumes are removed from either the chest or the abdomen.

Screening for congenital anomalies

Two to three per cent of infants will be born with a congenital anomaly that will require intervention soon after birth. Those that commonly require some form of immediate intervention include bilateral choanal atresia, congenital diaphragmatic hernia, or aspiration pneumonia as a complication of esophageal atresia or a high intestinal obstruction. A rapid screen for congenital defects can easily be performed by the delivery room staff to help identify many of these defects, as well as those that are not life-threatening but require recognition and intervention.

External physical examination

A rapid external physical examination will identify obvious abnormalities such as abnormal facies, and limb, abdominal wall or spinal column defects. A scaphoid abdomen may be a clue to the presence of a diaphragmatic hernia, whereas a two-vessel umbilical cord should alert the examiner to the increased probability of other congenital abnormalities.

Internal physical examination

Because infants are preferentially nose breathers, bilateral choanal atresia of the nares will present with respiratory distress and require a secure airway at birth. This defect can be quickly ruled in or out by assessing the infant's ability to breathe with its mouth held closed. Some infants with unilateral choanal atresia will appear normal and only exhibit respiratory distress when the mouth is held closed and the patent nostril is occluded. The inability to insert a soft nasogastric tube, with obstruction noted within 3–4 cm, suggests possible choanal atresia.

An examination of the mouth will reveal a cleft palate. Insertion of a nasogastric tube may help identify esophageal atresia or a high intestinal obstruction. If the tube does not reach the stomach, an esophageal atresia, commonly associated with a tracheoesophageal fistula, should be suspected. If the tube passes into the stomach, the contents of the stomach may be aspirated. The presence of 15–20 mL of gastric contents on initial aspiration raises the possibility of a high intestinal obstruction. The same tube can then be removed and inserted into the anal opening. Easy passage of the tube for 3 cm into the anus makes anal atresia unlikely. A minute or so spent screening for congenital defects in this way may help avert many future problems.

References

1 American Heart Association. 2005 American Heart Association (AHA) Guidelines for Cardiopulmonary Resuscitation (CPR) and Emergency Cardiovascular Care (ECC) of Pediatric and Neonatal Patients: Neonatal Resuscitation Guidelines. *Pediatrics* 2006. www.pediatrics.orgt/cgi/doi/10.1542/peds.2006–0349

2 Kattwinkel J, ed. *Textbook of Neonatal Resuscitation*, 5th edn. Elk Grove Village, IL: American Academy of Pediatrics, 2006.

3 Rudolph AM, Yuan S. Response of the pulmonary vasculature to hypoxia and H^+ ion concentration changes. *J Clin Invest* 1966; 45: 339–411.

4 Rudolph AM. Fetal cardiovascular response to stress. In: Wiknjosastro WH et al., eds. *Perinatology*. New York: Elsevier Science, 1988.

5 Morin CM, Weiss KI. Response of the fetal circulation to stress. In: Polin RA et al., eds. *Fetal and Neonatal Physiology*. Philadelphia: WB Saunders Co, 1992: 620.

6 Downing SE, Talner NS, Gardner TH. Influences of arterial oxygen tension and pH on cardiac function in the newborn lamb. *Am J Physiol* 1966; 211: 1203–1208.

7 Adamsons K, Behrman R, Dawes GS, James LS, Koford CO. Resuscitation by positive pressure ventilation and tris-hydroxy-methylaminomethane of rhesus monkeys asphyxiated at birth. *J Pediatr* 1964; 65: 807.

8 Dawes GS. Birth asphyxia, resuscitation, brain damage. In: *Foetal and Neonatal Physiology*. Chicago: Year Book Medical, 1968: 141.

9 Pearlman JM, Risser R. Cardiopulmonary resuscitation in the delivery room: Associated clinical events. *Arch Pediatr Adolesc Med* 1995; 149: 20–25.

10 Press S, Tellechea C, Prergen S. Cesarean delivery of full-term infants: identification of those at high risk for requiring resuscitation. *J Pediatr* 1985; 106: 477–479.

11 Miller DL, Oliver TK Jr. Body temperature in the immediate neonatal period: The effect of reducing thermal losses. *Am J Obstet Gynecol* 1966; 94: 964–969.

12 Bruck K. Temperature regulation in the newborn infant. *Biol Neonate* 1961; 3: 65.

13 Adamsons K, Gandy GM, James LS. The influence of thermal factors upon oxygen consumption of the newborn human infant. *J Pediatr* 1965; 66: 495.

14 Cordero L Jr, Hon EH. Neonatal bradycardia following nasopharyngeal stimulation. *J Pediatr* 1971; 78: 441–447.

15 Omar C, Kamlin F, Colm PF et al. Oxygen saturations in healthy infants immediately after birth. *J Pediatr* 2006; 148: 585–589.

16 Rabi Y, Yee W, Chen SY et al. Oxygen saturation trends immediately after birth. *J Pediatr* 2006; 148: 590–594.

17 Clark RH, Gerstmann DR, Jobe AH et al. Lung injury in neonates: causes, strategies for prevention and long-term consequences. *J Pediatr* 2001; 139: 478–86.

18 Dreyfuss D, Soler P, Basset G et al. High inflation pressure pulmonary edema. *Am Rev Respir Dis* 1988; 137: 1159–1164.

19 Wada K, Jobe AH, Ikegami M. Tidal volume effects on surfactant treatment responses with the initiation of ventilation in preterm lambs. *J Appl Physiol* 1997; 83(4): 1054–1061.

20 Bjorklund LJ, Ingimarsson J, Curstedt T et al. Manual ventilation with a few large breaths at birth compromises the therapeutic effect of surfactant replacement in immature lambs. *Pediatr Res* 1997; 42: 348–355.

21 Dreyfuss D, Saumon G. Ventilator-induced lung injury: lessons from experimental studies. *Am J Respir Crit Care Med* 1998; 157: 294–323.

22 American Heart Association. 2005 American Heart Association (AHA) Guidelines for Cardiopulmonary Resuscitation (CPR) and Emergency Cardiovascular Care (ECC) of Pediatric and Neonatal Patients: Neonatal Resuscitation Guidelines. *Pediatrics* 2006: 3–22. www.pediatrics.orgt/cgi/doi/10.1542/peds.2006-0349

23 Musceedere JG, Mullen JBM, Gan K, Slutsky AS. Tidal ventilation at low airway pressure can augment lung injury. *Am J Respir Crit Care Med* 1994; 149: 1327–1234.

24 Tremblay L, Valenza F, Ribeiro SP et al. Injurious ventilatory strategies increase cytokines and c-fos M-RNA expression in an isolated rat lung model. *J Clin Invest* 1997; 99: 944–952.

25 Dreyfuss D, Saumon G. Role of tidal volume, FRC and end-inspiratory volume in the development of pulmonary edema following mechanical ventilation. *Am Rev Respir Dis* 1993; 148: 1194–1203.

26 Frose AB, McCulloch P, Sugiura M et al. Optimizing alveolar expansion prolongs the effectiveness of exogenous surfactant theapy in athe adult rabbit. *Am Rev Respir Dis* 1993: 148: 569–577.

27 Michna J, Jobe AH, Ikegami M. Positive end-expiratory pressure preserves surfactant function in preterm lambs. *J Appl Physiol* 1999; 160: 634–649.

28 Jobe AH, Kramer BW, Moss TJ et al. Decreased indicators of lung injury with continuous positive expiratory pressure in preterm lambs. *Pediatr Res* 2002; 52: 387–392.

29 Avery ME, Tooley WH, Keller JB et al. Is chronic lung disease in low birth weight infants preventable? A survey of eight centers. *Pediatrics* 1987: 79: 26–30.

30 Van Marter LJ, Allred EN, Pagano M et al. Do clinical markers of barotrauma and oxygen toxicity explain interhospital variation in rates of chronic lung disease? *Pediatrics* 2000; 105: 1194–1201.

31 Halamek LP, Morley C. Continuous positive airway pressure during neonatal resuscitation. *Clin Perinatol* 2006; 33: 83–98.

32 Morley C. New Australian Neonatal Resuscitation Guidelines. *J Paediatr Child Health* 2007; 43: 6–8.

33 Saugstad OD, Ramji S, Vento M. Oxygen for neonatal resuscitation: How much is enough? *Pediatrics* 2006; 118: 789–792.

34 Richmond S, Goldsmith JP. Air or 100% oxygen in neonatal resuscitation? *Clin Perinatol* 2006; 33: 11–27.

35 Saugstad OD, Rootwelt T, Aalen O. Resuscitation of asphyxiated newborn infants with room air or oxygen: An international controlled trial: The Resair 2 Study. *Pediatrics* 1998; 102: el. www.pediatrics.org/cgi/contnet./full/102/1/el

36 Davis PG, Tan A O'Donnell CPF. Resuscitation of newborn infants with 100% oxygen or air: a systematic review and meta-analysis. *Lancet* 2004; 364: 1329–1333.

37 Canadian NRP Steering Committee. Addendum to the 2006 NRP Provider Textbook: Recommendations for specific treatment modifications in the Canadian Context. Updated: Nov 2006. www.cps.ca/english/proedu/nrp/addendum.pdf

38 Vain NE, Szyld EG, Prudent LM et al. Oropharyngeal and nasopharyngeal suctioning of meconium-stained neonates before delivery of their shoulders: multicentre, randomized controlled trial. *Lancet* 2004; 364: 597–602.

9 Ventilator Management in Critical Illness

Luis D. Pacheco[1] & Labib Ghulmiyyah[2]

[1]Departments of Obstetrics, Gynecology and Anesthesiology, Maternal-Fetal Medicine-Surgical Critical Care, University of Texas Medical Branch, Galveston, TX, USA

[2]Maternal–Fetal Medicine, Department of Obstetrics and Gynecology, University of Texas Medical Branch, Galveston, TX, USA

Introduction

Respiratory failure remains one of the leading causes of maternal mortality [1,2]. Thromboembolism, amniotic fluid embolism, and venous air embolism together account for approximately 20% of maternal deaths. Other causes of respiratory failure probably account for a further 10–15% of maternal deaths [1]. Not only does maternal respiratory failure affect the mother but it also contributes heavily to fetal morbidity and mortality. This chapter reviews the general principles of airway management in the gravid patient with respiratory failure. In addition, it will provide the reader with information to facilitate a timely recognition and management of respiratory compromise and describes the most recent advances in mechanical support.

Respiratory failure

Respiratory failure is a syndrome that develops when one or both functions of the respiratory system (oxygenation (O_2) and carbon dioxide (CO_2) elimination) fail. Respiratory failure is classified as either hypoxemic or hypercapnic. Hypoxemic respiratory failure is characterized by an arterial partial pressure oxygen (P_aO_2) of less than 60 mmHg with a normal or low arterial partial pressure of carbon dioxide (P_aCO_2). On the other hand, hypercapnic respiratory failure is characterized by a P_aCO_2 of more than 50 mmHg.

The most commonly encountered causes of acute respiratory failure in pregnancy are listed in Table 9.1. Hypoxemic respiratory failure is the most frequently seen of these. It is important to remember that respiratory failure during pregnancy leads to a decrease in oxygen delivery not only to the mother but also to the fetus.

Critical Care Obstetrics, 5th edition. Edited by M. Belfort, G. Saade, M. Foley, J. Phelan and G. Dildy. © 2010 Blackwell Publishing Ltd.

Ventilation/perfusion (V/Q) mismatch

Shunt (Q_S/Q_T)

The V/Q ratio, otherwise known as the alveolar ventilation/pulmonary perfusion ratio, determines the adequacy of gas exchange in the lung. When alveolar ventilation matches pulmonary blood flow, CO_2 is eliminated and the blood becomes fully saturated with oxygen. However, a mismatch of ventilation to perfusion (V_A/Q) is a major cause of lung dysfunction [3]. When the V/Q ratio decreases (<1), arterial hypoxemia occurs. As the mismatch worsens, the resultant hyperventilation produces either a low or normal arterial partial pressure of CO_2 (P_aCO_2). The hypoxemia caused by low V/Q areas is responsive to supplemental oxygen administration. The lower the V/Q ratio, the higher the inspired fraction of oxygen (F_iO_2) required to raise the arterial partial pressure of oxygen (P_aO_2). The most extreme case of V/Q mismatching (V/Q ratio = 0) is known as intrapulmonary shunting.

Oxygenation does not occur in an area of the lung without ventilation even in the face of normal perfusion. This perfused but non-ventilated area of the lung is known as a shunt. The shunt fraction (Q_S/Q_T) is the total amount of pulmonary blood flow that perfuses non-ventilated areas of the lung. In normal lungs, the value of the shunt fraction is 2–5% [4]. A shunt of 10–15% is evidence of significant impairment in oxygenation. A shunt fraction of >25%, in spite of therapy, suggests active acute respiratory distress syndrome (ARDS). The P_aO_2/F_iO_2 ratio is a sometimes used as indicator of gas exchange. A P_aO_2/F_iO_2 <200 correlates with a shunt fraction greater than 20% and is indicative of ARDS. A P_aO_2/F_iO_2 of between 200 and 300 is termed acute lung injury (ALI) and suggests marginal lung function.

The causes of pulmonary shunting include alveolar consolidation or edema, alveolar collapse and atelectasis, and anatomic right to left shunt (e.g. thebesian veins, septal defects). The shunt fraction (Q_S/Q_T) can be calculated using the following formula:

$$Q_S/Q_T = (C_cO_2 - C_aO_2)/(C_cO_2 - C_vO_2)$$

Table 9.1 Causes of lung injury and acute respiratory failure in pregnancy.

Hypoxic
Thromboembolism
Amniotic fluid embolism
Venous air embolism
Pulmonary edema
Aspiration of gastric contents
Pneumonia
Pneumothorax
Acute respiratory distress syndrome (ARDS)
Hypercapnic/hypoxic
Asthma
Drug overdose
Myasthenia gravis
Guillain–Barré syndrome

C_cO_2 is the oxygen content of pulmonary capillary blood. Directly measuring pulmonary capillary blood (CcO_2) is difficult; therefore, CcO_2 is assumed to be 100% when F_iO_2 equals 1. Therefore, using an F_iO_2 of 1.0 (100%) simplifies the calculation of the shunt fraction [3]. C_aO_2 is the oxygen content of arterial blood. C_vO_2 is the oxygen content of mixed venous blood.

Dead space

It is normal for a small percentage of air in the lungs not to reach the blood. The lung is ventilated but not perfused, creating what is known as "dead space". Air in the nasopharynx, trachea and bronchi does not reach the alveoli before exhalation. Too much dead space, however, can lead to hypoxia. The portion of tidal volume (V_t) that is dead space (V_d) is calculated as a ratio, V_d/V_t (~0.30) and can be calculated by the following formula:

$$V_d/V_t = (P_aCO_2 - P_eCO_2)/P_aCO_2$$

where P_eCO_2 is CO_2 in exhaled gas.

P_eCO_2 is measured by collecting expired gas in a large collection bag and using an infrared CO_2 analyzer to measure the PCO_2.

Causes of increased dead space include shallow breathing, vascular obstruction, pulmonary hypertension, pulmonary emboli, low cardiac output, hypovolemia, ARDS, impaired perfusion, positive-pressure ventilation, and increased airway pressure. Acute increases in physiologic dead space significantly increase ventilatory requirements and may result in respiratory acidosis and ventilatory failure. Increased dead space may impose higher minute ventilation, and hence higher work of breathing. A dead space to tidal volume ratio >0.6 usually requires mechanical ventilatory assistance [3].

Arterial oxygen tension (P_aO_2)

P_aO_2 is a measure of the amount of oxygen dissolved in plasma. P_aO_2 determines the percentage saturation of hemoglobin, which is the major factor in determining blood oxygen content. P_aO_2 changes with position and age, and is increased during pregnancy [5,6]. Pulmonary disorders that impair oxygen exchange affect P_aO_2. These include impaired diffusion, increased shunt, and ventilation/perfusion mismatch. The degree of mixed venous oxygen saturation also affects P_aO_2 especially in the presence of an increased shunt [3]. Hypercarbia also affects the P_aO_2 (especially when breathing room air), since CO_2 displaces oxygen.

Alveolar–arterial oxygen tension gradient

The alveolar–arterial oxygen tension gradient ($P_{(A-a)}O_2$) is a sensitive measure of impairment of oxygen exchange from lung to blood [3].

Alveolar–oxygen tension (P_aO_2) is estimated as:

$$P_aO_2 = (P_B - P_{H2O}) \times F_iO_2 - P_aCO_2/RQ$$

where P_B is barometric pressure, P_{H2O} is water vapor pressure, and RQ is the respiratory quotient.

The alveolar–arterial oxygen tension gradient ($P_{(A-a)}O_2$) is equal to:

$$P_aO_2 - P_aO_2$$

Under the clinical circumstances where the P_aO_2 value is less than 60 mmHg, and especially when oxygen therapy is administered, it is acceptable to discount the respiratory quotient disparity and use the simplified version of the ideal alveolar gas equation:

$$P_aO_2 = (P_B - P_{H2O}) \times F_iO_2 - P_aCO_2$$

This is best measured when the patient is breathing 100% oxygen [3]). Under these circumstances, the alveolar–arterial oxygen tension gradient is less than 50 torr on when the F_iO_2 is 1.0 (or less than 30 torr on room air).

Oxygen delivery and consumption

All tissues require oxygen for the combustion of organic compounds to fuel cellular metabolism. The cardiopulmonary system serves to deliver a continuous supply of oxygen and other essential substrates to tissues. Oxygen delivery is dependent upon oxygenation of blood in the lungs, the oxygen-carrying capacity of the blood, and the cardiac output [7]. Under normal conditions, oxygen delivery (DO_2) exceeds oxygen consumption (VO_2) by about 75% [8].

$$DO_2 = CO \times C_aO_2 \times 10 \text{ (normal range} = 700\text{–}1400 \text{ mL/min)}$$

Arterial oxygen content (C_aO_2) is determined by the amount of oxygen that is bound to hemoglobin (S_aO_2) and by the amount of oxygen that is dissolved in plasma ($P_aO_2 \times 0.0031$):

$$C_aO_2 = (Hgb \times 1.34 \times S_aO_2) + (P_aO_2 \times 0.0031)(\text{normal range} = 16\text{–}22\ \text{mL}\ O_2/\text{dL}).$$

It is clear from the above formula that the amount of oxygen dissolved in plasma is negligible (unless the patient is receiving hyperbaric oxygen therapy) and, therefore, the arterial oxygen content is largely dependent on the hemoglobin concentration and the arterial oxygen saturation. Oxygen delivery can be impaired by conditions that affect cardiac output (flow), arterial oxygen content, or both (Table 9.2). Anemia leads to a low arterial oxygen content because of a lack of hemoglobin binding sites for oxygen. Likewise, carbon monoxide poisoning will decrease oxyhemoglobin because of blockage of the oxygen binding sites. The patient with hypoxemic respiratory failure will not have sufficient oxygen available to saturate the hemoglobin molecule. Furthermore, it has been demonstrated that desaturated hemoglobin is altered structurally in such a fashion as to have a diminished affinity for oxygen [9].

Table 9.2 Causes of impaired oxygen delivery.

Low arterial oxygen content
Anemia
Hypoxemia
Carbon monoxide
Hypoperfusion
Shock
Hemorrhagic
Cardiogenic
Distributive
Septic
Anaphylactic
Neurogenic
Obstructive
Tamponade
Massive pulmonary emboli
Hypovolemia

It must be kept in mind that the amount of oxygen actually available to the tissues is also affected by the affinity of the hemoglobin molecule for oxygen. Thus, when attempts are made to maximize oxygen delivery one must consider the oxyhemoglobin dissociation curve (Figure 9.1) and those conditions that influence the binding of oxygen either negatively or positively must be considered [10]. An increase in the plasma pH level, a decrease in temperature or a decrease in 2,3-diphosphoglycerate (2,3-DPG) will increase hemoglobin affinity for oxygen, shifting the oxyhemoglobin dissociation curve to the left ("left shift") and resulting in diminished tissue oxygenation. If the plasma pH level falls or temperature rises, or if 2,3-DPG increases, hemoglobin affinity for oxygen will decrease ("right shift") and more oxygen will be available to tissues [10].

In certain clinical conditions, such as septic shock and ARDS, there is maldistribution of blood flow relative to oxygen demand, leading to diminished delivery and consumption of oxygen. The release of vasoactive substances is hypothesized to result in the loss of normal mechanisms of vascular autoregulation, producing regional and microcirculatory imbalances in blood flow [11]. This mismatching of blood flow with metabolic demand causes hyperperfusion to some areas, and relative hypoperfusion to others, limiting optimal systemic utilization of oxygen [11].

The patient with diminished cardiac output secondary to hypovolemia or pump failure is unable to distribute oxygenated blood to the tissues. Therapy directed at increasing volume with normal saline, or with blood if the hemoglobin level is less than 10 g/dL, increases oxygen delivery in the hypovolemic patient. The patient with pump failure may benefit from inotropic support and afterload reduction in addition to supplementation of intravascular volume. It is taken for granted that in such patients every effort will be made to ensure adequate oxygen saturation of the hemoglobin by optimizing ventilatory parameters.

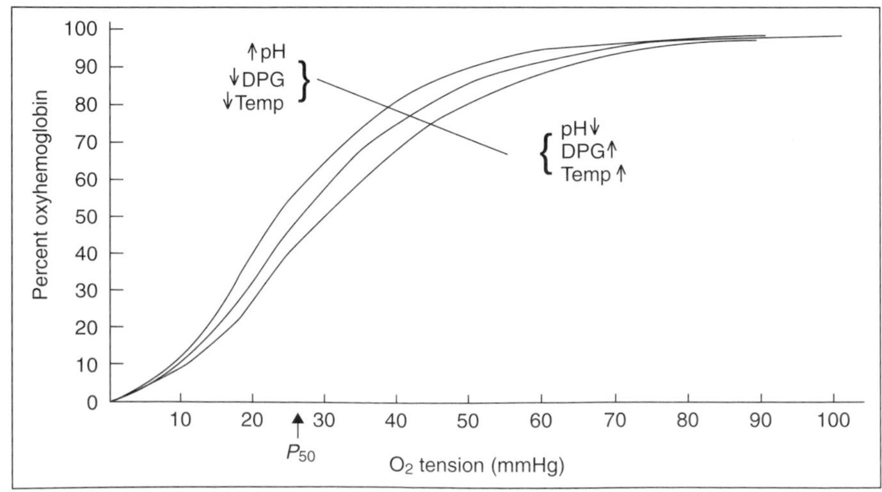

Figure 9.1 The oxygen-binding curve for human hemoglobin A under physiologic conditions (middle curve). The affinity is shifted by changes in pH, diphosphoglycerate (DPG) concentration, and temperature, as indicated. P_{50} represents the oxygen tension at half saturation. (Reproduced by permission from Bunn HF, Forget BG: *Hemoglobin: Molecular, Genetic, and Clinical Aspects*. Philadelphia, Saunders, 1986.)

Relationship of oxygen delivery to consumption

Oxygen consumption (VO_2) is the product of the arteriovenous oxygen content difference ($C_{a-v}O_2$) and cardiac output. Under normal conditions, oxygen consumption is a direct function of the metabolic rate [12].

$$VO_2 = C_{a-v}O_2 \times CO \times 10 \text{ (normal range} = 180\text{–}280 \text{ mL/min)}.$$

The oxygen extraction ratio (OER) is the fraction of delivered oxygen that actually is consumed:

$$OER = VO_2/DO_2$$

The normal oxygen extraction ratio is about 25%. A rise in OER is a compensatory mechanism employed when oxygen delivery is inadequate for the level of metabolic activity. A subnormal value suggests flow maldistribution, peripheral diffusion defects, or functional shunting [12]. As the supply of oxygen is reduced, the fraction extracted from the blood increases and oxygen consumption is maintained. If a severe reduction in oxygen delivery occurs, the limits of O_2 extraction are reached, tissues are unable to sustain aerobic energy production, and consumption decreases. The level of oxygen delivery at which oxygen consumption begins to decrease has been termed the "critical DO_2" [13,14]. At the critical DO_2, tissues begin to use anerobic glycolysis, with resultant lactate production and metabolic acidosis [13]. If this oxygen deprivation continues, irreversible tissue damage and death ensue.

Oxygen delivery and consumption in pregnancy

The physiologic anemia of pregnancy results in a reduction in the hemoglobin concentration and arterial oxygen content. Oxygen delivery is maintained at or above normal in spite of this because of the 50% increase that occurs in cardiac output. It is important to remember, therefore, that the pregnant woman is more dependent on cardiac output for maintenance of oxygen delivery than is the non-pregnant patient [15]. Oxygen consumption increases steadily throughout pregnancy and is greatest at term, reaching an average of 331 mL/min at rest and 1167 mL/min with exercise [16]. During labor, oxygen consumption increases by 40–60% and cardiac output increases by about 22% [17,18]. Because oxygen delivery normally far exceeds consumption, the normal pregnant patient is usually able to maintain adequate delivery of oxygen to herself and her fetus even during labor. When a pregnant patient has low oxygen delivery, however, she very quickly can reach the critical DO_2 during labor, compromising both herself and her fetus. Pre-eclampsia is known to have a significantly adverse effect on oxygen delivery and consumption, a condition that is believed to result from a tissue level disturbance that makes oxygen consumption dependent on oxygen delivery, i.e. there is loss of the normal reserve [19,20].

The obstetrician, therefore, must make every effort to optimize oxygen delivery before allowing labor to begin in the compromised patient.

Assessing oxygenation

Arterial blood gas (ABG) sampling is performed to obtain accurate measures of P_aO_2, P_aCO_2, blood pH and oxygen saturation. Usually, the radial artery is used. Arterial blood gas values differ in pregnancy compared with non-pregnant values [21] (Table 9.3). Interpreting the ABG is useful for identifying respiratory and metabolic derangements. Measuring P_aO_2 is required for calculating $P_{(A-a)}O_2$. In addition, acid–base disturbances can be diagnosed [22]. An indwelling arterial line is useful for obtaining arterial blood gas measurements and monitoring blood pressure when patients are receiving ventilatory support. However, arterial oxygen saturation can be assessed continuously and non-invasively by pulse oximetry. End-tidal CO_2 can also be measured non-invasively.

Pulse oximetry

Transcutaneous pulse oximetry estimates O_2 saturation (S_PO_2) of capillary blood based on the absorption of light from light-emitting diodes positioned in a finger clip or adhesive strip probe. The usual sites for measurement are the ear lobe or the finger nail bed.

Oxyhemoglobin absorbs much less red and slightly more infrared light than reduced hemoglobin. The degree of oxygen saturation of the hemoglobin thereby determines the ratio of red to infrared light absorption. The estimates are generally very accurate and correlate to within 2% of measured arterial O_2 saturation (S_aO_2) [23]. Results may be less accurate in patients with highly pigmented skin, those wearing nail polish, and those with arrhythmias or hypotension, in whom the amplitude of the signal may be dampened. Hyperbilirubinemia and severe anemia may lead to oximetry inconsistencies [3]. Carbon monoxide poisoning will lead to an overestimation of the P_aO_2. In addition, if methemoglobin levels reach greater than 5%, the pulse oximeter no longer accurately predicts oxygen saturation.

When assessing the accuracy of the arterial saturation measured by the pulse oximeter, correlation of the pulse rate determined by the oximeter and the patient's heart rate is an indication of proper placement of the electrode.

Pulse oximetry is ideal for non-invasive monitoring of the arterial oxygen saturation near the steep portion of the oxygen hemoglobin dissociation curve, namely at a P_aO_2 of 70 torr [3]. P_aO_2 levels of 80 torr result in very small changes in oxygen saturation, namely 97–99%. Large changes in the P_aO_2 value in the range of 90 torr to a possible 600 torr can occur without significant change in arterial oxygen saturation (Figure 9.1). This

Table 9.3 Arterial blood gas values in the pregnant and non-pregnant woman.

Status	pH	P_aO_2 (mmHg)	Pco_2 (mmHg)
Non-pregnant	7.4	93	35–40
Pregnant	7.4	100–105	30

technique, therefore, is useful as a continuous monitor of the adequacy of blood oxygenation and not as a method to quantitate the level of impaired gas exchange.

Mixed venous oxygenation

The mixed venous oxygen tension (P_VO_2) and mixed venous oxygen saturation (S_VO_2) are parameters of tissue oxygenation [12]. Normally, the P_VO_2 is 40 mmHg with a saturation of 73%. Saturations less than 60% are abnormally low. These parameters can be measured directly by obtaining a blood sample from the distal port of the pulmonary artery catheter when the catheter tip is well positioned for a wedge pressure reading and the balloon is not inflated (distal pulmonary artery branches). The S_VO_2 also can be measured continuously with a special fiberoptic pulmonary artery catheter.

Mixed venous oxygenation is a reliable parameter in the patient with hypoxemia or low cardiac output, but findings must be interpreted with caution. When the S_VO_2 is low, oxygen delivery can be assumed to be low. However, normal or high S_VO_2 does not guarantee that tissues are well oxygenated. In conditions such as septic shock and ARDS, the maldistribution of systemic flow may lead to abnormally high S_VO_2 in the face of severe tissue hypoxia [11]. The oxygen dissociation curve must be considered when interpreting the S_VO_2 as an indicator of tissue oxygenation [9] (Figure 9.1). Conditions that result in a left shift of the curve cause the venous oxygen saturation to be normal or high, even when the mixed venous oxygen content is low. The S_VO_2 is useful for monitoring trends in a particular patient, as a significant decrease will occur when oxygen delivery has decreased secondary to hypoxemia or a fall in cardiac output.

Impairment of oxygenation

A decrease in arterial oxygen saturation (P_aO_2) below 90% is one definition of hypoxemia. However, the degree to which the alveolar–arterial oxygen tension gradient is increased is a more accurate measurement of the degree of impairment. A shunt of greater than 20% reflects respiratory failure. This degree of shunt will result in an alveolar–arterial oxygen tension gradient of greater than 400 torr [3]. It is important to understand the interrelationship between shunt, the level of mixed venous oxygen saturation, and the arterial oxygen saturation. As more oxygen is extracted from the blood, the mixed venous oxygen saturation decreases resulting in a lower P_aO_2 (depending on the severity of the shunt). Therefore, a marked change in P_aO_2 can occur in the absence of any change in lung pathology [3].

Therapy

Hypoxemia is a major threat to normal organ function. Therefore, the first goal is to reverse and/or prevent tissue hypoxia. The goal is to assure adequate oxygen delivery to tissues, and this is generally achieved with a P_aO_2 of 60 mmHg or arterial oxygen saturation (S_aO_2) of greater than 90%. Isolated hypercapnia is usually well tolerated and is not a threat to the organs unless accompanied by severe acidosis (pH <7.2).

Hypoxemia is treated by increasing the fraction of inspired oxygen (F_iO_2) while attempting to correct the underlying problem. Disorders causing increased shunting, such as atelectasis and bronchial pneumonia, can usually be treated effectively with pulmonary toilet, position change, and antibiotic therapy. Since ventilation perfusion mismatching is frequently a component of hypoxemia, an increase in F_iO_2 usually results in some improvement in oxygenation [3]. Table 9.4 lists some available non-invasive oxygen delivery systems and the approximate F_iO_2 obtained with each [24]. When the shunt is large (>25%), increasing F_iO_2 does not significantly improve P_aO_2. This clinical situation usually arises in conditions such as ARDS or cardiogenic pulmonary edema, and in such cases mechanical ventilation is indicated.

Continuous positive airway pressure (CPAP)

Continuous positive airway pressure (CPAP) is the most widely used method of non-invasive positive pressure ventilatory support. This method consists of a continuous high flow of gas and an expiratory resistance valve attached to a tight-fitting mask. Airway pressure in CPAP is consistently higher than atmospheric pressure even though all of the patient's breaths are spontaneous. The flow of air creates enough pressure during inhalation to keep the airway patent. The best CPAP level is one in which oxygenation is adequate and there is no evidence of depressed cardiac function and carbon dioxide retention. CPAP prevents the development of alveolar collapse and increases the pressure in the small airways (including those in which the critical closing pressure has been elevated) thus increasing functional residual capacity. CPAP has the advantages of convenience, lower cost, and morbidity-sparing potential when compared with standard invasive positive-pressure ventilation. Unfortunately, CPAP also suffers from the disadvantage of a heightened risk of volutrauma and hypotension. An additional problem is the potential for developing pressure sores from the tight-fitting mask [25].

Non-invasive positive-pressure ventilation

Another type of non-invasive ventilation is called non-invasive positive-pressure ventilation (NPPV). In contrast to CPAP, which does not provide ventilatory assistance and which applies a sustained positive pressure, non-invasive positive-pressure ventilation delivers intermittent positive airway pressure through the upper airway and actively assists ventilation [25].

Non-invasive positive-pressure ventilation requires patient cooperation [26]. Patients must learn to coordinate their breathing efforts with the ventilator so that spontaneous breathing is assisted even during sleep. This type of ventilatory assistance is particularly efficacious in treating patients with chronic obstructive sleep apnea.

Non-invasive approaches have been most effective for managing episodes of acute respiratory failure in which rapid improvement is expected such as during episodes of cardiogenic

Table 9.4 Oxygen delivery systems.

Type	F_iO_2 capability	Comments
Nasal cannula		
Standard	True F_iO_2 uncertain and highly dependent on inspiratory flow rate	Flow rates should be limited to <5 L/min
Reservoir type	True F_iO_2 uncertain and highly dependent on inspiratory flow rate	Severalfold less flow required than with standard cannula
Transtracheal cannula	F_iO_2 less dependent on inspiratory flow rate	Usual flow rates of 0.25–3.0 L/min
Ventimask	Available at 24, 28, 31, 35, 40, and 50%	Less comfortable, but provides a relatively controlled F_iO_2. Poorly humidified gas at maximum F_iO_2
High humidity mask	Variable from 28 to nearly 100%	Levels >60% may require additional oxygen bleed-in. Flow rates should be 2–3 times minute ventilation. Excellent humidification
Reservoir mask		
Non-rebreathing	Not specified, but about 90% if well fitted	Reservoir fills during expiration and provides an additional source of gas during inspiration to decrease entrainment of room air
Partial rebreathing	Not specified, but about 60–80%	
Face tent	Variable; same as high humidity mask	Mixing with room air makes actual O_2 concentration inspired unpredictable
T-tube	Variable; same as high humidity mask	For spontaneous breathing through endotracheal or tracheostomy tube. Flow rates should be 2–3 times minute ventilation

Table 9.5 Selection guidelines for non-invasive positive-pressure ventilation use in acute respiratory failure.

Respiratory failure or insufficiency without need for immediate intubation with the following:
acute respiratory acidosis
respiratory distress
use of accessory muscles or abdominal paradox
Cooperative patient
Hemodynamic stability
No active cardiac arrhythmias or ischemia
No active upper gastrointestinal bleeding
No excessive secretions
Intact upper airway function
No acute facial trauma
Proper mask fit achieved

(Reproduced by permission from Meyer TJ, Hill NS. Non-invasive positive-pressure ventilation to treat respiratory failure. *Ann Intern Med* 1994; 120: 760.)

pulmonary edema or acute exacerbations of chronic obstructive pulmonary disease (COPD). In addition, NPPV has been associated with a significant reduction in endotracheal intubation in patients with hypoxemic acute respiratory failure. Recently, it was shown that NPPV applied as a first-line intervention in ARDS avoided intubation in 54% of treated patients [27]. Selection guidelines for NPPV in acute respiratory failure are presented in Table 9.5.

The pregnant patient suffering hypoxemia may respond positively to initial intervention with non-invasive means of increasing F_iO_2. However, clinical deterioration can be acute. Therefore, these gravida require intense surveillance with frequent evaluation of clinical status, S_pO_2 or S_aO_2. If viable (>24 weeks), the fetal status should also be frequently assessed. These assessments can be accomplished with continuous electronic fetal heart rate monitoring or intermittent non-stress testing or biophysical profile scoring as appropriate.

Mechanical ventilatory support in pregnancy

Clinical recognition of the gravida who is experiencing respiratory failure and needs mechanical ventilation is extremely important, because maternal and fetal reserve is likely impaired in the gravida who has been hypoxic. This is particularly important for the laboring patient, who may rapidly reach the "critical DO_2" level, i.e. that point at which oxygen consumption becomes directly dependent on oxygen delivery.

In addition to the parameters noted in Table 9.6, the onset of changes in the fetal heart rate pattern consistent with hypoxemia may signal respiratory failure in the pregnant patient. These fetal heart rate patterns include persistent late decelerations, tachycardia, bradycardia, and absent beat-to-beat variability [28]. One should not intervene on behalf of the fetus unless the maternal condition is stabilized. Intervention, in an unstable hypoxemic gravida, may lead to increased morbidity or even mortality for the patient as well as her fetus. One should also recognize that stabilization of the gravida and the institution of mechanical ventilatory support will likely rescue the fetus as well. However, if

Table 9.6 Definition of acute respiratory failure.

Parameter	Normal range	Indication for ventilatory assistance
Mechanics		
Respiratory rate (breaths/min)	12–20	>35
Vital capacity (mL/kg body weight)*	65–75	<15
Inspiratory force (cmH_2O)	(75–100)	<25
Compliance (mL/cmH_2O)	100	<25
FEV_1 (mL/kg body weight)*	50–60	<10
Oxygenation		
P_aO_2 (torr)†	80–95	<70
(kPa)	10.7–12/7	<9.3
$P_{(A-a)}O_2$‡(torr)	25–50	>450
(kPa)	3.3–6.7	>60
Q_s/Q_T (%)	5	>20
Ventilation		
P_aCO_2 (torr)	35–45	>55§
(kPa)	4.7–6.0	>7.3
V_D/V_T	0.2–0.3	>0.60

FEV_1, forced expiratory volume in 1 min; $P_{(A-a)}O_2$, alveolar–arterial oxygen tension gradient; Q_S/Q_T, shunt fraction; V_D/V_T, dead space to tidal volume ratio.
* Use ideal body weight;
† room air;
‡ $F_iO_2 = 1.0$; §exception is chronic lung disease.
(Reproduced by permission from Van Hook JW. Ventilator therapy and airway management. *Crit Care Obstet* 1997; 8: 143.)

maternal death appears imminent or cardiac arrest unresponsive to resuscitation occurs, the potentially viable fetus (>24 weeks) should be delivered abdominally within 5 minutes of the cardiac arrest. In this situation, delivery may actually improve maternal survival [29].

Intubation

In general, indications for intubation and mechanical ventilation do not vary with pregnancy. However, because of the reduced PCO_2 seen in normal pregnancy, intubation may be indicated once the PCO_2 reaches 35–40 mmHg since this may signal impending respiratory failure (especially in a patient with asthma). In addition to the criteria in Table 9.6, one should include: apnea, upper airway obstruction, inability to protect the airway, respiratory muscle fatigue, mental status deterioration, and hemodynamic instability.

Intubation of the pregnant patient should be accomplished by skilled personnel. Intubation in pregnancy differs somewhat from that of non-pregnant patients. Pregnancy, particularly at term, has been associated with slow gastric emptying and increased residual gastric volume [30]. This implies a slightly increased risk of aspiration of gastric contents during intubation of the gravid patient. The use of sodium bicarbonate preoperatively neutralizes gastric contents [31]. This should be administered before intubation if possible. In addition, intubation should proceed using techniques that preserve airway reflexes (e.g. awake intubation). Alternatively, use of "in rapid sequences," induction of general anesthesia and Sellick's maneuver (cricoid pressure) may be employed to prevent passive reflux of gastric contents into the pharynx [32]. Another difference is that hyperemia associated with pregnancy can narrow the upper airways sufficiently that patients are at increased risk for upper airway trauma during intubation [33]. Relatively small endotracheal tubes may be required (6–7 mm). Nasal tracheal intubation should probably be avoided as well unless no other way to secure an airway is available.

Decreased functional residual capacity in pregnancy may lower oxygen reserve such that, at the time of intubation, a short period of apnea may be associated with a precipitous decrease in the PO_2 [33]. Therefore, 100% oxygen should be administered either by mask or by ambubag when the patient requires intubation. Overenthusiastic hyperventilation should be avoided because the associated respiratory alkalosis may actually decrease uterine blood flow. In addition, if ambubreaths are given with too high a pressure, the stomach will fill with air and increase the risk of aspiration. In cases where intubation is not successful after 30 seconds, one should stop and resume ventilation with bag and mask before repeating the attempt in order to avoid prolonged hypoxemia [34]. Once the patient is intubated, the cuff should be inflated and the patient should be ventilated with the ambubag while auscultation over the chest and stomach is performed to ensure proper endotracheal tube placement. In addition, a chest X-ray should be ordered for confirmation of tube placement. Complications of endotracheal intubation are listed in Table 9.7.

The recommended initial ventilator settings are F_iO_2 0.9–1 and rate of 12–20 breaths per minute. Traditionally, a tidal volume (V_T) of 10–15 mL/kg was recommended. It has recently been recognized that these volumes result in abnormally high airway pressures and volutrauma. Therefore V_T should be instituted at 5–8 mL/kg to prevent excessive alveolar distention [35–37].

Ventilator modes

Controlled mechanical ventilation

When controlled mechanical ventilation (CMV) is instituted, the patient makes no effort and the ventilator assumes all respiratory work by delivering a preset volume of gas at a preset rate [38]. This mode of mechanical ventilation is typically used during general anesthesia, in certain drug overdoses, and when paralytic agents are used.

Assist control

In assist control (A/C) mode (Figure 9.2), every inspiratory effort by the patient triggers a ventilator-delivered breath at the selected

Table 9.7 Complications of endotracheal intubation.

During intubation: immediate
Failed intubations
Main stem bronchial or esophageal intubation
Laryngospasm
Trauma to naso/oropharynx or larynx
Perforation of trachea or esophagus
Cervical spine fracture
Aspiration
Bacteremia
Hypoxemia/hypercarbia
Arrhythmias
Hypertension
Increased intracranial/intraocular pressure
During intubation: later
Accidental extubation
Endobronchial intubation
Tube obstruction or kinking
Aspiration, sinusitis
Tracheoesophageal fistula
Vocal cord ulcers, granulomata
On extubation
Laryngospasm, laryngeal edema
Aspiration
Hoarseness, sore throat
Non-cardiogenic pulmonary edema
Laryngeal incompetence
Swallowing disorders
Soreness, dislocation of jaw
Delayed
Laryngeal stenosis
Tracheomalacia/tracheal stenosis

(Modified from Stehling LC. Management of the airway. In: Barash PG, Cullen BF, Stoelting RK, eds. Clinical Anesthesia, 2nd edn. Philadelphia: JB Lippincott, 1992: 685–708.)

tidal volume (volume control) or the selected pressure control level above PEEP (pressure control) [38]). If the patient does not trigger the ventilator, breaths will be delivered by the machine at a preset respiratory rate chosen by the clinician. All breaths are delivered by the ventilator, and therefore the work of breathing is minimized in this mode. Assist control ventilation may be volume control (every time the ventilator fires, spontaneously according to the preset rate or triggered by the patient, a preset tidal volume will be delivered), pressure control (each time the ventilator fires, according to the preset rate or triggered by the patient, a preset amount of pressure will be delivered), or pressure-regulated volume control (same principle as above, here a preset tidal volume will be delivered but the ventilator will deliver the minimal amount of pressure needed to supply the tidal volume). Because a full selected tidal volume or amount of pressure is delivered with each inspiratory effort initiated by the patient, respiratory alkalosis may develop in patients with tachypnea. Patients with rapid shallow respiration may generate very high minute ventilation leading to air trapping (auto-PEEP). This is easily recognized in the ventilator flow/time screen where the clinician will notice that a new tidal volume is being delivered before final exhalation is completed (see Figure 9.3). The resultant increase in intrathoracic pressure may compromise venous return and hemodynamics. In the majority of cases, this situation may be avoided by optimizing sedation.

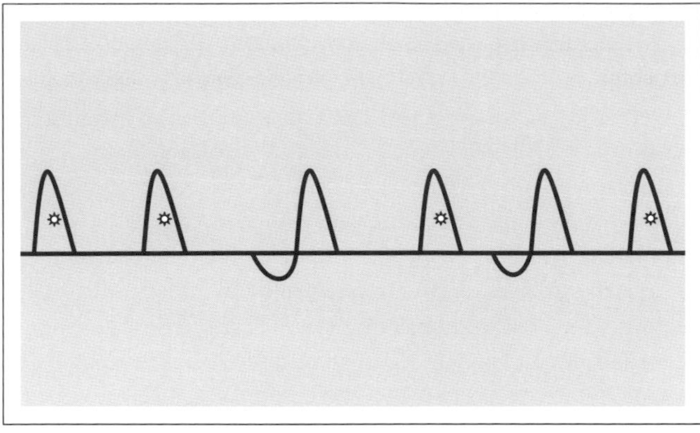

Figure 9.2 Assist control ventilation. Marked breaths are fired by the ventilator according to a preset rate. Each of these breaths may be volume controlled, pressure controlled, or pressure-regulated volume controlled. The two breaths not labeled are triggered by the patient. Note that unlike SIMV, when the patient triggers the ventilator she will receive a breath identical to the ones fired by the ventilator. In these modes of ventilation the work of breathing by the patient is minimized.

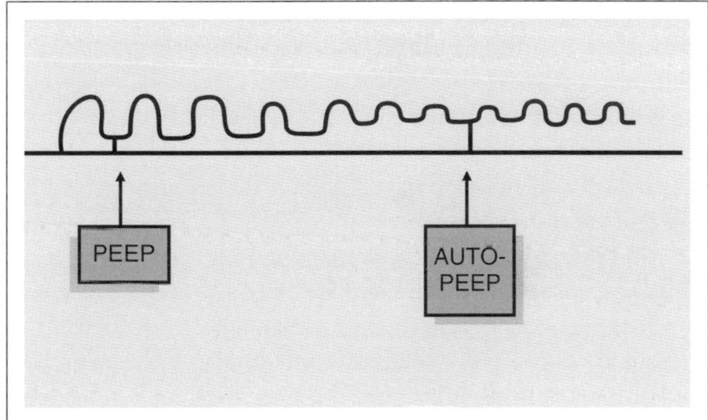

Figure 9.3 PEEP and auto-PEEP. Positive end-expiratory pressure (PEEP) refers to the amount of pressure that remains in the lungs after the end of expiration. Modern ventilatory strategies use PEEP to prevent ventilator-induced injury and favor lung recruitment. Auto-PEEP (intrinsic PEEP) may develop when the respiratory rate is fast enough to prevent full exhalation before the new breath is delivered. This will lead to air trapping that could compromise hemodynamics (see text for explanation).

In patients where limiting pressures is of paramount importance (e.g. bronchopleural fistulas), pressure control A/C is a good option. In this mode, a preset value of pressure control above PEEP is chosen (e.g. if PEEP is set at 10 cmH_2O, and the pressure control level is set at 20 cmH_2O, then each breath, spontaneous or triggered, will deliver 30 cmH_2O of pressure). This increase in pressure will be translated into a certain tidal volume. Importantly, if lung compliance decreases over the course of the disease, the ventilator will continue to deliver that pressure but obviously the tidal volume delivered will be less. Clinicians should be vigilant about changes in tidal volumes delivered when using this mode.

Synchronized intermittent mandatory ventilation

Synchronized intermittent mandatory ventilation (SIMV) (Figure 9.4) incorporates a demand valve that must be patient activated with each spontaneous breath and that allows a preset amount of pressure support to be delivered in concert with the patient's effort [38]. Every time the patient triggers the ventilator, she will receive a preset amount of pressure support. In most ventilators, the opening of the demand valve is triggered either by a fall in pressure or only by generating air flow. Once the ventilator senses air flow generated by the patient, it adds fresh gas into the circuit to meet the patient's ventilatory demand. When the patient does not trigger the ventilator, breaths will be delivered by the machine according to a preset respiratory rate. In SIMV, as discussed for A/C, ventilator-delivered breaths may be set in volume control, pressure control, or pressure-regulated volume control. The main difference with A/C is that when the patient triggers the ventilator in SIMV, she will only get the preset amount of pressure support and will be allowed to complete her breath. The patient determines the inspiratory time for that breath (in A/C, patient-triggered breaths will be identical to the preset machine breaths with a preset inspiratory time). Since machine and patient breaths are better synchronized, SIMV promotes greater patient comfort and tolerance. The SIMV system has a major drawback in that the work of breathing is increased.

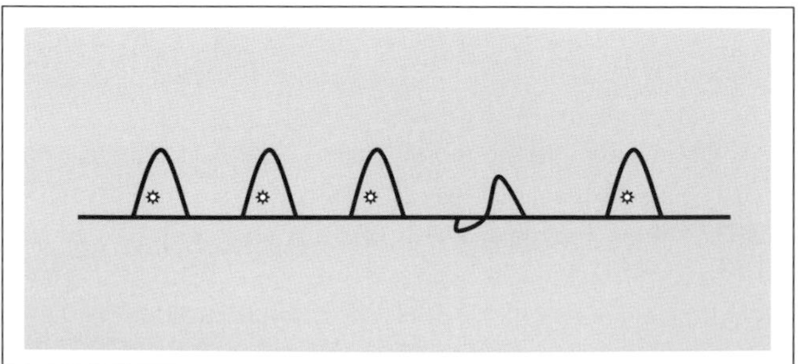

Figure 9.4 SIMV. Breaths marked with the star are fired by the ventilator at the preset respiratory rate. Each of these breaths may be volume controlled, pressure controlled, or pressure regulated volume controlled. The breath not labeled is a patient trigerred breath. Here, the tidal volume will be determined by the patient's effort and the preset amount of pressure support adjusted on the ventilator by the operator.

Pressure support ventilation

Pressure support ventilation (PSV) is used in awake patients who are assuming part of the work of breathing. In PSV, the ventilator provides a preset level of positive pressure in response to the patient's inspiratory effort [39]. Thus, PSV augments the patient's inspiratory effort with a pressure assist. A preselected pressure is held constant by gas flow from the ventilator for the duration of the patient's inspiratory effort. This is a flow cycled mode. This means that when the inspiratory flow drops below a certain value (depending on the ventilator it may be to less than 5 L/min or to less than 25% of the peak inspiratory flow), the pressure support given will finalize and expiration will follow. Pressure support ventilation is designed principally to reduce the work of breathing in a spontaneously breathing patient [40]. This allows for a larger tidal volume at a given level of work. This particular type of assisted ventilation may be especially useful for patients who have a small-diameter endotracheal tube in place and it helps reduce the fatigue often experienced with weaning from mechanical ventilation. Keep in mind that PSV differs from A/C ventilation and SIMV in that there is no set machine rate of breaths.

Since the patient decides the rate, and the tidal volume is determined by the amount of inflation pressure generated by the machine and the patient together, this modality may deliver a variable minute ventilation in a patient with an unreliable respiratory drive. PSV may be used as a primary mode or more frequently in combination with SIMV as discussed previously.

Pressure-regulated volume control ventilation

Pressure-regulated volume control (PRVC) is a mode in which breaths are delivered with a preset tidal volume (the operator sets the tidal volume desired) at a preset frequency. The ventilator will, breath by breath, adapt the inspiratory pressure control level to changes in lung/thorax compliance so that the lowest necessary pressure will be used to deliver the preset tidal volume. The inspiratory flow is decelerating so that the inspiratory pressure will be constant during the whole inspiratory time. Modern ventilators have PRVC as a control mode (every time the patient triggers the ventilator she will get a breath identical to the ones set by the operator) or as SIMV (the mandatory breaths will be on PRVC but when the patient triggers the ventilator he or she will receive the amount of pressure support preset by the operator and not the PRVC breath set previously).

Other ventilator modes

Because of limitations of the traditional forms of mechanical ventilation, alternative modes have been developed. Management of severe ARDS, which entails extremely non-compliant lungs with extensive shunting, has been particularly challenging [41].

Inverse ratio ventilation

Conventional mechanical ventilation devotes approximately one-third of the respiratory cycle to inspiration and two-thirds to expiration. In contrast, this ratio (I : E) is reversed in inverse ratio ventilation (IRV). The objective of IRV is to achieve better oxygenation as a result of higher mean alveolar pressure. The principle of IRV is to maintain alveoli open (recruited) for longer periods of time by prolonging the inspiratory period. In IRV, inspiration is set at longer duration than expiration. This results in slower inspiratory flow for a given tidal volume and therefore lower peak airway pressures [42]. This type of ventilation is used in patients with ARDS who are experiencing worsening compliance and refractory hypoxemia. Growing clinical experience with IRV suggests that it can be useful in improving gas exchange in patients with ARDS whose oxygenation cannot be maintained with more conventional approaches. In this type of ventilatory mode, oxygenation is improved as atelectatic areas are recruited and maintained as functional units, thereby lowering the dead space to tidal volume ratio.

There are a number of drawbacks associated with IRV [43]. It is a very unpleasant mode of ventilation, necessitating both sedation and paralysis when used in non-anesthetized patients. Neuromuscular blockade during the management of respiratory failure is associated with prolonged weakness and paralysis [44,45]. Also, expiratory time is encroached upon and air trapping and hyperinflation may occur which may result in volutrauma or hemodynamic compromise secondary to increased intrathoracic pressure [46]. This mode should be used only by experienced clinicians. If hypercapnia becomes an issue while on IRV, maneuvers to decrease the P_aCO_2 include a decrease in the respiratory rate (thus prolonging the expiratory time) and either a decrease in PEEP or an increase in the pressure control level above PEEP (if using a pressure control mode) in order to increase the gradient between both pressures.

With the advent of newer ventilatory modes, like airway pressure release ventilation, the use of IRV has declined in the last decade.

Airway pressure release ventilation

In airway pressure release ventilation (APRV) the patient receives continuous positive airway pressure that intermittently decreases from the preset value to a lower pressure as the airway pressure release valve opens [47]. Mean airway pressure is thereby lowered during an assisted breath. As in IRV, the I : E ratio is inverted in APRV. The theoretical utility of this strategy is based upon its ability to augment alveolar ventilation as well as opening, recruiting, and stabilizing previously collapsed alveoli without risk of volutrauma or detriment to the cardiac output [47]. APRV maintains alveolar recruitment during 80–95% of the total respiratory cycle time, optimizing V/Q matching and minimizing shear forces by preventing repetitive opening and closing of lung units with each tidal volume delivered [48]. The operator sets four critical parameters when using this mode. These include the pressure high (P high), time high (T high), pressure low (P low), and time low (T low) parameters. A reasonable starting point for P high is the plateau pressure obtained while the patient was on conventional mechanical ventilation. T high is usually set between 4 and 6 seconds. This means that for a period of 4–6 seconds, the patient will receive continuous positive airway pressure equal to the previous plateau pressure (e.g. 25 cmH_2O). Such prolonged T high provides a "stabilized open lung" [48]. After completion of T high, pressure release will follow and the pressure will drop shortly to the value set by the operator as P low. P low is usually set between 0 and 6 cmH_2O. A good starting time for T low (the time that the pressure will stay at P low) is 0.2–1.0 seconds. During this brief T low, released gas is exchanged with fresh oxygenated gas to regenerate the gradient for CO_2 diffusion. By limiting T low to a short period of time, derecruitment is prevented. Release time (T low) must be adjusted to maintain approximately 50% of lung recruitment before the next cycle begins. During APRV, patients can control the frequency and duration of spontaneous breaths. Spontaneous breathing may happen at any point in the respiratory cycle. The fact that patients may breathe and augment minute ventilation in response to changing metabolic demands promotes synchrony and diminishes the need for heavy sedation and use of neuromuscular blockers. Spontaneous breaths improve V/Q matching since they preferentially aerate well-perfused dependent lung areas; unlike mechanically delivered breaths which primarily ventilate lung areas with poor perfusion [49]. Finally, the presence of spontaneous breathing may have positive hemodynamic repercussions by augmenting preload through lowering intrathoracic pressures. Advocates of this mode have reported a mortality rate in patients with ARDS ventilated with APRV of 21.4%, lower than the mortality of 31% reported in the ARDS Network trial using low tidal volume lung protective strategies [48]. APRV physiology is summarized in Figure 9.5.

High-frequency oscillatory ventilation

Positive-pressure ventilation may injure the lung by overdistention (volutrauma), repeated opening and closing of collapsed alveoli (atelectrauma), excessive pressures (barotrauma), and biologic trauma induced by oxygen toxicity and inflammatory cytokines. High frequency oscillatory ventilation (HFOV) is a ventilation modality that uses high respiratory cycle frequencies (between 3and 9 Hz) with very low tidal volumes (1–4 mL/kg, depending on the frequency). Respiratory rates range between 200 and 900 breaths/minute [50]. By using high mean airway pressures, HFOV allows to maintain lung recruitment and prevents atelectrauma [51]. It has been used occasionally in ARDS refractory to conventional mechanical ventilation and in cases of bronchopleural fistulas. Mean airway pressure is usually set at 5 cmH_2O above the mean airway pressure measured during conventional ventilation. The initial frequency is usually set at 4–5 Hz and the bias flow between 20 and 40L/min. The F_iO_2 is also set by the operator. Unlike other forms of high frequency ventilation, expiration is active during HFOV. This is essential in preventing gas trapping [51]. Mean airway pressures may be titrated by 2–3 cmH_2O increments to allow lower F_iO_2 and prevent oxygen toxicity. P_aCO_2 values are adjusted by manipulating the pressure amplitude of oscillation and the oscillation frequency. Increases in pressure amplitude of oscillation and decreases in the

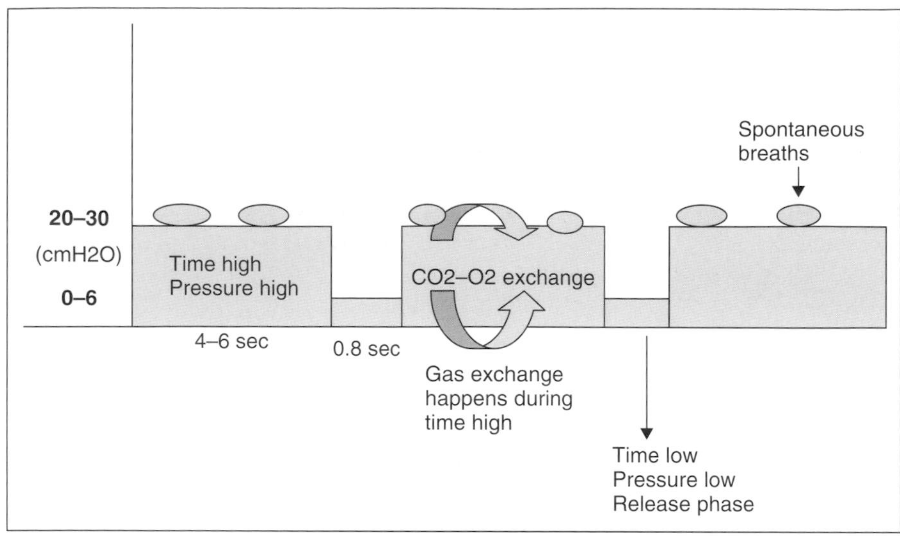

Figure 9.5 Airway pressure release ventilation. Typical starting values for time (high and low) and pressure (high and low) are shown. Ovals represent spontaneous breaths that may happen at any time during the respiratory cycle.

oscillation frequency lead to a decrease in serum P_aCO_2. Since use of higher mean airway pressures could compromise preload, patients in HFOV may require more fluid therapy to guarantee an adequate cardiac output. Other complications associated with this modality include barotrauma (higher prevalence of pneumothoraces) and mucus plugging leading to endotracheal tube obstruction [52].

In a prospective randomized study involving patients with ARDS, prone ventilation produced a greater increase in oxygenation than did HFOV in the supine position. Furthermore, HFOV in the prone position did not improve oxygenation further than the improvement seen with prone ventilation using conventional mechanical ventilation. Patients in the HOFV group had higher indexes of lung inflammation in samples obtained by bronchoalveolar lavage. The authors conclude by stating "HFOV is therefore not ready for prime time, and more needs to be learned before it can be safely used" [53]. Similarly, other recent reviews conclude that HFOV in adults with ARDS is still in its infancy [51]. HFOV should be reserved as a rescue therapy after lung protective strategies have failed. To date, no convincing evidence supports that HFOV improves mortality rates [54].

Positive end-expiratory pressure

"Physiologic PEEP" is the theoretical amount of residual end-expiratory pressure produced during normal exhalation as a byproduct of glottic closure. In an effort to reduce atelectasis, many clinicians will place ventilated patients using mechanical ventilators on 5 cmH_2O of baseline PEEP. Higher levels of PEEP have been used to promote airway recruitment in patients with significant pulmonary disease. Despite the potential disadvantages, the appropriate use of PEEP leads to airway recruitment, and reduction of intrapulmonary shunt, effecting an improvement in oxygenation [55]. Adequate use of PEEP allows the use of lower oxygen concentrations, minimizing the potential of oxygen-induced lung injury [54].

Critically ill patients with oxygenation problems, such as those with ARDS, frequently respond to the addition of positive end-expiratory pressure (PEEP) to a conventional method of ventilation, such as assist control [56] (Figure 9.4). Increased end-expiratory pressure is produced by placing a threshold resistor in the exhalation limb of the breathing circuit. Expiratory flow is unimpeded so long as expiratory pressure exceeds an arbitrary limit. Gas flow ceases when pressure reaches the predetermined value, thereby resulting in maintenance of PEEP without impedance of expiratory gas flow [56].

PEEP enhances oxygenation in patients by alleviating the V/Q inequality [57]. This is accomplished principally by an increase in the functional residual capacity (FRC). PEEP may increase the FRC by causing direct increases in alveolar volume when PEEP up to 10 cmH_2O is applied to normal alveoli. PEEP also recruits and re-expands alveoli that have previously collapsed (e.g. atelectasis) [58]. By opening previously collapsed alveoli, oxygen is delivered to such areas leading to pulmonary vasodilation with a subsequent improvement in the V/Q ratio and systemic oxygenation. With the patient in the supine position, PEEP usually recruits the regions of the lung closest to the sternum and the apex [59]. The use of PEEP decreases the constant opening and closing of recruitable alveoli which causes shear stress with disruption of the surfactant monolayer and release of inflammatory mediators leading to a systemic inflammatory response, a form of ventilator-induced lung injury known as atelectrauma [60]. Response to PEEP is dependent on the underlying disease. Patients with pulmonary causes of ALI/ARDS (e.g. pneumonia, aspiration, lung trauma) usually present with significant alveolar filling and respond less to PEEP. Patients with a non-pulmonary cause of ALI/ARDS (e.g. intraabdominal sepsis, extrathoracic trauma) predominantly present with interstitial edema and alveolar collapse and show a better response in systemic oxygenation when PEEP is applied [61].

Profound alterations in cardiovascular function may accompany PEEP therapy. PEEP will decrease preload with a subsequent decrease in cardiac output and systemic blood pressure. Such hemodynamic response is obviously more pronounced in patients with hypovolemia. High PEEP values could overstretch alveoli and "compress" pulmonary vessels with an increase in pulmonary vascular resistance leading to increased afterload of the right ventricle. Such high values also could potentially increase dead space ventilation (with increased P_aCO_2), worsen pulmonary edema, and increase tissue stress due to overstretching. In conditions with low pulmonary compliance, (e.g. ARDS) PEEP is usually well tolerated in the presence of adequate intravascular volume. The optimum level of PEEP ("best PEEP") is one that improves oxygenation without causing such adverse effects as reduced cardiac output and increased respiratory system compliance [55]. Some authors recommend measuring the lower inflection point of the pressure–volume curve and maintaining PEEP above such value. This is usually cumbersome and not performed in many centers. "Optimal PEEP" may be determined by performing a systemic PEEP trial, where respiratory parameters, such as arterial blood gases and respiratory system compliance, as well as cardiac parameters such as blood pressure and cardiac output, are measured at successive levels of PEEP. The key is to use the minimal amount of PEEP that attains the desirable outcome. The goal is not to maximize P_aO_2, but to maintain a P_aO_2 between 55 and 80 mmHg and oxygen saturation between 88 and 95% [60]. By accepting this relative low oxygen saturation the clinician will be able to use low tidal volumes and maintain low plateau pressures with minimal hemodynamic compromise and iatrogenic ventilator-induced lung injury. In a randomized trial involving 549 patients with ALI/ARDS receiving lung protective mechanical ventilation with a tidal volume of 6 mL/kg predicted body weight and plateau pressures below 30 cmH_2O, clinical outcomes were similar whether low PEEP (5–12 cmH_2O) or high PEEP (10–16 cmH_2O) levels were used [62]. Finding the "optimal" value of PEEP is still controversial. We recommend a clinical bedside approach with progressive increases in PEEP until acceptable oxygenation is achieved (P_aO_2 >55 mmHg and S_pO_2 >88%) while maintaining acceptable hemodynamics by optimizing intravascular volume status. The need for invasive hemodynamic monitoring in such patients should be individualized. The ARDS Network used PEEP–F_iO_2 tables to guide PEEP values according to oxygen requirements. Such values are depicted in Table 9.8.

Alternative maneuvers during mechanical ventilation

Prone ventilation

Considerable published experience documents that oxygenation improves when patients with ALI/ARDS are turned from supine to prone. Prone position-induced improvement in oxygenation may result from: (i) increases in the FRC; (ii) advantageous changes in diaphragm movement; (iii) improvement of ventilation and perfusion to the dorsal lung regions; (iv) improvements in cardiac output and, accordingly, in mixed venous partial pressure of oxygen; (v) better clearance of secretions; and (vi) anterior displacement of the heart with recruitment of alveolar units previously compressed by the mediastinum in the supine position [63,64]. In a randomized multicenter trial involving 304 patients with either ALI or ARDS, patients assigned to the prone position for a period of at least 6 hours every day for 10 days showed significant improvement in the ratio of the partial pressure of arterial oxygen to the fraction of inspired oxygen (P_aO_2/F_iO_2 ratio). However, no improvement in survival was found [65]. A post hoc analysis of subgroups in this study suggested that patients with the more severe forms of ARDS (P_aO_2/F_iO_2 ratio <89) may have had a survival advantage. Turning patients to the prone position may be associated with significant complications such as accidental displacement of the tracheal or thoracotomy tubes, loss of venous access, facial edema, and need for increased sedation. The routine use of this modality is certainly not recommended but may be considered in selected patients with severe hypoxemia refractory to conventional treatment modalities. If used, the period of prone ventilation should be at least of 12 hours per episode [66]. Some have used prone ventilation for up to 20 hours each day [67].

Extracorporeal membrane oxygenation

Extracorporeal membrane oxygenation (ECMO) was first used successfully in the treatment of ARDS in 1972 [68]. It evolved as a refinement of intraoperative cardiopulmonary bypass. Because ECMO involves perfusion as well as gas exchange, the term *extracorporeal life support* is probably a more apt description of the technique. This technique is administered in two broad categories: (i) venoarterial bypass which provides both cardiac output and oxygenation by removal of venous blood, which is then oxygenated and returned as arterial blood; and (ii) venovenous

Table 9.8 F_iO_2/PEEP combinations proposed to maintain oxygenation. (Reproduced with permission from The Acute Respiratory Distress Syndrome Network. Ventilation with lower tidal volumes as compared with traditional tidal volumes for acute lung injury and the acute respiratory distress syndrome. *N Engl J Med* 2000; 342: 1301–1308.)

F_iO_2	0.3	0.4	0.4	0.5	0.5	0.6	0.7	0.7	.7	0.8	0.9	0.9	0.9	1.0	1.0
PEEP	5	5	8	8	10	10	10	12	14	14	14	16	18	18	18–24

bypass, which provides respiratory support only (i.e. exchange of CO_2 but not O_2). To provide access, large-bore catheters are placed into the appropriate venous or arterial access sites. The internal jugular vein is the preferred venous site, while the common carotid artery is the preferred arterial site. In venovenous bypass, oxygenated blood is usually returned to the internal jugular, femoral, or iliac vein. In either method, full anticoagulation is required. The bypass circuit also can be used for ultrafiltration or hemodiafiltration [69].

The largest group to receive ECMO has been neonates with respiratory distress. Survival rates up to 90% have been reported by some investigators [70]. The efficacy of ECMO in treatment of acute respiratory disease in adults is less clear. The National Institutes of Health sponsored a multicenter investigation of ECMO in the treatment of adult ARDS [71]. Compared with conventional mechanical ventilation methods in use at the time, ECMO offered no advantage. Some, however, still feel that advances in both ECMO itself and in the mechanical ventilation techniques used in patients who would require ECMO hold promise. The extracorporeal life support organization reports adult ARDS survival rates of between 50% and 65% [72]. In one report, 62 out of 245 patients with ARDS were treated with ECMO [73]. The survival rate was 55% in ECMO patients and 61% in non-ECMO patients. The author concluded that ECMO was a therapeutic option likely to increase survival; however, a randomized controlled study proving benefit is still needed.

Nitric oxide

The selective pulmonary vasodilatory effects of inhaled nitric oxide (NO) have been demonstrated in various models of ALI including endotoxin and oleic acid exposure, and smoke inhalation [74]. In the pulmonary vasculature, nitric oxide increases cyclic guanosine 3′,5′-monophosphate (cGMP) which inhibits cellular calcium entrance. Because NO is inhaled, it is an effective vasodilator of well-ventilated regions of the lung, thus reducing intrapulmonary shunt and improving arterial oxygenation. Furthermore, NO is rapidly bound to hemoglobin, which thereby inactivates it and prevents systemic vasodilation. Evidence suggests that inhaled NO improves oxygenation and reduces pulmonary artery pressure in the majority of patients with ALI/ARDS. One multicenter study involving 268 adult patients with early acute lung injury evaluated the clinical reponse to NO therapy. The investigators concluded that oxygenation was improved by inhaled NO but that the frequency of reversal of acute lung injury was not increased. Additionally, use of inhaled NO did not alter mortality, although it did reduce the frequency of severe respiratory failure in patients developing hypoxemia [75]. In another study, NO was noted to decrease shunt and pulmonary vascular resistance index and improve oxygenation. Some evidence suggests that NO may also decrease inflammation in the alveolar–capillary membrane [76]. When used in patients with acute respiratory failure, a plateau effect is usually seen at doses between 1–10 parts per million (ppm). With prolonged use, inhaled NO may "leak" by collateral ventilation to adjacent non-ventilated alveoli with subsequent loss of efficacy. Prolonged administration is also associated with increasing sensitivity to NO and increased toxicity. Daily dose–response assessments are mandatory [76].

Since NO forms methemoglobin after interacting with oxyhemoglobin, it should not be administered to patients with methemoglobin reductase deficiency [77]. At doses lower than 40 ppm, the risk of this complication is rare. When mixed with high concentrations of inspired oxygen, NO-derived reactive nitrogen species (e.g. nitrogen dioxide) may cause pulmonary epithelial injury. Pulmonary toxicity is minimal if the dose is kept below 40 ppm. NO should not be used in patients with severe left ventricular failure since the predominantly pulmonary arterial vasodilation (as opposed to pulmonary venodilation) could lead to pulmonary edema [78]. To date, the benefits of inhaled NO in patients with ARDS are short-lived and mainly have shown a transient improvement in oxygenation without improving survival. It is not an effective therapy for ARDS and its routine use in this scenario cannot be recommended. It may be useful as a temporary short-term adjunct to respiratory support in patients with acute hypoxemia or life-threatening pulmonary hypertension [76].

Lung protective strategy mechanical ventilation

Since the year 2000, after The Acute Respiratory Distress Syndrome Network publication, a different view on mechanical ventilation has been adopted. More has been learned about the potential deleterious consequences of inappropriately high tidal volumes on lung function. High tidal volumes with low levels of PEEP may lead to volutrauma, barotrauma, atelectrauma, and biotrauma. This is known as ventilator-induced lung injury (VILI) and is discussed in detail in the next section of this chapter. In patients with ALI/ARDS the goal during mechanical ventilation should not be to achieve completely normal values of P_aO_2, P_aCO_2, and S_pO_2. On the contrary, one should focus on limiting VILI by using small tidal volumes, limiting F_iO_2, using adequate PEEP levels, and accepting P_aO_2 values of 55–80 mmHg and S_pO_2 values between 88 and 95%. Low tidal volumes will also result in high P_aCO_2 levels (permissive hypercapnia) and low arterial pH secondary to respiratory acidosis. This strategy is associated with reduced injurious lung stretch and consequently less release of inflammatory mediators [79]. In a randomized clinical trial involving 861 patients with ALI/ARDS, patients assigned to mechanical ventilation with tidal volumes of 6 mL/kg lean body weight in order to limit plateau pressures to less than 30 cmH$_2$O had a mortality of 31% compared to a mortality of 39.8% in the group receiving conventional mechanical ventilation with tidal volumes of 12 mL/kg lean body weight [80]. In the trial previously cited, arterial pH had to be kept above 7.15 at all times. In order to achieve this goal, the respiratory rate could be increased to a maximum of 35 breaths/minute, and if not effective, sodium bicarbonate infusions were permitted. Lung protective mechanical ventilation is the only therapy that has been shown to reduce mortality and the development of organ failure in patients with ALI/ARDS [67]. Patients with elevated intracranial pressures, severe pulmonary hypertension, severe hyperkalemia, and sickle cell disease are not candidates for permissive hypercapnia.

We recommend the use of lung protective mechanical ventilation in the critically ill pregnant patient with ALI/ARDS as an extrapolation from the general ARDS population. Concerns about maternal hypercapnia on the developing fetus are discussed in the section of permissive hypercapnia in this chapter. Due to decreased compliance of the chest wall during pregnancy, some have recommended that plateau pressures up to 35 cmH_2O could be accepted.

Special considerations during mechanical ventilation

Patients who undergo invasive mechanical ventilation experience complications caused by lung injury from oxygen toxicity; adverse effects from excessive ventilatory pressures, volumes, and flow rates; adverse effects from tracheal intubation; dangers from adjuvant drugs; stress related sequelae; altered enzyme and hormone systems; nutritional problems; and psychologic trauma [81].

Oxygen toxicity

A variety of gross and histopathologic lesions have been described in human and experimental animal lung tissues that have been exposed to increased concentrations of oxygen in the airways [81]. Free oxygen radicals generated by high concentrations of oxygen, in and along the airways and alveoli, attack intracellular enzyme systems, damage DNA, destroy lipid membranes, and increase microvascular permeability. The duration of exposure of the lungs to increased oxygen concentrations is directly related to the incidence and severity of any resultant lung injury. No definitive data are available to establish the upper limits of the concentration of oxygen in inspired air that can be considered safe [81]). However, the general consensus seems to be that oxygen concentrations greater than 60% in inspired air are undesirable and should be avoided if clinical circumstances permit. Therefore, one should institute measures to insure that the lowest possible concentration of oxygen is used during ventilatory support.

When oxygenation is inadequate, sedation, paralysis, and position change are possible therapeutic measures [82]. We recommend the use of adequate levels of PEEP in order to recruit alveoli and improve oxygenation. In many cases, the use of PEEP will allow the clinician to lower the oxygen requirements. When ventilating patients, one must remember that the goal should not necessarily be, in the majority of cases, to maximize P_aO_2, but to achieve an acceptable level of oxygenation (e.g. P_aO_2 of 55–80 mmHg and S_pO_2 of 88–95%) [60]. By accepting these "low values", application of lung protective mechanical ventilation with low tidal volumes and adequate levels of PEEP with the lowest possible F_iO_2 will be possible and thus VILI will be minimized.

Ventilator-induced lung injury (VILI)

It has become increasingly evident that gas delivery into the lungs by a mechanical ventilator at excessive and inappropriate pressures, volumes, and flow rates can be a two-edged sword and can result in significant lung damage. In some cases, this produces additional injury and functional impairment instead of assisting the failing, sick lung [83]. Ventilator-induced lung injury (VILI) includes volutrauma, barotrauma, atelectrauma, and biotrauma. Volutrauma refers to the use of large tidal volumes leading to overinflation and overstretching of alveoli [60]. Lung injury in ALI/ARDS is heterogeneous, this means that while some areas of the lung parenchyma are infiltrated with fluid and protein, others are not. A ventilator-induced breath will follow the path of least impediment, traveling to the better ventilated areas. This predisposes the "normal" areas of the lung to be exposed to high tidal volumes with resultant volutrauma [84]. Barotrauma is a form of VILI associated with pneumothorax, pneumomediastinum, pneumoperitoneum, and subcutaneous emphysema secondary to alveolar rupture [85]. Interestingly, several studies have shown that the incidence of barotrauma is independent of airway pressures [80,86]. Peak inspiratory pressure is influenced by resistance of the endotracheal tube and the airways. An increase in the peak inspiratory pressure without a concomitant increase in plateau pressure is unlikely to cause VILI [84]. The pressure that really matters is the transpulmonary pressure (pressure gradient between the alveoli and the pleural space). As a surrogate of the latter, the plateau pressure may be measured at the bedside easily. Plateau pressure reflects the peak alveolar pressure and it has been shown to be a better marker of the risk of VILI than peak airway pressures. Modern ventilation strategies target a plateau pressure under 30 cmH_2O [54]. Atelectrauma is caused by constant opening and closing of recruitable alveoli. Such injury results in shear stress with disruption of the surfactant monolayer [60]. Use of PEEP may prevent the constant recruitment–derecruitment of alveolar units. All three mechanisms described previously may induce biologic trauma (biotrauma). Either overstretching or repetitive opening and closing of alveolar units are associated with local inflammation with increased concentrations of interleukins, tumor necrosis factor-alpha, platelet-activating factors, and thromboxanes. Local inflammation in the lung leads to disruption of the capillary–alveolar membrane with worsening pulmonary edema. Translocation of these cytokines into the systemic circulation with secondary systemic inflammation and end-organ failure has been described [87]. VILI may be attenuated by using small tidal values and adequate PEEP levels to maintain alveoli open and keep a plateau pressure below 30 cmH_2O [80].

Permissive hypercapnia

Lung protective mechanical ventilation with the use of 6 mL/kg lean body weight tidal volumes and end-inspiratory plateau pressures of <30 cmH_2O has been shown to decrease mortality in patients with ALI/ARDS by avoiding ventilator-associated lung injury [80]. The trade-off of such approach is frequently an elevation in P_aCO_2 with subsequent development of respiratory acidosis. Hypercapnia (allowing P_aCO_2 to rise above normal levels) can be tolerated in patients with ALI/ARDS if required to minimize plateau pressures and tidal volumes [54]. Contraindications to such approach include intracranial hypertension, pulmonary hypertension, severe hyperkalemia, and sickle cell disease. No upper limit for P_aCO_2 has been established, some authorities recommend maintaining a pH above 7.20 [54]. In the Acute Respiratory Distress Syndrome Network trial comparing lower tidal volumes with traditional tidal volumes, the use of sodium bicarbonate infusions and respiratory rates up to 35/min were allowed in order to maintain a pH above 7.15. The theoretical concern that such iatrogenic acidemia could lead to increased requirements of fluid and vasopressor therapies secondary to acidosis-induced vasodilation and decreased cardiac performance was not confirmed in a recent trial [88].

Evidence is growing that hypercapnic acidosis may have anti-inflammatory and antioxidative effects at cellular and organ levels [89]. In a secondary analysis of a previous randomized clinical trial, hypercapnic acidosis was associated with a decreased 28-day mortality rate in the subgroup of patients exposed to mechanical ventilation with high tidal volumes. Patients already randomized to ventilation with a lung protective strategy (low tidal volumes) did not show a protective effect from hypercapnia [90].

Little is known about the effect of maternal hypercapnia on the fetus. Some data on neonates suggest that P_aCO_2 levels of 45–55 mmHg are tolerated [91]. Clearance of fetal CO_2 through the placenta requires a gradient of approximately 10 mmHg. Thus, it seems that limiting maternal P_aCO_2 values to less than 60 mmHg may be reasonable.

Critical illness polyneuropathy and myopathy

Critical illness polyneuropathy and myopathy is a neuromuscular disorder characterized by difficulty in weaning from the ventilator, severe weakness of limb muscles, and reduced or absent deep tendon reflexes [92]. Risk factors include sepsis, use of corticosteroids, hyperglycemia, female gender, and prolonged mechanical ventilation. Inconsistently, use of neuromuscular blockers has been associated with it. Axonal injury most likely results from alterations at the microcirculation level coupled with direct damage from cytokines. Muscle biopsy usually reveals severe atrophy with absent inflammatory changes [92]. Most patients improve after several weeks to months if they survive their critical illness. No specific treatment exists for this condition.

Gastrointestinal hemorrhage

Critically ill patients who present with non-gastrointestinal disease, such as acute respiratory failure, may develop gastrointestinal hemorrhage later in their intensive care course as a complication of critical illness [93]. Stress ulcerations predominately involve the stomach and are usually found in the fundus with sparing of the antrum [94]. Gastrointestinal bleeding due to stress ulcers was an important complication in critically ill patients 2 decades ago. With improvements in intensive care, the need for routine prophylaxis for GI bleeds has been questioned [95]. The incidence of GI hemorrhage in mechanically ventilated patients with no pharmacologic prophylaxis is 3.7% [96]. Some authors have advocated GI bleed prophylaxis only for those patients at the highest risk such as those with prolonged mechanical ventilation, coagulopathy, and hypotension [96].

Mucosal ischemia secondary to decreased gastric blood flow is one of the most important factors in stress ulceration. Increased concentrations of acid pepsin are not found in critically ill patients. The primary mechanism of ulceration is tissue acidosis or ischemia resulting in impaired mucosal handling of hydrogen ions that are already present [97]. Initial therapy of stress ulceration should be directed at correcting hypotension, shock, and acidosis.

Prophylactic measures have centered primarily on neutralizing gastric acidity with antacids or decreasing gastric acid secretion with histamine receptor blockers such as cimetidine, famotidine or ranitidine. Other agents used include proton pump inhibitors (PPIs) like omeprazole and pantoprazole. Sucralfate is a basic aluminum salt of sucrose octasulfate that appears to provide stress ulcer protection without reducing levels of gastric acid. Theoretically, by not alkalinizing the stomach, less colonization of gastric secretions by bacteria and consequently less incidence of ventilator-associated pneumonia due to aspiration of such contents would be expected with the use of this agent. Antacids require excessive nursing time and additionally may of themselves result in complications including diarrhea, hypophosphatemia, hypomagnesemia, and metabolic alkalosis [98].

In a randomized, blinded, multicenter, placebo-controlled trial, 1200 patients requiring mechanical ventilation for more than 48 hours were randomized to GI bleed prophylaxis with either sucralfate or ranitidine. Patients assigned to ranitidine had a significantly lower incidence of gastrointestinal hemorrhage. Interestingly, there was no difference in the incidence of ventilator-associated pneumonia between both groups [99].

If overt GI bleeding occurs, endoscopy with attempts to achieve hemostasis is indicated. After hemostasis, studies have shown that a gastric pH >6 is needed to maintain clotting in the stomach [100]). These patients will benefit from a continuous intravenous infusion of a PPI (pantoprazole) for 72 hours [101].

Thromboembolic complications

The actual frequency of pulmonary emboli complicating the course of patients with acute respiratory failure is unknown. Autopsy studies in respiratory ICU patients report an incidence of 8–27% [98]. The source of pulmonary emboli in critically ill patients is primarily due to deep vein thrombosis. Critically ill patients present many risk factors for deep vein thrombosis including prolonged venous stasis caused by bed rest, right and left ventricular failure, dehydration, obesity, and advanced age. In one study, deep vein thrombosis occurred in 13% of respiratory ICU patients during the first week of intensive care [102].

However, the precise risk of deep vein thrombosis in patients with acute respiratory failure is not known. Another source of pulmonary emboli in critically ill patients can be thrombosis associated with intravenous catheters [98]. One study found that 66% of 33 consecutive patients monitored for a mean of 3 days with a pulmonary artery catheter had internal jugular thrombosis as detected venographically or on autopsy [103]. Autopsy data suggest that pulmonary emboli are present in patients with catheter-associated thrombosis [104]. However, the relationship of pulmonary emboli to catheter-associated thrombosis is not clear.

Venous thromboembolism is both more common and more complex to diagnose in patients who are pregnant than in those who are not pregnant. The incidence of venous thromboembolism is estimated at 0.76 to 1.72 per 1000 pregnancies, which is four times as great as the risk in the nonpregnant population.A meta-analysis showed that two thirds of cases of deep-vein thrombosis occurred in the antepartum period and were distributed relatively equally among all three trimesters [105]. Needless to say, deep venous thrombosis prophylaxis is of paramount importance in the critically ill pregnant patient. Critically ill patients at very high risk for bleeding should receive mechanical prophylaxis (e.g. graduated compression stockings and/or intermittent pneumatic compression devices) until the bleeding risk decreases [106]. When the bleeding risk is moderate (e.g. postoperative patients or medically ill), either low-dose unfractionated heparin (UFH) or low-molecular-weight heparin (LMWH) may be used. In conditions associated with the highest risk of thromboembolic complications such as following major trauma and acute spinal cord injury, prophylaxis with LMWH is considered first-line therapy [106]. During pregnancy, if UFH is to be used, we recommend doses of 5000 U subcutaneously every 8 hours or 10 000 units every 12 hours for prophylaxis. Doses of 5000 U subcutaneously every 12 hours have been shown inadequate for prophylaxis during pregnancy. The use of early prophylaxis should be evaluated as soon as the patient is admitted to the intensive care unit. If no contraindications exist, we favor the use of low molecular weight heparin.

Renal complications

Mechanical ventilation can not only aggravate lung injury but also contribute to distant organ failure [82]. Ventilation with high tidal volumes and low values of PEEP has been noted to induce local and systemic cytokine responses that could lead to end-organ damage. Rat models have demonstrated increased lung, hepatic and renal concentrations of interleukin (IL) 6 in animals exposed to ventilation with high tidal volumes [107]. The use of a lung protective ventilatory strategy (small tidal volumes with adequate levels of PEEP) may attenuate ventilator-induced organ injury.

Acute renal failure secondary to acute tubular necrosis caused by mechanical ventilation may result from three different mechanisms [87]. The first one involves consequences directly related to arterial blood gas physiology. Hipoxemia leads to renal vasoconstriction and hypoperfusion. The same vasoconstrictive renal effect is seen with hypercapnia [108]. The second mechanism involves changes in cardiac output. Positive-pressure ventilation decreases cardiac output by diminishing preload and increasing right ventricular afterload. Studies have demonstrated an immediate decline in urine output after the institution of mechanical ventilation. This effect is more pronounced with the use of high PEEP values. Hormonal pathways at the kidney level are also altered during mechanical ventilation. Increased plasma renin activity leading to reduced renal blood flow has been described [109].Lastly, renal dysfunction during mechanical ventilation may be secondary to biotrauma associated with injurious ventilatory strategies (e.g. high tidal volumes). Cytokines may translocate from the lung to the bloodstream leading to tissue damage at the kidney level.

We favor the use of lung protective ventilation in order to diminish the risk of mechanical ventilation induced renal failure.

Ventilator-associated pneumonia

Ventilator-associated pneumonia (VAP) is the most common nosocomial infection in the intensive care unit. It is defined as pneumonia occurring more than 48 hours after initiation of mechanical ventilation [110]. The reported incidence varies in the literature between 10% to 40% with a mortality rate of 15–50% [111].

At least 50% of cases happen during the first 4 days of ventilation. The risk of developing VAP is 3%/day during the first 5 days after intubation, 2%/day from days 5–10 and 1%/day thereafter [112,113]. Clinically, VAP is suspected in the presence of new or progressive infiltrates in chest radiography together with other signs of infection such as new-onset fever, leukocytosis or leucopenia, purulent sputum or tracheal secretions or an otherwise unexplained decline in oxygenation. However, when compared with histologic analysis and cultures of lung biopsies obtained after death, the use of such criteria had only a 69% sensitivity and a specificity of 75% for the diagnosis of VAP [114]. If one relies on these criteria for diagnosis of VAP, overtreatment and unnecessary exposure to broad-spectrum antibiotics will result. Much controversy exists about the best way to confirm the diagnosis. One option includes non-bronchoscopic methods such as quantitative endotracheal tube aspirates or blind mini bronchoalveolar lavage. This techniques are easy to perform, non-expensive, and done by either nursing personnel or respiratory therapists. Another option includes the collection of samples by using a more invasive approach through bronchoscopy. Under direct visualization, samples are taken either by performing a bronchoalveolar lavage (BAL) or by collecting a sample with a protected specimen brush (PSB). Depending on the strategy used, different thresholds of bacterial growth are considered to be positive. If quantitative endotracheal aspirates (not qualitative) are done, a threshold of 10×6 colony-forming units (cfu)/mL achieves sensitivities and specificities comparable to bronchoscopic guided BAL using thresholds of 10×4 or 10×5 cfu/mL [115]. The American Thoracic Society Guidelines for the management of ventilator-associated pneumonia state that "quantitative cultures can be performed on endotracheal aspirates or samples collected either bronchoscopically or non-bronchoscopically. The choice of method depends on local expertise, experience, availability, and cost." [116].

Once cultures are taken, early broad-spectrum use of antibiotics is of paramount importance [117]. Initial coverage should include both Gram-negative bacteria and methicillin-resistant *Staphylococcus aureus*. Patients who either have received antimicrobial therapy or have been hospitalized in the last 90 days will need double coverage for *Pseudomonas aeruginosa*. The same coverage applies for patients with a current hospitalization of more than 5 days as well as patients from nursing homes, in extended care facilities or on chronic dialysis [116]. Once cultures are available, narrowing the spectrum of antibiotics is indicated according to sensitivities obtained. Traditionally, the duration of antimicrobial treatment has been 14 days. However, in the absence of immunosupression or infection by non-lactose-fermenting Gram-negative rods (e.g. *P. aeruginosa* or *Acinetobacter* spp.) therapy may be safely discontinued after 8 days of treatment in patients with uncomplicated VAP who initially received appropriate therapy and with good clinical response [111].

We cannot underscore the importance of incorporating prophylactic measures to prevent VAP. Ideally, ventilated patients should be in the semirecumbent position (30–45°) at all times, particularly while on enteral nutrition. Heavy sedation and paralysis should be limited if possible. We favor daily interruption or lightening of sedation in order to avoid unnecessary oversedation. The routine use of of oral chlorhexidine is not currently recommended by the American Thoracic Society Guidelines for prevention of VAP. The use of systemic antibiotics for the sole purpose of VAP prophylaxis is not recommended. The use of non-invasive positive-pressure ventilation in adequate candidates also reduces the incidence of VAP [118]. Continuous subglottic suctioning of endotracheal tubes has not shown clinical benefits. Finally, the endotracheal tube cuff pressure should be measured routinely; it should be kept ideally between 20 and 25 cmH_2O. Pressures below 20 cmH_2O may create a poor seal in the trachea with a higher probability of aspiration [119].

Nutritional implications

Nutritional complications in acute respiratory failure patients reflect the adverse effects of malnutrition upon the thoracic–pulmonary system, as well as complications associated with administration of nutritional support [98]. Nutritionally associated complications can occur with both enteral and total parenteral nutrition [120,121]. Malnourished patients who require mechanical ventilation have a significantly higher mortality rate than well-nourished patients requiring mechanical ventilation. Poor nutritional status can adversely affect thoracic–pulmonary function by impairment of respiratory muscle function, surfactant production, alveolar ventilation, and pulmonary defense mechanisms [122].

The diaphragm is the critical respiratory muscle, and malnutrition reduces diaphragmatic muscle mass [98]. Underweight patients with reduction of diaphragmatic mass may have contractile force reductions out of proportion to the reduction in muscle mass [98]. Hypophosphatemia and hypokalemia may also be responsible for respiratory muscle weakness. Nutritional repletion can improve altered respiratory muscle strength in some patients. Increase in maximal inspiratory pressure and body cell mass were noted in critically ill patients given parenteral nutrition for 2–4 weeks [123]. Malnutrition reduces ventilatory drive and influences the immune system. The systemic effects of malnutrition are most profound in cell-mediated immunity, as malnourished patients have suppressed delayed cutaneous hypersensitivity and impaired T-lymphocyte transformation in response to mitogens [124]. Nutritional support can be instituted either by the enteral route or with total parenteral nutrition. Nutritionally associated hypercapnia can occur in patients receiving enteral feeding or total parenteral nutrition. This develops when excess calories are given. Carbon dioxide production is increased because calories in excess of energy needs result in lipogenesis and a markedly increased respiratory quotient [98]. The respiratory quotient is defined as the ratio of carbon dioxide production to oxygen consumption during substrate utilization. Hypercapnia from increased CO_2 production is avoided in normal persons by a compensatory increase in ventilation. Patients with compromised ventilatory status may not be able to increase ventilation appropriately. The minimal amount of calories needed to achieve a substantial clinical benefit is unknown [125]. However, high energy feeding does not prevent protein catabolism, increases CO_2 production, induces hyperglycemia, and leads to development of fatty liver. Fat accumulation is associated with immune dysfunction and increased output of cytokines with a subsequent increase in mortality [126]. If adequate protein is provided with a relative calorie deficit, lean body mass maintenance could be achieved simultaneously with body fat loss. Studies have shown that in sedated ventilated patients, the resting energy expenditure may be as low as 1500 kcal/day [127]. Critically ill obese patients receiving 22 total kcal/kg ideal body weight /day (as opposed to 30 total kcal/kg ideal body weight/day) had a shorter ICU stay, decreased duration of antibiotic days, and a decrease in the number of ventilator days [125]. We recommend the use of hypocaloric (20–25 kcal/kg/day) high protein (1.5 g/kg/day) nutrition in the critically ill ventilated pregnant patient. Addition of an extra 300 kcal/day should be considered for singleton pregnancies (500 kcal/day if twins).

In the patient with severe respiratory compromise and receiving enteral nutrition, the use of formulas with high lipid content and low carbohydrates (e.g. Respalor®) should be considered in order to decrease CO_2 production. In a recent study involving patients with ALI/ARDS, patients receiving a high lipid–low carbohydrate formula had a significantly shorter length of ventilatory time compared to patients assigned to a control enteral formula [128]. If the patient is receiving total parenteral nutrition, it is reasonable to limit the amount of lipids. Lipids adversely affect gas exchange by coating the erythrocyte's membrane, decreasing gas diffusion secondary to lipid deposition in the alveolar–capillary space, and increasing blood viscosity with subsequent alterations in pulmonary microcirculation.

When feasible, early enteral feeding (within 48 hours of mechanical ventilation onset) should be started in the critically ill patient. Such intervention has been associated with a significant decrease in ICU and hospital mortality [129]. In patients with sepsis and ALI/ARDS undergoing mechanical ventilation, the use of anti-inflammatory acids such as γ-linolenic acid and fish oil plus antioxidant vitamins in enteral feeds increased the P_aO_2/F_iO_2 ratio, reduced mechanical ventilation time, and was associated with a 19.4% absolute risk reduction in mortality rate [130]. Recent literature has focused on the potential benefits of adding the amino acid glutamine to feeding regimens in patients with lung injury [131]. Numerous potential benefits have been associated with glutamine including induction of heat shock protein synthesis, improvement of ATP/ADP ratio, attenuation in cytokine release, increased IgA synthesis in both lung and intestinal tissues, improved nitrogen transport, decreases in gut bacterial translocation, and supporting synthesis of rapidly dividing cells such as enterocytes and lymphocytes. A recent meta-analysis indicated that the benefits of glutamine supplementation are greater when administered by the parenteral route and in doses of at least 0.5 g/kg/day [132].

Cardiovascular complications

Positive-pressure ventilation often impairs cardiac output by disturbing the loading conditions of the heart. Blood returns to the thorax along pressure gradients from peripheral vessels to the right atrium. To the extent that intrathoracic pressures affect right atrial pressure, it may alter the gradient for venous return. The negative effect of mechanical ventilation on preload is obviously more pronounced in patients with absolute or relative hypovolemia. Right ventricular output can also be affected by changes in right ventricular afterload. The latter is affected in a complex way by changes in lung volume. An increase in lung volume tends to increase the resistance of alveolar vessels while decreasing the resistance of extra-alveolar vessels. In patients with an increase in pulmonary vascular resistance (PVR) secondary to alveolar collapse and hypoxia (e.g. ARDS), initiation of mechanical ventilation with PEEP may actually diminish PVR due to the vasodilating effect of oxygen. However, overdistention of alveolar units by using excessive PEEP may collapse alveolar vessels with a significant increase in right ventricular afterload leading to a decrease in cardiac output. Positive-pressure ventilation also affects the performance of the left ventricle; it actually reduces left heart afterload. Where poor left ventricular function is limiting cardiac output, an increase in thoracic pressure may result in better left ventricular emptying. Provided adequate fluid resuscitation, such decrease in left ventricular afterload could improve coronary perfusion and favor cardiac output. When beginning mechanical ventilation in hypovolemic patients, the clinician should be ready to correct the volume status in order to maintain an adequate cardiac output.

As previously discussed, modern ventilatory management includes a strategy of small tidal volumes with adequate levels of PEEP. Some have argued that such strategy, which often leads to hypercapnia, could lead to respiratory acidosis with a deleterious effect on systemic hemodynamics and a concomitant increase in fluid and vasopressor requirements. In a recent publication, medical records of 111 patients enrolled in the National Heart, Lung, and Blood Institute ARDS Network randomized trial were reviewed [88]. Patients assigned to protective ventilatory strategies (mainly small tidal volumes and higher levels of PEEP) did not require more vasopressors or fluid compared to the control group. In fact, patients with the lower tidal volumes had significantly lower peak and plateau pressures, potentially improving venous return and cardiac output.

Fluid balance

Little controversy exists regarding the need for early aggressive fluid resuscitation in patients with either relative or absolute hypovolemia who are hemodynamically unstable. However, after the first hours or days of initial management, the fluid management strategy of mechanically ventilated patients with ALI or ARDS is more complex. In a recent randomized study, 1000 patients with ALI/ARDS were allocated to either a conservative or a liberal fluid management strategy [133]. All patients were intubated and had a P_aO_2/F_iO_2 ratio of less than 300. In the liberal strategy, a central venous pressure (CVP) of 10–14 mmHg and a pulmonary artery occlusion pressure (PAOP) of 14–18 mmHg were targeted. In the conservative strategy, the goal was a CVP of less than 4 mmHg and a PAOP of less than 8 mmHg. Patients in the latter group received more doses of furosemide and less fluid boluses.

Patients in the conservative group had improved lung function and shorter periods of mechanical ventilation without increasing non-pulmonary organ failures. All patients received their first protocol intervention on average 43 hours after admission to the ICU. The data suggests that after the initial acute resuscitation phase, once hemodynamically stable, patients with ALI/ARDS may benefit from a conservative fluid strategy. Other investigators have reported similar results [134]. Needless to say, when attempting fluid restriction the clinician should maintain stable hemodynamics and adequate tissue perfusion. In the previously cited study reported by Wiedemann et al. [52], the hemodynamic consequences of the fluid restriction strategy were of minimal clinical significance with no consequences on requirements of pressors, mixed venous oxygen saturation, or acute renal failure incidence.

Hypoproteinemic patients with sepsis have a higher risk of developing ALI/ARDS and are more likely to die from respiratory complications [135]. Some authors have studied the effects of fluid restriction on these patients. In a randomized double-blind placebo-controlled study, patients with hypoproteinemia on mechanical ventilation with ALI/ARDS who were hemodynamically stable had improved oxygenation and fluid balance when treated with albumin infusions and furosemide intravenous infusions [136]. Recently in another randomized, double-blind, placebo-controlled multicenter trial, patients with ALI/ARDS on mechanical ventilation with total protein concentrations <6 g/dL and who were hemodynamically stable were assigned to two different strategies [137]. One group received an intravenous infusion of furosemide without colloid replacement. The study group received 25% albumin boluses and a furosemide drip titrated to a negative fluid balance and a weight loss of at least 1 kg per day. Patients in the study group had improved oxygenation; however, there was no difference in duration of mechanical ventilation. The group assigned to albumin and furosemide achieved a greater net negative fluid balance and better maintenance of hemodynamic stability. We cannot recommend the use of this strategy during pregnancy or the early postpartum, but the concept of fluid restriction in the patient with ALI/ARDS after the initial resuscitation phase should be considered.

Pain control, sedation, and paralysis

Because of the discomfort inherent in receiving mechanical ventilation and intensive care, appropriate use of anxiolytics, analgesics, and sedatives is important to the welfare of the critically ill patient [138]. Simply having an endotracheal tube in the trachea causes discomfort and pain in some patients. Conversely, inappropriate use of sedatives, anxiolytics, and/or analgesics may delay extubation, produce hemodynamic instability, increase the incidence of ventilator-associated pneumonia or contribute to mental status abnormalities. Specific fetal side effects of these drugs have been referenced comprehensively [139,140].

Pain and agitation lead to increased endogenous catecholamine activity, myocardial ischemia, dysrhythmias, hypercoagulability, and depressed immunity [141].

Narcotics are useful for pain relief, sedation, and anxiolysis [142]. Morphine sulfate is used frequently as a primary agent for pain relief. Intravenous administration is preferred over other parenteral routes, either intermittently or by continuous administration. Side effects relating to histamine release and venodilation are uncommon in the normovolemic individual. In the patient with hemodynamic instability we favor the use of agents with less histamine release such as fentanyl or hydromorphone. Likewise, in presence of renal failure, the metabolite morphine-6-glucuronide may accumulate with use of continous infusions of morphine. In this setting, agents without active metabolites like fentanyl or hydromorphone have been favored [143]. Side effects of opioids include hypotension (mostly in hypovolemic patients), intestinal hypomotility, nausea, vomiting, pruritus, respiratory depression, urinary retention, delirium, and hallucinations.

Benzodiazepines like midazolam, lorazepam, and diazepam are useful anxiolytic/amnestic/hypnotics in long-term mechanical ventilation. Like opiates, benzodiazepines have minimal hemodynamic effects in euvolemic patients. All parenteral benzodiazepines are lipid soluble with large volumes of distribution and wide deposition throughout body tissues. This is particularly important in the critically ill patient with hypoalbulinemia, renal and/or hepatic dysfunction, or drug–drug interactions, where accumulation of these drugs in peripheral tissues is the rule [141]. While not singularly effective at providing pain relief, the hypnotic effects of the agents are additive with the effects of narcotics. Evidence suggests that they may enhance the analgesic effects of opiates [144]. Midazolam is useful for acute events because of its relatively short half-life and rapid onset of action (2–5 min). We do not recommend prolonged infusions of midazolam in the patient with renal impairment due to the accumulation of the active metabolite 1-hydroxylmethylmidazolam [141]. Lorazepam, due to its absence of active metabolites, may be a better option in this setting. Lorazepam (unlike midazolam which is metabolized by the liver cytochrome P450) carries the advantage of glucoronidase metabolism, which is well preserved and remains effective even in patients who have moderate degrees of liver disease. Diazepam has a rapid onset and a long half-life. For sporadic use, diazepam is an effective and inexpensive choice. For continued use, intermittent boluses or continuous infusions, midazolam or lorazepam are preferred [142]. In patients requiring mechanical ventilation for 3 days or more easier management of sedation was achieved at significant cost savings with the use of lorazepam as opposed to midazolam [143]. Infusions of lorazepam should be limited to a maximum of 10 mg/hour due to the potential accumulation of propylenglycol with subsequent development of metabolic acidosis.

Because of haloperidol's relatively large margin of safety and minimal hemodynamic and sedating side effects, it is the antipsychotic of choice in chronically long-term mechanically ventilated patients. Haloperidol has no significant effect on the ventilatory drive [145]. Agents such as haloperidol are useful for treatment of delirium and psychosis that is often a consequence of prolonged intensive care [146]. Rarely QT prolongation and even torsade de pointes have been described with its use.

Propofol is an effective sedative/anxiolytic that appears to act on the γ-aminobutyric acid (GABA) receptor. It has no analgesic properties. It is hydrophobic with high lipid solubility allowing rapid onset of action and rapid redistribution from peripheral tissues (within minutes) leading to a short duration of action [147]. Propofol clearance is not significantly affected by liver or renal failure. It should not be used in hemodynamically unstable patients since propofol induces myocardial depression and increases venocapacitance with a subsequent decrease in preload [148]. When used as a sedative during mechanical ventilation, propofol is used only as a continuous infusion and strict antiseptic techniques are of paramount importance since it is a lipid-rich solution with great potential for bacterial superinfection. Vials and tubings must be changed every 12 hours. Serum triglyceride measurements should be done periodically while receiving the infusion. It is an ideal agent for patients requiring frequent neurologic evaluations. In a randomized open-label trial patients requiring mechanical ventilation for >48 hours were randomized to intermittent bolus administration of lorazepam or a continous infusion of propofol with daily interruption of the infusion [149]. Patients in the propofol group had a significant reduction in ventilator days compared to the lorazepam group. We discourage the use of high doses of propofol for prolonged periods of time due to the risk of developing the "propofol infusion syndrome" [150]. This syndrome is characterized by myocardial depression, metabolic acidosis, dysrhythmias, hyperkalemia, rhabdomyolysis, pancreatitis, and liver steatosis.

Dexmedetomidine is a selective alpha-2 agonist that provides both sedation and analgesia. Rapid administration leads to hypertension and reflex bradycardia; prolonged administration leads to hypotension and bradycardia [143]. Interestingly, patients sedated with this medication are easily awaken with minimal stimulation, allowing frequent neurologic evaluations. No data exist yet regarding the prolonged use of dexmedetomidine infusions in mechanically ventilated patients. It is approved for use in the intensive care unit for periods shorter than 23 hours.

When continuous infusions of sedatives are used, daily interruption of the infusion with awakening and retitration (if necessary) is recommended in order to avoid oversedation. In a randomized controlled trial involving 128 adult patients receiving mechanical ventilation and continuous infusions of sedative drugs, those assigned to daily interruption of the infusions until patients were awake had decreased duration of mechanical ventilation and shorter length of stay in the intensive care unit [151]. Sedation should be assessed on a daily basis targeting predefined endpoints of sedation scales such as the Ramsay or the RASS (Richmond agitation and sedation scale) scales.

Skeletal muscle paralysis is necessary under two broad circumstances. The first circumstance is when temporary paralysis is required for intubation. The second situation is when paralysis is a necessary addition to sedation for advanced mechanical ventilation methods such as inversed I:E ratio ventilation [152]. Paralysis improves chest wall compliance, prevents respiratory dyssynchrony, reduces airway peak pressures, and reduces oxygen consumption by decreasing the work of breathing [153]. There is no evidence demonstrating benefits of one particular neuromuscular blocker over another [143]. Intermittent or continuous doses of non-depolarizing muscle relaxants are generally employed. A non-depolarizing block is produced when the post-junctional membrane receptors are reversibly bound with the drug. The duration of the block depends on the rate at which the relaxant is redistributed. The relaxant effects of non-depolarizing drugs are reversed by anticholinergic-blocking drugs such as neostigmine [154].

Of the several non-depolarizing agents available, pancuronium, vecuronium, cisatracurium and atracurium are most used. Pancuronium is effective for 60–90 minutes after an intubating dose is given. Anticholinergic effects of the drug may result in tachycardia and, rarely, hypotension [154,155]. Pancuronium should be avoided in patients with renal or liver impairment. Vecuronium produces a clinical effect for 30–60 minutes after an intubating dose. Hemodynamic effects are usually absent after typically used doses. Both vecuronium and pancuronium may have prolonged action in the presence of hepatic failure [156]. Atracurium has a relatively short duration of action and is degraded non-enzymatically (Hofmann reaction). It is, therefore, useful in patients with hepatic or renal failure. Cisatracurium is also degraded by the Hofmann reaction and it is a non-steroidal molecule. Any of the agents can be given by intermittent bolus or continuous infusion. Monitoring of the level for paralysis with peripheral nerve stimulator equipment ("twitch monitoring") is recommended during prolonged administration of paralytics. The American College of Critical Care Medicine recommends that one or two responses to a train-of-four stimulation be maintained. Because muscle relaxants paralyze without affording the patient any analgesia or sedation, appropriate monitoring for the adequacy of sedation is required any time a patient is pharmacologically paralyzed. The Bispectral Index may be used as a guide for sedation in the critically ill patient receiving pharmacologic paralysis. The appropriateness of this monitor in the ICU setting awaits further study [143].

Prolonged neuromuscular blockade may cause critical illness myopathy. Patients develop prolonged muscle weakness that involves also respiratory muscles leading to prolonged mechanical ventilation [157]. This syndrome is more frequent with concomitant sepsis, hyperglycemia, and use of steroids.

The use of modern lung protective strategies of mechanical ventilation is not associated with an increased need for sedation or neuromuscular blockade [88].

Table 9.9 lists agents commonly used for sedation, pain relief, and paralysis of the mechanically ventilated patient. Pain relief and sedation are very important components of the total care given to the ventilator "recipient." In many cases, otherwise difficult-to-ventilate patients have dramatically benefited from simple pain relief. Therefore, familiarity with the doses' interactions, side effects, and indications for analgesics, anxiolytics, non-depolarizing muscle relaxants, and antipsychotics is an important part of mechanical ventilation [152].

Acute asthma

The patient with severe acute asthma who requires intubation and mechanical ventilation is also at risk of barotrauma. Approximately 1–3% of patients with severe acute asthma attacks will require intubation and mechanical ventilation. The criteria for intubation of asthmatic patients include altered consciousness; apnea or severe respiratory distress; severe hypoxemia, hypercarbia, or respiratory acidosis; and arrhythmias [158]. Intubation may worsen bronchospasm or precipitate laryngospasm in asthmatics, and therefore, the airway should be managed by highly skilled individuals. Since the basic pathophysiology of asthma involves air trapping, asthmatics should be ventilated with caution to avoid barotrauma that may occur in the presence of elevated airway pressures [158]. Failure to ventilate adequately or no clinical improvement in mechanically ventilated patients with status asthmaticus receiving maximum medical therapy

Table 9.9 Sedation, analgesia, and paralysis in mechanical ventilation.

Agent	Infusion doses	Comments
Morphine	1–15 mg/h	Histamine release Careful in elderly patients Avoid in renal failure
Fentanyl	25–200 mcg/h	Minimal histamine release May use with renal failure
Hydromorphone	0.2–2.0 mg/h	Minimal histamine release May use with renal failure
Midazolam	1–15 mg/h	Avoid in renal failure Avoid prolonged infusions
Lorazepam	1–10 mg/h	Preferred in renal failure Delayed onset of action
Vecuronium	1–2 mcg/kg/min	Minimal hemodynamic effects Avoid in renal/liver impairment
Cisatracurium	2–4 mcg/kg/min	Hofmann reaction metabolism Minimal hemodynamic effects
Atracurium	4–12 mcg/kg/min	Hofmann reaction metabolism Dose-dependent histamine release
Propofol	5–50 mcg/kg/min	May cause hypotension Avoid prolonged infusions

should raise concern about severe extensive bronchial obstruction secondary to tenacious secretions. In this setting, flexible bronchoscopy by way of the endothracheal tube, for the removal of secretions may possibly be life saving [159]. General anesthesia, helium/oxygen inhalation, or ketamine sedation also may be useful adjuncts in the treatment of life-threatening status asthmaticus not responsive to conventional therapy [159].

A recent report documents survival of a pregnant woman with unresponsive status asthmaticus after mechanical ventilation with a helium–oxygen mixture [160]. Helium is an inert, nonflammable gas that possesses the lowest density of any gas other than hydrogen. Helium has no direct harmful effects or interactions with human tissues. The beneficial effects of a helium–oxygen mixture derive from its lower density when compared to either 100% oxygen or any concentration of oxygen in air/nitrogen. Helium–oxygen mixtures are usually used in ratios of 80 : 20 or 70 : 30. It should only be used in patients that tolerate such low oxygen concentrations. Therapy for severe asthma is primarily directed at relieving bronchospasm and increasing the radius of the airways. Using traditional methods, this effect may take hours to days to accomplish. The effect of lowering the density of the inhaled gas with the use of helium–oxygen mixture can be achieved within minutes, thereby allowing for decreased resistance to gas flow, improved gas exchange, and decreased peak inflating pressures [160]. In addition to decreasing resistance, administration of a gas mixture with a lower density and higher viscosity may improve gas flow by converting turbulent flow to laminar flow.

Small tidal volumes (6 mL/kg) and low respiratory frequencies are of paramount importance when applying mechanical ventilation to these patients. Inspiratory times as short as 0.8 seconds may be required to achieve I : E ratios near 1 : 4. Frequently, sedation and even the use of muscle relaxants will be needed. Paradoxically, the use of PEEP in patients with severe airway obstruction may relieve overinflation (auto-PEEP) [161]. In the latter trial, five out of eight patients with obstructive pulmonary disease demonstrated the occurrence of "paradoxic responses" to external PEEP. The application of PEEP in a sequential fashion lead to decreased functional residual capacity, plateau pressures, and total PEEP. Previous investigators have reported this response to external PEEP in severe asthma [162]. Theoretically, such external PEEP may prevent end-expiratory airway collapse promoting progressive lung deflation [161]. Response to this approach may be variable, so gradual application of PEEP at the bedside in order to determine the level resulting in the minimum plateau pressure may be warranted. Provided that the external PEEP level is below the initial intrinsic PEEP level, the possibility of overinflation is low [163].

Weaning from mechanical ventilation

Weaning has been defined as the process whereby mechanical ventilation is gradually withdrawn and the patient resumes spontaneous breathing [164]. The outcome of a trial of weaning from mechanical ventilation depends on the patient's underlying condition and the aggressiveness of the physician. The weaning process can be a difficult one. More than 40% of the total time that a patient spends in mechanical ventilation may be trying to wean from the ventilator [165]. In one study only 52% of 110 patients were successfully weaned on the first trial [166]. If mechanical ventilation is not discontinued as soon as possible, the patient will be exposed to unnecessary risks such as ventilator-associated pneumonia, ventilator-induced lung injury, and irreversible tracheal damage from artificial airway devices, to name just a few. On the other hand, premature extubation leading to reintubation within 48 hours after discontinuation of mechanical ventilation is associated with an 8-fold higher odds ratio for nosocomial pneumonia and a 6–12-fold increased mortality risk [167]. When deciding to discontinue mechanical ventilation, the clinician should perform a complete clinical assessment including the degree of resolution of the initial condition that required ventilatory support, ability to establish and protect the airway, nutritional status (including electrolyte values), and cardiovascular function (anticipating expected changes in preload and afterload that will occur with spontaneous breathing). Evaluation of "weaning predictors" measured at the bedside should also be taken into account. Even when all steps are followed and the patient is considered a good candidate for extubation, about 10–20% will require reintubation [61]. A fundamental concept that has been widely adopted in the last decade is the fact that many patients labeled as "ventilator dependent" may in fact not be. In one study, up to 66% of patients thought to be ventilator dependent were extubated after performing a spontaneous breathing trial (SBT) [165]. Patients that otherwise were not "thought to be ready for extubation" by the physician may in fact be ready for mechanical ventilation discontinuation. The most efficient way to identify these patients is to perform a SBT on a daily basis as soon as the patient has clinical improvement, is considered to be able to protect the airway, shows hemodynamic stability, and is receiving minimal ventilatory support (e.g. $F_iO_2 = 0.4$ and PEEP ≤5 mmHg). The implementation of daily SBT with weaning protocols in intensive care units do reduce the duration of mechanical ventilation [54].

Predicting weaning outcome

A wide variety of physiologic indices have been proposed to guide the process of discontinuing ventilator support. The most commonly used indices are listed in Table 9.10. In general, these indices evaluate a patient's ability to sustain spontaneous ventilation. The purpose of these indices is: (i) to identify the earliest time that ventilator support can be discontinued; and also (ii) to identify patients who are likely to fail a weaning trial and, thus, avoid cardiorespiratory and psychologic distress or collapse [164]. Some of these indices are useful while others not so much. Measurements of vital capacity, minute ventilation, and maximum negative inspiratory pressures show significant false-positive and false-negative results [61]. Other parameters like the ratio of respiratory frequency to tidal volume (f/V_t) have proven to be more reliable. This ratio is also known as the "rapid shallow breathing index". Some authors report that when this ratio is higher than 100, the probability of successful weaning is less than 5% [168]. In a recent publication, extubation failure (need for reintubation within 48–72 hours after extubation) was more frequent on patients with a f/V_t >57 breaths/L/min [169]. Out of all these parameters, we rely more on the f/V_t ratio and the negative inspiratory pressure (NIP) than any others.

Table 9.10 Variables used to predict weaning success.*

Tidal volume >5 mL/kg
Minute ventilation <10 L/min
Vital capacity >10 mL/kg
P_aO_2>60 mmHg on $F_iO_2 \leq 0.4$
Negative inspiratory pressure >–25 cmH$_2$O
P_aO_2/F_iO_2 ratio >200
f/V_t ratio <105

*All measurements must be obtained while on spontaneous breathing without any ventilatory support.

Weaning techniques

A variety of options for weaning from mechanical ventilation have been proposed and used over the past 25 years [170].

With the intermittent mandatory ventilation method, spontaneous breathing by the patient is assisted by a preset number of ventilatory-delivered breaths each minute. The intermittent mandatory ventilation rate is usually reduced in steps until a rate of 4 or close to 4 is reached. If the patient tolerates breathing with a mandatory rate of 4 and minimal pressure support (usually 5–7 cmH$_2$O) for a period of 30–120 minutes, she is extubated. In the pressure support ventilation method of weaning, each breath is initiated by the patient but supported in part by positive pressure delivered by the ventilator. In this method, weaning involves a progressive decrease in the magnitude of the pressure support delivered with each patient's breath. When the patient breathes comfortably with pressure support values of 5–7 cmH$_2$O for a period of 30–120 minutes, she is extubated.

Another technique for weaning mechanical ventilation is the "once-daily trial of spontaneous breathing" (SBT). In this technique, patients are disconnected from the ventilator and allowed to breathe spontaneously through a T-tube circuit for up to 2 hours each day. No evidence exists that "working the patient" for more than 2 hours a day has any benefits. In fact, it may lead to respiratory muscle fatigue. If signs of intolerance develop, assist controlled ventilation is reinstituted for 24 hours, at which time another trial is attempted. After failure of a SBT the clinician should actively look for reversible causes of the failure (e.g. development of pulmonary edema, electrolyte imbalances, metabolic acidosis, overfeeding). Patients who tolerate a SBT of at least 30 minutes and no more than 2 hours without signs of distress are extubated. These three methods of weaning were compared in a prospective, randomized, multicenter study [165]. The rate of success of weaning depended on the technique employed; a once-daily trial of spontaneous breathing led to extubation about three times faster than intermittent mandatory ventilation and about twice as quickly as pressure support ventilation. There were no significant differences in the rate of success between a once-daily trial and the multiple daily trials (T-tube trial) of spontaneous breathing, or between intermittent mandatory ventilation and pressure support ventilation.

Patients who tolerate a SBT of 30–120 minutes are successfully extubated at least 77% of the time [167]. Evidence-based guidelines for weaning and discontinuation of mechanical ventilation published by American College of Chest Physicians, the American Association for Respiratory Care, and The American College of Critical Care Medicine concluded that the daily SBT is the ideal method for ventilatory support weaning [167].

Failed weaning

The major underlying causes for ventilatory dependence are neurologic issues, respiratory system muscle/load/gas exchange interactions, cardiovascular factors, and psychologic factors [167]. When a patient fails a spontaneous breathing trial she should be evaluated closely and reversible causes should be corrected. If she is still a candidate for a weaning trial, it should be repeated in 24 hours. In between trials, the patient should receive a comfortable stable ventilatory support. No evidence supports the idea that slowly decreasing the level of ventilatory support will accelerate mechanical ventilation discontinuation [60].

Respiratory system interactions

Although mechanical ventilation is commonly instituted because of problems with oxygenation, this is rarely a cause of difficulty at the time that mechanical ventilation is being stopped. This is largely because ventilator discontinuation is not contemplated in patients who display significant problems with oxygenation. However, during a weaning trial, hypoxemia may occur as a result of hypoventilation, impaired pulmonary gas exchange, or decreased oxygen content of venous blood [164]. Impaired pulmonary gas exchange can be distinguished from pure hypoventilation by the presence of an elevated alveolar–arterial oxygen tension gradient. If the patient displays evidence of hypoxemic respiratory failure during weaning attempts, mechanical ventilation should be reinstituted until the cause of the hypoxemic respiratory failure has been identified and addressed. Impaired pulmonary gas exchange may be evidence of continuation of the initial precipitating illness or of other pathologic pulmonary processes such as pneumonia or pulmonary edema. These conditions should be treated before additional weaning attempts. Hypoventilation may occur secondary to extensive sedation or respiratory muscle fatigue.

As previously stated, respiratory muscle pump failure is a common cause of failure to wean from mechanical ventilation. This may result from decreased neuromuscular capacity, increased respiratory muscle pump load, or both [164] (Table 9.11). Evidence supports that in ventilator-dependent patients ventilatory muscles are weak, due to atrophy and remodeling from inactivity [167]. Decreased respiratory sensor output may result from neurologic structural damage, sedative agents, sleep deprivation, semistarvation, and metabolic alkalosis [164]. In addition, mechanical ventilation in itself may decrease respiratory center output by a number of mechanisms: lowering of arterial CO_2 tension, with a consequent reduction in chemoreceptor stimulation; activation of pulmonary stress receptors; and stimulation of muscle spindles or joint receptors in the chest wall.

Dynamic hyperinflation (e.g. asthma, COPD) poses a significant load to respiratory muscles and may be a cause of weaning failure. The increase in lung volume causes the inspiratory muscles to shorten with consequent decrease in the force of contraction. In the hyperinflated chest, thoracic elastic recoil is directed inward which poses an additional elastic load. Finally, increased diaphragmatic pressure secondary to lung overdistention may impair diaphragmatic blood supply. Adequate use of bronchodilators postextubation is of paramount importance in this population and in any patient who develops bronchospasm after mechanical ventilation is discontinued.

Underfeeding has a number of adverse effects on the respiratory system [170]. These adverse effects can interfere with weaning. It predisposes to nosocomial pneumonia and causes a decrease in the ventilatory response to hypoxia, decrease in diaphragmatic mass in thickness, and decrease in respiratory muscle strength and endurance. Malnutrition may be accompanied by metabolic abnormalities such as hypophosphatemia, hypokalemia, hypocalcemia, or hypomagnesemia that may adversely affect respiratory muscle function [164]. Overfeeding should also be avoided. It may impair the ventilator withdrawal process by increasing CO_2 production which further increases ventilatory demands [171]. Corticosteroid therapy [172] and thyroid disease [173] may also impair respiratory muscle function. Severe hypothyroidism impairs diaphragmatic function and blunts the brainstem response to hypoxia and hypercapnia [174]. Steroid use has been associated with an increased incidence of critical illness polyneuromyopathy. This entity is associated with prolonged periods of weaning from mechanical ventilation. However, adrenal insufficiency may also be a cause of suboptimal ventilatory muscle performance [167]. Another possibility is that respiratory muscle fatigue may be a primary cause of failure to wean. As discussed above, most evidence recommends that in between spontaneous breathing trials, the patient should receive comfortable stable ventilatory support in order to avoid muscle fatigue.

Increased ventilatory requirements may also lead to weaning failure. Factors that cause an increase in ventilatory requirements include increased CO_2 production (e.g. sepsis, fever, seizures, overfeeding), increased dead space ventilation, and an inappropriately elevated respiratory drive. Patients with a metabolic acidosis may not be able to adequately compensate their acid–base

Table 9.11 Causes of respiratory muscle pump failure.

Decreased neuromuscular capacity
Decreased respiratory center output
Phrenic nerve dysfunction
Decreased respiratory muscle strength and/or endurance
Hyperinflation
Malnutrition
Decreased oxygen supply
Respiratory acidosis
Mineral and electrolyte abnormalities
Endocrinopathy (hypothyroidism, adrenal insufficiency)
Disuse muscle atrophy
Respiratory muscle fatigue
Increased respiratory muscle pump load
Increased ventilatory requirements
Increased CO_2 production
Increased dead space ventilation
Inappropriately increased respiratory drive
Increased work of breathing

(Reproduced by permission from Tobin MJ, Yang K. Weaning from mechanical ventilation. *Crit Care Clin* 1990; 6(3): 725.)

disturbance by hyperventilating; correction of the primary disorder should be undertaken before starting the weaning process.

Neurologic issues

The ventilation pump controller is localized in the brainstem. This center receives feedback from cortical, chemoreceptive, and mechanoreceptive sensors. Ventilator dependence may be secondary to brainstem dysfunction due to structural damage (e.g. brainstem strokes) or metabolic conditions (e.g. electrolyte imbalances, sedation, narcotics) [175].

Cardiovascular factors

Patients with limited cardiac reserve (e.g. peripartum cardiomyopathy) may frequently fail attempts to withdraw mechanical ventilation secondary to heart failure and subsequent hydrostatic pulmonary edema. Spontaneous breathing generates negative intrathoracic pressure during inspiration; this translates into a significant increase in afterload for the left ventricle as well as preload as a pressure gradient develops between the abdomen and the thorax favoring venous return. Needless to say, the transition from mechanical ventilation to spontaneous breathing is associated with increased metabolic demands [164]. When performing a spontaneous breathing trial in patients with limited cardiac reserve, attention should be directed at changes in vascular filling pressures like the pulmonary artery occlusion pressure (if available) and central venous pressure, development of pulmonary edema, systemic blood pressure, and oxygen saturation. Bedside echocardiography during the breathing trial can provide valuable information regarding estimates of filling pressures. The use of diuretics and inotropes coupled with postextubation noninvasive positive-pressure ventilation could assist in liberating these patients from the ventilator.

Psychologic problems

Dependence on mechanical ventilation can be associated with feelings of insecurity, anxiety, fear, agony, and panic [176]. Many patients develop a fear that they will remain dependent on mechanical ventilation and that discontinuation of ventilator support will result in sudden death. These psychologic factors are major determinants of outcome of weaning trials in some patients, especially those patients who require prolonged ventilator support [177]. Stress can be minimized by frequent communication with the patient and family members. One should always keep in mind that in postoperative patients breathing may be impaired by pain associated with deep inspiration; pain control should always be adequate [60].

Conclusion

In summary, the management of the gravida with respiratory failure can be difficult. However, early recognition of respiratory failure and institution of ventilatory support, knowledge of the changes in the cardiorespiratory system that occurs in gestation, judicious therapy of underlying pathophysiologic aberrations, thoughtful measures to prevent known complications, and prudent attempts to release the patient from ventilator dependency may improve the outcome of pregnant patients who suffer respiratory failure.

References

1 Kaunitz AM, Hughes JM, Grimes DA et al. Causes of maternal mortality in the United States. *Obstet Gynecol* 1985; 65: 605–612.

2 United States Public Health Service. Progress toward achieving the 1990 objectives for pregnancy and infant health. *MMWR* 1988; 37: 405.

3 Demling RH, Knox JB. Basic concepts of lung function and dysfunction: oxygenation, ventilation, and mechanics. *New Horiz* 1993; 1: 362–370.

4 Pontoppidan H, Geffin B, Lowenstein E. Acute respiratory failure in the adult 2. *N Engl J Med* 1972; 287: 743–752.

5 Anderson GJ, James GB, Mathers NP et al. The maternal oxygen tension and acid-base status during pregnancy. *J Obstet Br Commonw* 1969; 76: 17.

6 Templeton A, Kelman GR. Maternal blood gases, (P_AO_2–P_aO_2), physiologic shunt, and V_DV_T in normal pregnancy. *Br J Anaesth* 1976; 48: 1001–1004.

7 Barcroft J. On anoxemia. *Lancet* 1920; 11: 485.

8 Cain SM. Peripheral oxygen uptake and delivery in health and disease. *Clin Chest Med* 1983; 4: 139–148.

9 Bryan-Brown CW, Baek SM, Makabali G et al. Consumable oxygen: oxygen availability in relation to oxyhemoglobin dissociation. *Crit Care Med* 1973; 1: 17–21.

10 Perutz MF. Hemoglobin structure and respiratory transport. *Sci Am* 1978; 239: 92–125.

11 Rackow EC, Astiz M. Pathophysiology and treatment of septic shock. *JAMA* 1991; 266: 548–554.

12 Shoemaker WC, Ayres S, Grenvik A et al. *Textbook of Critical Care*, 2nd edn. Philadelphia: WB Saunders, 1989.

13 Shibutani K, Komatsu T, Kubal K et al. Critical level of oxygen delivery in anesthetized man. *Crit Care Med* 1983; 11: 640–643.

14 Gutierrez G, Brown SD. Gastric tonometry: a new monitoring modality in the intensive care unit. *J Int Care Med* 1995; 10: 34–44.

15 Barron W, Lindheimer M. *Medical Disorders during Pregnancy*, 1st edn. St. Louis: Mosby-Year Book, 1991: 234.

16 Pernoll ML, Metcalf J, Schlenker TL et al. Oxygen consumption at rest and during exercise in pregnancy. *Respir Physiol* 1975; 25: 285–293.

17 Gemzell CA, Robbe H, Strom G et al. Observations on circulatory changes and muscular work in normal labor. *Acta Obstet Gynecol Scand* 1957; 36: 75–93.

18 Ueland K, Hansen JM. Maternal cardiovascular hemodynamics. II. Posture and uterine contractions. *Am J Obstet Gynecol* 1969; 103: 1–7.

19 Belfort MA, Anthony J, Kirshon B. Respiratory function in severe gestational proteinuric hypertension: the effects of rapid volume expansion and subsequent vasodilatation with verapamil. *Br J Obstet Gynaecol* 1991; 98(10): 964–972.

20 Belfort MA, Anthony J, Saade GR et al. The oxygen consumption: oxygen delivery curve in severe preeclampsia: evidence for a fixed oxygen extraction state. *Am J Obstet Gynecol* 1993; 169(6): 1448–1455.
21 ACOG. Pulmonary Disease in Pregnancy. ACOG Technical Bulletin 224: 2. Washington, DC: ACOG, 1996.
22 Shapiro BA, Peruzzi WT, Kozelowski-Templin R. *Clinical Application of Blood Gases*, 5th edn. Chicago: Mosby Year Book, 1994.
23 New W Jr. Pulse oximetry. *J Clin Monit* 1985; 1: 126–129.
24 Woodley M, Whelan A, eds. *The Washington Manual of Medical Therapeutics*. St Louis: Little, Brown and Company, 1993.
25 Meyer TJ, Hill NS. Non-invasive positive pressure ventilation to treat respiratory failure. *Ann Intern Med* 1994; 120: 760–770.
26 Carrey Z, Gottfried SB, Levy RD. Ventilatory muscle support in respiratory failure with nasal positive pressure ventilation. *Chest* 1990; 97: 150–158.
27 Antonelli M, Conti G, Esquinas A et al. A multiple-center survey on the use in clinical practice of noninvasive ventilation as a first-line intervention for acute respiratory distress syndrome. *Crit Care Med.* 2007; 35: 288–290.
28 Freeman RK, Garite TJ, Nageotte MP. *Fetal Heart Rate Monitoring*, 2nd edn. Baltimore: Williams & Wilkins, 1991.
29 Katz VL, Dotters DJ, Droegemueller W. Perimortem Cesarean delivery. *Obstet Gynecol* 1986; 68: 571–576.
30 Sutherland AD, Stock JG, Davies JM. Effects of preoperative fasting on morbidity and gastric contents in patients undergoing day-stay surgery. *Br J Anaesth* 1986; 58: 876–878.
31 Gibbs CP, Banner TC. Effectiveness of Bicitra as a preoperative antacid. *Anesthesiology* 1984; 61(1): 97–99.
32 Sellick BA. Cricoid pressure to control regurgitation of stomach contents during induction of anesthesia. *Lancet* 1961; 2: 404.
33 Cheek TG, Gutsche BB. Maternal physiologic alterations during pregnancy. In: *Anesthesia for Obstetrics*. Baltimore: Williams & Wilkins, 1987: 3.
34 Deem S, Bishop MJ. Evaluation and management of the difficult airway. *Crit Care Clin* 1995; 11: 1–27.
35 Bidani A, Tzouanakis AE, Cardenas VJ, Zwischenbergr JB. Permissive hypercapnia in acute respiratory failure. *JAMA* 1994; 272: 957–962.
36 Baudouin SV. Ventilator induced lung injury and infection in the critically ill. *Thorax* 2001; 56(2): 1150–1157.
37 Brower RG, Ware LB, Berthiaume Y, Matthay MA. Treatment of ARDS. *Chest* 2001; 120: 1347–1367.
38 Hinson JR, Marini JJ. Principles of mechanical ventilator use in respiratory failure. *Annu Rev Med* 1992; 43: 341–361.
39 MacIntyre N, Nishimura M, Usada Y, Tokioka H, Takezawa J, Shimada Y. The Nagoya conference on system design and patient-ventilator interactions during pressure support ventilation. *Chest* 1990; 97: 1463–1466.
40 Brochard L, Harf A, Lorino H, Lemaire F. Inspiratory pressure support prevents diaphragmatic fatigue during weaning from mechanical ventilation. *Am Rev Respir Dis* 1989; 139: 513–521.
41 Kollef MH, Schuster DP. The acute respiratory distress syndrome. *N Engl J Med* 1985; 332: 27–37.
42 Lain DC, DiBenedetto R, Morris SL et al. Pressure control inverse ratio ventilation as a method to reduce peak inspiratory pressure and provide adequate ventilation and oxygenation. *Chest* 1989; 95: 1081–1088.
43 Tharratt RS, Allen RP, Albertson TE. Pressure controlled inverse ratio ventilation in severe adult respiratory failure. *Chest* 1988; 94: 755–762.
44 Douglass JA, Tuxen DV, Horne M et al. Myopathy in severe asthma. *Am Rev Respir Dis* 1992; 146: 517–519.
45 Segredo V, Caldwell JE, Matthay MA et al. Persistent paralysis in critically ill patients after long-term administration of vecuronium. *N Engl J Med* 1992; 327: 524–528.
46 Biddle C. AANA Journal Course: Update for nurse anesthetists–Advances in ventilating the patient with severe lung disease. *J Am Assoc Nurse Anesthetists* 1993; 61(2): 170–174.
47 Stock MC, Downs JB, Frolicher DA. Airway pressure release ventilation. *Crit Care Med* 1987; 15: 462–466.
48 Habashi N. Other approaches to open-lung ventilation: Airway pressure release ventilation. *Crit Care Med* 2005; 33(3): S228–S240.
49 Frawley PM, Habashi NM. Airway pressure release ventilation: Theory and practice. AACN clinical issues. *Adv Pract Acute Crit Care* 2001; 12(2): 234–246.
50 Cole DE, Taylor TL, McCullough DM et al. Acute respiratory distress syndrome in pregnancy. *Crit Care Med* 2005; 33(10): S269–S278.
51 Chan KP, Stewart TE. Clinical use of high-frequency oscillatory ventilation in adult patients with acute respiratory distress syndrome. *Crit Care Med* 2005; 33(3): S170–S174.
52 Derdak S. High-frequency oscillatory ventilation for acute respiratory distress syndrome in adult patients. *Crit Care Med* 2003; 31(4): S317–S323.
53 Papazian L, Gainnier M, Valerie M et al. Comparison of prone positioning and high-frequency oscillatory ventilation in patients with acute respiratory distress syndrome. *Crit Care Med* 2005; 33(10): 2162–2171.
54 Sevransky JE, Levy MM, Marini JJ. Mechanical ventilation in sepsis-induced acute lung injury acute respiratory distress syndrome: An evidenced based review. *Crit Care Med* 2004; 32(11): S548–S553.
55 Suter PM, Fairley HB, Isenberg MD. Optimum end-expiratory pressure in patients with acute pulmonary failure. *N Engl J Med* 1975; 292: 284–289.
56 Shapiro BA, Cane RD, Harrison RA. Positive end-expiratory pressure therapy in adults with special reference to acute lung injury: A review of the literature and suggested clinical correlations. *Crit Care Med* 1984; 12: 127–141.
57 Ralph DD, Robertson HT, Weaver LJ et al. Distribution of ventilation and perfusion during positive end-expiratory pressure in the adult respiratory distress syndrome. *Am Rev Respir Dis* 1985; 131: 54–60.
58 Tyler DC, Cheney FW. Comparison of positive end-expiratory pressure and inspiratory positive plateau in ventilation of rabbits with experimental pulmonary edema. *Anesth Analg* 1979; 58: 288–292.
59 Puybasset L, Cluzel P, Chao N et al. A computed tomography scan assessment of regional lung volume in acute lung injury. *Am J Respir Crit Care Med* 1998; 158: 1644–1655.
60 MacIntyre NR. Current issues in mechanical ventilation for respiratory failure. *Chest* 2005; 128(5): S561–S567.
61 Tobin MJ. Advances in mechanical ventilation. *N Engl J Med* 2001; 344(26): 1986–1996.
62 Brower RG, Lanken PN, MacIntyre N et al. Higher versus lower positive end-expiratory pressures in patients with the acute respiratory distress syndrome. *N Engl J Med* 2004; 351(4): 327–336.

63 Piehl MA, Brown RS. Use of extreme position changes in acute respiratory failure. *Crit Care Med* 1976; 4: 13–14.
64 Douglas WW, Rehder K, Beynen FM et al. Improved oxygenation in patients with acute respiratory failure: The prone position. *Am Rev Respir Dis* 1977; 115: 559–566.
65 Gattinoni L, Tognoni G, Pesenti A et al. Effect of prone positioning on the survival of patients with acute respiratory failure. *N Engl J Med* 2001; 345(8): 568–573.
66 McAuley DF, Giles F, Fichter H et al. What is the optimal duration of ventilation in the prone position in acute lung injury and acute respiratory distress syndrome? *Intensive Care Med* 2002; 28: 414–418.
67 Anzueto A, Guntapalli K. Adjunctive therapy to mechanical ventilation: surfactant therapy, liquid ventilation, and prone position. *Clin Chest Med* 2006; 27: 637–654.
68 Hill JD, O'Brien TG, Murray JJ et al. Prolonged extracorporeal oxygenation for acute post-traumatic respiratory failure (shock-lung syndrome): use of the Bramson membrane lung. *N Engl J Med* 1972; 286: 629–634.
69 Prescenti A, Gattinoni L, Kolobow T et al. Extracorporeal circulation in adult respiratory failure. *ASAIO Trans* 1988; 34: 43–47.
70 ECMO. Quarterly Report. Ann Arbor, MI: ECMO Registry of the Extracorporeal Life Support Organization (ELSO), 1994.
71 Anderson HL III, Bartlett RH. Extracorporeal and intravascular gas exchange devices. In: Ayres SM, Grenvik A, Holbrook PR, Shoemaker WC, eds. *Textbook of Critical Care*, 3rd edn. Philadelphia: WB Saunders, 1995: 943–951.
72 Anderson HL III, Decius RE, Sinard JM et al. Early experience with adult extracorporeal membrane oxygenation in the modern era. *Ann Thorac Surg* 1992; 53: 553–563.
73 Mols G, Loop T, Geiger K, Farthmann E, Benzing A. Extracorporeal membrane oxygenation: a ten-year experience. *Am J Surg* 2000; 180: 144–154.
74 McIntyre RC, Pulido EJ, Bensard DD, Shames BD, Abraham E. Thirty years of clinical trials in acute respiratory distress syndrome. *Crit Care Med* 2000; 28(9): 3314–3331.
75 Lundin S, Mang H, Smithies M, Stenqvist O, Frostell C. Inhalation of nitric oxide in acute lung injury: results of a European multicentre study. The European Study Group of Inhaled Nitric Oxide. *Intensive Care Med* 1999; 25(9): 881–883.
76 Griffiths MJD, Evans TW. Inhaled nitric oxide therapy in adults. *N Engl J Med* 2005; 353(25): 2683–2695.
77 Young JD, Dyar O, Xiong L et al. Methaemoglobin production in normal adults inhaling low concentrations of nitric oxide. *Intensive Care Med* 1994; 20: 581–584.
78 Loh E, Stamler JS, Hare JM et al. Cardiovascular effects of inhaled nitric oxide in patients with left ventricular dysfunction. *Circulation* 1994; 90: 2780–2785.
79 Blanch L, Fernandez R, Valles J et al. Effect of two tidal volumes on oxygenation and respiratory system mechanics during the early stage of adult respiratory distress syndrome. *J Crit Care* 1994; 9: 151–158.
80 The Acute Respiratory Distress Syndrome Network. Ventilation with lower tidal volumes as compared with traditional tidal volumes for acute lung injury and the acute respiratory distress syndrome. *N Engl J Med* 2000; 342: 1301–1308.
81 Bezzant TB, Mortensen JD. Risks and hazards of mechanical ventilation: A collective review of published literature. *Dis Mon* 1994; 40: 581–638.
82 Slutsky AS, Tremblay LN. Multiple system organ failure. Is mechanical ventilation a contributing factor? *Am J Respir Crit Care Med* 1998; 157: 1721–1725.
83 Kolobow T. Acute respiratory failure. On how to injure healthy lungs (and prevent sick lungs from recovering). *ASAIO Trans* 1988; 34: 31–34.
84 Martin GS, Bernard GR. Acute respiratory distress syndrome: innovative therapies. *Semin Respir Crit Care Med.* 2001;2: 293–306.
85 Frutos-Vivar F, Esteban A, Apezteguia C et al. Outcome of mechanically ventilated patients who require a tracheostomy. *Crit Care Med* 2005; 33(2): 290–298.
86 Stewart TE, Meade MO, Cook DJ et al. Evaluation of a ventilation strategy to prevent barotraumas in patients at high risk for acute respiratory distress syndrome. *N Engl J Med* 1998; 338: 355–361.
87 Kuiper JW, Groeneveld ABJ, Slutsky AS et al. Mechanical ventilation and acute renal failure. *Crit Care Med* 2005; 33(6): 1408–1415.
88 Cheng IW, Eisner MD, Thompson BT et al. Acute effects of tidal volume strategy on hemodynamics, fluid balance, and sedation in acute lung injury. *Crit Care Med* 2005; 33(1): 63–70.
89 Caldwell-Kenkel JC, Currin RT, Coote A et al. Reperfusion injury to endothelial cells after cold storage of rat livers: protection by mildly acidic pH and lack of protection by antioxidants. *Transpl Int* 1995; 8: 77–85.
90 Kregenow DA, Rubenfeld GD, Hudson LD et al. Hypercapnic acidosis and mortality in acute lung injury. *Crit Care Med* 2006; 34(1): 1–7.
91 Varughese M, Patole S, Shama A et al. Permissive hypercapnia in neonates: The case of the good, the bad, and the ugly. *Pediatr Pulmonol* 2002; 33: 56–64.
92 Pastores SM. Critical illness polyneuropathy and myopathy in acute respiratory distress syndrome: More common than we realize! *Crit Care Med* 2005; 33(4): 895–896.
93 Lucas CE, Sugawa C, Riddle J, Rector F, Rosenberg B, Walt AJ. Natural history and surgical dilemma of stress gastric bleeding. *Arch Surg* 1971; 102: 266–273.
94 Skillman JJ, Bushnell LS, Goldman H, Silen W. Respiratory failure, hypotension, sepsis and jaundice: A clinical syndrome associated with lethal hemorrhage from acute stress ulceration of the stomach. *Am J Surg* 1969; 117: 523–530.
95 Kantorova I, Svoboda P, Scheer P et al. Stress ulcer prophylaxis in critically ill patients: A randomized controlled trial. *Hepat Gastroenterol* 2004; 51: 757–761.
96 Cook DJ, Fuller HD, Guyatt GH et al. Risk factors for gastrointestinal bleeding in critically ill patients. *N Engl J Med* 1994; 330: 377–381.
97 Kivilaakso E, Silen W. Pathogenesis of experimental gastric-mucosal injury. *N Engl J Med* 1979; 301: 364–369.
98 Pingleton SK. Complications of acute respiratory failure. *Am Rev Respir Dis* 1988; 137: 1463–1493.
99 Cook D, Guyatt G, Marshall J et al. A comparison of sucralfate and ranitidine for the prevention of upper gastrointestinal bleeding in patients requiring mechanical ventilation. *N Engl J Med* 1998; 338(12): 791–797.
100 Fennerty MB. Pathophysiology of the upper gastrointestinal tract in the critically ill patient: Rationale for the therapeutic benefits of acid suppression. *Crit Care Med* 2002; 30(6): S351–S355.
101 Morgan D. Intravenous proton pump inhibitors in the critical care setting. *Crit Care Med* 2002; 30(6): S369–S372.

102 Moser KM, LeMoine JR, Nachtwey FJ, Spragg RG. Deep venous thrombosis and pulmonary embolism. *JAMA* 1981; 246: 1422–1424.

103 Chastre J, Cornud F, Bouchama A et al. Thrombosis as a complication of pulmonary-artery catheterization via the internal jugular vein. Prospective evaluation by phlebography. *N Engl J Med* 1982; 306: 278–281.

104 Connors AF, Castele RJ, Farhaf NZ, Tomashefski JF. Complications of right heart catheterization. *Chest* 1985; 88: 567–572.

105 Marik PE, Plante LA. Venous Thromboembolic Disease and Pregnancy. *N Engl J Med.* 2008; 359: 2025–2033.

106 Geerts WH, Pineo GF, Heit JA et al. Prevention of Venous Thromboembolism: The Seventh ACCP Conference on Antithrombotic and Thrombolytic Therapy. *Chest* 2004; 126(3) Supplement: 338S–400S.

107 Gurkan OU, O'Donnell C, Brower R et al. Differential effects of mechanical ventilatory strategy on lung injury and systemic organ inflammation in mice. *Am J Physiol Lung Cell Mol Physiol* 2003; 285: L710–L718.

108 Anand IS, Chandrashekhar Y, Ferrari R et al. Pathogenesis of congestive state in chronic obstructive pulmonary disease. Studies of body water and sodium, renal function, hemodynamics, and plasma hormones during edema and after recovery. *Circulation* 1992; 86: 12–21.

109 Pannu N, Mehta RL. Effect of mechanical ventilation on the kidney. *Best Pract Res Clin Anaesthesiol* 2004; 18: 189–203.

110 Parker CM, Heyland DK. Aspiration and the risk of ventilator-associated pneumonia. *Nutr Clin Pract.* 2004; 19: 597–609.

111 Porzecanski I, Bowton DL. Diagnosis and treatment of ventilator-associated pneumonia. *Chest* 2006; 130: 597–604.

112 Cook D, De Jonghe B, Brochard L et al. Influence of airway management on ventilator-associated pneumonia: evidence from randomized trials. *JAMA* 1998; 279: 781–787.

113 Cook DJ, Walter SD, Cook RJ et al. Incidence of and risk factors for ventilator-associated pneumonia in critically ill patients. *Ann Intern Med* 1998; 129: 440.

114 Torres A, Ewig S. Diagnosing ventilator-associated pneumonia. *N Engl J Med* 2004; 350(5): 433–435.

115 Craven DE, De Rosa FG, Thornton D. Nosocomial pneumonia: emerging concepts in diagnosis, management, and prophylaxis. *Curr Opin Crit Care* 2002; 8: 421–429.

116 American Thoracic Society Documents. Guidelines for the management of adults with hospital-acquired, ventilator-associated, and health care-associated pneumonia. *Am J Respir Crit Care Med* 2005; 171: 388–416.

117 Shorr AF, Sherner JH, Jackson WL et al. Invasive approaches to the diagnosis of ventilator-associated pneumonia: A meta-analysis. *Crit Care Med* 2005; 33(1): 46–53.

118 Shorr AF, Kollef MH. Ventilator-associated pneumonia: insights from recent clinical trials. *Chest* 2005; 128(5): S583–S591.

119 Rello J, Sonora R, Jubert P et al. Pneumonia in intubated patients: role of respiratory airway care. *Am J Respir Crit Care Med* 1996; 154: 111–115.

120 Bernard EA, Weser E. Complications and prevention. In: Rombeau JL, Caldwell MD, eds. *Enteral and Tube Feeding*. Philadelphia: WB Saunders, 1984: 542.

121 Ang SD, Daly JM. Potential complications and monitoring of patients receiving total parenteral nutrition. In: Rombeau JL, Caldwell MD, eds. *Parenteral Nutrition*. Philadelphia: WB Saunders, 1986: 331.

122 Rochester DF, Esau SA. Malnutrition and respiratory system. *Chest* 1984; 85: 411–415.

123 Kelly SM, Rosa A, Field S et al. Inspiratory muscle strength and body composition in patients receiving total parenteral nutrition therapy. *Am Rev Respir Dis* 1984; 130: 33–37.

124 Martin TR. Relationship between malnutrition and lung infections. *Clin Chest Med* 1987; 8(3): 359–372.

125 Dickerson R. Hypocaloric feeding of obese patients in the intensive care unit. *Curr Opin Clin Nutr Met Care* 2005; 8(2): 189–196.

126 Jeejeebhoy KN. Permissive underfeeding of the critically ill patient. *Nutr Clin Pract* 2004; 19: 477–480.

127 Baker JP, Detsky AS, Stewart S, Whitwell J, Marliss EB, Jeejeebhoy KN. Randomized trial of TPN in critically ill patients: metabolic effects of varying glucose-lipid ratios as the energy source. *Gastroenterology* 1984; 87: 53–59.

128 Tehila M, Gibstein L, Gordgi D et al. Enteral fish oil, borage oil and antioxidants in patients with acute lung injury (ALI) [Abstract]. *Clin Nutr* 2003; 22 (Suppl): S20.

129 Artinian V, Krayem H, DiGiovine B. Effects of early enteral feeding on the outcome of critically ill mechanically ventilated medical patients. *Chest* 2006; 129: 960–967.

130 Pontes-Arruda A, Albuquerque AM, Albuquerque JD. Effects of enteral feeding with eicosapentacoic acid, γ-linolenic acid, and antioxidants in mechanically ventilated patients with severe sepsis and septic shock. *Crit Care Med* 2006; 34(9): 2325–2333.

131 Singleton KD, Serkova N, Beckey V, Wischmeyer P. Glutamine attenuates lung injury and improves survival after sepsis: Role of enhanced heat shock protein expression. *Crit Care Med* 2005; 33(6): 1206–1213.

132 Novak F, Heyland DK, Avenell A et al. Glutamine supplementation in serious illness: A systematic review of the evidence. *Crit Care Med* 2002; 30: 2022–2029.

133 The National Heart, Lung, and Blood Institute Acute Respiratory Distress Syndrome (ARDS) Clinical Trials Network. Comparison of two fluid-management strategies in acute lung injury. *N Engl J Med* 2006; 354.

134 Humphrey H, Hall J, Sznajder I et al. Improved survival in ARDS patients associated with a reduction in pulmonary capillary wedge pressure. *Chest* 1990; 97: 1176–1180.

135 Mangialardi RJ, Martin GS, Bernard GR et al. Hypoproteinemia predicts acute respiratory distress syndrome development, weight gain, and death in patients with sepsis. Ibuprofen in Sepsis Study Group. *Crit Care Med.* 2000; 28: 3137–3145.

136 Martin GS, Mangialardi RJ, Wheeler AP et al. Albumin and furosemide therapy in hypoproteinemic patients with acute lung injury. *Crit Care Med* 2002; 30(10): 2175–2182.

137 Martin GS, Moss M, Wheeler AP et al. A randomized, controlled trial of furosemide with or without albumin in hypoproteinemic patients with acute lung injury. *Crit Care Med* 2005; 33(8): 1681–1687.

138 Van Hook JW, Ventilator therapy and airway management. *Crit Care Obstet* 1997; 8: 143.

139 Rayburn WF, Zuspan FP, eds. *Drug Therapy in Obstetrics and Gynecology*, 3rd edn. St. Louis: Mosby Year Book, 1992.

140 Briggs GG, Freeman RK, Yaffe SJ. *Drugs in Pregnancy and Lactation*, 4th edn. Baltimore: Williams and Wilkins, 1994.

141 Kress JP, Hall JB. Sedation in the mechanically ventilated patient. *Crit Care Med* 2006; 34(10): 2541–2546.

142 Balestrieri F, Fisher S. Analgesics. In: Chernow B, ed. *The Pharmacologic Approach to the Critically Ill Patient*. Baltimore: Williams and Wilkins, 1995: 640–650.

143 Vender JS, Szokol JW, Murphy JS et al. Sedation, analgesia, and neuromuscular blockade in sepsis: An evidence-based review. *Crit Care Med* 2004; 32(11): S554–S561.

144 Bianchi M, Mantegazza P, Tammiso R et al. Peripherally administered benzodiazepines increase morphine induced analgesia in the rat. *Arch Int Pharmacodyn Ther* 1993; 322: 5–13.

145 Ward DS. Stimulation of the hypoxic pulmonary drive by droperidol. *Anesth Analg* 1984; 63: 106–110.

146 Ayd FJ Jr. Intravenous haloperidol therapy. *Int Drug Ther Newslett* 1978; 13: 20.

147 Shafer SL. Advances in propofol pharmacokinetics and pharmacodynamics. *J Clin Anesth.* 1993; 5: 14S–21S.

148 Goodchild CS. Cardiovascular effects of propofol and relevance to use in patients with compromised cardiovascular function. *Semin Anesth* 1992; 11: S37–S38.

149 Carson SS, Kress JP, Rodgers JE et al. A randomized trial of intermittent lorazepam versus propofol with daily interruption in mechanically ventilated patients. *Crit Care Med* 2006; 34(5): 1326–1332.

150 Cremer OL, Moons KG, Bouman EA et al. Long-term propofol infusion and cardiac failure in adult head-injured patients. *Lancet.* 200; 357: 117–118.

151 Kress JP, Pohlman AS, O'Connor MF et al. Daily interruption of sedative infusions in critically ill patients undergoing mechanical ventilation. *N Engl J Med* 2000; 342(20): 1471–1477.

152 Van Hook JW, Harvey CJ, Uckan E. Mechanical ventilation in pregnancy and postpartum minute ventilation and weaning. *Am J Obstet Gynecol* 1995; 172: 326(part 2). Abstract.

153 Murray MJ, Cowen J, DeBlock H, et al. Task Force of the American College of Critical Care Medicine (ACCM) of the Society of Critical Care Medicine (SCCM), American Society of Health-System Pharmacists, American College of Chest Physicians. *Crit Care Med.* 2002; 30(1): 142–156.

154 Cullen DJ, Bigatello LM, DeMonaco HJ. Anesthetic pharmacology and critical care. In: Chernow B, ed. *The Pharmacologic Approach to the Critically Ill Patient*, 3rd edn. Baltimore: Williams and Wilkins, 1994: 291–308.

155 Duvaldstein P, Agoston S, Henzel D et al. Pancouronium pharmacokinetics in patients with liver cirrhosis. *Br J Anaesth* 1978; 50: 1131–1136.

156 Miller RD, Rupp SM, Fisher DM et al. Clinical pharmacology of vecuronium and atracurium. *Anesthesiology* 1984; 61: 444–453.

157 Fletcher SN, Kennedy DD, Ghosh IR et al. Persistent neuromuscular and neurophysiologic abnormalities in long-term survivors of prolonged critical illness. *Crit Care Med* 2003; 31: 1012–1016.

158 Soler M, Imhof E, Perruchoud AP. Severe acute asthma. Pathophysiology, clinical assessment and treatment. *Respiration* 1990; 57: 114–121.

159 Einarsson O, Rochester CL, Rosenbaum S. Airway management in respiratory emergencies. *Clin Chest Med* 1994; 15(1): 13–34.

160 George R, Berkenbosch JW, Fraser RF II, Tobias JD. Mechanical ventilation during pregnancy using a helium-oxygen mixture in a patient with respiratory failure due to status asthmaticus. *J Perinatol* 2001; 21(6): 395–398.

161 Caramez MP, Borges JB, Tucci MR et al. Paradoxical responses to positive end-expiratory pressure in patients with airway obstruction during controlled ventilation. *Crit Care Med* 2005; 33(7): 1519–1528.

162 Qvist J, Penmberton M, Knud-age B. High-level PEEP in severe asthma. *N Engl J Med* 1982; 307: 1347–1348.

163 Ranieri VM, Dambrosio M, Brienza N. Intrinsic PEEP and cardiopulmonary interaction in patients with COPD and acute ventilatory failure. *Eur Respir J* 1996; 9: 1283–1292.

164 Tobin MJ, Yang K. Weaning from mechanical ventilation. *Crit Care Clin* 1990; 6(3): 725–747.

165 Esteban A, Frutos F, Tobin MJ et al. A comparison of our methods of weaning patients from mechanical ventilation. Spanish Lung Failure Collaborative Group. *N Engl J Med* 1995; 332: 345–350.

166 Pardee NE, Winterbauer RH, Allen JD. Bedside evaluation of respiratory distress. *Chest* 1984; 85(2): 203–206.

167 MacIntyre NR, Cook DJ, Guyatt GH. Evidence-based guidelines for weaning and discontinuing ventilatory support: A collective task force facilitated by the American College of Chest Physicians; the American Association for Respiratory Care; and the American College of Crit Care Med. *Chest* 2001; 120(6): S375–S395.

168 Jaeschke RZ, Meade MO, Guyatt GH et al. How to use diagnostic test articles in the intensive care unit: diagnosing weanability using fVt. *Crit Care Med* 1997; 25: 1514–1521.

169 Frutos-Vivar F, Ferguson ND, Esteban A et al. Risk factors for extubation failure in patients following a succesful spontaneous breathing trial. *Chest* 2006; 130(6): 1664–1671.

170 Tobin MJ, Alex CG. Discontinuation of mechanical ventilation. In: Tobin MJ, ed. *Principles and Practice of Mechanical Ventilation.* New York: McGraw-Hill, 1994: 1177.

171 Pingleton SK, Harmon GS. Nutritional management in acute respiratory failure. *JAMA* 1987; 257: 3094–3099.

172 Lewis MI, Belman MJ. Respiratory muscle involvement in malnutrition. In: Tobin MJ, ed. *The Respiratory Muscles.* Philadelphia: JB Lippincott Company, 1990.

173 Laroche CM, Moxham J, Green M. Respiratory muscle weakness and fatigue. *Q J Med* 1989; 71: 373–397.

174 Siafakas NM, Salesiotou V, Filaditaki V et al. Respiratory muscle strength in hypothyroidism. *Chest* 1992; 102: 189–194.

175 Barrientos-Vega R, Mar Sanchez-Soria M, Morales-Garcia C et al. Prolonged sedation of critically ill patients with midazolam or propofol: impact on weaning and costs. *Crit Care Med* 1997; 25: 33–40.

176 Bergbom-Enberg I, Haljamae H. Assessment of patient's experience of discomforts during respiratory therapy. *Crit Care Med* 1989; 17: 1068–1072.

177 Holliday JE, Heyers TM. The reduction of weaning time from mechanical ventilation using tidal volume and relaxation biofeed back. *Am Rev Respir Dis* 1990; 141(5 Pt 1): 1214–1220.

10 Vascular Access

Gayle Olson[1] & Aristides P. Koutrouvelis[2]

[1]Department of Obstetrics and Gynecology, Division of Maternal-Fetal Medicine, University of Texas Medical Branch, Galveston, TX, USA

[2]Department of Anesthesiology, University of Texas Medical Branch, Galveston, TX, USA

Introduction

Placement and maintenance of vascular access can be an important adjunct in the care of the critically ill obstetric patient. Arterial and venous access affords the clinician several advantages (Table 10.1). Long-term central intravenous (IV) access may also be indicated for gravidas with coexisting disease such as those illustrated in Table 10.2, for the administration of parenteral nutrition, drugs, or antibiotics [1–4].

Establishing central venous and arterial access are acquired skills that require knowledge of catheter types, access routes, insertion techniques and maintenance.

Catheter type

Choosing the venous catheter type and the site for insertion are influenced by indication (Table 10.2), duration of use, urgency of administration, and the composition of infusate (i.e., osmolarity, tonicity, crystalloid, colloid). Catheters with shorter lengths and larger diameters allow for more rapid flow rates. For example, coupling of tube diameter (0.71 mm or 22 gauge vs 1.65 mm or 16 gauge) results in almost a quadrupling of the flow rate (25 mL/min vs 96 mL/min) [5]. Multilumen catheters are routinely used for central venous cannulation (Figure 10.1). The more commonly used triple-lumen catheter has an outside diameter of 2.3 mm (6.9 French) and provides three channels (three 18-gauge, two 18-gauge plus one 16-gauge). The opening of each channel is separated from the other by 1 cm or more in order to reduce mixing of infusates.

Intravenous catheters are considered to be short- or long-term transcutaneous, or implantable subcutaneously (Table 10.3) as well as peripheral or central. A peripheral location is distal to a central vein and contains valves. In contrast, a centrally located catheter contains no valves and is considered to be at the level of the axillary or common femoral vein, and all other veins oriented toward the heart from this level. The use of the terminology "peripheral" and "central" is also based on the peripheral or central location of insertion and the location of the catheter tip. Central vein cannulation is required to accommodate the large-bore catheters necessary for high-volume administration rates. When administering highly osmolar, sclerotic, or thrombotic IV fluids, most clinicians agree that the catheter tip should be placed near the heart in the superior or inferior vena cava, although optimal placement has not been established in prospective human studies [6].

Short-term (less than 2 weeks) transcutaneous catheters are constructed of polyethylene, polyurethane, polycarbonate, vinyl chloride, or silicone and are available in multiple lengths, diameters, and lumen numbers. Short-term transcutaneous catheters are suitable for most obstetric patients in the "difficult access" group (i.e. history of IV drug abuse, IV chemotherapy, hypovolemia) and for others with rapidly resolvable clinical conditions. Because of the intended short duration of use, sites on the lower extremities, such as pedal, saphenous, and femoral veins, might be selected; however, decreased mobility and increased risk of catheter dislodgement are among the disadvantages of lower-extremity access locations.

Long-term (weeks to months) transcutaneous catheters are usually constructed of more flexible and less thrombogenic derivatives of silicone, and are passed through a subcutaneous tunnel between the points of venous insertion and exit from the skin [7,8]. Frequently, these catheters incorporate a Dacron cuff just proximal to the skin exit site. Catheter tunneling and the Dacron cuff promote tissue ingrowth and fixation and limit the spread of skin exit-site colonization or infection. Long-term catheters may incorporate a Groshong valve tip [9,10]. Such catheters are blind-ended, but incorporate a side slit near the catheter tip. Positive pressure exerted through the catheter blows the slit walls open outwardly for fluid or medication administration, while negative pressure draws the slit walls inward for blood sampling. At rest,

Critical Care Obstetrics, 5th edition. Edited by M. Belfort, G. Saade, M. Foley, J. Phelan and G. Dildy.

Table 10.1 Advantages of vascular access in the critically ill obstetric patient.

Vascular access site	Advantages
Artery	Continued access for: blood pressure monitoring frequent arterial sampling
Central venous	Rapid fluid and blood administration Hemodynamic monitoring

Table 10.2 Indications for prolonged venous access

Parenteral nutrition and drug therapy
Hyperemesis gravidarum
Inflammatory bowel disease
Gastroparesis
Pancreatitis
Cystic fibrosis
Short bowel syndrome
Heparin (heart valves, deep vein thrombosis)
Antibiotics (bacterial endocarditis, osteomyelitis)
Chemotherapeutic agents for malignancy
Magnesium sulfate
Lack of peripheral access
Previous intravenous drug abuse
Previous prolonged chemotherapy
Hemodialysis

the catheter is closed, theoretically obviating the need for heparinization between periods of catheter use. Venous sites commonly used for long-term catheter use include the subclavian, external and internal jugular, basilic, and greater saphenous veins. When the femoral, greater saphenous, or basilic veins are used, the catheter is tunneled to allow for port placement onto the lower chest, abdominal wall, thigh or forearm [11].

Peripherally inserted central venous catheters (PICCs), introduced in 1975 [12], are increasingly popular due to the ease of insertion compared with traditionally placed surgical catheters (e.g. Hickman ports, central venous ports) with potentially fewer complications [13].

Totally implantable venous access systems (TIVAs), generically known as portacath, utilize catheters attached to reservoirs placed into subcutaneous pockets. These systems are indicated for very long-term use (months to years), typically in patients requiring intermittent medications. During catheter use, the reservoir is accessed with the use of a special Huber-point needle that uses a non-coring tip. Though surgical insertion is required for implantable catheters, the early and late complications associated with venous access are reduced with implantable catheters [14]. Ideally, reservoirs for implantable catheters should be placed in a secure, flat, non-mobile area, preferably overlying a rib.

Arterial catheters should be used for specific purposes and for short time intervals. Arteries that are accessible to palpation and that can usually be cannulated include (in order of preference) the radial, dorsalis pedis, femoral, axillary, and brachial. In general, for an artery to be suitable for continuous monitoring of intraarterial pressures: (i) the diameter should be large enough to accommodate the catheter without occluding the lumen; (ii)

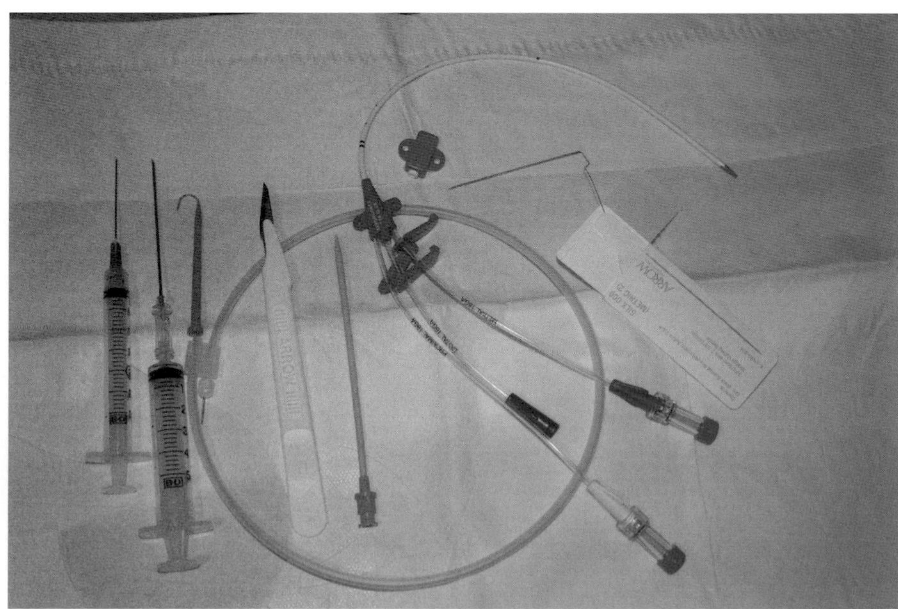

Figure 10.1 Multilumen catheter insertion set-up. From left to right: small finder needle, larger needle, guidewire, scalpel, dilator, triple lumen catheter, anchor and suture.

Table 10.3 Central venous catheter types.

Type	Short term	Long term	Implantable
Location	Transcutaneous	Transcutaneous	Subcutaneous
Duration	Less than 2 weeks	4 weeks or longer	Months to years
Venous site	Peripheral Pedal Saphenous Femoral	Central Subclavian External jugular Internal jugular Cephalic Facial Saphenous Femoral	Same as central long term. Huber point needle required for access to reservoir
Material	Polyethylene, polyurethane, vinyl chloride, silicone	Silicone	
Cuff	No cuff	Dacron	
Lumen	Varies		Single/double
Indication	Difficult access	Chronic illness	Chronic illness
Risks/benefits	Dislodgement of catheter Decreased patient mobility		Increased patient mobility
Tip	Open	Groshong valve	

there should be adequate collateral circulation; (iii) the site should be such that catheter care can be facilitated; and (iv) the site should not be prone to contamination.

Preparing for catheter insertion

Before cannulation of any vessel, it is necessary to assure patency of the vessel. Contraindications to vessel cannulation include infection or inflammation at the site, arterial–venous or aneurysmal malformations, and arterial graft. Coagulopathy is a relative contraindication to cannulation. In the presence of coagulopathy, the use of Doppler to identify the location of vessels reduces complications. Catheter insertion has been demonstrated in 242 patients with corrected coagulopathy and 88 with uncorrected coagulopathy. In these cases, most bleeding after cannulation was controlled with a suture at the catheter insertion site, and the only variable significantly associated with a bleeding complication was a platelet count $<50 \times 10^9$/L (P = 0.02) [15]. In addition, local pressure and use of topical thrombin spray may be used to control peripheral but not central bleeding.

Skin preparation

Cutaneous antisepsis is paramount. This includes but is not limited to handwashing, education of personnel, and the use of sterile technique to include large sterile drape, gown and gloves [16–19]. Antiseptic agents that reduce skin microflora for skin preparation include alcohol, iodine, chlorhexidine gluconate, and hexachlorophene. Alcohol has a broad spectrum of antibacterial activity but has no detergent action, and therefore may not work well on dirty skin [20,21]. The most popular antiseptic agents are chlorhexidine gluconate and the povidone-iodine preparation betadine. Betadine is a water-soluble complex of iodine with a carrier molecule. Iodine is slowly released from the carrier molecule, thus reducing any irritating effects. Due to this slow release, the preparation should be left in contact with the skin for at least 2 minutes [20–22]. In one study, a 2% aqueous solution of chorhexidine gluconate demonstrated superior antiseptic properties compared to 10% providone-iodine and 70% alcohol [16]. However, different concentrations of chorhexidine gluconate may not have the same efficacy. Shaving at catheter insertion sites is not recommended as it abrades the skin and promotes bacterial colonization. If hair removal is necessary, it should be clipped.

After the catheter has been inserted and secured, a dressing should be placed over the site. Gauze or transparent dressings may be used as both approaches have similar rates of catheter-related infection.

Catheterization techniques – general

Three catheterization techniques are available to obtain vascular access: direct, modified and classic Seldinger techniques. The direct approach involves palpation and direct needle puncture, usually with the advancement of a Teflon catheter over the needle and into the vessel. The Seldinger [23] technique involves the use of a guidewire. This approach is used to replace the needle during percutaneous arteriography. Once the vessel has been punctured and the return of blood flow (pulsatile in cases of arterial puncture) is achieved, needle advancement ceases and a fine, flexible wire is inserted through the needle and into the lumen of the vessel. The sharp needle is then removed and a polyurethane-type catheter is threaded over the wire and into the vessel. Commercially produced catheters that incorporate an integral guidewire and employ the modified Seldinger technique are also available. Beards and associates [24] compared these three insertion techniques in 69 critically ill patients. The direct puncture technique was associated with the highest failure rate, followed by the modified and classic Seldinger techniques, respectively. The direct puncture technique also took significantly longer, used more catheters, and required more punctures per successful insertion than did the modified or classic Seldinger techniques. These authors also observed that polyurethane catheters were significantly less likely to block and require reinsertion than were the Teflon catheters. As a result, they strongly endorsed use of the classic Seldinger technique and polyurethane catheters.

During catheterization, proper positioning of the patient is important. The patient should be in the Trendelenburg position and rolled slightly to the left in the later stages of pregnancy when the inferior vena cava is susceptible to compression by the enlarged uterus. If the patient is intolerant of the Trendelenburg position, the legs can be raised. Local anesthetic is infiltrated into the site for needle insertion, incisions or dissection for subcutaneous pockets. After venous puncture, the syringe is removed carefully, while the operator covers the needle hub to prevent excessive bleeding and entry of air. Covering the needle hub is especially important with central venous punctures. With the Seldinger technique a guidewire is placed through the needle, and the needle is withdrawn. Next, a stiff dilator is generally threaded over the wire and passed one or more times in order to dilate the tract to the vein, after which a dilator–catheter assembly is threaded over the wire into correct position, and the wire and dilator are removed. Correct placement is supported by confirming free aspiration of blood from the catheter and free flow (by gravity alone) of an appropriate crystalloid solution through the catheter.

Long-term transcutaneous catheters are generally placed using a peel-away sheath modification of the Seldinger technique. After dilation of the tract, a dilator–sheath assembly is advanced over the wire into the chosen vein, and the wire and dilator are removed. A Silastic catheter is then threaded through the peel-away sheath. Upon proper positioning, the handles on the peel-away sheath are rotated perpendicular to its long axis until the sheath cracks. Pulling the sheath handles apart, the sheath is then simultaneously peeled in half along its long axis and removed while the catheter is carefully held in place.

In cases of arterial cannulation, successful line placement can be confirmed by the appearance of pulsatile blood flow or, if any doubt exists, by blood gas analysis. Vessels suitable for cannulation include radial, femoral, brachial, axillary, dorsal pedis and superficial temporal arteries. For blood pressure monitoring, the catheter is connected to a transducer with a three-way stopcock and high-pressure tubing which is connected to a pressure bag containing normal saline and heparin (1500 U/500 mL). The high-pressure tubing is necessary to prevent damping of blood pressure readings. The heparinized saline is administered through the pressurized bag at a rate of approximately 2–5 mL/h to prevent the catheter from clotting off. It is critically important to purge all pressure lines and stopcocks before connecting the arterial line to prevent arterial air embolism. All set-ups should also have a purge or flush device that can be used to clear any blood that may back up into the pressure tubing as well as to clear the catheter itself and the stopcock after blood sampling. Complications of arterial cannulation include vessel spasm, infection, thrombosis, bleeding, and hematoma.

Special techniques for catheter insertion

Several authors have described utilizing real-time ultrasound to facilitate the location of a vein and to lessen the incidence of mechanical complications related to central catheter insertion [25,26]. The use of ultrasound during the central venous access placement, particularly in difficult patients, is becoming more commonplace. The placement of the transducer in the area of interest, whether internal jugular (Figure 10.2) or femoral, facilitates identification of the venous vessel. The dramatic enlargement of the superior vena cava during a Valsalva maneuver readily identifies the enlarged and yet compressible venous vessel as compared to the non-compressible, pulsating artery.

Schummer et al. conducted a study demonstrating a mechanical complication rate of 12% during catheter insertion using the Seldinger technique [27]. The complications encountered by this experienced group included inadvertent arterial puncture, pneumothorax, malposition, and failed cannulation. Ultrasound has the potential to decrease this complication rate. Fluoroscopic guidance has also been reported to be of assistance with catheter placement. Finally, right arterial electrocardiography can be used to facilitate proper catheter tip placement [6].

Complications – general

A wide range of immediate and delayed complications can be associated with central venous and arterial catheters (Tables 10.4 & 10.5). Specific complications related to catheter use are discussed individually within each subsection.

Catheter malposition

Catheter malposition can be a complication of any vascular cannulation. Optimal catheter tip location has not been established via prospective human studies but most practitioners believe the superior vena cava, proximal to the right atrium, to be the ideal location [6]. Catheter tips located in smaller, more proximal veins are more likely to be associated with venous thrombosis and stenosis, while catheter tips positioned in the heart may be associated with cardiac arrhythmias, perforation, tamponade, valvular injury, or endocarditis. PICC catheter tip malpositioning from an

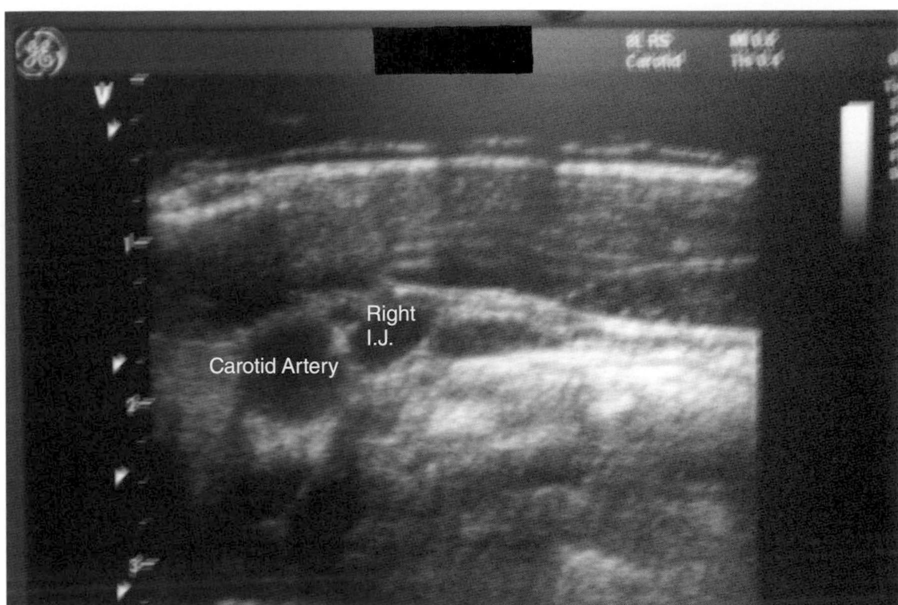

Figure 10.2 Ultrasound image of the IJV. The IJV can be visualized beneath the sternocleidomastoid muscle and adjacent to the carotid artery.

Table 10.4 Complications of central venous catheters.

Immediate	Delayed
Insertion failure	Venous thrombosis
Malposition	Pulmonary embolism
Air embolism	Superior vena caval syndrome
Catheter embolism	Venous stenosis
Cardiac arrhythmia	Arteriovenous fistula
Pneumothorax	Arterial pseudoaneurysm
Hemothorax	Catheter thrombosis
Hydrothorax/chylothorax	Catheter dislodgement/breakage
Tracheal/esophageal injury	Catheter-related infection
Femoral nerve injury	Endocarditis
Brachial plexus injury	Cardiac perforation
Phrenic nerve injury	Cardiac tamponade
Vagus nerve injury	Suppurative thrombophlebitis
Recurrent laryngeal nerve injury	Clavicular osteomyelitis
Stellate ganglion injury	

Table 10.5 Complications of arterial catheters.

Hematoma
Hemorrhage
Catheter occlusion
Catheter dislocation
Infection
Embolism
Ischemic injury
Thrombosis
Pseudoaneurysm
Arteriovenous fistula

antecubital approach is the most frequently seen with a rate of 21–55% [28]. Among the most devastating consequences of catheter malposition is cardiac tamponade. This uncommon yet potentially catastrophic complication must be considered after insertion of all central catheters. Postinsertion chest radiographs are universally recommended, with possibly the exception of the image-guided central venous catheter insertion [29–32]. These radiographic studies should demonstrate midline placement of the catheter tip in the center of the SVC, and not abutting the arterial or ventricular wall.

Thrombosis, stenosis and occlusion

Thrombosis of the great veins is frequently asymptomatic and therefore under-recognized and under-reported [33]. In SCV catheterization, the complication is clinically diagnosed with a frequency of less than 5%, but is diagnosed by contrast venography in 20–40% of patients [29]. Thrombosis appears to be related to several factors. The first consideration is the relative diameters of the catheters and vessel. Generally, the smaller the diameter of the catheter relative to the vessel size, the lower the incidence of thrombosis. Additional factors include duration of use, catheter material, shape of catheter tip, number of cannulation attempts, low cardiac output, hypotension, use of vasopressors, peripheral vaso-occlusive processes, and Raynaud's disease [24,34].

Catheter occlusion can result from the formation of a fibrin plug at the catheter tip. This is part of a fibrin sleeve that forms around essentially all IV catheters present for more than a week [29,35].

When withdrawing blood samples, the dead space in the system should be appreciated, and a sufficient quantity of blood to account for this should be withdrawn and discarded before actual specimen collection. It also is very important to purge the system after specimen collection, lest the line clot off. Clots adherent to the catheter tip, or even the vessel lumen, can be dislodged during flushing. Flushing protocols, with and without heparin, have been devised to reduce catheter thrombosis [33,36]. The use of a fibrinolytic agent administered through the catheter has also been shown to be successful in reopening thrombosed catheters [37–41]. Additional treatment of catheter-related deep vein thrombosis may also involve catheter removal [42,43].

Embolism

Air embolism is a rare but potentially fatal complication of central venous catheters with an estimated incidence of less than 1% but with a mortality rate as high as 50%. If the air embolus is of the magnitude of 50 mL or greater, the outcome is more likely to be fatal. Symptoms of an air embolus can include seizures, hemiparesis, and focal neurologic signs. An air embolus may be reduced by aspirating through the central line or placing the patient in Trendelenburg and in the left lateral decubitus position in the hopes of containing the air in the right ventricle until other measures can be enacted. In stable patients, treatment can be supportive and include administration of 100% oxygen. Rewiring central venous catheters can also be particularly hazardous. Attention to technique and position must also be employed during this seemingly innocuous procedure.

Vesely [44] reviewed complications for 11 583 central venous catheter insertions. Air embolism only occurred in 15 cases, the majority of which had undetectable, mild, or moderate symptoms that resolved with supplemental oxygen. Only one case in their series was fatal.

Specific venous access sites

Internal jugular vein (IJV)

The IJV is located under the sternocleidomastoid muscle (SCM), and, at its junction with the subclavian vein (SCV), helps form the brachiocephalic vein. Anatomic variation in the course of the IJV has been noted, and the relationship between the IJV and the carotid artery may be abnormal in 10% of the population [45]. Typically, when the head is turned away from the intended side of cannulation, the IJV forms a line from the pinna of the ear to the sternoclavicular joint and brings the IJV to a more anterior position relative to the carotid artery [8,46]. The IJV is a common route for central venous access. Its advantages include the ease by which this vessel can be compressed in the case of hemorrhage and the decreased risk of pneumothorax. The right IJV is preferred because the thoracic duct is avoided as well as providing a more direct course to the right atrium [45]. The anatomic relationship of the left IJV to the left brachiocephalic vein makes it difficult to negotiate vessel angles and increases the risk of stenosis and thrombosis.

Two insertion techniques, the median and posterior approaches are available for IJV cannulation. With the median approach the head is turned *away* from the cannulation site with the body maintained in a 20–30° Trendelenburg position. This maintains the head in a "down" position, distending the IJV and minimizing air entrapment. A trianglular region created by two heads of the SCM and the clavicle is then identified (Figure 10.3). The carotid artery is palpated medial to the IJV and medial and posterior to the SCM and is retracted medially. An 18-gauge cannulating needle, attached to a syringe, is inserted at the apex of the triangle, bevel facing up, and at a 30–45° angle to the skin (Figure 10.4). The needle is advanced toward the ipsilateral nipple. If the vein is not encountered by a depth of 5 cm, the needle is withdrawn 4 cm and advanced again in a more lateral direction. When a vessel is entered a flash of blood is noted at the catheter hub. If the blood is pulsating, you have entered the carotid artery. In this situation, remove the needle and tamponade the area for 5–10 minutes. When the carotid artery has been punctured, no further attempts should be made on either side because puncture of both arteries can have serious consequences.

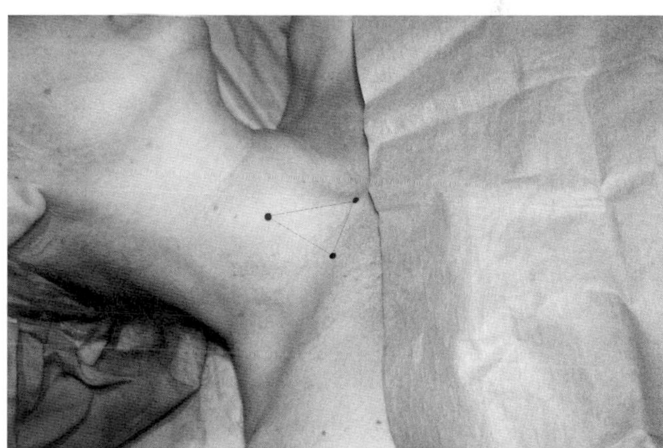

Figure 10.3 Positioning for internal jugular vein cannulation. The head is turned away from the insertion site. A triangle is formed by the junction of the heads of the SCM at the apex, and their insertions at the clavicle.

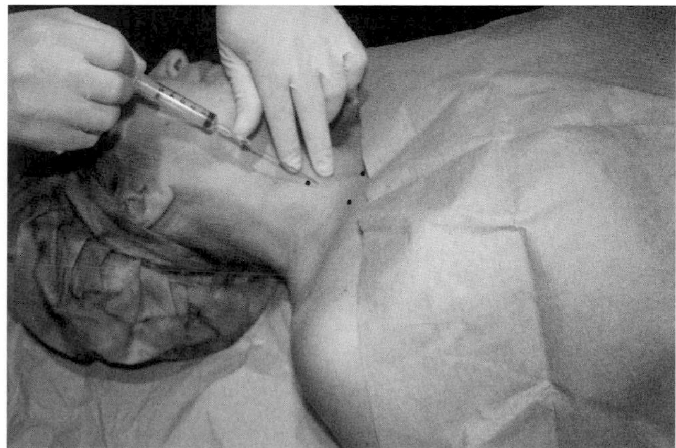

Figure 10.4 Anterior approach to internal jugular vein cannulation. The carotid artery is palpated and retracted medially while the needle is inserted at the tip of the triangle and advanced toward the ipsilateral nipple.

With the posterior approach, the body position is the same but the physician should plan an insertion site 1 cm superior to the point where the external jugular vein (EJV) crosses over the lateral edge of the SCM. In the posterior approach, the needle is then inserted at the 3 o'clock position, with the bevel up, and is advanced along the underbelly of the SCM and then aimed toward the SCM at its sternal insertion and the suprasternal notch (Figure 10.5). The IJV should be encountered 5–6 cm from the skin surface with this approach. If the advancing attempt does not produce a flash of blood in the hub of the needle, applying slow continuous negative pressure while withdrawing the needle potentiates identification of venous blood, thus identifying the vein. However, the absence of pulsatile blood flow does not necessarily ensure venous access has been achieved. Ideally, a pressure wave should be transduced to confirm a venous waveform [45,47].

In addition to the previously described approaches, tunneled central venous catheters have also been described using the IJV versus the SCV. The IJV approach was easier to perform with fewer complications [48]. Complications of IJV cannulation include hematoma, carotid artery puncture, nerve damage, air embolus, and cardiac tamponade.

As previously noted, ultrasound guidance for vessel location is favored by many physicians. Investigations utilizing ultrasound guidance for access of the IJV provide the most compelling evidence in support of this approach. Karakitsos et al. [49] performed a prospective randomized trial of 900 subjects, evaluating cannulation of the IJV using ultrasound guidance versus standard landmark methods. After controlling for multiple factors, real-time ultrasound-guided catheter insertion of the IJV was significantly associated with reductions in carotid puncture hematoma, hemothorax, pneumothorax, catheter-related infection, access time from skin to vein and number of attempts when compared to standard landmark methods.

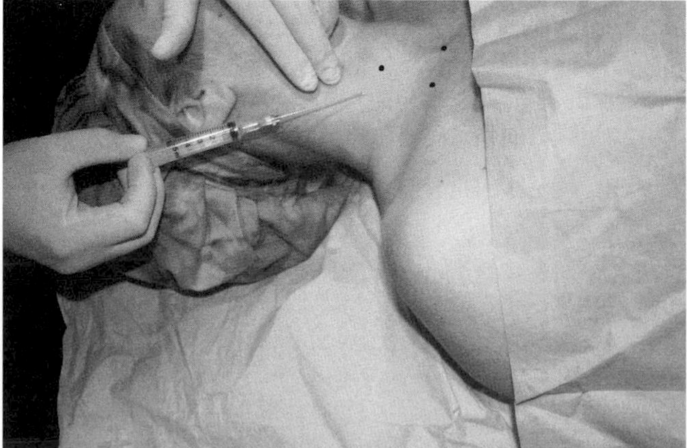

Figure 10.5 Posterior approach to internal jugular vein cannulation. In the posterior approach the needle is advanced along the underbelly of the SCM aiming at the suprasternal notch.

Neurologic complications are rare, but have been documented in association with IJV catheterization. The close anatomic relationship between the lower brachial plexus and the IJV can contribute to the potential for nerve damage, and is more commonly associated with a traumatic cannulation attempt [50].

External jugular vein (EJV)

The EJV is formed by the junction of the retromandibular and posterior auricular veins. It runs obliquely across the SCM along a line extending from the angle of the jaw to mid-clavicle. The EJV joins the SCV at an acute angle under the area of the clavicle [46]. The primary advantage of using the EJV for venous access is the decreased risk of pneumothorax. The disadvantages include difficulty in advancing a catheter, and vein perforation due to the acute angle with the SCV.

The patient is placed supine or in the Trendelenburg position and the head is turned *away* from the side of insertion. The vein can best be identified by applying pressure just above the clavicle and allowing the vein to engorge. Unfortunately, even under the best of conditions, 15% of patients will not have an identifiable EJV [51]. Once identified, the vein should be stabilized between the thumb and forefinger at a level midway between the clavicle and jaw and the catheter inserted with the bevel up. The length of the catheter should not exceed 15 cm. Undue force at the time of catheter insertion can result in perforation of the EJV at the angle in which is enters the SCV. Manipulation of the shoulder may facilitate passage of the J-wire past the clavicle without asserting undue pressure [52]. In addition, upon meeting resistance at the EJV-SCV junction, the J-wire can be withdrawn approximately 0.5 cm proximal to the junction. The triple-lumen catheter may then be slowly advanced over the J-wire. The success of this maneuver may lie in the smaller diameter of the catheter tip [53,54]. Complications of EJV cannulation include thrombosis, superior vena cava perforation, and hydrothorax [47,55].

Subclavian vein (SCV)

The SCV is often used to gain central access. As a continuation of the axillary vein, the course of the SCV runs underneath the clavicle and along the outer surface of the anterior scalene muscle. At the level of the thoracic inlet, the SCV joins the IJV to form the brachiocephalic vein [8,46]. To cannulate the vein, the patient is placed in the supine position, maintaining a 15% Trendelenburg position, with the head *facing toward* the site of insertion and the arms pronated, slightly flexed, and down at the sides. One helpful approach for catheter insertion is to place a rolled towel under the spine and shoulder. This type of positioning serves to widen the path between the first rib and the clavicle. Next, the operator should visualize the path of the subclavian artery divided into medial, middle, and lateral thirds along the clavicular line (Figure 10.6). Using this method, the junction of the medial and middle segment approximates the lateral aspect of the SCM insertion on the clavicle. Using this point for needle insertion may decrease the risk for pneumothorax. The bevel should initially be pointing upward. The catheter tip is "walked" along the underside of the

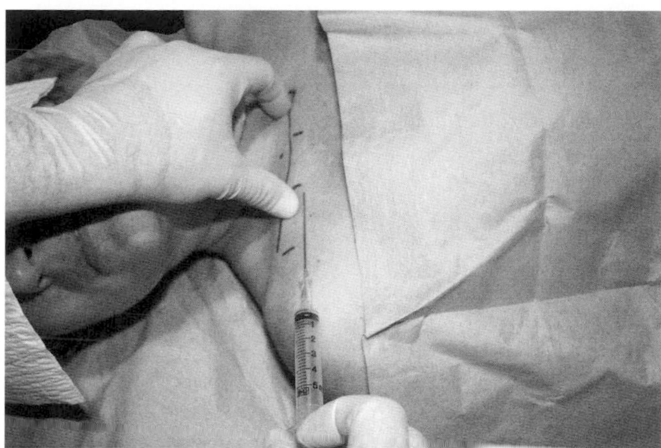

Figure 10.6 Landmarks for subclavian vein cannulation. Using the clavicle, the subclavian vein is divided into thirds. The junction of the middle and medial third identifies the location for needle insertion.

clavicle touching the bone itself as needed, pointing toward the suprasternal notch and parallel to the patient's back. Upon entering the vein, the bevel is turned to the 3 o'clock position to facilitate passing the catheter.

Immediate risks of SCV cannulation include pneumothorax, hemothorax, and catheter misplacement. The most common of these complications is pneumothorax with an incidence of 1–6%. Pneumothorax is primarily associated with direct subclavian or jugular vein catheterization. Collin and Clarke [56] reviewed the occurrence of delayed or late pneumothorax (48–72 h) following central venous catheterization and recommended that postinsertion chest radiographs be expiratory and upright. Expiration results in a decreased volume of air in the lung but not in the pleural space thus magnifying the radiographic appearance of the pneumothorax [57]. Finally, repeat or delayed chest radiographs are indicated following catheterizations requiring multiple attempts, persistent (pleuritic or back) pain and respiratory symptoms. The standard treatment for pneumothorax has traditionally consisted of placement of a thoracostomy tube. However in an investigation by Laronga [58], pneumothorax was managed by observation alone and/or the insertion of a pigtail catheter (8.5 French) with a Heimlich valve in the outpatient setting. Also, in spontaneous breathing patients who have developed a small pneumothorax, the use of 100% oxygen therapy for 60 minutes may denitrogenate and attenuate the pneumothorax, thus averting chest tube insertion.

Hemothorax is an infrequent complication of direct SCV catheterization. Because intrathoracic vascular structures are inaccessible for direct compression, subclavian and, to a lesser degree, IJV direct venous catheterization are contraindicated in patients with a coagulopathy.

A common location for misplacement of the catheter is in the ipsilateral IJV. Misplacement is most often detected by radiographic studies. Another technique has been described using the IJV occlusion test [59]. The occlusion test is performed by applying external pressure on the IJV in the supraclavicular area for 10 seconds. During the application of pressure, the central venous pressure and waveform were observed. In all cases of catheter misplacement into the IJV, the central venous pressure increased 3–5 mmHg. If the misplaced catheter was in another vessel, the central venous pressure did not change with this maneuver.

An attempt to compare IJV, SCV and femoral vein sites for subsequent thrombosis, stenosis and infection suggested that the SCV site is less often associated with infection, mechanical complications and thrombosis compared to the other sites [60].

Femoral vein

From lateral to medial, the femoral nerve, artery and vein traverse the femoral triangle by descending beneath the inguinal ligament [46]. The femoral vein can be located 1–2 cm medial to the palpated femoral artery pulse. If the femoral artery cannot be palpated, the location of the femoral vein can be estimated by imagining a line from the anterior superior iliac crest to the pubic tubercle and then dividing the line into equal thirds. The femoral artery lies at the junction of the middle and most medial segment and the femoral vein can be estimated as 1–2 cm medial to this point (Figure 10.7). The skin is punctured 2–3 cm caudal to the inguinal ligament to ensure the vein is cannulated in the area of the thigh. A catheter at least 15 cm in length can then be inserted into the femoral vein by directing the tip toward the vein at a 45° angle to the skin. Once in the vein, the angle of the catheter may be placed more parallel to the skin surface in order to align with the lumen of the vessel.

The advantage of using the femoral vein is its large size and the absence of risk of pneumothorax; however, cannulation is generally not recommended for cardiopulmonary resuscitation or in the presence of bleeding disorders [8]. Complications of femoral vein cannulation include arterial puncture, hematoma, bleeding, local inflammation, malposition of catheters tip, and thrombosis [61].

Cephalic vein

In its course away from the axillary vein, the cephalic vein travels below the clavipectoral fascia in the deltopectoral groove and descends down the lateral aspect of the arm [46]. The cephalic vein is most often used for central venous access via surgical cutdown.

Specific arterial access sites

Radial artery

The brachial artery divides into the radial and ulnar arteries in the forearm. The radial artery is a favored site for arterial cannulation due to its superficial location medial to the styloid process. The ulnar artery parallels the radial artery. Together, the radial and ulnar arteries form anastomosing palmar arches supplying blood to the hands [46]. Prior to cannulation of the radial artery, adequacy of collateral circulation must be established. The Allen

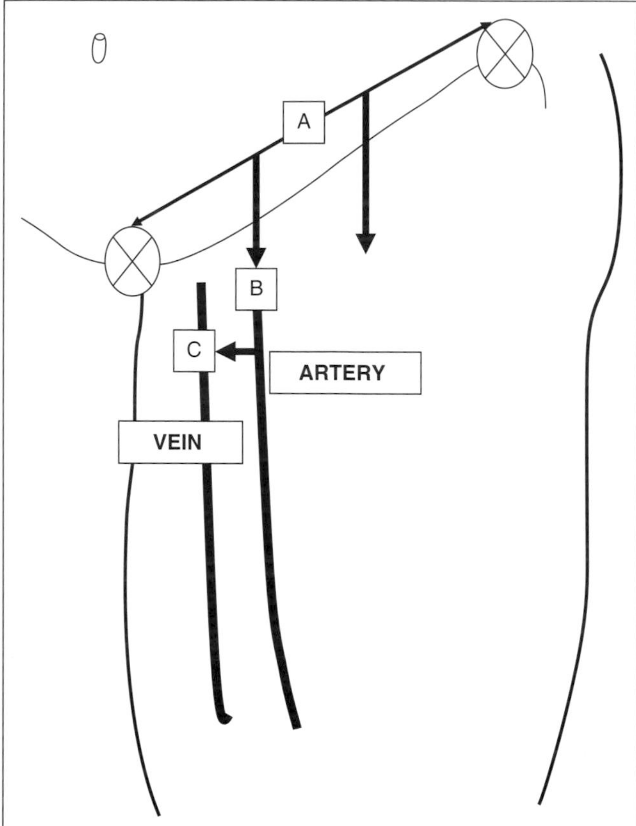

Figure 10.7 Estimating femoral vein location. When the femoral arterial pulsations cannot be appreciated, the location of the femoral vein can be estimated. (a) Draw a line from the anterior superior iliac crest to the public tubercle and (b) divide into equal thirds. The junction of the medial and middle segment approximates the femoral artery and the vein will lie 2–3 cm more medial (c).

test can be used in an attempt to document the adequacy of collateral flow. Even so, progressive delayed ischemia of the hand may occur, requiring amputation [62]. Blanching of the skin may occur with flushing of the catheter and indicate interference with skin circulation. In cases of radial line-induced ischemia where perfusion to the hand has been compromised, we have successfully used a stellate ganglion block to promote vasodilation and return perfusion to near necrotic fingers.

Allen test

The Allen test is performed in the following manner.

1 The radial and ulnar arteries are occluded simultaneously.

2 Continuing this occlusion, the patient elevates the hand above his or her head.

3 He or she repeatedly makes a fist until the hand blanches.

4 The pressure on the ulnar artery is then released.

The palm should regain its normal color within 6 seconds. Delay of color from 7 to 15 seconds indicates that ulnar artery filling is slow. Persistent blanching for up to 15 seconds or more indicates an incomplete or occluded ulnar arch. Failure to regain normal color promptly is presumptive evidence of inadequate collateral flow, and the radial artery should not be cannulated. In performing this test, care is taken not to hyperextend the wrist, which could falsely compromise ulnar flow.

Once adequate collateral circulation has been determined, preparation for cannulation of the radial artery can be undertaken. The wrist is dorsiflexed slightly to optimize exposure of the artery. This is best accomplished by use of an arm board and placement of a small gauze roll beneath the dorsal surface of the wrist, with tape placed across the patient's palm and upper forearm. When taping the upper forearm, care is taken not to constrict blood flow. Alternatively, an assistant may hold the patient's arm in place, but access to the puncture site is often obstructed in so doing. Once positioned, the area is prepped and anesthetized as described previously. We prefer using a 20–22-gauge Angiocath. The needle is advanced at a 30° angle to the artery until a flash of blood appears in the hub. If using the direct puncture technique, the angle of the needle is then slightly lowered and the catheter advanced while holding the needle stable. This can often be facilitated by rotating the catheter itself backward and forward, in a drilling motion. If the catheter fails to advance easily, the operator should avoid trying to force the catheter because of the risk of traumatic pseudoaneurysm. Often, both walls of the vessel will have been punctured and the catheter will lie posterior to the vessel. If the catheter has been advanced beyond the tip of the metal needle do not advance the needle farther because of the risk of damage to the catheter. Instead, completely remove the needle and then slowly withdraw the catheter until pulsatile flow is established. At that moment, one can gently reattempt to advance the catheter or pass a 25-gauge vascular wire through the catheter, followed by advancement over the wire. If neither of these maneuvers is met with success, the catheter should be removed and discarded. The procedure is then repeated with a new needle and catheter.

If the Seldinger technique (or a modification thereof) is used, the needle is advanced until a flash of blood is observed in the hub, after which the guidewire is advanced through the needle until it is 2–3 cm into the artery. The catheter can then be advanced over both guidewire and needle, or the needle can be removed and the catheter advanced over just the guidewire. Once the catheter has been advanced, the guidewire and/or needle are removed, pulsatile flow is established, and the line is secured and connected.

Rarely, cutdown and direct visualization will be required for radial artery catheterization. If a cutdown becomes medically necessary, a 2-cm transverse incision is made 2 cm proximal to the wrist fold, and the vessel is located by blunt dissection with small hemostats. The hemostats should separate the tissue in a plane parallel to the vessel to minimize vessel trauma. Skin hooks are helpful to hold the incision open. The dissection also is guided by intermittent palpation to maintain orientation to the vessel. Once exposed, a 1.0–1.5 cm length of vessel should be cleaned and mobilized, and 2-0 or 3-0 silk sutures are passed beneath the vessel with a right-angle clamp. To assist catheter insertion, one approach is to place one suture proximal and one distal to the site of vessel puncture. The distal suture can be used to elevate the vessel for direct visual puncture. If vessel puncture is not initially successful, traction on the proximal suture will stop the bleeding, providing visualization of the puncture site and thus allowing the catheter to be inserted without the necessity of another puncture. Once catheterized, both sutures are removed (not tied) and the skin is closed. Pressure should be maintained on the cutdown site for 5 or 10 minutes to prevent potential hematoma formation.

Brachial artery

The brachial artery is the continuation of the axillary artery. Collateral circulation is supplied by the ulnar collateral artery. This artery is best isolated just above the elbow crease medial to the biceps tendon. A 20-gauge, 2-inch catheter is inserted at a 30° angle to the skin until blood appears in the hub. The vessel is cannulated by either the direct, modified, or classic Seldinger technique. Use of an arm board prevents flexion at the elbow and kinking of the catheter.

Use of the brachial artery entails greater risks than use of the radial artery. These risks include, but are not limited to, the following: (i) adequacy of collateral circulation is much more difficult to ensure; (ii) embolization could occlude either of the major arterial supplies to the hand; and (iii) bleeding in the area of the median nerve may result in neuropathy and Volkmann's contracture. If bleeding does occur, a fasciotomy may be surgically necessary [63]. Cannulation of the brachial artery should not be attempted in patients with disorders of hemostasis.

Axillary artery

The axillary artery is a continuation of the subclavian artery. It enters the axilla from under the teres major and lies in the proximal groove between the biceps and triceps muscles medially in the arm. This artery is almost as large as the femoral artery and has significant collateral flow. As such, axillary artery thrombosis does not lead to distal ischemia. Since the right axillary artery arises from the right brachiocephalic trunk, which is itself in direct communication with the common carotid artery, air, clot, or particulate matter may embolize the brain during flushing. Thus, it may be safer to use the left axillary artery.

For cannulation, the patient can be positioned either with the palm of the hand beneath the occipital portion of the head or with the arm extended and externally rotated. After the vessel is located by palpation, an 18–20-gauge catheter, measuring at least 5 cm, is inserted into the artery until pulsatile blood is observed in the hub. The angle of insertion should initially be at about a 30° angle to the skin, and once blood return is noted, the angle is lowered for direct advancement or guidewire insertion. Because of the close proximity of the axillary artery and the brachial plexus, hematoma formation in this area could result in nerve compression. Additionally, direct injury to the cords of the brachial plexus may also occur during insertion attempts because of the vessel's relationship with the three cords of the brachial plexus. At this point, these cords form a neurovascular bundle within the axillary sheath. As for brachial cannulation, distal circulation should be checked regularly following axillary arterial line insertion.

Dorsalis pedis artery

The dorsalis pedis artery is located on the dorsal aspect of the foot and is usually easily palpated, but may be absent in 12% of the population. Collateral blood supply is usually good, and ischemia is uncommon following cannulation of this vessel. Collateral circulation, supplied by the lateral plantar artery, can be assessed by compression of the dorsalis pedis artery, followed by pressure on the nail bed of the great toe until it blanches. On release of pressure on the nail bed, color should return within 2–3 seconds.

To facilitate cannulation of the dorsalis pedis artery, hold the patient's foot in a neutral position, and introduce a 20- or 22-gauge needle into the artery at a shallow angle to the skin.

Femoral artery

The femoral artery as an extension of the external iliac artery lies just below the inguinal ligament midway along a line drawn from the superior iliac spine and symphysis pubis just lateral to the vein and medial to the nerve. The usual catheters employed range from 20 to 16 gauge, are 16 cm in length, and are attached to a 10-mL syringe. The needle is inserted about 2 cm below the inguinal ligament and at a 45° angle to the skin. The puncture of the vessel can often be felt by the operator and is heralded by the ability to rapidly aspirate bright red blood. Also, a gloved finger placed over the hub of the needle can usually feel the arterial pulsations. Once the vessel is punctured, the needle is lowered to an angle between 15–30° and a J-tipped guidewire is inserted into the vessel. The needle is removed, and direct pressure is applied to the insertion site to prevent bleeding or hematoma formation. The catheter is placed over the guidewire, but it is not advanced until the distal (external) tip of the guidewire itself has been secured. Care is also taken to ensure that the wire is straight, as any kinks will make passage of the catheter difficult. A scalpel nick of the skin may be required for ease of passage of the catheter through the skin. Once the catheter is in place, the wire is removed and the catheter connected and secured.

A complication peculiar to femoral vessel cannulation is puncture of the back wall of the vessel above the inguinal ligament. The resulting hemorrhage may dissect into the retroperitoneal space masking a hemorrhage of up to several liters. Because of the large size of the femoral artery, vein and the catheters used in these vessels, the chances of an AV fistula is higher than with smaller vessels, especially if both vessels have been penetrated during a single insertion. Similarly, the larger puncture site makes bleeding at the time of line removal an issue. Under these circumstances, pressure should be applied to the femoral site for 10–20 minutes following catheter removal.

Catheter-related infection

Catheter-related infections (CRIs) include exit-site and tunnel infections, catheter-associated bacteremia or sepsis, suppurative thrombophlebitis, endocarditis, and clavicular osteomyelitis. The exact incidence for catheter-related bloodstream infections (CRBSIs) is difficult to determine due to a number of factors. However, it is estimated that 80 000 cases occur annually in intensive care units alone; and, of these, there is a potential mortality rate of 35% [16]. Factors contributing to CRI include type of catheter and catheter material, number of insertion attempts, duration, location, type of dressing, experience of personnel, indication for catheter insertion and virulence of the infecting organism [16,64,65]. Upper extremity locations for catheter insertions are less often associated with infection compared with those inserted in the lower extremities. Coagulase-negative *Staphylococcus*, followed by *Enterococcus* and *Staphlococcus aureus* are the organisms most commonly associated with catheter-related bloodstream infection. Unfortunately, antibiotic resistance is also more frequently encountered with these organisms.

Catheter-related bloodstream infection is suspected clinically when signs of infection at the exit site are seen (e.g. erythema, tenderness, purulent drainage) or systemic signs of infection (e.g. fever, rigors, fluid sequestration, rising peripheral WBC count) are noted, particularly in patients lacking another likely source of infection. Historically, when signs of catheter-related bloodstream infection became manifest, the catheter was removed for culture of the catheter tip. Unfortunately, many catheter tip cultures returned as negative and only a small percentage of infections could actually be linked to the catheter. Catheter lumen colonization is a prerequisite to CRBSI. This knowledge has prompted the development of *in situ* techniques to determine catheter colonization and possibly avoid catheter removal.

Such techniques include the following.

1 Superficial, semiquantitative culture from the skin at the exit site and the catheter hub. A dry cotton swab is used to sample a 3-cm area around the exit site, and another dry cotton swab is introduced into the catheter hub.

2 Paired quantitative blood cultures from the peripheral blood and catheter. Peripheral blood (10 mL) is obtained and distributed into aerobic and anerobic culture media followed by blood from the catheter (10 mL from each lumen) which is likewise distributed.

3 Differential time to positivity of simultaneous samples from peripheral blood and the catheter hub. Again, 10 mL is obtained, simultaneously from the peripheral blood and catheter lumen.

4 Endoluminal brushing of the catheter. This technique was described as useful when blood could not be obtained from the catheter.

The superficial semiquantitative and differential time to positivity are sensitive and specific enough to be considered as first line in detecting CRBSI, while quantitative blood cultures are more difficult and expensive to perform and could be reserved as a confirmatory test when needed. The endoluminal brush seems best reserved for instances where blood cannot be withdrawn from the catheter [66,67].

Catheter removal is also generally recommended in catheterized patients whose presumed catheter-unrelated infections fail to rapidly improve with appropriate treatment. Others have investigated the efficacy of thrombolytic therapy in treating catheter colonization or infection [68].

The Centers for Disease Contol (CDC) have issued guidelines intended to minimize and monitor CRI [16]. These guidelines include, but are not limited to, the following:

- selection of insertion site (subclavian versus femoral)
- strict adherence to aseptic technique at the time of both insertion and dressing change
- changing gauze dressings every 2 days
- changing transparent dressings every 7 days
- not routinely replacing catheters or guidewires with the intent of preventing infection
- creating "catheter teams".

It is recommended that each patient care area that utilizes central catheters maintain a surveillance system whereby infection is documented by specifically using number of CRBSIs per 1000 catheter-days. Documenting infection in this manner can help facilitate interpretation of outcomes between patient care units. In previous studies, antimicrobial/antiseptic impregnated catheters were associated with a reduction in CRBSI [69–72]. However, in its latest recommendation the CDC suggests limiting the use of antimicrobial/antiseptic impregnated catheters to areas of the hospital with unacceptably high CRBSIs rates (in spite of implanting appropriate measures) or to patients expected to have the catheter in place for longer than 5 days. The National Nosocomial Infection Surveillance System (NNISS) compiles hospital data to issue benchmarks for CRBSI rates and these data can be used for comparisons. Though a specific obstetric category is not tracked by the NNISS, data could be extrapolated from Surgical and Medical Teaching categories with pooled mean infections/1000 catheter-days of 5.3.

Creating a surveillance system, standardizing catheter-related education and creating teams vested in catheter care cannot be emphasized enough. Frankel et al. [73] clearly demonstrated the importance of such measures in decreasing the CRBSI in their unit from 11 (well above national benchmarks) to 1.7 per 1000 catheter days by combining corporate performance improvement methodologies, changes in operating procedures, feedback and reviews.

Conclusion

Short- and long-term central venous access is a vital tool in women's healthcare. The proper and safe use of central catheters requires knowledge of indication, meticulous sterile technique, insertion techniques, competence in recognizing and treating complications, maintenance, and surveillance.

Acknowledgement

Special thanks to Maria D. Koutrouvelis for photography.

References

1 Wolk RA. Parenteral nutrition in obstetric patients. *Nutr Clin Pract* 1990; 5: 139.

2 Korelitz BI. Inflammatory bowel disease in pregnancy. *Clin Gastroenterol* 1992; 21: 827.

3 Wiedner LC, Fish J, Talabiska DG et al. Total parenteral nutrition in pregnant patient with hyperemesis gravidarum. *Nutrition* 1993; 9: 446.

4 Stewart R, Tuazon D, Olson GL, Duarte AG. Pregnancy and primary pulmonary hypertension: Successful outcome with prostacyclin therapy. *Chest* 2001; 119: 973–975.

5 De la Roche MRP, Gauthier L. Rapid transfusion of packed red blood cells: effects of dilution, pressure, and catheter size. *Ann Emerg Med* 1993; 22: 1551–1555.

6 McGee WT, Ackerman BL, Rouben LR et al. Accurate placement of central venous catheters: a prospective, randomized, multicenter trial. *Crit Care Med* 1993; 21: 1118.

7 Ray S, Stacey R, Imrie M, Filshie J. A review of 560 Hickman catheter insertions. *Anaesthesia* 1996; 51: 981.

8 Marino P. *The ICU Book*, 2nd edn. Williams & Wilkins, 1998.

9 Pasquale MD, Campbell JM, Magnant CM. Groshong versus Hickman catheters. *Surg Gynecol Obstet* 1992; 174: 408.

10 Delmore JE, Horbelt DV, Jack BL et al. Experience with the Groshung long-term central venous catheter. *Gynecol Oncol* 1989; 34: 216.

11 D'Angelo FA, Ramacciato G, Aurello P et al. Alternative insertion sites for permanent central venous access devices. *Eur J Surg Oncol* 1997; 23: 547–549.

12 Hoshal VL Jr. Total intravenous nutrition with peripherally inserted silicone elastomer central venous catheters. *Arch Surg* 1975; 110: 644.

13 Horattas MC, Trupiano J, Hopkins S et al. Changing concepts in long-term central venous access: catheter selection and cost savings. *Am J Infect Control* 2001; 29: 32.

14 Di Carlo I, Cordio S, Le Greca G, Privitera G et al. Totally implantable venous access devices implanted surgically: a retrospective study on early and late complications. *Arch Surg* 2001; 136: 1050–1053.

15 Mumtaz H, Williams V, Hauer-Jensen M et al. Central venous catheter placement in patients with disorders of hemostasis. *Am J Surg* 2000; 180: 503–505.

16 O'Grady NP, Alexander M, Dellinger EP et al. Guidelines for the prevention of intravascular catheter-related infections. *MMWR* 2002; 51: 1–29.

17 Parras F, Ena J, Bouza E et al. Impact of an educational program for the prevention of colonization of intravascular catheters. *Infect Control Hosp Epidemiol* 1994; 15: 239.

18 Puntis JWL, Holden CE, Finkel Y et al. Staff training: a key factor in reducing intravascular catheter sepsis. *Arch Dis Child* 1990; 65: 335.

19 Raad II, Hohn DC, Gilbreath BJ et al. Prevention of central venous catheter-related infections by using maximal sterile barrier precautions during insertion. *Infect Control Hosp Epidemiol* 1994; 15: 231.

20 Larson EL. Guidelines for use of topical antimicrobial agents. APIC Guidelines for Infection Control Practice. *Am J Infect Control* 1988; 16: 253–266.

21 Wyatt WJ, Beckett TA, Bonet V, Davis SM. Comparative efficacy of surgical scrub solutions on control of skin microflora. *Infect Surg* 1990; 9: 17–21.

22 Sheikh W. Comparative antibacterial efficacy of Hibiclens and Betadine in the presence of pus derived from human wounds. *Curr Ther Res* 1986; 40: 1096.

23 Seldinger SI. Catheter replacement of the needle in percutaneous arteriography. *Acta Radiol Diagn* 1953; 39: 368–376.

24 Beards SC, Doedens L, Jackson A, Lipman J. A comparison of arterial lines and insertion techniques in critically ill patients. *Anaesthesia* 1994; 49: 968–973.

25 Denys BG, Uretsky BF, Reddy PS et al. An ultrasound method for safe and rapid central venous access. *N Engl J Med* 1991; 324: 566.

26 Sherer DM, Abulafia O, DuBesher B et al. Ultrasonographically guided subclavian vein catheterization in critical care obstetrics and gynecologic oncology. *Am J Obstet Gynecol* 1993; 169: 1246.

27 Schummer W, Schummer C, Rose N et al. Mechanical complications and malpositions of central venous cannulations by experienced operators. A prospective study of 1794 catheterizations in critically ill patients. *Intensive Care Med* 2007; 33: 1055.

28 Goodwin ML, Carlson I. The peripherally inserted central catheter. *J Intravenous Nurs* 1993; 16: 92.

29 Nohr C. Vascular access, in Wilmore DW, Cheung LY, Harken AH, Holcroft JW, Meakins JL (eds): Scientific American Surgery, Surgical Technique Supplement 3. New York, NY, Scientific American, 1994, pp 1–28.

30 Agee KR, Balk RA. Central venous catheterization in the critically ill patient. *Crit Care Clin* 1992; 8: 677.

31 LaFortune S. The use of confirming x-rays to verify tip position for peripherally inserted catheters. *J Intravenous Nurs* 1993; 16: 246.

32 Lucey B, Verghese JC, Haslam P, Lee MJ. Routine chest radiographs after central line insertion: mandatory postprocedural evaluation or unnecessary waste of resources. *Cardiovasc Intervent Radiol* 1999; 22: 381–384.

33 Baranowsky L. Central venous access devices: current technologies, uses, and management strategies. *J Intravenous Nurs* 1993; 16: 167.

34 Kaye A. Invasive monitoring techniques: arteruak cannulation, bedside pulmonary artery catheterization and arterial puncture. *Heart Lung* 1983; 12: 395–427.

35 Lowell JA, Bothe Jr. A. Venous access: preoperative, operative, and postoperative dilemmas. *Surg Clin North Am* 1991; 71: 1231.

36 Fry B. Intermittent heparin flushing protocols. A standardization issue. *J Intravenous Nurs* 1992; 15: 160.

37 Lawson M. Partial occlusion of indwelling central venous catheters. *J Intravenous Nurs* 1991; 14: 157.

38 Wachs T. Urokinase administration in pediatric patients with occluded central venous catheters. *J Intravenous Nurs* 1990; 13: 100.

39 Holcombe BJ, Forloines-Lynn S, Garmhausen LW. Restoring patency of long-term central venous access devices. *J Intravenous Nurs* 7 A.D.; 15: 36.

40 Haire WD, Lieberman RP, Lund GB et al. Obstructed central venous catheters. Restoring function with a 12-hour infusion of low-dose urokinase. *Cancer* 1990; 66: 2279.

41 Atkinson JB, Bagnall HA, Gomperts E. Investigational use of tissue plasminogen activator (τ–PA) for occluded central venous catheters. *JPEN* 1990; 14: 310.
42 Clarke DE, Raffin TA. Infectious complications of in-dwelling long-term central venous catheters. *Chest* 1990; 97: 966.
43 Barclay GR, Allen K, Pennington CR. Tissue plasminogen activator in the treatment of superior vena caval thrombosis associated with parenteral nutrition. *Postgrad Med J* 1991; 66: 398.
44 Vesely TM. Air embolism during insertion of central venous catheters. *J Vasc Interv Radiol* 2001; 12: 1291–1295.
45 Fontes M. Complications of central venous cannulation. *Problems in Anesthesia* 1998; 10: 215–226.
46 Clemente C. *Anatomy: A Regional Atlas of the Human Body*, 4th edn. Lippincott, Williams & Wilkins, Philadelphia, PA, 1997.
47 Ho CM, Lui PW. Bilateral hydrothorax caused by left external jugular venous catheter perforation. *J Clin Anesth* 1994; 6: 243–246.
48 Macdonald S, Watt AJ, McNally D, Edwards RD, Moss JG. Comparison of technical success and outcome of tunneled catheters inserted via the jugular and subclavian approaches. *J Vasc Interv Radiol* 2000; 225.
49 Karakitsos D, Labropoulos N, DeGroot E et al. Real-time ultrasound-guided catheterization of the internal jugular vein: a prospective comparison with the landmark technique in critical care patients. *Crit Care Med* 2006; 10:R162.
50 DeMatteis J. Brachial plexus injury caused by internal jugular cannulation. *Hospital Physician* 1995; 52.
51 Seneff MG. Central venous catheterization. A comprehensive review. *Intensive Care Med* 1987; 40: 1096.
52 Sparks CJ, McSkimming I, George L. Shoulder manipulation to facilitate central vein catheterization from the external jugular vein. *Anaesth Intensive Care* 1991; 19: 567–568.
53 Segura-Vasi A, Suelto M, Boudreaux A. External jugular vein cannulation for central venous access. *Anesth Analg* 1999; 88: 692–693.
54 Belani KG, Buckley JJ, Gordon JR, Castaneda W. Percutaneous cervical central venous line placement: a comparison of the internal and external jugular vein routes. *Anesthesia and Analgesia* 1980; 59: 40–44.
55 Colomina MJ, Godet C, Bago J et al. Isolated thrombosis of the external jugular vein. *Surg Laparosc Percutan Tech* 2000; 10: 264–267.
56 Collin GR, Clarke LE. Delayed pneumothorax: a complication of central venous catheterization. *Surg Rounds* 1994; 17: 589.
57 Tocino IM, Miller MH, Fairfax WR. Distribution of pneumothorax in the supine and semirecumbent critically ill adult. *Am J Roentgenol* 1985; 144: 901–905.
58 Laronga C, Meric F, Truong M et al. A treatment algorithm for pneumothoraces complicating central venous catheter insertion. *Am J Surg* 2000; 180: 523.
59 Ambesh SP, Pandey JC, Dubey PK. Internal jugular vein occlusion test for rapid diagnosis of misplaced subclavian vein catheter into the internal jugular vein. *Anesthesiology* 2001; 95: 1377–1379.
60 Hamilton H, Foxcroft D. Central venous access sites for the prevention of venous thrombosis, stenosis and infection in patients requiring long-term intravenous therapy. *Cochrane Database Syst Rev* 2007; 3.
61 Durbee O, Viviand X, Potie F et al. A prospective evaluation of the use of femoral venous catheters in critically ill adults. *Crit Care Med* 1997; 25: 1943.
62 Mangar D, Laborde RS, Vu DN. Delayed ischaemia of the hand necessitating amputation after radial artery cannulation. *Can J Anaesth* 1993; 40: 247–250.
63 Hudson-Civetta J, Caruthers-Banner TE. Intra-vascular catheters: current guidelines for care and maintenance. *Heart Lung* 1983; 12: 466–476.
64 Egebo K, Toft P, Jakobsen CJ. Contamination of central venous catheters: The skin insertion wand is a major source of contamination. *J Hosp Infect* 1996; 32: 99.
65 Kruse JA, Shah NJ. Detection and prevention of central venous catheter-related infections. *Nutr Clin Pract* 1993; 8: 163.
66 Bouza E, Alvarado N, Alcala L et al. A randomized and prospective study of 3 procedures for the diagnosis of catheter-related bloodstream infection without catheter withdrawal. *CID* 2007; 44: 820.
67 Catton J, Dobbins B, Kite P et al. In situ diagnosis of intravascular catheter-related bloodstream infection: a comparison of quantitative culture, differential time to positivity, and endoluminal brushing. *Crit Care Med* 2005; 33: 787.
68 Fishbein HD, Friedman HS, Bennett BB et al. Catheter-related sepsis refractory to antibiotic treated successfully with adjunctive urokinase infusion. *Pediatr Infect Dis* 1990; 9: 676.
69 Maki DG, Wheeler SJ, Stolz SM et al. Study of a novel antiseptic-coated central venous catheter. *Crit Care Med* 1991; 19: S99.
70 Bach A, Bohrer H, Motsch J et al. Prevention of catheter-related infections by antiseptic coating. *Anesthesiology* 1992; 77: A259.
71 Mimoz O, Pleroni L, Lawrence C et al. Prospective randomized trial of two antiseptic solutions for prevention of central venous catheterization of arterial colonization and infection. *Crit Care Med* 1996; 24: 1818.
72 Rafkin HS, Hoyt JW, Crippen DW. Prevention of certified venous catheter-related infection with a silver-impregnated cuff. *Chest* 1990; 98: 117S.
73 Frankel H, Crede W, Topal J. Use of corporate six sigma performance-improvement strategies to reduce incidence of catheter-related bloodstream infections in a surgical ICU. *Am Coll Surg* 2005; 201: 349.

11 Blood Component Replacement

David A. Sacks
Department of Research, Southern California Permanente Medical Group, Pasadena, CA, USA

Introduction

Transfusion of blood components is a potentially life-saving procedure. Although meticulous care is taken in the selection of blood donors, processing, storage, and transfusion of blood products, serious transfusion-related complications may ensue. It is incumbent on the physician to be sure that a blood product is indicated, and that standard transfusion practices and precautions are observed [1]. This chapter is intended as an aid to understanding the preparation of, indications for, and potential complications of blood components for obstetric critical care.

Blood donation, collection, and storage

Blood donation

The prerequisites for blood donors are stringent, and require that the potential donor be in good health and not have been exposed to drugs which may have a deleterious effect on blood components (e.g. aspirin on platelet function). The donor must also be free of bloodborne bacterial, viral, and protozoal agents as well as not having had sexual contact with those who may be infected with these agents. A partial list of the American Association of Blood Banks' (AABB) requirements for donors is found in Table 11.1. Of note is the response to the 2003 FDA requirement for screening blood for West Nile virus. The bones of contention are that bloodborne West Nile viral infections are infrequent (0.44 per 10 000 donations in 2004 [2]), are of low infectious potential, and require costly testing. A strategy of testing "minipooled" blood samples from several donors during the half of the year when the incidence of infection is low, with individual testing reserved for those contributing to a positive minipool, has been proposed. The proposal includes individual testing during an outbreak [3].

Critical Care Obstetrics, 5th edition. Edited by M. Belfort, G. Saade, M. Foley, J. Phelan and G. Dildy.

Because the recipient is the same person as the donor, the requirements for an autologous donor are less stringent than those for allogeneic donors. Requirements include a hemoglobin of only 11 g/dL, deferral only when there is a possibility of bacteremia in the donor, and that the collection be performed no fewer than 72 hours before the anticipated transfusion [1].

Apheresis is a procedure wherein whole blood is withdrawn from a donor, a liquid (e.g. plasma) or solid (e.g. platelets) portion is retained, and the remainder of the blood reinfused. The time interval between donations is shorter for apheresis donors than for donors of whole blood. For example, donors of platelets may undergo apheresis up to twice a week, but no more than 24 times a year [1]. However, the other requirements for allogeneic donors also apply to apheresis donors (Table 11.1).

Blood collection and immediate storage

A unit of blood should be collected with a minimum of trauma and over a short time period (4–10 minutes) to decrease the likelihood of activation of coagulation factors. Each collection bag usually contains an average of 450 ± 45 mL of whole blood plus 63 mL of anticoagulant/preservative. The purpose of the anticoagulant/preservative is to prevent clotting and to maintain cell viability and function. Two commonly used storage solutions are CPD (citrate-phosphate-dextrose) and CP2D. The citrate chelates calcium, and prevents activation of the calcium-dependent steps of the coagulation process. Dextrose serves as a substrate for red cell glycolysis, while phosphate buffers lactic acid produced by metabolism. Storage of collected blood at 1–6°C slows glycolysis. If, however, platelets are to be separated from the whole blood the latter must be first cooled to no lower than 20°C and the platelets separated within 4 hours of phlebotomy. The United States Food and Drug Administration (FDA) approves storage of blood products containing red cells (RBCs) at 1–6°CC in CPD and CP2D for 21 days. The addition of adenine to the storage solution (e.g. in CPDA-1) to support RBC synthesis of ATP allows the blood to be stored for 35 days. Within 72 hours of collection and following removal of plasma (see below) 100 mL of an additive solution containing such substances as saline,

Table 11.1 Selected requirements for allogeneic blood donors, per AABB standards [1].

Age	Minimum 17 years
Volume of blood collected	Maximum 10.5 mL/kg of donor weight
Donation interval	8 weeks
Blood pressure	≤180 mmHg systolic ≤100 mmHg diastolic
Pulse	50–100 BPM non-athletic; <50 BPM in a healthy athlete
Temperature	≤37.5°C
Hemoglobin/hematocrit	≥12.5 g/dL/≥38%
Drugs taken	Aspirin: defer for 36 hours beyond last ingestion Isotretinoin: defer for one month after last dose Bovine insulin from the UK: defer indefinitely
Medical history	Family history of Creutzfeldt–Jakob disease: indefinite deferral Pregnancy: Defer for 6 weeks after pregnancy termination
Receipt of blood components	Defer for 12 months
Infectious disease	
Indefinite deferral	History of viral hepatitis ≥age 11 HBsAg [+] Repeated reactive test for anti-HBc antibody Present or past clinical or laboratory test for HIV, HCV, HTLV, or syphilis History of babesiosis or Chagas' disease Stigmata of parenteral drug use
12-month deferral from time of:	Sexual contact with an HIV-infected individual or one at high risk for HIV infection Sexual contact with an individual who has any form of clinically active viral hepatitis Sexual contact with an individual who is HBsAg [+] Sexual contact with an HCV [+] individual who has had clinical hepatitis within the past 12 months History of, or completion of therapy for syphilis or gonorrhea
Malaria	Diagnosis of, or symptoms of malaria after having lived in an endemic area: defer for 3 years after becoming asymptomatic Having lived in an endemic area for ≥5 years: defer for 3 years after departing the area Having traveled to an endemic area: defer for 12 months after departing the area
West Nile virus	Defer per FDA recommendations

adenine, mannitol, and dextrose to support red cell survival may be added from a satellite bag to the remaining red cells, thus prolonging the shelf life of the unit to 42 days [4].

Separation of whole blood into components

The term "blood component therapy" refers to the use of specific components of whole blood for a specific patient's needs. By using blood components, 1 donor unit can benefit several patients, as well as allowing conservation of unused components for future use. In addition, components may be used to manufacture such derivatives as individual coagulation factors and immune globulin. To maintain sterility, and thus shelf life, a unit of blood to be divided into components is collected into a primary bag to which up to three satellite bags are attached. Because red cells, plasma, and platelets have different specific gravities, they are separated and initially stored in these satellite bags by differential centrifugation [4]. While a detailed description of all available blood products is beyond the scope of this chapter, a brief description of those products used for obstetric critical care follows. For greater detail, interested readers are referred to appropriate texts [4,5].

Whole blood and components: description and indications

Whole blood

A unit of whole blood has a volume of approximately 500 mL and an additional 70 mL of anticoagulant/preservative. The hematocrit of the unit is from 36 to 44%. At the time of collection a unit of whole blood contains red cells, granulocytes, platelets, and plasma. After 24 hours of storage few platelets and granulocytes remain. Levels of labile coagulation factors V and VIII diminish progressively with storage, while stable clotting factors II, VII, IX, X, and fibrinogen are maintained. In addition, 2,3-diphosphoglyceric acid (2,3-DPG), an intracellular molecule that promotes dissociation between hemoglobin and oxygen, decreases with storage to a concentration of zero after 2 weeks [6]. Functionally, a decrease in 2,3-DPG in stored red cells results in less oxygen release to peripheral tissues than is released by fresh cells. However, 2,3-DPG is completely restored in blood 24 hours after transfusion [7]. Because whole blood provides both oxygen carriage and volume expansion, current indications for whole blood are limited to use for patients at risk for hemorrhagic shock, e.g. those who have lost 25% of their blood volume and who have persistent blood loss [5]. While an advantage of whole blood is the limited number of donors to whom the recipient is exposed, whole blood does not provide platelets and labile clotting factors. A unit of whole blood raises the hematocrit by 3–4%. Because of concerns for fluid overload, whole blood should not be used for normovolemic patients.

Red blood cells (RBCs)

RBCs are prepared by centrifuging whole blood followed by separation of the RBCs from plasma. A unit of RBCs collected in CPD or CPDA-1 has a hematocrit of 65–80%. Because of the greater volume of anticoagulant/preservative used, a unit stored in additive solution has a hematocrit of 55–65%. The indication for RBC transfusion is a need for oxygen carriage. Because a unit of RBCs contains the same number of red cells as does a unit of whole blood, it, too, will raise the hematocrit by about 3–4%.

Recently the collection of RBCs by apheresis has gained in popularity, partially in response to a shrinking donor base. Apheresis allows for the collection of 2 units of red cells at the same time. This has the benefit of exposing the recipient to fewer donors and to a lower transfusion risk while providing potential cost savings. However, the interval between red cell donations by apheresis lengthens to 16 weeks [1].

Red blood cells leukocyte reduced

A unit of RBCs contains 1–3 × 10^9 leukocytes. A unit of RBCs leukocyte reduced must contain no more than 5 × 10^6 leukocytes per unit and must contain 85% of the RBCs in the original unit [1]. Leukocytes may be removed from whole blood following addition of the anticoagulant/preservative by in-line filtration. By centrifugation of the filtered product both leukocyte-reduced RBCs and plasma may be retained. Alternatively, RBCs may be filtered after separation from plasma in the blood collection center or in the laboratory. Prestorage and laboratory leukocyte reduction is preferable to in-line leukocyte reduction at the time of transfusion. During storage leukocytes fragment, degranulate, or die, potentially releasing substances that result in febrile non-hemolytic transfusion reactions [8]. In addition, removal of leukocytes within 24 hours of phlebotomy may reduce the risk of bacterial contamination of the RBC product [9]. Antibodies to leukocyte antigens are responsible for febrile non-hemolytic transfusion reactions. Thus transfusion of RBCs leukocyte reduced is indicated for patients who have had recurrent febrile non-hemolytic transfusion reactions. Others who may benefit from receiving RBCs leukocyte reduced are those who are likely to have been previously exposed to leukocyte antigens. Included among the latter are women who have had several pregnancies and those who have received or who anticipate receiving several transfusions [10]. In addition, this product has been found to be as safe as cytomegalovirus-seronegative blood in preventing the transmission of this bloodborne viral pathogen [11].

Red blood cells washed

Washing red cells in 1–2 L of normal saline removes 99% of plasma proteins as well as electrolytes, some granulocytes, platelets, and cellular debris. Approximately 20% of the red cell volume is lost during washing. Washed cells are usually resuspended in normal saline to a hematocrit of 70–80%, in aliquots of about 180 mL. Cells may be obtained from banked blood at any time during the shelf life of the unit. Because washing takes place in an open system, and because washed cells are separated from their preservative solution, they must be used within 24 hours of washing to prevent bacterial contamination and maintain cell viability. Red cells washed are indicated for IgA-deficient recipients at risk for anaphylaxis due to exposure to IgA antibodies in donor plasma. They are not a substitute for red cells leukocyte depleted [5].

Red blood cells frozen; red blood cells deglycerolized

Long-term storage of frozen red cells may be indicated for those individuals who have rare blood types and for some autologous donors. In the process of cooling extracellular water freezes before intracellular water. The resultant osmotic egress of intracellular water results in red cell dehydration. To prevent this, glycerol, a cryoprotective agent to which the red cell membranes are permeable, is added to create an intracellular osmotic force preventing cellular dehydration. In addition, a high concentration (e.g. 40%) of glycerol prevents formation of ice crystals which may destroy cell membranes [4]. A unit of glycerolized red cells may be stored at –65°C for up to 10 years. Ordinarily red cells are frozen within 6 days of collection. However, cells stored at 1–6°C in CPD or CPDA-1 may have their ATP and 2,3-DPG restored by adding an FDA-approved solution of pyruvate, inosine, phosphate, and adenine within 3 days of expiration. These rejuvenated cells may then be glycerolized and frozen [1,4]. To prepare frozen cells for use they are washed in dextrose and saline solutions of progressively decreasing osmolarity, to maximize removal of glycerol and to minimize cell damage and loss. At least 80% of cells must be recovered following deglycerolyzation. Red cells deglycerolized in an open system must be transfused within 24 hours. Those deglycerolized in a closed system may be stored at 1–6°C for up to 14 days [1,4,5].

Platelets

Random donor platelets are separated from whole blood that has not been cooled below 20°C within 4 hours of phlebotomy. Following centrifugation the platelets are resuspended in 50–70 mL of plasma, an amount necessary to maintain stable clotting factors, and a pH of at least 6.2. To maintain viability and function they are stored at temperatures of 20–24°C with constant gentle agitation for up to 5 days. Platelets may also be obtained by apheresis. A unit of random donor platelets contains 5.5×10^{10} platelets. A unit obtained by apheresis contains 3×10^{10} platelets, or the equivalent of 5–6 random donor units. Platelet transfusions are indicated for bleeding associated with thrombocytopenia (platelet count less than 50 000/μL). They may be indicated in the face of thrombocytopenia associated with platelet destruction (e.g. autoimmune thrombocytopenia, disseminated intravascular coagulation) accompanied by bleeding. One unit of random donor platelets raises the platelet count by 5000, while an apheresed unit raises the count by 30–60 000. Because they express ABO antigens on their surface and because donor plasma may contain anti-A or -B antibodies, platelets ideally should be ABO-compatible with recipients' blood. Because a unit of platelets may contain red blood cell fragments, Rh-negative recipients should receive platelets from Rh-negative donors.

As a rule, apheresed platelets are preferable to random-donor platelets. Transfusing the same volume of platelets from a single donor as would be obtained from five or six donors limits the recipients' potential exposure to bloodborne pathogens and to alloimmunization. A specific indication for apheresed platelets is evidence of platelet refractoriness. This entity is defined by a failure to raise the recipient's platelet count by a calculated minimum number [12], and is usually due to recipient antibodies to Class I HLA antigens on donor platelets. These antigens are integral proteins within the platelet membranes. Apheresed HLA-matched platelets are indicated for such recipients [4,5].

Both random donor and apheresed platelets may be collected using leukocyte reduction filters. Platelets leukocyte reduced are indicated (as are red cells leukocyte reduced) for patients at risk for febrile non-hemolytic transfusion reactions. Controversy exists regarding whether of not their use is protective against platelet refractoriness [13]. Platelets leukocyte reduced are, however, useful in reducing transmission of CMV [14].

Fresh frozen plasma and thawed plasma

A unit of fresh frozen plasma (FFP) is prepared by first separating plasma from red cells in whole blood within 8 hours of phlebotomy. It may be banked for 1 year if then frozen to −18°C, and for 7 years frozen at –65°C [1]. Plasma may also be obtained by apheresis. As with apheresed red cells and platelets, apheresis offers the opportunity of collecting 2 units of plasma at the same collection from the same donor. A unit of FFP contains all clotting factors, including labile factors V and VIII. Likely the most common indication for FFP in obstetrics is in the face of sudden massive decrease of clotting factors, such as is seen in disseminated intravascular coagulation (DIC) and the dilutional coagulopathy accompanying volume replacement for hemorrhage. Once stabilized, the patient's need for further FFP transfusion should be based on laboratory testing, as clinical bleeding due to clotting factor deficiency is rarely seen if the International Normalized Ratio (INR) is below 1.6 for activated partial thromboplastin time and prothrombin time. An INR of 1.6 or greater indicates factor concentrations of 30% or lower [15]. FFP is also indicated for patients who have congenital factor deficiencies for which specific factor concentrates are not available, such as factors II, V, X, and XI [4,5]. While the volume of plasma transfused is a function of clinical response, 3–6 units will raise the concentration of coagulation factors in a factor-depleted patient by 20% [5]. While compatibility testing is not necessary, transfused plasma should be ABO compatible with recipient's blood [1]. Once thawed to 30–37°C it should be either immediately transfused or stored for no more than 24 hours at 1–6°C. From the time of thawing to 24 hours thereafter this product is renamed "FFP thawed". "Thawed plasma" is thawed FFP stored at 1–6°C days beyond the initial 24 hours of thawing and may be transfused for up to 5 days after thawing. While this product is deficient in factor VIII, it retains the minimum factor V activity (35%) required for coagulation [5].

Cryoprecipitated antihemophilic factor (CRYO)

A unit of CRYO is prepared by thawing a unit of FFP to 1–6°C. The supernatant plasma is then removed. The remaining insoluble portion (the precipitate) along with about 15 mL of plasma is refrozen to −18°C and may be stored for up to 1 year. A unit of CRYO contains concentrated factor VIII:C (procoagulant), factor VIII:vWF (von Willebrand's factor), factor XIII, and fibrinogen. Its major indication in obstetrics is for the replacement of concentrated fibrinogen in the presence of DIC. In addition, CRYO to which thrombin has been added (to convert the fibrinogen in CRYO to fibrin) has been found to form an effective plug in vitro for punctured amniotic membranes [16].

Transfusion practices

Administration of blood and blood components

Patient and donor unit identification

Because inadvertent administration of ABO-incompatible cells is the most common cause of fatal hemolytic transfusion reactions [17], meticulous attention to patient and unit identification is mandatory before initiating transfusion. The spelling of the patient's name and hospital identification number on the patient's wrist band must be identical with that on the blood unit's compatibility tag [1].

Warming of blood and duration of transfusion

Because blood administered at slower rates rapidly warms to the recipient's body temperature it is usually unnecessary to warm transfused blood, even in the recipient who has cold alloantibodies. However, cold stored red cells or plasma infused at a rate faster than 100 mL/min for 30 or more minutes has been associated with cardiac arrest [18]. Therefore, warming is necessary for recipients receiving large volumes of blood within short time periods and for those who have severe cold autoimmune hemolytic anemia. Contemporary blood warmers contain sensors to detect changes in rate of flow so that uniform temperature of administered blood may be maintained. Warming blood with a water bath or microwave is not permissible, as overheating of red cells may result in hemolysis [5]. Because of the risk of bacterial infection, blood which has been warmed to room temperature must be infused within 4 hours. A unit which has been warmed to 10°C or more may not be returned to the blood bank for reuse.

Filters

All infused blood products must be filtered. The standard in-line filter has a pore size of 170–260 microns and filters cellular debris, cell aggregates, and coagulated proteins. Because the aggregated proteins at room temperature foster bacterial growth as well as potentially slow the rate of transfusion, it is probably best to change the filter every 4 hours [4]. Microaggregate filters (pore size 20–40 microns) will filter fragments of degenerating leukocytes, platelets, and fibrin strands. Their primary use is cardiac bypass surgery. They are not routinely used for transfusions and should not be used for leukocyte reduction. Leukocyte reduction filters consist of layers of non-woven fibers that retain leukocytes but allow platelets and red blood cells to pass. Leukocyte reduction filters for red cells and for platelets use different technologies and therefore may be used only for retention of their intended component [4]. For reasons presented previously, in-line leukocyte reduction at the time of transfusion is less desirable than prestorage or laboratory leukocyte reduction.

Intravenous solutions used with transfusions

Only normal saline is compatible with transfused blood. It may be used to prime the infusion tubing. It may also be used to dilute concentrated red cells to decrease viscosity and increase flow. Hypotonic solutions (e.g. 5% glucose) are contraindicated because they may cause osmotic swelling and hemolysis of red cells as well as clumping of red cells in the tubing. Although not demonstrated clinically [19], in theory calcium-containing solutions (e.g. lactated Ringer's) may cause coagulation of blood stored in citrate preservatives. Finally, medications should not be added to transfused blood. Should a reaction occur, it will be impossible to determine if its etiology is the drug, the transfused blood, or both. In addition, the high pH of some medications may cause hemolysis, and if a transfusion is interrupted an unknown quantity of medication will have been infused [4,5].

Detecting red cell antigen–antibody interactions

Preparatory to a transfusion of red blood cells, it is essential to determine if transfused cells will be destroyed *in vivo* by antibodies in the potential recipient's serum. The first step in obtaining compatible blood is determining the ABO and Rh type of the recipient's red cells. This is followed by procedures to determine the presence of antibodies to RBC antigens in the potential recipient's serum. A *type and screen* is a three-step process to detect clinically significant antibodies (Figure 11.1). The latter are defined as those associated with a hemolytic transfusion reaction and/or a marked decrease in survival of transfused RBCs and/or hemolytic disease of the newborn. In the first step, also referred to as a "quick spin", two drops of recipient serum and one drop of reagent red cells are mixed and centrifuged at room temperature. The duration of centrifuging is dictated the calibration of the centrifuge (usually about 5 minutes). The reagent red cells are certified to contain all the clinically significant antigens. Agglutination or hemolysis following this step suggests the presence of an anti-A or anti-B antibody, a "cold" antibody, or both. ABO antibodies may be associated with hemolytic transfusion reactions, and thus pose a potential serious risk to the recipient. In contrast, cold antibodies are not likely of clinical significance. The second phase involves centrifugation of the RBC/recipient serum mix following incubation at body temperature. Hemolysis or agglutination at this phase is suggestive of the presence of a clinically significant antibody. In the third, or antiglobulin phase (e.g. rabbit), anti-human IgG is added to the cells which have been incubated and centrifuged in the previous step. If anti-RBC IgG molecules from the recipient's serum have attached to the reagent red cells, the anti-human IgG will form a bridge between those IgG molecules attached to the RBCs, and visible hemolysis or agglutination will occur. If an antibody is detected by this process, its specificity is identified by the blood bank. When needed, donor blood for the potential recipient that does not contain the antigen corresponding to the detected antibody will be reserved for that patient [4,5]. Because of the possibility of the development of new antibodies a new antibody screen must be performed within 3 days of a possible transfusion for a woman who is pregnant and for a person who has been previously transfused.

For a *type and cross-match*, the same steps as for typing and screening are performed, except that instead of reagent red cells

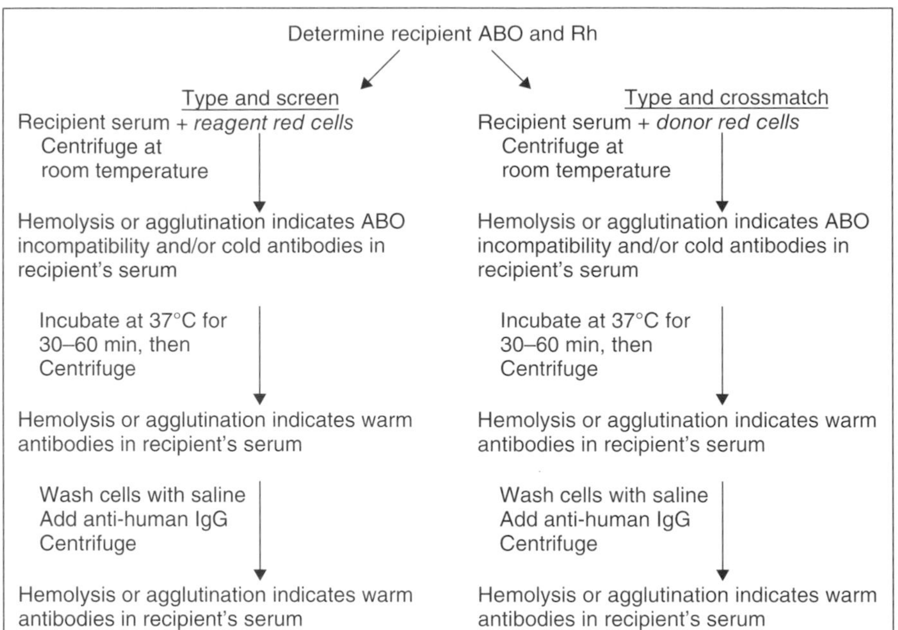

Figure 11.1 Laboratory procedures for type and screen and type and cross-match.

donor cells are used. Because the reagent red cells used for an antibody screen contain virtually all antigens associated with antibody-mediated *in vivo* RBC destruction, it is extremely unlikely that a recipient who has no detected antibodies will have a life-threatening transfusion reaction if given ABO-matched blood [20]. Therefore a quick spin cross-match for a recipient found to have no antibodies may be performed by centrifuging the donor cells with the recipient's serum at room temperature for 5 minutes. This procedure will detect any ABO incompatibility, and make cross-matched blood available within 15 minutes [5].

Computer cross-matching is a more recent technology which also may be used in lieu of the antiglobulin phase of a cross-match for a recipient found to have no detected antibodies. The requirements for allowing the computer to ABO match the unit of donor cells to the recipient are detailed and stringent. These include on-site validation of computer-generated ABO cross-matching, two determinations of the recipient's ABO type, and confirmatory testing of donor ABO group and Rh type; the latter in the instance of Rh-negative donor cells. Logic must be built in to the system to alert blood bank personnel to any discrepancies in these tests [1,4]. Published experience with over 270 000 computer cross-matched transfused units includes no instances of hemolytic transfusion reactions, a short turnaround time from ordering to issuing a unit, and a reduction in laboratory testing [21,22].

Advances in genetics have enabled molecular identification of blood groups. This is particularly advantageous for patients who have received recent transfusions, those who have received massive transfusions, and those who require multiple transfusions (e.g. sickle cell disease, autoimmune hemolytic anemia). For such patients serotyping is made difficult because their circulating blood contains both endogenous and donor cells and plasma. DNA prepared from a recipient who has received multiple transfusions will demonstrate the blood group of the recipient, and not the donor(s) [23]. Molecular blood typing is also of use in typing potential donors who have antigens for which the corresponding reagent antibodies either do not exist or are weakly reactive [24]. Finally, molecular identification has been used for some time in determining the RhD type of fetuses of women alloimmunized to this antigen from cells in amniotic fluid [24,25].

Maintaining blood inventory and blood ordering policies

The number of units of blood that a blood bank maintains is a function of hospital acuity [26] and patient volume. A minimum and ideal inventory level may be calculated from analyzing the number of emergency blood shipments, use of ABO-compatible in lieu of type-specific units, and outdate rates [4]. To optimize utilization of stored units a blood bank will have a policy of transfusion of the oldest banked unit first.

The proportion of cross-matched units that are transfused is a tool for utilization management. Whenever a unit of blood is cross-matched it is held for a specific patient for a time period determined by hospital policy. Until released, that unit may not be used for other potential recipients. Thus every time a unit of blood is cross-matched and goes unused its shelf life is decreased. One tool available to guide appropriate cross-matching is the cross-match to transfusion (C:T) ratio. A C:T ratio greater than 2.0 suggests excessive cross-matching [4]. C/T ratios may be calculated for individual physicians, procedures, or hospital services. Another tool is the Maximum Surgical Blood Order Schedule (MSBOS) [27]. Under MSBOS the number of units of blood to be cross-matched in advance of elective surgery is calculated by determining the number of units previously transfused at that hospital per patient per intended procedure. The MSBOS is procedure specific, and must be determined for each individual hospital. For those patients undergoing procedures that infrequently require transfusions a type and screen policy may be the appropriate guideline. The Standard Blood Order (SBO) is a variant of MSBOS [28]. Under the SBO a type and screen is recommended for those procedures requiring less than 0.5 units per patient per procedure.

Obstetric hemorrhage

The purpose of a red cell transfusion is to restore oxygen-carrying capacity in order to maintain adequacy of tissue oxygenation [4,29]. Maintaining adequate tissue oxygenation in the face of acute blood loss is a function of partial pressure of inspired oxygen, pulmonary gas exchange, oxygen delivery to the blood, cardiac performance, tissue oxygen demands, and red cell oxygen content. Oxygen content is the sum of the product of the hemoglobin concentration, the binding coefficient of oxygen for hemoglobin (1.39), and oxygen saturation, plus the small amount of oxygen dissolved in plasma. Oxygen consumption is calculated as the product of the difference in oxygen content between arterial and venous blood (Table 11.2). Normally as oxygen is extracted from blood as it passes through the tissues, the PO_2 falls from 100 mmHg in the arteries to 40 mmHg in the veins. Respective arterial and venous oxygen saturations are 100% and 75%. Thus the normal extraction ratio, or the proportion of delivered oxygen extracted by the tissues, is 25% [4]. Under conditions of decreased tissue oxygen supply such as occurs with acute blood loss tissue acidosis develops, and slowly 2,3-DPG in red cells increases, both allowing hemoglobin to desaturate at lower oxygen tensions and thus increase tissue oxygen extraction. An extraction ratio of 50% is considered critical [29].

The normal adult tolerates a 10–15% acute decrease in blood volume well. Once blood loss has reached 40% a sequence of physiologic changes whose purpose is to maintain tissue oxygenation rapidly comes into play [30]. In response to adrenergic stimuli, heart rate increases and systemic venules and small veins contract. Because 50% of blood volume resides in these capacitance vessels their constriction increases venous return to the heart, thus increasing stroke volume (preload). If rapid blood loss continues, catecholamines, increased vasopressin, and activation of the renin–angiotensin system cause arterial vasoconstriction of the skin, skeletal muscle, splanchnic organs, and kidneys. Systemic vascular resistance (afterload) increases. Blood is redistributed to the brain and heart. The net effect of these changes is a restoration of cardiac output unless the rapidity and volume of blood loss exceed compensatory mechanisms. Arterial vasoconstriction ultimately leads to tissue hypoxia and accumulation of fixed acids. Hyperventilation to compensate for the metabolic acidosis increases negative intrathoracic pressure, which in turn leads to increased venous return to the heart and increased stroke volume. The combination of increased systemic vascular resistance and systemic hypotension lead to increased transfer of interstitial fluid to the vascular space, which may in turn increase intravascular volume up to 50%. In addition, a slower osmotically induced transfer of intracellular fluid to the interstitial space occurs [31].

Table 11.2 Calculation of oxygen content and oxygen consumption.

O_2 content = (hgb × 1.39 × % saturation) + (pO_2 × 0.003) [in mL O_2/mL blood]
O_2 consumption = cardiac output × hgb × 1.39 × (% $sat_{arterial}$ − % sat_{venous})/100 [in mL O_2/min]

Deciding when red cell transfusion is necessary to maintain adequate tissue oxygenation in the face of acute hemorrhage is an extremely difficult task. Even if a patient is undergoing central monitoring, changes in pulmonary artery mixed venous oxygen tension reflect global changes in tissue oxygenation but not within critical organs [29,32]. Similarly, measurement of lactate levels may not be of use, because reasons in addition to tissue hypoxia are causal for elevation in serum lactate [32].

Hemoglobin concentration and hematocrit are usually readily accessible. Hemoglobin concentration is the product of the hematocrit and the mean corpuscular hemoglobin content (MCHC). Thus with the exception of diseases characterized by an altered MCHC (e.g. the thalessemias), hemoglobin and hematocrit are in an approximate 1:3 relationship [33]. Hemoglobin and hematocrit respectively reflect the volume of hemoglobin and red blood cells per unit volume of blood. Because of altered dynamics in red cell and plasma volume consequent to acute blood loss, measurement of either of these parameters may not accurately reflect the availability of oxygen carriage. In the hypovolemic patient the volume of red cells and plasma during the acute phase of blood loss are equivalent. Only after interstitial fluid is mobilized will a drop in hemoglobin or hematocrit be noted. Studies of controlled blood loss during blood donations have found that these fluid shifts take place in two phases; the first within minutes and the second over a period of days [34].

Normal changes in blood volume during pregnancy make utilization of hemoglobin or hematocrit during acute obstetric blood loss even more problematic. Plasma volume expansion begins at 6 weeks, accelerates to 24 weeks, and then continues to expand but at a slower rate. Red cell mass increase begins at 20 weeks, and progresses steadily to term [35]. During pregnancy red cell mass expands by about 20%, while plasma volume increases by approximately 40% [36]. The disproportionate expansion in plasma relative to red cell mass lowers the normal hemoglobin or hematocrit during pregnancy. The different rates of expansion in plasma and red cells throughout pregnancy make interpretation of these parameters gestational age dependent.

Acute obstetric blood loss is usually unpredictable, sudden, and voluminous, and therefore occurs under circumstances where sophisticated measurements of physiologic parameters are usually unavailable. The obstetrician must decide whether or not to transfuse based on observation of simple parameters such as heart rate, blood pressure, respiratory rate, and persistence of bleeding [29]. An arbitrary approach is to first restore circulating volume with a rapid infusion of 1–2 L of crystalloid (normal saline or lactated Ringer's solution) [37]. It must be remembered that only a third of the crystalloid remains in the intravascular space. Colloids (e.g. hydroxyethyl starch, Dextran, gelatins) remain within the intravascular space, but they are more expensive than crystalloids. They also carry the risks of serious side effects (e.g. anaphylaxis, fever, hypotension for Dextran; pruritus and prolongation of PT and PTT for hydroxyethyl starch [5]) and have not been demonstrated to have an advantage over crystalloids in the management of hypovolemic shock. If after attempted volume restoration signs of hemodynamic instability persist (e.g. tachycardia, tachypnea, hypotension, lowered pulse oxygen saturation) red cell transfusion should be administered until vital signs improve and bleeding is arrested.

The decision to infuse coagulation factors should be based on clinical and laboratory findings. If generalized capillary bleeding is observed and/or if the INR is 1.6 or greater, consideration should be given to transfusing an initial 2 units of FFP [38]. Platelet counts over 50 000/μL generally do not require platelet replacement [38]. Activated recombinant factor VIIa (rFVIIa) has been used as a coagulant for hemorrhage due to a variety of causes (trauma, platelet function disorders, liver disease) [39]. Its successful use in the treatment of postpartum hemorrhage has also been reported [40].

Massive transfusion

Massive transfusion is defined as the replacement of one or more blood volumes (generally 8–10 or more RBC units) within 24 hours. The selection of the units to be transfused depends upon whether the recipient's blood type is known, whether a current antibody screen has been performed, and whether the recipient has any special requirements (e.g. known antibodies, need for CMV-negative blood). In the selection of RBC units for emergency transfusion an effort should be made to transfuse type-specific blood when the recipient's type becomes known, as the consumption of type O cells by one patient will deplete inventory needs for other patients. Reproductive-age women should receive Rh-negative blood until their Rh type is known. Guidelines for coagulation components in the face of continued microvascular bleeding include the transfusion of the equivalent of one random donor platelet pack per 10 kg for the patient whose platelet count is less than 50 000/μL, of FFP or thawed plasma if the INR is over 1.5, and of cryoprecipitate if the fibrinogen concentration is less than 0.8 g/L [41]. While distinguishing between a dilutional coagulopathy and disseminated intravascular coagulation in a massively transfused patient is extremely difficult, it must be remembered that the former is much more common than the latter [41].

Massive transfusion is potentially accompanied by a number of complications. Citrate toxicity results from the chelation of calcium and magnesium. Toxicity may be manifest by decreased myocardial contractility and decreased systemic vascular resistance. Citrate is metabolized by liver mitochondria. When blood is transfused at a rate exceeding 30 mL/kg/h citrate loading may exceed citrate clearance, and hemodynamic instability may result. Although lactic acid accumulates with storage, metabolic acidosis in the massively transfused patient is usually the result of hypoperfusion. Because hypothermia below 30°C may result in ventricular arrhythmias massively transfused blood should pass through warmers which have adequate capacity but which do not cause thermal injury to RBCs [41].

Autologous blood

Autologous blood collection falls into two major categories: preoperative donation and perioperative collection. Included under the latter rubric are acute normovolemic hemodilution and intraoperative cell salvage and reinfusion.

Preoperative autologous donation

Preoperative autologous donation (PAD) has some advantages. A unit of autologous blood returned to the donor will not elicit an antibody response to a foreign antigen, will not elicit a transfusion reaction, and is unlikely to transmit most bloodborne infections. However, the transfusion of autologous blood does not protect against the most common cause of fatal transfusion reactions, namely the transfusion of ABO-incompatible blood due to administration error. Autologous blood may also transmit bacterial infections. The minimal hemoglobin required for autologous donation is 11 g/dL. One regimen for preoperative donation is to collect 1 unit of RBCs weekly for 3 weeks, with the last unit collected no later than 72 hours before surgery. Treatment of the donor with iron will help increase RBC production [4]. Recombinant erythropoietin may be used for patients requiring more than 3 units [42]. For a variety of reasons, PAD is rarely utilized in obstetrics. Bleeding requiring transfusion associated with the most common operative procedure (cesarean delivery) is rare. Obstetric bleeding is most often unpredictable, and massive. Women who have identifiable risk factors require transfusions [43]. One possible indication for PAD is placenta previa. The proportion of women who have this entity and who require RBC transfusion may be substantial [43–45]. A concern is that women who have a placenta previa and are phlebotomized for future autotransfusion may be more likely to be transfused when they start bleeding because of anemia incurred by PAD. One study of women with placenta previa and low-lying placentas found that after initiating routine autologous collection the rate of homologous transfusions decreased from 28 to 8.5% [45]. Changes in fetal hemodynamics during maternal phlebotomy have been reported [46,47,48]. One study found a decrease in middle cerebral artery pulsatility index [47] while another found no change in this parameter [48].

Acute normovolemic hemodilution

Acute normovolemic hemodilution (ANH) refers to the collection of 1 or more units of whole blood just before initiating surgery followed by the reinfusion of this blood at the end of surgery. Phlebotomy is followed immediately by volume replacement with crystalloid. Because of dilution, the volume of RBCs lost at surgery is less than would have been lost had the procedure not been performed. Transfusion of whole blood at the close of the procedure provides fresh RBCs, platelets, and clotting factors [5]. ANH has been used before cesarean delivery for women who have high-risk conditions such as placenta previa, placenta accreta, and large fibroids [49]. A case was reported of a woman undergoing ANH before a cesarean hysterectomy for placenta percreta. Her predonation hematocrit was 41%, her post-hemodilution hematocrit 31%, and her postoperative/post-retransfusion hematocrit 29.8% [50].

Intraoperative blood salvage

Intraoperative blood salvage (IBS) starts with aspiration of blood from the operative site. It then passes through a heparinized tube and a microfilter to a reservoir, and after the addition of normal saline the RBCs are separated by hemoconcentration and differential centrifugation. Subsequent washing in normal saline removes debris, microaggregates, fibrin, platelets, plasma, and complement as well as most of the heparin. In obstetrics, further filtration of washed blood is performed. Up to 250 mL of RBCs with a hematocrit of 55–80% may be reinfused to the patient within 3 minutes of aspiration [5,51].

Reinfusion of blood collected by IBS has been used extensively in non-pregnant patients undergoing traumatic blood loss or cardiovascular surgery. Although its use has been reported in over 400 obstetrics cases [51–53] its utilization in pregnancy remains controversial [51,54–6]. Two major concerns present, namely the possibility of an amniotic fluid embolus (AFE) and the infusion of Rh-positive fetal cells into an Rh-negative mother. Although it is unclear which elements of amniotic fluid are responsible for the cardiovascular collapse and DIC seen with an AFE, removal of amniotic fluid from IBS-retrieved blood seems prudent. The use of a small-pore microfiber filter after the washing phase of blood retrieved at cesarean delivery has been demonstrated to remove all fetal squames and lamellar bodies [57]. Use of a double-suction technique, in which amniotic fluid is drained upon opening the uterus via one suction apparatus followed by aspiration of blood from a second has also been reported [53,57]. While these measures may prevent reinfusion of amniotic fluid contents, separation of fetal from maternal erythrocytes during IBS has not been achieved. The suggestion has been made that following IBS a Kleihauer–Betke test be performed for Rh-negative women delivering Rh-positive fetuses followed by appropriate doses of Rh immune globulin [51,54]. Finally, the argument has been made that given the need for a dedicated technologist to run the cell saver, the time needed for set-up, and the unpredictability of obstetric hemorrhage this technology has limited application in obstetrics [54,56].

Directed donation

Patients with certain medical conditions may benefit from receiving transfusions from directed rather than anonymous donors. Included among these are patients who have rare blood types, those who may require numerous transfusions, and those who require cellular products (e.g. platelets) from HLA-compatible donors. The assumption that blood from family or friends provides a decreased risk of infectious disease transmission is not supported by data [5]. Furthermore, lymphocytes transfused from blood-related donors may pose an increased risk for graft-vs-host disease [58]. For that reason blood from these family members should be irradiated before transfusion [5,58].

Transfusion reactions

A transfusion reaction is defined as any untoward effect following and due to transfusion of a blood product. Up to 10% of all transfusions are complicated by transfusion reactions [5]. Fortunately, the three most common causes of transfusion-related mortality (acute hemolytic reaction, sepsis, and transfusion-related acute lung injury) are the least frequent post-transfusion events [59]. While there is significant overlap in symptoms of the different types of reaction it is important to endeavor to differentiate among them, as treatment and prognosis differ for each type.

Acute transfusion reactions

Acute hemolytic reactions

Acute transfusion reactions are defined as those which occur within 24 hours of the transfusion. Most fatal reactions occur early in the course of a transfusion. For this reason patients require constant surveillance while a blood product is being administered. A list of acute transfusion reactions is found in Table 11.3. Some of the clinically more important acute reactions will now be discussed.

Acute hemolytic transfusion reaction

An *acute hemolytic transfusion reaction* (AHTR) occurs when RBCs containing antigens to existing antibodies in recipient plasma are transfused. Transfusion of ABO-incompatible blood is the most common cause of hemolytic transfusion reaction-related mortality. This is most often due to patient misidentification during collection, during processing in the laboratory, or at the time of administration of blood. An AHTR typically begins within minutes of initiating the transfusion. The initial event is the binding of complement by anti-A and anti-B antibodies. The C5–9 component of complement (the membrane attack complex) then binds to the surface of the red cell, and causes the formation of a pore in the cell membrane. The plasma water entering the results in osmotic lysis of that cell. Laboratory evidence of these events include a decrease in hematocrit, detection of serum-free hemoglobin, a decrease in haptoglobin, increased lactate dehydrogenase, and hemoglobinuria. The release of inflammatory cytokines tumor necrosis factor-alpha and IL-1, -6, and -8 results in fever, hypotension, and disseminated intravascular coagulation (DIC). Hypotension also results from the release of anaphylaxis-precipitating complement fragments C3a and C5a. Renal

Table 11.3 Workup of an acute transfusion reaction.

If an acute transfusion reaction occurs:
1. Stop blood component transfusion immediately
2. Verify the correct unit was given to the correct patient
3. Maintain IV access and ensure adequate urine output with an appropriate crystalloid or colloid solution
4. Maintain blood pressure and pulse
5. Maintain adequate ventilation
6. Notify attending physician and blood bank
7. Obtain blood/urine for transfusion reaction workup
8. Send report of reaction, samples, blood bag, and administration j set to blood bank
9. Blood bank performs workup of suspected transfusion reaction as follows:
   A. Clerical check is performed to ensure correct blood \j" component was transfused to the right patient
   B. The plasma is visually evaluated for hemoglobinemia
   C. A direct antiglobulin test is performed
   D. Other serologic testing is repeated as needed (ABO, Rh, crossmatch)

If intravascular hemolytic reaction is confirmed:
1. Monitor renal status (BUN, creatinine)
2. Initiate diuresis; avoid fluid overload if renal failure is persent
3. Analyze urine for hemoglobinuria
4. Monitor coagulation status (PT, aPTT, fibrinogen, platelet count)
5. Monitor for signs of hemolysis (LDH, bilirubin, haptoglobin, plasma hemoglobin)
6. Monitor hemoglobin and hematocrit
7. Repeat compatibility testing (crossmatch)
8. **Consult with blood bank physician before further transfusion.**

If bacterial contamination is suspected:
1. Obtain blood culture of patient
2. Return unit or empty blood bag to blood bank for culture and Gram's stain
3. Maintain circulation and urine output
4. Initiate broad-spectrum antibiotic treatment as appropriate; revise antibiotic regimen on the basis of microbiological results
5. Monitor for signs of DIC, renal failure, respiratory failure

IV = intravenous; BUN = blood urea nitrogen; PT = prothrombin time; aPTT = activated partial thromboplastin time; LDH = lactate dehydrogenase; DIC = disseminated intravascular coagulation. Adapted from Snyder EL. Transfusion reactions. In: Hoffman R, Benz EF Jr, Shattil SJ, et al. Hematology: basic principles and practice. 2nd ed. New York: Churchill Livingstone, 1995;2045–53.

ischemia is exacerbated by the binding of nitric oxide, an endothelial relaxing factor, which may in turn lead to acute tubular necrosis and acute renal failure [5]. The first step in the treatment of a patient who acutely develops fever, hypotension, intravascular hemolysis, and renal failure, either alone or in combination, is cessation of the transfusion. After applying supportive measures careful evaluation seeking the cause of the reaction should follow (Table 11.4). If ABO incompatibility is not found then another source of this reaction should be sought.

Acute extravascular hemolytic transfusion reaction

In an *acute extravascular hemolytic transfusion reaction* (AEHTR) the antibody to the transfused incompatible cells does not fix complement, but does bind onto the corresponding antigens of the transfused cells. Fever, a positive direct antibody (Coombs) test, and a falling hematocrit characterize this reaction. Because of the marked diminution of complement and cytokine activation [60] the hypotension, DIC, hemoglobinuria and renal failure that characterize an AHTR are rarely found with an AEHTR [5].

Febrile non-hemolytic transfusion reactions

Fever is common to acute hemolytic transfusion reactions and sepsis. A febrile non-hemolytic transfusion reaction (FNHTR) is defined as a temperature elevation of 1°C or more within 2 hours of a blood transfusion and for which no cause can be found [4,5]. It is thus a diagnosis of exclusion, and occurs more commonly in patients who have previously been exposed to blood antigens, such as multiparous women and patients who have had previous transfusions. FNHTRs may develop by different pathways. One mechanism is the binding of recipient antibodies to (most often HLA) antigens on transfused leukocytes, lymphocytes, or platelets. These antibody–antigen complexes then cause phagocytes to release pyrogens. A second mechanism is the release of cytokines from leukocytes contained within units of stored cellular products (e.g. following leukocyte apoptosis). The transfusion of cellular blood products from which leukocytes have been filtered out at the time of blood collection has been reported to decrease the frequency of FNHRs [61,62]. FNHTRs occur more often following platelet transfusions than following transfusions of RBCs. Over 90% of FNHTRs accompanying platelet transfusions are due to the passive infusions of leukocyte-derived cytokines. The passage of platelet products through polyester filters has been shown to remove some cytokines and complement fragments [63]. A more efficient means of reducing the incidence of FNHTRs is the removal of supernatant plasma before transfusion of a platelet product [63]. The first step in the management of a suspected FNHTR is to rule out potentially life-threatening causes of transfusion-associated fever, i.e. AHTR and sepsis (Table 11.4). Once these entities have been ruled out, some feel that transfusion of the same unit may be resumed [4]. Antipyretics are the standard treatment for FNHTRs. For patients with thrombocytopenia acetaminophen or non-steroidal anti-inflammatory agents are preferable to aspirin [4,5].

Allergic reactions

Allergic reactions are seen more frequently in patients who have received multiple transfusions. While most are characterized by mild cutaneous manifestations (e.g. urticaria), they may be more severe, with systemic symptoms such as nausea, vomiting, diarrhea, and bronchospasm. Rarely a full-blown anaphylactic reaction may occur in response to a transfusion. Fever rarely accompanies an allergic reaction, a feature which distinguishes it from a hemolytic transfusion reaction and from sepsis. The mechanism of development of an allergic reaction is the binding

Table 11.4 Acute transfusion reactions.

Type	Signs and Symptoms	Usual Cause	Treatment	Prevention
Intravascular hemolytic (immune)	Hemoglobinemia and hemoglobinuria, fever, chills, anxiety, shock, DIC, dyspnea, chest pain, flank pain, oliguria	ABO incompatibility (clerical error) or other complement-fixing red cell antibody	Stop transfusion; hydrate, support blood pressure and respiration; induce diuresis; treat shock and DIC, if present	Ensure proper sample and recipient identification
Extravascular hemolytic (immune)	Fever, malaise, indirect hyperbilirubinemia, increased LDH, urine urobilinogen, falling hematocrit	IgG non-complement-fixing antibody	Monitor hematocrit, renal and hepatic function, coagulation profile; no acute treatment generally required	Review historical records; ensure proper sample and recipient identification; give antigen-negative units as appropriate; possible high-dose IVIG
Febrile	Fever, chills	Antibodies to leukocytes or plasma proteins; hemolysis; passive cytokine infusion; bacterial contamination; commonly due to patient's underlying condition	Stop transfusion; give antipyretics, eg, acetaminophen; for rigors in adults, use meperidine 25 to 50 mg IV or IM	Pretransfusion antipyretic; leukocyte-reduced blood components
Allergic (mild to severe)	Urticaria (hives), dyspnea, wheezing, throat tightening, rarely, hypotension or anaphylaxis	Antibodies to plasma proteins; rarely, antibodies to IgA	Stop transfusion; give antihistamine (PO or IM); if severe, epinephrine and/or steroids	Pretransfusion antihistamine; washed red cells, if recurrent or severe; check pretransfusion IgA levels in patients with a history of anaphylaxis to transfusion
Hypotension	Hypotension, tachycardia	Bradykinin generation; may be exacerbated by ACE inhibitor	Stop transfusion; fluids; Trendelenberg position	Discontinue ACE inhibitor; avoid bedside leukocyte-reduction filters
Hypervolemia	Dyspnea, hypertension, pulmonary edema, cardiac arrhythmias	Too rapid and/or excessive blood transfusion	Induce diuresis; phlebotomy; support cardio-respiratory system as needed	Avoid rapid or excessive transfusion
Transfusion-related acute lung injury (TRALI)	Dyspnea, fever, hypoxia, pulmonary edema, hypotension, normal pulmonary capillary wedge pressure	Donor HLA or leukocyte antibody transfused with plasma in component; neutrophil-priming lipid mediator; less commonly, recipient antibody to donor white cells	Support blood pressure and respiration (may require intubation)	Leukocyte-reduced red cells and platelets; notify transfusion service and blood center to test donors(s); quarantine remaining components from donor(s)
Bacterial contamination	Rigors, chills, fever, shock	Contaminated blood component	Stop transfusion; support blood pressure; culture patient and blood unit; give antibiotics; notify blood transfusion service	Care in donor selection, blood collection and storage; careful attention to arm preparation for phlebotomy

DIC = disseminated intravascular coagulation; IV = intravenous; IM = intramuscular; PO = by mouth; ACE = angiotensin-converting enzyme; LDH = lactate dehydrogenase; IVIG = intravenous immune globulin.

of soluble substances in transfused plasma with preformed IgE antibodies on mast cells, resulting in histamine release. IgA-deficient patients have an increased susceptibility to allergic reactions. These patients make anti-IgA antibodies to IgA-like substances in the environment. When challenged with IgA in transfused plasma protein, an allergic reaction may result. While IgE anti-IgA antibodies have been demonstrated, it must be noted that the majority of anti-IgA antibodies belong to the IgG or IgM classes. In addition, while anti-IgA antibodies are common, anaphylactic reactions in patients bearing these antibodies are not [4]. Thus the mechanism of development of most transfusion-related allergic reactions remains unexplained. The treatment of an allergic reaction depends on its severity. A mild reaction may be treated with antihistamines. If following medication administration the signs and symptoms abate, the transfusion may be resumed. A severe or anaphylactic reaction requires immediate cessation of the transfusion. Fluid resuscitation, epinephrine, steroids, vasopressors and intubation may be required either alone or in combination. Once a patient has had an allergic reaction to transfusion of a blood product preventative steps to avoid recurrence of such a reaction should be taken before a subsequent transfusion. Pretransfusion treatment with an antihistamine is usually sufficient for the patient who has had a mild reaction. IgA-deficient patients who have had severe reactions and who are found to have anti-IgA antibodies should be given blood products from IgA-deficient donors. They and others who have had severe reactions but are not IgA-deficient should be transfused with washed or thawed deglycerolized cells, to minimized the volume of transfused plasma. Autologous components are also appropriate for these transfusion recipients. Management of the rare patient who has had a severe allergic reaction but who requires transfusion of plasma products (e.g. the patient with thrombotic thrombocytopenic purpura) poses a serious challenge. Pretreatment with antihistamines, steroids, and epinephrine has been suggested for such cases [4,5].

Transfusion-related acute lung injury

Transfusion-related acute lung injury (TRALI) should be suspected by the development of acute pulmonary insufficiency within 1–6 hours of a transfusion that is unexplained by other cardiac or respiratory diseases. Its diagnosis is supported by oxygen saturation <90% on room air and clinical and X-ray evidence of bilateral pulmonary edema [4,5,64]. It is often accompanied by fever, chills, and hypotension. Although the respiratory signs and symptoms of TRALI closely resemble those of circulatory overload, the former is suggested by the absence of a response to diuresis, a pulmonary artery wedge pressure <18 mmHg, and alveolar fluid edema/protein concentration >0.65 at the onset of acute respiratory failure [64]. The treatment of TRALI requires cessation of the transfusion and support with oxygen and ventilation. While it has a mortality of about 10%, most patients recover within 2–4 days [4]. Although a variety of mechanisms for the development of this entity have been proposed, its root cause appears to be immunologic. Most commonly the binding of antibodies in donor plasma to recipient HLA or leukocyte (HNA and CD 16 [65]) antigens appear to be the precipitating event. These antibody–antigen interactions cause a sequence of events leading to the increased permeability of pulmonary capillaries to plasma proteins. These proteins then leak into the pulmonary interstitium and alveoli. Less common is the interaction between recipient antibodies and donor granulocytes. Complement activation, activation of anaphylaxotoxins C3a and C5a, the aggregation of leukoemboli in pulmonary capillaries and transfusion of cytokines specific for target antigens have also been proposed as precipitating mechanisms [4]. A "two-hit" theory has been proposed, in which the initial hit is an antecedent condition in the recipient (e.g. trauma) which initiates endothelial activation and neutrophil priming with sequestration of these neutrophils in the pulmonary capillaries. The second hit is caused by a donor factor such as antibodies, cytokines, or lipids from membranes of stored cells which then activates the neutrophils to cause the damage to the endothelium leading to a capillary leak [4,5]. Because donor antileukocyte antibodies are found in 65–85% of cases of TRALI [66], ascertainment of such antibodies precludes that individual as a future donor. Because women have been found to have a progressive increase in the frequency of HLA antibodies with each successive pregnancy [67], caution should be exercised in using multiparous blood donors for transfusions to critically ill patients.

Bacterial contamination

Bacterial contamination of transfused blood products results from contamination of phlebotomy sites, undetected asymptomatic bacteremia in a donor, or, rarely, while handling the product during processing [59]. Likely due to screening of potential donors for clinically significant bloodborne viral infections, the incidence of viral sepsis following transfusions has markedly decreased in recent years, while the incidence of bacterial sepsis has remained static. Because platelets are stored at room temperature and because many bacteria (e.g. staphylococcus and *Escherichia coli*) proliferate at these temperatures bacterial contamination of platelets occurs more frequently than bacterial contamination of stored RBCs. The organisms contaminating RBC products most commonly are those which proliferate at colder temperatures. *Yersinia* and *Pseudomonas* species, both of which thrive at the temperatures required for RBC storage and which require a source of iron, are the most and secondmost common organisms contaminating RBC products, respectively [68]. While a common perception is that HIV infection poses the greatest infectious risk from blood transfusion [69], bacterial sepsis by far exceeds the risk of any bloodborne viral infection. The incidence of transfusion-associated mortality due to bacterial contamination is exceeded only by that resulting from transfusion of ABO-incompatible RBCs [68]. Clinical findings common to bacterial sepsis and acute intravascular hemolysis include fever, chills, hypotension, and DIC. While AIHTR occurs early in the course of transfusion, signs of sepsis may become evident either during or following transfusion. Unlike AIHTR, bacterial contamination is rarely associated with hemoglobinemia or hemoglobinuria [5]. Immediate care of the recipient suspected of having received a bacterially-contaminated blood product includes discontinuation of that product and Gram stain and blood culture of both the transfused unit and the recipient. Broad-spectrum antibiotics as well as supportive measures should be initiated. The blood bank should be notified so that it may recall any other blood components from the same donor [5].

Delayed transfusion reactions

Delayed hemolytic transfusion reactions

Delayed hemolytic transfusion reactions (DHTRs) differ from acute intravascular hemolytic transfusion reactions in both mechanism and severity of clinical presentations. Those DHTRs that are due to an anemnistic antibody response to transfused RBCs may occur within days of transfusion, while those due to *de novo* antibodies may not manifest signs and symptoms for weeks or months. The destruction of donor RBCs that are coated with recipient IgG antibodies takes place extravascularly, i.e. within the reticuloendothelial system. However, anemnistic antibody production rarely results in hemolysis, and may be referred to as a "delayed serologic transfusion reaction". DHTRs antibodies rarely fix complement, and elicit a lower level of proinflammatory cytokines and C3a and C5a anaphylatoxins than do AIHTRs. The most common findings of a DHTR are decreased hemoglobin concentration and a positive antibody screen. Others include mild fever, leukocytosis, anemia, and jaundice. Laboratory findings include those consistent with antibody-mediated RBC destruction, e.g. decreased haptoglobin, increased LDH, and reticulocytosis. Hemoglobinuria is rarely found. Because DHTRs are rarely severe, treatment is rarely necessary. Observation of coagulation tests and urine output may be advisable. If additional transfusions are needed, units should be sought which do not contain the antigen corresponding to the recipient's antibody [4,5].

Transfusion-associated graft-vs-host disease

Transfusion-associated graft-vs-host disease (TA-GVHD) may occur when donor T lymphocytes escape immune destruction in the recipient, engraft, and then destroy host tissues. A predisposing factor is similarity in HLA antigens between donor and recipient, e.g. when blood is transfused from a related donor, or when the donor is homozygous for an HLA haplotype for which the recipient is heterozygous. While extremely rare in the US, it is seen more often in Japan, where a relative homogeneity of HLA haplotypes is found [4,70]. The disease characteristically is manifest 4–30 days following transfusion with findings of a maculopapular rash beginning on the face and trunk and progressing to the extremities, fever, diarrhea, hepatitis, and bone marrow aplasia. Death occurs in 90% of cases, most often from bone marrow failure leading to infection and pancytopenia [70,71]. While no treatment exists for TA-GVHD, radiation of cellular products before transfusion to susceptible individuals (e.g. blood from relatives and HLA-matched donors) will prevent TA-GVHD. A dose of at least 2500 cGy is mandated by the Food and Drug Administration (FDA) to render T lymphocytes incapable of replication. This dose of radiation does not affect platelets and granulocytes [4]. However, because the viability of RBCs is shortened by irradiation, the FDA advises that irradiated red cells be used no later than 28 days following treatment of these cells [71].

Post-transfusion purpura

Post-transfusion purpura (PTP) is a rare complication of transfusions, with only 200 cases having been reported [4,72]. It is characterized by the sudden onset of profound thrombocytopenia (e.g. <20 000/mm^3) within 1–2 weeks of transfusion of a blood product. Clinical findings include bleeding from virtually any site, including cutaneous purpura, bleeding from wounds, epistaxis, gastrointestinal hemorrhage, and hematuria. Although the disease usually resolves spontaneously within 1–8 weeks, between 10 and 15% of cases are fatal, most often from intracranial hemorrhage. The typical patient is a multiparous Caucasian woman who is among the 2% of the population whose platelets lack the HPA-1a antigen. Of interest is the observation that both donor platelets, which lack the antigen, and recipient platelets, which contain the antigen, are destroyed in PTP. A number of theories have been proposed to explain this phenomenon. One is that either antigen-containing fragments of destroyed transfused platelets or antibody–antigen complexes are adsorbed onto the recipient's platelets. The latter are then destroyed either by complement activation or by phagocytosis within the reticuloendothelial system. Another is that antigens common to donor and recipient platelets along with foreign platelet antigens elicit an autoantibody response parallel with the alloantibody response [72]. Although PTP is usually self-limited, treatment is indicated for patients whose low platelet counts are accompanied by active bleeding. Currently the treatment of choice is high-dose intravenous IgG, whose proposed mechanism of action is blockade of Fc receptors on autologous platelets and within the reticuloendothelial system [72]. The transfusion of antigen-matched platelets does not seem practical, in that finding matched donors is unlikely, and also because in PTP both donor and recipient platelets are destroyed [5,72].

Transfusion-transmitted disease

The routine screening of blood donors for hepatitis B surface antigen (HBsAg) and core antibody (HBcAb), hepatitis C (HCV) antibody, antibody to HIV 1 and 2, antibody to human T-lymphotropic virus types I and II (HTLV I/II), and syphilis have decreased, but not eliminated the possibility of transmission of these diseases by blood transfusion. Of concern is the window of time between donor infection and the ability to detect the disease [73]. In the past, the latter was possible only by antibody detection. The duration of the latency window has been narrowed by the ability to detect some of these viruses by nucleic acid testing (NAT). In the United States NAT testing is routinely performed for HIV, HCV, and West Nile virus. Current estimates of the risk of transfusion-related transmission of HIV and HCV are respectively 1 in 2 million units and 1 in 1.7 million units [74]. Because of its slow replication hepatitis B has a longer window of latency. Because the time from infection to the time of detection of HBsAg is 40 days, the risk of transfusion-associated hepatitis B infection is from 1 : 50 000 to 1 : 250 000 units. It has been estimated that latency period and thus the risk of transmission of this virus may be halved by routine NAT testing [74].

Other viruses may be transmitted by transfusions. Transfusion-associated transmission of West Nile virus is unusual. It has, however, caused serious febrile illness, encephalitis, and meningitis [5]. The scheme of seasonal testing for this virus has been previously discussed [3].

HTLV I/II are retroviruses unrelated to HIV. They are causal agents of adult T-cell lymphoma/leukemia (ATL) and peripheral neuropathy (HAM, or HTLV-associated myelopathy). These diseases are rarely reported in the United States.

Cytomegalovirus (CMV), a DNA virus of the herpesvirus family, usually causes a mononucleosis-like syndrome in susceptible adults. A woman who experiences a primary CMV infection stands a 40% chance of transmitting the virus to her fetus. Fetal infection may result in cerebral calcifications, mental retardation, deafness, motor retardation, thrombocytopenia, jaundice, and death. Approximately 40–90% of the population has anti-CMV antibodies. The risk of transfusion-associated transmission of CMV during pregnancy is unknown. While most pregnancy-related transfusions occur postpartum, it seems prudent to transfuse the pregnant seronegative woman or her fetus with blood from a seronegative donor [70]. Although controversial, the transfusion of leukoreduced RBCs is considered by some to be equivalent in risk of transmission of CMV to that of transfusion from CMV-seronegative donors [4,5,70].

Parvovirus B19 is a DNA virus that may attack and lyse RBC progenitor cells in the marrow. It is of particular concern in patients whose active erythropoiesis compensates for their chronic hemolytic anemia (e.g. hemoglobinopathies and pure red cell aplasias [75]). From 30 to 60% of blood donors have antibodies to parvovirus, and therefore will not transmit the disease. In addition, because the red cell P-antigen is the receptor for parvovirus B19 those deficient in the P-antigen are not susceptible to parvovirus infection [4]. Transfusion-associated transmission of parvovirus is rare [76]. However, a theoretical concern for pregnant recipients of blood products is that parvovirus B19 may cause a severe aplastic hemolytic anemia in the fetus, resulting in hydrops and fetal demise. Parvovirus is rarely transmitted by cellular components and plasma, but has been reported with transfusion of clotting factor concentrates. NAT screening for high-titer parvovirus B19 is currently classified as an in-process manufacturing control but not as a screening test [4].

Transmissible spongiform encephalopathies (TSEs) are degenerative brain disorders caused by protein particles called prions. Creutzfeldt–Jakob disease (CJD) is a TSE characterized by rapid progression to death once dementia is manifest. While 85% of cases are sporadic, another 15% are due to transmission of a mutated prion gene. To date, there have been no reports of CJD transmission by blood transfusions. In contrast, based on the demonstration of variant Creutzfeldt–Jakob disease (vCJD) by transfusion in a mouse model [77], human transmission of vCJD by blood products seems plausible [5]. While the prion responsible for vCJD is distinct from that of CJD, it appears identical with that which causes bovine spongiform encephalopathy (BSE). Following a cluster of cases of vCJD in the United Kingdom, all of which were likely due to consumption of animal products from cattle infected with BSE, the UK Department of Health instructed the UK Blood Transfusion Services to institute universal leukodepletion as a precautionary measure against vCJD transmission. Subsequently leukodepletion was demonstrated to decrease prion protein content in whole blood, RBCs, and plasma [77]. Because no cases of either BSE or vCJD have been reported in the US, universal leukodepletion of blood products has not been adopted. However, since 2002 donor deferrals for a cumulative stay in the UK since 1980 longer than 3 months, in Europe for longer than 5 years, or on a US military base in Europe for over 6 months have been instituted [78].

Concluding comments

The transfusion of blood or blood components is often lifesaving. Because blood products for obstetrical complications may be required with little notice and in massive amounts the mechanisms for obtaining and administering blood and its components rapidly should be maintained at any institution delivering care to pregnant women. The likelihood of a serious complication due to transfusion of a blood product is remote. However, despite standard precautions and blood banking and hospital procedures, serious immune and infectious complications during and following transfusions still occur. Therefore the practicing obstetrician should be prepared to rapidly decide the necessity for and quantity of blood products to be administered as well as to recognize and initiate care for transfusion complications.

References

1 American Association of Blood Banks. *Standards for Blood Banks and Transfusion Services*, 23rd edn. Bethesda, MD: AABB, 2004.
2 Kuehn B. Studies propose targeting screening of blood for West Nile Virus. *JAMA* 2005; 295: 1235–1236.
3 Custer B, Busch MP, Marfin AA, Petersen LR. The cost-effectiveness of screening the US blood supply for West Nile virus. *Ann Intern Med* 2005; 143: 486–492.
4 Brecher ME, ed. *American Association of Blood Banks. Technical Manual*, 15th edn. Bethesda, MD: AABB, 2005.
5 Gottschall J, ed. *Blood transfusion therapy. A physician's handbook*, 8th edn. Bethesda, MD: AABB, 2005.
6 Latham JT, Bove JR, Weirich FL. Chemical and hematologic changes in stored CPDA-1 blood. *Transfusion* 1982; 22: 158–159.
7 Heaton A, Keegan T, Holme S. In vivo regeneration of red cell 2,3-diphosphoglycerate following transfusion of DPG-depleted AS-1, AS-3 and CPDA-1red cells. *Br J Haematol* 1989; 71: 131–136.
8 Yazer MH, Podlosky L, Clarke G, Nahirniak SM. The effect of prestorage WBC reduction on the rates of febrile nonhemolytic transfusion reactions to platelet concentrates and RBC. *Transfusion* 2004; 44: 16–24.
9 Buckholz DH, AuBuchon JP, Snyder EL et al. Effects of white cell reduction on the resistance of blood components to bacterial multiplication. *Transfusion* 1994; 34: 852–857.
10 Lane TA, Anderson KC, Goodnough LT et al. Leukocyte reduction in blood component therapy. *Ann Intern Med* 1992; 117: 151–162.
11 Laupacis A, Brown J, Costello B et al. Prevention of posttransfusion CMV in the era of universal WBC reduction: A consensus statement. *Transfusion* 2001; 41: 560–569.
12 Daly PA, Schiffer CA, Aisner J, Wiernik PH. Platelet transfusion therapy: One hour posttransfusion increments are valuable in pre-

dicting the need for HLA-matched preparations. *JAMA* 1980; 243: 435–438.
13 Paglino JC, Pomper GJ, Fisch GS et al. Reduction of febrile but not allergic reactions to RBCs and platelets after conversion to universal prestorage leukoreduction. *Transfusion* 2004; 44: 16–24.
14 Bowden RA, Cays MJ, Schoch G et al. Comparison of filtered blood (FB) to seronegative blood products (SB) for prevention of cytomegalovirus (CMV) infection after marrow transplant. *Blood* 1995; 86: 3598–3603.
15 College of American Pathologists. Practice parameter for the use of fresh-frozen plasma, cryoprecipitate, and platelets. *JAMA* 1994; 271: 777–781.
16 Reddy UM, Shah SS, Nemiroff RL et al. In vitro sealing of punctured fetal membranes: potential treatment for midtrimester premature rupture of membranes. *Am J Obstet Gynecol* 2001; 185: 1090–1093.
17 Linden JV, Wagner K, Voytovich AE, Sheehan J. Transfusion errors in New York State: An analysis of 10 years experience. *Transfusion* 2000; 40: 1207–1213.
18 Boyan CP, Howland WS. Cardiac arrest and temperature of bank blood. *JAMA* 1963; 183: 58–60.
19 Lorenzo M, Davis JW, Negin S et al. Can Ringer's lactate be used safely with blood transfusions? *Am J Surg* 1998; 175: 308–310.
20 Boral LI, Henry JB. The type and screen: a safe alternative and supplement in selected surgical procedures *Transfusion* 1977; 17: 163 168.
21 Säfwenberg J, Högman CF, Cassemar B. Computerized delivery control–a useful and safe complement to the type and screen compatibility testing. *Vox Sang* 1997; 72: 162–168.
22 Wong KF, Kwan AMY. Virtual blood banking. A 7-year experience. *Am J Clin Pathol* 2005; 124: 124–128.
23 Daniels G. Molecular blood grouping. *Vox Sang* 2004; 87 (Suppl 1): 563–566.
24 Reid ME, Lomas-Francis C. Molecular approaches to blood group identification. *Curr Opin Hematol* 2002; 9: 152–159.
25 Daniels G, van der Schoot CE, Olsson BML. Report of the First International Workshop on molecular blood group genotyping. *Vox Sang* 2005; 88: 136–142.
26 van Klei WA, Moons KGM, Leyssius ATR, Knape JTA, Rutten CLG, Grobbee DE. A reduction in Type and Screen: preoperative prediction of RBC transfusion in surgery procedures with intermediate transfusion risks. *Br J Anaesth* 2001; 87: 250–257.
27 Friedman BA, Oberman HA, Chadwich AR, Kingdon KI. The maximum surgical blood ordering schedule and surgical blood use in the United States. *Transfusion* 1976; 16: 380–387.
28 Devine P, Linden JV, Hoffstadter L et al. Blood donor-, apheresis-, and transfusion-related activities. Results of the 1991 American Association of Blood Banks Institutional Membership Questionnaire. *Transfusion* 1993; 33: 779–782.
29 Simon TL, Alverson DC, AuBuchon J et al. Practice parameter for the use of red blood cell transfusions. *Arch Pathol Lab Med* 1998; 122: 130–138.
30 Hofmeyr GJ, Mohala BKF. Hypovolemic shock. *Best Pract Res Clin Obstet Gynaecol* 2001; 15: 645–662.
31 Stehling L, Simon T. The red blood cell transfusion trigger. *Arch Pathol Lab Med* 1994; 118: 429–434.
32 Sibbald WJ, Messmer K, Fink MP. Roundtable conference on tissue oxygenation in acute medicine, Brussels, Belgium, 14–16 March 1998. *Intensive Care Med* 2000; 26: 780–791.
33 Tan IKS, Lim JMJ. Anemia in the critically ill-the optimal hematocrit. *Ann Acad Med Singapore* 2001; 30: 293–299.
34 Valeri CR, Dennis RC, Ragno G et al. Limitations of the hematocrit to assess the need for red blood cell transfusion in hypovolemic anemic patients. *Transfusion* 2006; 46: 365–371.
35 de Leeuw NKM, Brunton L. Maternal hematologic changes, iron metabolism, and anemias in pregnancy. In: Goodwin JW, Godden JO, Chance GW, eds. *Perinatal Medicine*. Baltimore (MD): Williams & Wilkins, 1976: 425–447.
36 Chesley LC. Plasma and red cell volumes during pregnancy. *Am J Obstet Gynecol* 1972; 112: 440–450.
37 Martel M-J. Hemorrhagic shock. *J Obstet Gynaecol Can* 2002; 24: 504–511.
38 Santoso JT, Saunders BA, Grosshart K. Massive blood loss and transfusion in obstetrics and gynecology. *Obstet Gynecol Surv* 2005; 60: 827–837.
39 Jansen AJG, van Rhenen DJ, Steegers EAP, Duvekot JJ. Postpartum hemorrhage and transfusion of blood and blood components. *Obstet Gynecol Surv* 2005; 60: 663–671.
40 Ahonen J, Jokela R. Recombinant factor VIIa for life-threatening post-partum haemorrhage. *Br J Anaesth* 2005; 94: 592–595.
41 Bracey A, Harrison C, Weiskopf R, Sipherd B, Steiner EA. *Guidelines for Massive Transfusion*. Bethesda MD: AABB, 2005.
42 Goodnough LT, Skikne B, Brugnara C. Erythropoietin, iron, and erythropoiesis. *Blood* 2000; 96: 823–833.
43 Andres RL, Piaquadio KM, Resnik R. A reappraisal of the need for autologous blood donation in the obstetric patient. *Am J Obstet Gynecol* 1990; 163: 1551–1553.
44 Dinsmoor MJ, Hogg BB. Autologous blood donation with placenta previa: is it feasible? *Am J Perinatol* 1995; 12: 382–384.
45 Yamada T, Mori H, Ueki M. Autologous blood transfusion in patients with placenta previa. *Acta Obstet Gynecol Scand* 2005; 84: 255–259.
46 Droste S, Sorensen T, Price T, Sayers M, Benedetti T, Easterling T, Hendricks S. Maternal and fetal hemodynamic effects of autologous blood donation during pregnancy. *Am J Obstet Gynecol* 1992; 167: 89–93.
47 Suzuki S, Tataoka S, Yagi S et al. Fetal circulatory responses to maternal blood loss. *Gynecol Obstet Invest* 2001; 51: 157–159.
48 Yeo M, Tan HH, Choa LC, Ong YW, Liauw P. Autologous transfusion in obstetrics. *Singapore Med J* 1999; 49: 631–634.
49 Grange CS, Douglas MJ, Adams TJ, Wadsworth LD. The use of acute hemodilution in parturients undergoing cesarean section. *Am J Obstet Gynecol* 1998; 178: 156–160.
50 Estella NM, Berry DL, Baker BW, Wali A, Belfort MA. Normovolemic hemodilution before cesarean hysterectomy for placenta percreta. *Obstet Gynecol* 1997; 90: 669–670.
51 Catling S, Jocis L. Cell salvage in obstetrics: the time has come. *Br J Obstet Gynaecol* 2005; 112: 131–132.
52 Rebarber A, Lonser B, Jackson S, Copel JA, Sipes S. The safety of intraoperative autologous blood collection and autotransfusion during cesarean section. *Am J Obstet Gynecol* 1998; 179: 715–720.
53 Potter PS, Waters JH, Burger GA, Mraovic B. Application of cell-salvage during cesarean section. *Anesthesiology* 1999; 90: 619–621.
54 Weiskopf RB. Erythrocyte salvage during cesarean section. *Anesthesiology* 2000; 92: 1519.
55 Thomas D. Facilities for blood salvage (cell saver technique) must be available in every obstetric theatre. *Int J Obstet Anesth* 2005; 14: 48–50.
56 Clark V. Facilities for blood salvage (cell saver technique) must be available in every obstetric theatre. *Int J Obstet Anesth* 2005; 14: 50–52.

57 Waters JH, Biscotti C, Potter P, Phillipson E. Amniotic fluid removal during cell salvage in the cesarean section patient. *Anesthesiology* 2000; 92: 1531–1536.

58 Kantor MH. Transfusion-associated graft-versus host disease: do transfusions from second-degree relatives pose a greater risk than those from first-degree relatives? *Transfusion* 1992; 32: 323–327.

59 Kopko PM, Holland PV. Mechanisms of severe transfusion reactions. *Transfus Clin Biol* 2001; 8: 278–281.

60 Davenport RD, Burdick M, Moore SA, Kunkel SL. Cytokine production in IgG-mediated red cell incompatibility. *Transfusion* 1993; 33: 19–24.

61 King KE, Shirey RS, Thoman SK et al. Universal leukoreduction decreases the incidence of febrile nonhemolytic transfusion reactions to RBCs. *Transfusion* 2004; 44: 25–29.

62 Paglino JC, Pomper GJ, Fisch GS et al. Reduction of febrile but not allergic reactions to RBCs and platelets after conversion to universal prestorage leukoreduction. *Transfusion* 2004; 44: 16–24.

63 Heddle NM. Pathophysiology of febrile nonhemolytic transfusion reactions. *Curr Opin Hematol* 1999; 6: 420–426.

64 Gajic O, Gropper MA, Hubmayr RD. Pulmonary edema after transfusion: how to differentiate transfusion-associated circulatory overload from transfusion-related acute lung injury. *Crit Care Med* 2006; 34: S109–S113.

65 Odent-Malaure H, Quainon F, Ruyer-Dumontier P et al. Transfusion related acute lung injury (TRALI) caused by red cell transfusion involving residual plasma anti-HLA antibodies: a report on two cases and general considerations. *Clin Devel Immunol* 2005; 12: 243–248.

66 Holness L, Knippen MA, Simmons L, Lachenbruch PA. Fatalities caused by TRALI. *Transfus Med Rev* 2005; 18: 184–188.

67 Palfi M, Berg S, Ernerudh J, Berlin G. A randomized controlled trial of transfusion-related acute lung injury: is plasma from multiparous blood donors dangerous? *Transfusion* 2001; 41: 317–322.

68 Wagner SJ. Transfusion-transmitted bacterial infection: risks, sources and interventions. *Vox Sang* 2003; 86: 157–163.

69 Lee D. Perception of blood transfusion risk. *Transfus Med Rev* 2006; 20: 141–148.

70 Hume HA, Preiksaitis JB. Transfusion associated graft-versus-host disease, cytomegalovirus infection, and HLA alloimmunization in neonatal and pediatric patients. *Transfus Sci* 1999; 21: 73–95.

71 Williamson LM, Warwick RM. Transfusion-associated graft-versus-host disease and its prevention. *Blood Rev* 1995; 9: 251–261.

72 Gonzalez CE, Pengetze YM. Post-transfusion purpura. *Curr Hematol Rep* 2005; 4: 154–159.

73 Wang B, Schreiber GB, Glynn SA et al. Does prevalence of transfusion-transmissible viral infection reflect corresponding incidence in United States blood donors ? *Transfusion* 2005; 45: 1089–1096.

74 Goodnough L. Advances in hematology. *Clin Adv Hematol Oncol* 2005; 3: 614–616.

75 Prowse C, Ludlam CA, Yap PL. Human parvovirus B19 and blood products. *Vox Sang* 1997; 72: 1–10.

76 Dodd RY. Current viral risks of blood and blood products. *Ann Med* 2000; 32: 469–474.

77 Krailadsiri P, Seghatchian J, MacGregor I et al. The effects of leukodepletion on the generation and removal of microvesicles and prion protein in blood components. *Transfusion* 2006; 46: 407–417.

78 Goodnough LT, Shander A, Brecher ME. Transfusion medicine: looking to the future. *Transfusion* 2003; 261: 161–169.

12 Hyperalimentation

Jeffrey P. Phelan[1] & Kent A. Martyn[2]

[1]Department of Obstetrics and Gynecology, Citrus Valley Medical Center, West Covina *and* Clinical Research, Childbirth Injury Prevention Foundation, City of Industry, Pasadena, CA, USA
[2]Citrus Valley Medical Center, West Covina, CA, USA

Introduction

Pregnancy represents one of the most profound physiologic stresses that a woman will experience. The length of pregnancy as well as the unique nature of the fetomaternal unit requires that significant adaptation be made by the mother to assure optimal fetal and maternal outcomes (Table 12.1). Most women adapt physiologically with a minimal need for supplementation other than with a few minerals and vitamins. In rare circumstances, the mother may be unable to meet this nutritional challenge and requires medical intervention to overcome nutritional deficiencies. Often times, the deficiency is brief and readily ameliorated by dietary adjustment and/or pharmacotherapy. When these measures fail or the patient experiences a prolonged critical illness, nutritional support by the enteral or parenteral route will become obstetrically necessary.

In 1972, Lakoff and Feldman [1] published the first report of parenteral feeding during pregnancy in a woman with anorexia nervosa [2]. Since then, there have been several case reports of successful use of enteral and central venous nutrition (CVN) or peripheral venous nutrition (PVN) in pregnancy for various indications [3,4].

Normal nutrition in pregnancy

Our understanding of the crucial relationship between maternal nutritional status and perinatal outcome has improved substantially in the last three decades. Maternal prepregnancy weight and weight gain during pregnancy are important determinants of fetal growth and perinatal mortality. Low prepregancy weight and poor weight gain during pregnancy are associated with a lower birth weight and higher perinatal morbidity [5–8].

Critical Care Obstetrics, 5th edition. Edited by M. Belfort, G. Saade, M. Foley, J. Phelan and G. Dildy.

In the normal singleton pregnancy, the average total extra energy necessary to meet the metabolic demands of the fetus, placenta, and uterus is about 80 000 kcal or about 300 kcal/day above maternal basal needs [9]. In the pregnant adolescent, slightly more calories are required [9]. This should result in a total weight gain of about 11–14 kg.

Caloric requirements increase throughout pregnancy but not uniformly (Figure 12.1). For example, the first half of pregnancy is under the predominant influence of progesterone and aldosterone and is referred to as the anabolic phase. Here, the maternal accumulation and storage of fat, protein, minerals, and fluid account for most of the maternal weight gain [10]. The latter half of pregnancy is characterized by the catabolic phase. This phase is under the influence of human placental lactogen, cortisol, estrogen, and deoxycorticosterone. This leads to the depletion of maternal glycogen, fat, and protein stores to provide glucose, free fatty acids, and free amino acids for the fetal accumulation of fat, protein, and placental growth [10]. Fetal fat depots are important storage sites for high-calorie density tissue, fat-soluble vitamins, and essential fatty acids necessary for brain growth and metabolism in the perinatal period. In contrast, amino acids are fundamental building blocks for organ development and enzyme synthesis. Any aberration of this process may affect fetal growth.

The placenta plays a crucial role in fetomaternal nutrition and is more than a biologic pipeline passively directing nutrients from the mother to the fetus. For example, placental human chorionic gonadotropin (HCG) is important for the maintenance of the corpus luteum in early pregnancy. Progesterone, produced from the corpus luteum, induces a glucose-sparing effect in the placenta and makes more glucose available to the developing embryo. Human placental lactogen (HPL), by stimulating lipolysis, stimulates free fatty acid release into the maternal circulation to serve as a caloric source and thereby spare amino acids and glucose to be passed transplacentally to the actively growing fetus. Placental estrogen stimulates protein synthesis for uterine growth and systematic vasodilatation to help maintain uteroplacental blood flow.

Additionally, the placenta has well-developed mechanisms to control passage of substrate to the fetus (Table 12.2). The effectiveness of the passage of any substance across the syncytiotrophoblast depends on a number of factors listed in Table 12.3.

Malnutrition in pregnancy

Our knowledge of the effects of nutritional deprivation in pregnancy are based primarily on animal studies and unfortunate

Table 12.1 Changes in pregnancy that relate to nutrition.

Weight gain (11–14 kg)
Fetal and placental growth
Increased fat stores
Increased total body water (6–9 L)
Increased extracellular volume
Vascular space increased 40–55%
Red blood cell mass increased 25%
Dilutional anemia and normal MCV (normal hemoglobin >10 g/dL, hct >30%)
Dilutional hypoalbuminemia
Increased clotting factor production
Retention of sodium (1000 mEq) and potassium (350 mEq)
Increased cardiac output (50%), heart rate (20%), stroke volume (25–40%) with reduced systemic vascular resistance (20%)
Increased renal blood flow (50%) and glomerular filtration rate (50%) with increased clearance of glucose urea and protein
Creatinine clearance increased (100–180 mL/min)
Increased serum lipids
Increased total iron-binding capacity (40%)
Increased serum iron (30%)
Hypomotility of gastrointestinal tract
Delayed gastric emptying
Gastroesophageal reflux
Constipation

hct, hematocrit; MCV, mean corpuscular volume.

Table 12.2 Substances that cross the placenta and currently accepted mechanisms of transport [21].

Transport mechanism	Substances transported
Passive diffusion	Oxygen Carbon dioxide Fatty acids Steroids Nucleosides Electrolytes Fat-soluble vitamins
Facilitated diffusion	Sugars/carbohydrates
Active transport	Amino acids Some cations Water-soluble vitamins
Solvent drag	Electrolytes
Pinocytosis, breaks in membrane	Proteins

(Reproduced by permission from Martin R, Blackburn G. Hyperalimentation in pregnancy. In: Berkowitz R, ed. *Critical Care of the Obstetric Patient*. New York: Churchill Livingstone, 1983.)

Table 12.3 Factors responsible for the transport of substrates between the maternal–fetal units.

Maternal–fetal concentration gradient
Physical properties of the substrate
Placental surface area
Uteroplacental blood flow
Nature of transport mechanism (passive vs active transport)
Specific binding or carrier proteins in maternal or fetal circulation
Placenta metabolism of the substance

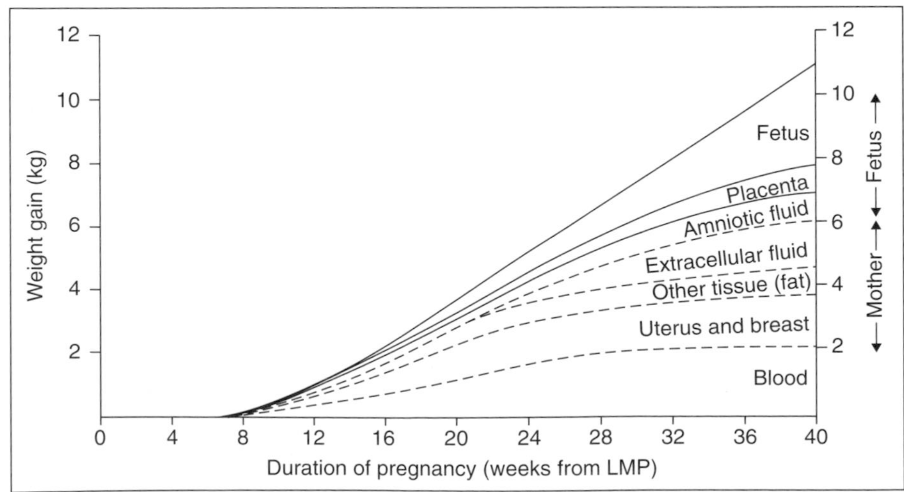

Figure 12.1 Patterns and components of maternal weight gain during pregnancy [38]. (From Pitkin RM. Obstetrics and gynecology. In: Schneider HA, Anderson CE, Cousin DB, eds. *Nutritional Support of Medical Practice*, 2nd edn. Hagerstown, MD: Harper & Row, 1983: 491–506.)

human circumstance. Although several well-designed experiments studying the effects of starvation in pregnant rats are available, the suitability of using the rodent model for studying the primate pregnancy has been questioned [11]. One would expect, intuitively, that the consequences of nutritional deprivation to the mother or fetus in a multifetal gestation of short duration (the typical rodent gestation) should differ from one of a singleton gestation of long duration (the typical human pregnancy). Pond [12], following their experiments in swine, concluded the following: "All gravidas fed protein-deficient diets lost weight. The earlier the protein deficiency began, the more severe the adverse effects." Protein deficiency during periods of fetal growth may affect DNA/RNA synthesis in vital organs (brain, liver) or enzyme systems. Maternal prepregnant labile protein reserve may mitigate the effect of protein deprivation in pregnancy. Riopelle [13] made the following observations of the rhesus monkey: "Although protein deficiency tends to increase fetal morbidity and mortality, the precise effect is dependent on several interacting factors. The improvement in metabolic efficiency in response to starvation is greater in the pregnant than the non-pregnant monkey." Antonov [14] reported that birth weight was reduced by 400–600 g when pregestational nutrition was poor during the war in Leningrad. Reporting on undernourished women during a famine in Holland, Smith and Stein and Susser [15,16] observed that birth weight declined 10% and placental weight 15% when poor nutrition and caloric intake less than 1500 g/day occurred in the third trimester.

Generalized caloric intake reduction, as well as specific deficiencies like protein, zinc, folate, and oxygen, have been implicated in the etiology of fetal growth restriction [17,18]. Winick's hypothesis is particularly helpful in understanding the effect of maternal malnutrition on fetal growth [19]. He suggests there are three phases of fetal growth: cellular hyperplasia, followed by both hyperplasia and hypertrophy, and then predominantly hypertrophy. Fetal malnutrition early in pregnancy is likely to cause a decrease in cell size and number and results in symmetric growth failure. A later insult affects only cell size and not number and results in an asymmetric growth failure. This difference is of prognostic importance because postnatal catch-up growth is more likely with asymmetric rather than symmetric intrauterine growth impairment. Even when low total fetal body weight suggests growth restriction, the severity varies with the organ system. The adrenals and heart are more severely affected than the brain or skeleton [20].

Nutritional assessment during pregnancy

Several protocols have been proposed to evaluate the nutritional status of women during pregnancy. Some are based on parameters including maternal morphometry, serum biochemistry, and provoked immune responses [21,22]. In practice, however, such techniques have limited utility for the following reasons.

1 Normal values obtained in non-pregnant women cannot be readily extrapolated to the hemodiluted pregnant patient.
2 Immune function is impaired in normal pregnancy.
3 Nutritional supplementation is initiated in pregnant patients whose food intake is inadequate before these observations are made.
4 Although nitrogen balance and creatinine clearance may be effective methods to assess protein status in the non-pregnant patient, both are altered markedly by the increased glomerular filtration rate in normal pregnancy.

Routes for nutritional support

The decision whether a given patient requires nutritional support is best determined by a multidisciplinary team composed of the obstetrician, intensivist, clinical nutritionist, and patient. Once the decision for nutritional support has been made, the goal of support must clearly be established. Two important issues relevant to this decision are the baseline nutritional status of the patient and whether the patient is able to ingest any "normal" nutrition. These determine whether the hyperalimentation goal will be to supplement, to maintain, or to build tissue (anabolic). This determination significantly influences the potential routes and formulations that can or need to be used. Two routes of hyperalimentation are available: enteral and parenteral.

The enteral route should be the first consideration unless it is impractical, ineffective, or intolerable. Enteral hyperalimentation is associated with fewer complications than parenteral and is more physiologic. Enteral, in contrast with parenteral, helps maintains bowel function, causes fewer maternal metabolic derangements, is more cost effective, and makes it easier to monitor maternal health. When using enteral hyperalimentation, the delayed gastric emptying typical of pregnancy should be taken into account. The maternal risks of regurgitation and aspiration can be reduced by simply adjusting the feeding solution delivery rates.

Parenteral hyperalimentation or total parenteral nutrition (TPN) may be given in a peripheral (PVN; peripheral venous nutrition) or a central (CVN; central venous nutrition) vessel. Watson [23] reported favorably on the tolerance and efficacy of hypercaloric, hyperosmotic 3-in-1 (carbohydrates, protein, and lipid in same solution) PVN in pregnant patients. While the precise indications and potential side effects had not been elucidated satisfactorily by 1990 [23], CVN does carry a greater risk than PVN. Most of those risks are related to the mechanical risks associated with central venous access. Nevertheless, PVN cannot be continued for more than 1–2 weeks because of the risk of phlebitis [4], it has limitations on substrate capacities that can be delivered through a peripheral vein, and it requires administration of significant volumes to meet the total nutritional needs of the patient. If though, as pointed out by Hamaoui and Hamaoui, PVN does meet the nutritional needs of the pregnant woman,

Table 12.4 Possible criteria for consideration of pregnant patients for total parenteral nutrition.

Inaccessible or inadequate gastrointestinal nutritional route for any reason
Maternal malnutrition
Weight loss greater than 1 kg/week for 4 weeks consecutively
Total weight loss of 6 kg or failure to gain weight
Underlying chronic disease that increases basal nutritional demands and/or precludes enteral feedings such as inflammatory bowel disease, unremitting pancreatitis
Prepregnancy malnutrition
Biochemical markers of malnutrition
Severe hypoalbuminemia less than 2.0 g/dL
Persistent ketosis
Hypocholesterolemia
Lymphocytopenia
Macrocytic anemia: diminished folic acid
Microcytic anemia and decreased serum Fe
Negative nitrogen balance
Anthropometric markers of malnutrition
Weight and height
Growth rate
Poor weight gain
Delayed growth of adolescent
Skin fold thickness
Head, chest, waist, and arm circumference
Intrauterine growth restriction of the fetus

(Reprinted by permission from the American College of Obstetricians and Gynecologists. *Obstet Gynecol* 1982; 59: 660–664.)

CVN may not be medically justifiable due to the greater maternal risks [4,24].

The majority of pregnant patients requiring nutritional support receive CVN. Some of the more common indications for its use in pregnant patients are shown in Table 12.4. CVN is generally well tolerated by the pregnant woman and is convenient for the medical staff. CVN delivers a precise mixture of nutrients directly into the maternal bloodstream and at the same time allows the parenteral administration of other potentially necessary medications such as insulin and heparin. The disadvantages include the necessity for central venous access, the possibility of maternal metabolic derangements, a costlier delivery system, and a more complicated method of maternal monitoring.

Calculation of nutritional requirements

To determine the nutritional needs of a pregnant woman, the first step is to estimate the woman's total caloric needs. Maintenance needs, described as basal energy expenditure (BEE), can be calculated using Wilmore's normogram [25] or the Harris–Benedict equation for women [26] and adjusted slightly for pregnancy [27].

$$\text{BEE (kcal)} = 655 + 9.563W + 1.85H - 4.676A$$

where W is weight in kilograms, H is height in cm and A is age in years.

During pregnancy this value is then multiplied by the "stress factor" of 1.25 to account for the caloric demands of pregnancy [28]. The recommended dietary allowance is an additional 300 kcal/day in singleton or 500 kcal/day in twin pregnancies in the second and third trimesters. A nutritionally deficient pregnant woman may require more than 300 kcal/day for supplementation in a singleton pregnancy. Therefore:

Maintenance therapy	BEE (kcal) × 1.25 + 300 kcal (singleton) or 500 kcal (twins)
Anabolic therapy	
Parenteral	BEE (kcal) × 1.75
Enteral	BEE (kcal) × 1.50

The estimation of caloric requirements should be individualized and tailored to the patient's current metabolic rate. Commercially available metabolic carts, which base estimation of caloric requirement on oxygen consumption and carbon dioxide production, have recently become available for clinical use. These systems are generally quite accurate except at very high F_iO_2 values (≥60%). A useful but imprecise rule to help a patient maintain a positive nitrogen balance [29] is 36 kcal/kg/day. Monitoring the effectiveness of maternal nutritional support is accomplished by plotting maternal weight gain against standard charts and serial sonographic estimates of fetal growth. The American Academy of Pediatrics and the American College of Obstetrics and Gynecology recommend a weight gain of 1–2 kg for the first trimester with 0.4 kg/week and 0.35 kg/week in the second and third trimesters, respectively [30]. Fetal growth can be evaluated against appropriate normograms. A sample calculation of CVN requirements for a 60-kg pregnant patient is described in Table 12.5.

Table 12.5 Sample calculation of total parenteral nutrition requirements for a 60-kg patient.

Total protein requirements	1.5 g/kg = 1.5 × 60 = 90 g/day
Total caloric requirements	36 kcal/kg = 36 × 60 = 2160 kcal/day
If calories are provided in a ratio of 70% : 30% dextrose : lipid:	
Daily dextrose requirement	(2160 × 0.7) (3.4 kcal/g) = 445 g
Daily lipid requirement	(2160 × 0.3) (9 kcal/g) = 72 g

Infusion is usually begun at about 50% of total estimated needs and increased gradually to target values at a rate that minimizes maternal metabolic derangement.

Amino acids

When the intake of other nutrients is adequate, nitrogen and energy intake are the dominant factors influencing positive nitrogen balance. Protein catabolism rises with an increase in the maternal metabolic rate, whereas total protein need is additionally dependent on the women's previous nutritional status, the provision of non-protein energy, and the rate of desired replacement. With the expansion of the maternal circulating blood volume and growth of the uterus, fetus, and placenta, maternal requirements for protein intake are increased during pregnancy. The minimum daily protein requirement throughout pregnancy is approximately 1 g/kg to meet maternal and fetal nutritional needs. The adequacy of maternal protein intake can be assessed by measuring maternal serum protein levels and urea nitrogen excretion. In certain situations such as maternal renal failure, protein and caloric requirements are increased significantly. Frequent dialysis may require even higher amounts. Under these circumstances, survival rates appear to correlate with the adequacy of maternal caloric and protein intake. For example, the protein requirements may reach 2 g/kg to maintain a normal nitrogen balance. Most commercially available amino acid products have been used successfully to maintain normal fetal growth.

Carbohydrates

Dextrose, the most common energy source, is easily metabolized, promotes nitrogen retention, is readily miscible with other additives, can be prepared in any relevant concentration, and is relatively inexpensive. The disadvantages may include increased oxygen consumption, increased carbon dioxide production, hyperglycemia, and its low caloric potency (3.4 kcal/kg) precluding its use as the sole source of energy. Dextrose in concentrations greater than 10% (600 mosm) should not be administered peripherally in order to minimize osmolarity-induced phlebitis and venospasm. Small amounts of amino acids and electrolytes can be added to the dextrose for peripheral solutions. Fat emulsions can also be added to increase calorie density and decrease the osmolarity. Aside from the concentration (osmolarity) limits, other limiting factors in the use of these solutions peripherally are the volume needed to meet patient needs, the time needed to infuse this volume, and the total fat limitations. To infuse hyperosmolar solutions of dextrose utilizing more concentrated energy and protein substrates, central venous access is medically necessary. Although infusion rates of 4–6 mg/kg/min of dextrose may reduce the severity and the likelihood of maternal complications, insulin may be necessary to maintain maternal euglycemia. Assuming maternal euglycemia can be maintained, no adverse fetal effects have been described.

Fat emulsions

Lipids are an important component of TPN in the pregnant patient for the following reasons.

1 They are an excellent energy source (approximately 9 kcal/g).

2 Essential fatty acids are utilized for fetal fat depot formation, brain development and myelination, and lung surfactant synthesis.

3 Fatty acid metabolism requires less oxygen and produces less carbon dioxide than glucose metabolism.

Most commercially available solutions are a suspension of chylomicrons of arachidonic acid precursors and essential fatty acids in a base of safflower or soybean oil. Emulsions are available in concentrations of 10% and 20%. Infusion is usually limited to 12 hours a day, because chylomicrons may remain in maternal circulation for up to 8–10 hours after administration and because of concern about possible bacterial contamination of the emulsion when infusion "hang time" is prolonged. Since the placental transport of fatty acids is primarily by passive diffusion, a high maternal fetal concentration gradient is necessary to ensure adequate lipid transfer. Essential fatty-acid deficiency usually requires 4 weeks or more of nutritional depletion to become clinically manifested [31]. Maternal serum hypertriglyceridemia and ketosis are important complications of lipid use that should be sought and corrected. Initial concerns about preterm labor and placental infarction from fat embolism [32] have failed to materialize with the concentrations of lipid commonly used for TPN (i.e., 30–40% of total caloric requirements) [33].

Fluids and electrolytes

Maternal fluid requirements over the course of a singleton term pregnancy are increased dramatically as total body water increases by about 8–9 L. This 8–9-L requirement for water is to compensate for the expansion of extracellular and intravascular volumes, fetal needs, and amniotic fluid formation. Inadequate plasma volume expansion adversely affects fetal well-being [34,35]. An additional 30 mL/day over standard maintenance fluids is considered sufficient to satisfy maternal fluid requirements [9].

Care should be taken to match any additional losses (e.g. gastrointestinal fluid from hyperemesis) with the appropriate solutions. Fluid replacement should be separate from the hyperalimentation solution to prevent complications due to changes in rate and contents of the TPN delivered. Suggested recommended dietary allowance for electrolytes and vitamins for pregnant and non-pregnant women are displayed in Table 12.6. These are based on estimates of oral recommended dietary allowances actually absorbed. Commercially available intravenous vitamin preparations have proven to be adequate for normal fetal growth.

Table 12.6 Recommended daily allowances for pregnant and non-pregnant women [4].

Nutrients (units)	Non-pregnant	Pregnant	% increase
Energy (kcal)	2200	2500	14
Protein (g)	44–45	60	20
Calcium (mg)	1200*	1200	50
Phosphorus (mg)	800	1200	50
Iron (mg)	15	30	100
Magnesium (mg)	280	320	14
Iodine (mg)	150	175	17
Zinc (mg)	12	15	25
Selenium (mg)	55	65	18
Vitamin A (mcg and RE)	800	800	0
Vitamin D (mg)	10†	10	0
Vitamin E (mg and TE)	8	10	25
Vitamin K (mg)	55	55	0
Vitamin C (mg)	60	70	17
Thiamine (mg)	1.1	1.5	36
Riboflavin (mg)	1.3	1.6	23
Niacin (mcg and NE)	15	17	13
Folate (mg)	180	400	122
Vitamin B6 (mg)	1.6	2.2	38
Vitamin B12 (mg)	2.0	2.2	10

*Above age 24, RDA is 800 mg (no further bone growth).
†Above age 24, RDA is 5 mg (no further bone growth).
NE, Niacin equivalent; MCG, micrograms; RDA, recommended dietary allowance; RE, Retinol equivalent; TE, Tocopherol equivalent.
(Reproduced by permission from Hamaoui E, Hamaoui M. Nutritional assessment and support during pregnancy. *Gastroenterol Clin N Am* 1998; 27(1): 90.)

Table 12.7 Monitoring during total parenteral nutrition.

Daily weights
Strict input/output
Urine sugar and ketones
Serum glucose monitoring (every 6–12 h)
Daily electrolytes
Liver function assessment, calcium
PO_4, magnesium, albumin (2–3 times/week)
Weekly nitrogen balance
Fetal growth assessment (every 2–4 weeks)

Monitoring and complications

A suggested protocol for monitoring the pregnant patient receiving TPN is outlined in Table 12.7. Commonly encountered complications of nutritional therapy [4,24] are detailed in Table 12.8. Catheter-related infections, including candidemia [36], are fairly common. Thus, an important part of any parenteral nutrition program during pregnancy is to minimize the risk of catheter-related infections through a program of frequent monitoring [37].

Table 12.8 Complications of total parenteral nutrition in the obstetric patient.

Catheter related
Pneumothorax
Arterial laceration
Mediastinal hematoma
Malposition
Brachial plexus/phrenic nerve palsy
Catheter sepsis
Subclavian vein thrombosis/right atrial thrombosis
Hydro-/chylothorax
Metabolic
Deficiencies of vitamins, minerals, electrolytes, trace metals, or essential fatty acids
Hyperglycemia
Hepatic dysfunction and fatty infiltration
Carbon dioxide retention
Over-/underhydration
Other
Bowel atrophy
Cholecystitis
Heparin-related complications (e.g. hemorrhage, thrombocytopenia, osteopenia)
Neonatal
Maternal diabetes syndrome (e.g. macrosomia, postnatal hypoglycemia)
Growth restriction

References

1 Lakoff KM, Feldman JD. Anorexia nervosa associated with pregnancy. *Obstet Gynecol* 1972; 36: 699.
2 Lee R, Rodger B, Young C et al. Total parenteral nutrition in pregnancy. *Obstet Gynecol* 1986; 68: 563–571.
3 Smith C, Refleth P, Phelan J et al. Long-term hyperalimentation in the pregnant woman with insulin-dependent diabetes: a report of two cases. *Am J Obstet Gynecol* 1981; 141: 180–183.
4 Hamaoui E, Hamaoui M. Nutritional Assessment and support during pregnancy. *Gastroenterol Clin N Am* 1998; 27(1): 89–121.
5 Taffell SM, National Center of Health Services. *Maternal weight gain and the outcome of pregnancy: United States; 1980.* Vital and Health Statistic Series 21-No.44. DHHS (PHS) 86, Public Health Service. Washington, DC: US Government Printing Office, 1986.
6 Abrams B, Newman V, Key T, Parker J. Maternal weight gain and preterm delivery. *Obstet Gynecol* 1989; 74: 577–583.
7 Abrams B, Newmann V. Small for gestational age birth: maternal predictors and comparison with risk factors of spontaneous preterm delivery in same cohort. *Am J Obstet Gynecol* 1991; 164: 785.
8 Institute of Medicine, Committee on Nutritional Status During Pregnancy and Lactation, National Academy of Sciences. *Nutrition During Pregnancy.* Washington, DC: National Academy Press, 1990.
9 National Research Council. *Subcommittee on the Tenth Edition of the RDA's Food and Nutrition Board.* Commission on Life Sciences. Washington DC: National Academy Press, 1989.
10 Dunnihoo D. *Fundamentals of Gynecology and Obstetrics.* Philadelphia: JB Lippincott, 1990: 164–176.

11 Payne PR, Wheeler EF. Comparative nutrition in pregnancy and lactation. *Proc Nutr Soc* 1968; 27: 129–138.

12 Pond WG, Strachan Dn, Sinha YN et al. Effect of protein deprivation of the swine during all or part of gestation on birth weight, postnatal growth rate, and nucleic acid content of brain and muscle of progeny. *J Nutr* 1969; 99: 61.

13 Riopelle AJ, Hill CW, Li SC. Protein deprivation in primates versus fetal mortality and neonatal status of infant monkeys born of deprived mothers. *Am J Clin Nutr* 1975; 28: 989–993.

14 Antonov AN. Children born during siege of Leningrad in 1942. *J Pediatr* 1947; 30: 250–259.

15 Smith CA. Effects of maternal undernutrition upon newborn infants in Holland: 1944–1945. *J Pediatr* 1947; 30: 229–243.

16 Stein Z, Susser M. The Dutch famine 1944–1945, and the productive process. I. Effects on six indices at birth. *Pediatr Res* 1975; 9: 70.

17 Goldenberg RL, Tamura T, Cliver SP et al. Serum folate and fetal growth retardation: a matter of compliance? *Obstet Gynecol* 1992; 79: 719–722.

18 Neggars YH, Cutter GR, Alvarez JO et al. The relationship between maternal serum zinc levels during pregnancy and birthweight. *Early Hum Dev* 1991; 25: 75–85.

19 Winick M. Cellular changes during placental and fetal growth. *Am J Obstet Gynecol* 1971; 109: 166–176.

20 Lafever HN, Jones CT, Rolph TP. Some of the consequences of intrauterine growth retardation. In: Visser HKA, ed. *Nutrition and Metabolism of the Fetus and Infant*. The Hague: Martinus Nijhoff, 1979: 43.

21 Martin R, Blackburn G. Hyperalimentation in pregnancy. In: Berkowitz R, ed. *Critical Care of the Obstetric Patient*. Edinburgh: Churchill Livingstone, 1983: 133–163.

22 Wolk RA, Rayburn WF. Parenteral nutrition in obstetric patients. *Nutr Clin Pract* 1990; 5: 139–152.

23 Watson LA, Bermarilo AA, Marshall JF. Total peripheral parenteral nutrition in pregnancy. *JPEN* 1990; 14: 485–489.

24 Turrentine MA, Smalling RW, Parisi V. Right atrial thrombus as a complication of total parenteral nutrition in pregnancy. *Obstet Gynecol* 1994; 84: 675–677.

25 Wilmore D. *The Metabolic Management of the Critically Ill*. New York: Plenum, 1980.

26 Harris J, Benedict F. *Biometric Studies of Basal Metabolism in Man*. Washington, DC: Carnegie Institute of Washington, 1919, publication no.279.

27 Driscoll DF, Blackburn GL. Total parenteral nutrition 1990. A review of its current status in hospitalized patients and the needs for patient-specific feeding. *Drugs* 1990; 40: 346–363.

28 Badgett T, Feingold M. Total parenteral nutrition in pregnancy. Case review and Guidelines for calculating requirements. *J Matern Fetal Med* 1997; 6: 215–217.

29 Oldham H, Shaft B. Effect of caloric intake on nitrogen utilization during pregnancy. *J Am Diet Assoc* 1957; 27: 847.

30 Little G, Frigoletto F, eds. *Guidelines for perinatal care*, 2nd edn. Washington, DC: American College of Obstetrics and Gynecologists, 1988.

31 Parenteral and Enteral Nutrition Team. *Parenteral and Enteral Nutrition Manual*, 5th edn. Ann Arbor, MI: University of Michigan Hospitals, 1988.

32 Heller L. Clinical and experimental studies in complete parenteral nutrition. *Scand J Gastroenterol* 1968; 4 (suppl): 4–7.

33 Elphick MC, Filshie GM, Hull D. The passage of fat emulsion across the human placenta. *Br J Obstet Gynaecol* 1978; 85: 610–618.

34 Daniel SS, James LS, Stark RI et al. Prevention of the normal expansion of maternal plasma volume: a model for chronic fetal hypoxemia. *J Dev Physiol* 1989; 11: 225 228.

35 Rosso P, Danose E, Braun S et al. Hemodynamic changes in underweight pregnant women. *Obstet Gynecol* 1992; 79: 908–912.

36 Paranyuk Y, Levine G, Figueroa R. Candida septicemia in a pregnant woman with hyperemesis receiving parenteral nutrition. *Obstet Gynecol* 2006; 107: 535–537.

37 O'Grady NP, Alexander M, Dellinger EP, Gerberding JL, Heard SO, Maki DG et al. Guidelines for the prevention of intravascular catheter-related infections. Center for Disease Control and Prevention. *MMWR Recomm Rep* 2002; 51: 1–29.

38 Pitkin RM. Obstetrics and gynecology. In: Schneider HA, Anderson CE, Coursin DB, eds. *Nutritional Support of Medical Practice*, 2nd edn. Hagerstown, MD: Harper & Row, 1983: 491–506.

13 Dialysis

Shad H. Deering[1] & Gail L. Seiken[2]

[1]Department of Obstetrics and Gynecology, Uniformed Services University of the Health Sciences, Old Madigan Army Medical Center, Tacoma, WA, USA

[2]Washington Nephrology Associates, Bethesda, MD, USA

Introduction

The need for dialytic support in pregnancy, while uncommon, is by no means a rarity and may be seen more often with the improvements in care of renal failure patient. Dialysis may be required in the setting of acute renal failure (ARF), end-stage renal disease (ESRD), or deterioration of chronic renal failure (CRF) during pregnancy. Furthermore, prophylactic dialysis has been instituted in the setting of CRF in the hopes of improving maternal and fetal outcomes.

Incidence of pregnancy in end-stage renal disease

The exact incidence of pregnancy in ESRD is difficult to estimate. For instance, a report by the National Registry documented a conception rate of 2.2% over a 4-year period, based on a survey of approximately 40% of all US dialysis units between 1992 and 1995 [1]. Among more than 6000 women of childbearing age, 73% of whom received hemodialysis, 135 pregnancies were reported (109 in hemodialysis patients, 18 in peritoneal dialysis patients, and 8 pregnancies in which the mode of dialysis was unknown). A comparable conception rate of 0.44% was described among nearly 40 000 women undergoing renal replacement therapy in Japan in 1997 [2]. Previously, the European Dialysis and Transplant Association (EDTA) had reported on 115 pregnancies in approximately 8500 women on dialysis between the ages of 15 and 44 through 1978 [3]. Similarly, Gadallah and colleagues reported an incidence of pregnancy of 3.6% in hemodialysis patients [4] and a retrospective survey of pregnancy in hemodialysis patients in Saudi Arabia between 1985 and 1990 revealed an incidence of less than 1% [5]. These statistics, however, are likely to underestimate the true incidence of conception in ESRD because many pregnancies in dialysis patients end in early miscarriage and therefore remain undetected, and many groups fail to report unsuccessful outcomes. A recent review article on the topic supports this theory and reported that the frequency of pregnancy in women on chronic dialysis appears to be increasing and ranges from 1% to 7% in the most current literature [6]. These numbers are higher than those previously reported. Additionally, the true number of women who are sexually active and do not use contraception is unknown.

Women with CRF or ESRD are often uninformed of the potential for conception and the need for birth control. Similarly, many physicians remain unaware of this possibility as well. Amenorrhea or irregular menses along with markedly decreased fertility are often seen in CRF, in part related to hyperprolactinemia. With administration of erythropoietin and correction of anemia, menses as well as fertility may be restored. Symptoms of early pregnancy may also be confused with uremia, thus delaying the diagnosis (Table 13.1). Furthermore, laboratory tests including serum pregnancy tests may be difficult to interpret in this population due to impaired excretion of human chorionic gonadotropin in renal failure [7]. Thus, confirmation of pregnancy and assessment of gestational age will often rely upon ultrasound. The mean gestational age at diagnosis of pregnancy is 16.5 weeks in women with ESRD [8]. There is little information regarding fertility differences among women utilizing peritoneal vs hemodialysis for ESRD, although registry data have suggested a higher rate of conception in women receiving the latter [1].

Overview of dialysis

Dialysis refers to renal replacement therapy designed to correct electrolyte abnormalities and remove excess fluids and toxic products of protein metabolism. In the setting of CRF, dialysis is usually initiated when the glomerular filtration rate (GFR), as determined by the 24-hour urine creatinine clearance, reaches 5–10 mL/min. At this level of renal function, biochemical abnormalities such as hyperkalemia and metabolic acidosis are likely to

Critical Care Obstetrics, 5th edition. Edited by M. Belfort, G. Saade, M. Foley, J. Phelan and G. Dildy.

develop, as are fluid overload and uremic complications (Table 13.2). In patients with diabetes who often have other end-organ damage, including autonomic neuropathy and vascular disease, dialytic support may be required even earlier, when the GFR reaches 15 mL/min.

Table 13.1 Signs and symptoms of uremia.

Organ involvement	Subjective complaints	Objective findings
Neurologic	Cognitive difficulties Sleep–wake reversal Dysesthesias	Hyperreflexia, asterixis Seizures, encephalopathy Peripheral neuropathy
Hematopoietic	Easy bruising and bleeding Fatigue	Anemia Prolonged bleeding time
Gastrointestinal	Metallic taste Constipation Nausea	Angiodysplasia
Musculoskeletal	Weakness Bone pain Myopathy	Carpal tunnel syndrome Bone fractures
Cardiovascular	Dyspnea Chest pain Pericarditis	Hypertension Pulmonary edema
Dermatologic	Pruritus	Cutaneous calcifications
Endocrine	Decreased libido Dysmenorrhea, amenorrhea	Decreased fertility

Table 13.2 Indications for initiation of dialysis.

Hyperkalemia
Metabolic acidosis
Volume overload
Uremic pericarditis
Uremic encephalopathy
Glomerular filtration rate (GFR) 5–10 mL/min

The physiology of dialysis is based on diffusive and convective transport. Diffusion refers to the random movement of a solute down its concentration gradient. It is by this means that the majority of urea and solute clearance is achieved. Convection is that solute movement that occurs by means of solvent drag as water is removed, either by hydrostatic or osmotic force. A lesser degree of clearance is obtained during fluid removal by ultrafiltration.

Modes of dialysis

Options for dialysis include hemodialysis and peritoneal dialysis, with the latter consisting of continuous ambulatory peritoneal dialysis (CAPD), continuous cycling peritoneal dialysis (CCPD), and nocturnal intermittent peritoneal dialysis (NIPD).

Hemodialysis

Hemodialysis requires a vascular access for extracorporeal therapy. This is usually a surgically created artificial arteriovenous (AV) shunt or a native AV fistula, although dual-lumen central venous catheters can be used temporarily (Figure 13.1). Products of protein metabolism, such as urea nitrogen, potassium, and phosphate, are removed by both diffusion and convection across a semipermeable dialyzer membrane, while ions such as bicarbonate and calcium diffuse into the blood. Fluid removal is accomplished by applying hydrostatic pressure across the dialyzer membrane. The dialysis prescription for non-pregnant patients generally consists of 3–4 hours of hemodialysis thrice weekly, depending on urea generation rate and dialyzer solute clearance. Heparinization is generally employed throughout the dialysis treatment.

Peritoneal dialysis

The various forms of peritoneal dialysis have in common the removal of these same metabolites and excess fluid, albeit by diffusion and convective flow across the peritoneal membrane. Surgical placement of a peritoneal catheter allows repeated access to the peritoneal cavity (Figure 13.2). Removal of fluid by osmotic force is achieved by instilling a hypertonic dialysate such as dextrose solution into the peritoneal cavity. Urea and other ions

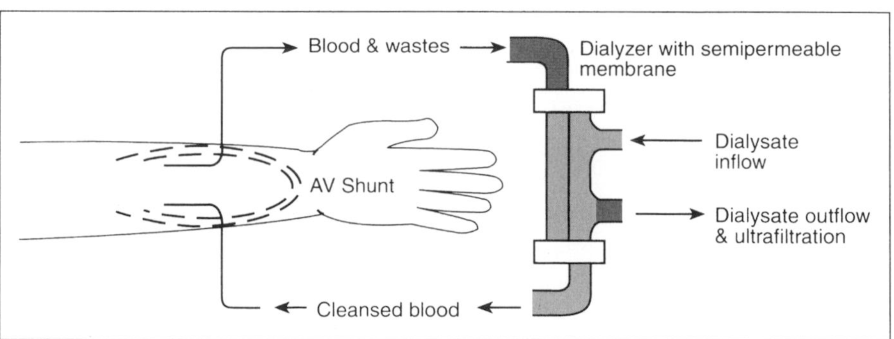

Figure 13.1 Hemodialysis.

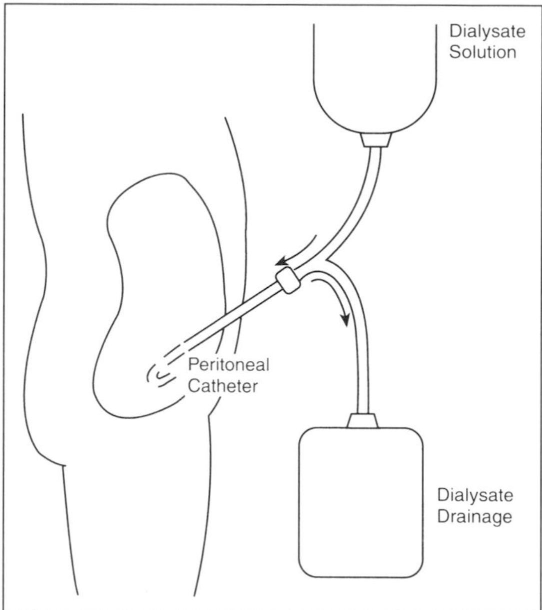

Figure 13.2 Peritoneal dialysis.

present in high concentrations diffuse from the peritoneal vasculature into the dialysate, while calcium and a bicarbonate source such as lactate move in the opposite direction. Depending on the mode of peritoneal dialysis selected, dialysate is instilled and drained either manually or automatically at repeated intervals throughout the day. CAPD consists of approximately four manual exchanges per day; the peritoneum is filled with several liters of dialysate with each exchange, and the fluid is drained 4–6 hours later. Both CCPD and NIPD utilize an automated cycler to repeatedly fill and drain the peritoneum at shorter intervals throughout the night. CCPD differs in that it also includes a daytime dwell for added clearance.

Dialysis and pregnancy

Hemodialysis vs peritoneal dialysis

Both hemodialysis and peritoneal dialysis have been used successfully in pregnancy, although randomized prospective trials to determine the optimal therapy have not been done. Early reports favored peritoneal dialysis, demonstrating greater fetal survival than with hemodialysis, although these studies were limited by small numbers of patients and the use of historical controls in some: 67% vs 20% [4], 83% vs 42% [9], and 63% vs 20% [10]. This benefit has not been borne out in more recent analyses and likely reflects improvement in outcome for pregnant patients on dialysis as a whole. The National Registry for Pregnancy in Dialysis Patients (NPDR) documented virtually identical fetal survival rates among 184 pregnancies for hemodialysis (39.5%) vs peritoneal dialysis (37%) [1]. Similar data are described by Chan and colleagues (82% vs 72%) in their review of all pregnancies in dialysis patients at their institution since 1965 [11], although nearly one-third of their patients conceived before the onset of dialysis.

Table 13.3 Mode of dialysis: advantages in pregnancy.

Hemodialysis	Peritoneal dialysis
Less work intensive for patient	Stable biochemical environment
No risk of peritoneal catheter-related complications	Continuous fluid removal avoids hypotension
Adequate clearances late in gestation readily obtained	Allows liberal fluid intake
No interruption in therapy needed after cesarean section	Permits continuous insulin administration in diabetes mellitus
	No anticoagulation necessary
	Permits administration of intraperitoneal $MgSO_4$ in pre-eclampsia
	Hypertension easier to control
	Less severe anemia

There are many theoretical reasons to utilize peritoneal dialysis in pregnancy, most notably of which is the steady-state removal of uremic toxins (Table 13.3). This, coupled with easier fluid removal, should minimize episodes of hypotension and thus placental insufficiency. Additional advantages of peritoneal dialysis often include less severe anemia, as well as better blood pressure control and more liberal dietary restrictions due to the continuous nature of the therapy [12–14]. Furthermore, peritoneal dialysis obviates the need for systemic anticoagulation. In diabetic patients, the use of intraperitoneal insulin can also facilitate strict glycemic control. There have also been several case reports of successful intraperitoneal magnesium administration for the treatment of pre-eclampsia, maintaining a steady-state magnesium serum level of approximately 5 mEq/L, although generally, alternative therapy may be recommended in renal failure to avoid magnesium toxicity [10,15].

Despite these apparent advantages of peritoneal dialysis, several unique complications exist, including catheter-related complications such as laceration of the uterine vessels [16] and peritonitis. Hou reported precipitation of preterm labor and delivery in two of three patients secondary to peritonitis, but other reports suggest that the incidence of peritonitis is not increased in pregnant versus non-pregnant patients [6]. Peritoneal dialysis catheters have been placed as late as 29 weeks gestation. In some patients, however, difficulties with catheter obstruction and failure to drain necessitate placement of multiple catheters or conversion to hemodialysis. It is also difficult to determine whether either method of dialysis actually precipitates preterm labor, because preterm labor has been described in the setting of both hemodialysis and peritoneal dialysis, as well as in CRF alone.

Intensive dialysis

Generally, modification of the dialysis prescription in pregnancy has been recommended for patients treated with both hemodialysis and peritoneal dialysis. Although there are no firm guidelines, it is the belief of most nephrologists that a more intensive dialysis regimen is required during pregnancy to minimize fetal exposure to uremic toxins and improve outcome. This is based in part on the fact that pregnancy outcome appears to be better in those women who require initiation of dialysis due to a deterioration of renal function during pregnancy, as well as among women with significant residual renal function who require dialysis before conception [9]. Infant survival as reported by the NPDR was 73% in the former group of women, although only 40% in those women who were already on dialysis at the time of pregnancy [1]. Similar pregnancy success rates in dialysis patients were reported by Bagon and colleagues based on a review of all pregnancies in Belgium extending beyond the first trimester [17]. Furthermore, pregnancy appears to be most common during the first year of dialysis, presumably related to the greater residual renal function often present at the initiation of renal replacement therapy. There are reports of successful pregnancies in severely uremic patients and patients on dialysis for more than 10 years, as well as pregnancy failures in women treated with intensive dialysis.

Intensive dialysis corresponds to initiation of dialysis at levels of BUN and creatinine approximately 60–70 mg/dL and 6–7 mg/dL, respectively, with a goal of maintaining predialysis BUN levels less than 50 mg/dL and 5 mg/dL, respectively [6,9]. To maintain such low levels of azotemia in pregnancy, dialysis patients may require a significant increase in total treatment time. This is especially true in the third trimester when fetal urea production increases and may account for as much as 540 mg/day [18], a 10% increase. For women on hemodialysis, daily treatments of 5 or more hours may be necessary to obtain adequate clearances late in gestation. As with hemodialysis, a patient's treatment requirements may increase markedly with peritoneal dialysis as well, especially because women in the latter half of gestation may be unable to tolerate the standard dwell volumes due to abdominal fullness. A switch to CCPD with an increased frequency of small volume exchanges and supplemental manual exchanges is often required late in gestation to obtain adequate clearance. A combination of hemodialysis and peritoneal dialysis may even be indicated.

Although the ideal dialysis prescription has yet to be established, the National Registry data suggest a trend towards greater infant survival and more advanced gestational age in those women receiving more than 20 hours of hemodialysis weekly [1,19]. Others have confirmed this finding, although no benefit was found in those women prescribed a higher dose of peritoneal dialysis [11]. Even though the number of weekly hemodialysis treatments had no effect on outcomes in some studies, performing dialysis 4 to 6 times per week may allow for better fluid and blood pressure management and may also decrease the risk of polyhydramnios which can lead to preterm labor and delivery. While no guidelines exist with regard to evaluating the adequacy of dialysis, a minimum combined renal and dialytic clearance of 15 mL/min is recommended.

An additional benefit of intensive dialysis is that a low level of azotemia should minimize the risk of polyhydramnios, although it is not known if this will lead to improved outcome or a decreased incidence of preterm labor. Polyhydramnios, seen in a high percentage of pregnancies, has been ascribed to the urea diuresis that normally occurs in utero due to high fetal levels of urea nitrogen, as well as to fluid shifts that accompany intermittent hemodialysis [20,21]. An increased frequency of hemodialysis in particular limits the large interdialytic weight gains often seen in hemodialysis patients, thus avoiding hypotension and enabling better blood pressure control by minimizing that component of hypertension that is volume mediated.

Modification of the dialysis prescription

With respect to hemodialysis, certain parameters of the dialysis prescription may warrant adjustment. Specifically, a lower sodium dialysate of 134 mEq/L is recommended due to the mild physiologic hyponatremia of pregnancy. Similarly, a bicarbonate concentration as low as 25 mEq/L may be necessary to avoid alkalemia, due to the repeated exposure to a bicarbonate dialysate and the concomitant respiratory alkalosis seen in pregnancy. Acetate dialysis is not generally recommended because it has been associated with an increased frequency of hypotension, although there are no data in pregnancy. A standard calcium dialysate can be used with both hemodialysis and peritoneal dialysis, thus ensuring a net positive calcium balance sufficient to meet fetal requirements. Due to placental production of calcitriol, however, there is augmented gastrointestinal absorption of calcium from calcium-containing antacids; thus, serum calcium levels must be monitored to avoid hypercalcemia [22]. With both methods of dialysis, one must also monitor closely for hypokalemia, which may develop with frequent dialysis.

Changes in the efficacy of peritoneal dialysis have not been noted during pregnancy. In one patient studied there was no apparent change in peritoneal physiology or peritoneal blood flow as assessed by the standard peritoneal equilibration test of glucose and creatinine [23]. Similarly, Redrow and colleagues reported excellent ultrafiltration in all patients throughout pregnancy, and less than a one-third decrease in peritoneal solute clearance in three patients studied [10].

Dialysis and uteroplacental perfusion

Doppler flow velocity measurements have been performed during and after hemodialysis in an attempt to assess the effect of hemodialysis on uteroplacental blood flow. Results have been conflicting, with studies reporting unchanged, worsened, and improved perfusion during dialysis as assessed by the systolic–diastolic ratio or resistance index [24–26]. In those patients studied, however, there was no evidence of uterine irritability or fetal distress as measured by external fetal monitoring during hemodialysis.

Maternal complications

In the past, women with severe renal disease were often advised to terminate pregnancies due to the belief that pregnancy carried

Table 13.4 Renal failure and pregnancy: maternal complications.

Accelerated decline in renal function
Accelerated hypertension
Superimposed pre-eclampsia
Preterm labor
Worsened anemia
Hemodialysis access thrombosis
Abruptio placentae
Spontaneous abortion and second-trimester fetal loss

Table 13.5 Renal failure and pregnancy: fetal complications.

Spontaneous abortion and fetal loss (50%)
Fetal/neonatal death (21–33%)
Preterm delivery (>80%)
Intrauterine growth restriction (20%)
Polyhydramnios (29–67%)
Maternal hypertension (35–72%)

a high risk of maternal complications and a low success rate. Because there are definite risks to both the mother and the fetus as a result of CRF requiring dialysis in pregnancy, these patients should be counseled before conception if at all possible. Potential complications include an accelerated decline in renal function, accelerated hypertension, an increased risk of superimposed pre-eclampsia, polyhydramnios, worsened anemia often requiring transfusion, hemodialysis access thrombosis, and an increased incidence of abruptio placentae (Table 13.4). The latter cannot be ascribed solely to the use of heparin during hemodialysis because it has been seen with greater than normal frequency in patients on peritoneal dialysis as well.

Pregnancy has been associated with a permanent decline in renal function in a relatively small percentage of patients with mild renal failure, defined by a serum creatinine of <1.4 mg/dL. This risk may be increased significantly in those women with moderate or severe renal failure, especially in the setting of uncontrolled hypertension. It is always important to rule out readily reversible causes of declining renal function, such as volume depletion, pyelonephritis, and obstruction. One report of 37 pregnant women with moderate or severe renal failure, defined as a serum creatinine greater than 1.4 mg/dL, demonstrated a deterioration in renal function, defined as greater than a 50% rise in creatinine, in 16% [27]. Five of these six women also suffered from poorly controlled chronic hypertension, and a clinical diagnosis of superimposed pre-eclampsia was established in nearly 60% overall. Similarly, a more recent review encompassing more than 80 pregnant women with renal failure demonstrated accelerated hypertension in nearly 50% and an accelerated decline in renal function in more than one-third [28]. Hou reviewed these studies along with five others, all of which confirmed the increased incidence of accelerated renal failure in women with a serum creatinine greater than 1.4 mg/dL at the time of conception [29]. Severe hypertension and proteinuria were predictive of an accelerated course in more than 20% of patients with moderate to severe renal failure due to a wide range of primary glomerular diseases [30]. Of interest, a review of pregnancy in patients with diabetic nephropathy, defined as nephrotic-range proteinuria and severe hypertension, failed to describe an accelerated loss of renal function during pregnancy, although nearly one-third of women had reached ESRD or died during the 3-year follow-up period [31]. Three maternal deaths have been reported to date, one of which was the result of lupus cerebritis [1].

Polyhydramnios is a common finding, reported in between 29% and 67% of pregnancies in CRF patients [6]. This may be caused by the rapid removal of solutes during hemodialysis and shifting of free water into the amniotic space or an increased fetal osmotic diuresis because of the increased maternal urea concentration.

Preterm delivery is an expected outcome in these patients as well, with the mean age of delivery being only 32 weeks gestation [32]. Early delivery may be because of spontaneous preterm labor, and polyhydramnios may contribute to this, the result of fetal distress, intrauterine growth restriction, pre-eclampsia, or placental abruption.

Fetal complications

The likelihood of fetal survival beyond the neonatal period is better than previously believed (Table 13.5). Surveys conducted by the EDTA [3], the American Nephrology Nursing Association [9], as well as a group in Saudi Arabia [5] reported a fetal viability of 20–30% in those pregnancies that were not electively terminated. The EDTA survey revealed that greater than 50% of pregnancies resulted in spontaneous abortion [3]. Hou et al noted a comparable incidence of 54% fetal loss, including spontaneous abortion, stillbirth, and neonatal death [21]). Virtually all infants delivered were premature, and approximately 20% were growth-restricted. When stratified according to year, however, survival was greater than 50% in those pregnancies occurring since 1990. Another study supports improved neonatal survival and summarized the outcomes of 111 pregnancies in patients receiving chronic hemodialysis and reported that 71% (79/111) of these infants who were born survived [6].

As noted previously, polyhydramnios, possibly attributed to the fetal urea diuresis, is seen with greater frequency in renal failure and may contribute to the high incidence of prematurity. Additionally, a urea-induced diuresis following delivery may result in volume depletion in the neonatal period.

Early reports failed to identify an increased incidence in congenital anomalies [3,9]. However, the NPDR reported on 11 infants with congenital anomalies among 55 live births [1]. Not surprisingly, there was also a high proportion of infants with developmental delays or long-term medical problems documented at follow-up, the latter possibly attributable to problems often encountered with premature birth. Unfortunately, there is little additional long-term follow-up on infants exposed to azotemia in utero with regard to physical and intellectual development.

Anemia

Anemia develops during pregnancy largely due to an increase in plasma volume of 3–4 L without a corresponding increase in red cell mass [6]. In patients with renal failure, the picture is complicated by a relative deficiency in erythropoietin production by the diseased kidneys, as well as shortened red cell survival, bone marrow suppression by uremic toxins, and possible superimposed nutritional deficiencies. The severe anemia that was typical of ESRD in the past is now treated successfully in most cases with recombinant human erythropoietin (rHuEpo). Furthermore, correction of the anemia of ESRD may result in return of regular menses due to resolution of hyperprolactinemia, and conception may follow [8].

Recombinant human erythropoietin has been studied in pregnant animals at doses used clinically without apparent complications. Hou reported on 11 patients with CRF treated with rHuEpo in whom no congenital anomalies were seen and no rHuEpo could be detected in the cord blood [9]. All of the women required an increase in their dose of rHuEpo, compared with prepregnancy, and three still required blood transfusions during pregnancy. Only one woman experienced severe hypertension complicating therapy, although several required additional antihypertensive medications. Additional reports have yielded similar results [1,17,33,34]. It is accepted by most obstetricians that a hemoglobin less than 6 g/dL is associated with increased perinatal mortality and maternal morbidity secondary to high-output failure. Given this fact, as well as the increased risk of bleeding complications in uremia due to platelet dysfunction, and the overwhelming likelihood of preterm delivery, the recommendation for women with renal disease is an empirical 50% increase in rHuEpo dose once the pregnancy is detected, with a goal of maintaining the hemoglobin at more than 10 g/dL [9]. Most patients require oral iron supplementation or intermittent intravenous iron, because iron deficiency eventually develops in most patients successfully treated with rHuEpo. Although intravenous iron has been used without incident in at least 20 patients, it is generally recommended only if iron deficiency persists despite oral therapy.

Dietary guidelines

Dietary restrictions in renal failure generally consist of modest protein restriction, as well as restriction of potassium, phosphate, and sodium intake. Fluids are restricted to 1 L daily, with more liberal intake permitted in those with substantial residual urine output. In pregnancy, however, protein intake is liberalized to allow for normal fetal development. The recommended protein intake is 1.5 g/kg/day in hemodialysis and 1.8 g/kg/day in peritoneal dialysis and daily caloric intake increased to 30–35 kcal/kg/day as well [29]. Increasing delivery of dialysis is recommended for worsening azotemia rather than strict protein restriction.

Supplementation of water-soluble vitamins, which are removed during dialysis, is recommended, as well as supplementation with folate, zinc, and iron. Specifically, it is important to monitor hemoglobin and iron stores on a regular basis as oral iron supplementation is often insufficient given the increased requirements during pregnancy. Intravenous iron has been given to pregnant dialysis patients without adverse outcomes as mentioned previously [35]. Standard prenatal vitamins, which may contain excess vitamin A, are best avoided.

Antepartum management

Care during pregnancy for patients on dialysis should include a multidisciplinary team with at least initially a nephrologist and maternal-fetal medicine specialist. Given the extremely high likelihood of a preterm delivery, it is also important to make the neonatologist and the neonatal intensive care unit aware of the patient as these infants may also demonstrate some degree of azotemia after delivery. In addition, the patient should be counseled on the likely complications and possibility of premature delivery.

Early in pregnancy, care should be focused on dating the pregnancy as accurately as possible, which is difficult given the advanced gestational age at which patients often present. Dialysis time should be increased and anemia monitored closely which will require increasing the dose of erythropoietin as discussed before. Dietary alterations, including increased folate supplementation and protein intake, should also be instituted.

Hypertension is a common comorbidity and is seen in up to 80% of pregnant dialysis patients [6]. Many antihypertensive medications are considered safe in pregnancy and may be utilized; however, the angiotension-converting enzyme inhibitors and angiotensin receptor blockers are contraindicated in pregnancy secondary to associations with renal dysplasia, neonatal anuria, and stillbirth [36,37]. Some of the older medications that have been described to treat hypertension in pregnancy include methyldopa and hydralazine and these are acceptable to use. Even though there have been reports of concerns about intrauterine growth restriction and neonatal bradycardia and hypoglycemia with the use of some beta-blockers, the best evidence for this was associated with atenolol. Other beta blockers, such as labetalol, are recommended by some as first-line therapy for treatment of hypertension in pregnancy [38]. Regardless of which medication is used, treatment of hypertension is essential during pregnancy for these patients.

In addition, the physician should monitor for urinary tract infections and aggressively treat even asymptomatic bacteruria as the risk of pyelonephritis is quite high when this is present and untreated. Generally, urine cultures can be done every 4–6 weeks and patients treated as appropriate.

A new approach to the prevention of recurrent preterm delivery may also have some benefit in dialysis patients. Two randomized trials have now demonstrated a significant reduction in the incidence of recurrent preterm birth with the administration of progesterone supplementation during pregnancy [39,40]. Given the extremely high risk of preterm delivery, as well as additional evidence that dialysis may significantly affect serum progesterone levels, it is not unreasonable to consider the administration of progesterone supplementation, either by injection or vaginal suppositories, beginning around 16–20 weeks [19].

After a sonogram for a complete anatomic survey between 18 and 20 weeks, the patient should be followed with serial growth scans approximately every 4 weeks. Unless indicated earlier, antepartum fetal testing should begin at 28–30 weeks and include twice weekly non-stress tests and at least a weekly measurement of the amniotic fluid index (AFI). If intrauterine growth restriction is diagnosed, then monitoring with serial umbilical artery Doppler measurements is appropriate as well.

If preterm labor occurs, then medical interventions may be undertaken in an effort to prolong the pregnancy and improve fetal outcomes. Steroids should be administered, either betamethasone or dexamethasone, according to standard protocols. Tocolytics may be given and, before 32 weeks, indomethacin can and has been used in women with renal disease [41]. It is important to note, however, that indomethacin is generally not continued for greater than 72 hours or given after 32 weeks secondary to the potential for premature closure of the fetal ductus arteriosus and fetal anuria. Magnesium sulfate may also be used for tocolysis with a target level of 5–7 mg/dL considered to be therapeutic. Care must be taken with the use of magnesium in renal failure patients because it is cleared though the kidney and the provider must monitor serum levels closely and watch for evidence of magnesium toxicity. Calcium channel blockers, such as nifedipine, may also be used in dialysis patients for tocolysis.

Delivery is often required for pregnant patients on dialysis for intrauterine growth restriction and preterm premature rupture of membranes (PPROM). In general, if PPROM occurs at 34 weeks or later, delivery is indicated as there is no significant benefit to prolonging the pregnancy and the risk of infection is more concerning.

There are no data to support preference for any difference in the mode of delivery in dialysis patients. Reported rates of cesarean section range from 24% to more than 60% [3,11,16,34,42]. Cesarean delivery should be performed for standard obstetric indications. In peritoneal dialysis patients requiring cesarean section, both standard and extraperitoneal approaches have been utilized [10,43]. In either case, it may be necessary to interrupt peritoneal dialysis for several days to allow healing of the abdominal wall and prevent dialysate leak or hernia formation. Peritoneal dialysis can be reinitiated using smaller dwell volumes initially, with a progressive increase in volume as tolerated. If necessary, temporary hemodialysis can be performed in the interim. In general, the route of delivery should be determined by the fetal status and cesarean section reserved for normal obstetric indications.

In the postpartum period, the patient must be monitored closely as the provider should anticipate significant fluid shifts in the first week after delivery.

Pregnancy and acute renal failure

Most of the literature pertaining to dialysis in pregnancy concerns those women with CRF or ESRD. There are, however, a number of case reports of dialysis for ARF in pregnancy. Hemodialysis has been the primary form of dialysis utilized, both for ARF and for acute ingestion of toxic substances [44–46]. Because the incidence of ARF itself has fallen to less than 1% of pregnancies in developed countries, the need for acute dialysis is rare [47]. This topic is addressed in more detail in Chapter 28.

Summary

Although pregnancy remains uncommon in women with severe CRF or ESRD, it is nevertheless a possibility, especially with modern treatment. With intensive management by the obstetrician and nephrologist, the likelihood of a favorable outcome can be maximized. This will generally entail early initiation of dialysis in women with CRF or intensified dialytic therapy in those already requiring renal replacement therapy.

References

1 Okundaye I, Abrinko P, Hou S. Registry of pregnancy in dialysis patients. *Am J Kidney Dis* 1998; 31: 766–773.

2 Toma H, Tanabe K, Tokumoto T et al. A nationwide survey on pregnancies in women on renal replacement therapy in Japan. *Nephrol Dial Transpl* 1998; 31: A163.

3 Registration Committee of the European Dialysis and Transplant Association. Successful pregnancies in women treated by dialysis and kidney transplantation. *Br J Obstet Gynaecol* 1980; 87: 839–845.

4 Gadallah MF, Ahmad B, Karubian F, Campese VM. Pregnancy in patients on chronic ambulatory peritoneal dialysis. *Am J Kidney Dis* 1992; 20: 407–410.

5 Souqiyyeh MZ, Huraib SO, Saleh AG, Aswad S. Pregnancy in chronic hemodialysis patients in the Kingdom of Saudi Arabia. *Am J Kidney Dis* 1992; 19: 235–238.

6 Reddy SS, Holley JL. Management of the pregnant chronic dialysis patient. *Adv Chronic Kid Dis* 2007; 14(2): 146–155.

7 Schwarz A, Post KG, Keller F, Molzahn M. Value of human chorionic gonadotropin measurements in blood as a pregnancy test in women on maintenance hemodialysis. *Nephron* 1985; 39: 341–343.

8 Hou SH, Orlowski J, Pahl M et al. Pregnancy in women with end-stage renal disease: treatment of anemia and premature labor. *Am J Kidney Dis* 1993; 21: 16–22.

9 Hou SH. Frequency and outcome of pregnancy in women on dialysis. *Am J Kidney Dis* 1994; 23: 60–63.

10 Redrow M, Lazaro C, Elliot J et al. Dialysis in the management of pregnant patients with renal insufficiency. *Medicine* 1988; 67: 199–208.

11 Chan WS, Okun N, Kjellstrand CM. Pregnancy in chronic dialysis: a review and analysis of the literature. *Int J Artif Organs* 1998; 21: 259–268.

12 Jakobi P, Ohel G, Szylman P, Levit A, Lewin M, Paldi E. Continuous ambulatory peritoneal dialysis as the primary approach in the management of severe renal insufficiency in pregnancy. *Obstet Gynecol* 1992; 79: 808–810.

13 Changs H, Miller MA, Bruns FJ. Tidal peritoneal dialysis during pregnancy improves clearance and abdominal symptoms. *Perit Dial Int* 2002; 22: 272–274.

14 Castillo AA, Lew SQ, Smith AM, Bosch JP. Women issues in female patients receiving peritoneal dialysis. *Adv Ren Replace Ther* 1999; 6: 327–334.

15 Elliot JP, O'Keeffe DF, Schon DA, Cherem LB. Dialysis in pregnancy: a critical review. *Obstet Gynecol Surv* 1991; 46: 319–324.

16 Hou SH. Pregnancy and birth control in CAPD patients. *Adv Perit Dial* 1993; 9: 173–176.

17 Bagon JA, Vernaeve H, de Muylder X et al. Pregnancy and dialysis. *Am J Kidney Dis* 1998; 31: 756–765.

18 Hou SH, Grossman SD. Pregnancy in chronic dialysis patients. *Semin Dial* 1990; 3: 224–229.

19 Hou S. Pregnancy in dialysis patients: Where do we go from here? *Semin Dial* 2003; 16(5): 376–378.

20 Nageotte MP, Grundy HO. Pregnancy outcome in women requiring chronic hemodialysis. *Obstet Gynecol* 1988; 72: 456–459.

21 Hou SH. Pregnancy in women on haemodialysis and peritoneal dialysis. *Bailliere's Clin Obstet Gynaecol* 1994; 8: 481–500.

22 Grossman S, Hou S. Obstetrics and gynecology. In: Daugirdas JT, Ing TS, eds. *Handbook of dialysis*. New York: Little, Brown, 1994: 649–661.

23 Lew SQ, Watson JA. Urea and creatinine generation and removal in a pregnant patient receiving peritoneal dialysis. *Adv Perit Dial* 1992; 8: 131–135.

24 Weiner Z, Thaler I, Ronen N, Brandes JM. Changes in flow velocity waveforms in umbilical and uterine artery following haemodialysis. *Br J Obstet Gynaecol* 1991; 98: 1172–1173.

25 Jakobi P, Weiner Z, Geri R, Zaidise I. Umbilical and arcuate uterine artery flow velocity measurements during acute hemodialysis. *Gynecol Obstet Invest* 1993; 37: 247–248.

26 Krakow D, Castro LC, Schwieger J. Effect of hemodialysis on uterine and umbilical artery Doppler flow velocity waveforms. *Am J Obstet Gynecol* 1993; 170: 1386–1388.

27 Cunningham FG, Cox SM, Harstad TW et al. Chronic renal disease and pregnancy outcome. *Am J Obstet Gynecol* 1990; 163: 453–459.

28 Imbasciati E, Ponticelli C. Pregnancy and renal disease: predictors for fetal and maternal outcome. *Am J Nephrol* 1991; 11: 353–362.

29 Hou S. Pregnancy in chronic renal insufficiency and end-stage renal disease. *Am J Kidney Dis* 1999; 33: 235–252.

30 Jungers P, Chauveau D, Choukroun G et al. Pregnancy in women with impaired renal function. *Clin Nephrol* 1997; 47: 281–288.

31 Reece EA, Leguizamon G, Homko C. Pregnancy performance and outcomes associated with diabetic nephropathy. *Am J Perinatol* 1998; 15: 413–421.

32 Holly J, Reddy S. Pregnancy in dialysis patients: A review of outcomes, complications, and management. *Semin Dial* 2003; 16: 389–402.

33 Barth W, Lacroix L, Goldberg M, Greene M. Recombinant human erythropoietin (rHEpo) for severe anemia in pregnancies complicated by renal disease. *Am J Obstet Gynecol* 1994; 170: 329A.

34 Scott LL, Ramin SM, Richey M et al. Erythropoietin use in pregnancy: two cases and a review of the literature. *Am J Perinatol* 1995; 12: 22–24.

35 Hou S, Firanek C. Management of the pregnant dialysis patient. *Adv Ren Replace Ther* 1998; 5: 24–30.

36 Pryde PG, Sedman AB, Nugent CE et al. Angiotensin-converting enzyme inhibitor fetopathy. *J Am Soc Nephrol* 1993; 3: 1575–1582.

37 Bhatt Mehta V, Deluga KS. Fetal exposure to lisinopril: Neonatal manifestations and management. *Pharmacotherapy* 1993; 13: 515–518.

38 Sibai BM. Hypertension. In: Gabbe SG, Niebyl JR, Simpson J, eds. *Obstetrics: Normal and Problem Pregnancies*, 5th edn. Philadelphia, PA: Elsevier, 2007: 903.

39 DaFonseca EB, Carvalho MHB, Zugaib M. Prophylactic administration of progesterone by vaginal suppository to reduce the incidence of spontaneous preterm birth in women at risk: a randomized, placebo-controlled double-blind study. *Am J Obstet Gynecol* 2003; 188: 419–424.

40 Meis PJ, Kleanoff M, Thorn E, Dombrowski MP, Sibai B, Moawad AH, Spong CY et al. Prevention of recurrent preterm delivery by 17 alpha-hydroxyprogesterone caproate. *N Engl J Med* 2003; 348: 2379–2385.

41 Reister F, Reister B, Heyl W et al. Dialysis and pregnancy – A case report and review of the literature. *Ren Fail* 1999; 21: 533–539.

42 Yasin SY, Bey Doun SN. Hemodialysis in pregnancy. *Obstet Gynecol Surv* 1988; 43: 655–668.

43 Hou SH. Pregnancy in continuous ambulatory peritoneal dialysis (CAPD) patients. *Perit Dial Int* 1990; 10: 201–204.

44 Trebbin WM. Hemodialysis and pregnancy. *JAMA* 1979; 241: 1811–1812.

45 Kleinman GE, Rodriquez H, Good MC, Caudle MR. Hypercalcemic crisis in pregnancy associated with excessive ingestion of calcium carbonate antacid (milk–alkali syndrome): successful treatment with hemodialysis. *Obstet Gynecol* 1991; 78: 496–499.

46 Devlin K. Pregnancy complicated by acute renal failure requiring hemodialysis. *Anna J* 1994; 27: 444–445.

47 Krane NK. Acute renal failure in pregnancy. *Arch Intern Med* 1988; 148: 2347–2357.

14 Cardiopulmonary Bypass

Katherine W. Arendt
Mayo Clinic, Rochester, MN, USA

Introduction

Cardiopulmonary bypass (CPB) is a commonly used and often necessary technique during cardiac surgery. It results in significant alterations in patient physiology with virtually every organ system affected. Some of the prominent adverse effects include: (i) profound alterations in coagulation (dilution of all clotting factors, intense heparinization, platelet dysfunction); (ii) disturbances in cardiovascular function (hypotension, non-pulsatile blood flow, myocardial ischemia and cardiac stunning, arrhythmias); and (iii) a significant generalized systemic inflammatory response. Systemic embolization of particulate material occurs, including marrow and fat spilled into the chest when the sternum is split. Air embolization also frequently occurs. Embolic phenomena are thought to be major contributors to the significant risk of cerebrovascular accident (2–6%) and neurocognitive dysfunction (20–60%) [1–3]. In addition, the management of patients requiring CPB frequently includes the use of hypothermic techniques, invasive monitoring, and the administration of a variety of cardiovascular drugs. Not infrequently, complications involving one or more major organ systems are experienced.

The application of "off-pump" coronary artery bypass for patients with coronary artery disease has become popular to a great degree because of the inherent risks of CPB [4]. However, off-pump approaches are not available for patients with cardiac valvular surgical disease, the cardiac pathology that most often affects the pregnant patient. Closed mitral valvotomy in order to avoid cardiopulmonary bypass (CPB) in pregnancy has been widely described [5–7]. Likewise, more and more cardiac procedures are being done without requiring CPB with percutaneous modalities. However, fetal radiation exposure during fluoroscopy remains a prohibitive factor for percutaneous techniques during pregnancy. Echocardiography imaging alone without fluoroscopy has been described in percutaneous balloon valvuloplasty [8,9], but experience in this technique is limited. For now, many cardiac procedures will continue to require parturients to undergo CPB for open heart or aorta surgeries.

The first reports of cardiac surgery during pregnancy were published in 1952 and involved 11 closed mitral commissurotomies performed during pregnancy [10–13]. In 1958, CPB was first performed on a pregnant woman [14]. Since this time, multiple cases and series have been published describing CPB in pregnancy [15]. Maternal mortality for cardiac surgeries does not appear to be affected by pregnancy, but the risk of fetal loss is significant.

Maternal and fetal risks of cardiopulmonary bypass

For understandable reasons, no well-controlled studies have been reported assessing the impact of CPB on the pregnant patient, the fetoplacental unit, or fetal outcome. In addition, many of the existing case series date back to the late 1950s and early 1960s. Approaches and techniques that cardiac patients receive continue to change. Thus, many conclusions regarding management and outcome must be viewed with caution.

From the data that are available, pregnant women do well during CPB with a variable mortality rate similar to that for non-pregnant patients: 1.4–13.3%. Fetal loss, however, is significant, with rates ranging from 16% to 38.5%. These quoted mortality rates are from multiple published series [16–22]. The first series of CPB in pregnancy was published in 1969 and described 20 cases with a single (5%) maternal death and 7 (33%) fetal deaths [16]. The highest fetal mortality was reported in a series of 15 parturients in Mexico undergoing open heart surgery from 1972 to 1998 with 2 (13.3%) maternal deaths and 5 (38.5%) fetal deaths [22]. In the most recent literature, Weiss et al. (1998) [23] describes 59 cases of CPB in pregnancy reported in the literature from 1984 to 1996 with 3 (5%) maternal deaths and a fetal/neonatal mortality rate of 29%. They also noted a 25% rate of premature births.

Critical Care Obstetrics, 5th edition. Edited by M. Belfort, G. Saade, M. Foley, J. Phelan and G. Dildy.

With such significant fetal death rates, it is likely that fetal morbidity is similarly high in the fetal survivors of CPB. At present, there are no long-term follow-up studies assessing the probable deleterious effects of CPB on those with fetal exposure to CPB. The confounding effects of fetal exposures to their mother's cardiac disease, pharmacologic management, and possibly other cardiac interventions would make such assessments difficult.

In spite of the significant number of series that have been published describing mortality rates associated with CPB in pregnancy, few correlations can be made with CPB techniques and reduction in maternal and fetal morbidity and mortality. The optimal gestational age at the time of surgery, fetal heart rate monitoring, high flow CPB, normothermic CPB, and possibly pulsatile CPB have all been proposed to improve outcome.

Cardiac procedures avoiding cardiopulmonary bypass

The physiologic changes of pregnancy involve increases in cardiac output. Because of this, left-sided obstructive lesions such as mitral or aortic valvular stenosis are more likely than other valvular lesions to cause complications during pregnancy [24]. Likewise, most available reports of cardiac surgery during pregnancy involve valve repair or replacement.

With the significant fetal risks CPB, parturients with mitral stenosis may be evaluated for candidacy for closed mitral commissurotomy. In this procedure, CPB is not necessary. Instead, the cardiothoracic surgeon performs an anterior lateral thoracotomy, places his or her finger inside the left atrium, guides a dilator across the mitral valve orifice and splits open the narrowed mitral valve. Early collective experience in over 500 patients undergoing closed mitral commissurotomy before 1965 was associated with maternal mortality of under 2% and fetal mortality under 10% [25]. Multiple more recent studies have confirmed that this procedure is lower risk for the fetus than open procedures requiring CPB [5,18,20].

Presently, a more common technique to avoid CPB in the parturient with mitral stenosis is percutaneous balloon mitral commissurotomy [26–30]. Mishra and colleagues (2001) [31] reported improved hemodynamics and symptoms in 81 out of 85 severely symptomatic pregnant women with critical mitral stenosis who underwent this procedure. They noted that although the procedure was safe and generally effective, mitral regurgitation increased by 1–2 grades in 18 of the 85 patients. Abouzied and coworkers (2001) [32] reported similar results in 16 pregnant women with severe mitral stenosis who underwent balloon mitral commissurotomy. They also reported no immediate detrimental effects of radiation exposure related to fluoroscopy on the fetuses. In order to avoid fetal radiation exposure, echocardiography imaging alone without fluoroscopy has been described for this procedure [8,9]. Few centers offer this technique.

Whether by thoracotomy or a percutaneous balloon technique, mitral commissurotomy instead of open valve repair or replacement is associated with a significant likelihood of patients requiring additional surgery at a later date. Mangione and coworkers [28] published favorable results with only 9% of their 23 patients requiring repeat valvuloplasty after 8 years of follow-up. Fawzy and colleagues [29] reported that 16% of their patients undergoing mitral balloon valvuloplasty developed restenosis over a follow-up period of 9 years. In the series of Vosloo and Reichart [5], 22% of patients receiving closed commissurotomy required an additional cardiac surgery during a follow-up period lasting from 5 to 17 years. These data led some to recommend that parturients undergo the open valve repair or replacement requiring CPB during pregnancy.

The performance of coronary artery bypass grafting (CABG) without CPB ('off-pump' CABG, beating heart CABG) avoids the risks of CPB. Silberman and coworkers [33] describe a case of coronary artery bypass grafting performed on a beating heart without the use of CPB on a patient at 22 weeks gestation status after spontaneous dissection of the left anterior descending artery. She subsequently gave birth to a healthy term baby. Although long-term (10 years) results of beating heart CABG are not yet known to be equal to that of traditional CABG techniques, it has gained wider acceptance. This is because studies to date indicate that off-pump CABG techniques provide complete revascularization, reduced myocardial injury, less coagulopathy, decreased transfusion requirements, higher hematocrit at discharge, and shorter hospital length of stay [34].

Timing cardiac surgery during pregnancy

Cardiologists who care for women with heart disease of childbearing age counsel these patients about the risks of pregnancy and optimizing their condition before conception. Such optimization is not always possible, pregnancy is not always planned, and often the existence or extent of cardiac disease is unmasked by the cardiovascular changes of the pregnancy itself. Therefore, cardiologists and cardiovascular surgeons are left trying to decide if surgical intervention is going to be necessary before term delivery and, if so, the optimal gestational age to intervene.

Typically, in obstetric medicine, what is in the best interest of maternal health is in the best interest of her fetus. This may not be the case when deciding the timing of surgery in the parturient with a deteriorating cardiac status. In a systematic review from 1984 to 1996, Weiss et al. compared maternal and fetal outcomes in cardiac surgeries performed during pregnancy, those performed immediately after delivery of the neonate, and those in which the surgery was delayed until after the postpartum period [23]. Fetal mortality was greatest (about 30%) in those surgeries performed during pregnancy, with two (5%) fetal deaths when the mother underwent surgery immediately after delivery, and no fetal deaths when the mother delayed surgery until the postpartum period. In contrast, however, the maternal mortality increased when the surgery was delayed until after birth. Therefore, it seems that the fetus benefits most from delaying maternal cardiac surgery until after birth, but the mother may benefit from an earlier intervention, while still pregnant. Clearly, these retrospective data may be confounded by the fact that the sickest parturients were unable to wait for surgery and had to be treated earlier. Nonetheless, the challenge of determining the optimal timing for a deteriorating parturient is difficult and this study illustrates the consequences of this important clinical judgment: decreasing maternal risk by intervening early may result in fetal demise while delaying until after delivery may result in maternal death.

In determining the optimal gestational timing for cardiac surgery, the effects of general anesthesia need to be considered separately from the effects of CPB. The most thorough evaluation of the risks of all types of anesthesia and surgery during pregnancy retrospectively evaluated a population of 720 000 pregnant women who underwent 5405 surgical procedures [35]. The incidence of congenital malformations or stillbirths was not increased in the offspring in the women who underwent surgery, regardless of gestational age at the time of surgery. The incidence of prematurity, low-birth-weight infants and the rate of infant death within 168 hours of birth was slightly increased. This increase, however, was not linked to the gestational age at the time of surgery. Further, patients who require surgery may have underlying illness that affects the health of their pregnancy. This confounds the results making it difficult to determine the singular risk of surgery during pregnancy. Very few of the cases in this series involved CPB. Therefore, although we can state that anesthesia at any time during pregnancy is probably safe, the risks of fetal exposure to CPB at various times during gestation are less clear.

No relationship between gestational age at the time of CPB surgery and fetal morbidity and mortality can be conclusively determined at this time. There is, however, a case report of a parturient undergoing mitral valve surgery at the 6th week of gestation with fetal hydrocephalus detected at 18 weeks gestation by ultrasound [36]. Some quote this case along with a case from the 1960s as reason to avoid surgery requiring CPB during the first trimester [37,38]. A case report of fetal hydrocephalus and hydrops has also been described after CPB at 19 weeks gestational age, illustrating that the second trimester is not free from fetal risk. [39] In retrospective series of parturients undergoing CPB, fetal mortality has been described during every trimester of gestation [16–18,22,23]. Therefore, although the risks of anesthesia and CPB during first trimester and organogenesis would theoretically increase fetal risks, there are no data to support this theory. None the less, many anesthesiologists, cardiologists, obstetricians and cardiothoracic surgeons recommend that surgery, especially surgery requiring CPB, be delayed until after organogenesis during the first trimester of pregnancy.

During late second trimester, the cardiac output of the parturient peaks. As a result, if the parturient is doing poorly at the beginning of the second trimester, she will likely further deteriorate depending upon the lesion. Therefore, if it is determined that a parturient may not survive into the third trimester, early second trimester may be the ideal time to perform surgery. This prevents further deterioration of cardiac status but exposes the fetus to anesthesia and CPB after organogenesis has occurred. Others suggest that cardiac surgery is best done between 24 and 28 weeks gestation after the attainment of fetal viability. With this timing, neonatal intensive care facilities should be available and if fetal distress is detected, cesarean delivery could occur perioperatively. Cesarean delivery *during* CPB should not occur because of the significant bleeding risk to the mother during heparinization. Successful cesarean delivery just before CPB has been described [16,40].

Uteroplacental perfusion and cardiopulmonary bypass

Uteroplacental blood flow (UPBF) is the major determinant of oxygen and other essential nutrient transport to the fetus. A direct correlation between uterine blood flow (UBF) and fetal oxygenation has been demonstrated in both animal models and humans [41,42]. UPBF is derived primarily from uterine arteries, with a smaller contribution (of unknown significance) coming from the ovarian arteries. The uterine arteries are branches of the internal iliac arteries. Uterine artery blood flow (UABF) increases two- to threefold in pregnancy and can represent up to 12% of the cardiac output. Increases in UBF during pregnancy are due to both physical (increased diameter of the uterine artery) and physiological (decreased responsiveness of the uterine artery to endogenous circulating vasoconstrictors) mechanisms. Selective uterine artery relaxation during pregnancy may be the result of vasodilators released from its endothelium, such as PGI_2 or nitric oxide, or local hormonal actions, which diminish the activity of certain intracellular enzymes that mediate vasoconstriction.

Therefore, under normal circumstances during pregnancy, the uterine arteries are maximally dilated and there is no autoregulation of UABF. Systemic hypotension results in vascular dilation to maintain blood flow for autoregulated organs such as the brain and kidneys. In contrast, the placental vasculature cannot further vasodilate in response to hypotension, and decreased uteroplacental perfusion and, if significant, fetal hypoxia results.

Fetoplacental sufficiency is related to fetal heart rate (FHR) with acute insufficiency resulting in fetal bradycardia and long-term insufficiency with subsequent fetal acidosis resulting in fetal tachycardia with minimal beat-to-beat variability on FHR tracing. An example of FHRs throughout CPB is provided in Figure 14.1. The onset of CPB is typically characterized by fetal bradycardia, while the conclusion of CPB demonstrates fetal tachycardia with minimal beat-to-beat variability [43,44].

The cause of this initial fetal bradycardia is thought to be secondary to placental hypoperfusion because it has been found reversible in most cases by increasing the perfusion rate. Other theories for this initial fetal bradycardia have included maternal

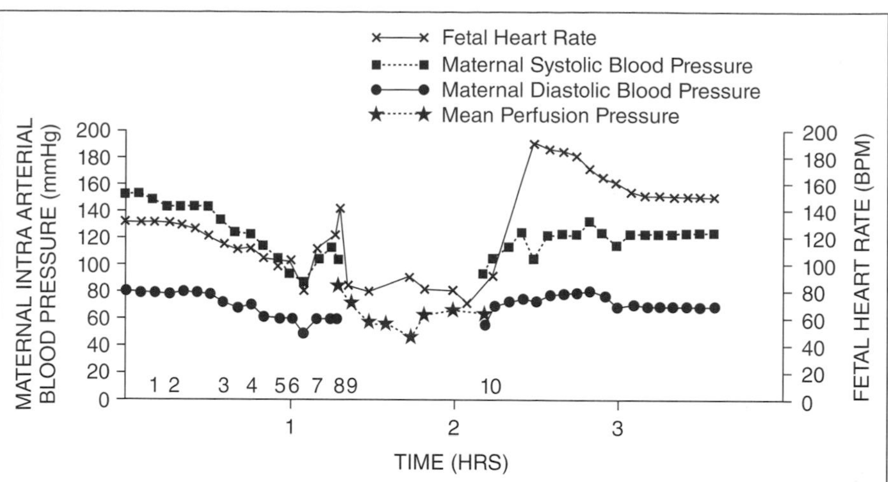

Figure 14.1 Fetal heart rate as related to maternal hemodynamics during cardiopulmonary bypass. 1, induction of anesthesia; 2, ventilatory rate adjustment; 3, median sternotomy; 4, pericardotomy; 5, heparin administration; 6, aortic cannulation and manipulation of the heart; 7, scopolamine and pancuronium administration; 8, start of cardiopulmonary bypass; 9, fall in maternal blood pressure and FHR with start of non-pulsatile flow; 10, cardiopulmonary bypass discontinued. (Reproduced by permission from Levy DL, Warriner RA, Burgess GE. Fetal response to cardiopiulmonary bypass. *Obstet Gynecol* 1980; 56: 112–115.)

hypothermia resulting in fetal bradycardia, fetal hypoxia from hemodilution acutely decreasing the maternal oxygen content, and uterine contractility at the onset of CPB increasing the uterine vascular resistance and decreasing placental sufficiency [45]. Whatever the cause of the initial fetal bradycardia seen with initiation of CPB, many reports indicate that FHR directly correlates with perfusion throughout CPB such that when flow rate is increased, the FHR is restored [19,38,46–50]. Thus, when the fetus is beyond about 25 weeks gestational age, most anesthesiologists monitor fetal heart rate throughout CPB and attempt to establish adequate flow to maintain a normal FHR (110–160 bpm).

Temperature manipulation during hypothermic CPB has also been thought responsible for the FHR changes [45]. It has been known for some time that maternal temperature change results in fetal heart rate changes with hyperthermia causing fetal tachycardia and hypothermia causing fetal bradycardia as shown in Figure 14.2 [51]. However, multiple cases of normothermic CPB demonstrate the characteristic initial bradycardia and post-CPB tachycardia, sustaining the theory that although temperature influences FHR, the typical changes observed during CPB are likely a result of uteroplacental insufficiency.

At the conclusion of CPB, the fetal heart rate often becomes tachycardic with minimal beat-to-beat variability which is presumed to be secondary to fetal acidosis developing from continuous uteroplacental insufficiency throughout CPB. The uteroplacental insufficiency throughout bypass is likely from multiple causes. Gas or debris could embolize to the placenta during CPB resulting in decreased perfusion. It is also known that CPB may cause regional alterations in flow in particular vascular beds. Studies are indicating that the non-pulsatile flow that occurs during non-pulsatile CPB incites placental vasoconstriction.

Animal studies researching placental function during CPB place an animal fetus on CPB and evaluate the effects of various bypass techniques on this exquisitely sensitive model. The bypass machine in these models does not have an oxygenator, but instead evaluates the placenta as an oxygenator as blood is pumped through it by the CPB machine. As the CPB techniques are changed, the blood gases of the fetus are evaluated. Some researchers believe that information gained from this model should translate to CPB techniques of the human parturient because placental function is still being evaluated, albeit from the other side [40].

By comparing the vasoactive effects of acetylcholine (endothelium dependent) and nitroprusside (endothelium independent), this model has shown that non-pulsatile flow bypass selectively inhibits endothelium-dependent vasodilation [52]. In other words, non-pulsatile flow and the absence of sheer stress on the vessel inhibits the placental endothelium's ability to synthesize nitric oxide. In contrast, pulsatile flow bypass preserves nitric oxide synthesis of the placental endothelium [53,54]. With the placental vasoconstriction that occurs with non-pulsatile CPB, higher flows and increased mean arterial pressures may be necessary to perfuse the placenta.

Myometrial activity during CPB

The onset of sustained contractions during CPB can lead to fetal distress and possible fetal death [20]. When the uterus contracts, placental vascular resistance increases, placental perfusion decreases, and if relaxation does not occur subsequent fetal hypoxia ensues. The mechanism(s) responsible for these uterine contractions have not been clearly delineated. The dilutional effect of CPB has been postulated to reduce the hormonal levels of progesterone resulting in increased uterine excitability [18,40,49]. Sabik and coworkers [55] have implicated the production of vasoactive prostaglandins. Further, both the cooling and rewarming phases of CPB are associated with sustained uterine contractions [18]. Normothermic (versus hypothermic) CPB demonstrates increased fetal survival which may partially be a result of preventing the contractions associated with temperature change [19].

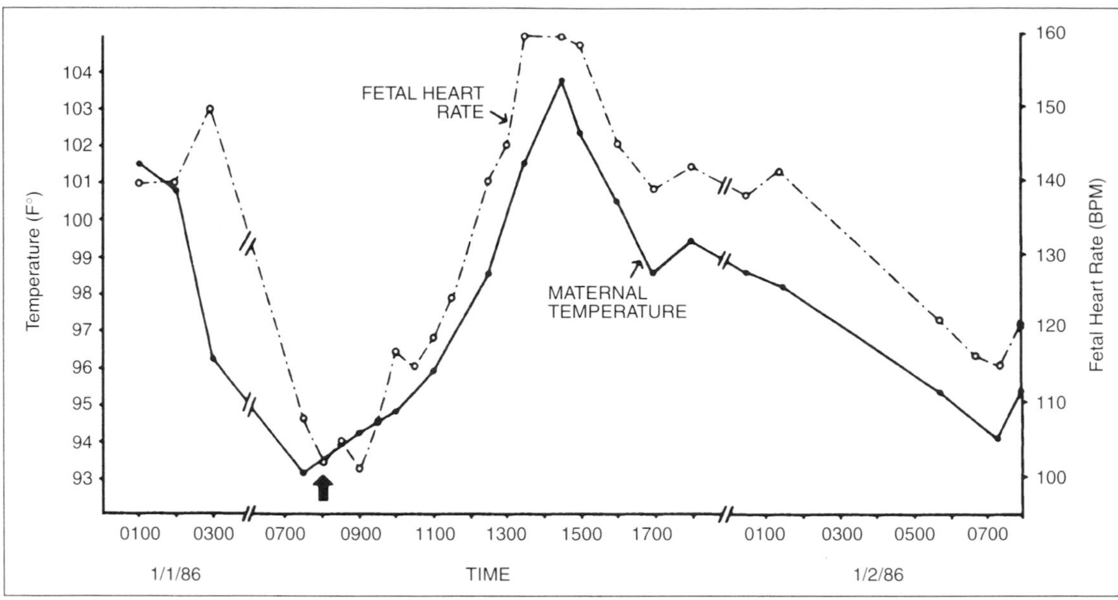

Figure 14.2 Maternal temperature and fetal heart rate (FHR). The FHR plot directly parallels the maternal temperature. The arrow at 0800, 1/1/86, represents the nadir of maternal BP: 87/46 mmHg (mean arterial pressure, 69). Within 20 minutes the BP was 94/57 mmHg (mean arterial pressure, 69). The mean arterial pressure during the rest of the illustrated time ranged from 64 to 76. Previous and subsequent pressures during this pregnancy ranged from 90/50 to 110/65 mmHg (mean arterial pressure, 63–80). BPM, beats per minute. (Reproduced by permission from Jadhon ME, Main EK. Fetal bradycardia associated with maternal hypothermia. *Obstet Gynecol* 1988; 72: 496.)

The anesthesiologist and obstetrician should monitor in order to detect uterine contractions so they can be treated immediately and appropriately. The routine prophylactic use of tocolysis before CPB surgery is controversial, especially because of the cardiac effect of the ß$_2$-sympathomimetic agents [50,56]. Progesterone, ß$_2$-sympathomimetic agents such as ritodrine or terbutaline, indomethacin, nitroglycerin, intravenous ethanol, and magnesium sulfate have all been described with some effect in decreasing uterine contractions associated with CPB [40,46,49,57]. In general, uterine contractions should be treated first with increased perfusion pressure and flow, then by increasing the potent volatile anesthetic agent to reduce uterine tone or by administering a tocolytic agent such as magnesium, nitroglycerin, ritodrine or terbutaline depending upon the hemodynamics at the time and recognizing the cardiac effects of the latter two ß$_2$-sympathomimetic agents.

Fetal monitoring during cardiopulmonary bypass

Consideration for fetal monitoring is important whether or not the fetus is viable. In the presence of bradycardia, alterations in pump flow, pressure or temperature may improve fetal status and outcome. Such monitoring is often most easily performed with continuous external electronic fetal heart rate monitoring, assuming fetal size, fetal movement and maternal habitus do not preclude such a technique. Otherwise, intermittent auscultation may allow the obstetric attendant to detect significant decreases in fetal heart rate and suggest the need for interventions [58].

Besides fetal bradycardia, other fetal heart rate features, such as diminished variability, fetal tachycardia and a sinusoidal-like pattern, have also been described in association with decreased perfusion during CPB and may be amenable to pump manipulation, as described previously [43,44,49,59]. Fetal decelerations or diminished variability occurring despite increased CPB flow in normothermic patients with normal acid–base status may be secondary to fetal exposure to drugs administered during anesthesia [48,60–62]. Such FHR changes will recover after anesthetic recovery and do not indicate fetal distress.

If technically feasible, uterine activity also should be monitored during CPB. Uterine contractile activity should be anticipated, especially during periods of reduced mean arterial pressure during and after CPB. If consistent uterine contractions or prolonged tetany of the uterus is detected, prompt treatment as previously discussed is warranted. Tocodynamometry should continue into the immediate postoperative days.

Anesthesia and surgery in the parturient

Lateral uterine displacement during surgery is essential to avoid aortocaval compression, and decreased cardiac output and uteroplacental perfusion [63]. A lateral tilt of at least 30–40° has been recommended during CPB [18,64]. This is especially crucial because CPB often involves periods of hypotension, and such compression is enhanced during periods of hypotension, further worsening a hypotensive episode. A combination of a wedge and table tilt is generally adequate to achieve appropriate lateral uterine displacement.

Anesthesiologists should also be aware that parturients have increased rates of failed intubation compared to non-pregnant patients [65,66]. Edema of the airway structures as pregnancy progresses may impede the anesthesiologist's laryngoscopic view. Because of reduction in functional residual capacity and an increase in oxygen consumption, an apneic parturient will drop their PaO_2 at twice the rate of a non-pregnant woman [67]. Therefore, careful attention should be paid to the obstetric airway.

Mechanical positive-pressure ventilation is instituted routinely in patients undergoing cardiac surgery, and various degrees of hyperventilation are frequently produced, either intentionally or inadvertently. Blood gas disturbances can affect sympathetic activity and thus indirectly affect UBF. In addition, hyperventilation may decrease uteroplacental perfusion either through mechanical means by increasing intrathoracic pressure and decreasing cardiac output, or through the induction of hypocapnia, which decreases UBF. Thus, hyperventilation should be minimized or avoided in the pregnant surgical patient unless specifically indicated.

The presence of pre-eclampsia and eclampsia complicate the anesthetic management of the parturient significantly. These patients are exquisitely sensitive to sympathetic stimulation, probably from impaired endothelial function. Cerebral vascular accident from malignant hypertension must be avoided with adequate antihypertension therapy, a deep induction for laryngoscopy, adequate anesthesia throughout surgery, and careful titration of sympathomimetic agents. This complex disease state and its anesthetic implications are reviewed elsewhere [68,69].

Cardiopulmonary bypass technique

Priming the pump

The various components of the CPB apparatus (e.g. tubing) require approximately 2 L of priming solution in most adult circuits. Priming of the CPB circuit produces hemodilution which is an important element of CPB. It decreases blood product utilization and its attendant costs and risks. Hemodilution also improves the rheology of blood by decreasing its viscosity, resulting in a lower arterial resistance and improved peripheral perfusion [70]. Other purported benefits of hemodilution during CPB include decreases in major organ complications, such as cerebral vascular accident, and renal and pulmonary dysfunction. In the pregnant cardiac surgical patient, or any anemic patient for that matter, CPB-associated hemodilution may result in severe anemia. This can compromise the oxygen-carrying capacity of blood as well as oxygen delivery. Anemic patients with poor cardiac function may not tolerate severe hemodilution. Whole blood or RBCs can be added to the prime of the CPB circuit so that the resultant hematocrit is no less than 21–26% [61]. Hemodilution and subsequent changes in hormone concentrations, such as a decrease in progesterone, may play a role in triggering uterine contractions [49]. Korsten and coworkers suggested that the addition of progesterone to the prime may be helpful in avoiding preterm uterine activity, but this approach requires further investigation before incorporation into clinical practice.

Mannitol is often added to the CPB prime in order to promote an osmotic diuresis and to scavenge oxygen free radicals from the circulation. For parturients, some recommend omitting mannitol in the CPB prime to decrease the risk of hemoconcentrating fetal blood [71]. As the osmotic pressure of the maternal blood increases, water would be pulled from the fetal into the maternal blood within the placenta. On the other hand, one case of fetal hydrocephalus and hydrops detected after CPB at 19 weeks gestation has been reported [39]. Perhaps the maternal hemodilution that occurs during CPB results in overhydration of fetal blood and resulting hydrops in some cases. Mannitol may prevent this. Further investigation is needed regarding the use of mannitol in CPB prime.

Hypothermia

Hypothermia was considered an important component of CPB for many years in order to decrease systemic and vital organ oxygen consumption and minimize organ damage. Animal studies initially demonstrated safety in the parturient, because the fetal sheep in pregnant ewes cooled to 29°C did not exhibit fetal distress as long as maternal acidosis and hypoxia were avoided [72]. Likewise, hypothermic CPB and even deep hypothermic circulatory arrest have been described with successful maternal fetal outcomes [56,73,74]. However, its use is now deemed less beneficial and perhaps unnecessary. It may also be harmful in the parturient, resulting in fetal bradycardia and possibly asystole, the provocation of uterine contractions, decreased placental blood flow and interference with placental function.

As maternal temperature decreases, FHR also decreases as demonstrated in Figure 13.2. Whether this is related to a decrease in fetal metabolism, changes in the placental vasculature, or fetal distress is not known. If hypothermic CPB is performed, decreases in FHR should be expected. An attempt to bring the FHR back into the normal range (110–160 bpm) by increasing flow may be prudent, but may not be successful as described in one case report in which the FHR decreased to 50 beats per minute [56]. The fetal heart rate in this case increased only after rewarming and the fetus survived. Two case reports describe the loss of fetal heart tones and presumed fetal asystole during hypothermia that were detected again after the surgery with subsequent fetal survival [62,74].

A fetal bypass study placed eight fetal ewes on CPB with the placenta working as an oxygenator [75]. Four fetuses had CPB performed at 37°C at various flow rates and four at 25°C at various flow rates. Although PCO_2 was lower in the hypothermic ewes, fetal oxygenation was significantly worse. This indicates that the placenta acts as a poor oxygenator during hypothermic CPB.

Hypothermia has been shown to decrease umbilical blood flow velocity in the human fetus. Goldstein et al. [45] measured umbilical artery flow velocities during hypothermic CPB (nadir 29°C) and found an absence of end-diastolic uterine artery blood flow from 10 minutes after initiation of CPB until the patient began rewarming. Because the diastolic flow returned after rewarming but before the end of CPB, he related the decrease in uterine blood flow to temperature, not just the effects of non-pulsatile CPB itself.

Rewarming is associated with increased frequency of uterine contractions [18] and reports of fetal heart rate decelerations have been reported in association with rewarming. Mahli and coworkers [62] suggest that these fetal decelerations may be secondary to deficient delivery of heat to the fetus during rewarming as a result of vasoconstriction of the umbilical vessels. Current knowledge and practice has been to avoid aggressive rewarming strategies. Such strategies were more often practiced in the past and have more recently been associated with increased CNS adverse effects [76].

The most influential study demonstrating the potential fetal benefit of normothermic CPB retrospectively evaluated 69 reports of CPB during pregnancy from 1958 to 1992 [19]. In evaluation of the 40 most recent cases, hypothermic CPB was associated with a fetal mortality of 24.0% while normothermic CPB was associated with no fetal losses. Because of this demonstrated improvement in fetal survival as well as the reports of fetal asystole, uterine contractions, and decreased placental blood flow during hypothermic CPB, normothermic CPB is preferred.

Pulsatility

Non-pulsatile flow is most commonly employed during CPB. It can be argued that pulsatile flow could be superior, providing a more normal physiologic milieu and better tissue and organ perfusion than non-pulsatile blood flow. For example, differences in vascular resistance, oxygen delivery, and myocardial lactate production indicate the superiority of pulsatile CPB [48,77,78]. As discussed earlier, non-pulsatile flow and the absence of sheer stress on the vessel inhibits the placental endothelium's ability to synthesize nitric oxide [52]. These same researchers also demonstrated that although the levels of endothelin-1, a potent vasoconstrictor, were increased after 60 minutes of both pulsatile and non-pulsatile CPB, the levels were significantly higher in the non-pulsatile group. Pulsatile flow has also been shown to maintain placental perfusion through decreasing the activation of the fetal renin–angiotensin–aldosterone axis, decreasing vasoconstriction of the fetal placental vasculature [78].

Non-pulsatile perfusion is performed during CPB at most institutions[79]. Pulsatile flow has been attempted in human parturients. In one case, a roller pump was used in a pulsed mode to produce maternal arterial pulse pressures of about 35 mmHg [80]. Two cases of intra-aortic balloon pump use in parturients have also been described [71]. In one case, the balloon pump was used to improve fetoplacental perfusion after CPB. In the second, the pump was inserted during the bypass period to produce pulsatility and thereby improve fetoplacental perfusion. Both patients did well. In spite of these potential benefits, clinical application of pulsatile flow during CPB is uncommon.

Flow and perfusion pressure

Because normal cardiac output in pregnant women is often greater than 6 L/min [81], the usual flows (~2.5 L/m^2) employed during CPB may be too little. Changes in baseline fetal heart rate have been identified after initial flow rates as high as 80 mL/kg/min, even in the absence of maternal hypotension [50]. Increases in CPB flows to 3.0–4.0 L/m^2 have been successfully (if only temporarily) employed during surgery in the pregnant patient, especially in response to fetal bradycardia [18,50,82]. For example, Koh and associates [43] were the first to describe improvement in fetal bradycardia by increasing flow rate by 16%. Other investigators have since confirmed the value of increasing pump flow rate to improve fetal bradycardia [20,46–49,82]. Further, fetal bypass animal models have shown that moderately high flow rates improve placental function [83].

The ideal mean arterial pressure (MAP) during CPB is not firmly established for cardiac surgical patients in general. In the pregnant patient, the use of moderate to high arterial pressures during CPB is recommended. Some recommend that MAP should initially be maintained at a level of 70 mmHg or greater. It is preferable to produce elevations in MAP with fluid volume administration and high flow rates as opposed to vasopressor administration, which could have an adverse effect on UPBF. It should be anticipated that on institution of CPB, transient but significant hypotension occurs and frequently produces fetal bradycardia [43,44,48,82]. This is generally correctable by appropriate manipulations of pump flow and pressure.

Cardioplegia

Myocardial protection during CPB is essential to reduce perioperative cardiac morbidity. Both cold and warm blood cardioplegia have been shown to reduce cardiac morbidity [84]. The application of cardioplegia may need to be more frequent with the maintenance of high flows during CPB, especially if normothermia or only mild hypothermia is employed. Normothermic perfusion often results in early rewarming of the left ventricle leading to difficulties with myocardial protection [40]. Cardiac activity may return as frequently as every 10 minutes under these circumstances. In one study, 3.5 L of cardioplegia was required to adequately suppress cardiac activity [49]. The use of cold cardioplegia has been associated with fetal bradycardia [85] and continuous cold pericardial irrigation or warm blood cardioplegia have been suggested as effective alternatives [86]. Concomitant tocolytic therapy may potentially also increase the need for cardioplegia and it is generally avoided as an elective prophylactic measure.

Anticoagulation and hematologic considerations

Anticoagulation is essential during CPB. It is generally accomplished with heparin therapy which has posed little risks to the fetus when used for CPB. Such anticoagulation is typically reversed with protamine sulfate following successful weaning and separation from the CPB pump. This drug has also not been shown to harm the fetus.

The use of antifibrinolytic agents to reduce blood loss in cardiac surgery during pregnancy has not been studied. Because pregnancy is associated with physiologic enhancement in clotting, the parturient likely relies upon fibrinolysis to prevent thrombotic adverse events such as placental infarction or deep venous thrombosis formation. Therefore, the use of antifibrinolytic therapy in pregnancy may not be prudent.

When transfusing red blood cells to the parturient, it is important to maintain the physiologic anemia of pregnancy (hemoglobin about 11.6 g/dL or hematocrit 35.5%). Teleologically, the decreased viscosity likely occurs to maintain uteroplacental perfusion. This is illustrated by the fact that elevations of maternal hematocrit are associated with placental infarction [87].

Acid–base status

Acid–base status may vary significantly during CPB. The most common approaches to the management of acid–base status during CPB are called alpha STAT and pH STAT. Briefly, alpha STAT management attempts to maintain a normal enzymatic milieu. This is accomplished by targeting normocarbia, as determined by blood gas analysis of a blood sample at a temperature of 37°C. pH STAT management attempts to maintain a pH of 7.4, no matter what the patient's temperature. This usually involves the addition of carbon dioxide to the CPB oxygenator to maintain a calculated patient blood PCO_2 of 40 mmHg at the patient's temperature during hypothermic CPB. While commonly practiced in the past, pH STAT approaches have become less popular in the adult cardiac surgical patient population.

During pregnancy, $PaCO_2$ decreases to 30 mmHg by week 12, bicarbonate concentration decreases to about 20 mEq/L, the base excess decreases to 2–3 mEq/L, and the blood pH increases by 0.02 to 0.06 units [88]. Normally, the fetal pH is 0.1 units lower than that of the mother. Maintenance of a normal acid–base balance is paramount for the parturient and her fetus. Maternal acidosis can result in fetal acidosis, and the fetus is unable to compensate for acidemia by compensatory respiratory and renal responses like the adult. Therefore, maternal pH should be kept as close to 7.44 as possible. Likewise, hyperventilation and alkalosis should be avoided because this shifts the oxyhemoglobin dissociation curve to the left with subsequent decreased unloading of oxygen from mother to fetus. In sheep, it has been demonstrated that maternal hyperventilation with hypocapnia and alkalemia decreases fetal oxygenation [89]. Therefore, maternal $PaCO_2$ should be kept as close to 30 mmHg as possible and maternal alkalosis or acidosis avoided.

Cardiopulmonary bypass duration

The technical proficiency and speed of the cardiac surgical team are two of the primary determinants of outcome in cardiac surgery. With regard to the pregnant cardiac patient, fetal morbidity and mortality also appear to increase with CPB duration. Thus, it is essential that CPB time be minimized in the pregnant patient.

Postoperative course

The most common problems cardiac surgery patients experience in the immediate postoperative period involve hemostasis, and cardiovascular and respiratory function. Less commonly, renal function may deteriorate and renal failure significantly worsens the prognosis. In the pregnant patient, such problems, if severe, may necessitate postoperative emergency cesarean delivery [90].

Patients undergoing CPB can suffer significant neurologic complications after heart surgery. Deficits can occur in up to 50% of patients, with a much smaller percentage (2–3%) experiencing permanent focal or cognitive problems [1–3]. In pregnant patients, these problems also are likely to be of concern for several reasons. Emergency procedures, and especially open heart operations, will increase neurologic complication rates. Systemic embolization and stroke will also be increased in pregnant patients if their condition includes rheumatic valvular disease with bacterial endocarditis and the presence of vegetations.

Once postoperative bleeding has resolved, and depending on the type of valvular prosthesis employed, mothers may require continued and consistent anticoagulation postoperatively. The complex issues surrounding the use of heparin versus warfarin derivatives in these patients is discussed elsewhere in this text.

Delivery of the fetus may take place several months after cardiac operation. At the time of delivery, the cardiac team should be made aware and complete evaluation of the mother's cardiovascular status should be undertaken even if maternal outcome after cardiac surgery has been excellent. The team should be prepared for treatment of any cardiac problems (e.g. hemorrhage) that may arise during or after delivery.

Summary

Cardiopulmonary bypass during pregnancy is safe for the parturient but poses significant risk to the fetus. If possible, delaying the surgery until after delivery is best for the neonate, but can result in increased morbidity and mortality for the mother. High-flow, normothermic, pulsatile cardiopulmonary bypass of the shortest length possible likely improves outcome for the fetus. Caution with the maternal airway and positioning the parturient in a left lateral tilt are paramount. If possible, fetal heart rate and uterine activity should be monitored throughout CPB. The anesthesiologist should be prepared to treat fetal bradycardia by increasing perfusion flow and to treat uterine activity with tocolytic drug administration as necessary. Fetal and uterine monitoring should continue postoperatively. The acid–base status of the parturient should be maintained to the normal values of pregnancy. Overall, meticulous management and careful monitoring can result in successful outcomes.

References

1 Shaw PJ, Bates D, Cartlidge NE et al. Neurologic and neuropsychological morbidity following major surgery: comparison of coronary artery bypass and peripheral vascular surgery. *Stroke* 1987; 18: 700–707.

2 Murkin JM, Martzke JS, Buchan AM, Bentley C, Wong CJ. A randomized study of the influence of perfusion technique and pH management strategy in 316 patients undergoing coronary artery bypass surgery. II. Neurologic and cognitive outcomes. *J Thorac Cardiovasc Surg* 1995; 110: 349–362.

3 Roach GW, Kanchuger M, Mangano CM et al. Adverse cerebral outcomes after coronary bypass surgery. Multicenter Study of Perioperative Ischemia Research Group and the Ischemia Research and Education Foundation Investigators. *N Engl J Med* 1996; 335: 1857–1863.

4 Plomondon ME, Cleveland JC, Jr., Ludwig ST et al. Off-pump coronary artery bypass is associated with improved risk-adjusted outcomes. *Ann Thorac Surg* 2001; 72: 114–119.

5 Vosloo S, Reichart B. The feasibility of closed mitral valvotomy in pregnancy. *J Thorac Cardiovasc Surg* 1987; 93: 675–679.

6 Pavankumar P, Venugopal P, Kaul U, Iyer KS, Das B, Sampathkumar A, Airon B, Rao IM, Sharma ML, Bhatia ML. Closed mitral valvotomy during pregnancy: A 20-year experience. *Scand Cardiovasc J* 1988; 22: 11–15.

7 Abid A, Abid F, Zargouni N, Khayati A. Closed mitral valvotomy in pregnancy–a study of seven cases. *Int Cardiol* 1990; 26: 319–321.

8 Kultursay H, Turkoglu C, Akin M, Payzin S, Soydas C, Akilli A. Mitral balloon valvuloplasty with transesophageal echocardiography without using fluoroscopy. *Cathet Cardiovasc Diagn* 1992; 27: 317–321.

9 Trehan V, Mukhopadhyay S, Nigam A, Yusuf J, Mehta V, Gupta MD, Girish MP, Tyagi S. Mitral valvuloplasty by inoue balloon under transthoracic echocardiographic guidance. *J Am Soc Echocardiogr* 2005; 18: 964–969.

10 Brock R. Valvulotomy in pregnancy. *Proc R Soc Med* 1952; 45: 538.

11 Cooley DA, Chapman DW. Mitral commissurotomy during pregnancy. *JAMA* 1952; 150: 1113.

12 Logan A, Turner RWD. Mitral valvulotomy during pregnancy. *Lancet* 1952; 1: 1286.

13 Mason J, Stable FE, Szekely PJ. Cardiac disease in pregnancy. *J Obstet Gyn Brit Em* 1952; 59: 569.

14 Dubourg G, Broustet P, Brigaud H et al. Correction complete d'une Triade de Fallot, en circulation extra-corporelle, chez une femme enceinte. *Arch Mal Coeur* 1959; 52: 1389–1391.

15 Harken DE, Taylor WJ. Cardiac surgery during pregnancy. *Clin Obstet Gynecol* 1961; 4: 697–709.

16 Zitnik RS, Brandenburg RO, Sheldon R, Wallace RB. Pregnancy and open-heart surgery. *Circulation* 1969; 39: 5(Suppl 1): 257–262.

17 Strickland RA, Oliver WC, Jr., Chantigian RC, Ney JA, Danielson GK. Anesthesia, cardiopulmonary bypass, and the pregnant patient. *Mayo Clin Proc* 1991; 66: 411–429.

18 Becker RM. Intracardiac surgery in pregnant women. *Ann Thorac Surg* 1983; 36: 453–458.

19 Pomini F, Mercogliano D, Cavalletti C, Caruso A, Pomini P. Cardiopulmonary bypass in pregnancy. *Ann Thorac Surg* 1996; 61: 259–268.

20 Bernal JM, Miralles PJ. Cardiac surgery with cardiopulmonary bypass during pregnancy. *Obstet Gynecol Surv* 1986; 41: 1–6.

21 Rossouw GJ, Knott-Craig CJ, Barnard PM, Macgregor LA, Van Zyl WP. Intracardiac operation in seven pregnant women. *Ann Thorac Surg* 1993; 55: 1172–1174.

22 Salazar E, Espinola N, Molina FJ, Reyes A, Barragan R. Heart surgery with cardiopulmonary bypass in pregnant women. *Arch Cardiol Mexico* 2001; 71: 20–27.

23 Weiss BM, von Segesser LK, Alon E, Seifert B, Turina MI. Outcome of cardiovascular surgery and pregnancy: a systematic review of the period 1984–1996. *Am J Obstet Gynecol* 1998; 179: 1643–1653.

24 Siu SC, Sermer M, Colman JM, Alvarez AN, Mercier LA, Morton BC, Kells CM, Bergin ML, Kiess MC, Marcotte F. Prospective multicenter study of pregnancy outcomes in women with heart disease. *Am Heart Assoc* 2001: 515–521.

25 Ueland K. Cardiac surgery and pregnancy. *Am J Obstet Gynecol* 1965; 92: 148.

26 Ben Farhat M, Gamra H, Betbout F et al. Percutaneous balloon mitral commissurotomy during pregnancy. *Heart* 1997; 77: 564–567.

27 Gupta A, Lokhandwala YY, Satoskar PR, Salvi VS. Balloon mitral valvotomy in pregnancy: maternal and fetal outcomes. *J Am Coll Surg* 1998; 187: 409–415.

28 Mangione JA, Lourenco RM, dos Santos ES et al. Long-term follow-up of pregnant women after percutaneous mitral valvuloplasty. *Catheter Cardiovasc Interv* 2000; 50: 413–417.

29 Fawzy ME, Kinsara AJ, Stefadouros M et al. Long-term outcome of mitral balloon valvotomy in pregnant women. *J Heart Valve Dis* 2001; 10: 153–157.

30 Uygur D, Beksac MS. Mitral balloon valvuloplasty during pregnancy in developing countries. *Eur J Obstet Gyn Reprod Biol* 2001; 96: 226–228.

31 Mishra S, Narang R, Sharma M et al. Percutaneous transseptal mitral commissurotomy in pregnant women with critical mitral stenosis. *Indian Heart J* 2001; 53: 192–196.

32 Abouzied AM, Al Abbady M, Al Gendy MF, Magdy A, Soliman H, Faheem F, Ramadan T, Yehia A. Percutaneous balloon mitral commissurotomy during pregnancy. *Angiology.* 2001; 52: 205–209.

33 Silberman S, Fink D, Berko RS, Mendzelevski B, Bitran D. Coronary artery bypass surgery during pregnancy. *Eur J Cardiothorac Surg* 1996; 10: 925–926.

34 Puskas JD, Williams WH, Duke PG, Staples JR, Glas KE, Marshall JJ, Leimbach M, Huber P, Garas S, Sammons BH, McCall SA, Petersen RJ, Bailey DE, Chu H, Mahoney EM, Weintraub WS, Guyton RA.

Off-pump coronary artery bypass grafting provides complete revascularization with reduced myocardial injury, transfusion requirements, and length of stay: A prospective randomized comparison of two hundred unselected patients undergoing off-pump versus conventional coronary artery bypass grafting. *J Thorac Cardiovasc Surg* 2003; 125: 797–808.

35 Mazze RI, Kallen B. Reproductive outcome after anesthesia and operation during pregnancy: a registry study of 5405 cases. *Am J Obstet Gynecol* 1989; 161: 1178–1185.

36 Lapiedra OJ, Bernal JM, Ninot S, Gonzalez I, Pastor E, Miralles PJ. Open heart surgery for thrombosis of a prosthetic mitral valve during pregnancy. Fetal hydrocephalus. *J Cardiovasc Surg (Torino)* 1986; 27: 217–220.

37 Leyse R, Ofstun M, Dillard DH, Merendino KA. Congenital aortic stenosis in pregnancy, corrected by extracorporeal circulation, offering a viable male infant at term but with anomalies eventuating in his death at four months of age–report of a case. *JAMA* 1961; 176: 1009–1012.

38 Westaby S, Parry AJ, Forfar JC. Reoperation for prosthetic valve endocarditis in the third trimester of pregnancy. *Ann Thorac Surg* 1992; 53: 263–265.

39 Khandelwal M, Rasanen J, Ludormirski A, Addonizio P, Reece EA. Evaluation of fetal and uterine hemodynamics during maternal cardiopulmonary bypass. *ACOG J* 1996; 88: 667–671.

40 Parry AJ, Westaby S. Cardiopulmonary bypass during pregnancy. *Ann Thorac Surg* 1996; 61: 1865–1869.

41 Skillman CA, Plessinger MA, Woods JR, Clark KE. Effect of graded reductions in uteroplacental blood flow on the fetal lamb. *Am J Physiol* 1985; 249: H1098–1105.

42 Bilardo CM, Nicolaides KH, Campbell S. Doppler measurements of fetal and uteroplacental circulations: relationship with umbilical venous blood gases measured at cordocentesis. *Am J Obstet Gynecol* 1990; 162: 115–120.

43 Koh KS, Friesen RM, Livingstone RA, Peddle LJ. Fetal monitoring during maternal cardiac surgery with cardiopulmonary bypass. *Can Med Assoc J* 1975; 112: 1102–1104.

44 Levy DL, Warriner RA, III, Burgess GE, III. Fetal response to cardiopulmonary bypass. *Obstet Gynecol* 1980; 56: 112–115.

45 Goldstein I, Jakobi P, Gutterman E, Milo S. Umbilical artery flow velocity during maternal cardiopulmonary bypass. *Ann Thorac Surg* 1995; 60: 1116–1118.

46 Werch A, Lambert HM, Cooley D, Reed CC. Fetal monitoring and maternal open heart surgery. *Southern Med J* 1977; 70: 1024.

47 Veray FX, Hernandez CJJ, Raffucci F, Pelegrina IA. Pregnancy after cardiac surgery. *Conn Med* 1970; 34: 496–499.

48 Trimakas AP, Maxwell KD, Berkay S, Gardner TJ, Achuff SC. Fetal monitoring during cardiopulmonary bypass for removal of a left atrial myxoma during pregnancy. *Johns Hopkins Med J* 1979; 144: 156–160.

49 Korsten HH, Van Zundert AA, Mooij PN, De Jong PA, Bavinck JH. Emergency aortic valve replacement in the 24th-week of pregnancy. *Acta Anaesth Belg* 1989; 40: 201–205.

50 Chambers CE, Clark SL. Cardiac surgery during pregnancy. *Clin Obstet Gynecol* 1994; 37: 316–323.

51 Jadhon ME, Main EK. Fetal bradycardia associated with maternal hypothermia. *Obstet Gynecol* 1988; 72: 496.

52 Reddy VM, McElhinney DB, Rajasinghe HA, Liddicoat JR, Hendricks-Munoz K, Fineman JR, Hanley FL. Role of the endothelium in placental dysfunction after fetal cardiac bypass. *AATS/WTSA* 1999: 343–351.

53 Champsaur G, Vedrinne C, Martinot S et al. Flow-induced release of endothelium-derived relaxing factor during pulsatile bypass: experimental study in the fetal lamb. *J Thorac Cardiovasc Surg* 1997; 114: 738–744.

54 Vedrinne C, Tronc F, Martinot S et al. Better preservation of endothelial function and decreased activation of the fetal renin-angiotensin pathway with the use of pulsatile flow during experimental fetal bypass. *J Thorac Cardiovasc Surg* 2000; 120: 770–777.

55 Sabik JF, Assad RS, Hanley FL. Prostaglandin synthesis inhibition prevents placental dysfunction after fetal cardiac bypass. *J Thorac Cardiovasc Surg* 1992; 103: 733–741.

56 Kawkabani N, Kawas N, Baraka A, Vogel T, Mangano CM. Case 3 – 1999. Severe fetal bradycardia in a pregnant woman undergoing hypothermic cardiopulmonary bypass. *J Cardiothorac Vasc Anesth* 1999; 13: 346–349.

57 Karahan N, Öztürk T, Yetkin U, Yilik L, Baloglu A, Gürbüz A. Managing severe heart failure in a pregnant patient undergoing cardiopulmonary bypass: case report and review of the literature. *J Cardiothorac Vasc Anesth* 2004; 18: 339–343.

58 Liu PL, Warren TM, Ostheimer GW, Weiss JB, Liu LM. Foetal monitoring in parturients undergoing surgery unrelated to pregnancy. *Can Anaesth Soc J* 1985; 32: 525–532.

59 Burke AB, Hur D, Bolan JC, Corso P, Resano FG. Sinusoidal fetal heart rate pattern during cardiopulmonary bypass. *Am J Obstet Gynecol* 1990; 163: 17–18.

60 Katz JD, Hook R, Barash PG. Fetal heart rate monitoring in pregnant patients undergoing surgery. *Am J Obstet Gynecol* 1976; 125: 267–269.

61 Eilen B, Kaiser IH, Becker RM, Cohen MN. Aortic valve replacement in the third trimester of pregnancy: case report and review of the literature. *Obstet Gynecol* 1981; 57: 119–121.

62 Mahli A, Izdes S, Coskun D. Cardiac operations during pregnancy: review of factors influencing fetal outcome. *Ann Thorac Surg* 2000; 69: 1622–1626.

63 Clark SL. Cardiac disease in pregnancy. *Crit Care Clin* 1991; 7: 777–797.

64 Nazarian M, McCullough GH, Fielder DL. Bacterial endocarditis in pregnancy: successful surgical correction. *J Thorac Cardiovasc Surg* 1976; 71: 880–883.

65 Lyons G. Six years' experience in a teaching maternity unit. *Anaesthesia* 1985; 40: 759–762.

66 Hawthorne L, Wilson R, Lyons G, Dresner M. Failed intubation revisited: 17-yr experience in a teaching maternity unit. *Br J Anaesth* 1996: 680–684.

67 Archer GW, Marx GF. Arterial oxygen tension during apnoea in parturient women. *Br J Anaesth* 1974: 358–360.

68 Connell H, Dalgleish JG, Downing JW. General anaesthesia in mothers with severe pre-eclampsia/eclampsia. *Br J Anaesth* 1987; 59: 1375–1380.

69 Von Dadelszen P, Menzies J, Gilgoff S, Xie F, Douglas MJ, Sawchuck D, Magee LA. Evidence-based management for pre-eclampsia. *Front Biosc* 2007; 12: 2876–2889.

70 Cooper JRJ, Slogoff S. *Hemodilution and Priming Solutions for Cardiopulmonary Bypass*. Baltimore: Williams and Wilkins, 1993: 124–137.

71 Willcox TW, Stone P, Milsom FP, Connell H. Cardiopulmonary bypass in pregnancy: Possible new role for the intra-aortic balloon pump. *J Extracorp Technol* 2005; 37: 189–91.

72 Matsuki A, Oyama T. Operation under hypothermia in a pregnant woman with an intracranial arteriovenous malformation. *Can Anaesth Soc J* 1972; 19: 184–191.

73 Plunkett MD, Bond LM, Geiss DM. Staged repair of acute type I aortic dissection and coarctation in pregnancy. *Ann Thorac Surg* 2000; 69: 1945–1947.

74 Buffolo E, Palma JH, Gomes WJ et al. Successful use of deep hypothermic circulatory arrest in pregnancy. *Ann Thorac Surg* 1994; 58: 1532–1534.

75 Hawkins JA, Paape KL, Adkins TP, Shaddy RE, Gay WA. Extracorporeal circulation in the fetal lamb. Effects of hypothermia and perfusion rate. *J Cardiovasc Surg* 1991; 32: 295–300.

76 Grigore AM, Grocott HP, Mathew JP et al., the Neurologic Outcome Research Group of the Duke Heart Center. The rewarming rate and increased peak temperature alter neurocognitive outcome after cardiac surgery. *Anesth Analg* 2002; 94: 4–10.

77 Philbin DM. *Pulsatile Blood Flow*. Baltimore: Williams and Wilkins, 1993: 323–337.

78 Vedrinne C, Tronc F, Martinot S et al. Effects of various flow types on maternal hemodynamics during fetal bypass: is there nitric oxide release during pulsatile perfusion? *J Thorac Cardiovasc Surg* 1998; 116: 432–439.

79 Farmakides G, Schulman H, Mohtashemi M, Ducey J, Fuss R, Mantell P. Uterine-umbilical velocimetry in open heart surgery. *Am J Obstet Gynecol* 1987; 156: 1221–1222.

80 Tripp HF, Stiegel RM, Coyle JP. The use of pulsatile perfusion during aortic valve replacement in pregnancy. *Ann Thorac Surg* 1999; 67: 1169–1171.

81 Clark SL, Cotton DB, Lee W et al. Central hemodynamic assessment of normal term pregnancy. *Am J Obstet Gynecol* 1989; 161: 1439–1442.

82 Lamb MP, Ross K, Johnstone AM, Manners JM. Fetal heart monitoring during open heart surgery. Two case reports. *Br J Obstet Gynaecol* 1981; 88: 669–674.

83 Hawkins JA, Clark SM, Shaddy RE, Gay WA, Jr. Fetal cardiac bypass: improved placental function with moderately high flow rates. *Ann Thorac Surg* 1994; 57: 293–296.

84 Fremes SE, Tamariz MG, Abramov D et al. Late results of the Warm Heart Trial: the influence of nonfatal cardiac events on late survival. *Circulation* 2000; 102: 19(Suppl 3): 339–345.

85 Garry D, Leikin E, Fleisher AG, Tejani N. Acute myocardial infarction in pregnancy with subsequent medical and surgical management. *Obstet Gynecol* 1996; 87: 802–804.

86 Lichtenstein SV, Abel JG, Panos A, Slutsky AS, Salerno TA. Warm heart surgery: experience with long cross-clamp times. *Ann Thorac Surg* 1991; 52: 1009–1013.

87 Naeye RL. Placental infarction leading to fetal or neonatal death. A prospective study. *ACOG J* 1977; 50: 583–588.

88 Templeton A, Kelman GR. Maternal blood gases, (PAO_2–PaO_2), physiological shunt, VD/VT in pregnancy. *Br J Anaesth* 1976; 48: 1001–1004.

89 Levinson G, Shnider SM, Delorimier AA, Steffenson JL. Effects of maternal hyperventilation on uterine blood flow and fetal oxygenation and acid-base status. *Anesthesiology* 1974; 40: 340–347.

90 Baraka A, Kawkabani N, Haroun-Bizri S. Hemodynamic deterioration after cardiopulmonary bypass during pregnancy: resuscitation by postoperative emergency Cesarean section. *J Cardiothorac Vasc Anesth* 2000; 14: 314–315.

15 Non-Invasive Monitoring

Michael Cackovic[1] & Michael A. Belfort[2]

[1]Division of Maternal-Fetal Medicine, Department of Obstetrics, Gynecology and Reproductive Sciences, Yale University School of Medicine, New Haven, CT, USA

[2]Department of Obstetrics and Gynecology, Division of Maternal-Fetal Medicine, University of Utah School of Medicine, Salt Lake City, UT *and* HCA Healthcare, Nashville, TN, USA

Introduction

The appropriate management of critically ill patients requires frequent observation of biophysical parameters. The most important of these parameters describe the delivery of oxygenated blood to the peripheral tissues. Peripheral oxygen saturation and markers of hemodynamic function are essential prerequisites in the provision of intensive care, the development of which was initially based upon the accuracy and utility of pulmonary artery catheters as an investigative tool. While this technology has remained synonymous with critical care practice it is now recognized that the invasive nature of this monitoring is associated with a range of complications. Newer, non-invasive technologies have been developed that now provide similar, or more extensive data with fewer risks.

Non-invasive hemodynamic assessment has permitted the collection of diagnostic and research data beyond the arena of critical care. Information derived from the use of echocardiography in particular has helped to expand our understanding of many conditions including the physiological events of normal pregnancy, the pathogenesis of pre-eclampsia, the abnormalities characteristic of various forms of heart disease, and a variety of medical disorders. In some circumstances, echocardiography has become an integral part of the prepregnancy and antenatal assessment of women with heart disease.

This chapter will review some aspects of this technology and the clinical issues associated with the use of non-invasive monitoring that may be encountered in obstetric practice.

The measurement of cardiac output

An adequate cardiac output is essential to deliver oxygenated blood to the peripheral tissues. Low output will reflect either hypovolemia or ventricular failure. Knowledge of the cardiac output will determine management and will also allow calculation of other derived hemodynamic values including vascular resistance and oxygen delivery and consumption indices.

In the past, cardiac output was measured using the Fick principle. This principle states that the amount of a substance taken up by the body per unit time equals the difference between the arterial and venous levels multiplied by the blood flow. Hence, oxygen consumption by the body divided by the arteriovenous oxygen difference equals the cardiac output.

$$CO = O_2\ \text{uptake}/([\text{arterial } O_2]-[\text{venous } O_2])$$

This principle has been modified to use other markers including dye dilution techniques and the thermodilution principle of the pulmonary artery catheter. In the latter case, iced water is the marker injected into the right atrium with a probe measuring the temperature of the blood flowing through the pulmonary artery thus allowing the derivation of the cardiac output from the area under the curve. This technique, although clinically sound, may produce results that are confounded by variations in catheter position, variations in injectate temperature and volume, and differences in the rate of saline injection.

These technologies have nevertheless contributed to our understanding of physiology and pathophysiology and remain the gold standard against which newer techniques are assessed. The need to cannulate peripheral and central vessels has been associated with some risk of injury and justified the search for safer technology.

Ultrasound in the form of echocardiography allows estimation of cardiac output by measuring changes in left ventricular dimensions during systole measured in the plane below the level of the mitral valve. By assuming that the ventricle is ellipsoid in shape and that the long axis is double the short axis, stroke volume can be calculated from the cube of the change in left ventricular dimension. This measurement is inaccurate when the assumptions upon which it is based are no longer true. Hence, the dilated ventricle and the pregnant woman with an increased volume and

Critical Care Obstetrics, 5th edition. Edited by M. Belfort, G. Saade, M. Foley, J. Phelan and G. Dildy.

end-diastolic dimensions violate these assumptions and may overestimate stroke volume and cardiac output.

Doppler ultrasound has added to the utility of echocardiography by allowing an estimation of blood velocity. The Doppler principle measures the frequency of a reflected ultrasound beam striking moving erythrocytes where the change in frequency detected is proportional to the velocity of the red cells moving in the axis of the beam. The velocity of a column of red cells multiplied by the period of ejection provides a measure of the distance traveled by a column of blood during systole. The use of ultrasound to measure the diameter of the vessels containing the blood will allow calculation of cross-sectional area with subsequent derivation of stroke volume and cardiac output. The velocity of blood flow can also be related to the pressure gradient down which the blood is moving thus providing a way of calculating intracardiac pressure gradients and pulmonary artery pressures.

Doppler probes may be pulsed (range-gated) to allow the measurement of a signal from a given depth of tissue. The pulsed Doppler signal usually allows simultaneous ultrasound imaging and estimation of the angle of insonation between the Doppler probe and the vessel. This latter measurement is important because the calculation of velocity from the reflected Doppler signal requires a knowledge of the angle between the ultrasound beam and the column of blood from which the signal is being reflected. Where the signal is perpendicular to the moving column of blood, no movement will be detected, and the closer the beam moves to being parallel to the vessel, the more completely the reflected vector represents the velocity of the cells in the path of the beam.

The combination of cross-sectional echocardiography and Doppler measurement of flow velocity at specific points in the heart and great vessels allows the determination of volumetric flow. The mitral and aortic valve orifices and the root or arch of the aorta have all been studied using both suprasternal and intra-esophageal Doppler probes. Potential for error exists in these techniques both in the calculation of the insonation angle and in the measurement of the cross-sectional area of the vessel. Of the different sites studied, the best correlation between the Doppler technique and thermodilution studies was documented in the aortic valve orifice measurements. Although transthoracic Doppler studies are the most widely accessible tool, transesophageal Doppler allows the posterior structures of the heart to be more clearly imaged with more accurate diagnosis of cardiac pathology and precise alignment to the aortic valve in both the long and short axis as well as providing long axis views of the ascending aorta [1]. The use of multiplanar transesophageal echocardiography allows precise measurements of asymmetric ventricles that cannot be reliably imaged using a transthoracic probe [2]. It provides high spatial resolution and access to structures such as the left atrial appendage, the thoracic aorta, and the pulmonary veins that are not well seen by transthoracic echocardiography on routine exam [3]. The probe has particular utility in the diagnosis of aortic dissection and thromboembolism [4] although the need for esophageal endoscopy limits the application of this technology to specific situations including intraoperative and postoperative care.

Other techniques of measuring cardiac output include impedance cardiography based upon changes in transthoracic electrical resistance associated with the ejection of blood into the pulmonary circulation. This technique has been shown to overestimate low cardiac output with the opposite error in high cardiac output states.

Doppler ultrasound and the physiology of pregnancy

Doppler techniques have confirmed the increased cardiac output and stroke volume of pregnancy associated with progressive increases in left atrial dimension and function.

Both filling phases of the left ventricle show increased filling velocities (E- and A-wave velocity). The increase in early wave velocity occurs by the end of the first trimester whereas the peak A-wave velocity changes occur in the third trimester. The E/A ratio increases in the first trimester but falls again as the A-wave velocity increases and is accompanied by decreasing left ventricular isovolumetric relaxation time [5,6].

Left ventricular mass increases significantly while fractional shortening and velocity of shortening diminish throughout pregnancy [7]. Systolic function is preserved by falling systemic (including uterine artery) resistance [5,6]. Peak left ventricular wall stress, an indicator of afterload, has been demonstrated in early pregnancy and normalizes as ventricular mass increases in the mid-trimester [5]. Geva et al. [8] similarly report a 45% increase in cardiac output in normal pregnancy accompanied by an increase in left ventricular end-diastolic volume and increased end-systolic wall stress accompanied by transient left ventricular hypertrophy. These authors also report a reversible decline in left ventricular function during the second and third trimesters.

Systemic arterial vascular compliance is thought to diminish because of reduced vascular tone [9].

The pulmonary circulation shows increased flow during pregnancy with some reduction in vascular resistance without any significant alteration in blood pressure. These changes are evident by 8 weeks gestation without any subsequent alteration and return to prepregnancy values by 6 months postpartum [10].

Doppler ultrasound and critical care

There are few studies that address this issue, and non-invasive techniques for the routine estimation of stroke volume and ventricular filling pressures have only been recently reported in the obstetric literature. Validation studies have, however, been conducted and show reliable correlation between non-invasive techniques and values derived by the use of pulmonary artery catheters. Two-dimensional and Doppler echocardiography was used to demonstrate this in a group of 11 critically ill obstetric patients. The findings of this study showed a high correlation between invasive and non-invasive techniques in the measurement of stroke volume and cardiac output. Ventricular filling pressures and pulmonary artery pressures also showed a similar significant correlation with invasive techniques [11].

The specific choice of echocardiographic technique for estimating stroke volume and ejection fraction was explored in the same group of patients. Comparisons between M-mode and two-dimensional Doppler techniques revealed similar findings, although M-mode echocardiography was not possible in 2 out of 11 subjects secondary to body habitus and paradoxical motion of the intraventricular septum. This study also allowed calculation of the ejection fraction by dividing the stroke volume by the end-diastolic volume. Using this equation, similar results were obtained by all the methods employed for estimating left ventricular function in pregnant women [12].

Belfort et al. have reported a series of 14 patients with an indication for invasive hemodynamic monitoring in whom Doppler ultrasound was used as a guide to clinical management. These 14 women had a spectrum of pathologies ranging from intractable hypertension to complex cardiac lesions and included women with oliguria and pulmonary edema. This pilot study concluded that the non-invasive monitoring had facilitated management and only two patients went on to have invasive monitoring in order to allow continuous monitoring. Large volumes of fluid were administered to some of these patients (up to 8 L of crystalloid) without the development of fluid overload or pulmonary edema. To date this is the only study that has indicated the potential utility of routine rapid echocardiographic assessment of left ventricular function in critically ill obstetric patients [13].

Doppler ultrasound and pre-eclampsia

Doppler echocardiography has provided a ready means of studying women at risk for developing hypertensive complications during pregnancy. Longitudinal studies have demonstrated that women with non-proteinuric or gestational hypertension maintain a hyperdynamic circulation with a high cardiac output throughout pregnancy. By contrast women destined to develop pre-eclampsia have significantly elevated cardiac output without any change in systemic resistance in the preclinical phase of the disease. This is followed by a fall in cardiac output and increasing resistance coincident with the onset of clinical disease [14].

More recently, studies have focused on echocardiographically described cardiac structure and function in pre-eclampsia, especially in relation to levels of atrial and brain natriuretic peptide (ANP, BNP). Initial work had related elevated ANP levels to increased left atrial dimensions following delivery in normal pregnancies. These increased ANP levels did not lead to any demonstrable diuresis in normal postpartum women. Women with pre-eclampsia had bigger atria and higher ANP levels in the early puerperium and these changes were associated with natriuresis and diuresis. The hypothesis related by these findings was that increased atrial distension in pre-eclampsia triggered a diuretic response.

These data have been contested. The most detailed study, to date, by Borghi et al. [15] described detailed cardiac findings among 40 women with mild pre-eclampsia compared to a control cohort of pregnant women and non-pregnant controls. This study showed a progressive rise in left ventricular mass between non-pregnant women compared to normal pregnancy with a further increase in mass among women with pre-eclampsia. Ejection fraction and fractional shortening decreased in normal pregnancy while not reaching statistical significance. However, women with pre-eclampsia had a significant reduction in both these parameters in comparison to non-pregnant women. In addition, left ventricular end-diastolic volume rose significantly in pre-eclampsia. Together with a fall in cardiac output in the pre-eclamptic group, these findings suggest a compensatory increase in ventricular size to maintain cardiac output against an elevated systemic vascular resistance.

The latter study also showed changes in the peak filling velocities of the left ventricle during diastole. The E/A ratio fell significantly during pregnancy, partly reflecting increased preload. In pre-eclamspsia further augmentation of the A-wave peak velocity resulted in further significant reduction in the ratio. Collectively these data support the notion of changes in both cardiac systolic and diastolic function. The authors also measured ANP levels. In keeping with previous studies elevated levels of ANP were found in pregnancy with further increments occurring in pre-eclampsia. These could not be accounted for by differences in atrial size although a significant correlation was found between left ventricular mass and volume in women with pre-eclampsia [15].

Doppler ultrasound and cardiomyopathy

Doppler ultrasound has an important role in the management and evaluation of women with impaired ventricular function.

Echocardiography is used to delineate impaired left ventricular systolic function in women with suspected peripartum cardiomyopathy. It plays a further role in the ongoing evaluation of women once this diagnosis has been made. Specifically the prognosis has been related to the normalization of left ventricular size and function within 6 months of delivery [16]. Currently accepted opinion is that approximately 50% of affected women will recover normal function. Those who have persistently impaired function face a significant risk of mortality [16].

Subsequent pregnancies in women with a prior diagnosis of cardiomyopathy demand careful echocardiographic assessment. Although no clear agreement exists regarding risk, those with persistently abnormal left ventricular function have been advised against pregnancy. Conflicting reports have been made concerning those who become pregnant. De Souza et al. report on the evaluation of seven women who became pregnant after developing peripartum cardiomyopathy in a previous pregnancy. All pregnancies were well tolerated without significant change in symptomatology. Echocardiographic studies showed no change in left ventricular end-diastolic diameters, with an increase occurring in left ventricular fractional shortening [17]. Other studies have reported similarly successful pregnancies [18]. However, there are papers suggesting a risk of recurrent cardiomyopathy and impaired contractile reserve, even in those with apparently normal left ventricular function before pregnancy [19,20].

Doppler ultrasound and other medical disorders

Echocardiocardiography is an essential investigation in women with structural heart disease due to valvular damage or congenital malformation [21–27]. Echocardiography will also contribute to the diagnosis of Libman–Sacks endocarditis, which occurs, though not frequently, among women suffering from systemic lupus erythematosus, with or without antiphospholipid antibodies [28,29].

The management of Marfan's syndrome also requires echocardiographic assessment because of the risk of catastrophic aortic dissection. Transesophageal echocardiography is the preferred method for evaluating the ascending aorta. The risk of dissection correlates with an aortic root diameter greater than 4 cm [30]. Aortic dissection may also occur under other circumstances and may follow the use of crack cocaine [31,32].

The role of transesophageal Doppler

Esophageal Doppler monitoring of hemodynamic data has been carried out in adult intensive care units and found to be equivalent to data derived from pulmonary artery catheter measurements [33]. Pregnancy data are few, and to date only one study has reported the use of transesophageal Doppler monitoring in pregnancy compared to pulmonary artery catheters. This study showed that the Doppler consistently underestimated cardiac output by 40% in women under the age of 35 years [34]. This error may be due to the assumptions implicit in the algorithm used to calculate output. These assumptions include a fixed aortic diameter during systole and a fixed percentage of blood perfusing upper and lower parts of the body. Pregnancy physiological changes probably invalidate these assumptions. The authors nevertheless conclude that esophageal Doppler may contribute to the estimation of trends in cardiac output over time in pregnancy.

Oximetry in the intensive care environment

Spectrophotometry is the detection of specific light frequencies reflected by a range of molecules. Specific molecules reflect specific frequencies and their reflective properties differ with changes in molecular conformation. Oximetry is the detection of oxygenated and deoxygenated blood. Deoxygenated hemoglobin absorbs more light at 660 nm whereas at 940 nm oxygenated hemoglobin

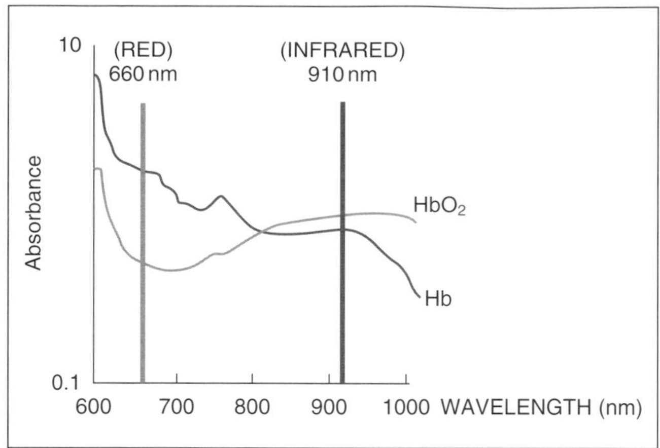

Figure 15.1 Oximetry in the intensive care environment. The oxygenated hemoglobin reflects more light at 660 nm whereas at 940 nm deoxyhemoglobin reflects infrared light more strongly.

abosorbs the infrared light more strongly (Figure 15.1). This allows the simultaneous acquisition of peripheral signals from which the ratio of oxy- to deoxyhemoglobin can be calculated and expressed as a percentage of oxyhemoglobin saturation.

Oximetry may be based on transcutaneous measurements or can be derived from mixed venous blood via a probe located in a pulmonary artery catheter. The peripheral pulse oximetry devices rely on detection of pulsed alterations in light transmitted between transmitter and a photodetector. This filtered signal is necessary to eliminate the signal arising from venous blood that would contain more deoxyhemoglobin.

Although oximetry is regarded as an effective method of monitoring oxygenation, some limitations are recognized. They include the assumptions that methemoglobin and carboxyhemoglobin are not present in significant concentrations. Mixed venous oxygen saturation monitoring is less frequently used than peripheral oxygen saturation monitoring. It also shows greater spontaneous variation than peripheral monitors but has a clinical role to play in determining the balance between peripheral oxygen delivery and peripheral oxygen consumption. This is a robust measurement that will reflect changes in cardiac output, hemoglobin concentration, arterial and venous hemoglobin oxygen saturation. This provides useful clinical information in many clinical circumstances. A number of the determinants of the ultimate mixed venous oxygen saturation value have the potential to change at any given moment (hemoglobin, oxygen saturation, and cardiac output). It is therefore important to understand that it is only when all other parameters remain stable that changes in the mixed venous oxygen saturation reflect changes in cardiac output.

Capnometery

Exhaled gas can be evaluated using an infrared probe and a photodetector set to detect carbon dioxide. This is usually found in the expiratory limb of a ventilator circuit. Expired gas shows a pattern of increasing carbon dioxide concentration related to the sequential expiration of air in the upper airway followed by air from the alveoli. The end-expiratory (or end-tidal) carbon dioxide concentration should approximate the partial pressure of carbon dioxide in arterial blood. The development of a gradient between these measurements reflects an increase in anatomical or physiological dead space. In the latter event, low cardiac output and pulmonary embolism may both affect the measurement. Changes in end-tidal partial pressure of carbon dioxide have been correlated to changes in cardiac output and may be used as a means of monitoring the efficacy of resuscitation.

Transcranial Doppler ultrasound

Compared to the physiologic alterations in other vascular beds during gestation the normal cerebral blood flow changes of pregnancy are poorly documented. This is due, partly, to technical difficulties associated with in vivo studies of blood flow in the human brain. Angiography, the gold standard in the evaluation of the cerebral vasculature, is an invasive test and presents obvious ethical concerns for its use in normal pregnant women. Very little data exist on the physiologic adaptations of the brain to pregnancy in the current literature and most texts dealing with the changes of pregnancy do not address this issue at all. There are also ethical problems with using angiography and other methodologies involving radiation, as well as magnetic resonance imaging during pregnancy. The advent of Doppler ultrasound, and in particular transcranial Doppler (TCD) ultrasound, has changed this. It is now possible to acquire Doppler-derived velocity information from most of the basal brain arteries (including almost all of the circle of Willis branches) using a non-invasive technique. Using these data, it is possible to diagnose arterial malformations, functional abnormalities, and physiological changes in brain blood velocity. One can detect direction and velocity of blood flow, and from this infer the presence of distal or proximal arterial constriction or dilatation. In addition, TCD can be used to determine real-time changes over very short time intervals and to continuously monitor cerebral blood velocity during surgical procedures, or experimental drug protocols. TCD has been extensively used in the clinical scenario by neurologists and neurosurgeons to detect and follow cerebral vasospasm in patients with subarachnoid hemorrhage [35]. TCD has also been used for neurological monitoring during cardiopulmonary bypass in pediatric cardiac surgeries [36]. Investigators are beginning to use TCD to define pregnancy-induced/associated changes in the cerebral circulation.

Belfort et al. [37] have recently defined the hemodynamic changes, specifically velocity, resistance indices, and cerebral perfusion pressure, in the middle cerebral artery distribution of the brain during normal pregnancy. TCD ultrasound was used to determine the systolic, diastolic, and mean blood velocities in the middle cerebral arteries in non-laboring women studied longitudinally (at 4-week intervals) during normal gestation. The resistance index (RI), pulsatility index (PI), and cerebral perfusion pressure (CPP) were calculated using the velocity and blood pressure data. The mean value, and the 5% and 95% percentiles, were defined and it was noted that the middle cerebral artery (MCA) velocities and the resistance and pulsatility indices decrease, while the CPP increases, during normal pregnancy. Figure 15.2 shows the CPP change during normal pregnancy. This study defined the normative ranges for middle cerebral artery velocity, resistance indices, and cerebral perfusion pressure during normal human pregnancy using longitudinally collected data.

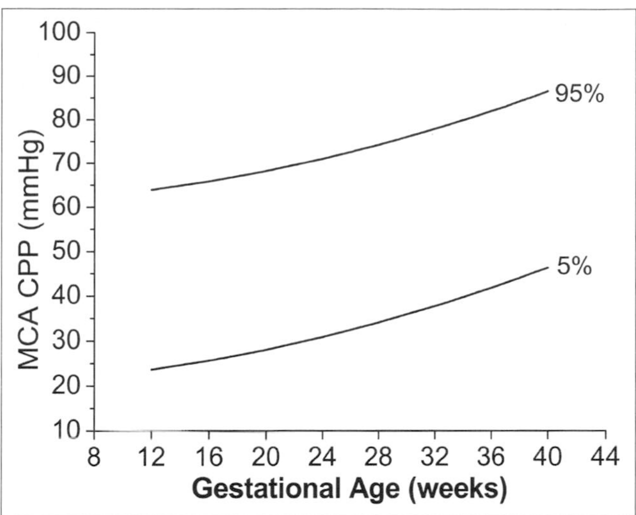

Figure 15.2 Cerebral perfusion pressure (CPP) changes during a normal pregnancy as detected by middle cerebral artery (MCA) velocity.

Women with pre-eclampsia and hypertensive women with superimposed pre-eclampsia have been studied using TCD ultrasound. Findings among these subjects include globally elevated cerebral perfusion pressures and lower cerebral vascular resistance compared to normotensive controls [38,39]. The increased pressures were not directly related to blood pressure alone [39].

Doppler ultrasound, bias and confounders

There are a number of confounding influences that can affect the interpretation of Doppler cerebral velocity data. These include any factors that may: (i) increase the CO_2 or H^+ tension in the cerebral circulation; (ii) decrease or increase the hemoglobin concentration; (iii) independently alter the diameter of the vessel being studied at the point of insonation; and (iv) introduce error, such as cigarette smoking and changes in posture. In pregnant women (v) gestational age is another important factor that requires consideration, since as the pregnancy progresses there are significant hemodynamic changes.

Increased CO_2 tension leads to cerebral vasodilation, as does acidosis. Patients undergoing cerebral Doppler studies should, ideally, be studied in a steady state or should have their end-tidal CO_2 tension measured in order to control for fluctuations. Even the minimal increases in tidal volume and respiratory rate associated with labor contractions may be of importance. Labor itself has been shown to be associated with decreases in mean middle cerebral artery flow velocity.

Hemoconcentration and hemodilution are also important and attention should be paid to the hematocrit level in studies where blood loss or volume infusion may have altered the hemoglobin content of the blood during the study period.

The segmental nature of the vasospasm seen in some conditions, notably pre-eclampsia, is of concern as well, since the same segment of artery can show completely different velocity profiles depending on its state of contraction. Thus, if the region of vessel being insonated is apt to change, its diameter velocity readings may be inaccurate, particularly if some indication of downstream vascular condition is being extrapolated. In this regard, the M1 portion of the middle cerebral artery has been shown to be unlikely to change diameter [40], since it is well supported by alveolar tissue in its bony canal. The angle of insonation is critical since the velocity is related to the cos of the angle of insonation (q). If q is less than 10° the error involved is almost negligible and quite acceptable for most purposes. Because of the anatomy of the bony canal through which the M1 portion of the MCA runs, the angle of insonation very rarely exceeds 10°. This ensures that, in almost all cases, once the optimum signal is obtained the angle of insonation is less than 10°.

The effect of maternal cigarette smoking on middle cerebral artery blood flow velocities during normal pregnancy was described by Irion et al. [41]. They found that the systolic, diastolic, and mean velocities of the middle cerebral artery, detected in both the left lateral decubitus and sitting positions, were significantly higher at 18 and 26 weeks gestation in women who smoked cigarettes. They determined that the number of cigarettes smoked positively correlated with increased middle cerebral artery velocities. This factor must be taken into account when studying women known to smoke, and is an important confounding factor in some of the earlier studies published. Posture should be taken into account when studying pregnant, and in particular, pre-eclamptic pregnant women. A change from lying to sitting has been shown to significantly increase both systolic and diastolic velocities in the middle cerebral artery in such patients.

Another important variable that must be taken into account when studying pregnant women is the gestational age. As pregnancy advances there is a reduction in middle cerebral artery velocity which should be controlled for when comparing women of different gestational ages.

Cerebral perfusion pressure

Under normal conditions, the arterioles in the cerebrovascular system are responsible for about 80% of the vascular resistance. Because arterioles have active smooth muscle tone, they do not behave simply like tubes of variable dimension. Smooth muscle tone in the arterioles reduces their diameter when systolic pressure is transmitted into them via the arteries. In addition, this tone also tends to close the arterioles when pressure falls during the pulse cycle. Under conditions of low vascular resistance, the arterioles remain open throughout the pulse cycle and the active smooth muscle tone never causes them to close completely. However, even a slight increase in arteriolar tone will narrow the diameter of open arterioles and, in some cases, cause them to close completely when the pressure within them falls at the end of the pulse cycle. The pressure at which an arteriole closes is called its "critical closing pressure" [35,42]. Critical closing pressure explains why arterioles close as pressure falls during the pulse cycle and why fewer arterioles are open at the end of the pulse cycle than earlier, when pressure is at its systolic maximum. Thus, pressure at the end of a pulse cycle is less effective in perfusing the capillary bed than that early in the cycle. In the brain, CPP is reduced as arteriolar resistance rises abruptly due to more and more arterioles reaching their critical closing pressure. Another feature of arteriolar tone is its effect in delaying the flow of blood from arteries to capillaries. When arteriolar tone is high it reduces the rate of blood flow from arteries to capillaries. This maintains the arterial blood pressure at a higher level for a longer portion of the pulse cycle than if the arteriolar tone was low and there was a rapid run-off of blood. Blood pressure distends the arterial segments and blood is effectively stored in the arteries while the pressure decays during the pulse cycle. The amount stored in each segment depends on the compliance of the artery and the pressure gradient between the lumen and the region outside the artery. The result of storing blood in the arteries and reducing the rate of flow through arterioles is to slow the deceleration of blood flow during the pulse cycle. The more compliant the arterial segment, the slower the deceleration during the pulse cycle. This feature of arteriolar tone interacting with arterial pressure and arterial compliance affects the shape of the velocity profile during the pulse cycle. When arteriolar tone is low, blood velocity rapidly rises to a maximum and falls quickly to a minimum. In contrast, when arteriolar tone is high, the blood flow velocity falls more slowly. The area under the pulsatile amplitude of the velocity waveform, and the height of the pulse velocity wave, may be used to estimate the proportion of blood flow stored in arterial segments during the peak of the pulse cycle and released when pressure falls during the cycle.

One of the major problems with the currently used Doppler indices is that they were initially developed for use in peripheral vascular examination of large-diameter arteries such as the femoral, dorsalis pedis, and brachial arteries. Indices such as the PI and RI focus on the systolic component of the velocity profile. The traditional Doppler indices of hemodynamics (i.e. the RI and PI) provide limited data regarding arteriolar tone when applied to the cerebral circulation. Both the RI, defined as:

$$(\text{velocity}_{\text{systolic}} - \text{velocity}_{\text{diastolic}})/(\text{velocity}_{\text{systolic}})$$

and the PI, defined as:

$$(\text{velocity}_{\text{systolic}} - \text{velocity}_{\text{diastolic}})/(\text{velocity}_{\text{mean}})$$

are significantly influenced by the systolic velocity which reflects large-caliber arterial constriction. These indices were originally developed using older technology and larger diameter arteries (femoral artery and aorta). The typical waveform shape from such arteries has a tall peaked systolic component, a steep diastolic slope, and a low/non-existent diastolic component. The smaller diameter arteries that are now easily visualized with modern equipment provide completely different waveforms from those seen in the larger diameter, higher velocity, and higher resistance vessels. Using indices that focus on the systolic velocity tends to ignore aspects of waveform shape peculiar to lower resistance vascular beds. Specifically, the typical waveform seen in low resistance, low velocity, smaller diameter arteries has a low systolic velocity, flatter diastolic downslope, and a proportionately higher diastolic velocity, than that seen in high-resistance, high-velocity arteries.

A further deficiency of the current cerebral Doppler assessment techniques is that they fail to take into account the systemic arterial pressure, a vital component of the cerebral perfusion pressure. In 1986 Aaslid et al. [43] validated a Doppler method of estimating CPP. They measured velocity in the middle cerebral artery (Doppler ultrasound), and intraventricular pressure and radial arterial blood pressure (direct strain gauge transducers) in 10 patients undergoing a supratentorial shunt procedure. They estimated CPP using the following ratio: (mean flow velocity)/(pulsatile amplitude of flow velocity) multiplied by the arterial blood pressure. To increase the accuracy, Fourier analysis was used and only the amplitude of the first harmonic of the pulsatility in both flow-velocity and arterial blood pressure recordings were used. They expressed their calculations as:

$$\mathrm{CPP} = \frac{V_0}{V_1} \times \mathrm{ABP}_1$$

where V_0 is the mean and V_1 is the amplitude of the first harmonic of the velocity waveform, and ABP_1 is the first harmonic of the arterial pressure wave. Their experimental results confirmed the validity of the method. The standard deviation between estimated CPP (CPP_e) and measured CPP (CPP_m) was 8.2 mmHg at a CPP of 40 mmHg, and the mean deviation was only 1 mmHg.

Belfort et al. [44] have adapted the method of Aaslid et al. [43] by altering the formula to reflect the area under the pulsatile amplitude of the flow velocity and arterial blood pressure waveforms rather than the first harmonic. Their equation, using areas under pulsatile amplitudes, is as follows [44]:

$$\mathrm{CPP} = \frac{\mathrm{Velocity}_{\mathrm{mean}}}{\mathrm{Velocity}_{\mathrm{mean}} - \mathrm{Velocity}_{\mathrm{diastolic}}} \times (\mathrm{BP}_{\mathrm{mean}} - \mathrm{BP}_{\mathrm{diastolic}})$$

Recently Belfort et al. [45] have suggested that elevated CPP, rather than decreased CBF, is the key determinant of cerebral injury in pre-eclampsia/eclampsia. Since this technology is still in its infancy as a non-invasive monitoring tool in severe pre-eclamptics routine use of this modality is not recommended until further research has confirmed the findings. However, in those cases of refractory seizure activity unresponsive to conventional therapy, TCD may offer another diagnostic option. In those cases where CPP is shown to be significantly elevated, drug therapy can be tailored to lowering the CPP (i.e. with labetalol) versus those rare cases where there is a low CPP and presumably cerebral ischemia from underperfusion, a cerebral vasodilator such as nimodipine can be used.

Conclusion

Non-invasive techniques of monitoring will become increasingly utilized as an alternative to the invasive techniques currently practiced in most intensive care units. This technology, however, requires expertise in the application and interpretation of data. Even correctly interpreted data are of unknown utility and stringent evaluation is necessary before this (often) expensive technology is incorporated into routine clinical practice.

References

1 Flachskampf FA, Hoffmann R, Verlande M, Schneider W, Ameling W, Hanrath P. Initial experience with a multiplane transoesophageal echo-transducer: assessment of diagnostic potential. *Eur Heart J* 1992; 13(9): 120–126.

2 Krebs W, Klues HG, Steinert S et al. Left ventricular volume calculations using a multiplanar transoesophageal echoprobe; in vitro validation and comparison with biplane angiography. *Eur Heart J* 1996; 17(8): 1279–1288.

3 Flachskampf FA. The standard TEE examination: procedure, safety, typical cross-sections and anatomic correlations, and statistical analysis. *Semin Cardiothorac Vasc Anesth* 2006; 10(1): 49–56.

4 Lee LC, Black IW, Hopkins A, Walsh WF. Transoesophageal echocardiography in heart disease – old technologies, new tricks. *Aust N Z J Med* 1992; 22(5 Suppl): 527–531.

5 Mesa A, Jessurun C, Hernandez A et al. Left ventricular diastolic function in normal human pregnancy. *Circulation* 1999; 99(4): 511–517.

6 Valensise H, Novelli GP, Vasapollo B et al. Maternal cardiac systolic and diastolic function: relationship with uteroplacental resistances. A Doppler and echocardiographic longitudinal study. *Ultrasound Obstet Gynecol* 2000; 15(6): 487–497.

7 Mone SM, Sanders SP, Colan SD. Control mechanisms for physiological hypertrophy of pregnancy. *Circulation* 1996; 94(4): 667–672.

8 Geva T, Mauer MB, Striker L, Kirshon B, Pivarnik JM. Effects of physiologic load of pregnancy on left ventricular contractility and remodelling. *Am Heart J* 1997; 133: 53–59.

9 Poppas A, Shroff SG, Korcarz CE et al. Serial assessment of the cardiovascular system in normal pregnancy. Role of arterial compliance and pulsatile arterial load. *Circulation* 1997; 95(10): 2407–2415.

10 Robson SC, Hunter S, Boys RJ, Dunlop W. Serial changes in pulmonary haemodynamics during human pregnancy: a non-invasive study using Doppler echocardiography. *Clin Sci (Colch)* 1991: 80(2): 113–117.

11 Belfort MA, Rokey R, Saade GR, Moise KJ Jr. Rapid echocardiographic assessment of left and right heart hemodynamics in critically ill obstetric patients. *Am J Obstet Gynecol* 1994; 171(4): 884–892.

12 Rokey R, Belfort MA, Saade GR. Quantitative echocardiographic assessment of left ventricular function in critically ill obstetric patients: a comparative study. *Am J Obstet Gynecol* 1995; 173(4): 1148–1152.

13 Belfort MA, Mares A, Saade GR, Wen T, Rokey R. Two-dimensional echocardiography and Doppler ultrasound in managing obstetric patients. *Obstet Gynecol* 1997; 90(3): 326–330.

14 Bosio PM, McKenna PJ, Conroy R, O'Herlihy C. Maternal central hemodynamics in hypertensive discorders of pregnancy. *Obstet Gynecol* 1999; 94(6): 978–984.

15 Borghi C, Esposti DD, Immordino V et al. Relationship of systemic hemodynamics, left ventricular structure and function, and plasma natriuretic peptide concentrations during pregnancy complicated by preeclampsia. *Am J Obstet Gynecol* 2000; 183(1): 140–147.

16 Pearson GD, Veille JC, Rahimtoola S et al. Peripartum cardiomyopathy: National Heart, Lung, and Blood Institute and Office of Rare Diseases (National Institutes of Health) workshop recommendations and review. *JAMA* 2000; 283(9): 1183–1188.

17 De Souza JL, de Carvalho Frimm C, Nastari L, Mady C. Left ventricular function after a new pregnancy in patients with peripartum cardiomyopathy. *J Card Fail* 2001; 7(1): 30–35.

18 Sutton MS, Cole P, Plappert M, Saltzman D, Goldhaber S. Effects of subsequent pregnancy on left ventricular function in peripartum cardiomyopathy. *Am Heart J* 1991; 121(6 Pt 1): 1776–1778.

19 Demakis JG, Rahimtoola SH, Sutton GC et al. Natural course of peripartum cardiomyopathy. *Circulation* 1971; 44: 1053–1061.

20 Lampert M, Weinert L, Hibbard J, Korcarz C, Lindheimer M, Lang RM. Contractile reserve in patients with peripartum cardiomyopathy and recovered left ventricular function. *Am J Obstet Gynecol* 1997; 176(1 Pt 1): 189–195.

21 Gultekin F, Baskin E, Gokalp A, Dogan K. A pregnant woman with Ebstein's anomaly. A case report. *Mater Med Pol* 1994; 26(4): 149–151.

22 Ben Farhat M, Gamra H, Betbout F et al. Percutaneous balloon mitral commissurotomy during pregnancy. *Heart* 1997; 77(6): 564–567.

23 Martinez Reding J, Cordero A, Kuri J, Martinez Rios MA, Salazar E. Treatment of severe mitral stenosis with percutaneous balloon valvotomy in pregnant patients. *Clin Cardiol* 1998; 21(9): 659–663.

24 Niwa K, Perloff JK, Kaplan S, Child JS, Miner PD. Eisenmenger syndrome in adults: ventricular septal defect, truncus arteriosus, univentricular heart. *J Am Coll Cardiol* 1999; 34(1): 223–232.

25 Wilansky S, Phan B, Adam K. Doppler echocardiography as a predictor of pregnancy outcome in the presence of aortic stenosis: A case report. *J Am Soc Echocardiogr* 1999; 12: 324–325.

26 Barbosa PJ, Lopes AA, Feitosa GS et al. Prognostic factors of reheumatic mitral stenosis during pregnancy and puerperium. *Arq Bras Cardiol* 2000; 75(3): 215–224.

27 Mangione JA, Lourenco RM, dos Santos ES et al. Long-term follow-up of pregnant women after percutaneous mitral valvuloplasty. *Catheter Cardiovasc Interv* 2000; 50(4): 413–417.

28 Gleason CB, Stoddard MF, Wagner SG, Longaker RA, Pierangeli S, Harris EN. A comparison of cardiac valvular involvement in the primary antiphospholipid syndrome versus anticardiolipin-negative systemic lupus erythematosus. *Am Heart J* 1993; 125(4): 1123–1129.

29 Hojnik M, George J, Ziporen L, Shoenfeld Y. Heart valve involvement (Libman–Sacks endocarditis) in the antiphospholipid syndrome. *Circulation* 1996; 93(8): 1579–1587.

30 Elkayam U, Ostrzega E, Shotan A, Hehra A. Cardiovascular problems in pregnant women with the Marfan syndrome. *Ann Intern Med* 1995; 123(2): 117–122.

31 Ecknauer E, Schmidlin D, Jenni R, Schmid ER. Emergency repair of incidentally diagnosed ascending aortic aneurysm immediately after caesarean section. *Br J Anaesth* 1999; 83(2): 343–345.

32 Madu EC, Shala B, Baugh D. Crack-cocaine-associated aortic dissection in early pregnancy – a case report. *Angiology* 1999; 50(2): 163–168.

33 Singer M, Clarke J, Bennet ED. Continuous hemodynamic monitoring by esophageal Doppler. *Crit Care Med* 1989; 17: 447–452.

34 Penny JA, Anthony J, Shennan AH, de Swiet M, Singer M. A comparison of hemodynamic data derived by pulmonary artery flotation catheter and the esophageal Doppler monitor in preeclampsia. *Am J Obstet Gynecol* 2000; 183: 658–661.

35 Aaslid R, Huber P, Nornes H. Evaluation of cerebrovascular spasm with transcranial Doppler ultrasound. *J Neurosurg* 1984; 60(10): 37–41.

36 Polito A, Ricci Z, Di Chiara L, Giorni C, Iacoella C, Sanders SP, Picardo S. Cerebral blood flow during cardiopulmonary bypass in pediatric cardiac surgery: the role of transcranial Doppler – a systematic review of the literature. *Cardiovasc Ultrasound* 2006; 4: 47.

37 Belfort MA, Tooke-Miller C, Allen JC et al. Changes in flow velocity, resistance indices, and cerebral perfusion pressure in the maternal middle cerebral artery distribution during normal pregnancy. *Acta Obstet Gynecol Scand* 2001; 80: 104–112.

38 Riskin-Mashiah S, Belfort MA. Preeclampsia is associated with global cerebral hemodynamic changes. *J Soc Gynecol Investig* 2005; 12(4): 253–256.

39 Belfort MA, Tooke-Miller C, Allen JC Jr, Varner MA, Grunewald C, Nisell H, Herd JA. Pregnant women with chronic hypertension and superimposed pre-eclampsia have high cerebral perfusion pressure. *BJOG* 2001; 108(11): 1141–1147.

40 Gibo H, Carver CC, Rhoton AL, Jr., Lenkey C, Mitchell RJ. Microsurgical anatomy of the middle cerebral artery. *J Neurosurg* 1981; 54(2): 151–169.

41 Irion O, Moutquin JM, Williams K, Forest JC. Reference values and influence of smoking on maternal middle cerebral artery blood flow. *Am J Obstet Gynecol* 1996; 174: 367A.

42 Dewey RC, Pieper HP, Hunt WE. Experimental cerebral hemodynamics. Vasomotor tone, critical closing pressure, and vascular bed resistance. *J Neurosurg* 1974; 41(5): 597–606.

43 Aaslid R, Lundar T, Lindegaard KF, Nornes H. Estimation of cerebral perfusion pressure from arterial blood pressure and transcranial Doppler recordings. In: Miller JD, Teasdale GM, Rowan JO, Galbraith SL, Mendelow AD, eds. *Intracranial Pressure VI*. Berlin, Heidelberg: Springer-Verlag, 1986: 226–229.

44 Belfort MA, Tooke-Miller C, Varner M et al. Evaluation of a non-invasive transcranial Doppler and blood pressure bases method for the assessment of cerebral perfusion pressure in pregnant women. *Hypertens Pregnancy* 2000; 19(3): 331–340.

45 Belfort MA, Varner MC, Dizon-Townson DS, Grunewald C, Nisell H. Cerebral perfusion pressure, and not cerebral blood flow, may be the critical determinant of intracranial injury in preeclampsia: a new hypothesis. *Am J Obstet Gynecol* 2002; 187: 626–634.

16 Pulmonary Artery Catheterization

Steven L. Clark[1] & Gary A. Dildy III[2]

[1]Women's and Children's Clinical Services, Hospital Corporation of America, Nashville, TN, USA
[2]Maternal-Fetal Medicine, Mountain Star Division, Hospital Corporation of America, Salt Lake City, UT *and* Department of Obstetrics and Gynecology, LSU Health Sciences Center, School of Medicine in New Orleans, New Orleans, LA, USA

Introduction

Following its introduction into clinical medicine three decades ago, the pulmonary artery catheter was shown to play an important role in the management of critically ill patients in a number of specialties, including obstetrics [1–6]. Several early prospective trials demonstrated the benefits of pulmonary artery catheterization in select critically ill patients. Such benefits include a reduction in operative morbidity and mortality in certain complicated surgical patients and a significant mortality reduction in patients in shock in whom catheter-obtained parameters led to changes in therapy [7,8]. In one study, management recommendations changed as a direct result of knowledge obtained by pulmonary artery catheter placement in 56% of patients admitted to an intensive care unit [9]. In patients with major burn injuries, survival is predicted by early response to pulmonary artery catheter-guided resuscitation [10]. This technique, however, was not without its critics [11]. In a non-randomized observational study, Califf and colleagues [12] demonstrated increased mortality and cost associated with pulmonary artery catheterization, and suggested that a randomized trial aimed at better patient selection was needed. An subsequent randomized controlled trial (n = 201) of the pulmonary artery catheter in critically ill patients concluded that its use is not associated with increased mortality [13].

In response to concerns of increased morbidity and mortality associated with the pulmonary catheter in observational studies, the National Heart, Lung, and Blood Institute (NHLBI) and the US Food and Drug Administration (FDA) conducted the Pulmonary Artery Catheterization and Clinical Outcomes workshop in 1997 to develop recommendations to improve pulmonary artery catheter utility and safety [14]. They concluded that a "need exists for collaborative education of physicians and nurses in performing, obtaining, and interpreting information from the use of pulmonary artery catheters. This effort should be led by professional societies, in collaboration with federal agencies, with the purpose of developing and disseminating standardized educational programs." Areas given high priority for clinical trials were pulmonary artery catheter use in persistent/refractory congestive heart failure, acute respiratory distress syndrome, severe sepsis and septic shock, and low-risk coronary artery bypass graft surgery.

Since this conference, several investigators have attempted to better define benefits and risks of pulmonary artery catheterization both in general categories of critical illness, and in specific subsets of critically ill patients. Most studies that used broad and non-specific patient inclusion criteria (such as "critically ill patients" or "high-risk surgical patients") have, not surprisingly, generally detected neither beneficial nor detrimental effects of pulmonary artery catheterization on mortality rates [15–17] and the use of pulmonary artery catheterization has decreased in the United States over the past decade [18]. On the other hand, studies directed at specific subsets of critically ill patients have proven much more informative. It would appear, for example, that such monitoring techniques are not typically associated with improved survival in patients with acute lung injury and acute respiratory distress syndrome [19,20]. On the other hand survival benefit has been demonstrated in patients with severe trauma or illness, those admitted in severe shock and in older trauma patients [21,22]. Another study demonstrating lack of benefit of pulmonary artery catheterization in patients with severe septic shock does not address the question of whether patients so managed before late or end-stage disease may benefit from the information provided by these techniques [23]. Interpretation of such data is further compounded by the general lack of uniform, evidence-based management protocols for most patients in whom pulmonary artery catheters are utilized. No diagnostic testing modality can improve outcomes in any disease in the absence of effective therapy [15,24]. Thus, at present, the pulmonary artery catheter should be viewed neither as a panacea for all seriously ill patients, nor as a technique lacking diagnostic value

Critical Care Obstetrics, 5th edition. Edited by M. Belfort, G. Saade, M. Foley, J. Phelan and G. Dildy.

in any patient. In a recent review article focusing on the use of this technique in pregnant patients, Fujitani and Baldisseri [25] concluded "Invasive monitoring remains useful when the pathophysiology of critically ill obstetric patients cannot be explained by non-invasive monitoring, and the patient fails to respond to conservative medical management; invasive hemodynamic monitoring may be helpul to guide management." As emphasized by Harvey et al, future studies will need to be adequately powered and focus on specific patient subsets receiving targeted therapies in order to better define the proper role of this technique in the management of critically ill patients [26].

This chapter provides an overview of placement techniques and complications; indications for the use of this diagnostic tool in the obstetric patient are examined in more detail in the ensuing chapters.

Catheter placement

The procedure for catheter placement involves two phases. The initial phase of pulmonary artery catheterization is establishing venous access with a large-bore sheath. Access is most commonly obtained via the internal jugular or subclavian veins; however, under certain circumstances (e.g. where access to the neck or thoracic region is difficult or in a patient with a coagulopathy where bleeding from a major artery could be hazardous), peripheral veins–including cephalic or femoral–can be used [27]. Insertion of the introducer sheath via the right internal jugular vein is described here.

Insertion of the sheath

To catheterize the internal jugular vein, the patient is placed supine in a mild Trendelenburg position with the head turned to the left. The landmark for insertion is the junction of the clavicular and sternal heads of the sternocleidomastoid muscle. When this junction is indistinct, its identification can be facilitated by having the patient raise her head slightly. When the landmark has been identified, 1% lidocaine is infiltrated into the skin and superficial subcutaneous tissue.

The internal jugular vein is entered first with a finder needle, consisting of a 21-gauge needle on a 10-mL syringe. The skin is punctured at the junction of the two clavicular heads, and the needle is directed with constant aspiration toward the ipsilateral nipple at an angle approximately 30° superior to the plane of the skin. Free flow of venous blood confirms the position of the internal jugular vein. Next, the needle is withdrawn and the vein once again entered with a 16-gauge needle and syringe. Then a guidewire is placed through the needle and into the jugular vein. This placement is perhaps the most crucial part of the entire procedure, and it is vital that the guidewire passes freely without any resistance whatsoever. Free passage confirms entrance into the vein.

Next, the needle is removed with the guidewire left in place. The incision is widened with a scalpel, and the introducer sheath/vein dilator apparatus is introduced over the guidewire. During introduction of the introducer sheath/vein dilator, it is crucial that the proximal tip of the guidewire be visible at all times, to avoid inadvertent loss of the guidewire into the central venous system. The introducer sheath/vein dilator apparatus is advanced with a slight turning motion along the guidewire. In general, the point of entry into the vein is felt clearly by a sudden decrease in resistance. The sheath apparatus then is advanced to the hilt. The conscious patient is instructed to hold her breath to prevent negative intrathoracic pressure and air embolism, and the guidewire and trocar are quickly removed with the sheath left in place. Occasionally, portable real-time sonography may be helpful in guiding central venous cannulation [28,29].

Most current introducer systems contain an accessory port, which attaches to the proximal end of the introducer sheath and includes a one-way valve that prevents air introduction into the central venous system during removal of the guidewire and trocar. To keep the line open, the sheath then is infused with a crystalloid solution containing 1 unit of heparin per milliliter and secured in place with suture.

Insertion of the catheter

Phase two involves the actual placement of the pulmonary artery catheter (Figure 16.1). Careful attention must be paid to maintaining sterile technique as the catheter is removed from the package. The distal and proximal ports are flushed to assure patency. The balloon then is tested with 1 mL of air. When the catheter has been attached to the physiologic monitor and the air

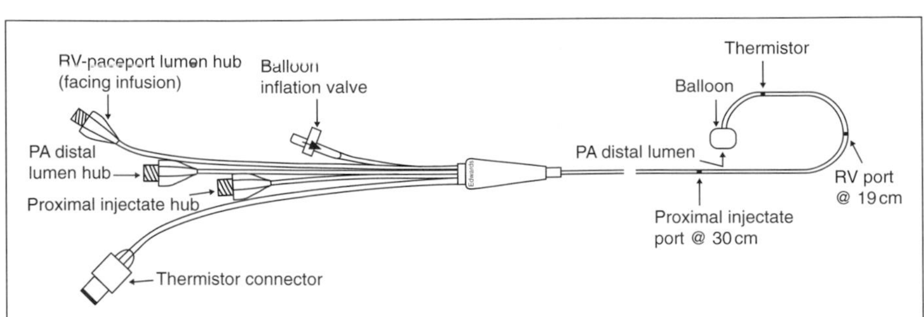

Figure 16.1 Pulmonary artery catheter. (Reproduced by permission from American Edwards Laboratories.)

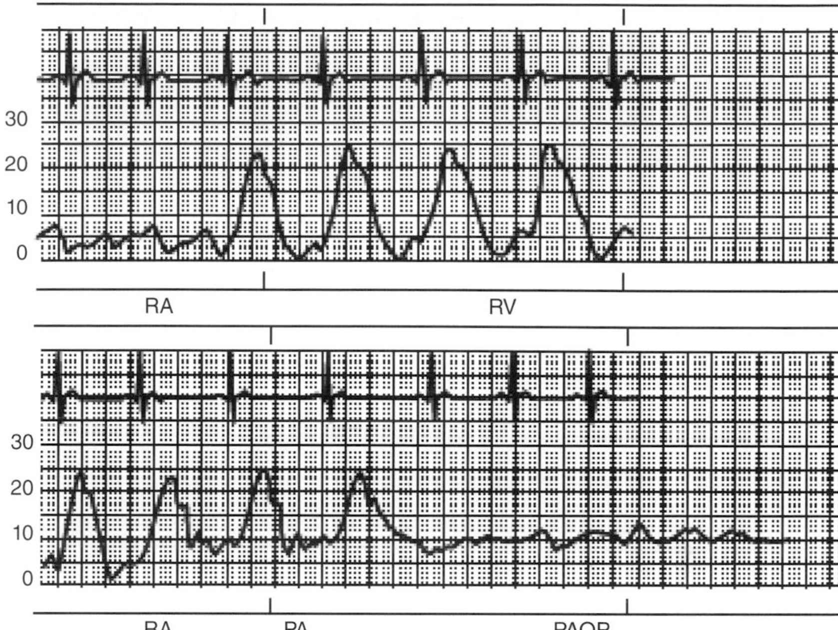

Figure 16.2 Pulmonary artery catheter placement. Catheter tip position, corresponding waveforms, and normal pressure ranges are demonstrated. (Reproduced by permission from American Edwards Laboratories.)

completely flushed from the system, minute movements in the catheter tip should produce corresponding oscillations on the monitor. The catheter tip is introduced through the sheath and advanced approximately 20 cm. At this point, the balloon is inflated and the catheter advanced through the introducer sheath into the central venous system. Occasionally, portable real-time sonography may be helpful in guiding central venous cannulation [29].

Waveforms and catheter placement

Once within the superior vena cava, the balloon on the tip of the catheter will advance with the flow of blood into the heart. Characteristic waveforms and pressures are observed (Figure 16.2). Entrance into the right ventricle is signaled by a high spiking waveform with diastolic pressures near zero. This is the time of maximum potential complications during catheter placement, because most arrhythmias occur as the catheter tip impinges on the interventricular septum. For this reason, the catheter must be advanced rapidly through the right ventricle and into the pulmonary artery. If premature ventricular contractions occur during this process and the catheter does not advance promptly out of the right ventricle, the balloon should be deflated and the catheter withdrawn to the right atrium.

As soon as the catheter enters the pulmonary artery, the waveform has two notable characteristics. First, and most important, is the rise in diastolic pressure from that seen in the right ventricle. Second, a notching of the peak systolic waveform often is seen and represents closure of the pulmonic valve. After entrance into the pulmonary artery has been confirmed (in most pregnant women, this occurs between 40 and 45 cm of catheter length), the catheter is advanced farther until the tip reaches a point within the pulmonary vasculature where the balloon diameter exceeds that of the corresponding pulmonary arterial branch. At this point, a wedge tracing is observed. If the balloon is deflated, the tracing should return to a pulmonary artery pattern.

Following catheter placement, it is essential that healthcare personnel skilled in the interpretation of these waveforms continuously monitor the waveforms for evidence of catheter migration (spontaneous advancement), which may lead to pulmonary infarction. This may be manifest by the appearance of a spontaneous "wedge" tracing at the distal port, rather than the pulmonary artery waveform, which should be continuously manifest on the display monitor. Alternately, the appearance of a pulmonary artery waveform in the central venous pressure port will alert the attendant to distal catheter migration and the need for adjustment [30]. Komadina et al. described disturbingly high interobserver variability in the interpretation of waveform tracings, although agreement on numerical wedge pressure readings was high [31]. In a similar manner, Iberti et al. reported a wide variation in the understanding of pulmonary artery catheter waveforms and techniques among critical care nurses using this device [32]. It would appear that graphic recording at end-expiration is the most reliable means of measuring hemodynamic pressures [33]. Clearly, continuous training and credentialing programs are essential for healthcare providers utilizing these techniques. Recently described digital output volumetric pulmonary artery catheters have been shown to reduce interoperator interpretation variability and to improve consistency of treatment decisions. [34] Normal ranges for hemodynamic parameters in term pregnancy have been described, and are useful in assessing and managing the pregnant woman requiring invasive monitoring techniques [35,36].

Caution also is advised during pulmonary artery catheter removal; techniques to avoid complications have been described [37].

Cardiac output determination

Once in place, cardiac output is obtained with the use of a cardiac output computer connected to a terminal on the pulmonary artery catheter. This instrument derives cardiac output from thermodilution curves created by the injection of cold or room-temperature saline into the proximal central venous port of the catheter. The resultant flow-related temperature changes detected at the distal thermistor are converted into cardiac output by the computer and correlate well in pregnant women with those obtained by the more precise, but clinically cumbersome, oxygen extraction (Fick) technique [35]. Nevertheless, it should be emphasized that cardiac output determinations are of most value in following trends in individual patients; caution is advised in relying on absolute cardiac output values, and sound clinical judgment is essential in data interpretation [38]. One study suggests that the thermodilution technique may overestimate cardiac output, especially with very low values [39]. In addition, meticulous attention must be paid to technique if reliable information regarding cardiac output is to be obtained. The exact injectate temperature must be known, the proximal injectate port must have advanced beyond the introducer sheath, and the introducer sheath sidearm must be closed [40]. If the central venous port line becomes non-functional, room-temperature thermodilution cardiac outputs can be used with saline injection into the sideport, with the understanding that a slight overestimation of cardiac output will occur [41]. Additional issues that affect the validity of cardiac output measurements include the rate of injection, the timing of injection during the respiratory cycle, the position of the patient, and the presence of other, concurrent infusions [42]. More recently, techniques have been evaluated for continuous cardiac output measurement, both by thermodilution and with the use of a special flow-directed Doppler pulmonary artery catheter [43,44]. Penny et al. [45] demonstrated that esophageal Doppler monitoring consistently underestimates cardiac output in patients with pre-eclampsia by approximately 40%, compared to direct measurements with pulmonary artery catheters.

With appropriate modification of technique, right ventricular ejection fraction measurements also may be obtained with the pulmonary artery catheter [46,47]. Specially designed fiberoptic catheters allow continuous assessment of mixed venous oxygen saturation in critically ill patients. Newer techniques for continuous thermodilution measurement compare well with conventional methods [48,49].

Complications

Most complications encountered in patients undergoing pulmonary artery catheterization are a result of obtaining central venous access. Such events include pneumothorax and insertion site infection and occur in 1–5% of patients undergoing this procedure [50–52]. Potential complications of pulmonary artery catheterization per se include air embolism, thromboembolism, pulmonary infarction, catheter-related sepsis, direct trauma to the heart or pulmonary artery, postganglionic Horner's syndrome, and catheter entrapment [53–58]. Such complications occur in 1% or less of patients. More recently, a pressure release balloon has been described to limit overinflation and potentially reduce the risk of vessel rupture [59]. Arrhythmias, consisting of transient premature ventricular contractions, occur during catheter insertion in 30–50% of patients and are generally of no clinical consequence.

The remaining complications can be minimized or eliminated by careful attention to proper insertion maintenance and removal techniques [37]). In patients with right-to-left shunts, the use of this catheter is hazardous; when its placement is deemed mandatory, the use of carbon dioxide instead of air for balloon inflation may minimize the risk of systemic air embolism [60]. A Food and Drug Administration task force has summarized recommendations regarding methods to minimize complications of central venous catheterization procedures [61]. A recent study suggested that with proper attention to aseptic technique of placement and catheter maintainance, a pulmonary artery catheter may be left in place for up to 7 days before replacement becomes mandatory [62].

Numerous studies have documented the frequent discrepancy between measurements of pulmonary capillary wedge pressure and central venous pressure during pregnancy [4,63–65]. In such circumstances, clinical use of the central venous pressure would be misleading. Both techniques entail the risks of obtaining central venous access, the principal source of complication for either procedure. For these reasons, in a modern perinatal intensive care unit, central venous monitoring is uncommonly utilized. Where proper equipment and personnel exist, the vast amount of additional information obtainable by pulmonary artery catheterization often outweighs the slight potential increase in risk attributable to catheter placement itself. When the hemodynamic status of the critically ill pregnant woman is unclear, pulmonary artery catheterization is nearly always preferable.

Non-invasive techniques

Despite the small risks associated with properly managed pulmonary artery catheterization, the search continues for non-invasive methods of central hemodynamic assessment of the critically ill patient. Such techniques generally focus on sonographic or bioimpedance techniques to estimate cardiac output, and have been described in both pregnant and non-pregnant patients [66–70]. In addition, investigation continues into techniques to allow non-invasive central pressure determination [71]. These techniques appear to be useful in a research setting or in patients requiring only a single evaluation of hemodynamics in order to classify their disease and initiate appropriate therapy. Invasive techniques, however, remain the mainstay of long-term management of complex, critically ill obstetric patients.

One area of non-invasive assessment warrents special mention. In non-pregnant patients, echocardiographic assessment of pulmonary artery pressures are commonly accepted, and generally valid. In the past three decades, clinicians with extensive experience in the management of pregnant women with pulmonary hypertension have commonly noted significant discrepancies between non-invasive assessment of pulmonary artery pressures and actual pressures measured directly with right heart catheterization. In 2001, this observation was validated by Penny et al. who found that pulmonary artery pressures were commonly overestimated in pregnant women with suspected pulmonary hypertension [72]. Based upon this data, and many years of clinical experience, we recommend that any pregnant woman with elevated pulmonary artery pressures by echocardiogram have this diagnosis confirmed by invasive right heart catheterization before counseling and critical clinical decisions are initiated.

References

1 Swan JHC, Ganz W, Forrester J et al. Catheterization of the heart in man with use of a flow-directed balloon-tipped catheter. *N Engl J Med* 1970; 283: 447–451.

2 Clark SL, Horenstein JM, Phelan JP et al. Experience with the pulmonary artery catheter in obstetrics and gynecology. *Am J Obstet Gynecol* 1985; 152: 374–378.

3 Clark SL, Greenspoon JS, Aldahl D, Phelan JP. Severe preeclampsia with persistent oliguria: management of hemodynamic subsets. *Am J Obstet Gynecol* 1986; 154(3): 490–494.

4 Clark SL, Cotton DB. Clinical opinion: clinical indications for pulmonary artery catheterization in the patient with severe preeclampsia. *Am J Obstet Gynecol* 1988; 158: 453–458.

5 European Society of *Intensive Care Medicine*. Expert panel: the use of the pulmonary artery catheter. *Intensive Care Med* 1991; 17: I–VIII.

6 Clark SL, Phelan JP, Greenspoon J, Aldahl D, Horenstein J. Labor and delivery in the presence of mitral stenosis: central hemodynamic observations. *Am J Obstet Gynecol* 1985; 152(8): 984–988.

7 Sola JE, Bender JS. Use of the pulmonary artery catheter to reduce operative complications. *Surg Clin North Am* 1993; 73: 253–264.

8 Mimoz O, Rauss A, Rekik N et al. Pulmonary artery catheterization in critically ill patients: a prospective analysis of outcome changes associated with catheter-prompted changes in therapy. *Crit Care Med* 1994; 22: 573–579.

9 Coles NA, Hibberd M, Russell M et al. Potential impact of pulmonary artery catheter placement on short term management decisions in the medical intensive care unit. *Am Heart J* 1993; 126: 815–819.

10 Schiller WR, Bay RC, McLachlan JG. Survival in major burn injuries is predicted by early response to Swan–Ganz-guided resuscitation. *Am J Surg* 1995; 170: 696–699.

11 Cruz K, Franklin C. The pulmonary artery catheter: uses and controversies. *Crit Care Clin*. 2001; 17(2): 271–291.

12 Califf RM, Fulkerson WJ, Jr, Vidaillet H et al. The effectiveness of right-heart catheterization in the initial case of critically ill patients. *JAMA* 1996; 18: 889.

13 Rhodes A, Cusack RJ, Newman PJ, Grounds RM, Bennett ED. A randomised, controlled trial of the pulmonary artery catheter in criticallyill patients. *Intensive Care Med* 2002; 28(3): 256–264.

14 Bernard GR, Sopko G, Cerra F et al. Pulmonary artery catheterization and clinical outcomes: National Heart, Lung,and Blood Institute and Food and Drug Administration Workshop Report. Consensus Statement. *JAMA* 2000; 283(19): 2568–2572.

15 Shah MR, Hasselblad V, Stevenson LW et al. Impact of the pulmonary artery catheter in critically ill patients: meta-analysis of randomized clinical trials. *JAMA* 2005; 294; 1664–1670.

16 Sandham JD, Hull RD, Brandt RF et al. A randomized controlled trial of the use of pulmonary artery catheters in high risk surgical patients. *N Engl J Med* 2003; 348: 5–14.

17 Harvey S, Harrison DA, Singer M, Ashcroft J et al. Assessment of the clinical effectiveness of pulmonary artery catheters in management of patients in intensive care (PAC-Man): a randomized controlled trial. *Lancet* 2005; 366: 472–477.

18 Weiner RS, Welch HG. Trends in the use of the pulmonary artery catheter in the United States, 1993–2004. *JAMA* 2007; 298(4): 423–429.

19 Wheeler AP, Bernard GR, Thompson BT et al. Pulmonary artery versus central venous catheter to guide treatment of acute lung injury. *N Engl J Med* 2006; 354: 2213–2224.

20 Richard C, Warszawski J, Anguel N et al. Early use of the pulmonary artery catheter and outcomes in patients with shock and acute respiratory distress syndrome: a randomized clinical trial. *JAMA* 2003; 290: 2713–2720.

21 Friese RS, Shafi S, Gentilello LM. Pulmonary artery catheter use is associated with reduced mortality in severely injured patients: A National Trauma Data Bank analysis of 53,312 patients. *Crit Care Med* 2006; 34: 1597–1601.

22 Chittock DR, Dhingra VK, Ronco JJ et al. Severity of illness and risk of death associated with pulmonary artery catheter use. *Crit Care Med* 2004; 32: 911–915.

23 Yu DT, Platt R, Lanken PN et al. Relationship of pulmonary artery catheter use to mortality and resource utilization in patients with severe sepsis. *Crit Care Med* 2003; 31: 2734–2741.

24 Pinsky MR, Vincent JL. Let us use the pulmonary artery catheter correctly and only when we need it. *Crit Care Med* 2005; 33: 1119–1122.

25 Fujitani S, Baldisseri MR. Hemodynamic assessment in a pregnant and peripartum patient. *Crit Care Med* 2005; 33: S354–S361.

26 Harvey SE, Welch CA, Harrison DA, Rowan KM, Singer M. Post hoc insights from PAC-Man –the UK pulmonary artery catheter trial. *Crit Care Med* 2008; 36: 1714–1721.

27 Findling R, Lipper B. Femoral vein pulmonary artery catheterization in the intensive care unit. *Chest* 1994; 105: 874–877.

28 Lee W, Leduc L, Cotton DB. Ultrasonographic guidance for central venous catheterization. *Am J Obstet Gynecol* 1989; 161: 1012–1013.

29 Sherer DM, Abulafia O, DuBeshter B et al. Ultrasonically guided subclavian vein catheterization in critical care obstetrics and gynecologic oncology. *Am J Obstet Gynecol* 1993; 169: 1246–1248.

30 Santora T, Ganz W, Gold J et al. New method for monitoring pulmonary artery catheter location. *Crit Care Med* 1991; 19: 422–426.

31 Komadina KH, Schenk DA, LaVeau P et al. Interobserver variability in the interpretation of pulmonary artery catheter pressure tracings. *Chest* 1991; 100: 1647–1654.

32 Iberti TJ, Daily EK, Leibowitz AB. Assessment of critical care nurses' knowledge of the pulmonary artery catheter. *Crit Care Med* 1994; 22: 1674–1678.

33 Johnson MK, Schumann L. Comparison of three methods of measurement of pulmonary artery catheter readings in critically ill patients. *Am J Crit Care* 1985; 4: 300–307.

34 Gracias VH, Horan Ad, Kim PK et al. Digital output volumetric pulmonary artery catheters eliminate intraoperator interpretation variability and improve consistency of treatment decisions. *J Am Coll Surg* 2007; 204: 209–215.

35 Clark SL, Cotton DB, Lee W et al. Central hemodynamic assessment of normal term pregnancy. *Am J Obstet Gynecol* 1989; 161: 1439–1442.

36 Clark SL, Cotton DB, Pivarnik JM, Lee W, Hankins DGV, Benedetti TJ, Phelan JP. Position change and central hemodynamic profile during normal third-trimester pregnancy and postpartum. *Am J Obstet Gynecol* 1991; 164(3): 883–887.

37 Wadas TM. Pulmonary artery catheter removal. *Crit Care Nurse* 1994; 14: 63–72.

38 Vender JS. Clinical utilization of pulmonary artery catheter monitoring. *Int Anesthesiol Clin* 1993; 31: 57–85.

39 Espersen K, Jensen EW, Rosenberg D et al. Comparison of cardiac output techniques: Thermodilution, Doppler CO_2 rebreathing and the direct Fick method. *Acta Anaesthesiol Scand* 1995; 39: 245–251.

40 Boyd O, Mackay CJ, Newman P et al. Effects of insertion depth and use of the sidearm of the introducer sheath of pulmonary artery catheters in cardiac output measurement. *Crit Care Med* 1994; 22: 1132–1135.

41 Pesola HR, Pesola GR. Room temperature thermodilution cardiac output. Central venous vs side port. *Chest* 1993; 103: 339–341.

42 Sommers MS, Woods SL, Courtade MA. Issues in methods and measurement of thermodilution cardiac output. *Nurs Res* 1993; 42: 228–223.

43 Segal J, Gaudiani V, Nishimura T. Continuous determination of cardiac output using a flow directed Doppler pulmonary artery catheter. *J Cardiothorac Vasc Anesth* 1991; 5: 309–315.

44 Mihaljevic T, von Segesser LK, Tonz M et al. Continuous thermodilution measurement of cardiac output: in-vitro and in-vivo evaluation. *Thorac Cardiovasc Surg* 1994; 42: 32–35.

45 Penny JA, Anthony J, Shennan AH, DeSwiet M, Singer M. A comparison of hemodynamic data derived by pulmonary artery floatation catheter and the esophageal Doppler monitor in preeclampsia. *Am J Obstet Gynecol* 2000; 183: 658–661.

46 Cockroft S, Withington PS. The measurement of right ventricular ejection fraction by thermodilution. A comparison of values obtained using differing injectate ports. *Anaesthesia* 1993; 48: 312–314.

47 Safcsak K, Nelson LD. Thermodilution right ventricular ejection fraction measurements: room temperature versus cold temperature injectate. *Crit Care Med* 1994; 22: 1136–1141.

48 Inomata S, Nishikawa T, Taguchi M. Continuous monitoring of mixed venous oxygen saturation for detecting alterations in cardiac output after discontinuation of cardiopulmonary bypass. *Br J Anaesth* 1994; 72: 11–16.

49 Lefrant JY, Bruelle P, Ripart J et al. Cardiac output measurement in critically ill patients: Comparison of continuous and conventional thermodilution techniques. *Can J Anesth* 1995; 42: 972–976.

50 Patel C, Laboy V, Venus B et al. Acute complications of pulmonary artery catheter insertion in critically ill patients. *Crit Care Med* 1986; 14: 195–197.

51 Scott WL. Complications associated with central venous catheters. *Chest* 1988; 91: 1221–1224.

52 Gilbert WM, Towner DR, Field NT, Anthony J. The safety and utility of pulmonary artery catheterization in severe preeclampsia and eclampsia. *Am J Obstet Gynecol* 2000; 182(6): 1397–403.

53 Soding PF, Klinck JR, Kong A et al. Infective endocarditis of the pulmonary valve following pulmonary artery catheterization. *Intensive Care Med* 1994; 20: 222–224.

54 Bernardin G, Milhaud D, Roger PM et al. Swan–Ganz catheter related pulmonary valve infective endocarditis: a case report. *Intensive Care Med* 1994; 20: 142–144.

55 Yellin LB, Filler JJ, Barnette RE. Nominal hemoptysis heralds pseudoaneurysm induced by a pulmonary artery catheter. *Anesthesiology* 1991; 74: 370–373.

56 Manager D, Connell GR, Lessin JL. Catheter induced pulmonary artery haemorrhage resulting from a pneumothorax. *Can J Anaesth* 1993; 40: 1069–1072.

57 Lanigan C, Cornwell E. Pulmonary artery catheter entrapment. *Anaesthesia* 1991; 46: 600–601.

58 Vaswani S, Garvin L, Matuschak GM. Postganglionic Horner's syndrome after insertion of a pulmonary artery catheter through the internal jugular vein. *Crit Care Med* 1991; 19: 1215–1216.

59 Shevde K, Raab R, Lee P. Decreasing the risk of pulmonary artery rupture with a pressure relief balloon. *J Cardiothorac Vasc Anesth* 1994; 8: 30–34.

60 Moorthy SS, Tisinai KA, Speiser BS et al. Cerebral air embolism during removal of a pulmonary artery catheter. *Crit Care Med* 1991; 19: 981–983.

61 U.S. Food and Drug Administration. Precautions necessary with central venous catheters. *FDA Drug Bulletin* July 1989; 15.

62 Chey YY, Yen DH, Yang YG et al. Comparison between replacement at 4 days and 7 days of the infection rate for pulmonary artery catheters in an intensive care unit. *Crit Care Med* 2003; 31: 1358–1358.

63 Benedetti TJ, Cotton DB, Read JC et al. Hemodynamic observations in severe preeclampsia with a flow-directed pulmonary artery catheter. *Am J Obstet Gynecol* 1980; 136: 465.

64 Cotton DB, Gonik B, Dorman K et al. Cardiovascular alterations in severe pregnancy induced hypertension: relationship of central venous pressure to pulmonary capillary wedge pressure. *Am J Obstet Gynecol* 1985; 151: 762–764.

65 Bolte AC, Dekker GA, van Eyck J, van Schijndel RS, van Geijn HP. Lack of agreement between central venous pressure and pulmonary capillary wedge pressure in preeclampsia. *Hypertens Pregnancy* 2000; 19(3): 261–271.

66 Clark SL, Southwick J, Pivarnik JM et al. A comparison of cardiac index in normal term pregnancy using thoracic electrical bioimpedance and oxygen extraction (Fick) technique. *Obstet Gynecol* 1994; 83: 669–672.

67 Belfort MA, Rokey R, Saade GR et al. Rapid echocardiographic assessment of left and right heart hemodynamics in critically ill obstetric patients. *Am J Obstet Gynecol* 1991; 171: 884–892.

68 Belfort MA, Mares A, Saade G et al. A re-evaluation of the indications for pulmonary artery catheters in obstetrics: the role of 2-D echocardiography and Doppler ultrasound. *Am J Obstet Gynecol* 1996; 174: 331.

69 Easterling T, Watts D, Schmucker B et al. Measurement of cardiac output during pregnancy: validation of Doppler technique and clinical observations in preeclamplsia. *Obstet Gynecol* 1987; 69: 845–850.

70 Weiss S, Calloway E, Cairo J et al. Comparison of cardiac output measurements by thermodilution and thoracic electrical bioimpedance in critically ill vs. noncritically ill patients. *Am J Emerg Med* 1995; 13: 626–631.

71 Ensing G, Seward J, Darragh R et al. Feasibility of generating hemodynamic pressure curves from noninvasive Doppler echocardiographic signals. *J Am Coll Cardiol* 1994; 23: 434–442.

72 Penning S, Robinson KD, Major CA, Garite TJ. A comparison of echocardiography and pulmonary artery catheterization for evaluation of pulmonary artery pressures in pregnant patients with suspected pulmonary hypertension. *Am J Obstet Gynecol* 2001; 184: 1568–1570.

17 Seizures and Status Epilepticus

Michael W. Varner
Department of Obstetrics and Gynecology, University of Utah Health Sciences Center, Salt Lake City, UT, USA

Introduction

Epilepsy is a common clinical disorder seen in women of reproductive age. The prevalence in the developed world is estimated at 5–10 per 1000, with an annual incidence of 50 per 100 000 people [1] and a lifetime incidence of a single seizure of 110 per 1000. There is no evidence to suggest that this distribution should be any different for women of reproductive age, making this condition among the more common concurrent neurological disorders seen in pregnant women.

Etiology

Epilepsy is a predisposition to recurrent seizures based on identified or suspected dysfunction of the central nervous system. The occurrence of seizures may represent a myriad of etiologies (Table 17.1). Because optimum treatment of seizures should be directed at their underlying etiology or etiologies, confirmation of this or these is important. Irrespective of etiology, generalized convulsive seizures, because of the potential for maternal physical injury, prolonged apnea and/or an unguarded airway, and for fetal injury and/or hypoxia/ischemia, require immediate and urgent attention. Partial seizures, unless followed by secondary generalized tonic–clonic seizures, pose much lower risks for mother and baby and thus require less emergent responses.

It is not clear that pregnancy increases seizure frequency. Engel and Perley [2] report that 22% of pregnant women had decreased seizure frequency, 24% had increased seizure frequency and 54% had no change. Of those women with increased seizure frequency, the most likely time for exacerbation was the first trimester. This most commonly reflects pregnancy-associated pharmacokinetic changes and/or decreased medication ingestion because of concerns about teratogenesis.

Critical Care Obstetrics, 5th edition. Edited by M. Belfort, G. Saade, M. Foley, J. Phelan and G. Dildy.

Seizure prophylaxis

The development of effective anticonvulsant medications has revolutionized the lives and prognoses of individuals with epilepsy. The options for treatment have expanded rapidly in recent years, although effects of these medications during pregnancy are still not well known. An extensive review of these options is beyond the scope of this chapter and recent reviews are available [3,4]. Pregnancy registries are available through the pharmaceutical companies for many of the newer anticonvulsant medications and patients are encouraged to enrol with these registries voluntarily. In general, pregnant women should take the medication that best controls their epilepsy. Switching medications during pregnancy is not recommended because of the risk of losing seizure control.

If the patient desires to discontinue the anticonvulsant medication, it ideally should be accomplished preconceptionally as the greatest risk to the fetus is during the first trimester of the pregnancy. In addition, it is optimal to determine whether seizures are going to recur or worsen after stopping the medication before the patient becomes pregnant. It is not recommended that the anticonvulsant medication be discontinued if the patient has a history of recurrent seizures in the past, even if they have been seizure free on medication for over a year. In some instances, if the patient discontinues the medication and loses complete seizure control, they are never again able to completely control their seizures with medication. If the patient still desires to try and stop the medication before or during the pregnancy, consultation with a neurologist or epileptologist is recommended for further counseling.

Because of the increases in maternal blood volume and hepatic metabolism during pregnancy, total levels of anticonvulsant medications, which are highly protein bound, will decline in almost all women. Monitoring total drug levels will be sufficient if the patient is clinically well controlled.

While free drug levels also decline during pregnancy, the percentage decline is much less than for total drug levels. Thus, if the woman is having recurrent or persistent seizures or side effects,

Table 17.1 International classification of seizures by mode of onset and spread.*

Type	Subtype	Characteristics	Medication(s)
Partial			
	Simple partial	Electrical abnormality confined to one localized area of the brain. The person remains conscious and fully aware.	Carbamazepine (begin at 200 mg bid), or dilantin (begin at 100 mg tid) Gabitril, neurontin (newer option – but therefore less clinical experience)
	Complex partial	Impaired consciousness, often exhibiting automatisms. The electrical abnormality usually starts in the temporal lobes. May spread to the rest of the brain and result in secondary generalized tonic-clonic seizures	Carbamazepine (see above) Dilantin (see above)
Generalized			
	Generalized tonic-clonic	Initial stiffness (tonic) and collapse followed by generalized jerking (clonic) movements, averaging several minutes in duration. Often apneic and involuntarily incontinent. Thereafter followed by relaxation and deep unconsciousness. Post-ictal confusion and fatigue may last for hours. Also known as "grand mal" seizures	Carbamazepine (see above) Dilantin (see above) Valproic acid (begin at 15 mg/kg/day in 3 divided doses)
	Absence	Brief episodes of unconsciousness, sometimes with fluttering of the eyelids. Rapid recovery. Also known as "petit mal" seizures.	Zarontin, valproic acid
	Myoclonic	Sudden symmetrical shock-like limb movements with or without loss of consciousness.	Valproic acid, ethosuximide
	Tonic	Stiffening of the whole body with or without loss of consciousness.	
	Atonic	Momentary loss of limb muscle tone causing sudden collapse, head drooping, etc.	

*Adapted from Commission on Classification and Terminology of the International League Against Epilepsy. Proposal for revised clinical and electroencephalographic classification of epileptic seizures. *Epilepsia* 1981; 22: 489.

then free (i.e. non-protein-bound) drug levels should be obtained and monitored.

In women whose seizures have been well controlled for at least the preceding year and whose therapeutic-free and total anticonvulsant levels have been determined preconceptionally, anticonvulsant drug levels need only be determined every trimester. However, if the woman has had uncontrolled seizures within the year before conception, recurrent seizure activity during the pregnancy, develops troublesome side-effects or is suspected of noncompliance, then monthly free anticonvulsant levels should be monitored. If total drug levels decrease by more than 60% or if free drug levels decrease by more than 30% and values fall out of the recommended therapeutic range, the dosage should be increased.

All anticonvulsant drugs have folic acid antagonist properties. As a result, women taking anticonvulsant medications are at a relative increased risk for having fetuses with a number of structural abnormalities, including cleft lip and palate, congenital heart defects and neural tube defects [5–7]. It is generally acknowledged that anticonvulsants double the risk of teratogenicity from baseline and that multiple anticonvulsants increase the risk still further. Of the anticonvulsant drugs that are currently widely utilized, valproic acid has a higher risk of neural tube defects and thus is not recommended in women planning a pregnancy whenever it can be avoided. Although it is not completely clear how much supplementation is truly needed in this population, all women of reproductive age should now be advised to ingest at least 4 mg folic acid per day for at least several months preconceptionally and through the first few months of pregnancy in order to reduce the risk of neural tube defects in pregnancy. Pregnant women on anticonvulsants should be continued on at least 1 mg/day of folic acid for the duration of their pregnancy and their reproductive careers.

They should also receive vitamin K (10 mg orally daily) beginning 4 weeks before expected delivery until birth in order to minimize the risk of neonatal hemorrhage [8]. Reports of increased risk of spontaneous hemorrhage in newborns suggest that the inhibition of vitamin K-dependent clotting factors (i.e. II, VII, IX, X) secondary to increased vitamin K metabolism and the inhibition of placental transport of vitamin K results from anticonvulsant use. Historically, most patients on anticonvulsant medications received oral vitamin K supplementation at the end of pregnancy. However, a recent study of 204 neonates born to mothers taking anticonvulsants who did not receive vitamin K supplementation showed no evidence of coagulopathy [9]. Upon delivery, clotting studies can be performed on the cord blood, and vitamin K should be routinely administered to the infant. If the cord blood is deficient in clotting factors, fresh frozen plasma may be required to protect the newborn.

Because of the rapid postpartum changes in maternal blood volume, women receiving anticonvulsant medications during pregnancy should have free and total drug levels assessed at 2 weeks postpartum. Serum levels commonly rise in the first few weeks after delivery in association with resolution of the hormonally mediated effects of pregnancy. If medication doses were increased during the pregnancy, the patient may develop symptoms of medication toxicity if doses are not appropriately lowered again in the postpartum period.

Evaluation of new-onset seizures in pregnancy

While most seizure disorders manifest themselves before pregnancy, the initial onset of seizures and of epilepsy can occur during pregnancy (Table 17.2). Acute etiologies (hemorrhage, thrombosis, etc.) must be ruled out and any underlying predisposing factors treated appropriately. A careful history is often very helpful in establishing a diagnosis. Witnesses, family members and the patient should be questioned. The onset, duration and characteristics of the seizure should be described. The setting in which the episode occurred should be defined. The possibility of precipitating factors must be pursued, including:

- infection (recent history of febrile illness with or without change in mental status, history of parenteral drug use, recent dental work, heart murmur or valvular heart disease)
- alcohol and/or drugs (consider cocaine, or amphetamine withdrawal) or toxin exposure
- mass lesions (history of malignancy, focal findings on examination)
- intracranial hemorrhage (sudden onset of "worst headache of my life")
- intracranial thrombosis (fluctuating neurologic deficits)
- trauma.

For much of the history witnesses are better sources than patients, but patients are the best source for presence and type of aura. Determine whether the patient completely lost consciousness and whether incontinence of bowel or bladder occurred. Determine whether there was an aura and whether there was antegrade amnesia or postictal confusion.

Vital signs should be promptly assessed and patients evaluated for orthostatic hypotension. Fetal heart rate monitoring should be undertaken if the woman is within the realm of potential viability. A complete physical examination should be performed, with particular attention to the neurologic (fundoscopy, cranial nerves, speech, mental status, neck, motor, sensory and deep tendon reflexes) and cardiovascular (heart murmur, arrhythmia) systems.

Initial laboratory evaluation should focus on a complete blood count, chemistry profile, liver function testing, toxicology screen and urinalysis.

If the patient has a normal neurologic examination, an electroencephalogram (EEG) and brain imaging study are still indicated. If intracranial hemorrhage is suspected a computed tomography (CT) scan should be considered, as the CT scan is the procedure of choice for detection of acute intracranial hemorrhage. If the clinical situation is less urgent, a magnetic resonance imaging (MRI) study would be preferable, as MRI technology is more sensitive for intracranial anatomy than is the CT scan. If intracranial infection is suspected, a lumbar puncture should be performed.

The most common differential diagnosis of a seizure is syncope. In contradistinction to seizures, syncope is *not* associated with

Table 17.2 Differential diagnosis of initial seizure(s) during pregnancy.

Condition	Clinical presentation	Diagnostic considerations
Brain tumor	Most likely to become symptomatic in the first trimester. Rare.	Papilledema should be prominent with supratentorial tumors.
Intracranial hemorrhage	Sudden severe headache or loss of consciousness. May have been preceded by a "sentinel" bleed	Arteriovenous malformations are more likely in younger, non-hypertensive women. Aneurysms are more likely in older, parous, hypertensive women.
Cerebral venous thrombosis	Fluctuating deficits and/or consciousness.	Most common in late pregnancy and the first few weeks after delivery.
Gestational epilepsy	Variable. Very rare.	A diagnosis of exclusion.
Eclampsia	Usually preceded by generalized headache, visual disturbances and/or abdominal pain.	Associated with hypertension, proteinuria and other symptoms and laboratory abnormalities (elevated liver function studies, decreased platelet counts; see Chapter 34)
Pseudoseizures	Often with atypical physical findings such as unresponsiveness without movement, asynchronous extremity movement, forward pelvic thrusting, and geotropic eye movements (a physical finding that indicates the eyes deviating toward the ground in a non-physiologic manner whether the head is turned left or right)	Past history of psychiatric disorders.

incontinence, tongue biting or confusion (before and/or after the episode).

Treatment of seizures

As previously emphasized, optimum treatment should be based on the known or presumed diagnosis. Although this information is often historical and available either from the patient, her friends or family or her medical records, the differential considerations outlined in Tables 17.1 and 17.2 must be considered, particularly in the seizing or postictal patient for whom no history is available.

Consultation with a neurologist is particularly important in the setting of an initial seizure (unless the diagnosis of eclampsia is reasonably certain), particularly if the neurologic examination is abnormal, the seizure is focal or the EEG is abnormal.

Providers must be familiar with and use the anticonvulsants that are considered the most effective for the individual seizure classifications (Table 17.1). Evidence strongly suggests that during pregnancy women should take the medication that best controls their epilepsy. Switching medications during pregnancy is not recommended because of the risk of losing seizure control.

Alternate treatment options for patients with medically refractory epilepsy include vagal nerve stimulation therapy, which has no known or suspected adverse effects on pregnancy, and epilepsy surgery. Surgical options, in general, should be addressed before or after pregnancy.

Status epilepticus

While uncommon (less than 1% of all pregnant epileptic women) major motor status epilepticus requires immediate intervention to prevent permanent brain damage or death to both mother and fetus. Although treatment will be administered to both mother and fetus, primary attention should be directed to the mother since maternal resuscitation and stabilization will optimally resuscitate her fetus. Initial attention must be paid to the maternal airway. As soon as the airway is secured, maternal oxygen saturation should be assessed and sufficient oxygen administered to return these values to normal, with intubation if necessary. Concurrent assessments should evaluate maternal blood pressure as well as forebrain and brain stem status.

Additional key initial evaluation should include a history (if available from accompanying persons) and baseline laboratory studies (CBC, glucose, calcium, electrolytes, phosphorus, arterial blood gases, urinalysis, and anticonvulsant levels when appropriate). Fetal wellbeing in the form of fetal heart rate monitoring (if the pregnancy has reached a viable gestational age) should then be undertaken.

Concurrent with this the patient must be admitted to an intensive care area, the maternal airway must be secured and intravenous access established for administration of normal saline, glucose, thiamine and anticonvulsant medication.

For women in whom imaging is considered, an initial CT without contrast is the procedure of choice because of the availability and the utility of the test in detecting acute hemorrhage. Additional neuroimaging could be considered if questions exist about the etiology of the status or if the episode is difficult to control. While MRI offers better anatomic detail than CT scan, but the longer test time, difficulties with patient management, and uneven availability all weigh against use of MRI in the acute setting. A chest X-ray could be considered to assess for aspiration or endotracheal tube positioning.

While seizure disorders can initially present as status epilepticus, the possibility of other underlying conditions must also be considered. One series of pseudoseizures reported that unresponsiveness without movement was the most common presentation [10]. If there is any question of recent exposure, serum or urine screens for substances of abuse should also be performed (within the informed consent guidelines of the individual jurisdiction). Other considerations should include infection (e.g. meningitis, brain abscess, encephalitis), electrolyte abnormalities (hyponatremia, hypernatremia, hypercalcemia), hepatic encephalopathy, tumor, hypoxic injury and subarachnoid hemorrhage.

Included in the differential diagnosis of status epilepticus are two conditions that can respond dramatically to therapeutic, and therefore diagnostic, IV infusions. These conditions are hypoglycemia and Wernicke's encephalopathy. Eclampsia must also be considered in the diagnosis, particularly if the pregnancy is beyond 20 weeks gestation and hypertension and proteinuria are present.

A glucose bolus should be initially administered – usually 50 ml of D50. If the woman is seizing because of hypoglycemia this administration can be life-saving. If the woman is hyperglycemic, the additional amount of glucose will not make her problem significantly worse.

Although Wernicke's encephalopathy (thiamine, or vitamin B_1, deficiency) is rare in women of reproductive age, the dramatic improvement that can be seen with thiamine administration warrants administration of thiamine, 100 mg IV, followed by 50–100 mg IM/IV daily if a significant response is seen.

If the woman is not responsive to these initial therapeutic measures, specific medical therapy should be promptly undertaken. This should consist of an intravenous benzodiazepine (10 mg diazepam or 4 mg lorazepam) which can be repeated in 10–15 minutes if seizure activity continues, followed by administration of an appropriate anticonvulsant (fosphenytoin or phenytoin) (Box 17.1). These medications are all short acting, which allows the patient to regain consciousness more rapidly and to therefore be more rapidly and thoroughly assessed from a neurologic perspective.

If seizures still persist at this point (≤60 min), the patient should be intubated and sedated, usually with phenobarbital (20–25 mg/kg, not to exceed 100 mg/min) (Box 17.1). If seizures

Box 17.1 Treatment of status epilepticus in pregnancy.

1 **Initial stabilization**
(a) Secure the airway.
(b) Establish intravenous access.
(c) Admit to intensive care unit.

2 **Therapeutic trials** (to be administered sequentially)

Medication	Dosage	Intent	Precautions
Glucose	50 ml of D50 IV	Correct hypoglycemia	
Thiamine (vitamin B_1)	100 mg IV, followed by 50–100 mg IM/IV qd	Correct Wernicke's encephalopathy	

3 **Initiate first-line anticonvulsants** – ONE from EACH drug class

Drug class	Specific drug	Dosage	Therapeutic levels	Precautions
Benzodiazepine				
	Diazepam	5–10 mg IV q 10–15 min		Maximum dosage 30 mg
	Lorazepam	4 mg IV; may repeat once in 10–15 min		Maximum dosage 8 mg/12 h
Anticonvulsant				
	Fosphenytoin	15–20 mg PE/kg IV × 1; begin maintenance dose 12 hours after loading dose	Total = 10–20 µg/mL Free = 1–2 µg/mL	Continuous EEG and blood pressure monitoring recommended during IV infusions. Use non-glucose-containing IV fluids
	Phenytoin	15–20 mg/kg IV q 30 minutes prn; begin maintenance dose 12 hours after loading dose.	Total = 10–20 µg/mL Free = 1–2 µg/mL	Continuous EEG and blood pressure monitoring recommended during IV infusions. Use non-glucose-containing IV fluids.

4 **Intubation and sedation**
(a) Intubation.
(b) Intravenous sedation:
(i) phenobarbital (20–25 mg/kg, administration not to exceed 100 mg/min)
(ii) midazolam (0.02–0.10 mg/kg/h)
(iii) propofol (5–50 µg/kg/min, start at 5 µg/kg/min IV × 5 min, then increase 5–10 µg/kg/min q5–10 min until desired effect).

5 **General anesthesia**
(a) If seizures still persist, institute general anesthesia with halothane and neuromuscular junction (NMJ) blockade.

PE, phenytoin sodium equivalent units.

still persist, the patient should be anesthetized using a general anesthetic while continuous EEG monitoring is performed under the supervision of a neurologist.

Significant physiologic changes also accompany status epilepticus. Many of these systemic responses are thought to result from the catecholamine surge that accompanies the seizures. Hypertension, tachycardia, and cardiac arrhythmias are examples of these systemic effects. Body temperature may increase in patients following the vigorous muscle activity that accompanies status epilepticus, but infection etiologies must first be excluded in such situations. Lactic acidosis can also occur.

Subsequent management and prognosis

With control of the seizures attention must be directed to the treatment of any underlying or predisposing conditions and to the prevention of recurrence. The most common cause of status epilepticus in the epileptic population is non-compliance with medication. Therefore it is critical to ascertain if the patient was taking the medication, and if they simply forget doses, then a pill box or other memory aids should be suggested. Medication dosing must be optimized. Ideally, preconceptional total and free anticonvulsant levels would be available so that medication dosage can be readjusted accordingly.

Establishment or resumption of a supportive lifestyle must also be emphasized. Women should be encouraged to eat regular meals, get adequate rest, nutrition and sleep and avoid stress where possible. They should be counseled to avoid hazardous situations as well as alcohol and other sedatives. Given the high frequency of unplanned pregnancy in the United States all women of reproductive age with a seizure disorder should be particularly encouraged to maintain their daily intake of folic acid (at least 1 mg daily) throughout the duration of their reproductive lifespan.

Well-controlled epilepsy is not a contraindication to breastfeeding. While most anticonvulsants do cross into breast milk, they achieve much lower levels than in maternal serum, ranging between 0.1 and 0.4 mcg/mL for phenytoin and carbamazepine, respectively [11]. Contraindications to breastfeeding would be increased seizure activity due to sleep deprivation or infant sedation from medication effect (mostly commonly a concern with phenobarbital).

Enzyme-inducing anticonvulsants, such as carbamazepine, phenytoin, phenobarbital, primidone, felbamate, lamotrigine, topiramate and oxcarbazepine, decrease the efficacy of birth control pills. Some anticonvulsants cause this drug interaction in a dose-dependent manner, with a negligible effect at low doses. Some providers use a high-dose estrogen–progesterone pill. An alternative and possibly preferred approach is to use a second method of contraception.

Providers should also be aware of the possibility of sudden unexpected death in individuals with seizure disorders. The incidence of sudden death in individuals with seizure disorders is about 2.3 times higher than the incidence of sudden death in the general population and occurs most commonly in individuals with longstanding partial-onset epilepsy. However, it is also seen in individuals with uncontrolled seizures and probably also in people with poor compliance. The mechanism of death in these cases is controversial but suggestions include cardiac arrhythmias, pulmonary edema, and suffocation during a convulsion.

References

1 Hauser AW, Annegers JF, Hurland LT. Incidence of epilepsy and unprovoked seizures in Rochester, Minnesota 1935–84. *Epilepsia* 1993; 34: 453–468.

2 Engel J, Perley T. Pregnancy and the mother. In: *Epilepsy: A Comprehensive Textbook.* Philadelphia: Lippincott, PA, 1998: 2029–2030.

3 Pschirrer ER, Monga M. Seizure disorders in pregnancy. *Obstet Gynecol Clin North Am* 2001; 28: 601–611.

4 Yerby MS. The use of anticonvulsants during pregnancy. *Semin Perinatol* 2001; 25: 153–158.

5 Kelly TE. Teratogenicity of anticonvulsant drugs. I. Review of the literature. *Am J Med Genet* 1984; 19: 413–434.

6 Rosa F. Spina bifida in infants of women treated with carbamazepine during pregnancy. *N Engl J Med* 1991; 324: 674–677.

7 Omtzigt JCG, Los FJ, Grobbee DE, Pijper L, Jahoda MG, Brandenberg H et al. The risk of spina bifida aperta after first-trimester exposure to valproate in a prenatal cohort. *Neurology* 1992; 42: 119–125.

8 Deblay FM, Vert P, Andre M, Marchal F. Transplacental vitamin K prevents hemorrhagic disease of infants of epileptic mothers. *Lancet* 1982; 1: 1247.

9 Choulika S, Grabowski E, Holmes LB. Is antenatal vitamin K prophylaxis needed for pregnant women taking anticonvulsants? *Am J Obstet Gynecol* 2004 190: 882–883.

10 Leis AA, Ross MA, Summers AK. Psychogenic seizures: ictal characteristics and diagnostic pitfalls. *Neurology* 1992; 42: 95–99.

11 American Academy of Pediatrics Committee on Drugs. The transfer of drugs and other chemicals into human milk. *Pediatrics* 2001; 108: 776–789.

18 Acute Spinal Cord Injury

Chad Kendall Klauser[1], Sheryl Rodts-Palenik[2] & James N. Martin, Jr[3]
[1]Mount Sinai School of Medicine, New York, NY, USA
[2]Acadiana Maternal-Fetal Medicine, Lafayette, LA, USA
[3]Department of Obstetrics and Gynecology, Division of Maternal-Fetal Medicine, University of Mississippi Medical Center, Jackson, MA, USA

Introduction

Spinal cord injury (SCI) affects approximately 11 000 Americans each year and is associated with significant loss of physical and personal independence. Since 20–30% of these patients are women at an average age between 16 and 45 years at the time of injury [1,2], consideration must be given to their reproductive potential. While amenorrhea occurs in a majority of women following SCI, 90% return to normal menstrual cycles within 12 months of their injury [3]. While 30% of these women will choose to use either temporary or permanent contraceptive methods secondary to the concern of possible pregnancy complications, many look forward to a rewarding life as a mother following their acute injury. A generalist obstetrician or subspecialist in maternal-fetal medicine may become involved as part of the team working to stabilize the pregnant patient in the critical first hours after an acute spinal cord injury, or managing the pregnancy, labor, and delivery of a patient years later when the sequelae of chronic spinal cord damage are present. Competent care in either setting requires the physician to be knowledgeable about the common and predictable complications specific to the acute and chronic forms of SCI.

Acute care of spinal cord injury: maternal considerations

The primary goal of emergent care of a pregnant patient with acute spinal cord trauma is to diagnose and treat life-threatening injuries, while preventing any unnecessary traction or motion of the spinal column (Table 18.1). As with any trauma patient, ensuring the survival of the pregnant patient and her fetus begins with a primary survey and prompt attention to the ABCs: *a*irway management, *b*reathing, and *c*irculation. The physiologic adaptations of the mother to her pregnancy and the autonomic dysfunction of neurogenic shock can obscure the detection of shock originating from other traumatic injuries. Thus, the contributions of the obstetric consultant are fundamental in elucidating the true clinical scenario.

Spinal immobilization

The importance of spinal immobilization cannot be overemphasized. In the patient with an SCI, the manner in which the spine is stabilized is of critical importance to prevent secondary extension of the damage. The necessity for immediate airway management often precludes the feasibility of a complete neurologic assessment (Table 18.2). The most common level of injury to the spinal cord is at the level of C5, followed by C4 and C6 [4]. As such, cervical spine immobilization is crucial before any attempts to intubate patients suspected of having cervical spine trauma. Injuries to C3 to C5 do require immediate assisted ventilation, secondary to damage to nerve roots to the diaphragm.

Orotracheal intubation

Orotracheal intubation employing rapid sequence induction using the jaw-thrust maneuver instead of head-tilt is considered to be the procedure of choice in SCI patients [5]. However, utilizing video fluoroscopy in cadavers with C5–6 instability, Donaldson and coworkers demonstrated that indirect nasal intubation techniques produced less spinal motion than direct oral intubation techniques [6]. Chin-lift/jaw-thrust and cricoid pressure cause more motion than some of the blind nasal intubation techniques. With instability at the level of C1–2, no difference in motion was detected between oral or nasal techniques, while the chin-lift/jaw-thrust maneuvers caused the most motion associated with intubation [7]. Ideally, intubation procedures should be performed by a minimum of three people in concert: one to perform the intubation, one to assist and provide cricoid pressure, and a third to insure in-line immobilization of the spine to prevent extension and rotation of the cervical spine [5]. While all trauma patients should be considered to have a full stomach, the

Critical Care Obstetrics, 5th edition. Edited by M. Belfort, G. Saade, M. Foley, J. Phelan and G. Dildy.

Table 18.1 Acute spinal cord injury: basics of emergent care.

Goals of therapy
Stabilize the patient
Immobilize the spine in an attempt to prevent further injuries
Evaluate and treat other injuries
Achieve early recognition, prevention, and management of frequently encountered complications.

Management protocol
Achieve initial patient stabilization including stabilization of the patient's neck, airway management, circulatory system assessment, and fetal monitoring.
Methylprednisolone should be considered within 8 hours of the SCI and given as a bolus dose of 30 mg/kg, followed by infusion at 5.4 mg/kg/h for 23–48 hours.
Hemodynamic monitoring may be required for optimum fluid management of neurogenic shock.
Adequate fluid and pressor support may be necessary during the period of neurogenic shock.
Delivery may be indicated for obstetric indications, to facilitate maternal resuscitation, or in conjunction with surgery for other injuries.

Table 18.2 Acute spinal cord injury: innervation of spinal segments and muscles and grading scale for evaluating motor function.

Spinal segment	Muscle	Action
C5, C6	Deltoid	Arm abduction
C5, **C6**	Biceps	Elbow flexion
C6, C7	Extensor carpi radialis	Wrist extension
C7, C8	Triceps	Elbow extension
C8, T1	Flexor digitorum profundus	Hand grasp
C8, **T1**	Hand intrinsics	Finger abduction
L1, **L2**, L3	Iliopsosas	Hip flexion
L2, **L3, L4**	Quadriceps	Knee extension
L4, **L5, S1**, S2	Hamstrings	Knee flexion
L4, **L5**	Tibialis anterior	Ankle dorsiflexion
L5, S1	Extensor hallucis longus	Great-toe extension
S1, S2	Gastrocnemius	Ankle plantar flexion
S2, S3, S4	Bladder, anal sphincter	Voluntary rectal tone
Grade	**Muscle strength**	
5	Normal strength	
4	Active power against both resistance and gravity	
3	Active power against gravity but not resistance	
2	Active movement only with gravity eliminated	
1	Flicker or trace of contraction	
0	No movement or contraction	

The predominant segments of innervation are shown in boldface type.
(Reproduced by permission from Chiles BW III, Cooper PR. Acute spinal injury. *N Engl J Med* 1996; 334: 514.

pregnant patient in late gestation has the additional risk of aspiration due to her reduced gastric sphincter tone compounded by the mechanical effects of increased gastric pressure from her gravid uterus. Consequently, appropriately applied cricoid pressure is essential to prevent reflux of gastric contents into the trachea. Once again, the importance of spinal immobilization cannot be overemphasized.

Relevant pregnancy physiology

A number of physiologic changes that occur in the pregnant patient can complicate intubation. There is significant capillary engorgement of the mucosa throughout the respiratory tract leading to swelling of the nasal and oral pharynx, larynx, and trachea, all of which can increase the challenge of intubating a patient involved in an acute spinal cord injury [8]. Additionally, pregnant patients have a decreased functional residual capacity, thus decreasing their oxygen reserves. The initiation of tracheal protective procedures such as jaw-thrust, bag-valve-mask ventilation, and cricoid pressure, while necessary, can inadvertently cause movement of the cervical spine and subsequent damage if meticulous stabilization is not practiced [5,6].

Circulatory system considerations

The evaluation of the circulatory system in a pregnant trauma patient with acute SCI can be very difficult. The typical assessment parameters may be obscured by the altered hemodynamics of pregnancy, the autonomic derangements of neurogenic shock, and cardiovascular instability from acute hemorrhage. The presence of hypotension, a common component of both hemorrhagic and neurogenic shock, can be confused with the normal reduction in blood pressure associated with pregnancy itself. Supine hypotension can further complicate assessment of trauma patients as aortocaval compression stimulates sympathetic output, increasing both blood pressure and heart rate. Even the normal dilutional anemia of pregnancy can be misinterpreted as a sign of acute blood loss.

Spinal neurogenic shock versus hypovolemic shock

If the patient has a cervical or high thoracic injury, the presence of neurogenic shock may obfuscate the assessment of circulatory status. The presenting signs and symptoms of spinal neurogenic shock are typically the exact opposite of those expected with hypovolemia. While both disorders present with hypotension, the classic stigmata of hypovolemia result from enhanced sympathetic output. Reflex sympathetic stimulation maximizes cardiac function and increases peripheral vasoconstriction, resulting in tachycardia, delayed capillary refill, and cool, clammy extremities. Conversely, spinal neurogenic shock is due to an acute loss of sympathetic input from below the injury. Subsequently, there is no shunting of blood from the periphery back toward the heart and other critical organs. In addition to warm, dry skin and preserved capillary refill, such patients exhibit a "paradoxical bradycardia" [9] when sympathetic input to the heart is lost, and vagal control predominates. Preserved vasodilation in the periphery promotes heat loss, leading to hypothermia and further exacerbation of the bradycardia.

Perils with hypotension and fluid resuscitation

The emergency team must be alert to the contradictory influences of pregnancy, hypovolemia, and neurogenic autonomic disruption while evaluating and stabilizing the pregnant trauma patient. Because of time constraints in deciphering these various factors, the presence of significant hypotension should be considered and treated as hypovolemia until safely proven otherwise. The primary survey should be accompanied by simultaneous intravenous fluid resuscitation through two large-bore IV cannulae, serial vital sign measurements, and the placement of a foley catheter [9]. While fluid resuscitation is imperative in the acute setting, providers must remain cognizant of the increased risk of pulmonary edema during pregnancy secondary to a low colloid oncotic pressure and hypoalbuminemia. Conventional wedging of the patient's back to avoid caval compression can result in exacerbation of spinal trauma. However, these same benefits may be achieved by a 15° tilt of the backboard if the patient is immobilized, or by simple manual displacement of the gravid uterus to the left. Obvious external bleeding is controlled, and a search is initiated for evidence of internal hemorrhage.

Use of ultrasound

Ultrasound provides rapid assessment for fluid in the cul de sac, abdominal cavity, renal gutters, and perisplenic, perihepatic, pericardial, and retroplacental areas and, if negative, may allow avoidance of peritoneal lavage and its associated risks [10,11]. If ultrasound is not immediately available, there is no other explanation for the patient's shocked state, or there is obvious severe abdominal/thoracic trauma, peritoneal lavage is required to rule out intra-abdominal hemorrhage. An open entry technique is recommended during the late second and third trimesters to minimize risk to the gravid uterus [10,12]. This is best performed with sharp dissection at or above the umbilicus while elevating the anterior wall away from the uterus. The anterior abdominal peritoneum can then be opened under direct visualization. The procedure is considered diagnostic if either greater than 100 000 RBCs per mL are detected or bowel contents are present in the effluent.

Fetal status reflects maternal status

The status of the fetus is not only important in its own right, but also serves as a marker of changes in maternal hemodynamics. A previously normal fetus can tolerate a remarkable diminution in uterine blood flow before abnormalities supervene in the fetal heart tracing [13]. The onset of tachycardia, late decelerations, bradycardia, or a sinusoidal pattern can herald a deleterious change in maternal oxygenation, acid–base balance, or hemodynamic status. Likewise, adequate correction of maternal metabolic or hemodynamic derangements may be signaled by a return to a reassuring fetal heart rate tracing. Placental abruption occurs in up to 50% of women involved in major trauma, contributing to both fetal compromise and further vascular insult to the pregnant patient [3].

Maternal hemodynamic status and assessment

Whether or not concurrent hypovolemia is present, placement of a pulmonary artery catheter and an arterial line may be advantageous in guiding fluid and pressor administration in the pregnant patient with neurogenic shock. Cardiac output and mean arterial pressure must be carefully monitored to prevent cardiopulmonary complications that often accompany spinal cord injury [4]. If an initial search for subclinical bleeding (chest and pelvic radiographs, pericardial and abdominal ultrasound, peritoneal lavage, or CT) fails to reveal evidence of hemorrhage, neurogenic shock is presumed to be the cause of the patient's hypotension [5]. Attention should then be directed toward countering the cardiopulmonary dysfunction associated with neurogenic shock, and measures to maximally preserve residual spinal cord function should be instituted. To this end, intravenous fluid administration is decreased to maintenance rates and therapy with pressor agents (dopamine and dobutamine) is started. The period of neurogenic shock can last weeks. During this time, sympathomimetics and occasionally atropine sulfate are essential to counter parasympathetic dominance and to facilitate restoration of vascular tone and cardiac performance. Maintaining perfusion of injured spinal tissue and oxygen supplementation reduces the threat of secondary ischemic damage to traumatized tissue. Consultation with an expert in blood pressure management under these circumstances is important.

Corticosteroids

In patients with blunt spinal cord injury, the administration of high-dose methylprednisolone early in treatment has been recommended as a proactive measure to reduce the extent of paralysis in the long term [4,9,10,14]. This recommendation is based on findings from two multicenter, double-blind, randomized trials in which patients received placebo, naloxone, or very high-dose methylprednisolone therapy within 8 hours of their injury. The methylprednisolone group experienced significantly greater improvement in sensation and motor function up to 1 year after injury [15,16]. Theorized mechanisms by which methylprednisolone improves neurological outcome include blocking PGF-2α-induced membrane lipid peroxidation [17], potentiating the neuroprotective/regenerative effects of taurine in the damaged cord [18], and suppressing expression of neurotropin receptors involved in secondary cell death [19]. Follow-up multicenter randomized trials by the same investigators verified efficacy and refined treatment protocols [20,21]. In the recommended regimens, all patients less than 8 hours from the occurrence of blunt spinal trauma receive a 30 mg/kg loading dose of methylprednisolone over 15 minutes. If the initial bolus was administered within 3 hours of injury, a continuous drip of 5.4 mg/kg/h methylprednisolone is infused for 23 hours. Patients loaded between 3 and 8 hours after injury receive the same postbolus infusion but it is extended over a longer interval (48 hours). There is no proven benefit to initiating high-dose steroid therapy to any patient beyond 8 hours from their injury.

Potential complications with corticosteroids

Although high-dose steroid therapy is approved by the Food and Drug Administration (FDA) and considered by many to be a best practice, discussion continues about the pros and cons of its use in part because the dosages employed are some of the highest used in any clinical scenario [22–24]. Patients receiving steroids have an increased incidence of pneumonia and require more ventilation and intensive care nursing [25]. Those receiving the 48-hour regimen are also more likely to have more severe sepsis and severe pneumonia than patients who receive the 24-hour regimen [21]. Thus, if steroids are administered, vigilance for, and prophylaxis of, anticipated steroid-related complications (infections, gastrointestinal bleeding, wound disruption, steroid myopathy, avascular necrosis, and glucose intolerance) are necessary.

Radiologic imaging considerations

The secondary survey of the pregnant patient with an acute SCI focuses on more precisely defining the nature and extent of the lesion and determining the status of the fetus. A thorough neurological exam is required and complete documentation is important so that improvement or deterioration of the lesion can be monitored with serial examinations. Once the lesion has been clinically identified, a number of radiological studies may be necessary to further define it and help with planning for appropriate treatment. Radiographs of the cervical spine are the standard initial studies used to assess the injury and dictate what further modalities may be needed. CT is best for bony detail and may become necessary to clarify fractures revealed by radiographs especially if: (i) neurologic injury is present; (ii) more extensive injury is clinically apparent than is seen on the radiograph; or (iii) injury detected on the radiograph suggests instability. If a neurologic lesion appears to be progressing, CT myelography may be required to exclude spinal cord compression by an extrinsic mass such as a hematoma [5]. As will be discussed later, ionizing radiation can have adverse fetal consequences. The input of the obstetrician may be helpful in minimizing fetal radiation exposure.

Acute care of spinal cord injury: fetal considerations

Mother first (usually) with exceptions

While it is important to remember that there are at least two individuals to be cared for in every pregnant trauma patient, initial efforts should be focused primarily on the stabilization of the mother. There are two exceptional circumstances where it may be more appropriate to attend to the fetus first: (i) a viable fetus in a dying mother; or (ii) a dying viable fetus in a stabilized mother. In either case, prompt cesarean delivery is indicated. Because 48% of SCI patients die as a result of their injuries [4], the possibility of perimortem cesarean delivery is very real in these patients. The procedure should be initiated if there is no response to CPR within 4 minutes, with the intent to complete delivery by 5 minutes [26]. Delivery relieves caval compression and also allows for a large autotransfusion of blood back into the circulation when the uterus is evacuated and contracts. These events, together with maintaining a leftward tilt, increase venous return, the efficacy of chest compressions, and ultimately survival. Direct access to the maternal aorta via the abdominal incision may also allow its compression above the renal arteries and optimization of blood flow to the brain and heart.

Cesarean delivery

If the mother is stable, cesarean delivery should also be performed as a rescue procedure for a stressed/distressed but viable fetus. Documentation of the fetal heart rate should ideally be included as part of the primary survey on a pregnant trauma patient ascertained to be in the third trimester of her pregnancy [27]. Continuous electronic fetal heart rate monitoring usually is initiated with completion of the primary survey in patients with a viable and potentially salvageable baby. When immediate delivery for fetal indications is necessary and no anesthesia is available, cesarean section without anesthesia has been reported in patients with neurogenic shock and a lesion above T10 [10]. However, anesthesia is generally required and recommended for all SCI patients undergoing cesarean delivery. The clinician should anticipate the possibility of uterine atony if dopamine is being used to treat neurogenic shock secondary to its uterine relaxant effect [10].

Potential fetal hazards with diagnostic radiography

The pregnant women with SCI may require many examinations involving radiation, both acutely and later in her care. Currently, a cumulative radiation exposure of up to 5 rad or less is regarded as unlikely to have significant teratogenic effects [28,29]. With the exception of CT, individual diagnostic procedures typically deliver radiation in the millirad range (Table 18.3) which will not

Table 18.3 Estimated radiation exposure (millirads) associated with commonly used trauma radiography.

Cervical spine	<1 mrad
Chest (two views)	0.02–0.07 mrad
Abdomen (one view)	100 mrad
Pelvis	200–500 mrad
Lumbar spine	600–1000 mrad
Hip (one view)	200 mrad
CT head/chest	<1000 mrad
CT abdomen/lumbar spine	3500 mrad
CT pelvis	3000–9000 mrad

(Derived from Jagoda A, Kessler SG. Trauma in pregnancy. In: Harwood-Nussa, ed. *The Clinical Practice of Emergency Medicine*, 3rd edn. Philadelphia, PA: Lippincott, Williams and Wilkins, 2001 and the American College of Obstetricians and Gynecologists Committee Opinion. *Guidelines for Diagnostic Imaging during Pregnancy*, no. 158, Sept 1995).

subject the fetus to enough ionizing radiation to inflict harm. However, the cumulative dose of the studies required to define and treat a patient with SCI may approach the critical threshold. The radiation exposure from numerous higher-dose studies, such as abdominal or pelvic CT scans, barium studies, and intravenous pyelography, can quickly add up to more than 5 rad [30]. In a study involving 114 pregnant patients admitted to a trauma center between 1995 and 1999, the mean initial radiation exposure was 4.5 rad. Cumulative radiation exposure exceeded 5 rad in 85% of patients [31]. Minimizing fetal exposure is a fundamental component of patient care. While there should be no hesitation to perform necessary radiological studies in patients with an acute SCI, one should insure that only those studies that are truly indicated are obtained. Whenever possible, the number of views obtained should be minimized and radiologic techniques employed to diminish the dose absorbed per view [28]. Monitoring devices such as personal radiation monitors or thermoluminescent dosimeters can be used to provide an accurate measure of cumulative radiation exposure [32].

Long term antepartum–intrapartum maternal concerns

Autonomic hyperreflexia

Long-term care of the pregnant patient with SCI requires cognizance of the specific, predictable medical complications that may occur in such pregnancies. The acute care of the SCI patient revolves around treatment of neurogenic shock and minimizing secondary injury to the cord. Of primary importance in managing the chronic SCI patient is the prevention, prompt recognition of, and treatment of, autonomic hyperreflexia (AH) [33]. This potentially life-threatening complication occurs in up to 85% of patients with lesions at or above T5–6, although it has been reported with lesions as low as T10 [34]. Reflex activity generally returns within 6 months of injury, at which time those patients with damage above the region of splanchnic sympathetic outflow (T6 to L2) become susceptible to the development of AH [35]. With this complication, noxious stimuli create impulses that enter the cord at different levels and progress upward until they are blocked by the lesion. Unable to ascend further, afferent impulses are channeled instead by interneurons to synapse with sympathetic nerves, resulting in an extensive, multilevel dispersal of sympathetic activity [35]. This explosive autonomic discharge can manifest suddenly and dramatically. The patient typically develops an intense, pounding headache, profuse sweating, facial flushing, and nausea. Nasal congestion, piloerection, and a blotchy rash above the level of the lesion are also frequently present.

Severe systolic hypertension

Impressive signs accompany the physical expressions of sympathetic discharge. In a matter of seconds, blood pressure can increase threefold to reach malignant levels. Systolic blood pressures as high as 260 mmHg and diastolic pressures in excess of 200 mmHg have been reported [35]. Left untreated, such hypertensive crises can quickly lead to retinal hemorrhage, cerebrovascular accidents, intracranial hemorrhage, seizures, encephalopathy, and death [36]. In addition, placental abruption is a significant fetal as well as maternal concern.

Paradoxical bradycardia

The same spinal cord lesion that blocks the ascent of sensory impulses that trigger sympathetic discharge also prevents the descent of central supraspinal inhibitory impulses. Intense compensatory reflex parasympathetic output is thus channeled outside of the spinal system via the vagus nerve. Consequently, the patient with autonomic hyperreflexia can present with paradoxical bradycardia and cardiac dysrhythmias in synchrony with the manifestations of unrestrained sympathetic activity.

Prevention

Recognition and prevention are paramount in avoiding the potentially lethal consequences of AH. It can occur in response to virtually any sensory stimulus below the level of the lesion, during any stage of pregnancy. It has been reported in conjunction with cervical examination, bladder and bowel distention, catheterization, rectal disimpaction, breastfeeding, and episiotomy [37]. Hence, any potentially noxious stimuli should be consciously avoided or minimized by employing topical anesthetic jelly for digital exams, catheterization, and fecal disimpaction [38]. While bladder distention is the most common precipitant of AH [39], labor is a potent stimulus for the pregnant SCI patient.

Confusion with pre-eclampsia

In AH-susceptible patients, it should be anticipated and differentiated from pre-eclampsia. Maternal death secondary to intracranial hemorrhage has been reported when AH was misdiagnosed as pre-eclampsia [36]. The hypertension of pre-eclampsia usually persists into the immediate puerperium, often resolving slowly in the first days postpartum. In contrast, the hypertension of AH crescendos with each contraction and subsides in the interim between contractions, with occasional patients actually becoming hypotensive between contractions. It abates abruptly with removal of the noxious stimulus. Patient familiarity and experience with AH is also helpful for rapid differentiation between these disease entities.

Treatment of autonomic hyperreflexia

Immediate management of AH is orientated towards identifying the inciting stimulus and normalization of blood pressure. The patient should be assessed for bladder distention from lack or obstruction of drainage, uterine contractions, perineal distention, and fecal impaction. Tight clothing, footwear, or external fetal monitoring straps can also cause AH. Blood pressure can be lowered quickly simply by changing the maternal position from supine to erect. Short-acting pharmacologic agents such as nifedipine or hydralazine are also useful for lowering the blood pressure until more definitive therapy with regional anesthesia is feasible. Short-acting agents are preferable to longer acting drugs since they allow avoidance of prolonged hypotension between contractions once the stimulus is removed or suppressed. Calcium channel blockers must be used judiciously, since common side effects include headache, flushing, and palpitations, symptoms that can easily be confused with those of AH. Additionally, it is recommended that an arterial line be placed to provide continuous evaluation of the extremely labile pressures associated with AH.

Regional anesthesia

Prophylactic and therapeutic administration of regional anesthesia is the cornerstone of labor management of the SCI patient at risk for AH. Epidural anesthesia effectively disrupts the propagation of sympathetic afferent impulses through the spine. Although obtaining a good regional block in patients with prior neurologic damage or back surgery can be technically difficult, it is nearly universally successful in preventing or aborting an episode of AH [37–40]. Failure of regional anesthesia to arrest ongoing AH is one of the few unique indications for cesarean section in a patient with SCI. The depth of general anesthesia typically required to suppress AH often results in neonatal suppression. When feasible, supplemental regional anesthesia should be employed for cesarean section patients with high spinal lesions [37]. Alternatively, if general anesthesia is used, adequate neonatal resuscitation expertise and equipment should be immediately available at the time of delivery.

Labor and delivery considerations

Given the potential for serious maternal morbidity and death, the possibility of AH should be anticipated in patients with SCI, and a plan for care should be established well in advance of labor [41]. Early antepartum anesthesia consultation is mandatory, not only for those parturients at risk for AH, but for all SCI patients. This allows for the risks and benefits of regional anesthesia to be discussed in a controlled setting, and alerts the patient to the possibility, and consequences, of AH in labor. It is recommended that an epidural be placed as soon as the patient presents in labor, as well as before induction or augmentation of labor [39]. Meticulous and frequent blood pressure monitoring is essential. Placement of an arterial line and continuous cardiac monitoring for dysrhythmia are recommended [38]. Continuous bladder drainage is also advisable. An early anesthesia consultation also provides an opportunity for pulmonary function assessment. Patients with cervical or high thoracic lesions can have compromised pulmonary capacity secondary to debilitated intercostal muscle function as well as an attenuated cough reflex. Patients with SCI often have baseline vital capacities measuring less than 2 L, predisposing them to atelectesis and pneumonia, and diminishing their capacity to satisfy oxygen requirements [37]. The burden of pregnancy-related decrements in functional reserve capacity and expired reserve volume, as well as increased oxygen consumption, can culminate in the need for assisted ventilation in SCI patients. Thus, ventilatory function should be monitored with serial vital capacity measurements [38] and ventilatory support initiated when the VC falls below 15 mL/kg [42].

Summary

Care of the acute spinal cord patient requires an awareness of commonly occurring serious or life-threatening complications. Immediate care consists of initial stabilization, treatment of neurogenic shock, and the avoidance of secondary cord damage by minimizing physical manipulation and cord hypoxia. Extended antepartum and intrapartum care is focused on prevention, recognition, and expeditious management of AH. Comprehensive management of pregnant SCI patients necessitates attention to the multitude of medical complications that accompany chronic SCI including urinary hygiene, frequent urinary tract infections, pressure sores, thromboembolic surveillance, pulmonary toilet, and the potential for unattended delivery secondary to unperceived labor. Additionally, muscle spasms may require specific medications for control, as well as altering the mode of delivery, depending on their severity.

References

1 Blackwell TL, Krause JS, Winkler T, Stiens S. *Spinal Cord Injury: Guidelines for Life. Care Planning and Case Management.* Appendix A: Demographic characteristics of spinal cord injury. New York: Demos Medical Publishing, Inc., 2001: 133–138.

2 National Spinal Cord Injury Statistic Center. *Spinal Cord Injury: Facts and Figures at a Glance.* Birmingham, Alabama: National Spinal Cord Injury Statistic Center, 2000.

3 Atterbury JL, Groome LJ. Pregnancy in women with spinal cord injuries. *Orthoped Nurs* 1998; 33(4): 603–613.

4 Marotta JT. Spinal injury. In: Rowland LP, ed. *Merritt's Neurology*, 10th edn. Philadelphia, PA: Lippincott Williams and Wilkins, 2000: 416–423.

5 Ward KR. Trauma airway management. In: Harwood-Nuss A, ed. *The Clinical Practice of Emergency Medicine*, 3rd edn. Philadelphia, PA: Lippincott Williams and Wilkins, 2001: 433–441.

6 Donaldson WF III, Towers JD, Doctor A, Brand A, Donaldson VP. A methodology to evaluate motion of the unstable spine during intubation techniques. *Spine* 1993; 18(14): 2020–2023.

7 Donaldson WF III, Heil BV, Donaldson VP, Silvaggio VJ. The effect of airway maneuvers on the unstable C1-C2 segment. A cadaver study. *Spine* 1997; 22(11): 1215–1218.

8 Munnur U, de Boisblanc B, Suresh MS. Airway problems in pregnancy. *Crit Care Med* 2005; 33(10): S259–S268.

9 Mahoney BD. Spinal cord injuries. In: Harwood-Nuss A, ed. *The Clinical Practice of Emergency Medicine*, 3rd edn. Philadelphia, PA: Lippincott Williams and Wilkins, 2001: 495–500.

10 Gilson GJ, Miller AC, Clevenger FW, Curet LB. Acute spinal cord injury and.neurogenic shock in pregnancy. *Obstet Gynecol Surv* 1995; 50(7): 556–560.

11 Goodwin H, Holmes JF, Wisner DH. Abdominal ultrasound examination in pregnant blunt trauma patients. *J Trauma* 2001; 50(4); 689–693.
12 American College of Obstetrics and Gynecology. *Obstetric Aspects of Trauma Management.* Educational Bulletin Number 251, September 1998.
13 Lucas W, Kirschbaum T, Assali NS. Spinal shock and fetal oxygenation. *Am J Obstet Gynecol* 1965; 93(4): 583–587.
14 Coleman WP, Benzel D, Cahill DW et al. A critical appraisal of the reporting of the National Acute Spinal Cord Injury Studies of methylprednisolone in acute spinal cord injury. *J Spinal Discord* 2000; 13(3): 185–199.
15 Bracken MB, Shepard MJ, Collins WF et al. A randomized, controlled trial of methylprednisolone or naloxone in the treatment of acute spinal cord injury. Results of the Second National Acute Spinal Cord Injury Study. *N Engl J Med* 1990; 322(20): 1405–1411.
16 Bracken MB, Shepard MJ, Collins WF Jr et al. Methylprednisolone or naloxone treatment after acute spinal cord injury: 1-year follow-up data. Results of the second National Acute Spinal Cord Injury Study. *J Neurosurg* 1992; 76(1): 23–31.
17 Liu D, Li L, Augustus L. Prostaglandin release by spinal cord injury mediates production of hydroxyl radical, malondialdehyde and cell death: a site of the neuroprotective action of methylprednisolone. *J Neurochem* 2001; 77(4): 1036–1047.
18 Benton RL, Ross CD, Miller KE. Spinal taurine levels are increased 7 and 30 days following methylprednisolone treatment of spinal cord injury in rats. *Brain Res* 2001; 893(1–2): 292–300.
19 Brandoli C, Shi B, Pflug B, Andrews P, Wrathall JR, Mocchetti I. Dexamethasone reduces the expression of p75 neurotrophin receptor and apoptosis in contused spinal cord. *Brain Res Mol Brain Res* 2001; 87(1): 61–70.
20 Bracken MD, Shepard MJ, Holford TR et al. Administration of methylprednisolone for 24 or 48 hours or tirilazad mesylate for 48 hours in the treatment of acute spinal cord injury. Results of the third National Acute Spinal Cord Injury Randomized Controlled Trial. National Acute Spinal Cord Injury Study. *JAMA* 1997; 277(20): 1597–1604.
21 Bracken MB, Shepard MJ, Holford TR et al. Methylprednisolone or tirilazadmesylate administration after acute spinal cord injury: 1 year follow-up. Results of the third National Acute Spinal Cord Injury randomized controlled trial. *J Neurosurg* 1998; 89(5): 699–706.
22 Nesathurai S. Steroids and spinal cord injury: revisiting the NASCIS 2 and NASCIS.3 trials. *J Trauma* 1998; 45(6): 1088–1093.
23 Hurlbert RJ. Methylprednisolone for acute spinal cord injury: an inappropriate standard of care. *J Neurosurg* 2000; 93(Suppl 1): 1–7.
24 Short DJ, El Masry WS, Jones PW. High dose methylprednisolone in the management of acute spinal cord injury – a systematic review from a clinical perspective. *Spinal Cord* 2000; 38(5): 273–286.
25 Gerndt SJ, Rodriguez JL, Pawlik JW et al. Consequences of high-dose steroid therapy for acute spinal cord injury. *J Trauma* 1997; 42(2): 279–284.
26 Katz VL, Dotters DJ, Droegemueller W. Perimortem cesarean delivery. *Obstet Gynecol* 1986; 68(4): 571–576.
27 Morris J A Jr, Rosenbower TJ, Jurkovich GJ et al. Infant survival after cesarean section for trauma. *Ann Surg* 1996; 223(5): 481–491.
28 International Commission on Radiological Protection. *Protection of the Patient in Diagnostic Radiology.* ICRP Publication 34. Oxford, England: Pergamon, 1983.
29 Brent RL. The effect of embryonic and fetal exposure to X-ray, microwaves, and ultrasound: counseling the pregnant and nonpregnant patient about these risks. *Semin Oncol* 1989; 16(5): 347–368.
30 Damilakis J, Perisinakis K, Voloudaki A, Gourtsoyiannis N. Estimation of fetal radiation dose from computed tomography scanning in late pregnancy: depth–dose data from routine examinations. *Invest Radiol* 2000; 35(9): 527–533.
31 Bochicchio GV, Napolitano LM, Haan J, Champion H, Scalea T. Incidental pregnancy in trauma patients. *J Am Coll Surg* 2001; 192(5): 566–569.
32 Goldman SM, Wagner LK. Radiologic ABCs of maternal and fetal survival after trauma: when minutes may count. *Radiographics* 1999; 19(5): 1349–1357.
33 McGregor JA, Meeuwsen J. Autonomic hyperreflexi: a mortal danger for spinal cord-damaged women in labor. *Am J Obstet Gynecol* 1985; 151(3): 330–333.
34 Gimovsky ML, Ojeda A, Ozaki R, Zerne S. Management of autonomic hyperreflexia associated with a low thoracic spinal cord lesion. *Am J Obstet Gynecol* 1985; 153(2); 223–224.
35 Colachis SC III. Autonomic hyperreflexia with spinal cord injury. *J Am Paraplegia Soc* 1992; 15(3): 171–186.
36 Abouleish E. Hypertension in a paraplegic parturient. *Anesthesiology* 1980; 53(4): 348.
37 Baker ER, Cardenas DD. Pregnancy in spinal cord injured women. *Arch Phys Med Rehabil* 1996; 77(5): 501–507.
38 Greenspoon JS, Paul RH. Paraplegia and quadriplegia: special considerations during pregnancy and labor and delivery. *Am J Obstet Gynecol* 1986; 155(4): 738–741.
39 Lindan R, Joiner B, Freehafer AA, Hazel C. Incidence and clinical features of autonomic dysreflexia in patients with spinal cord injury. *Paraplegia* 1980; 18(5): 285–292.
40 Crosby E, St-Jean B, Reid D, Elliot RD. Obstetrical anesthesia and analgesia in chronic spinal cord-injured women. *Can J Anaesth* 1992; 39(5 Pt 1): 487–494.
41 Cross LL, Meythaler JM, Tuel SM, Cross AL. Pregnancy, labor and delivery post spinal cord injury. *Paraplegia* 1992; 30(12): 890–902.
42 Macklem PT. Muscular weakness and respiratory function. *N Engl J Med* 1986; 314(12): 775–776.

19 Pregnancy-Related Stroke

Edward W. Veillon, Jr[1] & James N. Martin, Jr[2]

[1]Maternal-Fetal Medicine, University of Mississippi Medical Center, Jackson, MA, USA
[2]Department of Obstetrics and Gynecology, Division of Maternal-Fetal Medicine, University of Mississippi, Medical Center, Jackson, MA, USA

Introduction

Cerebrovascular accidents (CVAs), also termed "strokes", in the pregnant patient are infrequent but often catastrophic events which account for 12–14% of all maternal deaths [1–3]. CVA is usually classified as either hemorrhagic or ischemic. Most hemorrhagic strokes occur secondary to a ruptured aneurysm or arteriovenous malformation (AVM) or a ruptured blood vessel(s) in association with sustained, severe hypertension. On the other hand, most ischemic strokes occur in relation to thromboembolic phenomena or vasculopathies. Ischemic and hemorrhagic CVAs are further classified according to location within the central nervous system. CVA in the pregnant patient reflects overall the spectrum of stroke etiologies encountered in young adults [4–6], or they occur secondary to pregnancy-associated or induced disorders such as central venous thrombosis (CVT) and pre-eclampsia/eclampsia [5,7]. When a CVA affects a pregnant patient, the obstetrician-gynecologist and maternal-fetal medicine subspecialist physician managing the patient are challenged to collaborate with other specialties including anesthesia, neurology/neurosurgery and critical care while maintaining an awareness of pregnancy physiology, pathophysiology and practice critical to the patient's special disease circumstances and recommended obstetric treatment. *The concurrence of pregnancy and CVA must not in general alter diagnosis and management of the CVA.* A thorough search for less serious medical disorders which can mimic stroke – metabolic, migraine, seizure, toxicology or psychogenic – must be considered and ruled out by appropriate history taking, laboratory tests and imaging studies.

Causation and time of occurrence

When CVA occurs during the pregnancy (11%), the peripartum period immediately around labor and delivery (41%) or up to 6 weeks postpartum (48%), it is described as a pregnancy-related stroke or PRS [3]. A tabular presentation of PRS is listed in Table 19.1 and divided between types of stroke incited or induced by pregnancy and types incidental to pregnancy. These have been summarized and described recently in a number of excellent reviews that were used to create Table 19.1 [1–27]. Based on published collective reviews through 2006, the worldwide incidence of PRS ranges from 8.9 to 67.1 per 100 000 deliveries or an average of 21.3 per 100 000 [28]. Differences among study findings reflect the variations in study populations, study intervals, study design and methodologies, case definitions, case ascertainment, neuroimaging techniques and likely other factors. Using data collected from 8 million American women in the 2001–2002 Nationwide Inpatient Sample which includes all-payer inpatient care from more than 1000 general and university hospitals in the United States, a national PRS incidence of 34.2 events/100 000 women was derived [3]. Death occurred in 117 of the 2,850 women with PRS, a rate of 1.4 stroke deaths per 100 000 deliveries [3].

Worldwide except for Taiwan the incidence of PRS due to ischemia/infarction is slightly higher than that of hemorrhage [15,16,22,28–33]. Pre-eclampsia/eclampsia accounted for 47% of ischemic PRS in the French Study Group and 24% in the Baltimore-Washington Study Group [4,15]. Risk for ischemic PRS remains low throughout gestation until the 2-day period before delivery and the first day postpartum [11]. During the remainder of the puerperium (6 weeks postpartum), the risk of ischemic and hemorrhagic PRS remains elevated but less so than the peripartum period [11] and during gestation itself [8,15]. A number of factors in any given patient impact her risk of PRS including developments within the pregnancy itself (obstetric) as listed in Table 19.2.

Pregnancy physiology and pathophysiology

Compared with the non-pregnant state, pregnancy increases by as much as 12–13-fold the risk of CVA [34,35]. One reason for such an increase in stroke potential for the pregnant patient is

Critical Care Obstetrics, 5th edition. Edited by M. Belfort, G. Saade, M. Foley, J. Phelan and G. Dildy.

Table 19.1 Types of pregnancy-related stroke (PRS).

Pregnancy-induced stroke	Pregnancy-incidental stroke
Pre-eclampsia-Eclampsia	**Subarachnoid Hemorrhage**
Severe Gestational Hypertension	Aneurysm
HELLP Syndrome	Arteriovenous Malformation
Cerebral Vein Thrombosis	Takayasu's Disease
Cerebral Sinus Thrombosis	**Ischemic Arterial Infarction**
Dural Sinus Thrombosis	Hematologic
Sagittal Venous Thrombosis	TTP
Postpartum Cerebral Angiopathy/Vasculopathy	DIC
	Polycythemia
Postpartum Reversible Encephalopathy Syndrome	Thrombocythemia
	Sickle Cell Diseases
Metastatic Choriocarcinoma	Paroxysmal Nocturnal Hemoglobinuria
Embolism	**Thrombophilias/Prothrombotic States**
Amniotic Fluid	Antithrombin III Deficiency
Air	Prothrombin Mutation
Fat	Antiphospholipid Antibodies
Paradoxical	Protein S or C Deficiency
Peripartum Cardiomyopathy	Factor V Leiden
Vascular	Homocysteinemia
Arterial Dissection	Nephrotic Syndrome
Moyamoya	**Inflammatory Disease**
	Systemic Lupus Erythematosus
	Sarcoidosis
	Wegener's Granulomatosis
	Behcet's Syndrome
	Others
	Bacterial Endocarditis
	Cardiac Arrhythmia
	Cerebral Ischemia
	Cocaine/Vasoactive Drugs
	Head Injury
	Severe Dehydration
	Meningitis/Sinusitis/Mastoiditis
	Systemic Infectious Disease
	Fibromuscular Dysplasia
	Marfan's Syndrome
	Ehlers-Danlos Type IV
	Neurofibromatosis
	Tuberous Sclerosis
	Osler-Weber-Rendu Syndrome
	Autosomal-Dominant Inherited Polycystic Kidney

Table 19.2 Contributing risk factors for stroke during pregnancy.

1. AGE : PRS risk increases with maternal age [3]
   35–39 years old = 90% increase in risk
   40+ years old = 3.3 fold increase versus <20 years old
2. RACE : PRS risk varies by race [3]
   26.1 : 100 000 deliveries = Hispanics
   31.7 : 100 000 deliveries = Caucasians
   52.5 : 100 000 deliveries = African Americans
3. HYPERTENSION : PRS Risk varies by type of hypertension:
   Pre-existing Hypertension (OR 2.61)
   Gestational Hypertension (OR 2.41)
   Pre-eclampsia/Eclampsia (OR 10.39)
   Superimposed Pre-eclampsia/Eclampsia (OR 9.23)
   1993–2002 Nationwide Inpatient Database [25]
4. HEART DISEASE : Valvular-Arrhythmia-Infection-Infarction OR 13.2 [3]
5. ILLICIT DRUG USE : Cocaine-Amphetamine OR 2.3 [3]
6. TOBACCO USE/ABUSE : OR 1.95 [25]
7. MIGRAINE HEADACHES : OR 16.9 [3]
8. DIABETES : OR 2.5 [3]
9. THROMBOPHILIA : OR 16.0 [3]
10. LUPUS/SLE : OR 15.2 [3]
11. SICKLE CELL DISEASE : OR 9.1 [3]
12. THROMBOCYTOPENIA : OR 6.0 [3]
13. ANEMIA : OR 1.9 [3]
14. OBSTETRIC : POSTPARTUM HEMORRHAGE = OR 1.8
    FLUID & ELECTROLYTE IMBALANCE = OR 7.2
    TRANSFUSION = OR 10.3
    INFECTION = OR 25.0 [3]

that she is considered to be in a hypercoagulable state despite an expected decrease in hematocrit, blood viscosity and vascular resistance. Platelet hyperaggregability, decreased fibrinolysis, increases in some clotting proteins (fibrinogen and factors V, VII, VIII, IX, X and XII), decreases in naturally occurring anticoagulant proteins (C, S, antithrombin III) in late gestation, acquired increased resistance to protein C and decreased protein C inhibitor activity all contribute to a hypercoagulable state that extends several weeks into the puerperium. Blood coagulability may also be enhanced by pregnancy hormones estrogen and progesterone. Finally, hemodynamic changes inclusive of increases in blood volume, cardiac output and venous blood pressure are important factors especially around delivery and if anesthesia and cesarean surgery are employed.

General diagnostic considerations

Neuroimaging a pregnant patient raises questions of safety for the fetus. Because head computed tomography (CT) of the mother with the abdomen shielded exposes the fetus to less than 1 millirad, it is considered safe in pregnancy [36,37]. Because magnetic resonance imaging (MRI) involves no radiation exposure and most animal studies have shown no adverse effects on fetal development, the present consensus is that MRI (magnetic resonance arteriography (MRA) and magnetic resonance venography (MRV)) is probably safe in pregnancy [37]. Triiodinated compounds used as intravenous contrast agents for CT and fluoroscopy are class B pharmaceuticals probably safe for use during pregnancy because they are undetectable in the fetus and amniotic fluid, but gadolinium contrast is avoided because it crosses the placenta and has unknown effects on fetal development [38] Conventional head angiography also exposes the fetus to minimal radiation (<1 mrad) if fluoroscopy is short in duration. Cerebrospinal fluid studies are infrequently undertaken unless vasculitis, infection or subarachnoid hemorrhage is suspected. Echocardiogram is used to detect a patient foramen ovale or right to left shunt in the young pregnant patient since hemodynamic changes and a predisposition to venous thrombosis increase the likelihood of a paradoxical embolus [39]. Until recently, the use of tissue plasminogen activator (tPA) thrombolysis in pregnancy has been regarded as relatively contraindicated, but recent case reports and series have shown some limited use for late pregnancy stroke or life-threatening and potentially debilitating thromboembolic disease [40–42].

Cerebral blood flow

The autoregulatory system of the human brain ensures constant cerebral blood flow and tissue perfusion over a wide range of systemic pressures. During normal pregnancy, cerebral hemodynamics change over the course of gestation as measured by Doppler [43] and velocity-encoded phase contrast magnetic resonance imaging [44]. The systolic velocity and resistance index in the middle cerebral artery both decrease approximately 20% over gestation, whereas the cerebral perfusion pressure (CPP) is estimated to increase by 50% from early pregnancy to term [45,46] although the methodology used has been criticized [47,48]. A similar decrease in flow is seen by magnetic resonance imaging studies of the posterior cerebral artery with no change in the middle and posterior cerebral artery diameters during late normal pregnancy [43,44]. The cerebral blood flow index (CFI) reflecting overall cerebral perfusion also increases approximately 10% during pregnancy. Despite this increase, cerebral autoregulation in the normal pregnancy patient remains very efficient. A small decrease in cerebral resistance occurs as blood pressure increases within the normal range late in pregnancy; if blood pressure increases outside the normal range, a physiological increase in cerebral resistance occurs to limit perfusion [46]. If the upper limit of autoregulation is exceeded by elevated blood pressure and impairments to normal cerebrovascular health such as endothelial dysfunction and water homeostasis [48,49], the subacute neurologic syndrome of hypertensive encephalopathy can develop [50,51]. It is variably characterized by headache, seizure, altered mental status, visual disturbance and/or focal neurologic disturbances in a hypertensive patient with preferential localization of focal cerebral edema formation in the posterior cerebral circulation.

Categories of pregnancy-related stroke

As depicted in Table 19.1, PRS can be divided into CVAs which occur as a consequence of disorders or diseases unique to pregnancy (pregnancy-induced) or CVAs which occur during gestation that are not primarily due to pregnancy-associated (pregnancy-incidental) pathology. Examples of the former are pre-eclampsia/eclampsia, cerebral venous thrombosis, and postpartum cerebral vasculopathy. Because the spectrum of disease encountered in the stroke patient with gestational hypertension/pre-eclampsia/eclampsia/HELLP syndrome is broad, the clinician can be challenged in some patients to distinguish between a stroke caused primarily by a pregnancy-induced hypertensive disorder versus some other non-pregnancy specific cause of cerebral infarction or intracranial (subarachnoid or intracerebral) hemorrhage. The history and physical examination may provide important clues to type and etiology of stroke.

Pregnancy-induced stroke

Pre-eclampsia-eclampsia-HELLP syndrome and severe gestational hypertension

General

That patients with hypertensive complications of pregnancy such as gestational hypertension and pre-eclampsia are 2 to 4 times more likely than controls to later suffer a postpregnancy cardiovascular, thromboembolic or stroke event suggests that there are underlying factors which contribute to a proclivity toward CVA in these women [52–54]. Indeed, a strong family history for heart disease or stroke imparts a 3.2-fold elevation in the risk for pre-eclampsia [55]. CVA is the most common cause of death in patients with eclampsia [56,57] as well as patients with atypical severe pre-eclampsia expressed as HELLP syndrome (hemolysis, elevated liver enzymes, thrombocytopenia) who receive traditional non-steroid obstetric and medical management [58–60]. It is less appreciated by clinicians that stroke can occur in the patient with severe pre-eclampsia without HELLP syndrome and in the patient with severe gestational hypertension who at the time of stroke does not have measurable proteinuria to merit a diagnosis of pre-eclampsia.

Severe systolic hypertension

The importance of preventing severe systolic hypertension (<160 mmHg) in the pathogenesis of stroke in patients with a pre-eclampsia disorder has led to a call for a paradigm change in obstetric practice away from an emphasis on high diastolic

(>110 mmHg) or mean arterial blood pressures (>125–140 mmHg) as thresholds to guide antihypertensive therapy [61]. The importance of aggressively treating severe systolic hypertension to <160 mmHg has been emphasized also by Cunningham [62] and is consistent with recommendations published by the 2000 National Institutes of Health Working Group on High Blood Pressure in Pregnancy [63]. The development of a pulse pressure of more than 60 mmHg difference between systolic and diastolic readings, in association with a systolic blood pressure increase over baseline also of more than 60 mmHg could be as important in the pregnant patient with pre-eclampsia to place her at risk of cerebrovascular accident as exceeding a systolic blood pressure threshold of 160 mmHg [61].

Abnormal cerebral hemodynamics

Changes in the cerebral hemodynamics of the pregnant patient with severe pre-eclampsia explain in part the susceptibility of these patients to cerebrovascular accident [46]. Compared to normal pregnant patients or those with mild pre-eclampsia, the majority of patients with severe pre-eclampsia have high cerebral perfusion pressures and cerebral vascular resistance which may cause vascular (endothelial, muscularis, arterial wall stiffness) damage centrally [64–66] over time and headache [67]. Women destined to develop pre-eclampsia or superimposed pre-eclampsia have cerebral hemodynamic changes that predate by 7–10 weeks the development of overt pre-eclampsia [68–71]. Cerebral blood flow velocity increases significantly in the first 24–48 hours postpartum, possibly related to the higher frequency of stroke seen postpartum in women with pre-eclampsia than antepartum in some series [61,72]. These and other central hemodynamic changes can persist for 7 days to 12 weeks postpartum [73–74].

Defective cerebral autoregulation and sequelae

A number of investigators have advanced the hypothesis that a protracted period of increased cerebral perfusion pressure in patients with pre-eclampsia/eclampsia may cause barotrauma and vascular damage that causes cerebral autoregulation to fail with overperfusion injury, vasogenic edema [46,75–77] and the clinical syndrome of hypertensive encephalopathy. Support for this concept has also been found in small animal studies [48,78,79]. Oehm and colleagues in Germany have reported that a substantial disturbance of dynamic cerebral autoregulation occurs in patients who develop eclampsia [80]. Some patients with severe gestational hypertension/severe pre-eclampsia/HELLP syndrome develop only symptoms of advanced cerebral pathology and hypertensive encephalopathy [81–83], some manifest this as eclampsia with seizure [84–87], while still others instead progress to cerebral hemorrhage or thrombosis [88–91,61] during pregnancy or the puerperium.

Spectrum and characteristics of stroke

In the recent series of strokes in 28 severely pre-eclamptic patients reported by Martin, most were hemorrhagic in type, frequently in multiple sites (37%), and present in frontal and parietal lobes of the brain as well as the occipital area [61]. This is consistent with recent data showing magnetic resonance imaging abnormalities in the occipital and parietal lobes of patients with pre-eclampsia [92]. Hemorrhage can be either intracerebral or subarachnoid [93–95], rarely involving the brainstem [96]. When Doppler and CNS imaging abnormalities are observed in postpartum patients with headache, altered consciousness, vomiting, seizures and focal neurologic signs that is similar to the spectrum of eclampsia, the term "postpartum cerebral angiopathy" has been utilized and managed with supportive and antiseizure medications given while awaiting spontaneous resolution [81,86]. The rare complication of cortical blindness is usually reversible since it is due to vasogenic edema in the posterior cerebral circulation of the occipital lobes, but permanent blindness or complete amaurosis rarely follows infarcts of the lateral geniculate bodies [97–100].

Pharmacotherapy

Magnesium sulfate has been shown to significant reduce eclamptic seizures in the MAGPIE trial, although a small percentage of patients develop eclampsia nevertheless and its use does not prevent stroke. Magnesium sulfate's mechanism of action to prevent seizure is still undefined, but it has been shown to reduce cerebral perfusion pressure via vasodilatation of constricted cerebral vessels [46,101] in contrast to nimodipine, a dihydropyridine calcium channel blocker [102] which increases CPP. Recent data suggest that magnesium sulfate acts to maintain cerebral flow index while reducing cerebral perfusion pressure in women with elevated CPP, and that its effect is linearly related to the baseline CPP. In other words, patients with a higher starting CPP will demonstrate a greater reduction in CPP following $MgSO_4$ than women with lesser elevation of their CPP. In addition, women with lower CPP will tend to "normalize" their CPP within the 5–95% after $MgSO_4$ infusion. Labetalol has both selective, competitive alpha-1 *and* non-selective, competitive β-adrenergic blocking actions that produce rapid dose-dependent decreases in blood pressure without reflex tachycardia or significant reduction in heart rate [103]. In addition, it has been shown to be a membrane stabilizer [104] and it may reduce cerebral perfusion pressure more effectively than magnesium sulfate without affecting cerebral perfusion. Hence it is a candidate agent to replace magnesium sulfate as first-line therapy to control blood pressure and prevent cerebral sequelae [46]. Guidelines for the use of labetolol and hydralazine have been published [105,63]; great individual variation in dosage amount and frequency exist in practices around the United States, suggesting the need for further studies to validate effectiveness of therapy for achieving and maintaining therapeutic goals (ie, a systolic blood pressure <160 mmHg) by traditional oral and systemic routes or via intravenous infusions (i.e. labetolol, nicardipine). Immediate postpartum or poststroke diuretic therapy as furosemide is recommended for patients with hypertensive encephalopathy and to improve blood pressure control in the severely hypertensive parturient [106–108].

Corticosteroids

The potential place of corticosteroids for stroke prevention in the hypertensive pregnant patient particularly with severe pre-eclampsia or HELLP syndrome is a worthy consideration [61]. Intravenous high-dose dexamethasone has been shown to reduce significant maternal morbidity when given early or late during the course of disease development in patients with HELLP syndrome, and it probably reduces the likelihood of patients with this disorder developing cerebral sequelae to their disease [61]. Cerebral hemodynamic studies in patients with HELLP syndrome reveal similar findings to patients with pre-eclampsia [109]. Almost all deaths due to stroke in patients with HELLP syndrome occur in the absence of aggressive pre-emptive corticosteroid therapy for basic disease management [58,61]. A cornerstone of management for patients with hypertensive encephalopathy is the administration of this category of drugs in association with antihypertensive and diuretic agents. Experience with a recent patient who had severe gestational hypertension that quickly and repeatedly returned after treatment with small, frequent intravenous administrations of labetalol and who suffered a cerebral hemorrhage raises the question of whether obstetricians should be more aggressive with labetalol (or other agents) for blood pressure control or whether this approach alone is unlikely to succeed without another agent such as glucocorticoids to interrupt cerebral pathophysiology and thereby avert CVA. Because sudden hypertension can result from, rather than lead to, intracranial bleeding, the initiation of potent glucocorticoids or other agents may augment poorly effective antihypertensive therapy and potentially avoid adverse cerebral sequelae. It is important to recognize that steroid therapy in potential stroke patients is not believed to act through any effect on cerebral edema prevention or alleviation, as it does when used in the management of cerebral edema due to space occupying lesions.

Cerebral venous and sinus thrombosis

General

Thrombosis of the cerebral veins (CVT) and sinuses is a distinct cerebrovascular disorder that is more often encountered in females than males, most often late in gestation or during the early puerperium [110–115]. The diagnosis is to be considered in a peripartum patient with persistent headache [116]. Thought to be caused by changes in the coagulation process of normal gravid patients or less often in others who have underlying thrombophilias, either of which can be stressed by events and treatments surrounding delivery, CVT has been diagnosed as late as 3 months postpartum [117]. Almost 200 years ago Ménière [118] and Abercrombie [119] were the first to demonstrate the relationship between pregnancy/puerperium and CVT. It was not until the early 1940s that the relationship was better publicized using clinical and autopsy studies [120–123]. Within 40 years, 273 puerperal CVT cases were reported by two groups of investigators in India where the incidence was approximately 1:250 obstetric admissions and the most common cause of stroke in young women [124,125]. Until the mid-1980s, the diagnosis of CVT was usually made postmortem [126,127]. The development of better imaging techniques, particularly MRI/MRA, has considerably facilitated radiologic diagnosis in the patient suspected of the condition.

Pathogenesis

The cerebral venous system of the human brain is unique in that major veins are composed of dural folds called sinuses which lack muscular walls, valves or the ability to contract. Hence blood can pool and clots form in these veins in susceptible patients to cause a sinus thrombosis, occluding and obstructing venous return in the brain with variable degrees of increased venous pressure, impaired absorption of cerebrospinal fluid, increased intracranial pressure, ischemia, infarction, cytotoxic edema, bleeding, and vasogenic edema [128,110]. The superior and inferior sagittal sinuses drain sequentially into the confluence of sinuses, the cavernous sinus, the transverse sinus, the right and left sigmoid sinus and finally the internal jugular veins. The location and extent of the affected vein(s) contribute to the terminology used to describe the particular CVT in a given patient such as cortical venous thrombosis, cerebral sinus thrombosis, dural sinus thrombosis, and sagittal venous thrombosis. The most common sites involved in the pregnant patient are thrombosis of the sagittal sinus with secondary extension into the cortical veins or primary thrombosis of a cortical vein [129]. A prothrombotic risk factor (genetic or acquired such as pregnancy/puerperium) or a direct mechanical cause (head injury, lumbar puncture, jugular catheterization, neurosurgical procedure) led to 85% of CVT cases in one series of patients[111]. In another, all patients that developed a CVT during pregnancy or the puerperium had a hypercoagulable state identified which was most often associated with elevated factor VIII [130]. Other hyperviscous states that can precipitate CVT with pregnancy include sickle cell anemia, malignancy, polycythemia, and paroxysmal nocturnal hemoglobinuria. The higher prevalence of CVT in countries like India may be secondary to factors such as higher rates of systemic infection, anemia and severe dehydration [11].

Clinical presentation

Initial symptomatology is diverse and varied, sometimes sudden but more often vague and insidious in onset. Progressive, unusual headache that is resistant to analgesia develops in more than 90% of patients, usually increasing gradually over several days sometimes in association with nausea and/or vomiting. Headache may be the sole complaint in some patients. Rarely it can be misdiagnosed as a postdural puncture headache if spinal analgesia was used for delivery [131]. The average time interval between symptom onset and eventual diagnosis is 7 days [132]. If all patients with CVT are considered as a group, approximately 50% develop cerebral lesions and neurologic signs and about 40% develop seizures (sometimes misinterpreted as an eclamptic convulsion). If thrombosis extends into the deep venous system of the thalami, behavioral symptoms such as delirium, amnesia, mutism and sometimes coma can be manifested [133]. Visual impairment as diplopia and blindness can result from very high intracranial pressure and severe papilledema [110].

Diagnosis

The most sensitive examination technique is MRI with gadolinium in combination with magnetic resonance venography-MRV [112,134,135]. T1-weighted and T2-weighted MRI will show a hyperintense signal from the thrombosed sinuses especially if performed in the first 5 days of thrombosis or after 1 month. Conventional CT scanning results can be entirely normal in the presence of CVT and mislead the physician into missing the diagnosis 60% of the time at initial presentation [136,115,117]. CT venography, however, is a promising new imaging technique to investigate the cerebral venous system. Cerebral angiography in experienced hands can provide better details of the cerebral veins, showing dilated and tortuous ("corkscrew") veins that suggest downstream sinus thrombosis.

Treatment

Based upon the combined findings of three small randomized clinical trials [137–139] and a large multicenter prospective observational study of 624 patients with CVT [140], anticoagulation with intravenous heparin is usually recommended to arrest the thrombotic process and to prevent pulmonary embolism [141] despite the potential risk that a venous infarct might become hemorrhagic. However, in three small randomized clinical trials there were no new cerebral hemorrhages and no increase in already present ones following CVT treatment with heparin. Fixed high dose, subcutaneous heparin of low molecular weight might be a suitable alternative, but presently there are no studies comparing its effectiveness with fractionated heparin. Heparin therapy is generally continued during the acute phase "until the patient stabilizes" [126,127] which usually is 3–7 days of therapy. Oral anticoagulant therapy using vitamin K antagonists (coumarin derivatives) is usually continued for 6 months [130] after a first episode of CVT, or longer in the presence of predisposing factors, with a target international normalized ration of 2.5 [110]. Because of rare CVT recurrence in a subsequent pregnancy and insufficient data to suggest that prophylactic anticoagulation provides any patient benefit, it is not recommended.

Potential thrombolytic therapy

In pregnant patients with a high-risk/poor-prognosis CVT associated with significant neurologic deficits and decline, endovascular thrombolysis can be attempted by experienced interventional radiologists using a combination of a thrombolytic enzyme such as rt-PA infused into the dural sinus, and mechanical intervention techniques to aspirate, disrupt and/or dislodge the thrombus [142–146]. Although tissue plasminogen activator thrombolysis in pregnancy has been regarded as relatively contraindicated, a number of case reports and series have been published recently to clarify maternal safety and efficacy issues for the treatment of acute ischemic stroke during gestation (see discussion later in chapter). Because the diagnosis of CVT is usually made many hours after the initial development of symptomatology, the potential for thrombolytic therapy for the patient with CVT probably holds less promise than with arterial ischemic stroke.

Prognosis

Despite remaining a diagnostic challenge and a potentially disabling or lethal disease, CVT associated with pregnancy and the puerperium overall has an excellent prognosis with 90–93% survival and few persistent neurologic deficits [147,19].

Postpartum cerebral vasculopathy

General

Another potential masquerader or mimic of postpartum eclampsia is postpartum cerebral vasculopathy, a type of postpartum angiopathy caused by reversible multifocal brain ischemia and multilocular segmental narrowing of large and medium-sized cerebral arteries [148–151]. Affected patients develop severe generalized or occipital headaches with abrupt onset, altered mental status, generalized motor seizures, neurologic deficits and often some degree of visual impairment which if untreated can progress to ischemic or hemorrhagic stroke in the postpartum period [152].

Diagnosis

Angiography is crucial to the diagnosis, especially to be considered in a patient with what is thought to represent delayed postpartum eclampsia. Individuals with Call–Fleming syndrome (benign postpartum angiopathy) may have no abnormalities on a standard MRI but exhibit characteristic angiopathic findings on magnetic resonance angiography [153–155]. Patients with postpartum reversible encephalopathy syndrome have hyperintense lesions suggestive of vasogenic edema on both T2-weighted images and diffusion-weighted images [151]. Other reported patients with cerebral angiopathy exhibited features of a vasculitis. Postpartum cerebral angiopathy may represent a continuum of vascular pathology which begins with vasospasm and progresses over time to a true vasculitis [156], consistent with Varner's suggestion that patient presentations represent different manifestations of similar underlying pathophysiology [157].

Treatment and prognosis

Distinguishing among the various subtypes of cerebral vasculopathy can be problematic, but prompt treatment is advised with antihypertensives, anticonvulsants, corticosteroids and mannitol or furosemide to reduce cerebral edema if present and prevent cerebral herniation [158]. In rare instances pulsed cyclophosphamide is required to stop the process in patients that fail to respond to methylprednisolone. Prognosis is excellent for patients with evidence of a diffuse vasculopathy but is worse when there is clinical or laboratory evidence supportive of extracerebral or systemic vasculitis [159].

Miscellaneous causes of pregnancy-associated stroke

A variety of other CVA etiologies related to the pregnancy itself can be encountered in the pregnant or puerperal patient [5,7–9,11]. These include the following:

Cardioembolism

The heart can be a source for cerebrovascular accident in patients with underlying cardiac disease (prosthetic heart valve, atrial fibrillation, mitral valve prolapse, subacute bacterial endocarditis, myocardial infarction, coronary dissection) or peripartum cardiomyopathy [9,20,22]. Left ventricular thrombus formation in the diseased heart of a patient with peripartum cardiomyopathy can cause embolic stroke in 5–10% of patients [160,161,7].

Paradoxical embolism

The presence of a patient foramen ovale is a risk factor for embolic stroke in the pregnant or puerperal patient [162–164] who undergoes either vaginal or cesarean delivery.

Choriocarcinoma

Choriocarcinoma has been reported to develop in 1 of every 30 molar pregnancies, and frequently metastasize to the brain with thrombosis or aneurysm formation that results in ischemic stroke or intraparenchymal hemorrhage [165–168].

Amniotic fluid embolism

Acute hemodynamic collapse and consumptive coagulopathy in patients with amniotic fluid embolism can cause brain insult either directly (hemorrhage, thrombosis), indirectly (cerebral hypoperfusion) or rarely by amniotic fluid debris passage through a patent foramen ovale to the brain [169].

Air embolism

When air enters the maternal venous circulation during cesarean (or rarely vaginal) delivery, bubbles can occlude pulmonary capillaries and lead to cardiovascular compromise or collapse. In addition to the potential for hypoperfusion of the brain in this clinical setting, air bubbles traveling to brain arteries can also lead to focal stroke-like deficits [170].

Moyamoya disease

This rare cerebrovascular disease is characterized by bilateral steno-occlusion of the supraclinoid carotid arteries with formation of abnormal fine networks of collateral vessels at the base of the brain. Pregnancy, particularly during labor and delivery, places affected patients at increased risk for CVA with intracerebral hemorrhage [171–174].

Other stroke causation during pregnancy

Intracerebral hemorrhage

Hemorrhagic cerebrovascular accidents are categorized as either subarachnoid (SAH) or intracerebral (ICH). Intracerebral (or intraparenchymal) hemorrhage involves bleeding from small arteries or arterioles directly into the brain. Blood spreads along white matter pathways and localized hematoma formation is common. Accumulation of blood can be rapid, but is classically more insidious which coincides with its gradual symptom progression over a few hours. Symptoms typically include worsening headache and focal findings such as a progressively worsening unilateral hemiparesis. In pregnancy, ICH is most commonly due to severe hypertension associated with pre-eclampsia/eclampsia. Illicit drug use, especially cocaine and methamphetamines, bleeding diatheses, trauma, tumors, and small vessel vasculitides are other known causes of ICH [175,176]. Diagnosis and management of ICH is similar to that of SAH (see discussion to follow).

Subarachnoid hemorrhage

General

Subarachnoid hemorrhage (SAH) is bleeding into the subarachnoid space (anatomically the area between the arachnoid membrane and the pia mater) surrounding the brain. SAH can occur secondary to trauma, but is more commonly encountered due either to spontaneous leaking, ruptured aneurysm or an arteriovenous malformation (AVM). Aneurysms and AVMs develop secondary to congenital defects in cerebral vasculature formation at anatomically predictable sites [177]. An aneurysm is a sacular dilation of a blood vessel generally located at an angle of bifurcation in or near the circle of Willis – the internal carotid (37%), anterior communicating/anterior cerebral (23%), posterior communicating (23%), and vertebral/basilar (10%) arteries. An AVM develops as a tangled, interconnected complex of high pressure arteries and low pressure veins without an intervening capillary bed. Frequently weak and prone to bleeding, AVMs are most commonly located in the frontoparietal and temporal regions of the brain, but can be found at other sites in the brain and spinal cord. As many as 60% of patients with an AVM are found to have an aneurysm located within the AVM itself or nearby [178].

SAH during pregnancy

SAH occurs at a frequency which averages 20–30 cases per 100 000 deliveries [7,14]. Maternal mortality is 13–35% and fetal mortality is 7–25% [179]. Pregnancy does not appear to increase the risk of maternal death from SAH due to aneurysmal bleeding, but it does with AVM probably due to the poor neurologic condition of these patients at presentation [180–183]. Presumably related to gestation-induced physiologic and anatomic changes in the mother, the risk of SAH increases as pregnancy progresses such that one-third occur in the second trimester and more than 50% are detected during the third trimester [7,179,177,183–185]. The remainder occur in the 1st trimester and postpartum [177]. Interestingly aneurysm rupture during actual labor and delivery is a rare event [180,182,186–191,28,32] even though it is estimated that between 20 000 and 40 000 women deliver successfully each year in the United States despite harboring intracranial aneurysms [192]. Protracted and repeated episodes of valsalva-type straining during the second stage of labor would theoretically stress any area of cerebrovascular weakness, but normal cerebral autoregulatory changes may provide compensatory relief in the non-hypertensive, healthy parturient [193,194] that are further augmented by epidural anesthesia when used.

Clinical presentation

The signs and symptoms of SAH are neither altered by pregnancy nor specific to underlying cause. Intracerebral bleeding (ICH) in patients with hypertensive complications of severe pre-eclampsia (including HELLP syndrome) can present with clinically similar findings. Rupture of an aneurysm sends blood under arterial pressure directly into the cerebrospinal fluid that produces a rapid increase in intracranial pressure and immediate symptomatology. Although the initial bleed may last only seconds, rebleeding is common and if persistent can lead to deep coma and death. In contrast, bleeding from an AVM is typically less abrupt at onset and can continue over a longer period of time. The dominant symptom with SAH is sudden severe headache with associated immediate cessation of non-focal neurologic activity such as knees buckling, loss of memory and/or loss of focus. The maximal immediate symptoms of SAH at onset differ from ICH which is usually more of an insidious onset and frequently associated with unilateral or focal findings that worsen over time. Up to half of patients with SAH report a severe headache several days before the acute bleeding episode [195]. Other symptoms due to SAH include nausea and vomiting, meningeal signs, ocular hemorrhages, decreased level of consciousness, hypertension, and seizures. These latter two findings can obfuscate the diagnosis of SAH due to aneurysmal or AVM rupture because they may be ascribed to pre-eclampsia/eclampsia.

Neurologic status

An important prognostic indicator of outcome is the patient's neurologic condition at presentation. A number of scales have been developed to categorize neurologic status in order to guide management and determine prognosis. The Hunt and Hess (1968) scale as shown in Table 19.3 grades the patient's condition based on level of consciousness, presence of meningeal signs, and focal neurologic signs which is subject to significant intra-observer and inter-observer variation [196]. In addition, there is poor correlation between meningeal signs and neurologic outcome in the presence of normal consciousness [197]. To remedy these limitations, a committee of the World Federation of Neurologic Surgeons proposed the more objective WNFS Scale which combines the Glascow Coma Scale with the presence or absence of motor deficits. Despite its advantages, the WNFS scale has yet to be widely incorporated into practice [197]. Maternal mortality in relation to initial clinical grade of aneurysmal hemorrhage is discussed below in the Prognosis section.

Table 19.3 Systems to assess central nervous system.

A. Hunt & Hess Clinical Grading Scale [196]

Grade	Criteria
I	Asymptomatic, or minimal headache and slight nuchal rigidity
II	Moderate to severe headache, nuchal rigidity, no neurologic deficit other than cranial nerve palsy
III	Drowsiness, confusion, or mild focal deficit
IV	Stupor, moderate to severe hemiparesis, early decerebrate rigidity and vegetative disturbances
V	Deep coma, decerebrate rigidity, moribund

B. Glasgow Coma Scale [268]

Behavior	Patient Response	Component Score
Eye opening (E)	Spontaneous	4
	To speech/loud noise	3
	To pain	2
	None	1
Best verbal response (V)	Oriented	5
	Confused, disoriented	4
	Inappropriate words	3
	Incomprehensible	2
	Sounds-none	1
Best motor response (M)	Obeys	6
	Localizes	5
	Flexion/withdraws	4
	Abnormal flexion posturing	3
	Extension posturing	2
	None	1

Coma score = E+V+M. Patients scoring 3 or 4 have an 85% chance of dying or remaining vegetative; scores above 11 indicate only a 5–10% likelihood of death or vegetative state and 85% chance of moderate disability or good recovery. Intermediate scores correlate with proportional chances of recovery.

C. World Federation of Neurological Surgeons (WFNS) SAH Scale [269]

WFNS Grade	Glasgow Coma Scale	Motor Deficit
I	15	Absent
II	13–14	Absent
III	13–14	Present
IV	7–12	Present/Absent
V	3–6	Present/Absent

Diagnosis

Clinical

The diagnostic approach to the pregnant patient does not differ from a patient who is not pregnant. The rarity of SAH in pregnancy and its potential for confusion with eclampsia due to the presence of hypertension and seizure can lead to diagnostic delay which worsens the prognosis by increasing the chance for rebleeding and cerebral vasospasm, along with prolonging the interval before neurosurgical evaluation and intervention can occur. Strong clinical suspicion of SAH is crucial. Eclampsia itself is associated with an increased likelihood of intracranial events. Tonic-clonic seizures associated with eclampsia are often followed by a prolonged postictal period which can be potentiated by high serum concentrations of magnesium sulfate being administered to prevent seizure recurrence. Following an eclamptic seizure it is important to periodically assess the patient's neurological status in order to avoid magnesium toxicity *and* to determine that intracranial hemorrhage has neither occurred nor is being masked by the magnesium. Eclampsia without intracranial hemorrhage permits the patient to exhibit normal papillary reactivity and response to painful stimuli in the absence of magnesium toxicity. Also, nausea and vomiting, nuchal rigidity, and focal motor weakness are rarely encountered in the eclamptic patient.

Imaging

A non-contrasted CT scan of the head is typically the first step in radiologic diagnosis of SAH. No pregnant patient with a suspected intracranial bleed should be denied CT scanning regardless of gestational age or fear of potential adverse fetal effects from ionizing radiation scatter. Although shielding of the maternal abdomen and uterus is recommended during any radiographic examination especially during the first trimester, lack of abdominal shielding is not grounds for denial of CT scanning. A shielded CT scan results in 2 mrad of fetal exposure [7,10]. Use of the cerebral CT scanning facilitates prediction, with a high degree of accuracy, of the type of hemorrhage and its site of origin. In addition, cerebral CT can be useful in determining the presence of life-threatening hematomas that require surgical evacuation, as well as the development of hydrocephalus [195]. The ability of cerebral CT scanning to detect blood in the subarachnoid space decreases from up to 95% within 24 hours of acute hemorrhage to 50% 1 week later [198]. If the CT scan is normal and there is high clinical suspicion of SAH, lumbar puncture is performed to examine the cerebrospinal fluid (CSF) for blood or xanthochromia. Non-clearing bloody CSF found at lumbar puncture supports the diagnosis of SAH. Cerebral angiography, including magnetic resonance angiography (MRA), remains the best diagnostic tool for identifying any vascular abnormality. In addition, important anatomic (and therefore prognostic) information is usually obtained with these invasive techniques. However, angiography may fail to visualize the cause of SAH in 20% of patients [199]. In these cases, a repeat angiogram may be necessary to rule out false-negative results secondary to vasospasm or clot filling of the aneurysm. Some authors feel that MRI scanning lacks sensitivity to detect acute SAH [195], but it may be helpful in situations where the initial angiogram fails to identify the lesion. However with technological advances in MRI, newer evidence suggests that it may be as accurate as CT for the detection of acute hemorrhage in patients presenting with acute focal stroke symptoms [200]. This technique also can identify vascular lesions in the spinal cord [184].

Laboratory evaluation

Several laboratory tests are performed to help identify if a patients has a pregnancy-associated condition (such as pre-eclampsia/eclampsia/HELLP syndrome or thrombotic thrombocytopenic purpura (TTP)) or a predilection for a hemorrhagic or ischemic event. Initial testing includes a complete blood count, metabolic profile, erythrocyte sedimentation rate (ESR), peripheral blood smear, lipid and triglyceride profile, coagulation profile, urine drug screen, antinuclear antibody (ANA) screen, thrombophilia work-up, and serologic testing for syphilis. A magnesium serum level may be warranted if the patient is receiving magnesium sulfate therapy and toxicity is suspected.

Management issues

Transfer to a tertiary care center or one with neurosurgical and critical care services is a necessity in the presence of a strong suspicion or a definitive diagnosis of SAH. Prognosis is directly related to level of consciousness upon arrival and condition before neurosurgical intervention. Prognosis is also inversely proportional to the patient's age and the extent of hemorrhage on initial CT scan. An intensive care setting is crucial for constant hemodynamic monitoring. Immediate neurology/neurosurgical consultation and direction of care is imperative to assess the patient's grade, initiate medical management and decide on timing/technique of surgical therapy. Immediate obstetric evaluation is also important to assess gestational age, fetal viability and maternal-fetal status. Bedrest, stool softeners and analgesia to diminish hemodynamic fluctuations and lower the risk of rebleeding are appropriate [201]. All anticoagulant and antiplatelet agents are stopped [202]. Reversal of any residual anticoagulant effect may be required using appropriate agents such as vitamin K and fresh frozen plasma. DVT prophylaxis with pneumatic compressing devices should be initiated.

Nimodipine

The calcium channel blocker nimodipine has been used since the 1980s to vasodilate cerebral blood vessels and theoretically prevent vasospasm in the patient with SAH, although it has not been possible to demonstrate a drug effect on angiographic or symptomatic vasospasm. There is good evidence, however, that nimodipine improves outcomes by decreasing severe neurologic deficit and death [203–205]. Compared to placebo, nimodipine was associated with a 24% risk reduction of poor outcome [206]. Therapy should be initiated within 4 days of SAH at a recommended dose of 60 mg orally (by nasogastric tube or mouth); IV and SQ routes are contraindicated. Despite relative site selectivity for cerebral vessels, peripheral blood pressure fluctuations are common with nimodipine use which requires continuous monitoring to avoid hypotension that could cause underperfusion of the uteroplacental circulation as well as decreased cerebral perfusion pressure [207,208]. It is a category C medication without evidence of any fetal toxicity in humans. Nimodipine has been used in pregnancy for the treatment of cerebral vasospasm associated with severe pre-eclampsia or eclampsia [209–212]. In addition, it was studied in 800 patients with pre-eclampsia to compare its efficacy against magnesium sulfate for seizure prophylaxis [213]. There was no difference in adverse fetal outcomes between the two treatments. During the initial stages of the trial there was an increased incidence of eclamptic seizures in the nimodipine group when a dose of 30 mg every 4 hours was used. This difference disappeared when the dose was increased to that typically used for the prevention of vasospasm in SAH.

Mannitol

Hyperosmotic agents such as mannitol (pregnancy category C) are used to treat elevated intracranial pressure associated with intracranial hemorrhage [10], cerebral venous thrombosis, and other causes of stroke. It is administered as an initial bolus of 1 g/kg, followed by infusions of 0.25–0.5 g/kg every 6 hours. The primary goal of therapy is to achieve plasma hyperosmolality (300–310 mosmol/kg) while maintaining an adequate plasma volume.

Intracranial pressure

Additional medical measures are instituted in the patient with SAH to maintain adequate cerebral circulation and prevent both ischemia and rebleeding. Elevations in intracranial pressure (ICP) from vascular engorgement and acute hydrocephalus occur following SAH. As ICP increases, cerebral perfusion decreases. Cerebral perfusion pressure (CPP) equals the mean arterial pressure (MAP) minus the ICP [CPP = MAP – ICP] [201]. To counteract increases in ICP, MAP must increase to maintain adequate CPP using what is termed "triple-H" therapy – hypertension, hypervolemia, and hemodilution. Colloid solutions are preferred for volume expansion. Vasopressors or inotropic agents are used judiciously to elevate the systolic blood pressure into the 150–200 mmHg range [214–216]. Because sustained systolic blood pressures above this level can worsen SAH via rebleeding, triple-H thereby is withheld until indicated surgical intervention is completed. Labetolol is the preferred agent to lower high blood pressure in this setting.

Surgical management

The decision to operate upon a pregnant patient with an intracranial hemorrhage is a neurosurgical decision, while the decision to deliver and the type and timing of delivery is based upon obstetric considerations [177,8,9]. Lesion-specific neurosurgical management is addressed briefly in the sections that follow.

Preoperative/operative assessment and general management

If the decision is made to proceed with neurosurgical operative intervention and continuation of pregnancy is planned, certain preoperative assessments are important for both mother and fetus. Evaluation and correction of electrolyte imbalances is crucial since metabolic derangements such as cerebral salt-wasting syndrome and glucose intolerance are common following SAH. Hypokalemia and hypocalcemia occur in 50–75% of patients [217]. Replacement of blood and clotting factors should be performed as needed. Cardiac abnormalities manifested primarily as rhythm disturbances are seen in 50–80% of patients post aneurysm rupture, due to impaired neurogenic control of the cardiac electrical system [218]. Electrocardiographic changes in patients with SAH are more likely to be reflected in subsequent poor neurologic outcome than to poor cardiovascular outcome. Continous cardiac monitoring is necessary to monitor for more severe problems such as myocarditis, acute myocardial infarction, and left ventricular failure. Significant cardiac events are rare and aneurysm repair should not be delayed unless there is severe pulmonary edema from cardiogenic shock [218].

Anesthetic management

Both endovascular intervention and extravascular exclusion through craniotomy should be performed under general anesthesia. Vigilant control of systemic and cerebral hemodynamics is important while considering the action of administered drugs that may induce uterine relaxation or fetal depression.

Blood pressure control

Tight operative control is crucial for mother and fetus. Low blood pressures decrease uterine perfusion and place the mother at risk of recurrent cerebral ischemia, while acute hypertension increases the risk of rebleeding and placental abruption. Nicardipine, a dihydropyridine calcium channel blocker, and remifentanil, a synthetic opiod with rapid onset and duration, are two agents that may be particularly advantageous for treating periods of acute hypertension [218].

Avoid fetal depression

Adequate maternal oxygenation and left uterine displacement are important to reduce aortacaval compression and prevent fetal asphyxia. Halothane should be avoided due to its potent ability to relax the uterine musculature.

Avoid hyperventilation

Second and third trimester pregnancies are states of respiratory alkalosis due to increased minute ventilation and the resultant P_aCO_2 is typically 28–32 mmHg [219–220]. The combination of physiologic alkalosis with hyperventilation, which is commonly induced in neurosurgical procedures, may cause a blunted response of the cerebral vasculature to hypocarbia. Hyperventilation may also cause fetal hypoxia and acidosis by increasing uterine arterial vasoconstriction causing uteroplacental insufficiency [221].

SAH prognosis

Regardless of pregnancy status, patients in general with CVA due to SAH have a 33% chance to achieve a "good result" following treatment [222]. Prognosis can be altered according to numerous factors including type, location and extent of lesion. Hunt and Hess initial clinical grades I and II have a favorable prognosis following aneurysmal rupture with mortality rates less than 20% and 35% respectively. Maternal mortality increases significantly with grade III lesion mortality to over 60% with the highest mortality of >95% observed in association with patients having grade V lesions [7].

Subarachnoid hemorrhage: aneurysm

General

The natural history of unruptured cerebral aneurysms varies clinically according to the presence or absence of symptoms. Most cerebral aneurysms are asymptomatic (95%) and usually identified incidentally at the time of cerebral angiography (approximately 1% of adults) or autopsy (approximately 1–6% of adults) [195]. Asymptomatic cerebral aneurysms rupture at a rate of 1–2% per year [223–224]. Activities that reportedly precede aneurysm rupture include emotional strain, heavy lifting, coughing, coitus, urination, and defecation. These activities alter cerebral hemodynamics by increasing intracranial pressure. Symptomatic cerebral aneurysms present the greatest risk of rupture with an annual rupture rate of 6% [224]. Once bleeding occurs, mortality risk is high. More than 10% of patients will die before reaching the hospital and 40% of those who reach the hospital will die within the next 30 days. Approximately a third of survivors will sustain significant lasting neurologic morbidity [195]. Significant factors that impact eventual outcome include patient status at initial presentation, if rebleeding occurs, and if secondary vasospasm develops [224]. Patients with a history of autosomal dominant polycystic kidney disease are at increased risk for aneurysms [225–226].

Management

Early aneurysm repair (within 48–72 hours after rupture) is associated with improved long-term survival and less morbidity in patients with Hunt and Hess grades 1 to 3 lesions. Approximately 70–90% of pregnant or non-pregnant patients following early repair of grade 1–3 lesions have good neurological recovery with low mortality rates between 1.7% and 8% [227]. Early repair permits the initiation of aggressive medical measures (triple-H therapy) and minimizes the potential for rebleeding and vasospasm. Patients with Hunt and Hess grade 4 and 5 lesions have a poor prognosis with (high operative mortality) or without early surgical intervention.

Endovascular occlusion therapy

Either neurosurgical clipping or the endovascular approach using Guglielmi detachable coils can provide definitive treatment for ruptured or unruptured aneurysms. The former technique has been shown to reduce maternal mortality from 63% to 11% and fetal mortality from 27% to 5% in non-surgically treated patients although figures are not adjusted for maternal clinical grade [177,183]. Temporary neurosurgical clipping may be preferable during pregnancy in order to avoid hypotension and hypothermia which might cause placental insufficiency [228]. Endovascular occlusion therapy has become a promising and safe alternative technique to open clipping in the pregnant patient with reports of good maternal and fetal outcomes [229–233]. The procedure involves intravascular delivery of occlusive devices to the aneurysm or AVM. Metal coils are placed within the lesion in order accomplish thrombosis formation and occlusion. Recently two pregnant patients were treated successfully with endovascular coils, including one patient who went on to have a successful term vaginal delivery [231]. Coil embolization was studied in 1383 patients with complete and partial occlusion of a cerebral aneurysm in 54% and 90% respectively, while 3.7% experienced complications which led to permanent neurologic deficits [233]. In the International Subarachnoid Hemorrhage Trial, endovascular coiling was associated with a significant relative risk reduction (22.6%, 95% CI 8.9–34.2%) and absolute risk reduction (6.9%, 95% CI 2.5–11.3%) in dependency and death compared with neurosurgical clipping [234]. We are unaware of any data comparing treatment outcomes between neurosurgical clipping and endovascular approaches in the pregnant patient.

Obstetric considerations

If gestational age is <26 weeks at the time of aneurysm rupture, treatment is guided by neurosurgical recommendations that are based on clinical grade and prognosis of the lesion. If gestational age is ≥26 weeks, the aneurysm is treated in the context of need for delivery [179,235]. If the patient is not in labor and there is no evidence of fetal compromise, neurosurgical considerations take precedence over obstetric concerns [5]. If aneurysmal rupture has not been treated and there is risk of cerebral infarction, recurrent hemorrhage or hydrocephalus and delivery is imminent, cesarean delivery is recommended. Cesarean delivery is also recommended for delivery of a viable pregnancy in a pregnant patient with poor neurological status (Hunt and Hess grades 4,5], if there is concern for adequacy of prior aneurysm surgery, or if labor begins shortly after aneurysm surgery during the period at risk for symptomatic vasospasm and cerebral infarction [5]. In the patient in advanced labor for whom vaginal delivery is chosen, epidural anesthesia is recommended to shorten the second stage of labor and reduce the time spent "bearing down." If aneurysm rupture occurs during labor, the patient may require cesarean delivery in order to reduce fetal exposure to anesthetics and other treatments followed by definitive aneurysm treatment [5]. If the aneurysm is treated and the patient is in good neurological condition, there is no neurosurgical contraindication to vaginal delivery in the future. If an aneurysm ruptures postpartum, the patient is treated as if she were not pregnant [179].

Subarachoid hemorrhage: arteriovenous malformations (AVMs)

General

The prevalence of AVMs in the United States is estimated at 1/1000 [236]. Approximately 53% of patients with an AVM will present with a hemorrhage [5]. The crude annual risk of first hemorrhage from an unruptured AVM is approximately 2%, but the risk of recurrent hemorrhage may be as high as 18% the first year, with uncertain risk thereafter [237–238]. The long-term crude annual case fatality rate is 1–1.5%. In two series, the rate of AVM rupture during pregnancy varied from 3.5% [239] to 9.3% [240] with the greatest risk during the second trimester. The risk may extend into the third trimester and may be exaggerated by the hemodynamic stresses of parturition [241].

Management

Management of a ruptured AVM follow similar medical management issues as enumerated previously for SAH in general. Although rebleeding of an AVM occurs in an estimated 27% of pregnant patients following an initial bleed [242], there is no consensus guideline for the prevention of rebleeding with AVM during pregnancy [9] and the timing and mode of repair remain controversial. Before 1990 it was demonstrated that antepartum resection of AVM is not beneficial to mother or fetus, with maternal mortality rates of 23–32% and fetal mortality rates from 0% to 23% [177]. Subsequently some surgeons advocated operative intervention only to remove clinically significant hematomas [243,177]. At this time, indications for AVM treatment include the patient considered to be at significant risk of hemorrhage, medically refractory seizures, progressive neurologic deficit, and intractable headaches [5]. As advances in endovascular therapy are made to provide an alternative mode of thereapy, this approach might be used successfully in the pregnant patient. Both open surgical excision and endovascular embolization are options, and most patients will benefit from multimodal therapy. Neurosurgeons determine the most appropriate treatment strategy for a given patient by considering her age, neurologic status, lesion size and location, associated clinical risk factors, and angioarchitectural features of the lesion. Despite its success outside pregnancy, radiosurgery is not considered useful during gestation because obliteration of the AVM may require 2–3 years.

Ischemic stroke other than cerebral vein thrombosis

General

The pregnant patient can suffer ischemic stroke other than in the central venous sinuses around delivery and during the puerperium. Because pregnancy is considered to be a "hypercoagulable" state to some degree, the incidence of thromboembolic phenomenon is heightened. Cerebral infarctions from thromboses can therefore cause CVA theoretically at any time during pregnancy and the puerperium. The presence of a genetic or acquired thrombophilia further predisposes the gravid female to this type of event. The most common of these are antiphospholipid antibody syndrome; protein C, S, and antithrombin III deficiency; and the Factor V Leiden mutation leading to activated protein C deficiency. Elevated levels of homocysteine and a mutation in the prothrombin gene have been implicated in an increased risk of thrombosis.

Symptomatology

Presenting symptoms are non-specific and mimic those of pre-eclampsia which can delay diagnosis. As with hemorrhagic events, the most common symptom is headache. Sudden or progressively worsening focal neurological deficits, visual changes, and seizures are also common. Imaging considerations are similar to those outlined for patients with suspected CVT. Any pregnant patient who suffers an acute thrombotic stroke is a candidate for a thorough thrombophilia evaluation. EEG, echocardiography, and/or carotid dopplers can further help to elucidate the cause of embolic events. Importantly, the underlying cause of an ischemic CVA need not be known before consideration for, and initiation of, thrombolytic therapy.

Thrombolytic therapy

The rare and unpredictable nature of CVA during pregnancy prevents the undertaking of any controlled trials of the efficacy of thrombolytic therapy for ischemic stroke. Thus the scientific worth of even large numbers of recent case reports and case series related to this issue must be interpreted with caution because it is largely anecdotal. At this time, recombinant tissue plasminogen activator (rt-PA, Alteplase) is the most widely used drug for the treatment of acute ischemic stroke in the non-pregnant patient. It is FDA approved for this indication and the highest success rates are achieved when there is strict adherence to the recommendations promulgated by the National Institute of Neurological Disorders (NINDS) rt-PA Stroke Study Group [244]. The incidence of symptomatic intracranial hemorrhage was 11% when there were deviations of practice in contrast to only 4% in patients who were treated according to the NINDS guidelines [245]. Patients properly treated with rt-PA for acute ischemic stroke were at least 30% more likely to have minimal or absent disability at 3 months as compared to patients who received placebo. Other recognized uses of rt-PA include treatment of massive pulmonary emboli, myocardial infarction and thrombosis of prosthetic heart valves. rt-PA has become the preferred thrombolytic agent over other thrombolytics streptokinase and urokinase. This is due to its high fibrin specificity, absence of antigenicity, short serum half-life and its demonstrated potential to establish reperfusion [40]. The large molecular weight of the drug prevents transit across the placenta, a desirable characteristic in the pregnant patient. In the non-pregnant patient, the use of rt-PA for thrombolysis of acute ischemic stroke is well established. In a meta-analysis of 15 published, open label studies involving 2639 patients, the primary complication was infrequent intracerebral hemorrhage in 5.2% of cases [246]. In contrast to successful experience with rt-PA, three trials of streptokinase for treatment of ischemic stroke were halted prematurely because of an excess of poor outcomes or deaths among treated patients [247–250].

rt-PA utilization by protocol

The FDA lists rt-PA as a category C drug; its use is not contraindicated in pregnancy or within the first postpartum week. Patients must meet the established eligibility criteria in order to be considered as viable candidates for the administration of rt-PA (Table 19.4). In the case of ischemic stroke the drug should be administered within 3 hours of symptom onset at a typical dose of 0.9 mg/kg of maternal body weight (maximum, 90 mg). The first 10% of the dose is given as a bolus followed by delivery of the remaining 90% as a constant infusion over a period of 60 minutes [244]. Although rt-PA administration is typically intravenous, some experts advocate the microcatheter-directed intra-arterial route as reported recently during pregnancy with excellent maternal and fetal outcome [251–252]. Overall, a net benefit of

Table 19.4 Treatment considerations – rt-PA for acute ischemic stroke [270,271].

INCLUSION CRITERIA

* Clinical diagnosis of acute ischemic stroke causing a measurable neurologic deficit
* Onset of symptoms within 3 hours of the initiation of treatment
* Patient or family understand the potential risks and benefits from treatment

EXCLUSION CRITERIA

Head CT scan

* Reveals evidence of hemorrhage
* Reveals evidence of a multilobar infarction (hypodensity >1/3 cerebral hemisphere)

Clinical

* Neurological signs/symptoms are minor/ isolated/ clearing spontaneously
* Neurological signs/symptoms are suggestive of subarachnoid hemorrhage even if the CT is normal
* Seizure(s) with postictal residual neurologic impairments
* Evidence of active bleeding or acute trauma (fracture)
* Persistent blood pressure elevation (systolic ≥185 mmHg, diastolic ≥110 mmHg)

or requiring aggressive antihypertensive therapy

History

* Any history of a previous intracranial hemorrhage
* Myocardial infarction, head trauma, or prior stroke within the previous 3 months
* Gastrointestinal or urinary tract hemorrhage in the previous 21 days
* Major surgery in the previous 14 days
* Arterial puncture at a non-compressible site in the previous 7 days

Laboratory

* Platelet count <100 000 mm^3
* Blood glucose concentration <50 mg/dL (2.7 mmol/L)
* INR > 1.7 if taking an oral anticoagulant
* Elevated activated partial thromboplastin time (aPTT) if receiving heparin in the previous 48 hours

[Adapted from Adams [270] and Caplan [271]]

combined intravenous and intra-arterial thrombolysis has been demonstrated in patients with acute ischemic stroke [251,253]. Any physician(s) considering rt-PA administration should be familiar with its use and follow the American Heart Association/ American Stroke Association "Guidelines for the Early Management of Adults With Ischemic Stroke," recently updated at the website http://stroke.ahajournals.org/cgi/reprint/38/5/1655 [254].

Pregnancy utilization

The most recent review of rt-PA thrombolytic therapy in pregnancy included data from 28 patients who were treated for a variety of indications including CVA (n = 10), thrombosis of cardiac valve prosthesis (n = 7), pulmonary embolism (n = 7), deep vein thrombosis (n = 3), and myocardial infarction (n = 1) [40]. Thrombolysis was successful in 25 of the 28 patients and two patients died (7%), but their deaths were not directly related to the application of rt-PA. In one case the underlying disease and in the other case the mechanical manipulation with subsequent vascular lesions were fatal factors. This compares favorably to the case fatality rate of 6.1–6.3% in the large randomized rt-PA stroke trials involving non-pregnant patients [255,256]. Six of 25 progeny in the surviving patients were lost (24%), three due to pregnancy termination for maternal indications and one prematurity-related neonatal loss. Thus in only two cases at most (8%) is there potentially a causal relationship between fetal death and rt-PA utilization [40]. The complication rate for rt-PA thrombolysis in the pregnant gravid is comparable to that observed in large randomized controlled trials involving non-pregnant patients. Intracranial hemorrhage, something not yet reported in rt-PA treated pregnant patients, occurs in 10.8–19.8% of non-pregnant patients [255,256]. The rate of spontaneous abortion and stillbirth (8%) after thrombolytic therapy is slightly higher than the general population [257,258]. Permanent sequelae have not been observed in the surviving children and to this date there have been no postmarketing reports of teratogenicity associated with the rt-PA use.

There are multiple case reports albeit no controlled studies which nevertheless demonstrate that thrombolysis with rt-PA can be used for the treatment of acute ischemic stroke in the pregnant patient with apparent safety, good maternal-fetal outcome and a relatively low complication rate. Presently there is insufficient data of high quality from which to derive guidelines for pregnancy use. At this time however it may not be justified to withhold rt-PA thrombolytic therapy from the pregnant patient if effective alternatives are lacking [40]. As demonstrated by the recent report of successful use of intra-arterial urokinase to treat a CVA immediately postpartum following cesarean delivery, thrombolytic therapy for ischemic stroke clearly becomes an option after the fetus leaves the uterus [259].

Risk of recurrence in subsequent pregnancy

The risk of recurrent ischemic stroke in a subsequent pregnancy is very low. The French Study Group on Stroke in Pregnancy followed 441 women for 5 years following a pregnancy complicated by arterial ischemic stroke (n = 373) or CVT (n = 68) [260]. Approximately 50% of these women received antiplatelet therapy during at least a portion of the subsequent pregnancy. Women with a history of prior CVT received heparin in the postpartum period but no therapy during pregnancy itself. In 187 subsequent pregnancies there were only two recurrent strokes and no cases of recurrent CVT. Eleven CVAs occurred outside of pregnancy. Thus the absolute risk of recurrence outside of pregnancy was 0.5% (95% CI 0.3–0.9) and rose to 1.8% (95% CI 0.5–7.5) during subsequent pregnancy and the puerperium [260,11]. Similar results were reported for 23 women with a history of stroke who had 35 subsequent pregnancies without CVA recurrence despite only 11 patients receiving any form of anticoagulation during any portion of the subsequent pregnancy [261]. Pregnant patients with a history of thrombophilia, however, are at some risk of CVA recurrence as shown in one recent patient series of 20 patients with thrombophilia and a 20% recurrence rate of stroke [262]. Thus in the absence of a known thrombophilia, the risk of recurrent stroke in subsequent pregnancy is 0–1% and should not be considered a contraindication to repeat pregnancy [260,261].

Prevention of recurrent ischemic stroke in at-risk patients

There is no consensus on how thromboprophylaxis should be used in the pregnant patient with a prior ischemic stroke and a reason (thrombophilia) to consider risk reduction for potential recurrence [263]. If the patient had a prior arterial ischemic stroke without a high-risk cardiac source of embolism, low-dose aspirin therapy (<150 mg/day) is recommended [11]. A number of studies have demonstrated that low-dose aspirin is safe for both mother and fetus in the second and third trimester [263–265]. Use in the first trimester should only be undertaken after weighing the risks and benefits with the patient. Consideration should be given to continuing low-dose aspirin during the postpartum period. Although the efficacy of this in postpartum stroke prevention has not been studied, the use of low-dose aspirin has been found to be safe during the postpartum/breastfeeding period [266,267]. The efficacy of other antiplatelet agents such as ticlopidine, clopidigrel, and dypiridimole for recurrent stroke prevention has not been established.

References

1 Donaldson JO, Lee NS. Arterial and venous stroke associated with pregnancy. *Neurol Clin* 1994; 12(3): 583–599.

2 Witlin AG, Friedman SA, Egerman RS, Frangieh AY, Sibai BM. Cerebrovascular disorders complicating pregnancy – beyond eclampsia. *Am J Obstet Gynecol* 1997; 176: 139–148.

3 James AH, Bushnell CD, Jamison MG, Myers ER. Incidence and risk factors for stroke in pregnancy and the puerperium. *Obstet Gynecol* 2005; 106: 509–516.

4 Kittner SJ, Stern BJ, Wozniak M et al. Cerebral infarction in young adults: the Baltimore-Washington Cooperative Young Stroke Study. *Neurology* 1998; 50: 890–894.

5 Sloan MA, Stern BJ. Cerebrovascular disease in pregnancy. *Curr Treatment Options Neurol* 2003; 5: 391–407.

6 Pettiti DB, Sidney S, Quesenberry CP, Bernstein A. Incidence of stroke and myocardial infarction in women of reproductive age. *Stroke* 1997; 28: 280–283.

7 Mas JL, Lamy C. Stroke in pregnancy and the puerperium. *J Neurol* 1998; 245: 305–313.

8 Pathan M, Kittner SJ. Pregnancy and stroke. *Curr Neurol Neuroscience Rep* 2003; 3: 27–31.

9 Turan TN, Stern BJ. Stroke in pregnancy. *Neurol Clin* 2004; 22: 821–840.

10 Sibai BM, Coppage KH. Diagnosis and management of women with stroke during pregnancy/postpartum. *Clin Perinatol* 2004; 31: 853–868.

11 Helms AK, Kittner SJ. Pregnancy and stroke. *CNS Spectrums* 2005; 10: 580–587.

12 Hender J, Harris DG, Bu H, Richard B, Khanna PB. Stroke in pregnancy. *Brit J Hosp Med* 2006; 67: 129–131.

13 Cantu C, Baringarrementeria F. Cerebral venous thrombosis associated with pregnancy and the puerperium: review of 67 cases. *Stroke* 1993; 24: 1880–1884.

14 Grosset DG, Ebrahim S. Stroke in pregnancy and the puerperium: what magnitude of risk? *J Neurol Neurosurg Psych* 1995; 58: 129–131.

15 Sharshar T, Lamy C, Mas JL. Incidence and causes of strokes associated with pregnancy and puerperium: a study in public hospitals of Ile de France. Stroke in Pregnancy Study Group. *Stroke* 1995; 26: 930–936.

16 Kittner SJ, Stern BJ, Feeser BR et al. Pregnancy and the risk of stroke. *NEJM* 1996; 335: 768–774.

17 Lanska DJ, Kryscio RJ. Peripartum stroke and intracranial venous thrombosis in the national Hospital Discharge Hospital Survey. *Obstet Gynecol* 1997; 89: 413–418.

18 Lanska DJ, Kryscio RJ. Stroke and intracranial venous thrombosis during pregnancy and puerperium. *Neurology* 1998; 51: 1622–1628.

19 Lanska DJ, Kryscio RJ. Risk factors for peripartum and postpartum stroke and intracranial venous thrombosis. *Stroke* 2000; 31: 1274–1282.

20 Witlin AG, Mattar F, Sibai BM. Postpartum stroke: a twenty-year experience. *Am J Obstet Gynecol* 2000; 183: 83–88.

21 Quereshi AI, Giles WH, Croft JB, Stern BJ. Number of pregnancies and risk for stroke and stroke subtypes. *Arch Neurol* 1997; 54: 203–206.

22 Jaigobin C, Silver FL. Stroke and pregnancy. *Stroke* 2000; 31: 2948–2951.

23 Dias MS, Sekhar LN. Intracranial hemorrhage from aneurysms and arteriovenous malformations during pregnancy and the puerperium. *Neurosurgery* 1990; 27: 855–866.

24 Trivedi RA, Kirkpatrick PJ. Arteriovenous malformations of the cerebral circulation that rupture in pregnancy. *J Obstet Gynaecol* 2003; 23(5): 484–489.

25 Bateman BT, Schumacher HC, Bushnell CD, Pile-Spellman J, Simpson LL, Sacco RL, Berman MF. Intracerebral hemorrhage in pregnancy. *Neurology* 2006; 67: 424–429.

26 Skidmore FM, Williams LS, Fradkin KD, Alonso RJ, Biller J. Presentation, etiology, and outcome of stroke in pregnancy and puerperium. *J Stroke Cerebrovasc Dis* 2001; 10: 1–10.

27 Sadasivan B, Malik GM, Lee C, Ausman JI. Vascular malformations and pregnancy. *Surg Neurol* 1990; 33: 305–313.

28 Liang CC, Chang SD, Lai SL, Hsieh CC, Chueh HY, Lee TH. Stroke complicating pregnancy and the puerperium. *Eur J Neurol* 2005; 13: 1256–1260.

29 Awada A, Al Rajeh S, Duarte R, Russell N. Stroke and pregnancy. *Internat J Gynecol Obstet* 1995; 48: 157–161.

30 Bashiri A, Lazer T, Burstein E, Smolin A, Lazer S, Perry ZH, Mazor M. Maternal and neonatal otucome following cerebrovascular accidents during pregnancy. *J Maternal-Fetal Neonatal Med* 2007; 20(3): 241–247.

31 Simolke GA, Cox SM, Cunningham FG. Cerebrovascular accidents complicating pregnancy and the puerperium. *Obstet Gynecol* 1991; 78: 37–42.

32 Jeng JS, Tang SC, Yip PK. Stroke in women of reproductive age: comparison between stroke related and unrelated to pregnancy. *J Neurol Sci* 2004; 221: 25–29.

33 Jeng JS, Tang SC, Yip PK. Incidence and etiologies of stroke during pregnancy and puerperium as evidenced in Taiwanese women. *Cerebrovascular Dis* 2004; 18: 290–295.

34 Wiebers DO. Ischaemic cerebrovascular complications of pregnancy. *Arch Neurol* 1985; 24: 1106–1113.

35 Ros HS, Lichtenstein P, Bellocco R, Petersson G, Cnattingius S. Pulmonary embolism and stroke in relation to pregnancy: how can high-risk women be identified? *Am J Obstet Gynecol* 2002; 186: 198–203.

36 Schwartz RB. Neuroradiographic imaging: techniques and safety considerations. *Adv Neurol* 2002; 90: 1–8.

37 ACOG Committee Opinion Number 299: *Guidelines for diagnostic imaging during pregnancy*. September 2004.

38 Garel C, Brisse H, Sebag G, Elmaleh M, Oury JF, Hassan M. Magnetic resonance imaging of the fetus. *Pediatr Radiol* 1998; 28: 201–211.

39 Gilberti L, Bino G, Tanganelli P. Pregnancy, patient foramen ovale and stroke: a case of pseudoperipheral facial palsy. *Neurol Sci* 2005; 26: 43–45.

40 Leonhardt G, Gaul C, Nietsch HH, Buerke M, Schleussner E. Thrombolytic therapy in pregnancy. *J Thromb Thrombolysis* 2006; 21: 271–276.

41 Wiese KM, Talkad A, Mathews M, Wang D. Intravenous recombinant tissue plasminogen activator in a pregnant woman with cardioembolic stroke. *Stroke* 2006; 37: 168–169.

42 Johnson DM, Kramer DC, Cohen E, Rochon M, Rosner M, Weinberger J. Thrombolytic therapy for acute stroke in late pregnancy with intra-arterial recombinant tissue plasminogen activator. *Stroke* 2005; 36: 53–55.

43 Belfort MA, Allen J, Saade G et al. Changes in flow velocity, resistance indices, and cerebral perfusion pressure in the maternal middle cerebral artery distribution during normal pregnancy. *Acta Obstet Gynecol Scand* 2001; 80: 104–112.

44 Zeeman GG, Hatab MR, Twickler DM. Increased cerebral blood flow in preeclampsia with magnetic resonance imaging. *Am J Obstet Gynecol* 2004; 191: 1425–1429.

45 Belfort MA, Varner MW, Dizon-Townson DS et al. Cerebral perfusion pressure, and not cerebral blood flow, may be the critical determinant of intracranial injury in preeclampsia: a new hypothesis. *Am J Obstet Gynecol* 2002; 187: 626–634.

46 Belfort MA, Clark SL, Sibai B. Cerebral hemodynamics in preeclampsia: cerebral perfusion and the rationale for an alternative to magnesium sulfate. *Obstet Gynecol Surv* 2006; 61: 655–665.

47 Kontos HA. Validity of cerebral arterial blood flow calculations from velocity measurements. *Stroke* 1989; 20: 1–3.

48 Cipolla MJ. Cerebrovascular function in pregnancy and eclampsia. *Hypertension* 2007; 50: 14–24.

49 Strandgaard S, Paulson OB. Cerebral autoregulation. *Stroke* 1984; 15: 413–416.

50 Chester EM, Agamanolis DP, Banker BQ et al. Hypertensive encephalopathy: a clinicopathologic study of 20 cases. *Neurol* 1977; 28: 928–939.

51 Schwartz RB, Jones KM, Kalina P et al. Hypertensive encephalopathy: findings on CT, MR imaging, and SPECT imaging in 14 cases. *Am J Radiol* 1992; 159: 379–383.

52 Kestenbaum B, Seliger SL, Easterling TR, Gillen DL, Critchlow CW, Stehman-Breen CO, Schwartz SM. Cardiovascular and thromboembolic events following hypertensive pregnancy. *Am J Kidney Dis* 2003; 42: 982–989.

53 Wilson BJ, Watson MS, Prescott GJ, Sunderland S, Campbell DM, Hannaford P, Smith WCS. Hypertensive diseases of pregnancy and risk of hypertension and stroke in later life: results from cohort study. *Brit Med J* 2003; 326: 845–851.

54 Brown DW, Dueker N, Jamieson DJ, Cole JW, Wozniak MA, Stern BJ, Giles WH, Kittner SJ. Preeclampsia and the risk of ischemic stroke among young women: results from the Stroke Prevention in Young Women Study. *Stroke* 2006; 37: 1055–1059.

55 Ness RB, Markovic N, Bass D, Harger G, Roberts JM. Family history of hypertension, heart disease, and stroke among women who develop hypertension in pregnancy. *Obstet Gynecol* 2003; 102: 1366–1371.

56 Okanloma KA, Moodley J. Neurological complications associated with the preeclampsia/eclampsia syndrome. *Int J Gynaecol Obstet* 2000; 71: 223–225.

57 Moodley J. Preeclampsia/eclampsia syndrome. *S Afr J Contin Med Educ* 1997; 15: 31–41.

58 Isler CM, Rinehart BK, Terrone DA, Martin RW, Magann EF, Martin JN Jr. Maternal mortality associated with HELLP (hemolysis, elevated liver enzymes, and low platelets) syndrome. *Am J Obstet Gynecol* 1999; 181: 924–928.

59 Angulo-Vazquez J et al. Mortalidad maternal en el Hospital de Gineco Obstetrica del Centro Medico Nacional de Occidente: Revision de 12 anos. *Ginecol Obstet Mex* 1999; 67: 419–424.

60 Argueta Zuniga M et al. Sincrome HELLP. Siete anos de experience en al Instituto Nacional de Perinatologia. *Ginecol Obstet Mex* 1995; 63: 217–221.

61 Martin JN Jr, Thigpen BD, Moore RC, Rose CH, Cushman J, May W. Stroke and severe preeclampsia and eclampsia: a paradigm shift focusing on systolic blood pressure. *Obstet Gynecol* 2005; 105: 246–254.

62 Cunningham FG. Severe preeclampsia and eclampsia: systolic hypertension is also important. *Obstet Gynecol* 2005; 105(2): 237–238.

63 Report of the National High Blood Pressure Education Program Working Group on High Blood Pressure in Pregnancy. *Am J Obstet Gynecol* 2000; 183: S1–S22.

64 Belfort MA, Varner MW, Dizon-Townson DS et al. Cerebral perfusion pressure, and not cerebral blood flow, may be the critical determinant of intracranial injury in preeclampsia: a new hypothesis. *Am J Obstet Gynecol* 2002; 187: 626–634.

65 Riskin-Mashiah S, Belfort MA, Saade GR, Herd JA. Cerebrovascular reactivity in normal pregnancy and preeclampsia. *Obstet Gynecol* 2001; 98: 827–832.

66 Brackley KJ, Ramsay MM, Pipkin FB, Rubin PC. The maternal cerebral circulation in preeclampsia: investigations using Laplace transform analysis of Doppler waveforms. *Brit J Obstet Gynaecol* 2000; 107: 492–500.

67 Belfort MA, Saade GR, Grunewald C, Dildy GA, Abedejos P, Herd JA, Nisell H. Association of cerebral perfusion pressure with headache in women with preeclampsia. *BJOG* 1999; 106: 814–821.

68 Demarin V, Rundek T, Hodek B. Maternal cerebral circulation in normal and abnormal pregnancies. *Acta Obstet Gyn Scand* 1997; 76: 619–624.

69 Ohno Y, Kawai M, Wakahara Y, Kitagawa T, Kakihara M, Arii Y. Transcranial assessment of maternal cerebral blood flow velocity in patients with preeclampsia. *Acta Obstet Gynecol Scand* 1997; 76: 928–932.

70 Riskin-Mashiah S, Belfort MA, Saade GF, Herd JA. Transcranial Doppler measurement of cerebral velocity indices as a predictor of preeclampsia. *Am J Obstet Gynecol* 2002; 187: 1667–1672.

71 Riskin-Mashiah S, Belfort MA. Cerebrovascular hemodynamics in chronic hypertensive pregnant women who later develop superimposed preeclampsia. *J Soc Gynecol Investig* 2005; 12: 28–32.

72 Williams KP, McLean C. Peripartum changes in maternal cerebral blood flow velocity in normotensive and preeclamptic patients. *Obstet Gynecol* 1993; 82: 334–337.

73 Vliegen JHR, Muskens E, Keunen RWM, Smith SJ, Godfried WH, Gerretsen G. Abnormal cerebral hemodynamics in pregnancy-related hypertensive encephalopathy. *Eur J Ob Gyn Reprod Biol* 1993; 49: 198–200.

74 Giannina G, Belfort MA, Cruz AL, Herd JA. Persistent cerebrovascular changes in postpartum preeclamptic women: a Doppler evaluation. *Am J Obstet Gynecol* 1997; 177: 1213–1218.

75 Belfort MA, Grunewald C, Saade GR, Varner M, Nisell H. Preeclampsia may cause both overperfusion and underperfusion of the brain: a cerebral perfusion model. *Acta Obstet Gynecol Scand* 1999; 78: 586–591.

76 Zunker P, Happe S, Georgiadis AL, Louwen F, Georgiadis D, Ringelstein EB, Holzgreve W. Maternal cerebral hemodynamics in pregnancy-related hypertension. A prospective transcranial Doppler study. *Ultr Obstet Gynecol* 2000; 16: 179–187.

77 Williams KP, Wilson S. Persistence of cerebral hemodynamic changes in patients with eclampsia: a report of three cases. *Am J Obstet Gynecol* 1999; 181: 1162–1165.

78 Cipolla MJ, Delance N, Vitullo L. Pregnancy prevents hypertensive remodeling of cerebral arteries: a potential role in the development of eclampsia. *Hypertension* 2006; 47: 619–626.

79 Cipolla MJ, Vitullo L, DeLance N, Hammer E. The cerebral endothelium during pregnancy: a potential role in the development of eclampsia. *Endothelium* 2005; 12: 5–9.

80 Oehm E, Reinhard M, Keck C, Els T, Spreer J, Hetzel A. Impaired dynamic cerebral autoregulation in eclampsia. *Ultrasound Obstet Gynecol* 2003; 22(4): 395–398.

81 Zunker P, Golombeck K, Brossmann J, Georgiadis D, Deuschl G. Postpartum cerebral angiopathy: repetitive TCD, MRI, MRA and EEG examinations. *Neurol Res* 2002; 24: 570–572.

82 Knopp U, Kehler U, Rickmann H, Arnold H, Gliemroth J. Cerebral haemodynamic pathologies in HELLP syndrome. *Clin Neurol Neurosurg* 2003; 105: 256–261.

83 Feske SK, Sperling RA, Schwartz RB. Extensive reversible brain magnetic resonance lesions in a patient with HELLP syndrome. *J Neuroimag* 1997; 7: 247–250.

84 Imaizumi H, Nara S, Kaneko M, Chiba S, Tamakawa M. Magnetic resonance evaluation of brainstem dysfunction in eclampsia and the HELLP syndrome. *J Emer Med* 1995; 13: 191–194.

85 Marano E, Scuteri N, Vacca G, Orefice G. HELLP syndrome with reversible posterior leukoencephalopathy. *Neurol Sci* 2003; 24: 82–84.

86 Fujiwara Y, Higaki H, Yamada T, Nakata Y, Kato S, Yammamoto H, Ito R, Yamaki J. Two cases of reversible posterior leukoencephalopathy syndrome, one with and the other without pre-eclampsia. *J Obstet Gynaecol* 2005; 31: 520–526.

87 Bartynski WS, Sanghvi A. Neuroimaging of delayed eclampsia: report of 3 cases and review of the literature. *J Comput Assist Tomogr* 2003; 27: 699–713.

88 Gliemroth J, Knopp U, Kehler JU, Felberbaum R, Nowak G. HELLP syndrome with haemoglobin vasospasm. *J Clin Neurosci* 2000; 7: 59–62.

89 Altamara C, Vasapollo B, Tibuzzi F, Novelli GP, Valensise H, Rossini PM, Vernieri F. Postpartum cerebellar infarction and haemolysis, elevated liver enzymes, low platelet (HELLP) syndrome. *Neurol Sci* 2005; 26: 40–42.

90 Ziedman LA, Videnovic A, Bernstein LP, Pellar CA. Lethal pontine hemorrhage in postpartum syndrome of hemolysis, elevated liver enzyme levels, and low platelet count. *Arch Neurol* 2005; 62: 1150–1153.

91 Hashiguchi K, Inamura T, Irita K, Abe M, Noda E, Yanai S, Takahashi S, Fukui M. Late occurrence of diffuse cerebral swelling after intracranial hemorrhage in a patient with the HELLP syndrome. *Neurol Med Chir* 2001; 41: 144–148.

92 Osmanagaoglu MA, Dinc G, Osmanagaoglu S, Dinc H, Bozkaya H. Comparison of cerebral magnetic resonance and electroencephalogram findings in preeclamptic and eclamptic women. *Austr NZJ Obstet Gynaecol* 2005; 45: 384–390.

93 Ezri T, Abouleish E, Lee C, Evron S. Intracranial subdural hematoma following dural puncture in a parturient with HELLP syndrome. *Can J Anesth* 2002; 49: 820–823.

94 Shah AK. Non-aneurysmal primary subarachnoid hemorrhage inpregnancy-induced hypertension and eclampsia. *Neurology* 2003; 61: 117–120.

95 Giannina G, Smith D, Belfort MA, Moise KJ Jr. Atraumatic subdural hematoma associated with preeclampsia. *J Mat Fetal Med* 1997; 6: 93–95.

96 Housni B, Bayad R, Cherkab R, Salmi S, Miguil M. Brainstem ischemia and preeclampsia. *Hyperten Pregnancy* 2004; 23: 269–273.

97 Norwitz ER, Hsu CD, Repke JT. Acute complications of preeclampsia. *Clin Obstet Gynecol* 2002; 45: 308–329.

98 Do DV, Rismondo V, Nguyen QD. Reversible cortical blindness in preeclampsia. *Am J Ophthal* 2002; 134: 916–918.

99 Apollon KM, Robinson JN, Schwartz RB, Norwitz ER. Cortical blindness in severe preeclampsia: computed tomography, magnetic resonance imaging, and single photon emission computed tomography findings. *Obstet Gynecol* 2000; 95: 1017–1019.

100 Moseman CP, Shelton S. Permanent blindness as a complication of pregnancy-induced hypertension. *Obstet Gynecol* 2002; 100: 943–945.

101 Naidu S, Payne AJ, Moodley J, Hoffman M, Gouws E. Randomized study assessing the effect of phenytoin and magnesium sulphate on maternal cerebral circulation in eclampsia using transcranial Doppler ultrasound. *BJOG* 1996; 103: 111–116.

102 Belfort MA, Saade GR, Yared M, Grunewald C, Herd JA, Varner MA, Nisell H. Change in estimated cerebral perfusion pressure after treatment with nimodipine or magnesium sulfate in patients with preeclampsia. *Am J Obstet Gynecol* 1999; 181: 402–407.

103 Van Zwieten PA. An overview of the pharmacodynamic properties and therapeutic potential of combined alpha- and beta-adrenoceptor antagonists. *Drugs* 1993; 45: 509–517.

104 Blakeley AG, Summers RJ. The pharmacology of labetalol, an alpha and beta-adrenoreceptor blocking agent. *Gen Pharmacol* 1978; 9: 399–402.

105 ACOG Practice Bulletin Number 33: Diagnosis and management of preeclampsia and eclampsia. January 2002.

106 Ascarelli MH, Johnson V, McCreary H, Cushman J, May WL, Martin JN Jr. Postpartum preeclampsia management with furose-

mide: a randomized clinical trial. *Obstet Gynecol* 2005; 105(1): 29–33.

107 Carr DB, Bavrila D, Brateng D, Easterling TR. Maternal hemodynamic changes associated with furosemide treatment. *Hypertens Pregnancy* 2007; 26(2): 173–178.

108 Martin JN Jr, Rose CH, Briery CM. Understanding and managing HELLP syndrome: the integral role of aggressive glucocorticoids for mother and child. *Am J Obstet Gynecol* 2006; 195: 914–934.

109 Williams KP, Wilson S. Maternal middle cerebral artery velocity changes in HELLP syndrome versus preeclampsia. *Ultrasound Obstet Gynecol* 1998; 11: 195–198.

110 Stam J. Thrombosis of the cerebral veins and sinuses. *NEJM* 2005; 352: 1791–1798.

111 Cantu C, Barinagarrementeria F. Cerebral venous thrombosis associated with pregnancy and the puerperium: review of 67 cases. *Stroke* 1993; 24: 1880–1884.

112 Fink JN, McAuley DL. Cerebral venous sinus thrombosis: a diagnostic challenge. *Int Med J* 2001; 31: 384–390.

113 Sagduyu A, Sirin H, Mulayim S, Bademkiran F, Yunten N, Kitis O, Calli C, Dalbasti T, Kumral E. Cerebral cortical and deep venous thrombosis without sinus thrombosis: clinical MRI correlates. *Acta Neurol Scand* 2006; 114: 254–260.

114 Panagariya A, Maru A. Cerebral venous thrombosis in pregnancy and puerperium – a prospective study. *J Assoc Physicians India* 1997; 45: 857–859.

115 Appenzeller S, Zeller CB, Annichino-Bizzachi JM, Costallat LTL, Deus-Silva L, Voetsch B, Faria AV, Zanardi VA, Damasceno BP, Cendes F. Cerebral venous thrombosis: influence of risk factors and imaging findings on prognosis. *Clin Neurol Neurosurg* 2005; 107: 371–378.

116 Martin SR, Foley MR. Approach to the pregnant patient with headache. *Clin Obstet Gynecol* 2005; 48: 2–11.

117 Nazziola E. Dural sinus thrombosis presenting three months postpartum. *Ann Emerg Med* 2003; 42: 592–595.

118 Meniere P. Observations et reflexious sur l'hemorrhagie cerebrale consideree. Pendant la prossesse pendant et après l'accouchement. *Arch Gen Med* 1828; 16: 489.

119 Abercrombie J. *Pathological and Practical Researches on Diseases of the Brain and Spinal Cord*. Edinburgh: 1812, p83.

120 Symonds CP. Cerebral thrombophlebitis. *Brit Med J* 1940; 2: 348.

121 Martin JP, Sheehan HL. Primary thrombosis of cerebral veins following childbirth. *Brit Med J* 1941; 1: 349.

122 Martin JP. Thrombosis in the superior longitudinal sinus following childbirth. *Brit Med J* 1941; 2: 537.

123 Stansfield FR. Puerperal cerebral thrombophlebitis treated by heparin. *Brit Med J* 1942; 1: 436.

124 Bansal BC, Gupta RR, Prakash C. Stroke during pregnancy and puerperium in young females below the age of 40 years as a result of cerebral venous/venous sinus thrombosis. *Jap Heart J* 1980; 21: 171–183.

125 Srinivasan K. Cerebral venous and arterial thrombosis in pregnancy and puerperium: a study of 135 patients. *Angiology J Vasc Dis* 1983; 34: 731–746.

126 Bousser MG, Russell RR. *Cerebral Venous Thrombosis*. London: Saunders, 1997.

127 Bousser MG, Barnett HJM. Cerebral venous thrombosis. In: Barnett HJM, Mohr JP, Stein BM, Yatsu FM, eds. *Stroke: Pathophysiology, Diagnosis and Management*, 3rd edn. New York: Churchill Livingstone, 1997: 623–647.

128 Soleau SW, Schmidt R, Stevens S, Osborn A, MacDonald JD. Extensive experience with dural sinus thrombosis. *Neurosurg* 2003; 52: 542–544.

129 Wilterdink JL, Easton JD. Cerebral ischemia. In: Devinsky O, Feldmann E, Hainline B, eds. *Neurological complications of pregnancy*. New York: Raven Press, 1994: 1–11.

130 Cakmak S, Derex L, Betruyer M et al. Cerebral venous thrombosis: clinical outcome and systematic screening of prothrombotic factors. *Neurol* 2003; 60: 1175–1178.

131 Kapessidou Y, Vokaer M, Laureys M, Bier JC, Boogaerts JG. Case report: cerebral vein thrombosis after subarachnoid analgesia for labour. *Can J Anesth* 2006; 53: 1015–1019.

132 Ferro JM, Canhao P, Stam J, Bousser MG, Barinagarrementeria F. Prognosis of cerebral vein and dural sinus thrombosis: results of the International Study on Cerebral Vein and Dural Sinus Thrombosis (ISCVT). *Stroke* 2004; 35: 664–670.

133 Kothare SV, Ebb DH, Rosenberger PB, Buonanno F, Schaefer PW, Krishnamoorthy KS. Acute confusion and mutism as a presentation of thalamic strokes secondary to deep cerebral venous thrombosis. *J Child Neurol* 1998; 13: 300–303.

134 Lafitte F, Boukobza M, Guichard JP et al. MRI and MRA for diagnosis and follow-up of cerebral venous thrombosis (CVT). *Clin Radiol* 1997; 52: 672–679.

135 Dormont D, Anxionnat R, Evrard S, Louaille C, Chiras J, Marsault C. MRI in cerebral venous thrombosis. *J Neuroradiol* 1994; 21: 81–99.

136 Curmurciuc R, Crassard I, Sarov M, Valade D, Bousser MG. Headache as the only neurological sign of cerebral venous thrombosis: A series of 17 cases. *J Neurol Neurosurg Psych* 2005; 76: 1084–1087.

137 Einhaupl KM, Villringer A, Meister W et al. Heparin treatment in sinus venous thrombosis. *Lancet* 1991; 338: 597–600. (Erratum, *Lancet* 1991; 338: 958.)

138 De Bruijn SF, Stam J. Randomized, placebo-controlled trial of anticoagulant treatment with low-molecular-weight heparin for cerebral sinus thrombosis. *Stroke* 1999; 30: 484–488.

139 Nagaraja D, Rao BSS, Taly AB, Subhash MN. Randomized controlled trial of heparin in puerperal cerebral venous/sinus thrombosis. *Nimhans J* 1995; 13: 111–115.

140 Ferro JM, Canhao P, Stam J, Bousser MG, Barinagarrementeria F, ISCVT Investigators. Prognosis of cerebral vein and dural sinus thrombosis: results of the International Study on Cerebral Vein and Dural Sinus Thrombosis (ISCVT). *Stroke* 2004; 35: 664–670.

141 Diaz JM, Schiffman JS, Urban ES, Maccario M. Superior sagittal sinus thrombosis and pulmonary embolism: a syndrome rediscovered. *Acta Neurol Scand* 1992; 86: 390–396.

142 Cole B, Criddle LM. A case of postpartum cerebral venous thrombosis. *J Neurosc Nurs* 2006; 38: 350–353.

143 Baker MD, Opatowsky MJ, Wilson JA, LGlazier SS, Morris PP. Rheolytic catheter and thrombolysis of dural venous sinus thrombosis: a case series. *Neurosurg* 2001; 48: 487–493.

144 Johnson DM, Kramer DC, Cohen E, Rochon M, Rosner M, Weinberger J. Thrombolytic therapy for acute stroke in late pregnancy with intra-arterial recombinant tissue plasminogen activator. *Stroke* 2005; 36: e53–e55.

145 Murugappan A, Coplin WM, Al-Sadat AN, McAllen KJ, Schwamm LH, Wechsler LR, Kidwell CS, Saver JL, Starkman S, Gobin YP, Duckwiler G, Krueger M, Rordorf G, Broderick JP, Tietjen GE,

Levine SR. Thrombolytic therapy of acute ischemic stroke during pregnancy. *Neurol* 2006; 66: 768–770.

146 Shaltoni HM, Albright KC, Gonzales NR, Weir RU, Khaja AM, Sugg RM, Campbell MS III, Cacayorin ED, Grotter JC, Noser EA. Is intra-arterial thrombolysis safe after full-dose intravenous recombinant tissue plasminogen activator for acute ischemic stroke? *Stroke* 2007; 38: 80–84.

147 Van der Stege JG, Engelen MJA, van Eyck J. Uncomplicated pregnancy and puerperium after puerperal CVT. *Eur J Ob Gyn Reprod Biol* 1997; 71: 99–100.

148 Ursell MR, Marras CL, Farb R, Rowed DW, Black SE, Perry JR. Recurrent intracranial hemorrhage due to postpartum cerebral angiopathy: implications for management. *Stroke* 1998; 29: 1995–1998.

149 Al-Sous W, Bohlega S, Al-Kawi Z, McLean D, Shukri KI. Postpartum cerebral angiopathy: a rare cerebrovascular complication. *Eur J Neurol* 1998; 5: 411–416.

150 Hinchey J, Chaves C, Appignani B, Breen J, Pao L, Wang A et al. A reversible posterior leukoencephalopathy syndrome. *NEJM* 1996; 334: 494–500.

151 Servillo G, Striano P, Striano S, Tortora F, Boccella P, DeRobertis E et al. Posterior reversible encephalopathy syndrome (PRES) in critically ill obstetric patients. *Int Care Med* 2003; 29: 2323–2326.

152 Konstantinopoulos PA, Mousa S, Khairallah R, Mtanos G. Postpartum cerebral angiopathy: an important diagnostic consideration in the postpartum period. *Am J Obstet Gynecol* 2004; 191: 375–377.

153 Call GK, Fleming MC, Sealfon S, Levine H, Kistler JP, Fisher CM. Reversible cerebral segmental vasoconstriction. *Stroke* 1988; 19: 1159–1170.

154 Singhal AB, Koroshetz W, Caplan LR. Cerebral vasoconstriction syndromes. In: Bogousslavsky J, Caplan RL (eds). *Uncommon Causes of Stroke.* Cambridge (UK): Cambridge University Press, 2001: 114–123.

155 Neudecker S, Stock K, Krasnianski M. Call-Fleming postpartum angiopathy in the puerperium: a reversible cerebral vasoconstriction syndrome. *Obstet Gynecol* 2006; 107: 446–449.

156 Calabrese LH, Furlan AJ, Gragg LA, Ropos TJ. Primary angiitis of the central nervous system: diagnostic criteria and clinical approach. *Cleve Clin J Med* 1992; 59: 293–306.

157 Varner MW. Cerebral vasculopathies masquerading as eclampsia. *Obstet Gynecol* 2006; 107: 437–438.

158 Belogolovkin V, Levine SR, Fields MC, Stone JL. Postpartum eclampsia complicated by reversible cerebral herniation. *Obstet Gynecol* 2006; 107: 442–445.

159 Geocadin RG, Razumovsky AY, Wityk RJ, Bhardwaj A, Ulatowski JA. Intracerebral hemorrhage and postpartum cerebral vasculopathy. *J Neurol Sci* 2002; 205: 29–34.

160 Fett JD. Peripartum cardiomyopathy: Insights from Haiti regarding a disease of unknown etiology. *Minn Med* 2002; 85: 46–48.

161 Ford RF, Barton JR, O'Brien JM, Hollingsworth PW. Demographics, management and outcome of peripartum cardiomyopathy in a community hospital. *Am J Obstet Gynecol* 2000; 182: 1036–1038.

162 Kozelj M, Novak-Antolic Z, Grad A, Peternel P. Patent foramen ovale as a potential cause of paradoxical embolism in the postpartum period. *Eur J Obstet Gynecol Repro Biol* 1999; 84: 55–57.

163 Giberti L, Bino G, Tanganelli P. Pregnancy, patient foramen ovale and stroke: a case of pseudoperipheral facial palsy. *Neurol Sci* 2005; 26: 43–45.

164 Szydelko M, Kwolek A, Majka M. Stroke in young woman in the first day after delivery. *Wiad Lek* 2006; 59: 280–284.

165 Fox MW, Harms RW, Davis DH. Selected neurologic complications of pregnancy. *Mayo Clin Proc* 1990; 65: 1595–1618.

166 Momma F, Beck H, Miyamoto T, Nagao S. Intracranial aneurysm due to metastatic choriocarcinoma. *Surg Neurol* 1986; 25: 74–76.

167 Gurwitt LJ, Ling JM, Clark RE. Cerebral metastatic choriocarcinoma: a postpartum cause of stroke. *Obstet Gynecol* 1975; 45: 583–588.

168 Komeichi T, Igarashi K, Takigami M, Saito K, Isu T, Itamoto K et al. A case of metastatic choriocarcinoma associated with cerebral thrombosis and aneuysmal formation. *No Shinkei Geka* 1996; 24: 463–467.

169 Tuffnell DJ. Amniotic fluid embolism. *Curr Opin Obstet Gynecol* 2003; 15: 119–122.

170 Muth CM, Shank ES. Primary Care: Gas Embolism. *NEJM* 2000; 342: 476–482.

171 Numaguchi Y, Gonzalez CF, Davis PC et al. Moyamoya disease in the United States. *Clin Neurol Neurosurg* 1997; 99: S26–S30.

172 Komiyama M, Yasui T, Kitano S, Sakamoto H, Fujitani K, Matsuo S. Moyamoya disease and pregnancy:case report and review of the literature. *Neurosurg* 1998; 43: 360–369.

173 Williams DL, Martin IL, Gully RM. Intracerebral hemorrhage and Moyamoya disease in pregnancy. *Can J Anesth* 2000; 47: 996–1000.

174 Nakai Y, Hyodo A, Yanaka K, Nose T. Fatal cerebral infarction after intraventricular hemorrhage in a pregnant patient with moyamoya disease. *J Clin Neurosci* 2002; 9: 456–458.

175 Caplan LR. TIAs – we need to return to the question What is wrong with Mr Jones (editorial). *Neurology* 1988; 38: 791.

176 Kase CS, Caplan LR. *Intracerebral hemorrhage.* Boston: Butterworth-Heinemann, 1996.

177 Dias M, Sekhar L. Intracranial hemorrhage from aneurysms and arteriovenous malformations during pregnancy and the puerperium. *Neurosurg* 1990; 27: 855–865.

178 Redekop G, TerBrugge K, Montanera W, Wilinsky R. Arterial aneurysms associated with cerebral arteriovenous malformations: classification, incidence, and risk of hemorrhage. *J Neurosurg* 1998; 89: 539–546.

179 Stoodley MA, Macdonald RL, Weir BKA. Pregnancy and intracranial aneurysms. *Neurosurg Clin N Am* 1998; 9: 549–556.

180 Cannell DE, Botterell EH. Subarachnid hemorrhage and pregnancy. *Am J Obstet Gynecol* 1956; 72: 844.

181 Pedowitz P, Perrell A. Aneurysm complicated by pregnancy. *Am J Obstet Gynecol* 1957; 73: 736.

182 Amias AG. Cerebral vascular disease in pregnancy. I. Haemorrhage. *J Obstet Gynaecol Br Commonw* 1970; 77: 100–120.

183 Dias M. Neurovascular emergencies in pregnancy. *Clin Obstet Gynecol* 1994; 37: 337–354.

184 Wilterdink JL, Feldmann E, Cerebral hemorrhage. In: Devinsky O, Feldman E, Hainline B, eds. *Neurological Complications of Pregnancy.* New York: Raven, 1994: 13.

185 Reichman OH, Karlman RL. Berry aneurysm. *Surg Clin North Am* 1995; 75: 115–121.

186 Copelan EL, Mabon RF. Spontaneous intracranial bleeding in pregnancy. *Obstet Gynecol* 1962; 20: 373.

187 Robinson JL, Hall CJ, Sedzimir CB. Subarachnoid hemorrhage in pregnancy. *J Neurosurg* 1972; 36: 27–33.

188 Robinson JL, Hall CS, Sedzimir CB. Arteriovenous malformations, aneurysms, and pregnancy. *J Neurosurg* 1974; 41: 63–70.

189 Wiebers D, Whisnant J. The incidence of stroke among pregnant women in Rochester, Minn. 1955 through 1979. *JAMA* 1985; 254: 3055–3057.

190 Wiebers DO. Subarachnoid hemorrhage in pregnancy. *Semin Neurol* 1988; 8: 226–229.

191 Forster DMC, Kunkler IH, Hartland P. Risk of cerebral bleeding from arteriovenous malformations in pregnancy: the Sheffield experience. *Stereotacct Funct Neurosurg* 1993; 61(Suppl 1): 20–22.

192 Hunt HB, Schifrin BS, Suzuki K. Ruptured berry aneurysms and pregnancy. *Obstet Gynecol* 1974; 43: 827–837.

193 Williams KP, Wilson S. Maternal middle cerebral artery velocity changes in HELLP syndrome versus preeclampsia. *Ultrasound Obstet Gynecol* 1998; 11: 195–198.

194 Williams KP, Wilson S. Persistence of cerebral hemodynamic changes in patients with eclampsia: a report of three cases. *Am J Obstet Gynecol* 1999; 181: 1162–1165.

195 Schievink W. Intracranial aneurysms. *N Engl J Med* 1997; 336: 28–40.

196 Hunt WE, Hess RM. Surgical risk as related to time of intervention in the repair of intracranial aneurysms. *J Neurosurg* 1968; 28: 14–20.

197 van Gijn J, Bromberg JEC, Lindsay KW, Hasan D, Vermeulen M. Definition of initial grading, specific events, and overall outcome in patients with aneurismal subarachnoid hemorrhage. *Stroke* 1994; 25: 1623–1627.

198 van Gijn J, van Dongen KJ. The time course of aneurysmal haemorrhage on computed tomograms. *Neuroradiology* 1982; 23: 153–156.

199 Gianotta SL, Daniels J, Golde SH et al. Ruptured intracranial aneurysms during pregnancy: a report of four cases. *J Reprod Med* 1986; 31: 139–147.

200 Kidwell CS, Chalela JA, Saver JL, Starkman S, Hill MD, Demchuk AM, Butman JA, Patronas N, Alger JR, Latour LL, Luby ML, Baird AE, Leary MC, Tremwel M, Ovbiagele B, Fredieu A, Suzuki S, Villablanca JP, Davis S, Dunn B, Todd JW, Ezzeddine MA, Haymore J, Lynch JK, Davis L, Warach S. Comparison of MRI and CT for detection of acute intracerebral hemorrhage. *JAMA* 2004; 20; 292: 1823–1830.

201 Singer RJ, Ogilvy CS, Rordorf G. Treatment of aneurysmal subarachnoid hemorrhage. *Up To Date* 2006; ver 15.1.

202 Broderick J, Connolly S, Feldmann E, Hanley D, Kase C, Krieger D, Mayberg M, Morgenstern L, Ogilvy CS, Vespa P, Zuccarello M. Guidelines for the Management of Spontaneous Intracerebral Hemorrhage in Adults: 2007 Update: A Guideline From the American Heart Association/American Stroke Association Stroke Council, High Blood Pressure Research Council, and the Quality of Care and Outcomes in Research Interdisciplinary Working Group: The American Academy of Neurology affirms the value of this guideline as an educational tool for neurologists. *Stroke* 2007; 38: 2001–2023.

203 Allen GS, Ahn HS, Preziosi TJ et al. Cerebral arterial spasm: a controlled trial of nimodipine on patienst with subarachnoid hemorrhage. *N Engl J Med* 1983; 308: 619–624.

204 Al-Yamany M, Wallace MC. Management of cerebral vasospasm on patients with aneurysmal subarachnoid hemorrhage. *Intensive Care Med* 1999; 25: 1463–1466.

205 Treggiari-Venzi MM, Suter PM, Romand JA. Review of medical prevention of vasospasm after aneurysmal subarachnoid hemorrhage: a problem of neurointensive care. *Neurosurgery* 2001; 48: 249–261.

206 Feigin VL, Rinkel GJ, Algra A. Calcium antagonists in patients with aneurysmal subarachnoid hemorrhage: a systematic review. *Neurology* 1998; 50: 876.

207 Belfort MA, Saade GR, Moise KJ Jr. et al. Nimodipine in the management of preeclampsia: maternal and fetal effects. *Am J Obstet Gynecol* 1994; 171: 417–424.

208 Belfort MA, Saade GR, Suresh M, Johnson D, Vedernikov YP. Human umbilical vessels: responses to agents frequently used in obstetic patients. *Am J Obstet Gynecol* 1995; 1395–1403.

209 Horn EH, Filshie M, Kerslake RW, Jaspan T, Worthington BS, Rubin PC. Widespread cerebral ischemia treated with nimodipine in a patient with eclampsia. *BMJ* 1990; 301: 794.

210 Belfort MA, Carpenter RJ Jr. Kirshon B, Saade GR, Moise KJ Jr. The use of nimodipine in a patient with eclampsia: color flow Doppler demonstration of retinal artery relaxation. *Am J Obstet Gynecol* 1993; 169: 204–206.

211 Befort MA, Saade GR, Yared M et al. Change in estimated cerebral perfusion pressure after treatment with nimodipine or magnesium sulfate in patients with preeclampsia. *Am J Obstet Gynecol* 1999; 181: 402–407.

212 Anthony J, Mantel G, Johnson R, Dommisse J. The haemodynamic and respiratory effects of intravenous nimodipine used in the treatment of eclampsia. *Br J Obstet Gynaecol* 1996; 103: 518–522.

213 Belfort MA, Anthony J, Saade GR. Prevention of eclampsia. *Semin Perinatol* 1999; 23: 65–78.

214 Awad IA, Carter LP, Spetzler RF et al. Clinical vasospasm after subarachnoid hemorrhage. response to hypervolemic hemodilution and arterial hypertension. *Stroke* 1987; 18: 365–372.

215 Solomon RA, Fink ME, Lennihan L. Early aneurysm surgery and prophylactic hypervolemic hypertensive therapy for the treatmetn of aneurysmal subarachnoid hemorrhage. *Neurosurgery* 1988; 23: 699–704.

216 Levy ML, Giannotta SL. Induced hypertension and hypervolemia for treatment of cerebral vasospasm. *Neurosurg Clin North Am* 1990; 1: 357–365.

217 Rudehill A, Gordon E, Sundqvist K et al. A study of ECG abnormalities and myocardial specific enzymes in patients with subarachnoid haemorrhage. *Acta Anaesthesiol Scand* 1982; 26: 344–350.

218 Nelson LA. Ruptured cerebral aneurysm in the pregnant patient. *Internat Anesthesiol Clin* 2005; 43: 81–97.

219 Templeton A, Kelman GR. Maternal blood gases, P_aO_2-P_aO_2, physiological shunt and VD/VT in normal pregnancy. *Br J Anaesth* 1976; 48: 1001–1004.

220 Machida H. Influence of progesterone on arterial blood and CSF acid-base balance in women. *J Appl Physiol* 1981; 51: 1433–1436.

221 Levinson G, Shnider SM, DeLorimier AA et al. Effects of maternal hyperventilation on uterine blood flow and fetal oxygenation and acid-base status. *Anesthesiology* 1974; 40: 340–347.

222 Tidswell P, Dias PS, Sagar HJ et al. Cognitive outcome after aneurysm rupture: Relationship to aneurysm site and perioerative complications. *Neurology* 1995; 45: 875.

223 Jane JA, Kassell NF, Torner JC, Winn RH. The natural history of aneurysms and arteriovenous malformations. *J Neurosurg* 1985; 62: 321–323.

224 Barrow DL, Reisner A. natural history of intracranial aneurysms and vascular malformations. *Clin Neurosurg* 1993; 40: 3–39.

225 Chapman AB, Rubinstein D, Hughes R et al. Intracranial aneurysms in autosomal dominant polycystic kidney disease. *N Engl J Med* 1992; 327: 916–920.

226 Ruggeri PM, Poulos N, Masaryk TJ et al. Occult intracranial aneurysms in polycystic kidney disease: screening with MR angiography. *Radiology* 1994; 191: 33–39.

227 Le Roux PD, Elliott JP, Downey L et al. Imroved outcome after rupture of anterior circulation aneurysms: A retrospective 10-year review of 224 good grade patients. *J Neurosurg* 1995; 83: 394.

228 Weir B, Macdonald RL. Management of intracranial aneurysms and arteriovenous malformations during pregnancy. *Neurosurgery* 1996; 2421–2427.

229 Kizilkilic O, Albayram S, Adaletli I et al. Endovascular treatment of ruptures intracranial aneurysms during pregnancy. *Arch Gynecol Obstet* 2003; 268: 325–328.

230 Meyers PM, Halbach VV, Malek AM et al. Endovascular treatment of cerebral artery aneurysms during pregnancy: report of three cases. *Am J Neuroradiol* 2000; 21: 1306–1311.

231 Piotin M, de Souza Filho CB, Kothimbakam R, Moret J. Endovascular treatment of acutely ruptured intracranial aneurysms in pregnancy. *Am J Obstet Gynecol* 2001; 185: 1261–1262.

232 Shahabi S, Tecco L, Jani J et al. Management of a ruptured basilar artery aneurysm during pregnancy. *Acta Chir Belg* 2001; 101: 193–195.

233 Brilstra EH, Rinkel GJE, van Rooij WJJ et al. Treatment of intracranial aneurysms by embolization with coils: a systematic review. *Stroke* 1999; 30: 470–476.

234 International Subarachnoid Aneurysm Trial (ISAT) Collaborative Group: International Subarachnoid Aneurysm Trial (ISAT) of neurosurgical clipping versus endovascular coiling in 2143 patients with ruptured intracranial aneurysms: a randomized trial. *Lancet* 2002; 360: 1267–1274.

235 Bendok BR, Getch CC, Malisch TW et al. Treatment of aneurysmal subarachnoid hemorrhage. *Semin Neurol* 1998; 18: 521–531.

236 The Arteriovenous Malformation Study Group. Arteriovenous Malformations of the Brain in Adults. *N Engl J Med* 1999; 340: 1812–1818.

237 Al-Shahi R, Warlow C. A systematic review of the frequency and prognosis of arteriovenous malformations of the brain in adults. *Brain* 2001; 124: 1900–1926.

238 Fleetwood IG, Steinberg GK. Arteriovenous malformations. *Lancet* 2002; 359: 863–873.

239 Horton J, Chambers W, Lyons S et al. Pregnancy and the risk if hemorrhage from cerebral arteriovenous malformations. *Neurosurgery* 1990; 27: 867–872.

240 Forster D, Kunkler I, Hartland P. Risk of cerebral bleeding form arteriovenous malformations in pregnancy: the Sheffield experience. *Stereotact Funct Neurosurg* 1993; 61(suppl): 20–22.

241 Sawin PD. Spontaneous subarachnoid hemorrhage in pregnancy. In: Loftus CM, ed. *Neurosurgical Aspects of Pregnancy*, 1st edn. Park Ridge: American Association of Neurological Surgeons, 1996: 85–100.

242 Sadasivan B, Malik GM, Lee C, Ausman JI. Vascular malformations and pregnancy. *Surg Neurol* 1990; 33: 305–313.

243 Grenvik A, Safar P. *Brain Failure and Resuscitation*. New York: Churchill Livingstone, 1981.

244 The NINDS rt-PA Stroke Study Group. Tissue plasminogen activator for acute ischemic stroke. *N Engl J Med* 1995; 333: 1581–1587.

245 Tanne D, Bates VE, Verro P et al. Initial clinical experience with IV tissue plasminogen activator for acute ischemic stroke: a multicenter survey. *Neurology* 1999; 53: 424–427.

246 Graham GD. Tissue plasminogen activator for acute ischemic stroke in clinical practice: A meta-analysis of safety data. *Stroke* 2003; 34: 2847–2850.

247 Hommel M, Boissel JP, Cornu C et al. Termination of trial of streptokinase in severe acute ischaemic stroke: MAST Study Group. *Lancet* 1995; 345: 57.

248 Donnan GA, Davis SM, Chambers BR et al. Streptokinase for acute ischemic stroke with relationship to time of administration: Australian Streptokinase (ASK) Trial Study Group. *JAMA* 1996; 276: 961–966.

249 Multicenter Acute Stroke Trial–Europe Study Group. Thrombolytic therapy with streptokinase in acute ischemic stroke. *N Engl J Med* 1996; 335: 145–150.

250 Multicentre Acute Stroke Trial–Italy (MAST-I) Group. Randomised controlled trial of streptokinase, aspirin, and combination of both in treatment of acute ischaemic stroke. *Lancet* 1995; 346: 1509–1514.

251 Elford K, Leader A, Wee R, Stys PK. Stroke in ovarian hyperstimulation syndrome in early pregnancy treated with intraarterial rt-PA. *Neurology* 2002; 59: 1270–1272.

252 Johnson DM, Kramer DC, Cohen E et al. Thrombolytic therapy for acute stroke in late pregnancy with intra-arterial recombinant tissue plasminogen activator. *Stroke* 2005; 36: e53–e55.

253 Wardlaw J. Overview of Cochrane thrombolysis meta-analysis. *Neurology* 2001; 57: S69–S76.

254 Adams HP, del Zoppo G, Alberts MJ et al. Guidelines for the early management of adults with ischemic stroke: a guideline from the American Heart Association/American Stroke Association Stroke Council, Clinical Cardiology Council, Cardiovascular Radiology and Intervention Council, and the Atherosclerotic Peripheral Vascular Disease and Quality of Care Outcomes in Research Interdisciplinary Working Groups. *Stroke* 2007; 38: 1655–1711.

255 Hacke W, Kaste M, Fieschi C et al. Intravenous thrombolysis with recombinant tissue plasminogen activator for acute hemispheric stroke. The European Cooperative Acute Stroke Study (ECASS). *JAMA* 1995; 274: 1017–1025.

256 Hacke W, Kaste M, Fieschi C et al. Randomised double-blind placebo-controlled trial of thrombolytic therapy with intravenous alteplase in acute ischaemic stroke (ECASS II). Second European-Australasian Acute Stroke Study Investigators. *Lancet* 1998; 352: 1245–1251.

257 Ellish NJ, Saboda K, O'Connor J et al. A prospective study of early pregnancy loss. *Hum Reprod* 1996; 11: 406–412.

258 Zinaman MJ, Clegg ED, Brown CC et al. Estimates of human fertility and pregnancy loss. *Fertil Steril* 1996; 65: 503–509.

259 Mendez JC, Masjuan J, Garcia N, de Lecinana M. Successful intra-arterial thrombolysis for acute ischemic stroke in the immediate postpartum period: a case report. *Cardiovasc Intervent Radiol* Sep 2006.

260 Lamy C, Hamon JB, Coste J et al. Ischemic stroke in young women: Risk of recurrence during subsequent pregnancies. *Neurology* 2000; 55: 269–274.

261 Coppage KH, Hinton AC, Moldnhauer J et al. Maternal and perinatal outcome in women with a history of stroke. *Am J Obstet Gynecol* 2004; 190: 1331–1334.

262 Soriano D, Carp H, Seidman DS et al. Management and outcome of pregnancy in women with thrombophylic disorders and past cerebrovascular events. *Acta Obstet Gynecol Scand* 2002; 81: 204–207.

263 Bates SM, Greer IA, Hirsh J, Ginsberg JS. Use of antithrombotic agents during pregnancy: the Seventh ACCP Conference on Antithrombotic and Thrombolytic Therapy. *Chest* 2004; 126(3 suppl): 627S–644S.

264 Imperiale TF, Perrulis AS. A meta-analysis of low-dose aspirin for the prevention of pregnancy-induced hypertensive disease. *JAMA* 1991; 266: 260–264.

265 Low dose aspirin in pregnancy and early childhood development: follow-up of the collaborative group. *Br J Obstet Gynaecol* 1995; 102: 861–868.

266 Ito W, Blajchman A, Stephenson M et al. Prospective follow-up of adverse reactions in breast-fed infants exposed to maternal medication. *Am J Obstet Gynecol* 1993; 168: 1393–1399.

267 Bar-Oz B, Bulkowstein M, Benyamini L et al. use of antibiotic and analgesic drugs during lactation. *Drug Saf* 2003; 26: 925–929.

268 Teasdale G, Jennett B. Assessment of coma and impaired consciousness. *Lancet* 1974; 2: 81–84.

269 Drake CG. Report of World Federation of Neurological Surgeons Committee on a universal subarachnoid hemorrhage grading scale. *J Neurosurg* 1988; 68: 985.

270 Adams et al. Guidelines for the early management of adults with ischemic stroke. *Stroke* 2007; 38: 1676.

271 Caplan LR. The evaluation of stroke. *UpToDate* 2007; 15.1.

20 Cardiac Disease

Michael R. Foley[1], Roxann Rokey[2] & Michael A. Belfort[3]

[1]Scotsdale Healthcare, Scottsdale, Arizona *and* Department of Obstetrics and Gynecology, University of Arizona College of Medicine, Tucson, AZ, USA
[2]Department of Cardiology, Marshfield Clinic, Marshfield, WI, USA
[3]Department of Obstetrics and Gynecology, Division of Maternal-Fetal Medicine, University of Utah School of Medicine, Salt Lake City, UT *and* HCA Healthcare, Nashville, TN, USA

Introduction

Although cardiac disease complicates only 1–4% of all pregnancies in the United States, such conditions continue to account for up to 10–25% of maternal mortality [1–5]. Similar findings are seen elsewhere. In the recently published Confidential Enquiry into maternal deaths, *Why Mothers Die*, 2000–2002, heart disease has now become the leading cause of indirect maternal death in the UK. In contrast to the very distant past, rheumatic fever and its valvular sequelae of heart failure is no longer the most common cause of maternal mortality. Both maternal congenital heart disease and acquired maternal heart disease such as myocardial infarction and cardiomyopathy now are the predominant causes of maternal death. With advances in the treatment of congenital heart disease in newborns and children, more young women are reaching reproductive age and attempting pregnancy. As a consequence, congenital heart disease is a common form of heart disease complicating pregnancy in North American women. On the other end of the spectrum, more women are postponing pregnancy until the fourth or fifth decade of life – a time where underlying medical conditions such as hypertension and diabetes, coupled with advancing maternal age, may exacerbate the incidence of acquired heart disease (such as myocardial infarction or cadiomyopathy) complicating pregnancy. Indeed, in the UK, maternal mortality rates from congenital causes have remained stable but those from ischemia/cardiomyopathy have risen.

The long held belief that pregnancy is absolutely contraindicated in maternal cardiovascular diasease is no longer justifiable using evidenced-based medicine. There are some conditions in which pregnancy is contraindicated and a high maternal risk and poor fetal outcome can be predicted. However, in many women with heart disease a more favorable maternal and fetal outcome will be expected.This chapter, therefore, will focus on the precarious interaction between cardiac disease and pregnancy.

Critical Care Obstetrics, 5th edition. Edited by M. Belfort, G. Saade, M. Foley, J. Phelan and G. Dildy.

Counseling the pregnant cardiac patient

Maternal outcome in the cardiac patient is dependent upon the type of cardiac disease, myocardial function, maternal functional status, presence and severity of cyanosis, pulmonary vascular pressures/resistance and prior surgical procedures along with any uncorrected lesions and residuae or sequelae of repair. Of these, maternal functional status, the degree of cyanosis along with accompanying pulmonary vascular pressure/resistance, and the type of current maternal cardiac disease are the most predictive of an adverse outcome. Siu et al [6] have reported a method of assessing risk and outcomes in women with cardiac disease using (i) functional status, (ii) left heart dysfunction, (iii) prior cardiac events, and (iv) left heart obstruction as indicators of who is at a level of risk that can safely allow delivery at a community hospital.

Before 1973, the Criteria Committee of the New York Heart Association (NYHA) recommended a classification of cardiac disease based on clinical function (classes I–IV). Table 20.1 outlines the specifics of the NYHA classification system. Such a classification is useful in discussing the pregnant cardiac patient, although patients who begin pregnancy as functional class I may develop congestive heart failure and pulmonary edema during the course of gestation. Other classifications including the Canadian Cardiovascular Society Functional Classification (classes I–IV) and Specific Activity Scale have been used in other countries and have similar grades of disability.

This functional classification system, although somewhat antiquated, remains most useful when comparing the performance of individuals with uniform etiologic and anatomic defects. In general, most women who begin pregnancy as a functional class NYHA I or II have an improved outcome as compared with those classified as class III or IV [7].

Counseling the pregnant cardiac patient regarding her prognosis for successful pregnancy is further complicated by recent advances in medical and surgical therapy, fetal surveillance, and neonatal care. Such advances render invalid many older estimates of maternal mortality and fetal wastage. Table 20.2 represents a

Table 20.1 New York Heart Association (NYHA) functional classification system.

Class I	No limitations of physical activity, ordinary physical activity does not precipitate cardiovascular symptoms such as dyspnea, angina, fatigue, or palpitations
Class II	Slight limitation of physical activity. Ordinary physical activity will precipitate cardiovascular symptoms. Patients are comfortable at rest
Class III	Less than ordinary physical activity precipitates symptoms that markedly limit activity. Patients are comfortable at rest
Class IV	Patients have discomfort with any physical activity. Symptoms are present at rest

Table 20.2 Maternal risk associated with pregnancy.

Group I: Minimal risk of complications (mortality <1%)
Atrial septal defect*
Ventricular septal defect*
Patent ductus arteriosus*
Pulmonic/tricuspid disease
Corrected tetralogy of Fallot
Bioprosthetic valve
Mitral stenosis, New York Heart Association (NYHA) classes I and II
Marfan syndrome with normal aorta
Group II: Moderate risk of complications (mortality 5–15%)
Mitral stenosis with atrial fibrillation†
Artificial valve*†
Mitral stenosis, NYHA classes III and IV
Aortic stenosis
Coarctation of aorta, uncomplicated
Uncorrected tetralogy of Fallot
Previous myocardial infarction
Group III: Major risk of complications or death (mortality >25%)
Pulmonary hypertension
Coarctation of aorta, complicated
Marfan syndrome with aortic involvement

* If unassociated with pulmonary hypertension.
† If anticoagulation with heparin, rather than coumadin, is elected.

synthesis of maternal risk estimates for various types of cardiac disease that was initially developed for the first edition of this text in 1987. Counseling of the pregnant cardiac patient, as well as general management approaches, were based on this classification [8]. Category I included conditions that, with proper management, were associated with negligible maternal mortality (1%). Cardiac lesions in category II traditionally carried a 5–15% risk of maternal mortality. Patients with cardiac lesions in group III were, and probably remain, subject to a mortality risk exceeding 25%. In all but exceptional cases, this risk is unacceptable, and prevention or interruption of pregnancy is generally recommended.

Currently available data suggest that today maternal mortality is almost exclusively seen in patients with pulmonary hypertension, cardiac valvular disease (acquired or congenital) and including endocarditis, coronary artery disease, cardiomyopathy, and sudden cardiac arrhythmia death. DeSwiet, reporting on maternal mortality from heart disease in the United Kingdom between 1985 and 1987, stated that all deaths occurred due to endocarditis (22%), pulmonary hypertension (30%), coronary artery disease (39%), and cardiomyopathy or myocarditis (9%) [2]. Similarly, a review of maternal mortality in Utah from 1982 to 1994 revealed 13 cardiac deaths, 4 (31%) due to pulmonary hypertension, 4 secondary to cardiomyopathy (31%), 2 due to coronary artery disease (15%), and 3 (23%) due to sudden arrhythmia [9]. In a smaller series of maternal deaths from West Virginia between 1985 and 1989, the two cardiac deaths described were due to cardiomyopathy [10]. Clark et al [11] reported on 95 maternal deaths within a large USA community hospital system in which 1.46 million deliveries occurred over a 6-year period (2000–2006). Cardiac disease accounted for 11% of all deaths (n = 10) and was the fourth most common cause of death after complications of pre-eclampsia, amniotic fluid embolism, and obstetric hemorrhage). Of interest is that 50% of the cardiac deaths were associated with myocardial infarction in women with no prior history of ischemic heart disease.

In a study of 252 pregnancies in women with cardiac disease the following independent predictors of cardiac events (congestive heart failure, arrhythmia, and stroke) were identified [12]:
- NYHA functional class III or IV
- maternal cyanosis
- history of prior arrhythmia
- pulmonary vascular disease
- myocardial dysfunction (ejection fraction <40%)
- left heart obstruction.

The same authors then prospectively applied these risk predictors to another cohort of women with congenital or acquired cardiac disease and found that the four predictors of having cardiac events were:
- left ventricular systolic dysfunction (LVEF <40%)
- poor functional status/cyanosis
- previous cardiac event (heart failure, stroke, transient ischemic attack)
- left-sided cardiac valvular lesions (mitral valve area <2.0 cm^2, aortic valve area <1.5 cm^2).

One point was given for each finding. Not suprisingly, those with scores of 0 and no specific risk issue had the lowest risk of developing pulmonary edema, stroke, arrhythmia necessitating treatment, cardiac arrest or death.

In a study by Presbitero et al. [13], looking at the outcome of the mother and the fetus in pregnancies complicated by cyanotic congenital heart disease, the adverse impact of low maternal oxygen saturation was clearly illustrated. The likelihood of a live birth was less frequent (12%) if the mother's resting oxygen saturation was below 85% as compared to a resting oxygen saturation of greater than 85% (63%). It would appear, however, that with appropriate obstetric care, the presence or absence of the aforementioned secondary complications of cardiomyopathy, pulmonary hypertension, endocarditis, and sudden arrhythmias play a much more important role in determining ultimate maternal outcome than the primary structural nature of the cardiac lesion itself.

Physiologic considerations

The unique problems encountered by the pregnant woman with cardiac disease are secondary to four principal physiologic changes [14].

1 *A 50% increase in intravascular volume* is seen in normal pregnancy. Figure 20.1 illustrates the changes in total blood volume, plasma volume, and red cell volume during normal pregnancy. In patients whose cardiac output is limited by intrinsic myocardial dysfunction, valvular lesions, or ischemic cardiac disease, volume overload will be poorly tolerated and may lead to congestive failure or worsening ischemia. In patients with an anatomic predisposition, such volume expansion may result in aneurysm formation or dissection (e.g. Marfan syndrome). Even in women with multiple pregnancies, the heart is able to withstand repetitive episodes of gestational volume overload without lasting detrimental structural or functional changes [15].

2 *Decreased systemic vascular resistance* (SVR) becomes especially important in patients with the potential for right to left shunts, which will invariably be increased by a falling SVR during pregnancy. Such alterations in cardiac afterload also complicate adaptation to pregnancy in patients with certain types of valvular disease. Table 20.3 summarizes the central hemodynamic changes associated with normal term pregnancy.

3 *The hypercoagulability associated with pregnancy* heightens the need for adequate anticoagulation in patients at risk for arterial thrombosis (artificial valves and some subsets of atrial fibrillation) at a time when optimum anticoagulation with coumarin derivatives may have adverse fetal consequences. Table 20.4 outlines the relative changes in the coagulation factors and inhibitors associated with normal pregnancy. For women receiving any type of therapeutic anticoagulation, the risk of serious postpartum hemorrhage is also increased.

4 *Marked fluctuations in cardiac output* normally occur in pregnancy, particularly during labor and delivery [16]. Such changes increase progressively from the first stage of labor, reaching, in

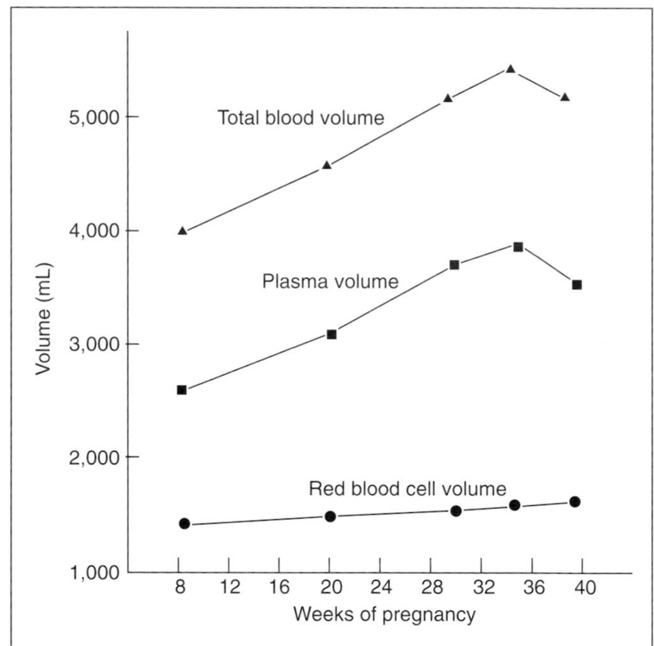

Figure 20.1 Changes in total blood volume, plasma volume, and red cell volume in normal pregnancy (Reproduced by permission from Shnider SM, Levinson G. *Anesthesia for Obstetrics*, 3rd edn. Lippincott, Williams & Wilkins, 1993.)

Table 20.3 Central hemodynamic changes associated with normal term pregnancy.

	Non-pregnant	Pregnant	Percent change*
Cardiac output (L/min)	4.3 ± 0.9	6.2 ± 1.0	+43
Heart rate (bpm)	71 ± 10.0	83 ± 1.0	+17
Systemic vascular resistance (dyne/cm/sec^5)	1,530 ± 520	1,210 ± 266	−21
Pulmonary vascular resistance (dyne/cm/sec^5)	119 ± 47.0	78 ± 22	−34
Colloid oncotic pressure (mmHg)	20.8 ± 1.0	18.0 ± 1.5	−14
COP − PCWP (mmHg)	14.5 ± 2.5	10.5 ± 2.7	−28
Mean arterial pressure (mmHg)	86.4 ± 7.5	90.3 ± 5.8	−NSC
Pulmonary capillary wedge pressure (mmHg)	6.3 ± 2.1	7.5 ± 1.8	−NSC
Central venous pressure (mmHg)	3.7 ± 2.6	3.6 ± 2.5	NSC
Left ventricular stroke work index (g/m/m^2)	41 ± 8	48 ± 6	+NSC

* NSC = no statistically significant change.

COP − PCWP = colloid oncotic pressure − pulmonary capillary wedge pressure (mmHg).

(Reproduced by permission from Clark SL, et al: Central hemodynamic assessment of normal term pregnancy. Am J Obstet Gynecol 1989;161:1439.)

some cases, an additional 50% by the late second stage. The potential for further dramatic volume shifts occurs around the time of delivery, both secondary to postpartum hemorrhage and as the result of an "autotransfusion" occurring with release of vena caval obstruction and sustained uterine contraction. Such volume shifts may be poorly tolerated by women whose cardiac output is highly dependent on adequate preload (pulmonary hypertension) or in those with fixed cardiac output (mitral stenosis). Figure 20.2 illustrates the marked fluctuations in cardiac output associated with normal labor, delivery, and postpartum [17].

The risk classification presented in Table 20.2 assumes clean delineation of various cardiovascular lesions. Unfortunately, in actual practice this is only rarely the case. Optimal management of a patient with any specific combination of lesions requires a thorough assessment of the anatomic and functional capacity of the heart, followed by an analysis of how the physiologic changes described previously will impact on the specific anatomic or physiologic limitations imposed by the intrinsic disease. Such an analysis will allow a prioritization of often conflicting physiologic demands and greatly assist the clinician in avoiding or managing potential complications.

Table 20.4 Coagulation factors and inhibitors during normal pregnancy.

Factor	Non-pregnant	Late pregnancy
Factor I (fibrinogen)	200–450mg/dL	400–650mg/dL
Factor II (prothrombin)	75–125%	100–125%
Factor V	75–125%	100–150%
Factor VII	75–125%	150–250%
Factor VIII	75–150%	200–500%
Factor IX	75–125%	100–150%
Factor X	75–125%	150–250%
Factor XI	5–125%	50–100%
Factor XII	75–125%	100–200%
Factor XIII	75–125%	35–75%
Antithrombin III	85–110%	75–100%
Antifactor Xa	85–110%	75–100%

(Reprinted by permission from Hathaway WE, Bonnar J. Coagulation in pregnancy. In: Hathaway WE, Bonnar I, eds. Perinatal Coagulation. New York: Grune & Stratton, 1978.)

Certain management principles generally apply to most patients with cardiac disease. These include the judicious use of antepartum bed rest and meticulous prenatal care. Intrapartum management principles include laboring in the lateral position; the use of epidural anesthesia, which will minimize intrapartum fluctuations in cardiac output (although the use of epidural narcotic rather than epidural local anesthesia may be more appropriate for patients with certain types of cardiac lesions); the administration of oxygen; and endocarditis prophylaxis, when appropriate. Positional effects on maternal cardiac output during labor with epidural analgesia have recently been detailed [18]. Additional management recommendations may vary according to the specific lesion present. For patients with significant cardiac disease, management and delivery in a referral center is recommended. In many cases, management with peripheral pulse oximetry is replacing invasive hemodynamic monitoring.

Congenital cardiac lesions

As previously discussed, the relative frequency of congenital as opposed to acquired heart disease is changing [2,7,19,20]. Rheumatic fever is less common in the United States, and more patients with congenital cardiac disease now survive to reproduc-

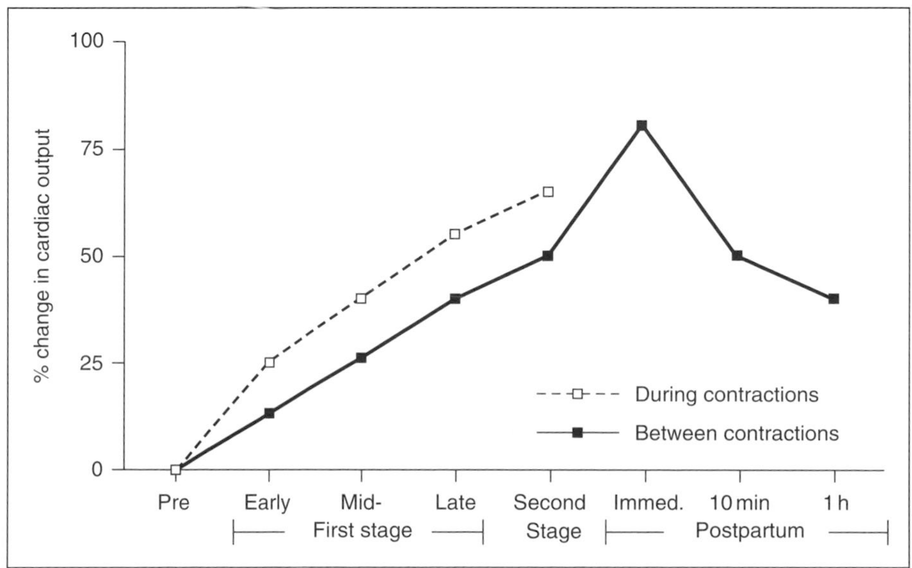

Figure 20.2 Fluctuations in cardiac output associated with normal labor, delivery, and postpartum. (Reproduced by permission from Bonica JJ, McDonald JS. *Principles and Practice of Obstetrics Analgesia and Anesthesia*, 2nd edn. Lippincott, Williams & Wilkins, 1994.)

tive age. In a review in 1954, the ratio of rheumatic to congenital heart disease seen during pregnancy was 16:1; by 1967, this ratio had changed to 3:1 [19–21]. A more recent report from Taiwan suggested a rheumatic/congenital cardiac ratio of 1:1.5 during pregnancy [7]. Similarly, in the United Kingdom between 1973 and 1987, the number of deaths from congenital heart disease has doubled, whereas the number of deaths from rhuematic heart disease has halved [2]. In the subsequent discussion of specific cardiac lesions, no attempt will be made to duplicate existing comprehensive texts regarding physical diagnostic, electrocardiographic, and radiographic findings of specific cardiac lesions. Rather, the discussion presented here focuses on aspects of cardiac disease that are unique to pregnancy.

Atrial septal defect

Secundum atrial septal defect (ASD) is the most common repaired and unrepaired congenital lesion that occurs in pregnant woment, and, in general, it is asymptomatic and well tolerated even in those with large left to right shunts [22–24]. The three significant potential complications seen with ASD are arrhythmias, heart failure and "paradoxical embolism". Although atrial arrhythmias are not uncommon in patients with ASD, their onset generally occurs after the fourth decade of life; thus, such arrhythmias, however unlikely, are becoming more of a concern with the recent prevalence of delayed childbearing. In patients with ASD, atrial fibrillation is the most common arrhythmia encountered; however, supraventricular tachycardia and atrial flutter also may occur. Antiarrythmic or rate-controlling agents or other medications may be indicated for symptomatic patients with these arrhythmias and in some, cardioversion may be necessary (see section on dysrrhythmia).

The hypervolemia associated with pregnancy results in an increased left to right shunt through the ASD, and, thus, a significant burden is imposed on the right atrium, right ventricle and pulmonary vasculature. Although this additional burden is tolerated well by most patients, congestive heart failure and death with ASD have been reported [25–27]. In contrast to VSD or PDA, large left to right shunts at the atrial level do not usually result in pulmonary hypertension or even irreversible pulmonary hypertension at childbearing age.

An extremely rare and unusual potential complication that exists with ASD is "paradoxical embolization." If this occurs, it is most likely as a result of venous thrombosis but can be air or amniotic in the pregnant woman. Thromboemboli from leg or pelvic veins may be directed across the ASD into the systemic circulation, "paradoxically," resulting in ischemic neurologic complications such as transient ischemic attack (TIA) or stroke or other arterial ischemic complications.

The vast majority of patients with ASD, however, tolerate pregnancy, labor, and delivery without complication. Neilson et al. [26] reported 70 pregnancies in 24 patients with ASD; all patients had an uncomplicated ante- and intrapartum course. During labor, avoidance of fluid overload, oxygen administration, labor in the lateral recumbent position, and pain relief with epidural anesthesia are means to reduce cardiac work. All ASDs have some degree of right to left shunting, particularly with valsalva-type maneuvers. Hence, consideration of air trap filters applied to IV lines should be considered to reduce this possibility. New recommendations regarding the use of antiobiotic prophylaxis for prevention of bacterial endocarditis have recently been published [28]. The American Heart Association does not recommend antibiotic prophylaxis for secundum atrial septal defects. Further discussion regarding the latest recommendations antiobiotic prophylaxis against bacterial endocarditis for congenital heart defects is found later in this chapter and in Table 20.5.

Table 20.5 Guidelines from the AHA 2007 Prevetion of infective endocarditis: Patients with highest risk of adverse outcomes from endocarditis.

1. Prosthetic cardiac valves (mechanical, bioprosthetic, homograft)
2. Previous history of infective endocarditis
3. Unrepaired cyanotic congenital heart disease, including palliative shunts and conduits
4. Completely repaired congenital heart defects with prosthetic material or device, surgically or interventionally placed, during the first 6 months after the procedure
5. Repaired CHD with residual defects at the site or adjacent to the site of a prosthetic patch or prosthetic device
6. Cardiac transplanted heart with significant valvulopathy (leaflet pathology and regurgitation)

Adapted from: Wilson W. et al. 2007.

Ventricular septal defect

Ventricular septal defect may occur as an isolated lesion or in conjunction with other congenital cardiac anomalies, including tetralogy of Fallot, transposition of the great vessels, and coarctation of the aorta. The size and location of the septal defect is the most important determinant of clinical prognosis during pregnancy. Small defects are tolerated well, while larger defects are associated more frequently with congestive failure, arrhythmias, or the development of pulmonary hypertension. Those VSDs that are associated with other congenital anomalies may be much more complicated and can be associated with much higher risk of heart failure, arrhythmia, cyanosis or pulmonary hypertension, depending on the lesion type, prior surgery and residual lesions after surgical repair. In general, pregnancy, labor, and delivery are generally well tolerated by patients with an uncomplicated VSD. Schaefer et al. [25] compiled a series of 141 pregnancies in 56 women with VSD. The only two maternal deaths were in women whose VSD was complicated by pulmonary hypertension (Eisenmenger's syndrome). Because of the high risk of death associated with unrecognized pulmonary hypertension, echocardiography or cardiac catheterization is essential in any adult patient in whom persistent VSD is suspected, or in whom the quality or success of the previous repair is uncertain [29,30].

The primary closure of a moderately restrictive or non-restrictive VSD in early childhood usually prevents the subsequent development of secondary pulmonary vascular hypertension and therefore permits an uneventful pregnancy. Fortunately, significant postoperative electrophysiologic conduction abnormalities are rarely encountered.

Although very rarely indicated, successful primary closures of VSDs during pregnancy have been reported. Intrapartum management considerations for patients with uncomplicated VSD or PDA are similar to those outlined for ASD. In general, invasive hemodynamic monitoring is usually unnecessary.

Patent ductus arteriosus

Although patent ductus arteriosus (PDA) is one of the most common congenital cardiac anomalies, its almost universal detection and closure in the newborn period makes it uncommon during pregnancy [20]. As with uncomplicated ASD and VSD, most patients are asymptomatic, and PDA is generally well tolerated during pregnancy, labor, and delivery. As with a large VSD, however, the high-pressure–high-flow left to right shunt associated with a large, uncorrected PDA can lead to pulmonary hypertension. In such cases, the prognosis becomes much worse since shunt reversal can occur with fall in systemic vascular resistance during pregnancy, delivery and early postpartum leading to a spiraling cycle of cyanosis, acidosis and hypotension. In one study of 18 pregnant women who died of congenital heart disease, three had PDA; however, all of these patients had severe secondary pulmonary hypertension [27]. In most circumstances, however, an asymptomatic young woman with a small or moderate-sized PDA, without pulmonary hypertension, will have a relatively uncomplicated pregnancy. Apart from a single case report of a spontaneous postpartum rupture of a PDA, in a patient with normal pulmonary pressure and without ductal aneurysm [31], the risks are minimal.

Pulmonary hypertension and Eisenmenger's syndrome

As discussed in the previous section, women with secundum ASD rarely manifest pulmonary hypertension in the childbearing age range and those with VSD or PDA are more likely to develop pulmonary hypertension compared to those with ASD. Patients with left to right shunts may have a continuum of progressive pulmonary artery pressure elevation and varying degrees of reversibility. It should be of note that with large left to right shunts, echocardiographic studies may suggest the presence of pulmonary artery systolic hypertension. Elevated pulmonary artery systolic pressures can be seen with high flow states in left to right shunts and should not be confused with irreversible pulmonary hypertension. Degree of left to right shunting and degree of pulmonary artery hypertension reversibility can usually be assessed before pregnancy or even during pregnancy with clinical evaluation, echocardiography along with other laboratory tests. A general rule of thumb is that pulmonary artery systolic hypertension in association with a left to right shunt of 1:5:1 or higher has some reversibility, otherwise, there would be no capcity for shunting. In these patients, in the absence of profound uncompensated left heart failure from volume overload, maternal outcomes are generally favorable. However, in those patients found to have irreversible pulmonary hypertension such as those with equivalent systemic and pulmonary artery pressures, cyanosis or bidirectional shunting, the prognosis during pregnancy is extremely grave.

Eisenmenger's syndrome consists of congenital systemic arterial to systemic venous shunt (left to right shunt), development of pulmonary hypertension and shunt reversal with bidirectional shunting/or cyanosis. This syndrome may occur from a variety of common congenital lesions including VSD, ASD, PDA and more complex anatomic disorders. The risk of developing pulmononary hypertension and Eisenmenger's syndrome from congenital shunts is determined by the the type of shunt and degree of left to right shunt as noted above. Whatever the etiology, development of irreversible pulmonary hypertension or Eisenmenger's syndrome during prengnacy portends a poor prognosis. During the antepartun period, decreased systemic vascular resistance increases right to left shunting, acidosis and hypotension. With systemic hypotension against a fixed pulmonary vascular resistance the degree of right to left shunting and hypoxia further increases, with a vicious spiraling circle of hypotension, cyanosis, hypoxia and ultimate death.

Such hypotension can result from hemorrhage or complications of conduction anesthesia and may result in sudden death [32–35]. Avoidance of such hypotension is the principal clinical concern in the intrapartum management of patients with pulmonary hypertension of any etiology.

Maternal mortality in the presence of Eisenmenger's syndrome is reported as 30–50% [26,27,30,31]. In a review of the subject, Gleicher et al. [33] reported a 34% mortality associated with vaginal delivery and a 75% mortality associated with cesarean section. In a more recent report, Weiss et al. [36] reviewed the published literature from 1978 to 1996 investigating Eisenmenger's syndrome, primary pulmonary hypertension and secondary pulmonary hypertension during pregnancy. Despite advances in maternal and cardiac care during this interval, the overall composite mortality rate for Eisenmenger's syndrome during pregnancy remained 36% – relatively unchanged for the last two decades [37–41]. In this series, however, there appeared to be little difference in mortality when comparing vaginal delivery (48%) to cesarean section (52%). These investigators also concluded that maternal prognosis depended on the early diagnosis of pulmonary vascular disease during pregnancy, early hospital admission, and individually tailored treatment during pregnancy with specific attention focused on the postpartum period. Table 20.6 reviews the management and outcome of pregnant women with Eisenmenger's syndrome [36]. In addition to the previously discussed problems associated with hemorrhage and hypovolemia, thromboembolic phenomena have been associated with up to 43% of all maternal deaths in Eisenmenger's syndrome [33]. In the more recent report by Weiss et al. [36], however, pulmonary thromboembolism accounted for only 3 of the 26 (12%) maternal deaths in this composite analysis. Sudden delayed postpartum death, occurring 4–6 weeks after delivery, also has been

Table 20.6 Management and outcome of pregnant women with Eisenmenger's syndrome ($n = 73$).

	Maternal survival	Maternal mortality
Number (%)	47 (64%)	26 (36%)
Age (years)	26.4 ± 4.8	24.9 ± 4.5
Hospital admission (weeks of pregnancy)	26.7 ± 6.5	31.4 ± 5.9
Toxemia of pregnancy	2 (4%)	3 (12%)
Delivery (weeks of pregnancy)	35.1 ± 3.5	34.4 ± 4.4
Vaginal delivery	27 (57%)	11 (48%)
Operative delivery	20 (43%)	12 (52%)
Monitoring		
Non-invasive, not reported	24 (51%)	15 (63%)
Invasive SAP and/or CVP	23 (49%)	9 (37%)
Invasive PAP	8 (17%)	6 (25%)
Anesthesia/analgesia		
Not reported	13 (28%)	5 (22%)
Regional techniques	22 (47%)	8 (35%)
General anesthesia	12 (25%)	7 (30%)
Local anesthesia/analgesia	0	3 (13%)
Oxytocic drugs	14 (30%)	4 (17%)
Antithrombotic therapy	28 (60%)	12 (46%)
Neonatal survival	43 (96%)*	20 (77%)
Maternal death, days postpartum	–	5 (0–30)

Data presented are mean value; ± SD, number (%) of patients, or median (range).

* In two cases neonatal outcome was not reported. Three patients died before delivery and 23 died after delivery.

CI, confidence interval; CVP, central venous pressure; PAP, pulmonary artery pressure; SAP, systemic arterial pressure.

(From Weiss BM, Zemp L, Burkhardt S, Hess O. Outcome of pulmonary vascular disease in pregnancy: a systemic overview from 1978 through 1996. J Am Coll Cardio 1998;31:1650–1657.)

reported [33,36,42]. Such deaths may involve a rebound worsening of pulmonary hypertension associated with the loss of pregnancy-associated hormones, which leads to decreased pulmonary vascular resistance during gestation [17].

Caution should be exercised when evaluating for the presence of pulmonary hypertension with non-invasive techniques such as Doppler/two-dimensional echocardiogram. The assumptions used by many cardiologists for assessment of pulmonary pressures do not take into account viscosity (Hb) nor pregnant state when assessing the tricuspid jet or estimating the right atrial pressure based on IVC size. The ordering physician should directly communicate with the interpreting physician these issues when trying to determine pulmonary artery pressures since other methods to assess these values may be available. Otherwise, these techniques have a clear tendency to significantly overestimate the degree of pulmonary hypertension during pregnancy and may incorrectly diagnose the presence of pulmonary hypertension in up to 32% of cases when compared with cardiac catheterization [43]. If any question exists regarding the presence of pulmonary hypertension, and the pregnancy is desired, pulmonary artery catheterization with direct measurement of pulmonary artery pressures may be performed on an outpatient basis in early pregnancy. This can be done with no to minimal radiation exposure in experienced hands using a brachial or internal jugular approach. Where significant fixed irreversible pulmonary hypertension exists, pregnancy termination in either the first or second trimester appears to be safer than allowing the pregnancy to progress to term [44]. Dilation and curettage in the first trimester or dilation and evacuation in the second trimester are the methods of choice. Hypertonic saline and F-series prostaglandins are contraindicated, the latter due to arterial oxygen desaturation seen with the use of this agent [45]. Prostaglandin E_2 suppositories appear to be safe under these circumstances.

It is highly recommended that the woman with significant pulmonary hypertension/Eisenmenger's syndrome who elects to continue pregnancy undergoes hospitalization for the duration of pregnancy. Alternatively very close clinical follow-up and early hospitalization at a center specialized in treatment of this condition at the first sign or detection of clinical deterioration may be considered on a case-by-case basis. Continuous administration of oxygen, the pulmonary vasodilator of choice, is suggested and may improve perinatal outcome. Consideration of anticoagulation in the peripartum period has been suggested as a method to lower this risk but there has been concern that this may instead contribute to a fatal outcome. Patients with Eisenmenger's syndrome have abnormalities with coagulation factors, and with platelet function and number. The very real possibility of fatal intrapulmonary hemorrhage and hemoptysis while on anticoagulants has to be weighed against the possible risk of suspected peripartum thromboembolism as the cause of death in these patients during the third trimester and postpartum. Since death has been reported with fatal hemorrhaging while on anticoagulants and benefit of this therapy is not proven, routine endorsement of this treatment modality cannot be given.

In cyanotic heart disease of any etiology, fetal outcome correlates well with maternal hemoglobin, and successful pregnancy is unlikely with a hemoglobin greater than 20 g/dL [13]. Maternal P_aO_2 should be maintained at a level of 70 mmHg or above [46]. Third-trimester fetal surveillance with antepartum testing is important because at least 30% of the fetuses will suffer growth restriction [33]. Although the overall fetal wastage with Eisenmenger's syndrome is reported to be up to 75%, more recent information suggests a more favorable outcome. Weiss et al. reported a neonatal survival rate of nearly 90% in cases of Eisenmenger's syndrome. Unfortunately, since only late pregnancy cases were reviewed, no conclusions can be drawn about the rate of early fetal wastage.

For pregnant patients with Eisenmenger's syndrome some experts previously advocated placement of a Swan–Ganz catheter in the intrapartum period in an effort to minimize changes in cardiovascular hemodynamics, cyanosis and the shunt that occurs with uterine contractions [47]. However, placement and stabilization of a right heart catheter in a pulmonary artery branch can be quite difficult in the presence of markedly elevated pulmonary pressures. These patients require ICU monitoring, and are increased risk of pulmonary artery rupture, pulmonary infarction, and dysrhythmia. They also require suspension of any oral anticoagulation before placement,with increased risk of pulmonary artery thrombosis. Many now believe the risk of this technique far outweighs the its benefits in patients with cyanotic heart disease [48] and its use is rare. In many cases, pulse oximetry may offer appropriate guidance in the intrapartum management of these patients without the need for and/or the associated risks of, pulmonary artery catheterization. Because the primary concern in such patients is the avoidance of hypotension, any attempt at preload reduction (i.e. diuresis) must be undertaken with great caution, even in the face of initial fluid overload. We prefer to manage such patients on the "wet" side, maintaining a preload margin of safety against unexpected blood loss, even at the expense of mild pulmonary edema. Recently, the use of inhaled nitric oxide and intravenous prostacyclin therapy have shown promise as potentially helpful agents in reducing the pulmonary vascular resistance while relatively sparing the systemic vascular resistance [49,50].

Anesthesia for patients with pulmonary hypertension is controversial. Theoretically, conduction anesthesia, with its accompanying risk of hypotension, should be avoided. However, there are several reports of its successful use in patients with pulmonary hypertension of different etiologies [51,52]. The use of epidural or intrathecal morphine sulfate, a technique devoid of effect on systemic BP, represents perhaps the best approach to anesthetic management of these difficult patients.

Although the AHA recommendations for antibiotic prophylaxis to prevent endocarditis have been extensively revised, the recommendations regarding cyanotic congenital heart disease have not. Endocarditis prophylaxis continues to be recommended for cyanotic congenital heart disease [28].

Ebstein's anomaly

Because it accounts for less than 1% of all congenital cardiac disease, Ebstein's anomaly is uncommonly encountered during pregnancy [53–55]. This anomaly consists of apical displacement of the tricuspid valve into the right ventricle, sometimes markedly so, with secondary tricuspid regurgitation of varying degrees, and enlargement of the right atrium by incorporation of the right ventricle situated above the tricuspid valve (the so called "atrialized right ventricle"). A patent foramen ovale may be present in the interatrial septum and thus these patients may have non-cyanotic or cyanotic form of the anomaly. The presence or absence of cyanosis and hemodynamic consequences of Ebstein anomaly result from the degree of displacement of the tricuspid valve leaflets and extent of atrialization of the right ventricle. The severity of tricuspid regurgitation and hence shunting across the patent foramen ovale depends on the extent of leaflet displacement, ranging from mild regurgitation with minimal displacement to severe tricuspid regurgitation with more apical displacement and atrialization of the right ventricle. Usually the functional right ventricle beyond the apically displaced tricuspid valve provides effective forward pulmonary blood flow. However, at times the functional right ventricle may be extremely small and barely able to produce enough forward pulmonary flow to sustain adequate blood pressure. Those women who reach childbearing years may have either the acyanotic or cyanotic form of Ebstein's anomaly. Since pulmonary hypertension is not seen in this anomaly, as noted, the cyanosis is determined by the degree of right to left shunting across the patent foramen ovale from tricuspid regurgitation. Fetal prematurity, loss and low birth weight are more common in the cynanotic form of Ebstein's anomaly, reflecting this finding. It is extremely unusual for the non-cyanotic form of Ebstein's anomaly to convert to a cyanotic form once patients have reached maturity. However, this is dependent upon the degree of tricuspid regurgitation and the functional capacity of the non-atrialized portion of the right ventricle. Therefore, evaluation of oxygen and volume status is an important consideration during gestation, labor and delivery.

Paroxysmal atrial arrhythmias have been reported to occur in up to one-third of non-pregnant women with Ebstein's anomaly and represent a potential concern during pregnancy. The Wolff–Parkinson–White syndrome is an arrhythymia classically associated with Ebstein's anomaly and may represent a risk factor for excessively rapid ventricular rates in response to the increased incidence of atrial arrhythmias that are associated with Ebstein's anomaly [56].

Despite these concerns, in a review of 111 pregnancies in 44 women, no serious maternal complications were noted. Seventy-six per cent of pregnancies ended in live births, with a 6% incidence of congenital heart disease in the offspring of these women [55].

Coarctation of the aorta

Coarctation of the aorta accounts for approximately 10% of all congenital cardiac disease. The most common site of coarctation is usually at the origin of the left subclavian artery. Associated anomalies of the aorta and left heart, including VSD and PDA, are common, as are intracranial aneurysms in the circle of Willis [57]. Coarctation is often asymptomatic. Its presence is suggested by hypertension confined to the upper extremities, although Goodwin [58] cites data suggesting a generalized increase in peripheral resistance throughout the body. Resting cardiac output may be increased; however, increased left atrial pressure with exercise suggests occult left ventricular dysfunction. Aneurysms also may develop below the coarctation or involve the intercostal arteries and may lead to rupture. In addition, ruptures without prior aneurysm formation have been reported [59].

Over 150 patients with uncorrected and corrected coarctation of the aorta have been reported during pregnancy, with maternal mortality ranging from 0% to 17% [25,59,60]. In a 1940 review of 200 pregnant women with coarctation of the aorta, Mendelson [61] reported 14 maternal deaths and recommended routine abortion and sterilization for these patients. Deaths in this series were from aortic dissection and rupture, congestive heart failure, cerebral vascular accidents, and bacterial endocarditis. Six of the 14 deaths occurred in women with associated lesions. In contrast to this dismal prognosis, a more recent series by Deal and Wooley [60] reported 83 pregnancies in 23 women with uncomplicated coarctation of the aorta. All were NYHA class I or II before pregnancy. In these women, there were no maternal deaths or permanent cardiovascular complications. In one review, aortic rupture was more likely to occur in the third trimester, before labor and delivery [62]. More recent reviews have also supported the finding that improved surgical and percutaneous techniques, medical therapy for hypertension, and improvement in the management of these women during pregnancy have resulted in more favorable maternal outcomes [63–65].

Thus, it appears that today, patients with coarctation of the aorta uncomplicated by aneurysmal dilation or hemodynamically significant associated cardiac lesions who enter pregnancy as class I or II have a good prognosis and a minimal risk of complications or death. Even if uncorrected, uncomplicated coarctation has historically carried with it a risk of maternal mortality of only 3–4% [58]. These unrepaired patients should be considered for repair of their coarctation after the postpartum period is concluded and before contemplation of a next pregnancy. Those pregnant women who have uncontrolled symptomatic hypertension attributable to coarctation despite maximal medical therapy should have a stent placed at the coarctation site. This procedure is 90% successful with <20 mmHg residual gradient. The risk of fetal irradiation is low compared to the high maternal risk of death from heart failure, arrhythmia, dissection, stroke, and myocardial infarction. The fetal risk can further be reduced by involving a radiation physicist from the hospital who can help calculate the radiation dose based on the distance of the X-ray tube from the mother's abdomen, by shielding the mother's abdomen with lead (both anterior and posterior), and by performing the procedure after the second trimester. Surgical intervention for coarctation of the aorta in a pregnant woman is not ideal.

For those with previously surgically repaired coarctation of the aorta, the maternal outcome appears good [63,65]. Surgical repair of the coarctation, often accomplished in early childhood, usually results in long-term normalization of blood pressure. However, those who have surgeries done at an early age require ongoing surveillance since the site of surgical intervention does not typically "grow" with the child and further intervention may be necessary for redevelopment of hypertension, aneurysm at the site of the surgical repair, or other issues related to the repair. Percutaneous catheter-based interventional techniques for treatment of coarctation are also being widely used as well, for management of both children and older patients. Weakness in the aortic wall, both proximal and distal to the repair, is histologically similar (cystic medial necrosis) to the aortic weakness exhibited in Marfan syndrome and bicuspid aortic valve. This abnormality can be amplified during pregnancy. For women who have unrepaired coarctation of the aorta, who have residual coarctation after surgical or interventional therapy, or who have a residual gradient, β-blockade therapy seems reasonable, although unproven, to decrease the force of left ventricular ejection into the aorta and to reduce aortic wall stress. Despite these concerns, most patients with a successfully repaired coarctation of the aorta have a relatively unremarkable pregnancy. Saidi, et al [63] followed 18 pregnancies in women who had undergone a successful repair of their aortic coarctations. All 18 women had uneventful pregnancies. Interestingly, the incidence of pre-eclampsia in this series was no different than that reported in the normal population. Maternal risk, however, is clearly increased if pre-eclampsia develops [66]. In a recent retrospective study of 100 women [65], a higher incidence of hypertension and pre-eclampsia was found in women who had previously had a repair of coarctation of the aorta. Interestingly, 80% had had end-to-end surgical resection at a median age of 6 years, 13% had required intervention for recoarctation and 30% were noted to have hypertension at the time of the review. This supports the contention that children often outgrow their initial surgery and that hypertension is quite common even after successful repair of coarctation of the aorta.

In the presence of aortic or intervertebral aneurysm, known as aneurysm of the circle of Willis, or associated cardiac lesions, the risk of death may approach 15%; therefore, termination of pregnancy should be strongly considered.

Tetralogy of Fallot

Tetralogy of Fallot refers to four key anatomic features which lead to cyanosis: VSD, overriding aorta, right ventricular hypertrophy, and pulmonary stenosis. In the United States, most cases of tetralogy of Fallot are corrected during infancy or childhood. Most of the women with this condition at childbearing age have had it surgically corrected but many have residual lesions such as ongoing VSD through a VSD patch, pulmonary insufficiency of varying degrees with right heart enlargement, prosthetic pulmonary valve, residual right ventricular outflow tract obstruction, or a combination of these. A few will have only had palliative procedures and are cyanotic [67]. Rarely do they present in the cyanotic state without any prior surgical correction.

Several published reports attest to the relatively successful outcome of pregnancy in patients with totally or partially corrected tetralogy of Fallot [66,68]. For the totally corrected patient, pregnancy outcome is similar to that of the general population. For those with residual lesions including mild pulmonic and/or tricuspid regurgitation, mild pulmonary stenosis, or small VSD patch leak, the maternal and fetal risk is minimal. If there is significant right heart enlargement from residual pulmonary insufficiency, right ventricular outflow obstruction or pulmonic stenosis, the risk is higher for development of arrhythmias or heart failure during pregnancy. However, these patients still can be managed successfully if they first present during pregnancy. Women with uncorrected tetralogy of Fallot do not fare as well. In a review of 55 pregnancies in 46 patients, there were no maternal deaths among nine patients with correction of this lesion before pregnancy; in patients with an uncorrected lesion, however, maternal mortality has traditionally ranged from 4% to 15%, with a 30% fetal mortality due to hypoxia [66,69]. In patients with uncorrected VSD and right ventricular outflow tract obstruction or pulmonic stenosis, the decline in SVR that accompanies pregnancy can lead to worsening of the right to left shunt. This condition can be aggravated further by systemic hypotension as a result of peripartum blood loss. A poor prognosis for successful pregnancy has been related to several prepregnancy parameters, including a hemoglobin exceeding 20 g/dL, a history of syncope or congestive failure, electrocardiographic evidence of right ventricular strain, cardiomegaly, right ventricular pressure in excess of 120 mmHg, and peripheral oxygen saturation below 85%. Women who present with a palliative shunt procedure only from childhood may be cyanotic and/or have pulmonary hypertension with the same attendant problems as outlined in the section on pulmonary hypertension/Eisenmenger's syndrome. If they are found to have this problem they should be discouraged from attempting or continuing pregnancy.

Transposition of the great vessels

Transposition of the great vessels consists of two types:

- L-transposition; the so-called congenitally corrected transposition of the great arteries
- D-transposition: the complete transposition.

L-transposition (L-TGA)

In L-transposition, or congenitally corrected transposition, the great arteries are transposed. This accounts for less than 1% of all congenital cardiac defects. In this defect, the atria and ventricles are also transposed. Hence there is a double discordance of the atrial-ventricular and ventricular-arterial connections. The right ventricle is attached to the aorta and acts as the systemic arterial ventricle receiving oxygenated blood from the lungs and left atrium. The morphologic left ventricle is attached to the pulmonary artery and acts as the systemic venous ventricle receiving venous blood from the right atrium, IVC and SVC. Although the morphologic right ventricle is not designed to accommodate systemic arterial pressures, it may accommodate this pressure well for years. Ventricular dysfunction and AV valve regurgitation are recognized and important complications of patients with L-TGA but this may present slowly and insidiously and does not happen in all L-TGA patients. Although RV dilation is common, few develop evidence of symptomatic heart failure. Serial studies do not indicate that there is an inevitable progressive downward and progressive deterioration of function with time. Heart failure symptoms are typical, as one would expect, with pulmonary edema, increasing pulmonary pressures and decreased forward systemic arterial output. This condition is detected later in life usually when the morphologic right ventricle can no longer accommodate systemic arterial pressures or the AV valve becomes regurgitant and symptoms of shortness of breath, palpitations, and arrhythmia become manifest. Disconcertingly, the diagnostic anatomic features of this congenital defect may be missed on echocardiography by adult cardiologists not trained in congenital heart disease.

For those in whom the diagnosis is established, both maternal outcome and pregnancy is generally well tolerated with NYHA class I or II symptoms [70]. It is still difficult to quantify RV function due to the lack of a suitable control group for comparison, and because of the dependence on shape assumptions and loading conditions of the commonly used systolic indices. Nevertheless, those with severe AV valve regurgitation or severely depressed morphologic RV function should be counseled against pregnancy regardless of functional class. Lessons being learned from those who have had atrial switch operations for D-TGA (see below) and similar systemic arterial RV functional issues may be of help in this group of patients.

D-transposition (D-TGA)

D-transposition or complete transposition of the great vessels is incompatible with prolonged life after birth. In this condition, the transposed aorta is connected to the RV and the pulmonary artery to the LV. The atria and ventricles are not transposed so that systemic venous return to the RV is ejected into the aorta. This defect requires urgent surgical palliation and then subsequent complete repair. The first complete repair involved the "atrial switch" operation. Both the Mustard and Senning operations in the late 1950s and early 1960s revolutionized the management of babies with D-TGA and became the treatment of choice. In this operation, the systemic venous flow from the RA is redirected into the LV and PA, while the systemic arterial flow is redirected from the pulmonary veins into the morphologic RV to the aorta. Since the morphologic RV serves as the systemic arterial ventricle, similar issues arise to those seen with L-TGA, and the key to long-term outcome is the fate of the RV. In addition, because of the extensive surgical intervention to the atria in redirection of flow, significant arrhythmias have been described in both types of surgeries. This procedure has been largely abandoned in favor of the arterial switch begun in the 1980s [71] because of these concerns. This procedure appears to reduce the late morbidity rates that have been described with the atrial repairs [72,73]. Women that have had successful arterial switch procedures are now entering reproductive ages. The arterial switch procedure is done within days of birth. Both great arteries are transected and reanastomosed above the sinuses of Valsalva, and the coronary arteries are translocated. The native pulmonary valve becomes the systemic outflow valve, and the anatomic pulmonary root is subjected to systemic blood pressure. The native valves are not touched. Short- and midterm follow-up of these patients have shown coronary artery narrowing, pulmonary artery stenosis, neoaortic valve aortic insufficiency, and neoaortic root dilation [74,75]

The risk of pregnancy in patients with D-transposition who have had the Mustard or Senning procedure is related to the severity of any heart failure present, the degree of AV valve regurgitation, the degree of resultant pulmonary hypertension and the presence of arrhythmias. A series of pregnant patients who were followed subsequent to the Mustard (atrial switch) operation reported 12 of 15 live births and no maternal deaths [76]. In a similar series of seven patients with transposition having undergone the Mustard procedure, no maternal deaths were reported [77]. In one case, however, pregnancy termination was necessary due to maternal deterioration. In the largest series described thus far, using a retrospective nationwide registry in the Netherlands, outcomes of 70 women with D-transposition and Mustard or Senning operations were reported [78]. Forty-two were childless of whom 35 wished to bear children in the future. Of the 28 patients who completed 49 pregnancies, all were in NYHA class I or II before pregnancy. There was clinical deterioration in NYHA in one-third of pregnancies and development of clinically significant arrhythmias in 20% of these pregnancies. No maternal deaths occurred. The cardiac issues were manageable. However, there was a high incidence of obstetric complications. The authors indicated that in contrast to what is generally assumed, pregnancy is not always well tolerated in these patients. They also estimate that approximately 4500 women with this congenital lesion and surgical procedure will enter childbearing age in the USA over the next few years.

Women who have had the Jatene (arterial switch) procedure are only now entering their childbearing years. There has been a case report, cited frequently, of a successful pregnancy and delivery in a patient with D-transposition and arterial switch [79].

Pulmonic stenosis

Pulmonic stenosis is a common congenital defect. Although obstruction can be valvular, supravalvular, or subvalvular, the degree of obstruction, rather than its site, is the principal determinant of clinical performance [8]. Maternal well-being is rarely significantly affected by pulmonic stenosis. Even 30 years ago, a compilation (totaling 106 pregnancies) of three series of patients with pulmonic stenosis revealed no maternal deaths [25–27]. With severe stenosis, right heart failure can occur; fortunately, this is usually less clinically severe than is the left heart failure associated with mitral or aortic valve lesions. Symptoms of dyspnea, angina, syncope or presyncope can occur in those with markedly stentotic lesions. Severe pulmonic stenosis is defined by a peak valvular gradient of more than 80 mmHg. Because this degree of obstruction imposes a significant load on the right ventricle, patients with severe pulmonic stenosis usually benefit from balloon valvuloplasty even in the absence of symptoms. In these women with severe pulmonic stenosis, pregnancy may be associated with increased risk during labor, delivery, and the puerperium. The first balloon valvuloplast was performed in 1982. Balloon valvuloplasty in pregnancy has since been performed successfully and with relatively low complication rates [80]. The incidence of fetal congenital heart disease in patients with pulmonic valve stenosis appears to be approximately 20%, with a 55% concordance rate [81].

Aortic stenosis

Congenital and rheumatic aortic valvular disease are important causes of aortic stenosis. The impact of aortic stenosis on pregnancy will be discussed in Acquired cardiac lesions.

Functional single ventricle and Fontan procedure

Some of the anomalies described as a functional single ventricle that will ultimately undergo staged reconstructive procedures resulting in a "Fontan circulation" are tricuspid atresia, hypoplastic left heart, double-inlet left ventricle, and some variations of double-outlet right ventricle. Given the variety of lesions and the infrequency of this procedure, data on pregnancy outcomes after Fontan operation are limited [82,83]. In the small numbers reported in the United States, no maternal deaths have occurred. Pregnancies in these patients have been associated with an increased incidence of spontaneous abortions, however. In a small survey from the Netherlands, 10 pregnancies in 6 women were associated with a 50% miscarriage rate and one aborted ectopic pregnancy. In the four live births, NYHA class deterioration, atrial fibrillation and premature delivery were reported. There were no maternal deaths. Thus, at this early stage, although maternal death does not appear to be prominent in patients who have undergone a Fontan repair with their specific underlying congenital lesion and who have elected to proceed with pregnancy, there appears to be a substantial risk for spontaneous abortion, as well as other significant obstetric and cardiac issues.

Fetal considerations

Perinatal outcome in patients with cyanotic congenital cardiac disease correlates best with hematocrit; successful outcome in patients with a hematocrit exceeding 65% or hemoglobin exceeding 20 g/dL is unlikely. Presbitero and associates [13] described outcome in 96 pregnancies complicated by cyanotic congenital heart disease. Patients with Eisenmenger's syndrome were excluded from this analysis. Although only one maternal death was seen (from endocarditis 2 months postpartum), the pregnancy loss rate was 51%. Functional class III or IV, hemoglobin greater than 20 g/dL, and a prepregnancy oxygen saturation less than 85% all were associated with a high risk for poor pregnancy outcome. Such patients have an increased risk of spontaneous abortion, intrauterine growth restriction, and stillbirth. Maternal P_aO_2 below 70 mmHg results in decreased fetal oxygen saturation; thus, P_aO_2 should be kept above this level during pregnancy, labor, and delivery. In the presence of maternal cardiovascular disease, the growth-restricted fetus is especially sensitive to intrapartum hypoxia, and fetal decompensation may occur more rapidly [7,84]. During the antepartum period, serial antepartum sonography for the detection of growth restriction and antepartum fetal heart rate testing are recommended in any patient with significant cardiac disease. Fetal activity counting also may be of value in patients with severe disease [85]. In a series of six patients with cyanotic cardiac disease, every pregnancy was eventually delivered secondary to fetal, rather than maternal, deterioration [86].

Of equal concern in patients with congenital heart disease is the risk of fetal congenital cardiac anomalies. This risk appears to be of the order of 5%, although one older study suggested that the actual risk may be as high as 10%, or even higher in women whose congenital lesion involves ventricular outflow obstruction [13,81,87,88] (see Figure 20.3). In such patients, fetal echocardiography is indicated for prenatal diagnosis of congenital cardiac defects [89]. Of special interest is that affected fetuses appear to be concordant for the maternal lesion in approximately 50% of cases. The genetics and embryologic development of congenital cardiac defects have been reviewed by Clark [90].

Acquired cardiac lesions

Many common complaints associated with normal pregnancy including dyspnea, fatigue, orthopnea, palpitations, presyncope and pedal edema mimic the symptoms of valvular heart disease making the clinical diagnosis difficult. Jugular venous distention, brisk and collapsing pulses, and a diffuse and laterally displaced left ventricular impulse, all normal physiologic adaptations to pregnancy, further confound the clinical assessment. On auscultation of the normal heart during pregnancy, it is not unusual to hear an accentuated first heart sound (S1) or a systolic flow murmur that peaks in midsystole and is best appreciated along the left sternal border. A third heart sound (S3), a fourth heart sound (S4), or a diastolic murmur are uncommon in normal pregnancy and require an echocardiographic assessment.

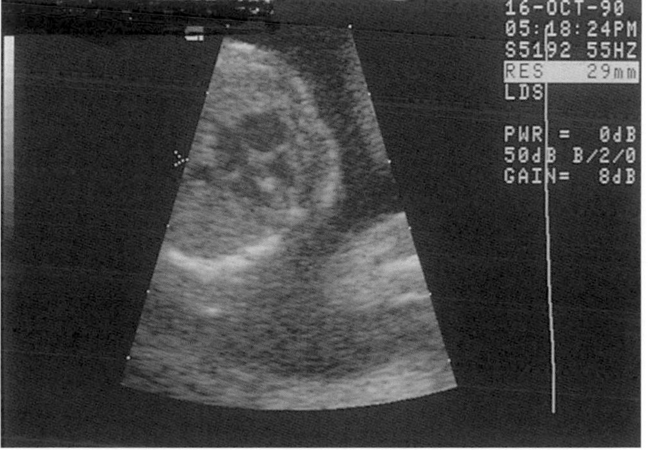

Figure 20.3 Echocardiographic image of a fetus at 19 weeks in a mother with a ventricular septal defect (VSD). A similar VSD is demonstrated in this fetus.

Doppler echocardiography in normal pregnancy reflects the physiologic consequences of the increased intravascular volume and blood flow on the cardiac chambers and valves. There is an increase in the left ventricular end-diastolic dimension and a decrease in the left ventricular end-systolic dimension representing an increase in both the stroke volume and ejection fraction. The aortic root dimension, as well as the mitral and tricuspid annuli, are slightly increased. The left ventricular mass increases by as much as 30% with minimal changes in wall thickness [91]. Flow velocities across the aortic valve are minimally increased but rarely exceed 1.5 m/s by Doppler assessment. Campos et al. [92] studied 18 pregnant women longitudinally throughout pregnancy utilizing Doppler echocardiogram. Mild valvular regurgitation was detected consistently throughout pregnancy. Aortic regurgitation was rarely detected; however, mitral (0–28%) tricuspid (39–94%), and pulmonic regurgitation (22–94%) were found to increase substantially from early to late gestation. Table 20.7 reviews the effect of pregnancy on the clinical and echocardiographic findings associated with cardiac valvular abnormalities [81].

Acquired valvular lesions generally are rheumatic in origin, although endocarditis secondary to intravenous drug abuse may

Table 20.7 The effect of pregnancy on the clinical and echocardiographic findings associated with cardiac valvular abnormalities.

	Heart sounds	Murmur	Other	Doppler echocardiography
Aortic stenosis (AS)	Diminished or single S2 – unchanged	Increase in intensity and duration	Systolic ejection click unchanged	Increase in Doppler gradient; AVA unchanged
Aortic insufficiency (AI)	Diminished S2 – unchanged	Decreased or unchanged	Wide pulse pressure – increased or unchanged	LV dimensions may increase secondary to pregnancy not AI
Mitral stenosis (MS)	Loud 1 – increased; P2 – increased	Increased decrease or unchanged	S2–OS interval gradient, decrease in pressure half-time and increase in calculated MVA	Increase in Doppler
Mitral regurgitation (MR)	Diminished S1 – unchanged	Decreased or unchanged	S3 – unchanged to pregnancy not MR	LV dimensions may increase secondary
Pulmonic stenosis (PS)	Diminished P2 – unchanged	Increase in intensity and duration	Systolic ejection click unchanged	Increase in Doppler gradient
Pulmonic insufficiency (PI)	Diminished P2 – unchanged	Decreased or unchanged	N/A secondary to pregnancy not PI	RV dimensions may increase
Tricuspid stenosis (TS)	N/A	Increased	N/A	N/A
Tricuspid regurgitation (TR)	N/A unchanged	Decreased or secondary to pregnancy not TR	N/A	RV dimensions may increase

AVA, arteriovenous anastomosis; LV, left ventricle; MVA, mitral valve anastomosis; RV, right ventricle.

occasionally occur, especially with right heart lesions. During pregnancy, maternal morbidity and mortality with such lesions result from congestive failure with pulmonary edema or arrhythmias. Szekely et al. [93] found the risk of pulmonary edema in pregnant patients with rheumatic heart disease to increase with increasing age and with increasing length of gestation. The onset of atrial fibrillation during pregnancy carries with it a higher risk of right and left ventricular failure (63%) than does fibrillation with onset before gestation (22%). In addition, the risk of systemic embolization after the onset of atrial fibrillation during pregnancy appears to exceed that associated with onset in the non-pregnant state. In counseling the patient with severe rheumatic cardiac disease on the advisability of initiating or continuing pregnancy, the physician must also consider the long-term prognosis of the underlying disease. Chesley [94] followed 134 women who had functionally severe rheumatic heart disease and who had completed pregnancy for up to 44 years. He reported a mortality of 6.3% per year but concluded that in patients who survived the gestation, maternal life expectancy was not shortened by pregnancy. Thus, in general, pregnancy does not appear to introduce long-term sequelae for patients who survive the pregnancy [44].

Pulmonic and tricuspid lesions

Isolated right-sided valvular lesions of rheumatic origin are uncommon; however, such lesions are seen with increased frequency in intravenous drug abusers, where they are secondary to valvular endocarditis. Pregnancy-associated hypervolemia is far less likely to be symptomatic with right-sided lesions than with those involving the mitral or aortic valves. In a review of 77 maternal cardiac deaths, Hibbard [27] reported no deaths associated with isolated right-sided lesions. In a more recent review, congestive heart failure occurred in only 2.8% of women with pulmonic stenosis [87]. Even following complete tricuspid valvectomy for endocarditis, pregnancy, labor, and delivery are generally well tolerated. Cautious fluid administration is the mainstay of labor and delivery management in such patients. In general, invasive hemodynamic monitoring during labor and delivery is not necessary.

Mitral stenosis

Mitral stenosis is the most common rheumatic valvular lesion encountered during pregnancy [42]. It can occur as an isolated lesion or in conjunction with aortic or right-sided lesions. When mitral stenosis is significant (valve area $<1.0\,cm^2$) the principal hemodynamic aberration involves a left ventricular diastolic filling obstruction, resulting in a relatively fixed cardiac output. Marked increases in cardiac output accompany normal pregnancy, labor, and delivery. If the pregnant patient is unable to accommodate such volume fluctuations, atrial arrhythmias and/or pulmonary edema may result.

Ideally it is best to treat significant mitral stenosis before pregnancy with balloon and/or surgical commissurotomy. Often the diagnosis of mitral stenosis will be discovered for the first time during pregnancy, illustrating what is frequently referred to as "occult" mitral stenosis. The hemodynamic changes accompanying normal pregnancy may represent the first time the patient's cardiovascular system has been significantly stressed. These patients may present with "acute" pulmonary edema and/or atrial fibrillation as the initial diagnostic clue to the presence of mitral stenosis. When clinical symptoms persist despite attentive medical management, interventional therapy may be prudent. Percutaneous balloon mitral valvuloplasty during pregnancy has become increasingly prevalent. More than 100 pregnant women have undergone percutaneous balloon mitral valvuloplasty without periprocedural maternal or fetal mortality. Multiple case reports [95–97] and case series [98–105] support the relative safety of this procedure during pregnancy. Procedural complications include cardiac tamponade, maternal arrhythmias, transient uterine contractions, and systemic thromboembolism. Transesophageal echocardiography can be used as the sole imaging modality, thereby eliminating the undesired radiation exposure associated with fluoroscopy.

Cardiac output in patients with mitral stenosis is largely dependent on two factors. First, these patients are dependent on adequate diastolic filling time. Thus, while in most patients tachycardia is a clinical sign of underlying hemodynamic instability, in patients with mitral stenosis, the tachycardia itself, regardless of etiology, may contribute significantly to hemodynamic decompensation. During labor, such tachycardia may accompany the exertion of pushing or be secondary to pain or anxiety. Such a patient may exhibit a rapid and dramatic fall in cardiac output and BP in response to tachycardia. This fall compromises maternal as well as fetal well-being. To avoid hazardous tachycardia, the physician should consider intravenous β-blocker therapy for any patient with severe mitral stenosis who enters labor with a pulse exceeding 90–100 bpm. A short acting β-blocker, such as esmolol, is ideal in that minute-to-minute heart rate control can be achieved without the undesired prolonged beat-blockade that is associated with more conventional agents such as propranolol. Another consideration is use of intravenous calcium channel blocking agents such as diltiazem with which the cardiologists and nursing personnel are generally familiar and for which administration is easier. In patients who are not initially tachycardic, acute control of tachycardia with an intravenous β-blocking agent is only rarely necessary [42].

A second important consideration in patients with mitral stenosis is left ventricular preload. In the presence of mitral stenosis, pulmonary capillary wedge pressure is not an accurate reflection of left ventricular filling pressures. Such patients often require high-normal or elevated pulmonary capillary wedge pressures to maintain adequate ventricular filling pressure and cardiac output. Any preload manipulation (i.e. diuresis), therefore, must be undertaken with extreme caution and careful attention to maintenance of cardiac output.

Potentially dangerous intrapartum fluctuations in cardiac output can be minimized by using epidural anesthesia [106];

however, the most hazardous time for these women appears to be the immediate postpartum period. Such patients often enter the postpartum period already operating at maximum cardiac output and cannot accommodate the volume shifts that follow delivery. In a series of patients with severe mitral stenosis, Clark and colleagues found that a postpartum rise in wedge pressure of up to 16 mmHg could be expected in the immediate postpartum period (Figure 20.4) [42]. Because frank pulmonary edema is infrequent with wedge pressures below 28–30 mmHg [184], it follows that the optimal predelivery wedge pressure for such patients is approximately 14 mmHg or lower, as indicated by pulmonary artery catheterization [107]. Such a preload may be approached by cautious intrapartum diuresis and with careful attention to the maintenance of adequate cardiac output. Active diuresis is not always necessary in patients who enter labor with evidence of only mild fluid overload. In such patients, simple fluid restriction and the associated sensible and insensible fluid losses that accompany labor can result in a significant fall in wedge pressure before delivery.

Previous recommendations for delivery in patients with cardiac disease have also included the liberal use of midforceps to shorten the second stage of labor. In cases of severe disease, cesarean section with general anesthesia also has been advocated as the preferred mode of delivery [108]. If intensive monitoring of intrapartum cardiac patients cannot be carried out in the manner described here, such recommendations for elective cesarean delivery may be valid. With the aggressive management scheme presented, however, our experience suggests that vaginal delivery is safe, even in patients with severe disease and pulmonary hypertension. Midforceps deliveries are rarely appropriate in modern obstetrics [109] and should be reserved for standard obstetric indications only.

Mitral insufficiency

Hemodynamically significant mitral insufficiency was usually of rheumatic origin in the past and most commonly occurred in conjunction with other valvular lesions. Now, however, cardiomopathy and other disease processes causing secondary mitral regurgitation have become the most common causes. Regardless of etiology, mitral regurgitation itself is generally well tolerated during pregnancy, and congestive failure is an unusual occurrence. A more significant risk is the development of atrial enlargement and fibrillation. There is some evidence to suggest that the risk of developing atrial fibrillation may be increased during pregnancy [93]. In Hibbard's review of 28 maternal deaths associated with rheumatic valvular lesions, no patient died with complications of mitral insufficiency unless there was coexisting mitral stenosis [27].

Mitral valve prolapse

Congenital mitral valve prolapse is more commonly seen during pregnancy than is rheumatic mitral insufficiency and can occur in up to 17% of young healthy women. This condition is generally asymptomatic [110]. The mid-systolic click and murmur associated with congenital mitral valve prolapse are characteristic; however, the intensity of this murmur, as well as that associated with rheumatic mitral insufficiency, may decrease during pregnancy because of decreased SVR [111]. As noted later in a separate section, the AHA no longer recommends antiobiotic prophylaxis in women with mitral valve prolapse [28].

Aortic stenosis

Congenital aortic stenosis (bicuspid aortic valve) has replaced rheumatic fever as the most common cause of aortic stenosis. The congenitally malformed aortic (bicuspid valve) represents 5% of all congenital cardiac lesions. In several series of pregnancies in women with cardiac disease, no maternal deaths due to aortic stenosis have been observed [2,5,66]. In contrast to mitral valve stenosis, aortic stenosis generally does not become hemodynamically significant until the orifice has diminished to one-third or less of normal. Based on the ACC/AHA 2006 guidelines for management of patients with valvular heart disease, patients with a mean gradient of 25–40 mmHg, and/or a calculated valve area of 1.0–1.5 cm^2 by echocardiographic criteria are considered to have

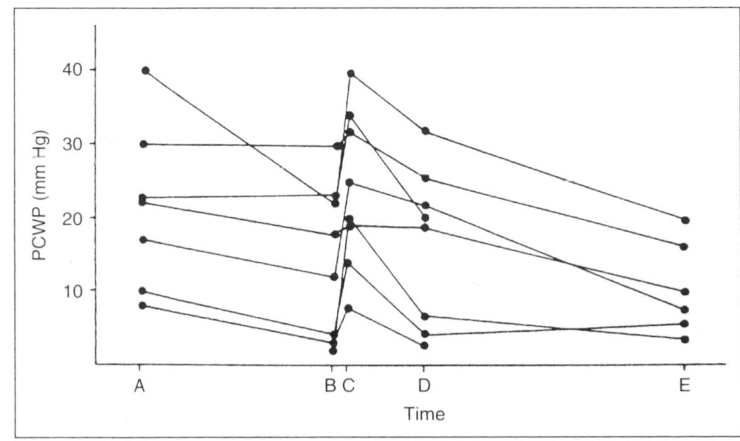

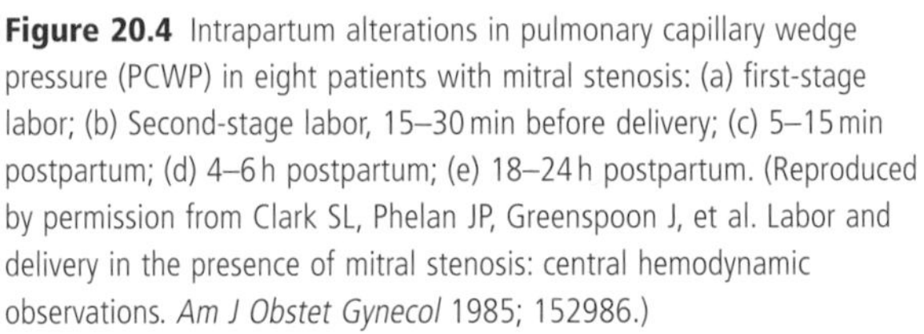
Figure 20.4 Intrapartum alterations in pulmonary capillary wedge pressure (PCWP) in eight patients with mitral stenosis: (a) first-stage labor; (b) Second-stage labor, 15–30 min before delivery; (c) 5–15 min postpartum; (d) 4–6 h postpartum; (e) 18–24 h postpartum. (Reproduced by permission from Clark SL, Phelan JP, Greenspoon J, et al. Labor and delivery in the presence of mitral stenosis: central hemodynamic observations. *Am J Obstet Gynecol* 1985; 152986.)

moderate stenosis [112]. Those with a jet velocity of >5 m/s (corresponding to 100 mmHg), are considered to be critical. However, the decision for valve replacement is not based solely on hemodynamics since some who meet the criteria are asymptomatic while others are not. For those with symptoms attributed to severe aortic stenosis, it is preferred to intervene before pregnancy. The options are either balloon valvuloplasty or, for those who are unsuitable due to valve calcification or age, valve replacement. There appears to be a window of opportunity for percutaneous balloon valvuloplasty in younger patients that unfortunately closes with increasing age. Younger patients have a lack of calcification of the valves and better relative mobility. For those requiring surgery, there are different types of valves that may be implanted including bioprosthetic, homograft, pulmonary autograft or mechanical. For practical purposes, pulmonary autograft and homografts are not widely available, leaving the bioprosthetic and mechanical valves as the two most common options for valve replacement. While bioprosthetic grafts do not require anticoagulation like mechanical valves, they do have a high risk of structural failure and need for reoperation within 15 years after implantation. For those who chose to have AVR with mechanical valve, the issue of anticoagulation will be discussed in a later section.

For those continuing pregnancy in the face of aortic stenosis, the severity will be dictated by the degree of symptoms and by echocardiographic assessment. In cases with severe aortic stenosis by all major echocardiographic criteria (including anatomic and Doppler criteria) some advocate consideration of termination of pregnancy even in an asymptomatic patient. We feel that before the decision for termination is undertaken in such cases, a second opinion at a center with a team experienced in the management of pregnant women with congenital heart disease should be considered. In women who decide to become pregnant, or who present in pregnancy, medical management is preferred and surgery resorted to for refractory NYHA class III or IV.

In aortic stenosis, the major problem experienced by patients with valvular aortic stenosis is maintenance of cardiac output. Because of the relative hypervolemia associated with gestation, such patients generally tolerate pregnancy well. With severe disease, however, cardiac output will be relatively fixed, and during exertion it may be inadequate to maintain coronary artery or cerebral perfusion. This inadequacy can result in angina, myocardial infarction, syncope, or sudden death. Thus, marked limitation of physical activity is vital to patients with severe disease. If activity is limited and the mitral valve is competent, pulmonary edema will be rare during pregnancy.

Delivery and pregnancy termination appear to be the times of greatest risk for patients with aortic stenosis [113]. The maintenance of cardiac output is crucial; any factor leading to diminished venous return will cause an increase in the valvular gradient and diminished cardiac output. Hypotension resulting from blood loss, ganglionic blockade from epidural anesthesia, or supine vena caval occlusion by the pregnant uterus may result in sudden death. Such problems are similar to those encountered in patients with pulmonary hypertension, discussed previously. Differences of opinion exist comparing the latest antibiotic prophylaxis recommendations for aortic stenosis in the United States when compared with those published abroad. The most recent recommendations by the AHA indicate that antibiotic prophylaxis for endocarditis is unnecessary in aortic stenosis unless the valve has previously been infected [28]. However, The Working Party of the British Society for Antimicrobial Chemotherapy propose that all patients with abnormalities of the aortic valve and bicuspid aortic receive antibiotic prophylaxis [114] Careful monitoring of these divergent recommendations will be needed. Further discussion regarding these recommendations are found in the section on antiobiotc prophylaxis.

The cardiovascular status of patients with aortic stenosis is complicated further by the frequent coexistence of ischemic heart disease; thus, death associated with aortic stenosis often occurs secondary to myocardial infarction rather than as a direct complication of the valvular lesion itself [113]. The overall reported mortality associated with aortic stenosis in pregnancy has been as high as 17%. Today, it would appear that with appropriate care and in the absence of coronary artery disease, however, the risk of death is minimal [2,5,115]. Pulmonary artery catheterization, particularly with the availability of continuous cardiac output and mixed venous oxygen monitoring, may allow more precise hemodynamic assessment and control during labor and delivery. Because hypovolemia is a far greater threat to the patient than is pulmonary edema, the wedge pressure should be maintained in the range of 15–17 mmHg to maintain a margin of safety against unexpected peripartum blood loss.

For those who require intervention for refractory class III or IV heart failure balloon valvuloplasty can reduce both the maternal and fetal the risks of surgical valve replacement [80]. After delivery definitive intervention can be undertaken. Aortic valve replacement during pregnancy is risky and it is preferable to intervene after delivery if at all possible.

Aortic insufficiency

Aortic insufficiency from a malformed aortic valve may be congenital or rheumatic in origin, and may be associated with a dilated aortic root or prior endocarditis. Aortic insufficiency generally is well tolerated during pregnancy because of the decreased systemic vascular resistance and the increased heart rate seen with advancing gestation. This decreases the time available for regurgitant flow during diastole. In Hibbard's series of 28 maternal rheumatic cardiac deaths, only one was associated with aortic insufficiency in the absence of concurrent mitral stenosis [27]. Endocarditis prophylaxis during labor and delivery is now only indicated for those who have had prior endocarditis [28].

Peripartum cardiomyopathy

Peripartum cardiomyopathy is defined as cardiomyopathy developing in the last month of pregnancy or the first 5 months post-

Table 20.8 Criteria for diagnosis of peripartum cardiomyopathy.

Classic

1 Development of cardiac failure in the last month of pregnancy or within 5 months of delivery
2 Absence of an identifiable cause for the cardiac failure
3 Absence of recognizable heart disease before the last month of pregnancy

Additional

4 Left ventricular systolic dysfunction demonstrated by classic echocardiographic criteria, such as depressed shortening fraction (less than 30%), ejection fraction (less than 45%), and a left ventricular end-diastolic dimension of more than 2.7cm per m^2 of body surface area (Hibbard et al. 1999)

partum in a woman without previous cardiac disease and after exclusion of other causes of cardiac failure [116–120] (Table 20.8). It is a separate entity from other known existing cardiomyopathies and can be associated with a high rate of mortality. It is, therefore, a diagnosis of exclusion that should not be made without a concerted effort to identify valvular, metabolic, infectious, or toxic causes of cardiomyopathy. Much of the current controversy surrounding this condition is the result of many older reports in which these causes of cardiomyopathy were not investigated adequately. Other peripartum complications, such as amniotic fluid embolism, severe pre-eclampsia, and arrhythmogenic, corticosteroid or sympathomimetic-induced pulmonary edema, also must be considered before making the diagnosis of peripartum cardiomyopathy. Sympathomimetic agents also may unmask underlying peripartum cardiomyopathy [121].

The incidence of peripartum cardiomyopathy is estimated to be between 1 in 3000 and 1 in 4000 live births, which would translate to 1,000–1300 women affected each year in the United States [117,122,123]. An incidence as high as 1% has been suggested in women of certain African tribes; however, idiopathic heart failure in these women may be primarily a result of unusual culturally mandated peripartum customs involving excessive sodium intake and may represent, as such, simple fluid overload [122,124,125]. In the United States, the peak incidence of peripartum cardiomyopathy occurs in the second postpartum month, and there appears to be a higher incidence among older, multiparous black females [125,126]. Other suggested risk factors include twinning and pregnancy-induced hypertension [125,127]. In rare cases, a familial recurrence pattern has been reported. The condition is manifest clinically by the gradual onset of increasing fatigue, dyspnea, and peripheral or pulmonary edema. Physical examination reveals classic evidence of congestive heart failure, including jugular venous distention, rales, and an S3 gallop. Cardiomegaly and pulmonary edema are found on chest X-ray, and the ECG often demonstrates left ventricular and atrial dilatation and diminished ventricular performance. In addition, up to 50% of patients with peripartum cardiomyopathy may manifest evidence of pulmonary or systemic embolic phenomena. Overall mortality ranges from 25% to 50% [122,125].

The histologic picture of peripartum cardiomyopathy involves non-specific cellular hypertrophy, degeneration, fibrosis, and increased lipid deposition. Many reports have documented the presence of a diffuse myocarditis and currently more evidence exists for myocarditis as a cause of peripartum cardiomyopathy than for any other purported etiology [118]. Because of the non-specific clinical and pathologic nature of peripartum cardiomyopathy, however, its existence as a distinct entity has been questioned [127]. Its existence as a distinct entity is supported primarily by epidemiologic evidence suggesting that 80% of cases of idiopathic cardiomyopathy in women of childbearing age occur in the peripartum period. Such an epidemiologic distribution also could be attributed to an exacerbation of underlying subclinical cardiac disease related to the hemodynamic changes accompanying normal pregnancy. Because such changes are maximal in the third trimester of pregnancy and return to normal within a few weeks postpartum, however, such a pattern does not explain the peak incidence of peripartum cardiomyopathy occurring, in most reports, during the second month postpartum. The National Heart, Lung and Blood Institute and Office of Rare Diseases (National Institute of Health) Workshop Recommendation and Review on peripartum cardiomyopathy continues to support the disease as a distinct entity [118,119]. It cannot be emphasized enough that the diagnosis of peripartum cardiomyopathy remains primarily a diagnosis of exclusion and cannot be made until underlying conditions, including chronic hypertension, valvular disease, and viral myocarditis, have been excluded.

Standard therapy for heart failure patients includes β-blockers, diuretics, afterload reduction with angiotensin-converting enzyme inhibitors (ACE)/angiotensin II receptor blockers (ARB)/hydralazine sodium restriction. The ACE/ARB agents should be avoided prenatally, but are a mainstay of therapy otherwise. In the pregnant patient with acute heart failure, oxygen, diuretics, and hydralazine should be used. Although digioxin is no longer considered first line therapy in the treatment of heart failure for non-pregnant patients, it is appropriate to use this drug in heart failure patients who have persistence of symptoms despite maximal use of other available agents. This agent is generally safe in pregnant women and is dosed to achieve therapeutic effect. It is not uncommon to see doses of 0.375–0.5 mg/day since the metabolism of the drug is increased in the pregnant state. Therapeutic anticoagulation should be considered when the ejection fraction is less than 35% to prevent intracardiac thrombosis and emboli. Beta-blockers should be withheld until acute heart failure is improving. If clinical worsening of CHF occurs or clear improvement is not seen despite maximal treatment with the above agents, referral to a tertiary center for evaluation and management of the cardiac condition and consideration of transplantation may be in order. The use of inotropes, vasopressors, aldosterone antagonists, and nesiritide should be reserved for the critically ill woman in whom any fetal risks can be justified. For pregnant patients who have improvement in heart failure symptoms or do not have acute heart failure, β-blockers should be added to the drug regimen. Up to two-thirds of patients with peripartum cardiomyopathy will normalize left ventricular function within 1 year. The remainder will either have persistently depressed function or (a small percentage) will require transplantation. A notable feature of peripartum cardiomyopathy is its tendency to recur with subsequent pregnancies. Several older reports have suggested that a prognosis for future pregnancies is related to heart size. Patients whose cardiac size returned to normal within 6–12 months had an 11–14% mortality in subsequent pregnancies; those patients with persistent cardiomegaly had a 40–80% mortality [116]. Lampert [128], however, demonstrated persistent decreased contractile reserve even in women who had regained normal resting left ventricular size. Witlin [126], in a series of 28 patients with peripartum cardiomyopathy, reported that only 7% had regression; in those undertaking subsequent pregnancy, two-thirds decompensated earlier than in the index pregnancy. A reported 19% mortality was seen in those who had persistently depressed left ventricular ejection fraction [129]. The available data justify recommendations to avoid additional pregnancies in those peripartum cardiomyopathy patients who have persistent left ventricular dysfunction. Elkayam published the results of surveys carried out by the ACC and in South Africa. He found that in women who had recovered satisfactory systolic function there was sometimes deterioration in function in a subsequent pregnancy. There was no maternal mortality (0/40) reported in the 2001 survey and 1/43 women in the 1995 survey. This resulted in the statement, "these results suggest a low likelihood of mortality as a result of subsequent pregnancies in peripartum cardiomyopathy women with recovered left ventricular function" [130]. However, this information should be shared with the patient and her family, and they should know that recurrence of cardiomyopathy is possible, and that the cardiac risks of pregnancy are not absent despite the fact that the risk of maternal mortality is small.

Hypertrophic obstructive cardiomyopathy

Hypertrophic cardiomyopathy (HOCM) is a condition with a variable manifestation of hypertrophy which can be obstructive or non-obstuctive to left ventricular outflow. There is thickening of the heart muscle with left ventricular stiffness leading to abnormalities of relaxation, and at times mitral valve changes. The incidence of HOCM is about 1 in 500, (previously thought to be much lower). The myocardial wall thickening is most commonly isolated and occurs in the septum below the aortic valve. Thickening can occur globally, or it can be isolated at the apex, in the lateral wall or in the RV. If there is obstruction to left ventricular outflow the condition may be called hypertrophic obstructive cardiomyopathy (HOCM) or idiopathic hypertrophic subaortic stenosis (IHSS). In cases without obstruction to flow it is known as non-obstructive HCM.

Hypertrophic cardiomyopathy is an autosomal dominantly inherited condition with variable penetrance. Serial echocardiographic studies of children who have the gene but who have a normal heart show that the asymmetric hypertrophy and obstructive features may not develop for many years or even decades. Thus, occult HOCM in spontaneous or unidentified cases often may be first manifest during pregnancy. Detailed physical and echocardiographic diagnostic criteria have been described elsewhere. Primarily, HOCM involves asymmetric left ventricular hypertrophy, typically involving the septum to a greater extent than the free wall. The hypertrophy results in obstruction to left ventricular outflow and secondary mitral regurgitation, the two principal hemodynamic concerns of the clinician [131]. Although the increased blood volume associated with normal pregnancy should enhance left ventricular filling and improve hemodynamic performance, this positive effect of pregnancy is counterbalanced by a fall in systemic vascular resistance and an increase in heart rate with reduced LV diastolic filling time, and myocardial contractility. In addition, tachycardia resulting from pain or anxiety during labor further diminishes left ventricular filling and aggravates the relative outflow obsuction, an effect also resulting from the second-stage Valsalva maneuver.

The keys to successful management of the peripartum period in patients with HOCM involve avoidance of hypotension (resulting from conduction anesthesia or blood loss) and tachycardia, as well as conducting labor in the left lateral recumbent position. The use of forceps to shorten the second stage also has been recommended. As with most other cardiac disease, cesarean section for HOCM patients should be reserved for obstetric indications only. General management principles for these patients have been reviewed by Spirito et al. [132].

Despite the potential hazards, maternal and fetal outcomes in HOCM patients are generally good. In a report of 54 pregnancies in 23 patients with HOCM, no maternal or neonatal deaths occurred [133]. Symptoms of heart failure are usually the result of diastolic dysfunction and elevated left ventricular filling pressures rather than from severe mitral regurgitation in pregnant women with HOCM. In these cases, β-blocking agents are indicated. Judicious use of diuretics, addition of calcium channel blocking agents and β-adrenergic agents may also be necessary. Atrial fibrillation is the most common worrisome atrial arrhythmia that occurs during pregnancy and can be treated with β-blockers, and if necessary, calcium channel blockers. Ideally, an automatic implantable cardiac defibrillator should be placed before conception for those at high risk for sudden death [134]. Studies have shown that the presence of an ICD does not increase maternal risk or frequency of ICD discharges [135].

Marfan syndrome

Marfan syndrome is an autosomal dominant disorder characterized by generalized weakness of connective tissue; the weakness results in skeletal, ocular, and cardiovascular abnormalities. The increased risk of maternal mortality during pregnancy stems from aortic root and wall involvement, which may result in aneurysm formation, rupture, or aortic dissection. Fifty per cent of aortic aneurysm ruptures in women under age 40 occur during pregnancy [59]. Rupture of splenic artery aneurysms also occurs more frequently during pregnancy. Sixty per cent of patients with Marfan syndrome have associated mitral or aortic regurgitation [136]. Although some authors feel pregnancy is contraindicated in any woman with documented Marfan syndrome, prognosis is best individualized and should be based on echocardiographic assessment of aortic root diameter and postvalvular dilation. It is important to note that enlargement of the aortic root is not demonstrable by chest X-ray until dilation has become pronounced.

Women with an abnormal aortic valve or aortic dilation may have up to a 50% pregnancy-associated mortality; women without these changes and having an aortic root diameter less than 40 mm have a mortality less than 5% [137]. Such patients do not appear to have evidence of aggravated aortic root dilatation over time [138]. Even in patients meeting these echocardiographic criteria, however, special attention must be given to signs or symptoms of aortic dissection, since serial echocardiographic assessments may not be predictive of complications [139]. In counseling women with Marfan syndrome, the genetics of this condition and the shortened maternal lifespan must be considered, in addition to the immediate maternal risk. The routine use of oral β-blocking agents to decrease pulsatile pressure on the aortic wall has been recommended [140]. If cesarean section is performed, retention sutures should be considered because of generalized connective tissue weakness.

Myocardial infarction

Coronary artery disease is uncommon in women of reproductive age; therefore, acute myocardial infarction in conjunction with pregnancy is rare [141–143]. However, as noted in the beginning of this chapter, this condition is becoming increasingly recognized as a cause of death in young pregnant women [11]. In addition, more women are postponing pregnancy until the fourth or fifth decade of life – a time where underlying medical conditions such as hypertension and diabetes, coupled with advancing maternal age, may exacerbate the incidence of acquired heart disease coronary artery disease and acute myocardial infarction. Cardiovascular risk factors for development of coronary artery disease include smoking, diabetes mellitus, elevated plasma cholesterol (total cholesterol), low levels of high-density lipoprotein (HDL), elevated LDL, family history of premature coronary artery disease in a first-degree relative aged less than 55, and use of oral contraceptives. Acute myocardial infarction during pregnancy can be a catastrophic event, associated with significant maternal morbidity and mortality. In one of the first comprehensive reviews of its type, 123 pregnancies with 125 well documented cases of acute myocardial infarction suggested that those most at risk were multigravidas older than 33 years of age [144] (Table 20.9). The most common anatomic location for the infarct was the anterior wall and the overall maternal death rate was 21%. Maternal death most often occurred at the time of the infarct or within 2 weeks of the infarct, often associated with the labor and delivery process. Similar findings were described in a similar study published the same year [145]. Subsequent to that, two publications with large populations of patients from both state and national administrative databases have also been culled to review the characteristics of pregnant women with acute myocardial infarction during pregnancy and postpartum [146,147]. Advancing maternal age, hypertension, and diabetes were also found as risk factors for acute myocardial infarction in these studies. Anterior wall infarction was also seen more commonly. In addition it appears that there may be other risk factors for pregnancy-related acute myocardial infarction since the majority of women do not have atherosclerotic disease. These include coronary artery dissection and thrombosis in the absence of atherosclerosis. In contrast. ruptured plaque with thrombus formation accounts for the majority of acute myocardial infarction in the non-pregnant state. Regardless of the cause, the risk of acute myocardial infarction appear to be about 3–4 times higher in pregnancy.

For pregnant women with prior myocardial infarction and who have preserved left ventricular function with no evidence of ischemia on cardiac evaluation, careful monitoring is indicated. For those with severe ischemia or heart failure early in gestation, termination of pregnancy should be considered. If a woman presents later in gestation the diagnostic and therapeutic options are much more limited. An ECG should be obtained to determine if active ischemia or acute infarction is present. Although minor electrocardiographic changes are often seen in pregnant women, evaluation of the ECG in women with suspected ischemic heart disease should not vary significantly because of pregnancy [148]. Laboratory tests and an echocardiogram will also help in the diagnosis. Echocardiography is especially valuable in defining abnormalities in wall motion. Non-invasive stress testing with radiologic or echocardiographic imaging techniques may be useful in specific circumstances. In women with angina, β-blockers are the drugs of choice because of their relative safety for the fetus. Low-dose aspirin should be used but for the shortest period of time as possible. Nitrates have also been used without adverse fetal effect.

For patients presenting with acute myocardial infarction who need revascularization, the two options are thrombolytic therapy or primary percutaneous intervention with balloon angioplasty/stent. Schumacher [149] reported successful treatment of acute myocardial infarction during pregnancy with tissue plasminogen activator. Because of the obvious issues of potential bleeding associated with systemic thrombolytic therapy to the mother or fetus, PTCA or stent placement would now be more ideal [150]. The use of a radial artery approach and limiting the procedure to a PTCA (which does not need complete platelet inhibition for a prolonged period like stent placement) has been described in pregnancy [151]. This

Table 20.9 Selected data in 123 pregnancies complicated by 125 myocardial infarctions.

Variable	Antepartum group (*n* = 78)*	Peripartum group (*n* = 17)†	Postpartum group (*n* = 30)‡	All groups (*n* = 125)
Maternal age (years)	33 ± 6	34 ± 5	29 ± 6	32 ± 6
Age range (years)	16–45	23–44	17–42	16–45
Anterior MI location (%)§	50/77 (65)	14/16 (87)	25/29 (86)	89/122 (73)
Multiparous (%)§	64/73 (88)	13/16 (81)	16/22 (73)	93/111 (84)
Hypertension (%)	21	24	17	19
Diabetes mellitus (%)	6	0	3	5
Ischemic heart disease (%)	10	0	7	–
Smoking (%)	32	12	26	–
Family history of MI (%)	12	0	8	–
Hyperlipidemia (%)	1	0	2	–
Pre-eclampsia (%)	10	18	11	–
Elective cesarean (%)	15	6	14	–
Semiselective or emergency cesarean (%)	14	12	12	–
CHF after MI (%)	12 (15)	7 (41)	6 (20)	25 (19)
Coronary anatomy available (%)	36 (46)	8 (47)	24 (80)	68 (54)
Stenosis	21 (58)‖	1 (12)	7 (29)¶	29 (43)
Thrombus	8 (22)	1 (12)	5 (21)	14 (21)
Dissection	3 (8)	0 (0)	(33)	11 (16)
Aneurysm	2 (6)	0 (0)	1 (4)	3 (4)
Spasm	1 (3)	0 (0)	0 (0)	1 (1)
Normal	9 (25)	6 (75)	20 (29)	–
Death				
Mothers (%)	11 (14)	6 (35)	9 (30)	26 (21)
Infants (%)	12 (15)	3 (18)	1 (3)	16 (13)
Infant death associated with maternal death (%)	8/12 (67)	1/3 (33)	1/1 (100)	10/16 (62)

CHF, congestive heart failure; MI, myocardial infarction.
* Includes patients who had myocardial infarctions that occurred 24 hours or more before labor.
† Includes patients who had myocardial infarctions that occurred within 24 hours before or after labor.
‡ Includes patients who had myocardial infarctions that occurred between 24 hours before and 3 months after labor.
§ The number in the denominator is the number of relevant patients.
‖ Associated thrombus in seven cases.
¶ Associated thrombus in one case.
(Reproduced by permission from Roth A, Elkayam U. Acute myocardial infarction associated with pregnancy. Annals of Internal Medicine 1996;125(9):751–762.)

approach has the potential to minimize radiation to the fetus and prolonged maternal/fetal platelet inhibition if all goes well. Delivery within 2 weeks of infarction is associated with increased mortality; therefore, if possible, attempts should be made to allow adequate convalescence before delivery. If the cervix is favorable, cautious induction under controlled circumstances after a period of hemodynamic stabilization is optimal. Labor in the lateral recumbent position, the administration of oxygen, pain relief with epidural anesthesia, and, in selected cases, hemodynamic monitoring with a pulmonary artery catheter are important management considerations.

In two prospective American studies, having six or more pregnancies was associated with a small but significant increase in the risk of subsequent coronary artery disease [152].

Anticoagulation and prosthetic heart valves

Any patient who requires anticoagulation when not pregnant should also be anticoagulated during pregnancy, although the anticoagulant used may be different. The presence of a prosthetic heart valve(s) in pregnancy adds a level of complexity in management for both the mother and the fetus. The main risks are associated with anticoagulation issues. These include maternal thromboembolic events due to insufficient anticoagulation, maternal valve thrombosis, fetal complications due to the effects of the anticoagulant used and the timing of administration, maternal bleeding from anticoagulation during (i) gestation, (ii) labor and especially (iii) during delivery [153]. The biologic tissue valves such as porcine valves, pericardial valves and homografts are the ideal valves for use during pregnancy since they do not require anticoagulation in the arterial systemic position during the childbearing years. However, these valves have a high rate of structural failure requiring reoperation, the biologic valves having a higher rate of failure compared to the homografts [154]. Mechanical valves have a high risk of thrombosis and thromboemboli without concomitant anticoagulation. The risk is further increased if there is atrial fibrillation or if the valve is one of the older models, particularly in the mitral position. Pregnancy increases the risks of thromboembolic disease as well as the risks of anticoagulation for mother and fetus in patients with mechanical valves [155]. The usual agents used for anticoagulation of mechanical prosthetic valves in the pregnant and non pregnant patient include warfarin, unfractionated heparin (UFH) and low molecular weight heparin (LMWH).

Anticoagulation in the patient with an artificial heart valve and/or atrial fibrillation during pregnancy remains controversial [156] becauseof the lack of an ideal agent for anticoagulation during pregnancy. Warfarin is the mainstay of anticoagulation in the non-pregnant population, and pregnant patients with prosthetic valves have the lowest risk of valve thrombosis and thomboembolic events when appropriately anticoagulated. For the fetus, warfarin (coumadin) is relatively contraindicated at all stages of gestation due to its association with fetal warfarin syndrome in weeks 6–9 and its relationship to fetal intracranial hemorrhage and secondary scarring at later stages [157,158]. The attractiveness of UFH and LMWH is that they do not cross the placenta and the risk to the fetus is less. The maternal effects of long-term administration of UFH include thrombocytopenia, bone loss and uneven therapeutic attainment of aPTT. These issues are not seen as commonly with LMWH which led to a preference of this agent over UFH in pregnant women with prosthetic valves. However, in comparison to warfarin, when used for long-term therapy, UFH and LMWH are much less effective in prevention of prosthetic valve thrombosis [159–165]. Earlier reports of valve thrombosis may have in part been due to inadequate dosing and/or monitoring of the aPTT for UFH or anti-factor Xa level for LMWH. Nevertheless sufficient concern was raised that in 2002 the FDA issued a warning stating that enoxaparin, an LMWH, should not be used for thromboprophylaxis in pregnant women with prosthetic heart valves [166]. Since that time, several societies have issued their own recommendations regarding anticoagulation of prosthetic valves during pregnancy. The recommendation against LMWH exnoxaparin was endorsed early on by the American College of Obstetrics and Gynecology in an Opinion statement in 2002. The European Society of Cardiology continues to advise against the use of LMWH for anticoagulation during pregnancy [167]. However several other societies have incorporated LMWH and UFH with warfarin as alternative strategies for anticoagulation during pregnancy, This is in part due to the consensus that valve thrombosis in these earlier cases could have occurred due to inadequate dosing and undermonitoring of the LMWH anticoagulant effects. All societies that endorse use of UFH or LMWH suggest frequent surveillance of appropriate blood studies to assess adequacy of the anticoagulation [112,168].

The recommendations/suggestions of each society vary with regard to the manner and timing of anticoagulation. With regard to manner of anticoagulation, warfarin can be used throughout pregnancy until about the 36th week. However, during the first trimester due to fetal concerns, if used, the dose should be ≤5 mg/day. INR should be maintained between 2.5 and 3.5 and should be tested frequently. Alternatively, IV UFH, SQ UFH or LMW heparin can be used throughout most of pregnancy either continuously or in a staged manner. If subcutaneous UFH or LMWH is used during pregnancy, a twice-daily dosing regimen with mid-interval testing of aPTT or anti-factor Xa should be aggressively followed. The aPTT should be at least twice control and the anti Xa level at at least 0.7–1.2. This should be checked at least weekly.

Women should be informed of both the maternal and fetal risk associated with anticoagulant regimen choices and they should fully participate in the decision process of anticoagulation. Because of warfarin-associated fetal embryopathy early in pregnancy, many suggest a staged approach to anticoagulation. During the first trimester, warfarin is withheld and subcutaneous UFH or LMWH is used. During weeks 12–36, IV heparin, SQ UFH or LMWH, or warfarin can be used. At approximately 36 weeks gestation, if warfarin is being used, the patient should be switched to an UFH or LMWH dosing route.

Ideally, delivery should be planned. SQ LMWH/UFH should be changed to IV UFH at least 24 hours before planned delivery and IV UFH stopped at least 4 hours before expected delivery. In the absence of significant bleeding, UFH or LMWH can be resumed 4–6 hours after the delivery, and the warfarin can be started within 24 hours. Bridging anticoagulation should continue until the INR is in therapeutic range for at least 24 hours.

Because not all deliveries occur as planned, there may be some women who present in labor or who need urgent delivery and who are fully anticoagulated either on UFH/LMWH or warfarin. If at all possible, we would attempt to delay delivery for 4–6 hours to minimize the effects of UFH/LMWH in such cases. For those on warfarin, fresh frozen plasma, and if time allows, vitamin K in small doses, can be given. The fetus is at increased risk of hemorrhage since it is anticoagulated if the mother has been receiving warfarin. Therefore, fresh frozen plasma and vitamin K may need to be administered to the infant after delivery.

Because of issues related to the uncertainty of the timing of delivery and the risks of maternal hemorrhage, the potential complications of emergent reversal of warfarin anticoagulation with attendant risks of valve thrombosis, and because of the risk of fetal embryopathy in early pregnancy and fetal bleeding throughout pregnancy, many favor use of UFH /LMWH over warfarin during pregnancy. The issue of anticoagulation in a mother with a mechanical valve clearly requires detailed explanation and an informed consent from the patient.

Prevention of bacterial endocarditis

Major revisions to the American Heart Association (AHA) recommendations for endocarditis prophylaxis were made in 2007 [28]. These revisions replaced the 1997 AHA guidelines and the 2006 ACC/AHA guidelines on the management of valvular heart disease. Antibiotic prophylaxis is limited now to those with cardiac conditions with the highest risk of adverse outcome from infective endocarditis. These include the following.

1 Prosthetic cardiac valves (mechanical, bioprosthetic, homograft).
2 Previous history of infective endocarditis.
3 Unrepaired cyanotic congenital heart disease, including palliative shunts and conduits.
4 Completely repaired congenital heart defects with prosthetic material or device, surgically or interventionally placed, during the first 6 months after the procedure.
5 Repaired CHD with residual defects at the site or adjacent to the site of a prosthetic patch or prosthetic device.
6 Cardiac transplanted heart with significant valvulopathy (leaflet pathology and regurgitation).

These 2007 AHA guidelines excluded previously treated conditions such as aortic stenosis, bicuspid aortic valve and other LV outflow tract conditions such as HOCM. Paradoxically, at the same time, in the UK, new antibiotic prophylaxis guidelines narrowing groups for antibiotic prophylaxis included these conditions but excluded transplant valvulopathy [114]. Given the divergence of these recommendations, it should be emphasized that the prophylaxis strategy for each case must be individualized taking into consideration the type of cardiac lesion and type of delivery that is anticipated.

The AHA now states that neither routine vaginal nor cesarean delivery is an indication for antibiotic prophylaxis because of the low rate of bacteremia. However, women with the highest cardiac risk conditions should be given the option of antibiotic prophylaxis. In addition, the AHA recommend giving antibiotic prophylaxis to patients with the highest-risk cardiac conditions if bacteremia is suspected during vaginal or cesarean delivery.

To be most effective, antibiotic administration is recommended from half to 1 hour before the anticipated bacteremia. Given the difficulty in reliably predicting half to 1 hour before birth, that the delivery will be "uncomplicated" and not involve vaginal or rectal lacerations or the need for manual exploration of the uterus, we suggest a policy of routinely giving antibiotic therapy to high-risk cardiac patients at the appropriate time before delivery. The most commonly used drugs for antimicrobial prophylaxis are similar to those used in the non-pregnant state. These include ampicillin or amoxicillin, and for penicillin-allergic women, azithromycin or clindamycin.

Dysrhythmias

While minor ECG changes are commonly seen during pregnancy, significant dysrhythmias are rare [148]. Atrial fibrillation, atrial flutter, atrial tachycardia, SVT, and WPW with rapid rhythm are more likely to occur in patients with congenital heart disease (both repaired and unrepaired) compared to those with structurally normal hearts. The first four arrhythmia types mentioned above can also be seen with thyroid abnormalities. Ventricular arrhythmias, both sustained and non-sustained, merit work-up for metabolic derangements, thyrotoxicosis, HOCM, myocardial ischemia, and congenital heart disease with a 12-lead ECG, thyroid tests, potassium and magnesium evaluation as well as echocardiogram as a minimum. On occasion, patients may also present with first-, second- or third-degree AV block. These are rarely seen in normal pregnancy and are usually due to either repaired or unrepaired congenital disease, acute rheumatic disease (extremely rare these days), digoxin treatment or ischemic heart disease. Again, evaluation is warranted to determine the cause and if it is potentially due to medication that medication should be stopped if at all possible. Patients with congenital heart block usually do quite well and do not need pacemaker treatment during gestation, labor or delivery.

The use of antiarrhythmic therapy has been reviewed extensively by Rotmensch et al. [169]. Many of these medications have been used to treat fetal dysrrhythmias as well [170]. For acute arrhythmias associated with hypotension unresponsive to medical therapy, electrical cardioversion is the treatment of choice and is safely done during pregnancy. In most cases, patients do not require such an aggressive approach. For SVT, adenosine is the drug of choice. For wide complex tachycardia of unknown etiology which could represent WPW with a bypass tract, after a trial of lidocaine, procainamide is the IV drug of choice. Ibutilide has been recently reported to be successful in terminating (without adverse maternal or fetal effect) atrial fibrillation and HOCM, atrial flutter, and atrial fibrillation with WPW. Digoxin procainamide, and quinidine have been used for treatment of maternal and fetal atrial fibrillation/flutter and SVT without significant adverse maternal or fetal effects. Atenolol should be avoided in the first trimester due to fetal concerns. Calcium channel blockers appear to have a safe maternal profile in treatment of appropriate maternal arrhythmias.

Because of its rather slow onset of action in the acute setting, and its inability to control heart rate at anything except a resting state, digoxin is less than desirable as a single rate control medication for maternal atrial fibrillation or flutter. The metabolism of digoxin has been reported to increase during pregnancy, decreasing its bioavailability. In addition, a digoxin-like immunoreactive substance appears in some normal and pre-eclamptic patients during the second trimester and can be identified in many patients during the third trimester [171]. Thus some have advocated increasing the dose of digoxin to 0.375–0.5 mg twice daily and adjusting the dosage based on closely monitored blood levels.

If serum monitoring of digoxin levels is anticipated, a pretreatment level should be obtained to improve interpretation of results.

Beta-blockers such metoprolol are used extensively for treatment atrial fibrillation/flutter in the older adult population with arrhythmias. However, in many pregnant patients who already have decreased SVR, larger doses of β-blocker to control atrial fibrillation/flutter rates may not be tolerated due to hypotension. The best combination seems to be that of digoxin and metoprolol. If this combination does not work then consideration of other antiarrhythmics such as procainamide or quinidine may come into play.

All efforts should be made to treat pregnant women with serious arrhythmias medically and delay potential electrophysiologic evaluation until after delivery. Women with recurrent atrial flutter or SVT should consider radiofrequency ablation before any pregnancy. Women with HOCM who are desirous of pregnancy and at risk for sudden death, should consider ICD before contemplated pregnancy. The issue of anticoagulation for atrial fibrillation in pregnancy has not been addressed specifically. It seems reasonable, however, to anticoagulate a pregnant patient if she meets the criteria described for non-pregnant patients. These include atrial fibrillation with a history of thromboembolic complications, atrial fibrillation in the presence of valvular disease such as mitral stenosis or regurgitation, atrial fibrillation in cardiomyopathy, or atrial fibrillation with thyrotoxic heart disease. Anticoagulation is recommended for 3 weeks before cardioversion of atrial fibrillation and for 4 weeks after conversion to sinus rhythm. Anticoagulation should be considered in the patient with atrial fibrillation and congestive heart failure.

Cardioversion appears safe for the fetus [172]. The presence of an artificial pacemaker, similarly, does not affect the course of pregnancy [173].

Pregnancy after cardiac transplantation

The number of pregnant women who have undergone cardiac transplantation is small; nevertheless, from a compilation of 47 pregnancies from 35 heart transplant recipients generalizations can be made [174,175]. First, most patients are maintained on cyclosporine and azathioprine; often, prednisone is added to the regimen. While theoretic concerns may exist regarding potential teratogenesis of these agents, limited experience with heart transplant patients and more extensive experience with patients having undergone renal transplant suggest that such fears are unfounded [176,177]. Patients should be counseled that these agents appear to pose minimal, if any, risk of adverse fetal effects.

Second, with regard to maternal risk, patients with cardiac transplants who have no evidence of rejection and have normal cardiac function at the onset of pregnancy appear to tolerate pregnancy, labor, and delivery well [174,175,177–180]. The denervated heart retains normal systolic function and contractile reserve [181–183]. Such patients undergo the normal hemodynamic response to pregnancy, as well as the expected intrapartum hemodynamic changes [177,183]. Central hemodynamic changes associated with pregnancy in a stable cardiac transplant recipient were described by Kim et al. [183], and were not significantly different from those expected during normal pregnancy.

To date, no reported cases exist of maternal death during pregnancy in cardiac transplant recipients. While three cases have been reported of delayed death following pregnancy, in two of these, voluntary withdrawal from the immunosuppressive agents and/or inappropriate medical care was implicated; there is no evidence that the antecedent pregnancy was related to the death of these women.

During pregnancy, meticulous prenatal care is essential, as is careful cardiology follow-up with frequent ECG, echocardiogram and monitoring of medications. Close attention must be paid to symptoms or signs of transplant rejection, which generally may be successfully managed by adjustments in medication. There appears to be an increased risk of pregnancy-induced hypertension, preterm delivery and low birth weight babies in these patients. Serial sonography to assess for adequate fetal growth and third-trimester antepartum fetal testing are recommended. There is no convincing evidence that the use of a pulmonary artery catheter will favorably influence the intrapartum management of these patients. Cesarean section and all but outlet instrumental vaginal deliveries should be reserved for standard obstetric indications.

References

1 Koonin LM, Atrash HK, Lawson HW, et al. Maternal mortality surveillance, United States 1979–1986. *MMWR CDC Surveill Summ* 1991; 40: 1–13.

2 DeSwiet M. Maternal mortality from heart disease in pregnancy. *Br Heart J* 1993; 69: 524.

3 Hogberg U, Innala E, Sandstrom S. Maternal mortality in Sweden, 1980–1988. *Obstet Gynecol* 1994; 84: 240–244.

4 Berg CJ, Atrash HK, Koonin LM, et al. Pregnancy related mortality in the United States, 1987–1990. *Obstet Gynecol* 1996; 88: 161–167.

5 Jacob S, Bloebaum L, Shah G, Varner MW. Maternal mortality in Utah. *Obstet Gynecol* 1998; 91: 187–191.

6 Sui SC, Sermer M, Colman JM, et al. Prospective multicenter study of pregnancy outcomes in women with heart disease. *Circulation* 2001; 104: 115.

7 Hsieh TT, Chen KC, Soong JH. Outcome of pregnancy in patients with organic heart disease in Taiwan. *Asia Oceania J Obstet Gynecol* 1993; 19: 21–27.

8 Clark SL. Structural cardiac disease in pregnancy. In: Clark SL, Cotton DB, Phelan JP, eds. *Critical Care Obstetrics*. Oradell, NJ: Medical Economics Books, 1987: 192.

9 Jacob S, Bloebaum L, Varner MW. Maternal mortality in Utah. *Obstet Gynecol.* 1998; 91: 187–191.

10 Dye TD, Gordon H, Held B, et al. Retrospective maternal mortality case ascertainment in West Virginia. *Obstet Gynecol* 1992; 167: 72–76.

11 Clark SL, Belfort MA, Dildy GA, et al. Maternal death in the 21st century: causes, prevention and relationship to cesarean delivery. *Am J Obstet Gynecol* 2008; 199(1): 36; discussion 91–92.
12 Siu SC, Sermer M, Harrison DA, et al. Risk and predictors for pregnancy-related complications in women with heart disease. *Circulation* 1997; 96: 2789–2794.
13 Presbitero P, Somerville J, Stone S, et al. Pregnancy in cyanotic congenital heart disease. Outcome of mother and fetus. *Circulation* 1994; 89: 2673–2676.
14 American College of Obsteticians and Gynecologists. Operative Vaginal Delivery. Practice Bulletin 17, June 2000. (Replaces Operative vaginal delivery. ACOG Technical Bulletin Number 196, August 1994)
15 Sandaniantz A, Saint Laurent L, Parisi AF. Long-term effects of multiple pregnancies on cardiac dimensions and systolic and diastolic function. *Am J Obstet Gynecol* 1996; 174: 1061–1064.
16 Van Oppen ACC, Stigter RH, Bruinse HW. Cardiac output in normal pregnancy: a critical review. *Obstet Gynecol* 1996; 87: 310–318.
17 Clark SL, Cotton DB, Lee W, et al. Central hemodynamic assessment of normal term pregnancy. *Am J Obstet Gynecol* 1989; 161: 1439–1442.
18 Danilenko-Dixon DR, Tefft L, Cohen RA, et al. Positional effects on maternal cardiac output during labor with epidural analgesia. *Am J Obstet Gynecol* 1996; 175: 867–872.
19 Ullery JC. Management of pregnancy complicated by heart disease. *Am J Obstet Gynecol* 1954; 67: 834.
20 Szekely P, Julian DG. Heart disease and pregnancy. *Curr Probl Cardiol* 1979; 4: 1–74.
21 Niswander KR, Berendes H, Dentschberger J, et al. Fetal morbidity following potential anoxigenic obstetric conditions: V. Organic heart disease. *Am J Obstet Gynecol* 1967; 98: 871–876.
22 Veran FX, Cibes-Hernandez JJ, Pelegrina I. Heart disease in pregnancy. *Obstet Gynecol* 1968; 34: 424.
23 Etheridge MJ, Pepperell RJ. Heart disease and pregnancy at the Royal Women's Hospital. *Med J Aust* 1971; 2: 277–281.
24 Rush RW, Verjans M, Spraklen FH. Incidence of heart disease in pregnancy. A study done at Peninsula Maternity Services hospitals. *S Afr Med J* 1979; 55: 808–810.
25 Schaefer G, Arditi LI, Solomon HA, et al. Congenital heart disease and pregnancy. *Clin Obstet Gynecol* 1968; 11: 1048–1063.
26 Neilson G, Galea EG, Blunt A. Congenital heart disease and pregnancy. *Med J Aust* 1970; 30: 1086–1088.
27 Hibbard LT. Maternal mortality due to cardiac disease. *Clin Obstet Gynecol* 1975; 18: 27–36.
28 Wilson W, Taubert KA, Gewitz M, et al. Prevention of infective endocarditis. Guidelines from the American Heart Association. *Circulation* 2007; 116: 1736–1754.
29 Gilman DH. Cesarean section in undiagnosed Eisenmenger's syndrome. Report of a patient with a fatal outcome. *Anesthesia* 1991; 46: 371–373.
30 Jackson GM, Dildy GA, Varner MW, et al. Severe pulmonary hypertension in pregnancy following successful repair of ventricular septal defect in childhood. *Obstet Gynecol* 1993; 82(Suppl): 680–682.
31 Jayakrishnan AG, Loftus B, Kelly P, et al. Spontaneous postpartum rupture of a patent ductus arteriosus. *Histopathology* 1921; 21: 383.
32 Knapp RC, Arditi LI. Pregnancy complicated by patent ductus arteriosus with reversal of flow. *NY J Med* 1967; 67: 573.
33 Gleicher N, Midwall J, Hochberger D, et al. Eisenmenger's syndrome and pregnancy. *Obstet Gynecol Surv* 1979; 34: 721–741.
34 Pirlo A, Herren AL. Eisenmenger's syndrome and pregnancy. *Anesth Rev* 1979; 6: 9.
35 Sinnenberg RJ. Pulmonary hypertension in pregnancy. *South Med J* 1980; 73: 1529–1531.
36 Weiss BM, Zemp L, Seifert B, Hess O. Outcome of pulmonary vascular disease in pregnancy: a systemic overview from 1978 through 1996. *J Am Coll Cardiol* 1998; 31: 1650–1657.
37 Meyer NL, Mercer B, Khoury A, Sibai B. Pregnancy complicated by cardiac disease: maternal and perinatal outcome. *J Matern Fetal Med* 1994; 3: 31–36.
38 Saha A, Balakrishnan KG, Jaiswal PK, et al. Prognosis for patients with Eisenmenger syndrome of various aetiology. *Int J Cardiol* 1994; 45: 199–207.
39 Smedstad K, Cramb R, Morison DH. Pulmonary hypertension and pregnancy: a series of eight cases. *Can J Anaesth* 1994; 41: 502–512.
40 Avila WS, Grinberg M, Snitcowsky R, et al. Maternal and fetal outcome in pregnant women with Eisenmenger's syndrome. *Eur Heart J* 1995; 16: 460–464.
41 Presbitero P, Rabajoli F, Somerville J. Pregnancy in patients with congenital heart disease. *Schweiz Med Wochenschr* 1995; 125: 311–315.
42 Clark SL, Phelan JP, Greenspoon J, et al. Labor and delivery in the presence of mitral stenosis: central hemodynamic observations. *Am J Obstet Gynecol* 1985; 152: 984–988.
43 Penning S, Robinson D, Major C, Garite. A comparison of echocardiography and pulmonary artery catheterization for evaluation of pulmonary artery pressure in pregnant patients with suspected pulmonary hypertension. *Am J Obstet Gynecol* 2001; 18: 1568–1570.
44 Gleicher N, Midwall J, Hocberger D, et al. Eisenmenger's syndrome and pregnancy. *Obstet Gynecol Surv.* 1979; 34: 721–741.
45 Hankins GDV, Berryman GK, Scott RT, et al. Maternal arterial desaturation with 15 methyl prostaglandin F2 alpha for uterine atony. *Obstet Gynecol* 1988; 72: 367–370.
46 Sobrevilla LA, Cassinelli MT, Carcelen A, et al. Human fetal and maternal oxygen tension and acid–base status during delivery at high altitude. *Am J Obstet Gynecol* 1971; 111: 1111–1118.
47 Midwall J, Jaffin H, Herman MV, et al. Shunt flow and pulmonary hemodynamics during labor and delivery in the Eisenmenger syndrome. *Am J Cardiol* 1978; 42(2): L299–303.
48 Weiss BM, Atanassoff PG. Cyanotic congenital heart disease and pregnancy: natural selection, pulmonary hypertension and anesthesia. *J Clin Anesth* 1993; 5: 332.
49 Sitbon O, Brenot F, Denjean A, et al. Inhaled nitric oxide as a screening vasodilator agent in primary pulmonary hypertension: a dose-response study and comparison with prostacyclin. *Am J Respir Crit Care Med* 1995; 151: 384–389.
50 Shapiro SM, Oudiz RJ, Cao T, et al. Primary pulmonary hypertension: improved long term effects and survival with continuous intravenous epoprostenol infusion. *J Am Coll Cardiol* 1997; 30: 343–349.
51 Spinnato JA, Kraynack BJ, Cooper MW. Eisenmenger's syndrome in pregnancy: epidural anesthesia for elective cesarean section. *N Engl J Med* 1981; 304: 1215–1217.
52 Abboud JK, Raya J, Noueihed R, et al. Intrathecal morphine for relief of labor pain in a parturient with severe pulmonary hypertension. *Anesthesiology* 1983; 59: 477–479.

53 Waickman LA, Skorton DJ, Varner MW, et al. Ebstein's anomaly and pregnancy. *Am J Cardiol* 1984; 53: 357–358.

54 Donnolly JE, Brown JM, Radford DJ. Pregnancy outcome and Ebstein's anomaly. *Br Heart J* 1991; 66: 368–371.

55 Connolly HM, Warnes CA. Ebstein's anomaly: outcome of pregnancy. *J Am Coll Cardiol* 1994; 23: 1194–1198.

56 Kounis NG, Zavras GM, Papadaki PJ, et al. Pregnancy induced increase of supraventricular arrhythmias in Wolff-Parkinson-White syndrome. *Clin Cardiol* 1995; 18: 137–140.

57 Taylor SH, Donald KW. Circulatory studies at rest and during exercise in coarctation, before and after correction. *Br Heart J* 1960; 22: 117.

58 Goodwin JF. Pregnancy and coarctation of the aorta. *Clin Obstet Gynecol* 1961; 4: 645.

59 Barrett JM, van Hooydonk JE, Boehm FH. Pregnancy-related rupture of arterial aneurysms. *Obstet Gynecol Surv* 1982; 37: 557–566.

60 Deal K, Wooley CF. Coarctation of the aorta and pregnancy. *Ann Intern Med* 1973; 78: 706–710.

61 Mendelson CL. Pregnancy and coarctation of the aorta. *Am J Obstet Gynecol* 1940; 39: 1014.

62 Barash PG, Hobbins JC, Hook R, et al. Management of coarctation of the aorta during pregnancy. *J Thorac Cardiovasc Surg* 1975; 69: 781–784.

63 Saidi A, Bezold LI, Altman CA, et al. Outcome of pregnancy following intervention for coarctation of the aorta. *Am J Cardiol* 1998; 82: 786–788.

64 Beauchesne LM, Connolly HM, Ammash NM, et al. Coarctation of the aorta: outcome of pregnancy. *J Am Coll Cardiol* 2001; 38: 1728–1733.

65 Vriend JW, Drenthen D, Pieper PG, et al. Outcome of pregnancy in patients after repair of aortic Coarctation. *Eur Heart J* 2005; 26: 2173–2178.

66 Shime J, Mocarski EJM, Hastings D, et al. Congenital heart disease in pregnancy: short- and long-term implications. *Am J Obstet Gynecol* 1987; 156: 313–322.

67 Rammohan M, Airan B, Bhan A, et al. Total correction of tetralogy of Fallot in adults – surgical experience. *Int J Cardiol* 1998; 63: 121–128.

68 Loh TF, Tan NC. Fallot's tetralogy and pregnancy: a report of a successful pregnancy after complete correction. *Med J Aust* 1975; 2: 141.

69 Meyer EC, Tulsky AS, Sigman P, et al. Pregnancy in the presence of tetralogy of Fallot. *Am J Cardiol* 1964; 14: 874.

70 Connolly HM, Grogan M, Warnes CA. Pregnancy among women with congenitally corrected transposition of great arteries. *J Am Coll Cardiol* 1999; 33: 1692–1695.

71 Jatene AD, Fontes VF, Souza LC, et al. Anatomic correction of transposition of the great arteries. *J Thorac Cardiovasc Surg* 1982; 83: 20–26.

72 Gutgesell HP, Massaro TA, Kron IL. The arterial switch operation for transposition of the great arteries in a consortium of university hospitals. *Am J Cardiol.* 1994; 74: 959–960.

73 Losay J, Hougen TJ. Treatment of transposition of the great arteries. *Curr Opin Cardiol.* 1997; 12: 84–90.

74 Formigari R, Santoro G, Guccione P, et al. Treatment of pulmonary artery stenosis after arterial switch operation: stent implantation vs. balloon angioplasty. *Catheteriz Cardiovasc Intervent* 2000; 50: 207–211.

75 Prifti E, Crucean A, Bonacchi M. Early and long term outcome of the arterial switch operation for transposition of the great arteries: predictors and functional evaluation. *Eur J Cardiothorac Surg* 2002; 22: 864–873.

76 Clarkson PM, Wilson NJ, Neutze JM, et al. Outcome of pregnancy after the Mustard operation for transposition of the great arteries with intact ventricular septum. *J Am Coll Cardiol* 1994; 24: 190–193.

77 Lao TT, Sermer M, Colman JM. Pregnancy following surgical correction for transposition of the great arteries. *Obstet Gynecol* 1994; 83: 665–668.

78 Drenthen W, Pieper PG, Ploeg M, et al. Risk of complications during pregnancy after Senning or Mustard (atrial) repair of complete transposition of the great arteries. *Eur Heart J* 2005; 26: 2588–2595.

79 Ploeg M, Drenthen W, van Dijk A, et al. Successful pregnancy after an arterial switch procedure for complete transposition of the great arteries. *Br J Obstet Gynaecol* 2006; 113: 243–244.

80 Presbitero P, Prever SB, Brusca A. Interventional cardiology in pregnancy. *Eur Heart J* 1996; 17: 182–188.

81 Teerlink JR, Foster E. Valvular heart disease in pregnancy: a contemporary perspective. *Cardiol Clin* 1998; 16: 573–598.

82 Canobbio MM, Mair DD, van der Velde M, et al. Prengnacy outcomes after the Fontan repair. *J Am Coll Cardiol* 1996; 28: 763–767.

83 Drenthen W, Pieper PG, Roos-Hesselin JW, et al. Pregnancy and delivery in women after Fontan palliation. *Heart* 2006; 92: 1290–1296.

84 Block BSB, Llanos AJ, Creasy RK. Responses of the growth-retarded fetus to acute hypoxemia. *Am J Obstet Gynecol* 1984; 148: 878–885.

85 Simon A, Sadovsky E, Aboulatia Y, et al. Fetal activity in pregnancies complicated by rheumatic heart disease. *J Perinat Med* 1986; 14: 331.

86 Patton DE, Lee W, Cotton DB, et al. Cyanotic maternal heart disease in pregnancy. *Obstet Gynecol Surv* 1990; 45: 594–600.

87 Whittemore R, Hobbins JC, Engle MA. Pregnancy and its outcome in women with and without surgical treatment of congenital heart disease. *Am J Cardiol* 1982; 50: 641–651.

88 Driscoll DJ, Michels VV, Gesony WM, et al. Occurrence risk for congenital heart defects in relatives of patients with aortic stenosis, pulmonary stenosis, or ventricular septal defect. *Circulation* 1993; 87(Suppl 2): 114–120.

89 Allan LD, Sharland GK, Milburn A, et al. Prospective diagnosis of 1006 consecutive cases of congenital heart disease in the fetus. *J Am Coll Cardiol* 1994; 23: 1452–1458.

90 Clark EB. Pathogenic mechanisms of congenital cardiovascular malformations revisited. *Semin Perinatol* 1996; 20: 465–472.

91 Otto CM, Easterling TR, Beneditti TJ. Role of echocardiography in the diagnosis and management of heart disease in pregnancy. In: Otto CM, ed. *The Practice of Clinical Echocardiography*. Philadelphia: WB Saunders, 1997: 495–519.

92 Campos O, Andrade JL, Bocanegra J, et al. Physiologic multivalvular regurgitation during pregnancy: a longitudinal Doppler echocardiographic study. *Int J Cardiol* 1993; 40: 265–272.

93 Szekely P, Turner R, Snaith L. Pregnancy and the changing pattern of rheumatic heart disease. *Br Heart J* 1973; 35: 1293–1303.

94 Chesley LC. Severe rheumatic cardiac disease and pregnancy: the ultimate prognosis. *Am J Obstet Gynecol* 1980; 126: 552–558.

95 Palacios IF, Block PC, Wilkins GT, et al. Percutaneous mitral balloon valvotomy during pregnancy in a patient with severe mitral stenosis. *Cathet Cardiovasc Diagn* 1988; 15: 109–111.

96 Smith R, Brender D, McCredie M. Percutaneous transluminal balloon dilation of the mitral valve in pregnancy. *Br Heart J* 1989; 61: 551–553.

97 Glanz JC, Pomerantz RM, Cunningham MJ, et al. Percutaneous balloon valvuloplasty for severe mitral stenosis during pregnancy: a review of therapeutic options. *Obstet Gynecol Surv* 1993; 48: 503–508.

98 Esteves CA, Ramos AI, Braya SL, et al. Effectiveness of percutaneous balloon mitral valvotomy during pregnancy. *Am J Cardiol* 1991; 68: 930–934.

99 BenFarhat M, Maatouk F, Betbout F, et al. Percutaneous balloon mitral valvuloplasty in eight pregnant women with severe mitral stenosis. *Eur Heart J* 1992; 13: 1659–1664.

100 Chow WH, Chow TC, Wat MS, et al. Percutaneous balloon mitral valvotomy in pregnancy using the Inoue balloon catheter. *Cardiology* 1992; 81: 182–185.

101 Gangbar EW, Watson KR, Howard RJ, et al. Mitral balloon valvuloplasty in pregnancy: advantages of a unique balloon. *Cathet Cardiovasc Diagn* 1992; 25: 313–316.

102 Ribeiro PA, Fawzy ME, Awad M, et al. Balloon valvotomy for pregnant patients with severe pliable mitral stenosis using the Inoue technique with total abdominal and pelvic shielding. *Am Heart J* 1992; 124: 1558–1562.

103 Patel JJ, Mitha AS, Hussen F, et al. Percutaneous mitral valvotomy in pregnant patients with tight pliable mitral stenosis. *Am Heart J* 1993; 125: 1106–1109.

104 Iung B, Cormier B, Elias J, et al. Usefulness of percutaneous balloon commissurotomy for mitral stenosis during pregnancy. *Am J Cardiol* 1994; 73: 398–400.

105 Kalra GS, Arora R, Khan JA, et al. Percutaneous mitral commissurotomy for severe mitral stenosis during pregnancy. *Cathet Cardiovasc Diagn* 1994; 33: 28–30; discussion 31.

106 Ueland K, Akamatsu TJ, Eng M, et al. Maternal cardiovascular dynamics: VI: Cesarean section under epidural anesthesia without epinephrine. *Am J Obstet Gynecol* 1972; 114: 775–780.

107 Clark SL, Horenstein JM, Phelan JP, et al. Experience with the pulmonary artery catheter in obstetrics and gynecology. *Am J Obstet Gynecol* 1985; 152: 374–378.

108 Ueland K, Hansen J, Eng M, et al. Maternal cardiovascular dynamics. V. Cesarean section under thiopental, nitrous oxide and succinylcholine anesthesia. *Am J Obstet Gynecol* 1970; 108: 615–622.

109 Operative vaginal delivery. ACOG Technical Bulletin Number 196–August 1994 (replaces No. 152, February 1991). *Int J Gynaecol Obstet.* 1994; 179–185.

110 Markiewicz W, Stoner J, London E, et al. Mitral valve prolapse in one hundred presumably healthy young females. *Circulation* 1976; 53: 464–473.

111 Haas JM. The effect of pregnancy on the midsystolic click and murmur of the prolapsing posterior leaflet of the mitral valve. *Am Heart J* 1976; 92: 407–408.

112 Bono RO, Carabello BA, Kanau C, et al. ACC/AHA 2006 guidelines for the management of patients with vavlular heart disease: a report of the American College of Cardiology/American Heart Association Task Force on Practice Guidelines. *J Am Coll Cardiol* 2006; 48: e1–148.

113 Arias F, Pineda J. Aortic stenosis and pregnancy. *J Reprod Med* 1978; 20: 229–232.

114 Gould FK, Elliott TS, Foweraker J, et al. Guidelines for the prevention of endocarditis: report of the Working Party of the British Society for Antimicrobial Chemotherapy. *J Antimicrob Chemother* 2006; 57: 1035–1042.

115 Lao TT, Sermer M, MaGee L, et al. Congenital aortic stenosis and pregnancy – a reappraisal. *Am J Obstet Gynecol* 1993; 169: 540–545.

116 Demakis JG, Rahimtoola SH, Sutton GC, et al. Natural course of peripartum cardiomyopathy. *Circulation* 1971; 44: 1053–1061.

117 Lampert MD, Lang RM. Peripartum cardiomyopathy. *Am Heart J* 1995; 180: 860–870.

118 Pearson GD, Veille JC, Rahimtoola S, et al. Peripartum cardiomyopathy – National Heart, Lung and Blood Institute and Office of Rare Diseases (National Institute of Health) workshop recommendations and review. *JAMA* 2000; 283: 1183–1188.

119 Ro A, Frishman WH. Peripartum cardiomyopathy. *Cardiol Rev* 2006; 14: 35–42.

120 Hibbard JU, Lindheimer M, Lang RM. A modified definition for peripartum cardiomyopathy and prognosis based on echocardiography. *Obstet Gynecol* 1999; 94: 311–316.

121 Blickstein I, Zalel Y, Katz Z, et al. Ritodrine-induced pulmonary edema unmasking underlying peripartum cardiomyopathy. *Am J Obstet Gynecol* 1988; 159: 332–333.

122 Homans DC. Peripartum cardiomyopathy. *N Engl J Med* 1985; 312: 1432–1437.

123 Ventura SJ, Peters KD, Martin JA, Maurer JD. Births and deaths: united states, 1996. *Mon Vital Stat Rep* 1997; 46(1 Suppl 2): 1–40.

124 Seftel H, Susser M. Maternity and myocardial failure in African women. *Br Heart J* 1961; 23: 43.

125 Veille JC. Peripartum cardiomyopathies: a review. *Am J Obstet Gynecol* 1984; 148: 805–818.

126 Witlin AG, Mabie WC, Sibai BM. Peripartum cardiomyopathy: an ominous diagnosis. *Am J Obstet Gynecol* 1997; 176: 182–188.

127 Cunningham FG, Pritchard JA, Hankins GD, et al. Peripartum heart failure: idiopathic cardiomyopathy or compounding cardiovascular events? *Obstet Gynecol* 1986; 67: 157–168.

128 Lampert MB, Weinert L, Hibbard J, et al. Contractile reserve in patients with peripartum cardiomyopathy and recovered left ventricular function. *Am J Obstet Gynecol* 1997; 176: 189–195.

129 Elkyam U, Tummala PP, Rao K, et al. Maternal complications associated with subsequent pregnancy in women with history of peripartum cardiomyopathy who did not have an abortion. *N Engl J Med* 2001; 344: 1567–1571.

130 Elkyam U. Pregnant again after peripartum cardiomyopathy: to be or not to be? *Eur Heart J* 2002; 23: 753–756.

131 Kolibash AJ, Ruiz DE, Lewis RP. Idiopathic hypertrophic subaortic stenosis in pregnancy. *Ann Intern Med* 1975; 82: 791.

132 Spirito P, Seidman CE, McKenna WJ, Maron BJ. The management of hypertrophic cardiomyopathy. *N Engl J Med* 1997; 336: 775–785.

133 Oakley GDG, McGarry K, Limb DG, et al. Management of pregnancy in patients with hypertropic cardiomyopathy. *BMJ* 1979; 1: 1749–1750.

134 Boriani G, Maron BJ, Shen W–K, et al. Prevention of sudden death in hypertrophic cardiomyopathy but which defibrillator for which patient? *Circulation* 2004; 110: e438–e442.

135 Natale A, Davidson T, Geiger MJ, et al. Implantable cardioverter-defibrillators and pregnancy. *Circulation* 1997; 96: 2808–2812.

136 Pyeritz RE, McKusick VA. The Marfan syndrome: diagnosis and management. *N Engl J Med* 1979; 300: 772–777.

137 Pyeritz RE. Maternal and fetal complications of pregnancy in the Marfan syndrome. *Am J Med* 1984; 71: 784–790.

138 Rossiter JP, Repke JT, Morales AJ, et al. A prospective, longitudinal evaluation of pregnancy in the Marfan syndrome. *Am J Obstet Gynecol* 1995; 173: 1599–1606.

139 Rosenblum NG, Grossman AR, Gabbe SG, et al. Failure of serial echocardiographic studies to predict aortic dissection in a pregnant patient with Marfan's syndrome. *Am J Obstet Gynecol* 1983; 146: 470–471.

140 Slater EE, DeSanctis RW. Dissection of the aorta. *Med Clin North Am* 1979; 63: 141–154.

141 Hankins GD, Wendel GD, Leveno KJ, et al. Mocardial infarction during pregnancy: a review. *Obstet Gynecol.* 1985; 65: 139–146.

142 Sheikh AU, Harper MA. Myocardial infarction during pregnancy: Management and outcome of two pregnancies. *Am J Obstet Gynecol.* 1993; 169: 279–284.

143 Badui E, Rangel A, Enciso R. Acute myocardial infarction during pregnancy and puerperium in athletic women. Two case reports. *Angiology* 1994; 45: 897–902.

144 Roth A, Elkayam U. Acute myocardial infarction associated with pregnancy. *Ann Intern Med* 1996; 125: 751–762.

145 Badui E, Rangel A, Enciso R. Acute myocardial infarction during pregnancy and puerperium review. *Angiology* 1996; 47(8): 739–756.

146 Ladner HE, Danielsen B, Gilbert W. Acute myocardial infarction in pregnancy and the puerperium: a population-based study, *Obstet Gynecol* 2005; 105: 480–484.

147 Andra HJ, Jamison MG, Biswas MS, et al. Acute myocardial infarction in pregnancy: a United States population-based study. *Circulation* 2006; 113: 1564–1571.

148 Veille JC, Kitzman DW, Bacevice AE. Effects of pregnancy on the electrocardiogram in healthy subjects during strenuous exercise. *Am J Obstet Gynecol* 1996; 175: 1360–1364.

149 Schumacher B, Belfort MA, Card RJ. Successful treatment of acute myocardial infarction during pregnancy with tissue plasminogen activator. *Am J Obstet Gynecol* 1997; 176: 716–719.

150 Sebastian C, Scherlag M, Kugelmass A, et al. Primary stent implantation for acute myocardial infarction during pregnancy: use of abciximab, ticlopidine and aspirin. *Cathet Cardiovasc Diagn* 1998; 45: 275–279.

151 Sharma GL, Loubeyre C, Morice MC, et al. Safety and feasibility of the radial approach for primary angioplasty in acute myocardial infarction during pregnancy. *J Invas Cardiol* 2002; 14: 359–362.

152 Ness RB, Harris T, Cobb J, et al. Number of pregnancies and the subsequent risk of cardiovascular disease. *N Engl J Med* 1993; 328: 1528–1533.

153 Chan WS, Anand S, Ginsberg JS. Anticoagulation of pregnant women with mechanical heart valves: a systematic review of the literature. *Arch Intern Med* 2000; 160: 191–196.

154 North RA, Sadler L, Stewart AW, et al. Long term survival and valve-related complications in young women with cardiac valve replacement. *Circulation* 1999; 999: 2669–2676.

155 Elkayam U, Bitar F. Valvular heart disease and pregnancy: part II: prosthetic valves. *J Am Coll Cardiol* 2005; 46: 403–410.

156 Ginsberg JS, Barron WM. Pregnancy and prosthetic heart valves. *Lancet* 1994; 344: 1170–1172.

157 Hall JG, Pauli RM, Wilson KM. Maternal and fetal sequelae of anticoagulation during pregnancy. *Am J Med* 1980; 68: 122–140.

158 Briggs GB, Bodendorfer JW, Freeman RK, Yaffe SJ, eds. *Drugs in Pregnancy and Lactation.* Baltimore, MD: Williams and Wilkins, 1994.

159 Oakley CM, Doherty P. Pregnancy in patients after heart valve replacement. *Br Heart J* 1976; 38: 1140–1148.

160 Antunes MJ, Myer IG, Santos LP. Thrombosis of mitral valve prosthesis in pregnancy: management by simultaneous caesarean section and mitral valve replacement. Case report. *Br J Obstet Gynaecol* 1984; 91: 716–718.

161 Golby AJ, Bush EC, DeRook FA, et al. Failure of high-dose heparin to prevent recurrent cardioembolic strokes in a pregnancy patient with a mechanical heart valve. *Neurology* 1992; 42: 2204–2206.

162 Lev Ran O, Kramer A, Gurevitch J, et al. Low-molecular-weight heparin for prosthetic heart valves: treatment failure. *Ann Thorac Surg* 2000; 69: 264–265.

163 Ginsberg JS, Chan WS, Bates SM, et al. Anticoagulation of pregnant women with mechanical heart valves. *Arch Intern Med* 2003; 16: 694–698.

164 Leyh RG, Fischer S, Ruhparwar A, et al. Anticoagulation for prosthetic heart valves during pregnancy: is low-molecular-weight heparin an alternative? *Eur J Cardiothorac Surg* 2002; 21: 577–579.

165 American College of Obstetricians and Gynecologists. Committee Opinion: safety of Lovenox in pregnancy. *Obstet Gynecol* 2002; 100: 845–846.

166 Medwatch Safety Alert 2002. www.fda.gov/medwatch/SAFETY/2002/lovenox.htm.

167 Vahanian A, Baumgartner H, Bas J, et al. Guidelines on the management of valvular heart disease: the task force on the management of valvular heart disease of the European Society of Cardiology. *Eur Heart J* 2007; 28: 230–268.

168 Bates SM, Greer IA, Hirsh J, et al. Use of antithrombotic agents during prengnacy: the seventh ACCP conference on antithrombotic agents and thrombolytic therapy. *Chest* 2004; 126: 627–644.

169 Rotmensch HH, Rotmensch S, Elkayam U. Management of cardiac arrhythmias during pregnancy: current concepts. *Drugs* 1987; 33: 623–633.

170 Kleinman CS, Copel JA, Weinstein EM, et al. In-utero diagnosis and treatment of fetal supraventricular tachycardia. *Semin Perinatol* 1985; 9: 113–129.

171 Phelps SJ, Cochran EC, Gonzalez-Ruiz A, et al. The influence of gestational age and preeclampsia on the presence and magnitude of serum endogenous digoxin-like immunoreactive substance(s). *Am J Obstet Gynecol* 1988; 158: 34–39.

172 Schroeder JS, Harrison DC. Repeated cardioversion during pregnancy. Treatment of refractory paroxysmal atrial tachycardia during three successive pregnancies. *Am J Cardiol* 1971; 27: 445–446.

173 Jaffe R, Gruber A, Fejgin M, et al. Pregnancy with an artificial pacemaker. *Obstet Gynecol Surv* 1987; 42: 137–139.

174 Scott JR, Wagoner LE, Olsen SL, et al. Pregnancy in heart transplant recipients: management and outcome. *Obstet Gynecol* 1993; 82: 324–327.

175 Branch KR, Wagoner LE, McGrory CH, et al. Risks of subsequent pregnancies on mother and newborn in female heart transplant recipients. *J Heart Lung Transplant* 1998; 17: 698–702.

176 Kossoy LR, Herbert CM, Wentz AC. Management of heart transplant recipients: guidelines for the obstetrician gynecologist. *Am J Obstet Gynecol* 1988; 159: 490–499.

177 Key TG, Resnik R, Dittrich HC, et al. Successful pregnancy after cardiac transplantation. *Am J Obstet Gynecol* 1989; 160: 367–371.

178 Lowenstein BR, Vain NW, Perrone SV, et al. Successful pregnancy and vaginal delivery after heart transplantation. *Am J Obstet Gynecol* 1988; 158: 589–590.

179 Hedon B, Montoya F, Cabrol A. Twin pregnancy and vaginal birth after heart transplantation. *Lancet* 1990; 335: 476–477.

180 Camann WR, Jarcho J, Mintz KJ, et al. Uncomplicated vaginal delivery 14 months after cardiac transplantation. *Am Heart J* 1991; 121: 939–941.

181 Borrow KM, Neumann A, Arensman FW, et al. Left ventricular contractility and contractile reserve in humans after cardiac transplantation. *Circulation* 1985; 71: 866–872.

182 Greenberg ML, Uretsky BF, Reddy PS, et al. Long-term hemodynamic follow-up of cardiac transplant patients treated with cyclosporin and prednisone. *Circulation* 1985; 71: 487–494.

183 Kim KM, Sukhani R, Slogoff S, Tomich PG. Central hemodynamic changes associated with pregnancy in a long term cardiac transplant recipient. *Am J Obstet Gynecol* 1996; 174: 1651–1653.

184 Forrester JS, Swan HJC. Acute myocardial infarction: a physiological basis for therapy. *Crit Care Med* 1974; 2: 283–292.

21 Thromboembolic Disease

Donna Dizon-Townson

Department of Obstetrics and Gynecology, University of Utah Health Sciences Center, Salt Lake City, UT *and* Intermountain Healthcare, Department of Maternal-Fetal Medicine, Provo, UT, USA

Pulmonary embolism (PE), albeit a rare event, remains the leading cause of maternal mortality in the United States [1,2]. Furthermore, deep venous thrombosis (DVT) can cause significant morbidity [3]. Pregnancy-related venous thromboembolism (VTE) has been reported to occur in approximately 0.5–3.0 per 1000 pregnancies based on studies using radiographic documentation [4–6]. Clinical symptomatology should be confirmed with objective testing. Almost 75% of patients who present with suspected thromboembolic disease, and are then subjected to testing such as Doppler ultrasound or venography, are found not to have the condition [7]. When DVT is diagnosed and heparin treatment instituted, the incidence of PE and maternal mortality can be decreased by threefold and 18-fold, respectively. The goal of this review is to facilitate the recognition of the clinical signs and symptoms of VTE disorders, describe a rational approach to the work-up of a suspected hypercoagulable state, and review the use of various diagnostic and treatment modalities.

Incidence and risk factors

Although many studies about maternal mortality cite PE as the leading cause, they do not distinguish VTE from amniotic fluid or air embolism [8–10]. At least half of these deaths are due to thrombotic embolism [9,11–15]. During 1991–1999, a total of 4200 deaths were determined to be pregnancy related. The overall pregnancy-related mortality ratio was 11.8 deaths per 100,000 live births and ranged from 10.3 in 1991 to 13.2 in 1999. The leading causes of pregnancy-related death were embolism (20%), hemorrhage (17%), and pregnancy-induced hypertension (16%). The leading causes of death among women who died after a live birth (60% of all pregnancy-related deaths) were embolism (21%), pregnancy-induced hypertension (19%), and other medical conditions (17%) 2 (Table 21.1).

Critical Care Obstetrics, 5th edition. Edited by M. Belfort, G. Saade, M. Foley, J. Phelan and G. Dildy. © 2010 Blackwell Publishing Ltd.

As illustrated in Figure 21.1, from 1970 to 1985, maternal mortality rates from PE declined by 50% [9]. The traditionally held view is that the maternal risk for VTE is greater in the immediate puerperium, especially following cesarean delivery. Postpartum DVT has been reported to occur 3–5 times more often than antepartum DVT, and 3–16 times more frequently after cesarean as opposed to vaginal delivery [16,17]. In contrast, Rutherford and associates found that the highest incidence of pregnancy-related VTE was not in the puerperium but in the first trimester of pregnancy [18,19] (Figure 21.2). These authors also found that the risk of DVT did not increase with advancing gestational age but stayed relatively constant (see Figure 21.2). In contrast, PE (Figure 21.3) was almost twice as likely to occur in the postpartum patient and appeared to be related to the route of delivery. More recently, Gerhardt and colleagues reported on 119 women with a pregnancy-related VTE [20]. Approximately half (62 women) experienced a DVT during pregnancy: 14 (23%) in the first trimester, 13 (21%) in the second trimester, and 35 (56%) in the third trimester. The other half (57 women) experienced a DVT in the immediate puerperium: 38 (68%) following vaginal delivery and 19 (32%) following cesarean section. In summary, pregnancy-related VTE may occur at any time during pregnancy or the immediate puerperium. A recent 30-year population-based study of trends in the incidence of VTE during pregnancy and post partum confirmed the significant riks of VTE during the puerperium [21]. Although the incidence of PE has decreased over time, the incidence of DVT is unchanged. Therefore, regardless of gestational age, the clinician should have a heightened awareness for the diagnosis when a gravid or postpartum woman presents with clinical symptomatology suspicious for VTE.

Important risk factors for VTE during pregnancy are immobility and bed rest. "Bed rest" is often recommended for a variety of obstetric disease such as threatened preterm labor or preeclampsia. The clinician should keep in mind the increased risk for VTE when making recommendations for limited maternal physical activity or long distance travel. Traveling long distances by air may also increase a pregnant woman's risk of a PE.

Table 21.1 Causes of pregnancy-related death, by outcome of pregnancy and pregnancy-related mortality ratios (PRMR*). United States, 1991–1999.

Cause of death	Outcome of pregnancy (% distribution)							All outcomes	
	Live birth (n = 2519)	Stillbirth (n = 275)	Ectopic (n = 237)	Abortion† (n = 165)	Molar (n = 14)	Undelivered (n = 438)	Unknown (n = 552)	% (n = 4200)	PRMR
Embolism	21.0	18.6	2.1	13.9	28.6	25.1	18.3	**19.6**	**2.3**
Hemorrhage	2.7	21.1	93.3	21.8	7.1	8.7	8.7	**17.2**	**2.0**
PIH§	19.3	20.0	0	0.6	0	12.3	11.8	**15.7**	**1.8**
Infection	11.7	18.9	2.5	33.9	14.3	11.0	12.9	**12.6**	**1.5**
Cardiomyopathy	10.1	5.1	0.4	1.8	0	3.4	11.2	**8.3**	**1.0**
CVA¶	5.7	0.7	0	1.2	0	3.9	8.5	**5.0**	**0.6**
Anesthesia	1.8	0.7	1.3	9.7	0	0	0.4	**1.6**	**0.2**
Other**	17.1	14.9	0.4	16.4	50.0	33.6	27.9	**19.2**	**2.3**
Unknown	0.6	0	0	0.6	0	2.1	0.4	**0.7**	**0.1**
Total††	**100.0**	**100.0**	**100.0**	**100.0**	**100.0**	**100.0**	**100.0**	**100.0**	**11.8**

* Pregnancy-related deaths per 100 000 live births.
† Includes spontaneous and induced abortions.
§ Pregnancy-induced hypertension.
¶ Cerebrovascular accident.
** The majority of the other medical conditions were cardiovascular, pulmonary, and neurologic problems.
†† Percentages might not add to 100.0 because of rounding.
Reproduced by permission from Chang J, Elam-Evans LD, Berg CJ, et al. Pregnancy-related mortality surveillance – United States 1991–1999. *MMWR* 2003; 52(SSO2): 1–8.

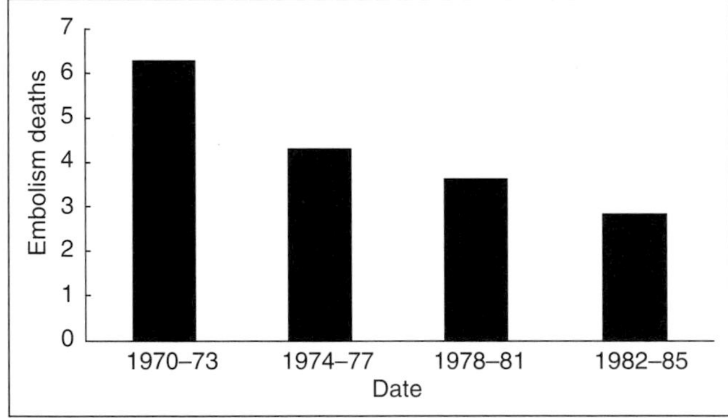

Figure 21.1 Maternal deaths due to pulmonary embolism per 100,000 births from 1970 to 1985. (Reproduced by permission from Franks AL, Atrash AK, Lawson, et al. Obstetrical pulmonary embolism mortality. United States 1970–1985. *Am J Publ Health* 1990; 80: 720–722.)

Additional risk factors in the gravid woman include surgery, trauma or a prior history of superficial vein thrombosis [22].

Ethnic background and maternal age are important risk factors for PE. The overall mortality rate for black women was 3.2 times higher than for white women. In addition, women 40 years or older were at a 10 times greater risk of mortality than women under 25 for both ethnic groups [9] (Figure 21.4). Recent pregnancy surveillance has confirmed that pregnancy-related mortality ratios continued to be 3–4 times higher for black women than

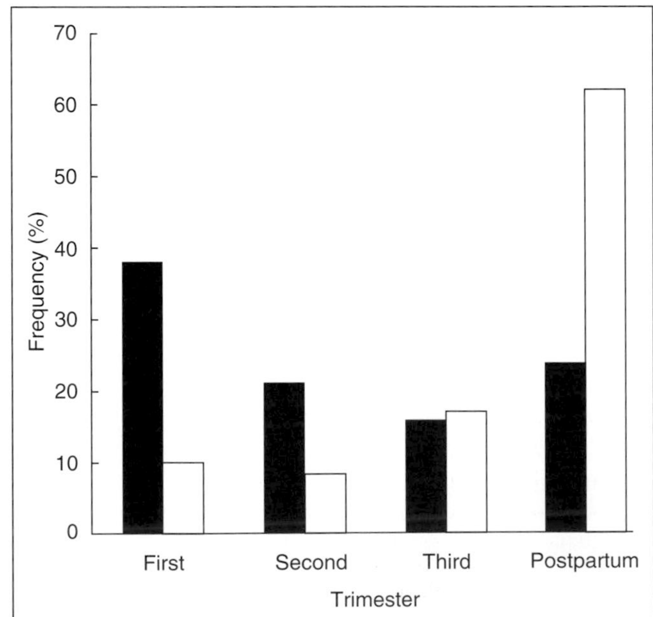

Figure 21.2 Distribution of deep venous thrombosis and pulmonary embolism during each trimester of pregnancy: an 11-year review. (Reproduced by permission from Rutherford SE, Montoro M, McGehee W, et al. Thromboembolic disease associated with pregnancy: an 11-year review, SPO Abstract 139. *Am J Obstet Gynecol* 1991; 164: 286.)

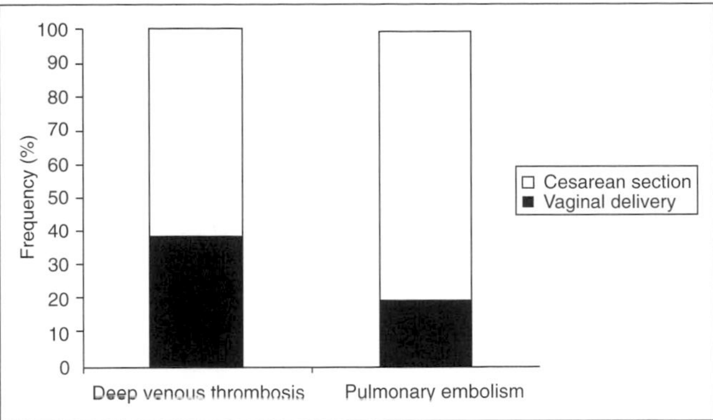

Figure 21.3 The frequency of postpartum deep venous thrombosis and pulmonary embolism according to route of delivery. (Reproduced by permission from Rutherford SE, Montoro M, McGehee W, et al. Thromboembolic disease associated with pregnancy: an 11-year review. *Am J Obstet Gynecol* 1991;164:286.)

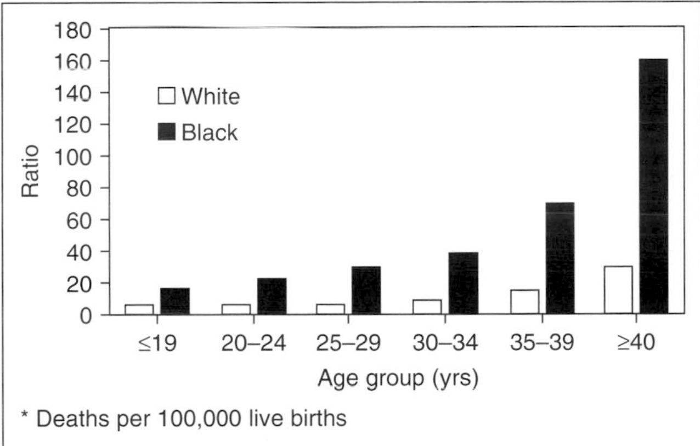

Figure 21.4 Pregnancy-related mortality ration, by age and race – United States, 1991–1999. (Reproduced by permission from Chang J, Elam-Evans LD, Berg CJ, et al. Pregnancy-related mortality surveillance – United States 1991–1999. *MMWR* 2003; 52(SS02): 1–8.)

for white women [2]. In addition, the pregnancy-related mortality ratios for black women aged >39 years were particularly high in comparison with white women in the same age group [2]. Blood groups A and AB may be associated with an increased risk for VTE during pregnancy [23].

A prior history of a VTE confers a greater risk for recurrence especially if the initial event was idiopathic or associated with a hereditary or acquired thrombophilia [24]. In a prospective cohort study investigating the risk of recurrence of pregnancy-related VTE in 125 women who had a history of VTE, heparin was withheld antepartum but administered 6 weeks postpartum in all women. The antepartum recurrence rate was 2.4% (95% CI 0.2–6.9%). There were no recurrences in the 44 patients (0%: 95% CI 0.0–8.0%) who did not have thrombophilia and had a previous episode of thrombosis that was associated with a temporary risk factor. Patients with a positive result for thrombophilia and/or a previous episode of thrombosis that was idiopathic

Table 21.2 Factors associated with a higher risk of pulmonary embolism.

Maternal age
Ethnic background
Operative delivery
Prior thromboembolism
Prolonged immobilization
Inherited/acquired coagulation disorders
Trauma

(unprovoked) had an antepartum recurrence rate of 5.9% (95% CI 1.2–16%). It is assumed that the risk of recurrence diminishes as the time from initial event increases. The mean time from initial event to enrollment in the study was 4 years. In another study, on a cohort of 1104 women with previous VTE, 88 of them became pregnant and did not receive thromboprophylaxis. There were nine recurrences during pregnancy and 10 during the puerperium, with a rate of 5.8% (95% CI 3.0–10.6). In pregnancy, the recurrence rate was 7.5% (95% CI 4.0–13.7) if the first VTE was unprovoked, related to pregnancy or to oral contraceptive use, whereas no recurrence occurred if the first VTE related to other transient risk factors [25].

Inherited and acquired thrombophilias are additional risk factors for VTE. The inherited thrombophilias include deficiencies of protein C, protein S, and antithrombin III, factor V Leiden, prothrombin G20210A, and the 5,10-methylenetetrahydrofolate reductase mutations. The most commonly investigated acquired thrombophilia is the antiphospholipid syndrome.

In summary, the risk of VTE varies among pregnant women, therefore individualization of management must be emphasized. This risk will depend not only on the pregnancy, but also on additional clinical factors such as a prior history of thromboembolism, mode of delivery, prolonged immobilization, age, and ethnicity (Table 21.2). In the presence of a personal or familial history of VTE, testing for thrombophilia should be accomplished to better define the specific risk. A comprehensive thrombophilia work-up should include testing for functional deficiencies of protein C, protein S, and antithrombin III. These tests should be performed preferably when the patient is not pregnant and prior to anticoagulation. In addition, molecular tests for factor V Leiden and the prothrombin G20210A mutation, which are unaffected by pregnancy or anticoagulation, should also be performed. To complete the evaluation, screening for antiphospholipid syndrome with testing for IgG and IgM anticardiolipin antibodies and lupus anticoagulant should be included. A positive test for antiphospholipid syndrome appears to carry the greatest impact on maternal and fetal outcome in subsequent pregnancies.

Normal hemostasis

Few systems are more complex than hemostasis. Interactions among the vessel wall, platelets, and soluble molecules in the vicinity of an injury work to repair the vessel defect without sacrificing nearby vessel patency. The key processes are: (i) vasoconstriction; (ii) formation of a platelet plug; (iii) formation of a stable "seal" by coagulation factors; (iv) prevention of spread of the clot along the vessel wall; (v) prevention of occlusion of the vessel by clots when possible; and (vi) remodeling and gradual degradation of the clot after it is no longer needed.

The maintenance of normal blood flow requires intact, patent blood vessels. After an injury, the hemostatic and fibrinolytic systems work together to protect vascular integrity and assist in repair. Vessel wall integrity, platelet aggregation, normal function of the coagulation cascade, and fibrinolysis are all vital to this process. The initial response to injury is vasoconstriction, which reduces local blood flow and limits the size of the defect that the thrombus is required to seal [26]. After platelets begin to adhere to the exposed vessel wall, they change shape and secrete the contents of their granules. This action leads to further platelet accumulation or aggregation, and results in the formation of a platelet plug.

The numerous substances released by platelets include thromboxane A_2 (TxA_2), a potent vasoconstrictor and preaggregatory agent [27,28]; serotonin, a vasoconstrictor [28]; and adenosine diphosphate (ADP), which enhances platelet aggregation. Platelets also produce vascular permeability factor and platelet growth factor, which stimulate fibroblasts and vascular smooth muscles [17,26]. Released platelet factor 4 (PF_4) and β-thromboglobulin are used as markers of platelet activity [29,30]. The platelet contractile protein, thrombasthenin, enables secretion of these substances and also enhances clot retraction [17]. A platelet surface phospholipoprotein, platelet factor 3 (PF_3), becomes available to bind factor V to catalyze the formation of thrombin. Thrombin, in turn, potentiates platelet aggregation [30].

Whereas TxA_2 is the result of platelet arachidonic acid metabolism, arachidonic acid in endothelial cells is metabolized to prostacyclin (PGI_2). Prostacyclin inhibits aggregation and stimulates vasodilation, and thus counteracts TxA_2 by increasing cyclic adenosine monophosphate (AMP) [26]. Because PGI_2 is concentrated within the vessel wall, the greater the distance from the lumen, the lower the concentration of PGI_2 and the higher the concentration of proaggregatory substances. As platelets begin to seal a vascular defect, the coagulation cascade produces fibrin, which is polymerized as clot and incorporated into the platelet plug.

Proteolytic cleavage or conformational changes activate the circulating clotting factors at the site of injury. Factors II, VII, IX, and X require a vitamin K-dependent reaction in the liver in which γ-carboxyglutamic acid residues are attached to the protein structure. This action provides a location to form a complex with calcium ion and phospholipid receptors on the platelet or endothelial cell membranes. Subsequent steps in the clotting cascade occur at those sites and include the formation of thrombin. Once formed, this is released into the fluid phase.

The intrinsic and extrinsic pathways lead to the final common clotting pathway. Both pathways are activated by components of the vessel wall and lead to activation of progressive exponential increase in subsequent factors. In the intrinsic pathway, high molecular weight kininogen and kallikrein are cofactors for the initial step of the process, the activation of factor XII (XIIa). By catalyzing the formation of kallikrein from prekallikreins, factor XIIa also helps to initiate fibrinolysis, activate the complement system, and produce kinins [26]. Factor XI is activated by XIIa and then cleaves factor IX to form IXa. In comparison, the extrinsic pathway is so named because this pathway relies on tissue thromboplastin as a cofactor. Tissue thromboplastin is released into the circulation following membrane damage or proteolysis [26]. Factor VII is then activated to VIIa which, with tissue thromboplastin, can activate factors IX or X. The common pathway begins with activation of factor X by either VIIa or IXa, in combination with the protein cofactor VIII:C (the antihemophilic factor) and the calcium ion, on the platelet surface (to form PF_3). Factor Xa, assisted by cofactor Va, enzymatically divides prothrombin into thrombin and a peptide activation fragment, F_{1+2}. Separation from this fragment liberates thrombin into the fluid phase. Thrombin catalyzes the formation of fibrin monomers from fibrinogen and, thus, releases fibrinopeptides A and B and facilitates activation of V, VIII:C, and XIII. A fibrin gel is created by the hydrophobic and electrostatic interactions of the fibrin α and γ chains. Subsequently, factor XIIIa forms covalent bonds linking nearby α and γ chains to form a stable polymerized fibrin clot into which water is also incorporated.

Trapped within the clot are proteins that contribute to the enzymatic digestion of the fibrin matrix: plasminogen and plasminogen activators. A variety of substances can activate plasminogen. Plasma plasminogen activator is activated by factor XIIa. Release of tissue activators (tissue plasminogen activator) from blood vessel epithelium (especially venous) is stimulated by exercise, emotional stress, trauma, surgery, hypotensive shock, pharmacologic agents, and activated protein C [17,26,31]. The fibrinolytic enzymes streptokinase and urokinase also activate plasminogen [32]. Having been activated from plasminogen, plasmin cleaves arginyl-lysine bonds in many substrates, including fibrogen, fibrin, factor VIII, and complement [32,33]. The result of plasmin action on fibrin and fibrinogen is release of protein fragments, referred to as fibrinogen degradation products (or fibrin split products). The larger fragments, which may have slow clotting activity, are further divided by plasmin. These fragments have anticoagulant activity, in that they inhibit the formation and cross-linking of fibrin [26]. Measurement of fibrin degradation products provides an indirect measurement of fibrinolysis. $\alpha 2$ antiplasmin, a specific plasmin inhibitor that binds to fibrin and fibrinogen, is found in serum, platelets, and within the clot, along with other inhibitors of plasmin or plasminogen activity [32].

As a potent inhibitor of thrombin, antithrombin III (AT III) is important in the regulation of hemostasis. In decreasing affinity, AT III binds and inactivates factors IXa, Xa, XIa, and XIIa.

AT III acts as a substrate for these serine proteases but forms stable intermediate bonds with the active portion and, thus, neutralizes the respective enzyme [34]. Heparin binds to AT III and induces a conformational change that increases the affinity of AT III for thrombin. The otherwise slow inactivation of thrombin by AT III is accelerated greatly by even small amounts of heparin. After a stable thrombin–AT III complex is formed, heparin is released and available for repetitive catalysis. Excess amounts of AT III are normally present in the circulation, and some are bound to endothelial cell membranes via heparan, a sulfated mucopolysaccharide with a function similar to heparin. The presence of heparan on intact endothelial cell surfaces and its binding to AT III, which neutralizes thrombin, help to prevent local extension of the thrombus beyond the sites of vessel injury [35]. Deficiency of AT III leads to a substantially higher incidence of thrombotic events [36].

Proteins C and S are normally part of the protein C anticoagulant system. Like certain clotting factors, their synthesis depends on vitamin K and involves addition of γ-carboxyglutamic acid residues that enable binding, via calcium ions, to cell surfaces. Protein C is attached to endothelial cells, and protein S is attached to endothelial and platelet membranes. Endothelial cell surfaces also have a specific protein receptor for thrombin – thrombomodulin. The binding of thrombin to thrombomodulin, in the presence of protein S, activates protein C (APC) and promotes anticoagulation. Complexes of APC and adjacently bound protein S cofactor proteolyze the phospholipid-bound factors VIII:Ca and Va. This action results in a second mechanism to prevent extension of the thrombus beyond the area of vessel injury [35]. Deficiencies of either protein C or S are associated with an increase in thromboembolic events [35,37]. Homozygosity of protein C deficiency leads to fatal neonatal purpura fulminans [38].

Changes in hemostasis in pregnancy

A century ago, Virchow described the triad of blood hypercoagulability, venous stasis, and vascular damage conferring an increased risk for thrombosis. All these conditions occur during pregnancy, thus conferring an increased risk for pregnancy-related VTE (Table 21.3). Estrogen stimulation of hepatic synthesis of several procoagulant proteins increases with pregnancy. Levels of factors V, VII, VIII, IX, X, XII, and fibrinogen increase. Venous stasis secondary to progesterone-mediated smooth muscle vascular relaxation and mechanical compression by the gravid uterus occurs. Placental separation and operative delivery can cause endothelial vascular damage.

Compensatory mechanisms such as concomitant rise in fibrinolytic activity help to maintain coagulation equilibrium [39]. As pregnancy progresses, a low-grade chronic intravascular coagulation results in fibrin deposition in the internal elastic lamina and smooth muscle cells of the spiral arteries of the placental bed [40]. Increased fibrin split products and D-dimers during this period suggest ongoing increased fibrinolytic activity [40]. Within an hour of delivery, this fibrinolytic potential decreases, as a result of placental inhibitors [41], and returns to normal. These changes are believed to contribute to the hypercoagulability of the puerperium [18,19]. Levels of factors XI and XIII decrease. When the placenta separates, tissue thromboplastin is released into the circulation, increasing the chance for thrombosis [42]. Additional factors balancing the increased tendency toward coagulation may be a pregnancy-specific protein (PAPP-A) which, like heparin, facilitates neutralization of thrombin by AT III [34]. Platelet counts appear to remain in the normal range during pregnancy, but have been documented to be significantly higher than predelivery on days 8 and 12 after vaginal delivery, and continued to rise 16 days after a cesarean delivery [43]. The platelet count remained significantly higher than predelivery values for 24 days after cesarean delivery [43].

Table 21.3 Hemostatic changes during pregnancy.

Hemostatic changes promoting thrombosis
Increased levels of factor V, VII, VIII, IX, X, XII, fibrinogen
Placental inhibitors of fibrinolysis
Tissue thromboplastin released into the circulation at placental separation
Venous stasis of the lower extremities
Endothelial damage associated with parturition
Hemostatic changes countering thrombosis
Decreased levels of factor XI, XIII
Pregnancy-specific protein neutralizing AT III

Thrombophilias

Approximately half of the women who have a pregnancy-related VTE possess an underlying congenital or acquired thrombophilia [44]. In almost 50% of patients with a hereditary thrombophilia, the initial thrombotic event occurs in the presence of an additional risk factor such as pregnancy, oral contraceptive use, orthopedic trauma, immobilization or surgery [45,46].

Antithrombin III deficiency, although the most rare of the congenital thrombophilias, is the most thrombogenic conferring a 50% lifetime and pregnancy-related risk for thrombosis [47]. AT III deficiency occurs in approximately 0.02–0.17% of the general population and 1.1% of individuals with a history of VTE. Deficiencies of protein C and protein S, although less thrombogenic than AT III deficiency, are more common [47]. Carrier rates for deficiencies of protein C and S are 0.14–0.5% in the general population. In individuals who have had a history of VTE, 3.2% will have either protein C or protein S deficiency.

As a result of the Human Genome Project and major advances in gene identification, common genetic predispositions to thrombophilia, including factor V Leiden and the prothrombin G20210A mutation, have been described. Resistance to APC is now known to be the most common genetic predisposition to thrombosis [48–50]. Eighty to 100% of cases of resistance to APC are due to the factor V Leiden mutation. This is a missense mutation in the gene encoding factor V protein. Individuals with factor V Leiden have normal levels of factor V protein, but this protein is resistant to the normal degradation by APC. The abnormal factor V protein fails to undergo the normal conformation change required for the proteolytic degradation by APC. Heterozygous carriers have a sevenfold increase in the risk for venous thrombosis, whereas homozygous carriers have an 80-fold increased risk. Carrier rates for factor V Leiden are 6–8% in northern Europeans and 4–6% in US Caucasians [51,52]. In the largest prospective observational study, 134 heterozygous carriers for the FVL mutation were identified among 4885 gravidas (2.7%) with both FVL mutation status and pregnancy outcomes available. No thromboembolic events occurred among the FVL mutation carriers (0%, 95% CI 2.7%). Three pulmonary emoboli and one deep venous thrombosis occurred (0.08%, 95% CI 0.02–0.21%), all in FVL non-carriers. Thus, although the FVL is a rather common mutation in the Caucasian population, the relative risk of a pregnancy-related thromboembolic event in a heterozygote carrier is low [53]. Another mutation in the 3′ untranslated region of the prothrombin gene, prothrombin G20210A, leads to elevated prothrombin levels (>155%) and a 2.1-fold increase in the risk for thrombosis. The prevalence of the mutation in the Caucasian population is 2%. The prevalence of the mutation is 6% among unselected patients with thrombosis and about 18% in families with unexplained thrombophilia.

Deep venous thrombosis

Clinical diagnosis

In the gravid patient, DVT appears to occur more often in the deep proximal veins and has a predilection for the left leg [15,54,55]. The clinical diagnosis of DVT [56] is difficult and requires objective testing. Of those patients with clinically suspected DVT, half will not be confirmed by objective testing. Due to the long-term implications of anticoagulant therapy and the expense of a hypercoagulable work-up, clinical symptomatology of VTE should usually be confirmed with objective testing before a diagnosis is rendered.

Symptoms and signs of DVT are illustrated in Table 21.4. Swelling is considered whenever there is at least a 2 cm measured difference in circumference between the affected and normal limbs. Homan's sign is present when passive dorsiflexion of the foot in a relaxed leg leads to pain, presumably in the calf or popliteal areas. The Lowenberg test is positive if pain occurs distal to a BP cuff rapidly inflated to 180 mmHg. The presence of marked swelling, cyanosis or paleness, a cold extremity or diminished pulses signals the rare obstructive iliofemoral vein thrombosis. DVT has also significant long-term implications, and a prior history of DVT may affect the patient's symptomatology. Years after a severe obstructive DVT, patients may experience postphlebitic syndrome (skin stasis dermatitis or ulcers). An investigation of 104 women with a median postthrombosis interval of 11 years revealed that 4% had ulceration, and only 22% were without complaints [57]. Finally, it is important to remember that pregnant patients commonly complain of swelling and leg discomfort and, as such, do not require objective testing in every instance. It is important to remember that the first sign of DVT may be the occurrence of a PE. In a similar manner, silent DVT has been found in 70% of patients with angiographically proven PE [58]. During the initial evaluation in a pregnant patient with clinical symptomatology suspicious for a pregnancy-related VTE, risk factors as described above should be sought. Again "bed rest" or limited physical activity, which is frequently recommended for a variety of obstetric diseases, is a common risk factor for VTE events.

Table 21.4 Clinical symptoms and signs of lower extremity deep venous thrombosis.

Unilateral pain, swelling, tenderness, and/or edema
Limb color changes
Palpable cord
Positive Homan's sign
Positive Löwenberg test
Limb size difference >2 cm

Diagnostic studies

Ultrasound

Non-invasive testing is usually the first step in confirming the diagnosis of DVT. Real-time imaging with compression ultrasound (CUS), including duplex Doppler, is the method of choice. CUS uses firm compression with the ultrasound transducer probe to detect an intraluminal defect. Experience is required for accurate interpretation, and the affected leg should be compared with the unaffected one. Maneuvers such as Valsalva (which distends the vein and slows proximal flow), release of pressure over a distal vein (which causes a rapid proximal flow of blood), and squeezing of the muscles all cause changes in Doppler shift. Real-time imaging in the presence of DVT may detect a mass in the vessel lumen, a failure of the lumen diameter to increase with Valsalva or a failure of the vein to compress with pressure [59]. Alternatively, imaging may identify a hematoma, popliteal cyst or other pathology to explain the patient's symptoms. In a symptomatic non-pregnant individual, CUS has a sensitivity of 95% for proximal DVT (73% for distal DVT) and specificity of 96% for detecting all DVT, with a negative predictive value of 98% and a positive predictive value for 97% in the non-pregnant symptomatic patient [60]. At least 50% of small calf thrombi are missed due to collateral venous channels [61,62]. Repeating the examination within 2–3 days may reveal a previously latent clot.

During pregnancy, the iliac vessels are especially difficult to image. This is due to pressure from the gravid uterus on the inferior vena cava. As a result, Doppler findings must be interpreted cautiously. In the puerperal patient, imaging may visualize a clot in the iliac vessels as well as pelvic thrombophlebitis or ovarian vein thrombosis. The use of computed tomography (CT) or magnetic resonance imaging (MRI), however, may be more helpful in these latter conditions. MRI is now being used more frequently for the diagnosis of DVT in the pregnant patient and may eventually become the imaging modality of choice [63].

Ascending venography

Venography is the gold standard for the diagnosis of DVT in pregnancy. If the clinical suspicion is high and non-invasive tests are negative, limited venography with abdominal shielding should be done. With the patient at an approximate 40° incline and bearing weight on her unaffected leg, radiographic contrast dye is injected into a dorsal vein of the involved foot. This position allows for the gradual and complete filling of the leg veins without layering of the dye and reduces the likelihood of a false-positive test. Nonetheless, false-positive tests may result from poor technique, poor choice of injection site, contraction of the leg muscles or extravascular pathology such as a Baker's (popliteal) cyst, hematoma, cellulites, edema or muscle rupture. In addition, the larger diameter of the deep femoral and iliac veins can lead to incomplete filling with the dye and unreliable results. Positive identification of a thrombus requires visualization of a well-defined filling defect in more than one radiography view (Figure 21.5). Suggestive signs of a DVT include abrupt termination of a vessel, absence of opacification or diversion of blood flow.

Unlike ultrasonography and Doppler procedures, venography is associated with significant side effects. Twenty-four percent of patients will experience minor side effects of muscle pain, leg swelling, tenderness or erythema [64]. Five percent will develop an allergic reaction. There exists a 1–2% risk of thrombophlebitis after the procedure. These side effects can be reduced by 70% by lowering the concentration of contrast medium [61]. Using a heparinized saline flush after dye injection and the concomitant use of corticosteroids can minimize the risks of phlebitis and clot formation. Radiation exposure to the fetus has been estimated at less than 1.0 rad for unilateral venography including fluoroscopy and spot films without an abdominal shield [65]. This is well below the minimum level of radiation exposure considered teratogenic [66,67].

Impedance plethysmography

Though infrequently used during pregnancy, other methods for diagnosis of DVT include impedance plethysmography (IPG), thermography, iodine 125 fibrinogen scanning, and radionuclide venography. To assess blood flow in the lower extremities, IPG uses changes in electrical resistance in response to changes in fluid volume. It is highly sensitive to proximal thrombosis but frequently fails to detect those below the knee. With inflation of a thigh cuff, blood is retained in the leg. In the absence of venous obstruction, sudden deflation results in immediate outflow of blood and a concomitant sudden increase in electrical resistance. A much slower change is associated with impaired outflow, which indirectly implies venous thrombosis [68]. In the symptomatic non-pregnant patient, IPG has a sensitivity of 83% and specificity of 92% for detecting proximal DVT. Because DVT confined to the calf rarely results in PE, anticoagulation for such DVT is not mandatory. In patients with suspected calf vein thrombosis, IPG may allow the clinician to avoid anticoagulation or venography by excluding extension of the clot above the knee over a 2-week period while the presumed calf thrombosis is treated with heat and elevation [69–73]. In pregnancy, compression of the inferior vena cava by the gravid uterus can yield falsely positive results [74] and confirmation of DVT with venography may be necessary.

Thermography

Thermography detects DVT by an increase in skin temperature. Infrared radiation emission is increased when blood flow is diverted to superficial collaterals or when inflammation is present. Changes are more likely to occur with extensive disease. False-negative results can occur with early or limited thrombosis.

Iodine 125 fibrinogen scanning

This technique is contraindicated during pregnancy because unbound radioactive iodine 125 (^{125}I) crosses the placental barrier [75,76]. Unbound ^{125}I also enters breast milk. In both instances,

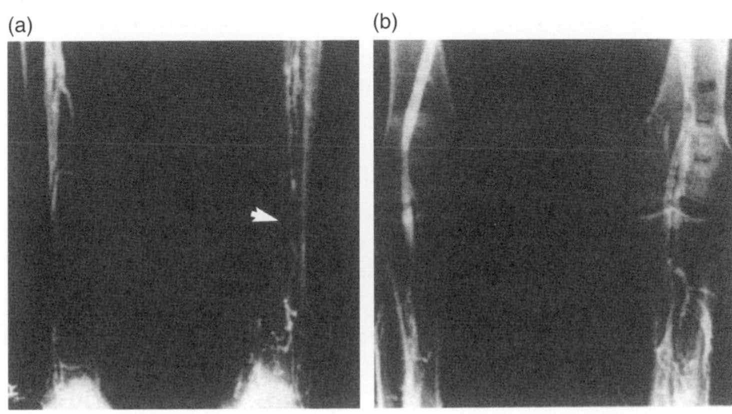

Figure 21.5 A contrast venogram shows each of two legs: (a) a cut-off sign in the posterior tibial vein and filling defects in the popliteal vein in one leg, (b) a normal study in the other leg.

^{125}I can be concentrated in the fetal or neonatal thyroid and produce goiter. Because ^{125}I has a half-life of 60.2 days [61], temporary interruption of lactation is impractical. Thus, the preferred approach, if this radiographic technique is medically necessary, is to avoid breastfeeding. To avoid the small risk of hypothyroidism, non-radioactive iodine should be administered orally for 24 hours prior to and for 2 weeks after the procedure.

In non-lactating postpartum patients, ^{125}I-labeled fibrinogen can be used to identify DVT. Iodine 125 has a longer half-life and gives a smaller radiation dose than the previously used ^{131}I. After intravenous (IV) injection, ^{125}I fibrinogen is incorporated like normal fibrinogen into developing thrombi. Sequential scintillation scanning is performed at any time between 4 and 72 hours. With each scan, radioactivity is compared with background precordial values in the search for a hot spot. For the lower thigh and calf, accuracy can be as high as 92%. Higher background counts in the femoral artery, bladder, and overlying muscle mass make detection of thrombi in the common femoral and pelvic veins difficult. False positives can be due to hematoma, inflammation or surgical wound uptake. Alternatively, if an old thrombus is no longer taking up fibrinogen or forms after the ^{125}I has been cleared from the circulation, a false-negative study may result.

Radionuclide venography

Radionuclide venography using technetium 99m (^{99m}Tc) particles is of low risk to the fetus and can be used to obtain leg studies as well as perfusion lung scans. When performed with a rapid-sequence gamma camera, which may not be available in many institutions, this technique is more than 90% accurate for DVT above the knee [75,76]. Sequential, staged imaging using BP cuffs on the legs to delay flow is an alternative. Correlations with conventional venography of 95% in the thigh and 100% in the pelvis have been reported [76].

D-Dimers and thrombin assay

Recent evidence supports the utility of D-dimer and measurements of thrombin in the assessment of VTE in the non-pregnant setting. Studies during pregnancy are needed before relying on these assays in the obstetric population. D-Dimer fragments are produced during degradation of thrombin-generated fibrin clots by plasmin. The presence of D-dimer is evidence that the blood clotting cascade has been initiated. Three tests for assessment of D-dimers exist: the enzyme-linked immunosorbent assay (ELISA), the latex agglutination assay, and whole-blood agglutination. The whole-blood agglutin assays involve monoclonal antibody that is specific for D-dimer linked to monoclonal antibody that binds to red cells. The advantage of this D-dimer assay is its high negative predictive value. Patients with a low clinical probability of DVT and a negative result on D-dimer testing could safely forego additional diagnostic testing for DVT [77,78]. Normal pregnancy has been shown to cause a progressive increase in circulating D-dimer. Thresholds for D-dimer levels to rule out VTE during each trimester of pregnancy are needed [79]. A serial postpartum evaluation of D-dimer with the Vidas DD assay showed that by using a cut-off of 500 ng/mL, the test was useful for ruling out VTE 4 weeks after delivery [80].

Thrombin generation is additional evidence of ongoing hemostasis. Individuals with thrombin generations <400 nM had a lower risk of recurrent VTE than those with greater values (RR 0.40; 95% CI 0.27–0.60; $p < 0.001$) [81].

Pulmonary embolus

Clinical diagnosis

The sudden onset of unexplained dyspnea and tachypnea is the most common clinical finding that suggests a PE (Table 21.5) [71,82,83]. Other signs and symptoms include tachycardia, cough, pleuritic chest pain, apprehension, atelectatic rales, hemoptysis, fever, diaphoreses, friction rub, cyanosis, and changes in the heart sounds (accentuated second heart sound, gallop or murmur). The clinical manifestations of PE are influenced primarily by the number, size, and location of the emboli. Pre-existing health problems, such as pneumonia, congestive heart failure or cancer, may also confuse the clinical interpretation. If an infarction of the lung occurs after a PE, the patient will typically complain of pleuritic chest pain and hemoptysis and will have a friction rub.

Signs of right-sided heart failure, such as jugular venous distension, liver enlargement, left parasternal heave, and fixed

Table 21.5 Clinical symptoms and signs associated with pulmonary thromboembolism.

	Frequency
Symptoms	
Tachypnea	90%
Tachycardia	40%
Hemoptysis	Less common
Diaphoresis	Less common
Fever	Less common
Rales	Less common
Wheezing	Less common
Syncope	Less common
Signs	
Dyspnea	80%
Pleuritic chest pain	70%
Apprehension	60%
Non-productive cough	50%

From Leclerc JR. Pulmonary embolism. In: Rake RE, ed. *Conn's Current Therapy – 1994.* Philadelphia: WB Saunders, 1994: 199–205; Rosenow EC III, Osmundson PJ, Brown ML. Pulmonary embolism. *Mayo Clin Proc* 1981; 56: 161–178; and Kohn H, Konig B, Mostbeck A. Incidence and clinical features of pulmonary embolism in patients with deep venous thrombosis. A prospective study. *Eur J Nucl Med* 1987; 13: S11–S13.

splitting of the second heart sound, can be seen when at least 50% of the pulmonary circulation has been obstructed. This may be caused by large emboli or multiple small ones, and is termed massive pulmonary embolism [84]. Of note, while multiple small pulmonary emboli can mimic massive pulmonary emboli, they can also present with no symptoms at all or resemble common pregnancy discomforts.

Not only does silent DVT sometimes lead to symptomatic PE, but some patients with clinical DVT can develop silent PE. In a group of 105 patients with objectively confirmed DVT, 60 (57%) were felt to have PE by lung scanning; 59% of these were asymptomatic [71]. In 49 patients with proximal DVT and no symptoms of PE, 35% had high-probability lung scans [85]. Thus, although non-invasive tests for DVT have been proposed as screening tools for PE, sensitivity and negative predictive values are poor (38% and 53%, respectively) [86]. Once DVT diagnosis is confirmed, the occurrence of silent PE is of diminished clinical importance because the treatment in pregnancy is similar.

Diagnostic studies

Laboratory studies

In addition to clinical examination, an arterial blood gas obtained on room air is the first step in confirming the diagnosis. An arterial P_aO_2 greater than 85 mmHg is reassuring but does not exclude PE. In one study [87], 14% of 43 patients with angiographically proven PE had a P_aO_2 greater than or equal to 85 mmHg. If the P_aO_2 is low and PE is suspected, anticoagulation should be considered while definitive diagnostic tests are performed (Table 21.6).

Electrocardiogram

The most common ECG finding is tachycardia. Unfortunately, this sign is often transient and may not be observed. In cases of massive PE, the ECG signs of acute cor pulmonale may be seen. These include a right axis shift with an S1 Q3 T3 pattern and non-specific T-wave inversion. The "classic" S1 Q3 T3 pattern is encountered in only 10% of patients with confirmed PE [83].

Table 21.6 Commonly used laboratory and radiographic techniques for assisting in the diagnosis of pulmonary embolism.

Arterial blood gas	$P_aO_2 < 85$ mmHg
Electrocardiogram	Sinus tachycardia Right axis shift S1 Q3 T3 pattern
Chest X-ray	Focal oligemia Atelectasis Pleural effusion Hemidiaphragm elevation

Chest X-ray

Chest radiographs are abnormal in 70% of patients with PE [82] but are mostly useful in excluding other causes for pulmonary symptoms. Elevation of the hemidiaphragm, atelectasis, and pleural effusion are the most common radiographic abnormalities. Focal oligemia (an area of increased radiolucency and decreased vascular marking) is seen in 2% of cases [88]. Massive PE can lead to a change in cardiac size or shape, increased filling of a pulmonary artery or a sudden termination of a vessel. Infiltrates or plural effusion are later signs of pulmonary infarction. In summary, the primary role of the chest radiograph is to eliminate other causes of the patient's symptoms and to assist in the interpretation of the lung scans.

Alveolar–arterial oxygen gradient

Pulmonary embolism causes decreased perfusion and increases mismatching and shunting. In cases of PE, the disparity between alveolar and arterial oxygen is often exaggerated. As such, alveolar–arterial oxygen gradient has been suggested as a simple screening test to exclude a pulmonary embolus. An alveolar–arterial oxygen gradient of 15 mmHg or greater is considered abnormal. In non-pregnant patients, few patients with documented PE had a normal alveolar–arterial oxygen gradient [61,89]. However, studies in pregnant patients by Powrie et al. concluded that the alveolar–arterial gradient should not be used because more than 50% of women with a documented pulmonary embolus would have been missed [90]. Thus, the role of the alveolar–arterial oxygen gradient as a screening test for PE may be limited to non-pregnant adults.

Ventilation-perfusion lung scan

The gold standard for the diagnosis of PE remains pulmonary arteriography. However, either ventilation perfusion (*V*/*Q*) lung scan or spiral CT, two non-invasive methods for diagnosis of PE, may be considered prior to invasive pulmonary arteriography. The costs of both tests are similar. The advantage of the *V*/*Q* scan is the accumulation of research establishing sensitivities and specificities for results of the procedure. The *V*/*Q* scan is useful in the presence of a very low probability scan result and low clinical suspicion or high probability scan result and high clinical suspicion. Unfortunately, 40–60% are intermediate and therefore additional testing is required.

The lung perfusion scan is performed by IV injection of ^{99m}Tc-labeled albumin microspheres or macroaggregates. These particles are trapped within the pulmonary precapillary arteriolar bed and occlude less than 0.2% of the vessels [91]. Pulmonary function does not change, except in patients with severe pulmonary hypertension [92,93]. Injection is performed with the patient supine in order to increase apical perfusion; imaging is performed with the patient upright to better visualize the lung bases. The following views should be obtained: anterior, posterior, right and left lateral, and right and left posterior oblique. Perfusion lung scans are highly sensitive, and a normal study virtually excludes PE [18,94]. Altered pulmonary perfusion from any source, such

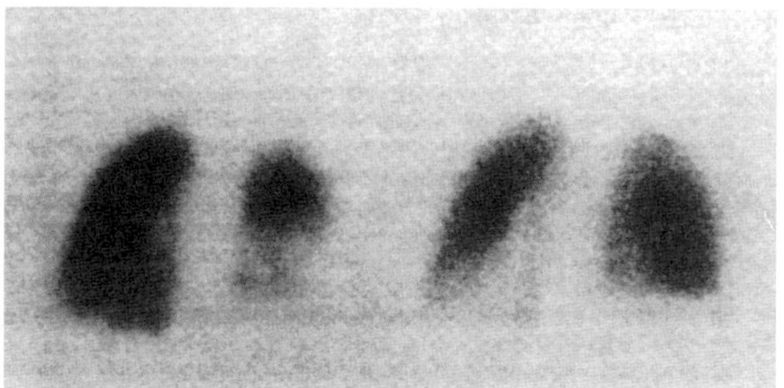

Figure 21.6 In these posterior views, the perfusion lung scan (left) reveals segmental defects, which are not "matched" in the normal.

as pneumonia, tumor, atelectasis or effusion, can result in a false-positive scan. For example, separate investigations revealed normal pulmonary arteriograms in 38% of patients with segmental perfusion defects [68] and in 83% of those with a high probability of PE by perfusion lung scan [95].

In the Prospective Investigation on Pulmonary Embolism Diagnosis (PIOPED) study, 755 individuals had both *V*/*Q* scan and pulmonary angiogram [61]. Two hundred and fifty-one of the 755 (33%) had a PE confirmed by angiogram. When a high probability scan was reported 102/116 (88%) had a PE confirmed by angiogram. For an intermediate, low probability, normal to near normal scan 33%, 12%, and 4% respectively had a PE confirmed on angiogram. The overall sensitivity was 98% and specificity was 10%. When chest X-ray opacification corresponds with perfusion defects, the scan is considered non-diagnostic. Subsequent angiography has shown that the likelihood of PE is low with isolated subsegmental defects or matching ventilation/perfusion defects and high in the presence of ventilation/perfusion mismatching or multiple defects (Figure 21.6). Chronic obstructive pulmonary disease, though infrequent during pregnancy, is the most common confounding factor in evaluation of the scans. In such cases, arteriography is often recommended.

No adverse fetal effects of xenon 133 (^{133}Xe) or ^{99m}Tc lung scanning have been reported, and the exposure dose has been estimated to be significantly less than that received with pulmonary arteriography [96]. The absorbed radiation dose to the lung is approximately 50–75 mrad with ^{99m}Tc aerosol versus 300 mrad with ^{133}Xe (the highest does of the ventilation agents mentioned) [97]. Even if both *V*/*Q* scanning and pulmonary angiography are performed, the total dose (<0.1 rad) will be far less than the lowest dose associated with a teratogenic effect in the human fetus [98].

Nevertheless, oxygen-15 (^{15}O)-labeled carbon dioxide inhalation may, in the future, be useful in pregnancy, due to an even lower radiation dose. The ^{15}O is incorporated rapidly in $H_2{}^{15}O$, which fails to clear the pulmonary circulation in areas of underperfusion. Resulting hot spots are visualized scintigraphically. The major disadvantage is the requirement for a cyclotron in order to produce the ^{15}O, which has a half-life of 2.1 minutes [99].

Spiral CT

The spiral CT is an alternative to the *V*/*Q* scan. This procedure is a chest CT scan with contrast administered via a peripheral IV. The chest CT is performed with narrow collimation during rapid administration of IV contrast. The examination is completed in approximately 15–20 minutes. Both sensitivity and specificity of spiral CT in non-pregnant patients for central pulmonary embolus are approximately 94%. The primary advantage of spiral CT is that it is non-invasive and provides direct visualization of an embolus at a segmental level or higher, as well as visualization of other disease pathology (pleural effusions, consolidation, emphysema, pulmonary masses) which may cause similar respiratory symptomatology [100–102]. In comparison to the *V*/*Q* scan, only 5% are indeterminate, requiring additional testing. The disadvantage is that the procedure is operator dependent. Its availability is becoming more widespread.

Pulmonary artery catheterization

A number of findings can suggest PE on pulmonary artery catheterization. Failure to wedge or the inability to obtain the appropriate waveform can occur in the case of completely occlusive embolism distal to the catheter tip. If the failure to wedge is combined with pulmonary hypertension, further investigation to rule out PE is warranted [103]. Using a minimal amount of contrast material, in conjunction with fluoroscopy, can be useful. Occlusion of the distal port of the catheter [104] or inability to measure cardiac output because of embedding of the catheter tip in the clot [105] are also clues to the presence of a PE. Elevated central venous pressures (>10 mmHg) may suggest a massive PE [106].

Pulmonary arteriography

Pulmonary arteriography is the definitive technique for confirming the diagnosis of PE, but can be indeterminate. Injection of contrast medium selectively into lobar or segmental branches of the pulmonary artery yields clear visualization of vessels greater than 2.5 mm in diameter [58]. A clot may be seen as a filling defect that does not obstruct flow or as an abruptly terminated vessel, possibly with a trailing edge of dye where the clot incompletely fills the lumen (Figure 21.7). Multiple views may be needed to exclude PE. Risks are related to the use of catheterization and contrast dye. With pulmonary arteriography, morbidity has been reported to be as high as 4–5% and mortality rates are 0.2–0.3% [93,107]. Most serious complications, however, occur in patients with underlying pulmonary hypertension and right ventricular end-diastolic pressure exceeding 20 mmHg [93].

Pulmonary arteriography is recommended when initial non-invasive lung scanning is indeterminate, does not correlate with clinical suspicion or indicates moderate probability of PE. The physician should take into account corresponding *V*/*Q* defects and/or chest X-ray findings [61]. The risks of thrombolytic therapy (e.g. streptokinase) or surgical interruption of the vena cava necessitate angiographic confirmation prior to consideration of these measures.

Digital subtraction pulmonary angiography

This relatively non-invasive tool involves the injection of a contrast medium into a peripheral vein and computerized subtraction of the preinjection chest X-ray from the postinjection film. Theoretically, an image of the pulmonary arterial vasculature, as exemplified by contrast filling, is obtained. However, poor imaging often results from respiratory and cardiac motion, and resolution with this technique is not as good as with conventional arteriography. In addition, it is difficult to obtain multiple projection views, and non-selective filling can cause vessel overlap. Digital subtraction angiography may be promising, given continued technologic improvement.

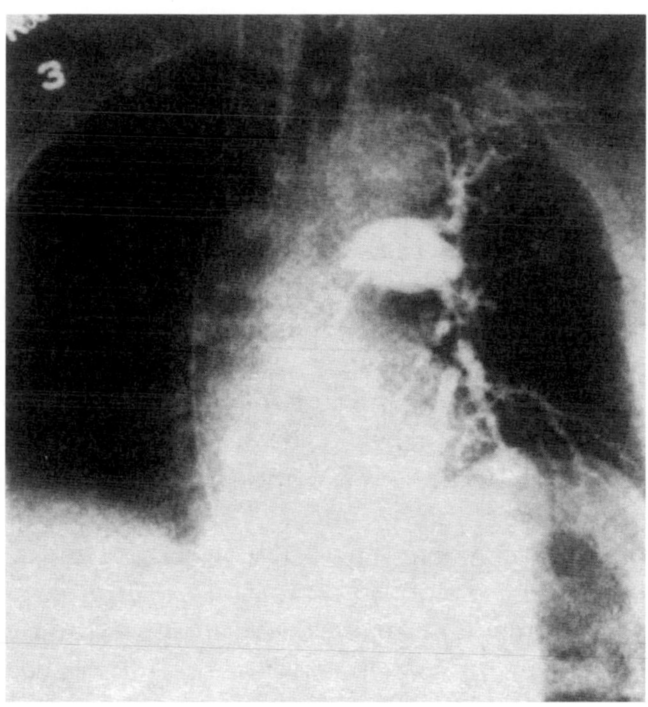

Figure 21.7 Arteriogram of the left pulmonary artery shows filling defects and an unperfused segment of lung as shown by the absence of contrast dye.

Indium 111 platelet imaging

This technique is not yet available for widespread clinical use but shows promise in the diagnosis and management of patients with thromboembolic disease. Platelets are extracted from venous blood, labeled, and reinjected into the donor. The platelets then accumulate at sites of active thrombosis. Heparin blocks the incorporation of these platelets into an established non-expanding thrombus. Images are obtained with gamma camera scintigraphy. For DVT, sensitivity is 90–95% and specificity is 95–100% [108]. Hematomas, wound infection, and prostheses can give false-positive results. Few data are available regarding the usefulness of this technique in PE. Since it relies on the presence of active thrombosis, it may permit anticoagulation to be monitored more effectively.

Anticoagulant therapy

Heparin therapy

Heparin is a heterogeneous acidic mucopolysaccharide with a high molecular weight, a property that prevents it from crossing the placenta [109] (Table 21.7). The molecular weight in commercial preparations of standard unfractionated heparin (UFH) ranges from 4000 to 40,000 daltons, and biologic activities of the different fractions also vary. Separation and use of the lower molecular weight molecules (4000–6000 daltons) provide a preparation of higher, more uniform activity [110–119]. Low molecular weight heparin (LMWH) differs slightly in its anticoagulant activity from UFH, and has a greater bioavailability and longer antifactor Xa activity [111,118,119].

Heparin exerts its primary anticoagulant activity by binding to plasma AT III. Once bound, the configuration of AT III is changed. This facilitates binding to and neutralization of factor Xa and thrombin primarily, and to a lesser extent factors IXa, XIa, and XIIa. Its antifactor Xa activity is inversely proportional to the molecular weight of the heparin fragment [113]. Once released, heparin can then interact similarly with other AT III molecules. Small amounts of heparin can inhibit the initial steps of the clotting cascade. After a thrombus has been formed,

Table 21.7 The distinguishing pharmacologic features of heparin and warfarin.

	Heparin	Warfarin
Molecular weight (daltons)*	12,000–15,000	1000
Mechanism of action	Binds AT III	Vitamin K-dependent factors
Administration	Intravenous, subcutaneous	Oral
Half-life	1.0–2.5 h	2.5 days
Anticoagulant effect	Immediate	36–72 h
Laboratory monitoring	Heparin levels, aPTT antifactor Xa	Prothrombin time, INR
Reversal	Protamine sulfate	Vitamin K
Placental transfer	None	Crosses

* Mean molecular weight.
INR, international normalized ratio.

however, much more heparin is needed to neutralize the larger amounts of already formed thrombin and prevent extension of the clot [120]. As thrombin production diminishes, the heparin dose needed may decrease.

A disadvantage of heparin is the need for parenteral administration via an IV or subcutaneous route. Heparin is not absorbed via the gastrointestinal tract, and intramuscular injections result in erratic absorption and carry a risk of hematoma formation. The half-life of heparin varies with the dose, the type of heparin, and the extent of active thrombosis. For example, higher doses result in both a higher peak and a longer half-life [121]. Half-lives of less than 1 hour to more than 2.5 hours have been found. Moreover, heparin levels may become abnormally elevated in cases of hepatic or renal failure [122]. Continuous IV infusion has been shown to result in more consistent levels and fewer hemorrhagic events than does administration via intermittent IV boluses. Subcutaneous administration also gives a steadier effect, but slower absorption results in a 2–4 hour delay in peak levels.

Another difficulty associated with heparin is adequate monitoring of its bioeffect in order to ensure an adequate yet safe dose. Laboratories vary in the type of tests they can offer, partly because the procedures are technique sensitive, and skill is required for consistent results. The activated partial thromboplastin time (aPTT) is the most commonly available test. Prolongation of the aPTT to 1.5–2.5 times the control value has been shown to be useful in monitoring patients [123,124]. There is a significant increase in clot extension with aPTT levels below 1.5, but no increase in bleeding complications as 2.5 is approached. Thus, anticoagulation in the upper range of 1.5–2.5 times control appears to be ideal.

Although no single laboratory test appears clearly superior in predicting bleeding, heparin assay may be the most helpful [125]. Heparin levels are measured indirectly using the protamine sulfate neutralization test in which the amount of protamine sulfate needed to reverse the effects of heparin on the thrombin clotting time is measured. Plasma heparin levels of 0.2–0.5 IU/mL are desirable for full therapeutic anticoagulation.

Low-molecular-weight heparin

Low molecular weight heparin is distinguishable pharmacologically from UFH by its preferential inactivation of factor Xa (Table 21.8). Antifactor Xa activity is inversely related to the molecular weight of the fragment. This means that LMWH has a greater anti-Xa activity than UFH. While any heparin will inactivate factor Xa by binding to AT III, UFH, by virtue of its longer saccharide chain and pentasaccharide sequence, also inactivates thrombin by forming a ternary complex with AT III and thrombin. In this way, UFH inhibits the activity of both factor Xa and thrombin. Because LMWH lacks the longer saccharide chains, this agent does not inhibit thrombin and its associated potential for bleeding is therefore less.

Low molecular weight heparin offers additional advantages over UFH [113,117]. For example, LMWH has a plasma half-life 2–4 times longer and a more predictable anticoagulant response than UFH. LMWH has less pronounced effects on platelet function and vascular permeability (with significantly less risk of heparin-induced thrombocytopenia). Unlike UFH, LMWH can resist inhibition by PF_4.

Low molecular weight heparin and UFH are similar in that neither crosses the placenta and both are administered either IV or subcutaneously. Protamine sulfate is used to reverse both heparins, although LMWH is less affected by the action of protamine sulfate [113]. Further, LMWH is administered as a weight-dependent dose, and because of its predictable effect, no monitoring of levels is necessary in the non-pregnant state. However, during pregnancy, periodic evaluation with anti-factor Xa levels with dosing of LMWH to achieve a peak antifactor Xa level of 0.5–1.2 U/mL is recommended [55].

Low molecular weight heparin has been shown to be effective when administered on an outpatient basis for the treatment of

Table 21.8 The distinguishing pharmacologic features of standard (unfractionated) heparin and low molecular weight heparin (L-heparin).

	UFH	LMWH
Molecular weight (daltons)*	12,000–15,000	4000–6000
Mechanism of action	Binds ATP III	Binds ATP III
Inhibitory activity	Factor Xa	Factor Xa
Thrombin administration	IV	IV
	SQ	SQ
Half-life (h)	1	4
	3	4
Laboratory monitoring	APTT	None needed; may be measured by anti-factor Xa
Heparin levels		
Anti-factor Xa		
Reversal	Protamine sulfate	Protamine sulfate
Placental transfer	None	None

* Mean molecular weight.
IV, intravenous; SQ, subcutaneous.

DVT [126,127]. Thus, the higher initial cost of the drug may be outweighed by the absence of need for hospitalization. However, caution should be exercised when using outpatient anticoagulation for the acute treatment of VTE during pregnancy [126]. Numerous studies have demonstrated the equivalence or superiority of LMWH to UFH for a variety of prophylactic and therapeutic indications [118,119,127–130]. Although not yet approved for therapeutic anticoagulation in pregnancy, this agent is increasingly prescribed for this indication, and most authorities believe LMWH will soon completely replace UFH for the prophylaxis and treatment of thromboembolic disorders. Although the ideal dosage for the pregnant patient has not been established, standard doses in non-pregnant women are enoxaparin 1 mg/kg subcutaneously twice a day for therapeutic purposes, and 30–40 mg subcutaneously twice a day for prophylaxis.

Heparin side effects

The primary risk of heparin anticoagulation (Table 21.9) is bleeding, which occurs in approximately 5–10% of patients [42,131,132] but can affect as many as one-third. Bleeding may present at the uteroplacental interface as a subchorionic hemorrhage [132]. Prior to initiating anticoagulation, the physician should request a baseline clotting profile to identify those patients with an underlying coagulation defect. The number of bleeding episodes appears to relate to the total daily dose of heparin and the prolongation of the aPTT. Unlike continuous infusion or subcutaneous injection, bolus infusion is associated with a higher total dose of heparin and a much greater risk of bleeding. When needed, as in the case of overdose or to prevent bleeding at the time of emergency surgery, rapid reversal of heparinization with either UFH or LMWH can be accomplished with protamine sulfate.

Because the primary hemostatic defense in heparinized patients is platelet aggregation, drugs such as non-steroidal anti-inflammatory agents or dextran, which interfere with platelet number or function, may induce bleeding. For example, patients receiving aspirin have twice the risk of bleeding [133]. Because heparin is an acidic molecule and incompatible with many solutions containing medications (e.g. aminoglycosides), heparin activity may be affected. However, there should be no loss of heparin activity when such drugs are administered at separate sites [109].

Another side effect of heparin therapy is thrombocytopenia. Estimates of the incidence of thrombocytopenia for UFH vary from 1% to 30% [15,134] and are around 2% for LMWH [113]. However, according to Fausett et al. [135], heparin-induced

Table 21.9 Side effects of heparin anticoagulation.

Side effect	Incidence (%)
Bleeding	5–10
Thrombocytopenia	5–10
Osteoporotic changes	2–17
Anaphylaxis	Rare

thrombocytopenia during pregnancy is rare when compared with non-pregnant women. Thrombocytopenia typically occurs, if at all, within hours to 15 days after the initiation of full-dose heparin therapy [15,109]. Clinically, the thrombocytopenia may be mild (platelet count >100,000/mm^3). With the mild form, treatment can be continued without an undue risk of bleeding. The severe form, however, requires discontinuation of heparin therapy, due to a paradoxic increase in risk for VTE, and is reversible. In the latter circumstance, heparinoids have been found to be 93% efficacious [136]. For patients receiving heparin therapy, maternal platelet counts should be determined weekly during the first 4 weeks of therapy. Thereafter, platelet counts are probably unnecessary [15].

The mechanism involved in the thrombocytopenia is incompletely understood but appears to be platelet clumping and sequestration, immune-mediated destruction, and consumption through low-grade disseminated intravascular coagulation. While heparin-associated thrombocytopenia is most frequently encountered in patients receiving high-dose heparin, patients on prophylactic low-dose heparin have a lower risk of this condition [137–139]. Patients on LMWH have been noted to occasionally experience thrombocytopenia [116,126]. Heparin derived from bovine lung rather than porcine gut is more often associated with thrombocytopenia [140].

Hypersensitivity to heparin therapy can result in chills, fever, and urticaria. Allergic skin reactions to both UFH and LMWH can occur. These take the form of itchy, erythematous infiltrated plaques, which may resolve when preparations are switched. However, cross-reactivity between the two preparations may occur. Because heparin-induced thrombocytopenia may manifest as cutaneous lesions, it is important that this be excluded. Fondaparinux, a synthetic pentasaccharide which binds to antithrombin and inhibits factor Xa without inhibiting thrombin, has been successfuuly used during pregnancy in patient with cutaneous intolerance to heparins [141,142]. Rarely, anaphylactic reactions to heparin have occurred.

Osteoporosis and symptomatic fractures are another side effect of prolonged heparin therapy [143–148]. These changes in bone density have ranged from demineralization changes observed in the spine, hip, and femur radiographs to overt fractures [114,146–148] and occur in patients who receive both UFH and LMWH. In 184 women given long-term heparin prophylaxis during pregnancy, symptomatic vertebral fractures occurred in four post partum. The mean dose in those with symptomatic vertebral fractures ranged from 15,000 to 30,000 units/day. In one such patient, the mean dose received was as little as 15,000 units/day for 7 weeks [147]. Radiographic changes have been observed in up to one-third of women receiving heparin therapy for longer than a month [116]. Reversal after discontinuing therapy can be slow [144,145] but there is reassuring evidence that reversal of osteopenia does occur and that treatment in consecutive pregnancies may not increase a woman's risk of this complication [148]. Pregnant women receiving heparin therapy should be advised to take at least one additional gram (should not exceed

2 g total per day) of supplemental calcium and encouraged to perform daily weight-bearing exercises.

The risk of spinal hematoma from regional anesthesia is an intrapartum consideration in the anticoagulated patient. Patient management is based on the timing of needle insertion, catheter removal, and anticoagulant drug administration [149,150]. The American Society of Regional Anesthesia has made the following recommendations. In individuals receiving subcutaneous mini-dose prophylaxis, there is no contraindication to neuraxial techniques. Concurrent use of other medications, such as antiplatelet medications (ASA), that affect other components of the clotting cascade may affect risk of bleeding complications. In individuals receiving LMWH, monitoring of anti-Xa levels is not recommended. For patients receiving thromboprophylaxis with LMWH, a wait period of at least 10 hours prior to needle insertion or catheter placement is recommended. Patients on therapeutic doses of LMWH (enoxaparin 1 g/kg twice daily) require 24 hours from time of last dose to needle insertion or catheter placement.

The careful administration of subcutaneous heparin prevents erratic absorption and local bruising. Preferably, the subcutaneous fat of the anterior flank (lateral abdominal wall) should be used rather than sites in the arms and legs. These latter sites are more painful and are subject to rapid absorption of heparin in association with movement. A small needle is fully inserted vertically into a raised fold of skin and withdrawn atraumatically after injection. Patients should be advised against massaging the injection sites as this increases absorption. Overall, heparin is safe for use in pregnancy; the perinatal outcome among heparin users is comparable to that for non-users [151].

Warfarin

Warfarin, a coumarin derivative, is the most commonly used oral anticoagulant (see Table 21.7). It inhibits regeneration of active vitamin K in the liver. Vitamin K is required to carboxylate the glutamic acid residues on factors II, VII, IX, and X and protein C. These factors are otherwise inactive and unable to complex normally with calcium and phospholipid receptors.

Except in the rare situation in which heparin cannot or should not be used, warfarin is contraindicated in pregnancy (Table 21.10). With a molecular weight of 1000 daltons, warfarin easily crosses the placenta. Administration in the first 6–9 weeks of gestation has been associated with warfarin embryopathy. This syndrome may include nasal hypoplasia, depression of the bridge of the nose, and epiphyseal stippling, such as is seen in Conradi-Hunermann chondrodysplasia punctata [131,152–154]. Exposure during the second and third trimesters is associated with a variety of CNS and ophthalmologic abnormalities. It is suspected that some of these abnormalities are related to fetal hemorrhage and scar tissue formation. In a retrospective review of published reports, abnormal live-born infants occurred in 13% of pregnancies in which warfarin or related substances were used. Approximately 4% resulted in infants with warfarin embryopathy. Of patients with warfarin embryopathy, approximately 30% may be developmentally retarded [131]. In those infants with CNS abnormalities, dorsal midline dysplasia (e.g. agenesis of the corpus callosum), Dandy–Walker malformation, midline cerebellar atrophy and ventral midline dysplasia (e.g. optic atrophy) have been described [155]. Such literature reviews, however, may be skewed in favor of abnormal outcomes. A review of 22 children of mothers who took warfarin during pregnancy revealed no significant difference when compared with controls; this outcome suggests that the incidence of abnormalities may be lower than previously reported [156]. Because of the anticoagulant effect in the fetus, there is also a higher risk of fetal hemorrhage at delivery. Thus, women who are treated with coumarin derivatives and contemplate pregnancy should be switched to heparin prior to conception. In select patients with cardiac disease at risk of arterial thromboembolic events, the apparent increased effectiveness of warfarin may justify the associated fetal risks. There appears, however, to be little justification for the use of coumarin derivatives in the treatment or prophylaxis of venous thromboembolism.

Table 21.10 Maternal and fetal side effects of warfarin therapy during pregnancy.

Maternal
Bleeding
Skin necrosis/gangrene
Purple toes syndrome
Hypersensitivity
Fetal
Hemorrhage
Warfarin embryopathy
CNS abnormalities
Optic atrophy
Mental retardation

The major maternal complication (see Table 21.10) of warfarin use is bleeding, which occurs more often with warfarin than with subcutaneous heparin [157]. Warfarin anticoagulation is also more sensitive to fluctuations in clotting factors and plasma volume and requires more frequent monitoring and adjustments. Numerous medications [158], including some antibiotics, can augment or inhibit warfarin (coumarin derivative) activity (Table 21.11).

Less common side effects of warfarin therapy are skin necrosis and gangrene [159]. Once an underlying disease is excluded as a cause of such dermatologic changes, warfarin should be discontinued and appropriate medical and/or surgical therapy instituted. The purple toes syndrome [160,161], an infrequent complication of warfarin therapy, is characterized by dark, purplish, mottled toes and occurs 3–10 weeks after the initiation of coumarin therapy. In most instances, this condition is reversible, but a few patients will progress to necrosis or gangrene. In rare circumstances, amputation may be necessary.

Table 21.11 Selected drugs that interact with coumarin derivative anticoagulants.

May potentiate oral anticoagulants	May antagonize oral anticoagulants
Alcohol, dose dependent	Antacids
Chlorpromazine	Antihistamines
Cimetidine	Barbiturates
Danocrine	Carbamazepine
Metronidazole	Corticosteroids
Neomycin	Oral contraceptives
Non-steroidal anti-inflammatory drugs	Primidone
Salicylates, large doses	Rifampin
Thyroxine	Vitamin K
Trimethoprim	
Phenytoin	

Reproduced by permission from Standing Advisory Committee for Haematology of the Royal College of Pathologists. Drug interaction with coumarin derivative anticoagulants. *BMJ* 1982; 185: 274–275.

Measurement of the prothrombin time (PT) is used to monitor the anticoagulant effect of warfarin. Therapeutic levels can be reached after 3–5 days and should yield a PT of 1.5–2.5 times control (international normalized ratio, INR) [162]. In a study of 266 non-pregnant patients with PE, early treatment with warfarin (begun during days 1–3) was found to be as effective as continuous IV heparin in preventing recurrences, with similar rates of bleeding complications. The major advantage with warfarin was a 30% decrease in hospital time [163].

Reversal of anticoagulation depends on regeneration of clotting factors and is slow. Administration of parenteral vitamin K can lead to reversal in 6–12 hours. In an acute situation, fresh frozen plasma can be given to provide clotting factors.

Selective factor Xa inhibitors

Fondaparinux (Arixtra, Sanofi-Synthelabo, Paris, France) is a pentasaccharide that selectively inhibits factor Xa. This is the first of a new class of synthetic antithrombotic agents. Due to its linear pharmacokinetic profile, a once-daily subcutaneous administration is recommended. This new medication has been approved for use in the prophylaxis of VTE following orthopedic surgery. It was found to reduce VTE risk by more than 50% as compared to LMWH without an increased risk for signficant bleeding [164]. Two case reports of the use of fondaparinux during pregnancy in the setting of cutaneous heparin intolerance during pregnancy have been published [141,142]. Although this novel medication shows promise, heparin, with UFH or LMWH, remains the first-line agent for treatment and prevention of VTE during pregnancy.

Antepartum management

Patients at high risk for thromboembolic disease require consideration for anticoagulation or prophylactic therapy during pregnancy and the puerperium. Such patients are those with hereditary thrombophilia, prior history of VTE, mechanical heart valve, atrial fibrillation, trauma/prolonged immobilization/major surgery, other familial hypercoagulable states, and antiphospholipid syndrome [165]. Patients with the following conditions are at highest risk and should be considered for therapeutic heparin anticoagulation: artificial heart valves, AT III deficiency, antiphospholipid syndrome (prior VTE), history of rheumatic heart disease with current atrial fibrillation, homozygosity for factor V Leiden or prothrombin G20210A, and receiving chronic anticoagulation for recurrent thromboembolism [165].

If the patient's clinical picture strongly suggests VTE, anticoagulation with heparin should be considered prior to diagnostic studies to minimize the risk of an embolic event while awaiting confirmation of the diagnosis. After obtaining a baseline clotting profile and a complete hypercoagulable evaluation, the physician can most easily achieve rapid anticoagulation by using an initial IV bolus of 70–100 units/kg or 5000–10,000 units [109]. For massive PE, an initial IV bolus as high as 15,000 units has been recommended [166]. Initial continuous infusion rates can be calculated at 15–20 units/kg/h. Doses that prolong the aPTT 1.5–2.5 times normal or give a plasma heparin level of 0.2–0.5 units/mL are considered therapeutic. Adequate and rapid initial anticoagulation is essential to minimize the risk of PE. The heparin dose is ideally adjusted every 4 hours until adequate anticoagulation has been achieved. Excessive doses that prolong the aPTT beyond 2.5 times normal or result in plasma heparin levels above 0.5 units/mL are associated with a greater likelihood of maternal bleeding [41,109]. In pregnancy, the required dose is related more closely to the maternal circulating blood volume than to maternal body weight [167]. To ensure accurate results, blood samples should be drawn remote from the site of heparin infusion. After initial adjustment and stabilization of the heparin dose, once-daily laboratory testing is sufficient. The infusion dose required may change as active thrombosis abates. A useful protocol for the adjustment to the dose of IV heparin is presented in Table 21.12 [4].

There is no difference between patients with DVT and PE as to the amount of heparin required to achieve therapeutic anticoagulation [168]. However, recommendations for duration of IV infusion vary. A *minimum* of 2 days with DVT and 5 days with PE are suggested [17,42]. Most authors recommend IV therapy for 5–7 days. The most recent statement by the Amercian College of Chest Physicians (ACCP) recommends that in women with an acute VTE, adjusted dose LMWH throughout pregnancy or IV UFH for at least 5 days, followed by adjusted-dose UFH or LMWH for the remainder of pregnancy and at least 6 weeks post partum. Adjusted dose defined as following: UFH SQ q12 hours in doses adjusted to a target midinterval aPTT into therapeutic range, LMWH weight adjusted, full treatment doses administered once or twice daily (e.g. dalteparin 200 U/kg or tinzaparin 175 U/kg, qd, or dalteparin 100 U/kg q12 hours or enoxaparin 1 mg/kg q12 h) [55]. Historically, the goal was to continue IV heparin until: (i) active thrombosis has stopped; (ii) thrombi are firmly

Table 21.12 Protocol for adjustment of the dose of intravenous heparin.*

Activated partial thromboplastin time (sec)†	Repeat bolus?	Stop infusion?	New rate of infusion	Repeat measurement of activated partial thromboplastin time
<50	Yes (5000 IU)	No	+3 mL/h (+2880 IU/24 h)	6 h
50–59	No	No	+3 mL/h (+2880 IU/24 h)	6 h
60–85‡	No	No	Unchanged	Next morning
86–95	No	No	−2 mL/h (−1920 IU/24 h)	Next morning
69–120	No	Yes (for 30 min)	−2 mL/h (−1920 IU/24 h)	6 h
>120	No	Yes (for 60 min)	−4 mL/h (−3840 IU/24 h)	6 h

* A starting dose of 5000 IU is given as an intravenous bolus, followed by 31,000 IU per 24 hours, given as a continuous infusion in a concentration of 40 IU/mL. The activated partial thromboplastin time is first measured 6 hours after the bolus injection, adjustments are made according to the protocol, and the activated partial thromboplastin time is measured again as indicated. Adapted from Hirsch J. Heparin. *N Engl J Med* 1991; 324: 1565.

† The normal range, measured with the Dade-Actin-FS reagent, is 27–35 seconds.

‡ The therapeutic range of 60–85 seconds is equivalent to a heparin level of 0.2–0.4 IU/mL by protamine titration or 0.35–0.7 IU/mL according to the level of inhibition of factor Xa. The therapeutic range varies with the responsiveness of the reagent used to measure the activated partial thromboplastin time to heparin.

Reproduced by permission from Toglia MR, Weg JG. Venous thromboembolism during pregnancy. *N Engl J Med* 1996; 335: 108.

attached to the vessel wall; and (iii) organization has begun [17]. A recent comparison of fixed-dose weight-adjusted UFH compared to LMWH for acute treatment of VTE in the non-pregnant state showed them to be equally effective and safe [127]. Seven hundred and eight patients with acute VTE were randomized to either UFH subcutaneously as an initial dose of 333 U/kg, followed by a fixed dose of 250 U/kg every 12 hours (n = 345), LMWH was administered subcutaneously at a dose of 110 IU/kg every 12 hours (n = 352). Recurrent VTE within 3 months and major bleeding within 10 days of randomization were the main outcome measures. Recurrent VTE occurred in 13 patients receiving UFH (3.8%) compared to 12 patients receiving LMWH (3.4%; absolute difference 0.4%; 95% CI −2.6% to 3.3%). There was no significant difference in major bleeding events between the two groups. The period of continuous IV infusion is followed in pregnancy by therapeutic subcutaneous heparin for the duration of the pregnancy [55,169]. Postpartum anticoagulation will need to be continued for 6–12 weeks in most patients. According to Schulman and associates, 6 months, not 6 weeks, of prophylactic anticoagulation after a first episode of venous thromboembolism may be required to lower the recurrence rate [170]. In contrast, Hirsch suggests that duration of anticoagulant therapy depends on whether the patient has a reversible risk factor for DVT, such as DVT after surgery or trauma, or a permanent risk factor, such as idiopathic DVT (the absence of any risk factors) [171]. With the Hirsch classification [172], prolonged anticoagulant therapy would be 6 weeks for the reversible group and 6 months for idiopathic DVT.

Monitoring of therapy in patients receiving adjusted-dose (therapeutic) subcutaneous heparin is more complex than with the IV route. With respect to the timing of aPTT in relationship to intermittent injection, some authorities recommend monitoring the mid-dose aPTT (i.e. drawn at 6 h for patients receiving 12-h injections), while an increasing number of physicians favor adjusting the heparin dose to achieve a level near 2.5 times control just prior to the next dose. Data to document the superiority of the approach are lacking; it is hoped that the use of LMWH will, in the near future, make such discussion moot.

Reported alternatives to long-term intermittent injections in pregnancy have included continuous infusions of heparin via a Hickman catheter [173] or subcutaneous pump [174]. In one series, six patients received continuous subcutaneous infusion to reach therapeutic PTTs of 1.5–2.0 times controls. Although there were no recurrences of thrombosis, five of the patients experienced major or minor bleeding complications [174].

A goal for antepartum care should also be to maximize a pregnant woman's candidacy for regional anesthesia. The American Society of Regional Anesthesia has recommended that patients receiving therapeutic doses of LMWH (specifically enoxaparin, 1 mg/kg twice daily) should not receive neuraxial blocks for 24 hours from the last dose [149,150]. Furthermore, obtaining an anti-factor Xa level before placing the block was not recommended since it did not adequately predict the risk of bleeding. Switching to UFH at approximately 37 weeks should be considered due to the shorter half-life. A normal aPTT usually is sufficient to ensure the safety of epidural anesthesia in a patient anticoagulated with UFH, as long as the platelet count is normal.

Intrapartum management

The risk of significant hemorrhage is minimal for patients receiving anticoagulants who deliver vaginally, as long as the platelet count and function are normal and uterine atony is avoided. Regional anesthetics (epidural and spinal), however, are not recommended in a fully anticoagulated patient because of the potential risk of epidural or spinal cord hematoma formation. For patients requiring cesarean delivery, therapeutic anticoagulation becomes more complex. On admission to labor and delivery, a clotting profile and hematocrit should be drawn. There are three basic choices in the approach to anticoagulant management in such patients.

1 *Continue therapeutic anticoagulation.* This approach is recommended for particularly high-risk patients, such as those with recent PE, iliofemoral thrombosis or mechanical heart valve prostheses. Because a more uniform therapeutic heparin level is desirable, the patient may be changed from subcutaneous injection to continuous IV infusion. A heparin level of 0.4 units/mL or a low therapeutic aPTT (close to 1.5 times normal) may be desirable in these surgical patients.

2 *Reduce the subcutaneous heparin dose.* In patients at lower risk of thromboembolism, the heparin dose can be reduced to a prophylactic level (5000 units every 12 hours); this dose is not associated with increased surgical bleeding.

3 *Stop or withhold heparin administration.* For patients at increased risk for operative bleeding (i.e. suspected placenta accreta) and at relatively low risk of clot propagation, heparin may be temporarily withheld or its effects reversed with protamine sulfate. Non-pharmacologic prophylaxis (e.g. pneumatic compression stockings) may be substituted during the intraoperative period.

With patients who are anticoagulated and in whom rapid reversal is deemed essential, protamine sulfate can be used to reverse either UFH or LMWH. One milligram of protamine sulfate neutralizes 100 units of heparin. To determine the proper dose of protamine, several approaches are available. One is to calculate the amount of circulating heparin by estimating the plasma volume at 50 mL/kg of body weight and multiplying the plasma volume by the heparin concentration [17]. In most institutions, however, this procedure may not be technically feasible. If heparin level is not available, the amount of protamine sulfate to give should be underestimated or slowly titrated to the whole-blood clotting time because of the short half-life (rapid metabolism) of heparin and the irreversible anticoagulant effect of excess protamine. No single dose should exceed 50 mg. A 50 mg dose is almost never needed because it would neutralize 5000 units of circulating heparin, an amount highly unlikely to be present. Protamine sulfate should be administered IV over 20–30 minutes to prevent hypotension. In patients receiving adjusted-dose subcutaneous heparin, a dose of 5–10 mg of protamine sulfate is often sufficient; further doses may be given, depending on the aPTT value. It should be emphasized that for vaginal delivery, even significantly prolonged aPTT values rarely result in clinical hemorrhage, and thus do not require protamine sulfate therapy.

Patients who present for delivery on warfarin anticoagulant are at heightened risk for bleeding with either vaginal or operative delivery. Parental vitamin K can help to regenerate the clotting factors within 12 hours. If there is little time or reversal is not adequate, fresh frozen plasma can be given to supply clotting factors. Regardless, the pregnant woman should be stabilized and be sufficiently able to clot before operative delivery is initiated.

Postpartum management

Conversion from heparin to warfarin anticoagulation should be initiated post partum in the hospital to minimize the maternal risk of complications. Once the patient has delivered and is sufficiently stable, full heparin anticoagulation should be resumed. Then, oral warfarin therapy should be started with 10–15 mg orally per day for 2–4 days, followed by 2–15 mg/day as indicated by the INR or PT [109]. Heparin and warfarin therapy should be overlapped for the first 5–7 days post partum until an INR of approximately 2. 0–3.0 has been achieved. One approach is to give the warfarin sodium at 6 p.m., then draw an INR or PT at 6 a.m. the following day, adjusting the dose for the subsequent day's warfarin according to that morning's results. Once the patient is therapeutically anticoagulated, heparin is discontinued. Postpartum suppression of lactation with estrogen is associated with a much higher incidence of thromboembolic complications and is contraindicated [175,176].

Prophylaxis of thromboembolism

The dosage of heparin needed during pregnancy appears to increase because of increases in heparin-binding proteins, plasma volume, renal clearance, and heparin degradation by the placenta. All contribute to a decreased bioavailability of heparin. Due to a lack of adequate prospective trials, a number of different prophylactic regimens have been proposed. Low-dose prophylaxis with UFH may be administered via 5000–7500 units every 12 hours during the first trimester, 7500–10,000 units every 12 hours during the second trimester, followed by 10,000 units every 12 hours during the third trimester unless the aPTT is elevated. Alternatively, LMWH may be used. For low-dose prophylaxis, dalteparin 5000 units once or twice daily or enoxaparin 40 mg once or twice daily may be used. Adjusted-dose prophylaxis may be accomplished with either dalteparin 5000–10,000 units every 12 hours or enoxaparin, 30–80 mg every 12 hours [165]. An increase from 5000 units to 7500–10,000 units in the third trimester [42] is often recommended [177]. Except for doses exceeding 8000 units, laboratory monitoring is not usually required [42]. Caution should be used in the patient with diminished renal function, such as seen during pre-eclampsia, which may elevate heparin levels.

Employing perioperative (cesarean) prophylaxis may be considered for certain patients, such as individuals who are obese, have difficulty ambulating or have been at prolonged bed rest. Conservative mechanical methods, such as intermittent pneumatic compression boots or graduated elastic compression stockings, may be used. A recent decision analysis investigated the use of thromboprophylaxis after cesarean delivery. The authors compared four methods: universal subcutaneous heparin prophylaxis, heparin prophylaxis only for patients with a genetic thrombophilia, use of pneumatic compression stockings, and no thromboprophylaxis. Use of pneumatic compression stockings after cesarean delivery was the strategy with the lowest numbers of adverse events. Universal prophylaxis with heparin was associated with an excess risk of heparin-induced thrombocytopenia induced thrombosis and bleeding per VTE [178]. Another group performed a decision analysis comparing no thromboprophylaxis to intermittent pneumatic compression and confirmed that mechanical thromboprophylaxis is estimated to a cost-effective strategy [179]. Early postoperative ambulation is also important in preventing thromboembolism. Low-dose heparin is accepted as prophylaxis for a variety of surgical procedures [180]. Although in some general surgical or orthopedic patients dihydroergotamine in combination with heparin is felt to be more effective than heparin alone [181,182], its use in pregnant or parturient women has not been studied. Thus, its use cannot be recommended. The combination of mechanical methods, especially pneumatic compression, and low-dose heparin may be the optimal approach for high-risk patients [183,184]. LMWH has been found useful in abdominal surgery; one dose is given preoperatively, followed by additional doses once every 24 hours [185,186].

According to the ACCP recommendations, patients with a history of a single episode of VTE, associated with a transient risk factor that is no longer present, should undergo antepartum clinical surveillance and postpartum anticoagulation [55]. In patients with a history of a single episode of VTE and thrombophilia or a strong family history and not currently on lifelong anticoagulation, antepartum prophylactic or intermediate-dose LMWH or minidose or moderate-dose UFH, plus postpartum anticoagulation is recommended. Intermediate-dose LMWH is defined as dalteparin 5000 U SC q12 h or enoxaparin 40 mg SC q12 h. Minidose heparin is UFH 5000 U SC q12 h and moderate-dose UFH is UFH SC q12 h in doses adjusted to target an anti-Xa level of 0.1–0.3 U/mL [55]. Therapeutic anticoagulation is necessary during pregnancy for those patients with mechanical heart valves [187] or inherited deficiency of a natural anticoagulant such as AT III [188]. In women with AT III deficiency, successful outcomes have been achieved with the use of subcutaneous and IV heparinization, accompanied by infusion of AT III concentrate at the time of abortion or delivery [188]. AT III deficiency should be considered when heparin requirements increase beyond typical dosages. Without such therapy, maternal morbidity or mortality and fetal loss are extremely high. Deficiencies of proteins C and S are also associated with thrombotic tendency [189]. In patients with medical histories remarkable for VTE, a systematic comprehensive approach to thrombophilic screening should be pursued. Knowledge of an individual's thrombophilic status can be used to better predict VTE recurrence risk [24].

Antiplatelet agents such as aspirin and dipyridamole may be helpful in preventing thrombosis in the arterial circulation and with some prosthetic heart valves. There is no known role for these agents in the prevention of pregnancy-associated VTE disease. Perioperative prophylaxis with dextran appears beneficial in some surgical patients, but the risk of bleeding is higher than with heparin, and dextran's usefulness in pregnant patients has not been established [187].

A potential but currently unproven approach in pregnancy for intrapartum prophylaxis in patients without an active thrombotic process is ultra-low-dose IV heparin [190]. In a randomized study to prevent postoperative DVT in non-pregnant patients, a dose of 1 IU/kg/h reduced the incidence of DVT from 22% to 4%.

Thrombolytic therapy

Defibrinating agents may be indicated in cases of life-threatening thromboembolism [191–194]. Streptokinase, urokinase, and tissue plasminogen activator activate plasminogen, which sets in motion the body's natural fibrinolytic system. Although helpful in early management of massive PE, thrombolysis plus heparin may not yield improved mortality over heparin alone [191]. Because of the potential risk of bleeding, thrombolytic therapy has not been recommended within 10 days of surgery or parturition [193]. Recommended treatment schedules vary, but all consist of an IV loading dose followed by continuous infusion for 12–72 hours, depending on the clinical situation [192]. Thrombolytic therapy is followed by anticoagulant therapy to prevent recurrence. A review of 172 patients by Turrentine et al. demonstrated that thrombolytic therapy could be used relatively safely during pregnancy in selected clinical situations (Table 21.13) and that these agents were partially or completely successful in 86–90% of recipients [194]. Nonetheless, the authors suggested that traditional therapies should be used first and, if unsuccessful, thrombolytic agents should be reserved for life- or limb-threatening VTE with the understanding of the increased risk of bleeding complications.

Ancrod, derived from Malayan pit viper venom, is contraindicated in pregnancy. Animal studies have shown a high incidence of fetal death. Postpartum hemorrhage from the placental site also occurs at a greater frequency.

Inferior vena cava filter placement

The safe placement of inferior vena cava filters to prevent PE has been reported during pregnancy. Eleven patients with DVT and who were presumed to have an increased risk of PE underwent placement of a temporary inferior vena cava filter between 1998 and 2004. All the filters were placed at the suprarenal inferior vena cava prior to delivery. During filter placement, anticoagulant therapy was continued and then stopped intrapartum. No

Table 21.13 Maternal and perinatal outcome in 172 patients who received thrombolytic therapy during pregnancy.

	n	%
Hemorrhage	14	8
Preterm birth	10	6
Perinatal deaths	10	6
Maternal deaths	2	1

Reproduced by permission from Turrentine MA, Braeems G, Ramirez MM. Use of thrombolytics for the treatment of thromboembolic disease during pregnancy. *Obstet Gynecol* 1995; 50: 534–541.

complications occurred at time of filter placement. No symptomatic PE occurred during or after delivery. Subsequently, all the filters were removed [195]. Placement of a vena cava filter has also been successfully performed during early labor followed by vaginal delivery without incident [196].

Surgical intervention

With pregnancy, surgical intervention may be indicated in some clinical situations, such as replacement of a thrombosed cardiac valve prosthesis, thrombectomy for acute iliofemoral thrombosis, embolectomy of a life-threatening massive PE, vena cava interruption for recurrent venous emboli despite adequate anticoagulation, or when anticoagulation is absolutely contraindicated. Embolectomy is a heroic measure, which may occasionally be life saving. Transvenous catheter embolectomy has been performed successfully for expeditious management of massive PE with cardiovascular collapse [197]. There are a variety of methods for interruption of the vena cava. These include complete ligation, Teflon clips, and devices inserted transvenously, such as the umbrella filter or the Greenfield filter [198].

Special considerations

Antithrombin III deficiency

The first evidence of an inherited AT III defect is frequently a thromboembolic event. Pregnant patients with inherited AT III deficiency often require therapeutic anticoagulation through the pregnancy and the puerperium [188,189,199–204]. In addition to heparin therapy throughout pregnancy [199,201,202,204], IV administration of AT III concentrate may be necessary to minimize the patient's risk of a thromboembolism [188,189]. This can be accomplished with fresh frozen plasma, but AT III concentrate is preferable [199,201,202]. The loading dose of AT III is 50–70 units/kg. This is followed by 20–30 units/kg/day to maintain an AT III level of 80% of normal [200]. The higher the AT III level, the less heparin will be required for therapeutic anticoagulation. If these patients remain untreated during pregnancy, 68% will develop thromboembolism [188,200,203,204]. In patients who require high doses of heparin to achieve anticoagulation, prophylactic biweekly doses of AT III concentrate may be necessary [203]. Many patients require lifelong anticoagulation, which is best achieved by oral anticoagulants when not pregnant and heparin throughout pregnancy.

Protein C or S deficiencies

In contrast to patients with AT III deficiency, patients with protein C or S deficiency carry a lower risk of antepartum thrombosis [35,37,38,204–211]. The incidences of antepartum thrombosis in the untreated patient with protein C and protein S deficiency in one series were 17% and 0% respectively. The postpartum risks, however, were similar [204]. While there is a split of opinion regarding heparin prophylaxis during pregnancy, there is uniform agreement that anticoagulant therapy is warranted in the puerperium [35,37,38,205–211]. For patients with recurrent thromboembolism or a family history of these deficiencies, prenatal screening for AT III, protein C, and protein S appears reasonable.

Antiphospholipid syndrome (APS)

Individuals presenting with clinical signs of thrombosis or embolism which is objectively confirmed should receive heparin, either unfractionated or low molecular weight, according to accepted therapeutic regimens. Since minimal doses of heparin may prolong the aPTT without a therapeutic level being achieved, it is best to follow these patients with anti-factor Xa levels to ensure adequacy of therapy. Patients with APS and a prior thrombosis appear to have a risk of recurrent thrombosis that is substantially higher than the recurrent risk with most other thrombophilias. Retrospective studies have shown that up to 70% of APS patients have recurrent thrombotic events during the 5–6 years following their initial thrombosis [212,213]. Prospective studies have confirmed a high risk of recurrent thrombosis among APS patients [214]. As such, most experts recommend long-term thromboprophylaxis in patients with APS who have experienced a thrombotic event.

References

1 Berg CJ, Atrash HK, Koonin LM, Tucker M. Pregnancy-related mortality in the United States, 1997–1990. *Obstet Gynecol* 1996; 88: 161–167.

2 Chang J, Elam-Evans LD, Berg CJ, et al. Pregnancy-Related Mortality Surveillance – United States 1991–1999. *MMWR* 2003; 52(SSO2): 1 8.

3 Bonnar J. Can more be done in obstetric and gynecologic practice to reduce morbidity and mortality associated with venous thromboemblism? *Am J Obstet Gynecol* 1999; 180(4): 784–791.

4 Toglia MR, Weg JG. Venous thromboembolism during pregnancy. *N Engl J Med* 1996; 335: 108–114.

5 Gherman RB, Goodwin TM, Leung B, Byrne JD, Hethumumi R, Montoro M. Incidence, clinical characteristics, and timing of objectively diagnosed venous thromboembolism during pregnancy. *Obstet Gynecol* 1999; 94: 730–734.

6 Lindqvist P, Dahlback B, Marsal K. Thrombotic risk during pregnancy: a population study. *Obstet Gynecol* 1999; 94: 595–599.

7 Ginsberg JS. Management of venous thromboembolism. *N Engl J Med* 1996; 334: 1816–1828.

8 Rochat RW, Koonin LM, Atrash HK, et al. Maternal mortality in the United States: report from the Maternal Mortality Collaborative. *Obstet Gynecol* 1988; 72: 91–97.

9 Franks AL, Atrash HK, Lawson HW, et al. Obstetrical pulmonary embolism mortality, United States, 1970–85. *Am J Pub Health* 1990; 80: 720–722.

10 Lawson HW, Atrash HK, Franks AL. Fatal pulmonary embolism during legal induced abortion in the United States from 1972 to 1985. *Am J Obstet Gynecol* 1990; 162: 986–990.

11 McLean R, Mattison ET, Cochrane NE. Maternal mortality study annual report 1970–1976. *NY State J Med* 1979; 79: 39–43.
12 Kaunitz AM, Hughes JM, Grimes DA, et al. Causes of maternal mortality in the United States. *Obstet Gynecol* 1985; 65: 605–612.
13 Gabel HD. Maternal mortality in South Carolina from 1970 to 1984: an analysis. *Obstet Gynecol* 1987; 69: 307–311.
14 Sachs BP, Yeh J, Acher D, et al. Cesarean section related maternal mortality in Massachusetts, 1954–1985. *Obstet Gynecol* 1988; 71: 385–388.
15 Barbour LA, Pickard J. Controversies in thromboembolic disease during pregnancy: a critical review. *Obstet Gynecol* 1995; 86: 621–633.
16 Bergqvist A, Bergqvist D, Hallbook T. Acute deep vein thrombosis (DVT) after cesarean section. *Acta Obstet Gynecol Scand* 1983; 62: 473–477.
17 Letsky EA. Coagulation problems during pregnancy. In: Lind T, ed. *Current Review in Obstetrics and Gynecology*. Edinburgh: Churchill Livingstone, 1985.
18 Rutherford SE, Phelan JP. Deep venous thrombosis and pulmonary embolism in pregnancy. *Obstet Gynecol Clin North Am* 1991; 18: 345–370.
19 Rutherford SE, Montoro M, McGehee W, et al. Thromboembolic disease associated with pregnancy: an 11-year review, SPO Abstract 139. *Am J Obstet Gynecol* 1991; 164: 286.
20 Gerhardt A, Scharf RE, Beckmann MW, et al. Prothrombin and factor V mutations in women with a history of thrombosis during pregnancy and the puerperium. *N Engl J Med* 2000; 342: 374–380.
21 Heit JA, Kobbervig CE, James AH, Petterson TM, Bailey KR, Melton LJ. Trends in the incidence of venous thromboembolism during pregnancy or postpartum: a 30-year population-based study. *Ann Intern Med* 2005; 143(10): 697–706.
22 Danilenko-Dixon DR, Heit JA, Silverstein MD, et al. Risk factors for deep vein thrombosis and pulmonary embolism during pregnancy or post partum: a population-based, case control study. *Am J Obstet Gynecol* 2001; 184(2): 104–110.
23 Larsen TB, Johnsen SP, Gislum M, Moller CA, Larsen H, Sorensen HT. ABO blood groups and risk of venous thromboembolism during pregnancy and the puerperium. A population-based, nested case-control study. *J Thromb Haemost* 2005; 3(2): 300–304.
24 Brill-Edwards P, Ginsberg J, Gent M, et al. For the recurrence of clot in this pregnancy study group. *N Engl J Med* 2000; 343: 1439–1444.
25 De Stefano V, Martinelli I, Rossi E, et al. The risk of recurrent venous thromboembolism in pregnancy and puerperium without antithrombotic prophylaxis. *Br J Haematol* 2006; 135(3): 386–391.
26 Stead RB. Regulation of hemostasis. In: Goldhaber SZ, ed. *Pulmonary Embolism and Deep Venous Thrombosis*. Philadelphia: WB Saunders, 1985: 27–40.
27 Needleman P, Minkes M, Raz A. Thromboxanes: selected biosynthesis and distinct biological properties. *Science* 1976; 193: 163–165.
28 Thompson AR, Harker CA. *Manual of Thrombosis and Hemostasis*. Philadelphia: FA Davis, 1983.
29 Files JC, Malpass TW, Yee EK, et al. Studies of human platelet alpha-granule release in vivo. *Blood* 1981; 58: 607–618.
30 Kaplan KL, Owen J. Plasma levels of B-thromboglobulin and platelet factor 4 and indices of platelet activation in vivo. *Blood* 1981; 57: 199–202.
31 Comp PC, Esman CT. Generation of fibrinolytic activity by infusion of activated protein C in dogs. *J Clin Invest* 1981; 68: 1221–1228.
32 Robbins KC. The plasminogen-plasmin enzyme system. In: Colman RW, Hirsh J, Marder VJ, et al., eds. *Hemostasis and Thrombosis*. Philadelphia: JB Lippincott, 1982.
33 Bonnar J, McNichol GP, Douglas AS. Coagulation mechanisms during and after normal childbirth. *BMJ* 1970; 2: 200–203.
34 Brandt JT. Current concepts of coagulation. *Clin Obstet Gynecol* 1985; 28: 3–14.
35 Comp PC, Clouse L. Plasma proteins C and S: the function and assay of two natural anticoagulants. *Lab Management* 1985; 23: 29–32.
36 Megha A, Finzi G, Poli T, et al. Pregnancy, antithrombin III deficiency and venous thrombosis: report of another case. *Acta Heamatol* 1990; 83: 111–114.
37 Broekmans AW, Bertina RM, Reinalda-Poot J, et al. Hereditary protein-S deficiency and venous thromboembolism. *Thromb Haemost* 1985; 53: 273–277.
38 Marciniak E, Wilson HD, Marlar RA. Neonatal purpura fulminans: a genetic disorder related to the absence of protein C in blood. *Blood* 1985; 65: 15–20.
39 Woodhams BJ, Candotti G, Shaw R, et al. Changes in coagulation and fibrinolysis during pregnancy: evidence of activation of coagulation preceding spontaneous abortion. *Thromb Res* 1989; 88: 26–30.
40 Hathaway WE, Bonnar J. *Perinatal Coagulation*. New York: Grune and Stratton, 1978.
41 Bonnar J, McNichol GP, Douglas AS. Fibrinolytic enzyme system and pregnancy. *BMJ* 1969; 3: 387–389.
42 Bonnar J. Venous thromboembolism and pregnancy. *Clin Obstet Gynecol* 1981; 8: 445–473.
43 Atalla RK, Thompson JR, Oppenheimer CA, Bell SC, Taylor DJ. Reactive thrombocytosis after caesarean section and vaginal delivery: implications for maternal thromboembolism and its prevention. *Br J Obstet Gynaecol* 2000; 107(3): 411–414.
44 Grandone E, Margaglione M, Colaizzo D, et al. Genetic susceptibility to pregnancy-related venous thromboembolism: roles of factor V Leiden, prothrombin G20210A, and methylenetetrahydrofolate reductase C677T mutations. *Am J Obstet Gynecol* 1998; 179: 1324–1328.
45 De Stefano V, Leone G, Mastrangelo S, et al. Clinical manifestations and management of inherited thrombophilia: retrospective analysis and follow-up after diagnosis of 238 patients with congenital deficiency of antithrombin III, protein C, protein S. *Thromb Haemost* 1994; 72: 352–358.
46 Middeldorp S, Henkens CM, Koopman MM, et al. The incidence of venous thromboembolism in family members of patients with factor V Leiden mutation and venous thrombosis. *Ann Intern Med* 1998; 128: 15–20.
47 Eldor A. Thrombophilia, thrombosis and pregnancy. *Thromb Haemost* 2001; 86: 104–111.
48 Bertina RM, Koeleman BPC, Koster T, et al. Mutation in blood coagulation factor V associated with resistance to activated protein C. *Nature* 1994; 396: 64–67.
49 Dahlback B. Inherited resistance to activated protein C, a major cause of venous thrombosis, is due to a mutation in the factor V gene. *Haemostasis* 1994; 24: 139–151.
50 Zoller B, Dahlback BD. Linkage between inherited resistance to activated protein c and factor v gene mutation in venous thrombosis. *Lancet* 1994; 343: 1536–1538.

51 Dizon-Townson DS, Nelson LM, Jang H, Varner MW, Ward K. The incidence of the factor V Leiden mutation in an obstetric population and its relationship to deep vein thrombosis. *Am J Obstet Gynecol* 1997; 176: 883–886.

52 Ridker PM, Miletich JP, Hennekens CH, Buring JE. Ethnic distribution of factor V Leiden in 4047 men and women. Implications for venous thromboembolism screening. *JAMA* 1997; 277(16): 1305–1307.

53 Dizon-Townson D, Miller C, Sibai BM, et al. The relationship of factor V Leiden mutation and pregnancy outcomes for mother and fetus. *Obstet Gynecol* 2005; 106: 517–524.

54 Dahlman TC, Hellgren M, Blomback M. Thrombosis prophylaxis in pregnancy with use of subcutaneous heparin adjusted by monitoring heparin concentration in plasma. *Am J Obstet Gynecol* 1989; 161: 420–425.

55 Bates SM, Greer IA, Hirsh J, Ginsberg JS. Use of antithrombotic agents during pregnancy. The Seventh ACCP Conference on antithrombotic and thrombolytic therapy. *Chest* 2004; 126: 627S–644S.

56 Barnes RW, Wu KK, Hoak JC. Fallibility of the clinical diagnosis of venous thrombosis. *JAMA* 1975; 234: 605–608.

57 Bergqvist A, Bergqvist D, Lindhagen A, et al. Late symptoms after pregnancy-related deep vein thrombosis. *Br J Obstet Gynaecol* 1990; 97: 338–344.

58 Hull RD, Hirsh J, Carter CJ, et al. Pulmonary angiography, ventilation lung scanning, and venography for clinically suspected pulmonary embolism with abnormal perfusion lung scan. *Ann Intern Med* 1983; 98: 891–899.

59 Raghavendra BN, Rosen RJ, Lam S, et al. Deep venous thrombosis: detection by high-resolution real-time ultrasonography. *Radiology* 1984; 152: 789–792.

60 Douketis JD, Ginsberg JS. Diagnostic problems with venous thromboembolic disease in pregnancy. *Haemostasis* 1995; 25: 58–71.

61 PIOPED Investigators. Value of the ventilation/perfusion scan in acute pulmonary embolism: results of the prospective investigation of pulmonary embolism diagnosis (PIOPED). *JAMA* 1990; 263: 2753–2759.

62 Gottlieb RH, Widjaja J, Tian L, Rubens DJ, Voci SL. Calf sonography for detecting deep vein thrombosis in symptomatic patients: experience and review of the literature. *J Clin Ultrasound* 1999; 27(8): 415–420.

63 Spritzer CE, Evans AC, Kay HH. Magnetic resonance imaging of deep venous thrombosis in pregnant women with lower extremity edema. *Obstet Gynecol* 1995; 85: 603–607.

64 Bettman MA, Paulin S. Leg phlebography: the incidence, nature and modifications of undesireable side effects. *Radiology* 1977; 122: 101–108.

65 Ginsberg JSA, Hirsh J, Rainbow AJ, et al. Risks to the fetus of radio-logic procedures used in the diagnosis of maternal venous thromboembolic disease. *Thromb Haemost* 1989; 61: 189–196.

66 American College of Obstetricians and Gynecologists. *Education Bulletin Number 233. Teratology.* Washington, DC: American College of Obstetricians and Gynecologists, 1997.

67 American College of Obstetricians and Gynecologists. *Committee Opinion Number 299. Guidelines for Diagnostic Imaging During Pregnancy.* Washington, DC: American College of Obstetricians and Gynecologists, 2004.

68 Markisz JA. Radiologic and nuclear medicine diagnosis. In: Goldhaber SZ, ed. *Pulmonary Embolism and Deep Venous Thrombosis.* Philadelphia: WB Saunders, 1985: 41–72.

69 Moser KM, LeMoine JR. Is embolic risk continued by location of deep venous thrombosis? *Ann Intern Med* 1981; 94: 439–444.

70 Huisman MV, Buller HR, ten Case JW, Vreeken JR. Seriel impedance plethysmography for suspected deep venous thrombosis in outpatients: the Amsterdam General Partitions Study. *N Engl J Med* 1986; 314: 823–882.

71 Kohn H, Konig B, Mostbeck A. Incidence and clinical feature of pulmonary embolism in patients with deep vein thrombosis: a prospective study. *Eur J Nucl Med* 1987; 13: S11–S13.

72 Mohr DN, Ryu JH, Litin SC, Rosenow EC III. Recent advances in the management of venous thromboembolism. *Mayo Clin Proc* 1988; 63: 281–290.

73 Monreal M, Salvador R, Ruiz J. Below-knee deep venous thrombosis and pulmonary embolism (letter). *AJR* 1987; 149: 860.

74 Nicholas GG, Lorenz RP, Botti JJ, et al. The frequent occurrence of false-positive results in phleborrheography during pregnancy. *Surg Gynecol Obstet* 1985; 161: 133–136.

75 Kakkar V. The diagnosis of deep vein thrombosis using the 125I fibrinogen test. *Arch Surg* 1972; 104: 152–159.

76 Bentley PG, Kakkar VV. Radionuclide venography for the demonstrations of the proximal deep venous system. *Br J Surg* 1979; 66: 687–690.

77 Wells PS, Anderson DR, Roger M, et al. Evaluation of D-dimer in the diagnosis of suspected deep vein thrombosis. *N Engl J Med* 349(13): 1227–1235.

78 Bockenstedt P. D-Dimer in venous thromboembolism. *N Engl J Med* 349; 13: 1203–1204.

79 Epiney M, Boehlen F, Boulvain M, et al. D-dimer levels during delivery and the postpartum. *J Thromb Haemost* 2005; 3(2): 268–271.

80 Kline JA, Williams GW, Hernandez-Nino J. D-dimer concentrations in normal pregnancy: new diagnostic thresholds are needed. *Clin Chem* 2005; 51(5): 825–829.

81 Hron G, Kollars M, Binder BR, Eichinger S, Kyrle PA. Identification of patients at low risk for recurrent venous thromboembolism by measuring thrombin generation. *JAMA* 2006; 296: 397–402.

82 Rosenow EC III, Osmundson PJ, Brown ML. Pulmonary embolism. *Mayo Clin Proc* 1981; 56: 161–178.

83 Leclerc JR. Pulmonary embolism. In: Rakel RE, ed. *Conn's Current Therapy – 1994.* Philadelphia: WB Saunders, 1994: 199–205.

84 Bell WR, Simon TL, DeMets DL. The clinical features of submassive pulmonary emboli. *Am J Med* 1977; 62: 355–360.

85 Dorfman GS, Cronan JJ, Tupper TB, et al. Occult pulmonary embolism: a common occurrence in deep venous thrombosis. *AJR* 1987; 148: 263–267.

86 Schiff MJ, Feinberg AW, Naidich JB. Noninvasive venous examinations as a screening test for pulmonary embolism. *Arch Intern Med* 1987; 147: 505–507.

87 Robin ED. Overdiagnosis and overtreatment of pulmonary embolism: the emperor may have no clothes. *Ann Intern Med* 1977; 87: 775–776.

88 Moses DC, Silver TM, Bookstein JJ. The complementary roles of chest radiography, lung scanning and selective pulmonary angiography in the diagnosis of pulmonary embolism. *Circulation* 1974; 44: 179–185.

89 McFarlane MJ, Imperiale TF. Use of the alveolar-arterial oxygen gradient in the diagnosis of pulmonary embolism. *Am J Med* 1994; 96: 57–62.

90 Powrie R, Star JA, Rosene-Montella K. Deep venous thrombosis and pulmonary embolism in pregnancy. *Med Health RI* 1998; 81(4): 141–143.

91 Gold WM, McCormack KR. Pulmonary function response to radiosotope scanning of the lungs. *JAMA* 1966; 197: 146–148.

92 Vincent WR, Goldberg SJ, Desilets D. Fatality immediately following rapid infusion of macroaggregates of 99mTc albumin (MAA) for lung scan. *Radiology* 1968; 91: 1181–1184.

93 Mills SR, Jackson DC, Older RA, et al. The incidence, etiologies, and avoidance of complications of pulmonary angiography in a large series. *Radiology* 1980; 136: 295–299.

94 Kipper MS, Moser KM, Kortman KE, et al. Long-term follow-up of patients with suspected pulmonary embolism and a normal lung scan. Perfusion scans in embolic subjects. *Chest* 1982; 82: 411–415.

95 Urokinase Pulmonary Embolism Trial. A national cooperative study. *Circulation* 1973; 43(suppl II): 47.

96 Henkin RE. Radionuclide detection of thromboembolic disease. In: Kwaan HC, Bowie EJQ, eds. *Thrombosis*. Philadelphia: WB Saunders, 1982: 236–252.

97 Alderson PO. Scintigraphic evaluation of pulmonary embolism. *Eur J Nucl Med* 1987; 13: S6–S10.

98 National Council on Radiation Protection and Measurements. *Medical Radiation Exposure of Pregnant and Potentially Pregnant Women*. Bethesda, MD: National Council on Radiation Protection and Measurements, 1977.

99 Nichols AB, Beller BA, Cochari S, et al. Detection of pulmonary embolism by positron imaging of inhaled 15O-labeled carbon dioxide. *Semin Nucl Med* 1980; 10: 252–258.

100 Cross JJ, Kemp PM, Walsh CG, Flower CD, Dixon AK. A randomized trial of spiral CT and ventilation perfusion scintigraphy for the diagnosis of pulmonary embolism. *Clin Radiol* 1998; 53: 177–182.

101 Lipchik RJ, Goodman LR. Spiral computed tomography in the evalution of pulmonary embolism. *Clin Chest Med* 1999; 20: 731–738.

102 Kim KL, Muller NL, Mayo JR. Clinically suspected pulmonary embolism: utility of spiral CT. *Radiology* 1999; 210: 693–697.

103 Traeger SM. Failure to wedge pulmonary hypertension during pulmonary artery catheterization: a sign of totally occlusive pulmonary embolism. *Crit Care Med* 1985; 13: 544–547.

104 Fairfax WR, Thomas F, Orme JF. Pulmonary artery catheter occlusion as an indication of pulmonary embolism. *Chest* 1984; 86: 270–272.

105 Lewis JF, Anderson TW, Fennel WH, et al. A clue to pulmonary embolism obtained during Swan-Ganz catheterization. *Chest* 1982; 81: 257–529.

106 Dalen JE, Banas JS, Brooks HC, et al. Resolution rate of acute pulmonary embolism in man. *N Engl J Med* 1969; 280: 1194–1199.

107 Dalen JE, Brooks HL, Johnson LW, et al. Pulmonary angiography in acute pulmonary embolism: indications, techniques, and results in 367 patients. *Am Heart J* 1971; 81: 175–185.

108 Ezekowitz MD, Pope CF, Smith EO. Indium-111 platelet imaging. In: Goldhaber SE, ed. *Pulmonary Embolism and Deep Vein Thrombosis*. Philadelphia: WB Saunders, 1985: 261–267.

109 Hirsch J. Heparin. *N Engl J Med* 1991; 324: 1565.

110 Bratt G, Tornebohm E, Lockner D, et al. A human pharmacological study comparing conventional heparin and a low molecular weight heparin fragment. *Thromb Haemost* 1985; 53: 208–211.

111 Samama M. [The new heparins.] *Presse Med* 1986; 15: 1631–1635.

112 Gillis S, Shushan A, Eldor A. Use of low molecular weight heparin for prophylaxis and treatment of thromboembolism in pregnancy. *Int J Gynecol Obstet* 1992; 39: 297–301.

113 Fejgin MD, Lourwood DL. Low molecular weight heparins and their use in the obstetrics and gynecology. *Obstet Gynecol Surv* 1994; 49: 424–431.

114 Rasmussen C, Wadt J, Jacobsen B. Thromboembolic prophylaxis with low molecular weight heparin during pregnancy. *Int J Obstet Gynecol* 1994; 47: 121–125.

115 Sturridge F, Letsky E. The use of low molecular weight heparin for thrombophylaxis in pregnancy. *Br J Obstet Gynaecol* 1994; 101: 69–71.

116 Ginsberg JS, Hirsh J. Use of antithrombotic agents during pregnancy. *Chest* 1995; 108: 3055–3115.

117 Lensing AW, Prins MH, Davidson BE, et al. Treatment of deep-venous thrombosis with low molecular weight heparins: a meta-ananlysis. *Arch Intern Med* 1995; 155: 601–607.

118 Koopman MMW, Prandoni P, Piovella F. Treatment of venous thrombosis with intravenous unfractionated heparin administered in the hospital as compared with subcutaneous low-molecular weight heparin administered at home. *N Engl J Med* 1996; 334: 682–687.

119 Levine M, Gent M, Hirsh J, et al. A comparison of low-molecular weight heparin administered primarily at home with unfractionated heparin administered in the hospital for proximal deep-vein thrombosis. *N Engl J Med* 1996; 334: 677–681.

120 White TM, Bernene JL, Marino AM. Continuous heparin infusion requirements: diagnostic and therapeutic implications. *JAMA* 1979; 241: 2717–2720.

121 DeSwart CAM, Nijmeter B, Roelofs JMM, et al. Kinetics of intravenously administered heparin in normal humans. *Blood* 1982; 60: 1251–1258.

122 Perry PJ, Herron GR, King JC. Heparin half-life in normal and impaired renal function. *Clin Pharmacol Res* 1974; 16: 514–519.

123 Basu D, Gallus A, Hirsh J, et al. A prospective study of the value of monitoring heparin treatment with the activated partial thromboplastin time. *N Engl J Med* 1972; 287: 324–327.

124 Hyers TM, Hull RD, Weg JG. Antithrombotic therapy for venous thromboembolic disease. *Chest* 1986; 89: 265–355.

125 Holm HA, Abildgaard U, Kalvenes S. Heparin assays and bleeding complications in treatment of deep venous thrombosis with particular reference to retroperitoneal bleeding. *Thromb Haemost* 1985; 53: 278–281.

126 Lepercq J, Conard J, Borel-Derlon A, et al. Venous thromboembolism during pregnancy: a retrospective study of enoxaparin safety in 624 pregnancies. *Br J Obstet Gynaecol* 2001; 108(11): 1134–1140.

127 Kearon C, Ginsberg J, Julian JA. Comparison of fixed-dose weight-adjuested unfractionated heparin and low-molecular-weight heparin for acute treatment of venous thromboembolism. *JAMA* 2006; 296: 935–942.

128 Clagett GP, Anderson FA, Heit J, et al. Prevention of venous thromboembolism. *Chest* 1995; 108(suppl 4): S312–334.

129 Bergqvist D, Benoni G, Bjorgell O, et al. Low molecular-weight heparin (enoxaparin) as prophylaxis against venous thromboembolism after total hip replacement. *N Engl J Med* 1996; 335: 696–700.

130 Geerts WH, Jay RM, Code K, et al. A comparison of low-dose heparin with low-molecular-weight heparin as prophylaxis against

venous thromboembolism after major trauma. *N Engl J Med* 1996; 355: 701–707.

131 Hall JG, Pauli RM, Wilson KM. Maternal and fetal sequelae of anticoagulation during pregnancy. *Am J Med* 1980; 68(1): 122–140.

132 Walker AM, Jick H. Predictors of bleeding during heparin therapy. *JAMA* 1980; 244: 1209–1212.

133 Lee RH, Goodwin TM. Massive subchorionic hematoma associated with enoxaparin. *Obstet Gynecol* 2006 ep; 108(3 Pt 2): 787–789.

134 Chong BH, Pitney WR, Castaldi PA. Heparin-induced thrombocytopenia: association of thrombotic complications with heparin-dependent IgG antibody that induces thromboxane synthesis and platelet aggregation. *Lancet* 1982; 2: 1246–1249.

135 Fausett MB, Vogtlander M, Lee RM, et al. Heparin-induced thrombocytopenia is rare in pregnancy. *Am J Obstet Gynecol* 2001; 185(1): 148–152.

136 Magnani HN. Heparin induced thrombocytopenia (HIT): an overview of 230 patients treated with orgaran (Org 10172). *Thromb Haemost* 1993; 70: 554–561.

137 Galle PC, Muss HB, McGrath KM, et al. Thrombocytopenia in two patients treated with low-dose heparin. *Obstet Gynecol* 1978; 52(suppl): 95–115.

138 Phillips YY, Copley JB, Stor RA. Thrombocytopenia and low dose heparin. *South Med J* 1983; 76: 526–528.

139 Hirsch J, Daeln JE, Deykin D, Poller L. Heparin: mechanisms of action, dosing considerations, monitoring, efficacy, and safety. *Chest* 1992; 102: 337–350.

140 Rao AK, White GC, Sherman L, et al. Low incidence of thrombocytopenia with porcine mucosal heparin. A prospective multicenter study. *Arch Intern Med* 1989; 149: 1285–1288.

141 Harenberg J. Letter to the Editors-in-Chief. Treatment of a woman with lupus and thromboembolism and cutaneous intolerance to heparins using fondaparinux during pregnancy. *Thromb Res* 2007; 119: 385–388.

142 Mazzolai L, Hohlfeld P, Spertini f, Hayoz D, Schapira M, Duchosal MA. Fondaparinux is a safe alternative in case of heparin intolerance during pregnancy. *Blood* 2006; 108(5): 1569–1570.

143 Griffith GC. Heparin osteoporosis. *JAMA* 1965; 143: 85–88.

144 De Swiet M, Ward PD, Fidler J, et al. Prolonged heparin therapy in pregnancy causes bone demineralization. *Br J Obstet Gynaecol* 1983; 90: 1129–1134.

145 Zimran A, Shilo S, Fisher D, et al. Histomorphometric evaluation of reversible heparin-induced osteoporosis in pregnancy. *Arch Intern Med* 1986; 146: 386–388.

146 Dahlman T, Lindvall N, Hellgren M. Osteopenia in pregnancy during long-term heparin treatment: a radiologic study postpartum. *Br J Obstet Gynaecol* 1990; 97: 221–224.

147 Dahlman TC. Osteoporotic fractures and the recurrence of thromboembolism during pregnancy and the puerperium in 184 women undergoing thromboprophylaxis with heparin. *Am J Obstet Gynecol* 1993; 168: 1265–1270.

148 Dahlman TC, Sjoberg HE, Ringertz H. Bone mineral density during long-term prophylaxis with heparin in pregnancy. *Am J Obstet Gynecol* 1994; 170: 1315–1320.

149 American Society of Regional Anesthesia. *Recommendations for Neuraxial Anesthesia and Anticoagulation*. Park Ridge, IL: American Society of Regional Anesthesia, 1998.

150 Horlocker TT, Wedel DJ, Benzon H, et al. Regional anesthesia in the anticoagulated patient: defining risk (the second ASRA consensus conference on neuraxial anesthesia and anticoagulation). *Reg Anesth Pain Med* 2003; 28(3): 172–197.

151 Ginsberg JS, Kowalchuck G, Brill-Edwards P, et al. Heparin therapy in pregnancy: effects on the fetus. *Clin Res* 1988; 36: A410.

152 Ginsberg JS, Hirsh J, Tuner C, et al. Risks to the fetus of anticoagulant therapy during pregnancy. *Thromb Haemost* 1989; 61: 197–203.

153 Ginsberg JS, Hirsh J. Use of antithrombotic agents during pregnancy. *Chest* 1992; 315: 1109–1114.

154 Colvin BT, Machin SJ, Barrowcliffe TW, et al. Audit of oral anticoagulant treatment. The BCHS British Haemostasis and Thrombosis Task Force of the British Society for Haematology. *J Clin Pathol* 1993; 46(12): 1069–1070.

155 Stevenson RE, Burton OM, Ferlauto GJ, Taylor HA. Hazards of oral anticoagulants during pregnancy. *JAMA* 1980; 243: 1549–1551.

156 Chang MKB, Harvey D, de Swiet M. Follow-up study of children whose mothers were treated with warfarin during pregnancy. *Br J Obstet Gynaecol* 1984; 91: 70–73.

157 Hull R, Delmore T, Carter C, et al. Adjusted subcutaneous heparin versus warfarin sodium in the long-term treatment of venous thrombosis. *N Engl J Med* 1982; 306: 189–194.

158 Standing Advisory Committee for Haematology of the Royal College of Pathologists. Drug interaction with coumarin derivative anticoagulants. *BMJ* 1982; 185: 274–275.

159 Horn JR, Danzinger LH, Davis RJ. Warfarin-induced skin necrosis: report of four cases. *Am J Hosp Pharm* 1981; 38: 1763–1768.

160 Lebsack CS, Weibert RT. "Purple toes" syndrome. *Postgrad Med* 1982; 71: 81–84.

161 Park S, Schroeter AL, Park YS, Fortson J. Purple toes and livido reticularis in a patient with cardiovascular disease taking coumadin. *Arch Dermatol* 1993; 129: 775–780.

162 Hirsch J. The treatment of venous thromboembolism. *Nouv Rev Fr Hematol* 1988; 30: 149–153.

163 Gallus A, Jackaman J, Tillet J, et al. Safety and efficacy of warfarin started early after submassive venous thrombosis or pulmonary embolism. *Lancet* 1986; 2: 1293 1296.

164 Turpis AG, Eriksson BI, Lassen MR, Bauer KA. Fondaparinux, the first selective factor Xa inhibitor. *Curr Opin Haematol* 2003; 10(5): 327–332.

165 American College of Obstetricians and Gynecologists. *Education Bulletin Number 19. Thromboembolism in Pregnancy*. Washington, DC: American College of Obstetricians and Gynecologists, 2000.

166 Moser KM, Fedullo PE. Venous thromboembolism: threes simple decisions (part 2). *Chest* 1983; 83: 256–260.

167 Ellison MJ, Sawyer WT, Mills TC. Calculation of heparin dosage in a morbidly obese woman. *Clin Pharm* 1989; 8: 65–68.

168 Tenero DM, Bell HE, Deitz PA, Bertino JS Jr. Comparative dosage and toxicity of heparin sodium in the treatment of patients with pulmonary embolism versus deep-vein thrombosis. *Clin Pharm* 1989; 8: 40–43.

169 Anderson G, Fagrell B, Holmgren K, et al. Subcutaneous administration of heparin: a randomized comparison with intravenous administration of heparin to patients with deep-vein thrombosis. *Thromb Res* 1982; 27: 631–639.

170 Schulman S, Rhedin A, Lindmarker P, et al. A comparison of six weeks with six months of oral anticoagulant therapy after a first episode of venous thromboembolism. *N Engl J Med* 1995; 332: 1661–1665.

171 Hirsch J. The optimal duration of anticoagulant therapy for venous thrombosis. *N Engl J Med* 1995; 332: 1710–1711.
172 Barbour LA, Smith JM, Marar RA. Heparin levels to guide thromboembolism prophylaxis during pregnancy. *Am J Obstet Gynecol* 1995; 173: 1869–1873.
173 Nelson DM, Stempel LE, Fabri PJ, et al. Hickman catheter use in a pregnant patient requiring therapeutic heparin antiocoagulation. *Am J Obstet Gynecol* 1984; 149: 461–462.
174 Barss VA, Schwartz PA, Greene MF, et al. Use of the subcutaneous heparin pump during pregnancy. *J Reprod Med* 1985; 30: 899–901.
175 Daniel DG, Campbell H, Turnbull AC. Puerperal thromboembolism and suppression of lactation. *Lancet* 1967; 2: 287–289.
176 Jeffcoate TNA, Miller J, Roos RF, Tindall VR. Puerperal thromboembolism in relation to the inhibition of lactation by oestrogen therapy. *BMJ* 1968; 4: 19–22.
177 Howell R, Fidler J, Letsky E, de Swiet M. The risks of antenatal subcutaneous heparin prophylaxis: a controlled trial. *Br J Obstet Gynaecol* 1983; 90: 1124–1128.
178 Quinones JN, James DN, Stamilio DM, Cleary KL, Macones GA. Thromboprophylaxis after cesarean delivery: a decision analysis. *Obstet Gynecol* 2005; 106(4): 733–740.
179 Casele H, Grobman WA. Cost-effectiveness of thromboprophylaxis with intermittent pneumatic compression at cesarean delivery. *Obstet Gynecol* 2006; 108(3 Pt 1): 535–540.
180 Collins R, Scrimgeour A, Peto R. Reduction in fatal pulmonary embolism and venous thrombosis by perioperative administration of subcutaneous heparin. *N Engl J Med* 1988; 318: 1162–1173.
181 Kakkar VV, Stamatatkis JD, Bentley PG, et al. Prophylaxis for postoperative deep-vein thrombosis: synergistic effect of heparin and dihydroergotamine. *JAMA* 1979; 241: 39–42.
182 Salzman EW, Hirsh J. Prevention of venous thromboembolism. In: Colman RW, Hirsh J, Marder VJ, Slazman EW, eds. *Hemostasis and Thrombosis: Basic Principles and Clinical Practice*, 2nd edn. Philadelphia: JB Lippincott, 1987: 1252–1264.
183 Stringer MD, Kakkar VV. Prevention of venous thromboembolism. *Herz* 1989; 14: 135–147.
184 Clark-Peterson DL, Synan IS, Dodge R, et al. A randomized trial of low-dose heparin and intermittent pneumatic calf compression for the prevention of deep venous thrombosis after gynecologic oncology surgery. *Am J Obstet Gynecol* 1993; 168: 1146–1154.
185 European Fraxiparin Study (EFS) Group. Comparison of a low molecular weight heparin and unfractionated heparin for the prevention of deep vein thrombosis in patients undergoing abdominal surgery. *Br J Surg* 1988; 75: 1058–1063.
186 Hirsch J, Barrowcliffe TW. Standardization and clinical use of LMW heparin. *Thromb Haemost* 1988; 59: 333–337.
187 Salazar E, Zajarias A, Gutierrez N, et al. The problem of cardiac valve prostheses, anticoagulants, and pregnancy. *Circulation* 1984; 70(suppl I): 169–177.
188 Nelson DM, Stempel LE, Brandt JT. Hereditary antithrombin III deficiency and pregnancy: report of two cases and review of the literature. *Obstet Gynecol* 1985; 65: 848–853.
189 De Stefano V, Leone G, DeCarolis S, et al. Management of pregnancy in women with antithrombin III congenital defect: report of four cases. *Thromb Haemost* 1988; 59: 193–196.
190 Negus D, Friedgood A, Cox SJ, et al. Ultra-low dose intravenous heparin in the prevention of postoperative deep-vein thrombosis. *Lancet* 1980; 1: 891–894.
191 Urokinase-Streptokinase Pulmonary Embolism Trial. Phase 2 results. A cooperative study. *JAMA* 1974; 229: 1606–1613.
192 Sharma GVRK, Cella, G, Parisi AF, et al. Thrombolytic therapy. *N Engl J Med* 1985; 306: 1268–1276.
193 Moran KT, Jewell ER, Persson AV. The role of thrombolytic therapy in surgical practice. *Br J Surg* 1989; 76: 298–304.
194 Turrentine MA, Braems G, Ramirez MM. Use of thrombolytics for the treatment of thromboembolic disease during pregnancy. *Obstet Gynecol Surv* 1995; 50: 534–541.
195 Kawamata K, Chiba Y, Tanaka R, Higashi M, Nishigami K. Experience of temporary inferior vena cava filters inserted in the perinatal period to prevent pulmonary embolism in pregnant women with deep vein thrombosis. *J Vasc Surg* 2005; 41(4): 652–656.
196 Clark SL, Blatter DD, Jackson GM. Placement of a temporary vena cava filter during labor. *Am J Obstet Gynecol* 2005; 193(5): 1746–1747.
197 Kramer FL, Teitelbaum G, Merli GJ. Panvenography and pulmonary angiography in the diagnosis of deep venous thrombosis and pulmonary thromboembolism. *Radiol Clin North Am* 1986; 24: 397–418.
198 Hux CH, Wagner R, Rattan P, et al. Surgical treatment of thromboembolic disease in pregnancy. Proceedings of the Society of Perinatal Obstetricians, January 30–February 1, 1986: 62.
199 Brandt P. Observations during the treatment of antithrombin III deficient women with heparin and antithrombin concentrate during pregnancy, parturition, and abortion. *Thromb Res* 1981; 22: 15–24.
200 Hellgren M, Tengborn L, Abildgaard U. Pregnancy in women with congenital antithrombin III deficiency: experience of treatment with heparin and antithrombin. *Obstet Gynecol Invest* 1982; 14: 127–130.
201 Samson D, Stirling Y, Woolf L, et al. Management of planned pregnancy in a patient with congenital antithrombin III deficiency. *Br J Haematol* 1984; 56: 243–249.
202 Leclerc JR, Geerts W, Panju A, et al. Management of antithrombin III deficiency during pregnancy without administration of antithrombin III. *Thromb Res* 1986; 41: 567–573.
203 Schwartz RS, Bauer KA, Rosenberg RD, et al. Clinical experience with antithrombin III concentrate in treatment of congenital and acquired deficiency of antithrombin. *Am J Med* 1989; 87(suppl 3B): 535–605.
204 Conrad J, Horellou MH, van Dredan P, et al. Thrombosis and pregnancy in congenital deficiencies in antithrombin III, protein C or protein S: study of 78 women. *Thromb Haemost* 1990; 63: 319–320.
205 Rose PG, de Moerloose PA, Bounameaux H. Protein S deficiency in pregnancy. *Am J Obstet Gynecol* 1986; 155: 140–141.
206 Malm J, Laurell M, Dahlbeck B. Changes in the plasma levels of vitamin K dependent protein C and S and of C4b-binding protein during pregnancy and oral contraception. *Br J Haematol* 1988; 68: 437–443.
207 Lao TT, Yuen PMP, Yin JA. Protein S and protein C levels in Chinese women during pregnancy, delivery, and puerperium. *Br J Obstet Gynaecol* 1989; 96: 167–170.
208 Lao TT, Yin JA, Ng WK, Yuen PMP. Relationship between maternal antithrombin III and protein C/protein S levels before, during, and after delivery. *Gynecol Obstet Invest* 1990; 30: 87–90.
209 Tharakan T, Baxi LV, Dinguid D. Protein S deficiency in pregnancy. A case report. *Am J Obstet Gynecol* 1993; 168: 141–142.

210 Faught W, Garner P, Jones G, Ivey B. Changes in protein C and protein S levels in normal pregnancy. *Am J Obstet Gynecol* 1995; 172: 147–150.

211 Goodwin TM, Gazit G, Gordon EM. Heterozygous protein C deficiency presenting as severe protein C deficiency and peripartum thrombosis: successful treatment with protein C concentrate. *Obstet Gynecol* 1995; 86: 662–664.

212 Rosove MH, Brewer PM. Antiphospholipid thrombosis: clinical course after the first thrombotic event in 70 patients. *Ann Intern Med* 1992; 117: 303–308.

213 Khamastha MA, Cuadrado MJ, Mujic F, et al. The management of thrombosis in antiphospholipid antibody syndrome. *N Engl J Med* 1995; 332: 993–997.

214 Schulman S, Svenungsson E, Granqvist S. Duration of Anticoagulation Study Group. Anticardiolipin antibodies predict early recurrence of thromboembolism and death among patients with venous thromboembolism following anticoagulant therapy. *Am J Med* 1998; 104: 332–338.

22 Etiology and Management of Hemorrhage

Irene Stafford[1], Michael A. Belfort[2] & Gary A. Dildy III[3]

[1]Maternal-Fetal Medicine, University of Texas Southwestern Medical Center, Dallas, TX, USA

[2]Department of Obstetrics and Gynecology, Division of Maternal-Fetal Medicine, University of Utah School of Medicine, Salt Lake City, UT *and* HCA Healthcare, Nashville, TN, USA

[3]Maternal-Fetal Medicine, Mountain Star Division, Hospital Corporation of America, Salt Lake City, UT *and* Department of Obstetrics and Gynecology, LSU Health Sciences Center, School of Medicine in New Orleans, New Orleans, LA, USA

In patients with major obstetric hemorrhage, three measures must be promptly taken: identify the cause, arrest the bleeding and management of hypovolemia, anemia and coagulopathy. Continued hemorrhage, particularly if concealed or underestimated, may result in the onset of irreversible shock. Although the percentage of death caused by hemorrhage decreased by approximately one-third between 1979–1986 and 1991–1997, it continues to be a leading cause of pregnancy-related mortality [1–3]. An estimated 140,000 women worldwide die every year from postpartum hemorrhage, with over 50% of these occurring within the first 24 hours after delivery [4]. Postpartum hemorrhage remains among the top three causes of maternal deaths in the United States, with life-threatening hemorrhage occurring in 1 in 1000 deliveries [5]. The major obstetric causes for antepartum hemorrhage are placental abruption and placenta previa, while postpartum hemorrhage is most commonly caused by uterine atony, retained placenta, and genital tract lacerations. Other less common but sometimes more serious causes include uterine rupture, uterine inversion and abnormal placental invasion (placenta accreta, increta, and percreta). Management of these conditions along with management of hemorrhage related to inherited or acquired bleeding disorders will be discussed in this chapter. Conditions caused by pregnancy (HELLP syndrome, acute fatty liver of pregnancy, amniotic fluid embolism) and disseminated intravascular coagulation are discussed in other chapters.

Massive hemorrhage may also result from surgical causes in pregnant or postpartum women. These include liver rupture in HELLP syndrome, and rupture of aortic, splenic, and renal artery aneurysms. Although rare, these should be considered in patients with hemorrhagic shock and concealed bleeding in whom an obstetric cause such as abruption, pelvic hematoma or uterine rupture is unlikely.

Critical Care Obstetrics, 5th edition. Edited by M. Belfort, G. Saade, M. Foley, J. Phelan and G. Dildy.

Placental abruption

Placental abruption is defined as the premature separation of a normally situated placenta, and may be partial or complete. The underlying mechanism is unknown, but most explanations center around vascular or placental abnormalities, including increased fragility of vessels, vascular malformations or abnormal placentation [6,7]. Often, in the acute setting, the etiology of abruption may be clear. For example, shearing forces are most likely responsible for abruption resulting from trauma. There is strong evidence linking abruption to abnormal first-trimester changes, suggesting that abruption may be chronic in nature. Abnormal serum analytes and placental biology studies support this notion [8].

Hemorrhage occurs into the decidua basalis, forming a hematoma which splits the decidua [9]. As the hematoma expands, further placental separation ensues. Large *Epidemiol*ogic studies report an incidence ranging from 5.9 to 6.5 per 1000 singleton births and 12.2 per 1000 twin births [10]. Discrepancies in rates of abruption are reported, mainly because abruption can also be discovered upon histologic examination of the placenta in otherwise normal pregnancies. Pre-eclampsia is the most common risk factor and is found in approximately 50% of women with placental abruption [11]. Other risk factors include preterm premature rupture of membranes, polyhydramnios, advanced maternal age, cocaine use, smoking, multiparity, chorioamnionitis, blunt trauma and possibly thrombophilias. Black women are more at risk than other population groups [12,13]. Bleeding in the first trimester has been linked with increased rates of abruption later in pregnancy [14,15] and there is approximately a 10% recurrence rate during a subsequent pregnancy. Placental abruption is associated with multiple adverse perinatal outcomes including a ninefold increased risk of intrauterine fetal demise, a threefold rise in preterm birth and a twofold increase in growth restriction. The risk of stillbirth has been found to correlate with the extent of placental separation, with higher rates of death associated with

>50% separation [16]. Infants born after abruption have increased rates of cystic periventricular leukomalacia and intraventricular hemorrhage compared to age-matched controls, most likely a result of oxygen and nutrient deprivation prior to delivery [17].

The classic signs and symptoms of placental abruption include vaginal bleeding accompanied by uterine tenderness, painful tetanic contractions and non-reassuring fetal heart rate patterns. However, not all signs may be present simultaneously. Vaginal bleeding may be concealed, leading to delays in seeking medical help by the woman as well as in diagnosis by the physician. Abruption can even present as simple unexplained preterm labor.

Sonographic evaluation of the placenta will fail to reveal over 50% of abruptions. The appearance of hemorrhage changes over the course of acute hemorrhage to stable hematoma, making the diagnosis more challenging [18]. In cases where bleeding is visualized sonographically, the likelihood of abruption is very high. A thickened placenta (>5 cm) may also suggest the presence of abruption. Retroplacental hemorrhage confers a worse prognosis for the fetus [18]. The Kleihaur–Betke (KB) test has not been proven to be clinically useful in the evaluation of abruption. In one study where over 25 placentas with histologic evidence of abruption were analyzed, there were no positive maternal KB tests. In the same study, there was a 9% false-positive rate [19]. The clinical utility of the KB test is mainly to help formulate the appropriate dosage of Rh immune globulin for the Rh-negative woman.

In a major abruption blood extravasates into the myometrium and the uterus becomes "woody hard" with fetal parts no longer palpable – the Couvelaire uterus. Hemorrhagic shock and coagulopathy may be present. Blood loss may be over 50% of maternal blood volume with abruption severe enough to kill the fetus [20]. Coagulation defects appear to develop rapidly after the occurrence of a severe abruption, within a few hours or even in minutes [11]. Upon presentation, evaluation of hematologic parameters including coagulation studies should be completed after immediate intravenous access has been obtained and resuscitation has begun. The blood bank should be informed about the need for blood and blood products, keeping several units ahead. If available, whole blood is preferred in these cases secondary to the additional benefit of volume expansion. A Foley catheter should be placed for hourly urine output measurement. Particular attention should be given to vital sign determination and coagulation studies should be performed regularly.

Anesthesia should be involved early with patient care. Coordinated efforts involving blood and product replacement in the operating room in the event of a cesarean or vaginal delivery will maximize resuscitative efforts in these as well as other cases involving hemorrhage.

Invasive monitoring may be necessary. Women with preeclampsia complicated by placental abruption need particular care in resuscitation. These patients tolerate hypovolemia poorly because of the contracted intravascular volume and low cardiac output, and are also highly susceptible to pulmonary edema due to volume overload [21]. Coagulopathy is uncommon with a surviving fetus; prompt delivery prevents further decompensation of both mother and fetus [11]. If the fetus is alive and of a viable gestational age at presentation, urgent delivery by cesarean section is indicated unless vaginal delivery is imminent. If severe fetal distress is suspected prior to cesarean, presence of fetal heart activity should be verified before anesthesia is commenced.

Major abruption sufficient to cause fetal death is life threatening for the mother. Blood loss is frequently 50% or more of blood volume [20]; up to 5 L of blood may extravasate into the myometrium, with little or no revealed bleeding [22]. Thromboplastin release is a powerful trigger for disseminated intravascular coagulation and is strongly uterotonic. In a series of 141 cases of abruption severe enough to kill the fetus, plasma fibrinogen concentration was below 150 mg/dL in 38%, and below 100 mg/dL in 28%, and in all cases developed within 8 hours of the onset of symptoms [20]. Delivery must be expedited, with vaginal delivery the preferred route unless contraindications exist. Cesarean delivery in patients with coagulopathy leads to difficulty in achieving surgical hemostasis, but is indicated in the presence of fetal jeopardy, prior classic cesarean delivery, fetal malpresentation or if the patient is remote from delivery with worsening coagulopathy. While the fetus is undelivered, correction of hypovolemia, blood loss, and coagulopathy must continue. In the presence of fetal demise, all efforts should be made for a successful vaginal delivery unless a contraindication exists or the mother becomes increasingly unstable. In the preterm infant, delivery can be postponed in the absence of profound hemorrhage or coagulopathic abnormalities and steroids for fetal lung maturity can be administered as long as maternal and fetal well-being are assured. This may require close follow-up or a prolonged hospital admission. The use of tocolytics is controversial, with data suggesting a prolongation of pregnancy with the use of magnesium sulfate [23]. The β-sympathomimetics cause tachycardia, masking the clinical signs of hemorrhage, and should not be used. Thus tocolysis should be used with caution in select, stable patients with no evidence of acute hemorrhage [23]. The major determinant of maternal outcome is adequate replacement of fluid and blood, rather than time to delivery [11].

Postpartum hemorrhage must be anticipated following a severe placental abruption, and prophylactic uterotonic drugs should be considered. Uterine atony may occur since myometrial contractility is impaired by fibrin degradation products [22]. Persistent uterine atony despite the administration of uterotonics may require hysterectomy. Maternal deaths from abruption are frequently post partum, when ongoing blood loss occurs in patients with inadequate correction of hemorrhagic shock and coagulopathy prior to delivery. Acute renal tubular and cortical necrosis may result from the products of the coagulation cascade in addition to renal ischemia due to hypovolemia.

Uterine rupture

Uterine rupture may occur in an unscarred uterus, at the site of a previous uterine scar from a cesarean section or a full-thickness incision secondary to gynecologic surgery. The overall rate varies from 2 to 8 per 10,000 deliveries [24]. Asymptomatic and bloodless dehiscence of a previous cesarean section scar may occur during subsequent vaginal delivery, and may also be seen at repeat cesarean section in women who have not labored. Uterine rupture is generally considered to include only cases with complete separation of the wall of the pregnant uterus, with or without expulsion of the fetus, that may endanger the life of the mother and/or fetus [25].

Rupture may occur antenatally or intrapartum; however, it is commonly first suspected post partum. The most common clinical sign in labor is the sudden onset of fetal distress, reported in 81% of cases [24]. The most common fetal heart rate disturbance is prolonged bradycardia [26]. Abdominal pain, cessation of contractions, and recession of the presenting part are less common. Data regarding the placement of an intrauterine catheter monitor to predict impending uterine rupture have revealed no correlation between uterine contractility patterns and rupture [27,28]. Bleeding may be intraperitoneal and into the broad ligament rather than revealed vaginally. Over 50% of cases are first diagnosed after delivery, when intractable hemorrhage follows precipitate, spontaneous or instrumental vaginal delivery. Alternatively, if bleeding is concealed, profound shock may occur before rupture is suspected. Uterine rupture should be considered in every obstetric patient with hemorrhagic shock in whom the cause is not immediately apparent.

Rupture of an unscarred uterus is frequently related to obstetric intervention. This includes use of uterotonic drugs for induction or augmentation of labor, mid-cavity forceps delivery or breech extraction with internal podalic version [25]. Prolonged labor in the presence of cephalopelvic disproportion or malpresentation may also cause uterine rupture; this is most common in underdeveloped countries with poor access to medical care, but also occurs due to inappropriate management of labor in industrialized nations. External trauma may cause uterine rupture at any gestation. Grand multiparity also increases the risk. Increased blood loss, transfusion rates, and fetal mortality are clinically significant with rupture of an intact uterus.

Rupture of a previously scarred uterus is more common than rupture of the intact uterus. Of 23 cases of uterine rupture reported from New Orleans between 1975 and 1983, 61.3% (14/23) involved rupture of a previous cesarean section scar, with six cases occurring prior to labor, five during labor, and the remaining three unknown [25]. The overall risk of uterine rupture for women attempting a trial of labor following lower segment cesarean section is 1%, but higher if the trial of labor is unsuccessful [29]. A previous classic cesarean section has a risk of rupture of 3–6%, increased to 12% if a trial of labor takes place. Spontaneous rupture of a classic cesarean section scar has been reported as early as 15 weeks of gestation [30]. Use of uterotonic drugs (prostaglandins, oxytocin, and misoprostol) in the presence of a cesarean section scar is associated with an increased risk of rupture. The risks are difficult to quantify, and use of these drugs in patients undergoing vaginal delivery after cesarean section is controversial. Data indicate that induction of labor and cervical ripening with prostaglandins (PGE-1 and PGE-2) may carry a high risk of uterine rupture [31]. Gynecologic uterine surgery including laparoscopic myometomy is also considered a strong risk factor for uterine rupture. Rates of rupture after myomectomy have been found to be as high as 1.5% [32]. Risk of rupture may have been minimized in this series since >50% of these patients underwent cesarean delivery before labor. Although the posterior fundus is considered the weakest part of the uterus, most ruptures occur in the lower anterior segment during labor and at the fundus during prelabor-associated ruptures [33]. Late complications of uterine hysteroscopy include uterine rupture [34].

Spontaneous uterine rupture has been documented in multiparous women with placenta accreta. Although rare, this has also been found in primiparous women with placenta accreta [35,36]. Congenital uterine anomalies are also a risk factor for uterine rupture, including those related to DES exposure. In one series, five cases of rupture were discovered in primiparous women with bicornuate uteri [32]. Literature suggests that an interdelivery interval of <24 months of gestation was associated wth a 2–3-fold increase in the risk of uterine rupture compared with an interval of greater than 24 months [37]. The same study demonstrated a twofold increase in rupture rates when single-layer closure was used to reapproximate the uterine incision in the previous cesarean delivery. Conversely, there are other studies demonstrating no difference in maternal or neonatal outcomes with single- or double-layer closure techniques [38–40].

The role of postpartum fever has been invested as a risk factor for rupture as well. In one study, the odds of rupture were four times greater than controls in women with postpartum febrile morbidity [41]. Although fetal macrosomia decreases the likelihood of successful vaginal delivery after cesarean delivery, multiple studies report no difference in rates of uterine rupture [42–44].

Management options consist of surgical repair and hysterectomy. Published case series, many spanning several decades, vary widely in reported use of each technique, with hysterectomy rates of 26–83% [24]. Most authors consider hysterectomy to be the procedure of choice for uterine rupture [25,45]. Subtotal hysterectomy may be performed if the rupture is confined to the uterine corpus. Evidence has shown that subtotal hysterectomy is associated with decreased operating time, lower morbidity and mortality and shorter hospital stay when compared to surgical repair [46]. Suture repair may be considered when technically feasible and there is a desire for future fertility. However, there is an increased risk of recurrence, which may be fatal. A meta-analysis from 1971 provides the most comprehensive data [47]. This analysis includes 194 women, with a total of 253 pregnancies following uterine rupture; two maternal deaths occurred. Overall, repeat rupture occurred in 6% with a previous lower segment rupture, 32% with a previous upper segment rupture, and 14% where the site of previous rupture was unknown. Of note, three women in this series had repeated rupture in two or three subsequent pregnancies. Other women had an uneventful pregnancy following uterine rupture, but with a repeat (even fatal) rupture in a subsequent pregnancy.

If suture repair is performed, elective cesarean section has been advocated as soon as evidence of fetal lung maturity is obtained in a future pregnancy. Repair has also been advocated if successful control of hemorrhage can be attained in hemodynamically unstable patients, avoiding further blood loss and prolonged surgery during hysterectomy. Bilateral tubal ligation should be considered in these cases. The need for massive transfusion usually accompanies operative management of uterine rupture. In a study evaluating over 25 peripartum hysterectomies, 98% of cases required multiple units of blood and blood products. Coordinated efforts with anesthesia and blood bank are of vital importance when the diagnosis of uterine rupture is suspected.

Table 22.1 Causes of primary postpartum hemorrhage.

Causes
Uterine atony
Retained placental tissue
Genital tract trauma
Vaginal lacerations
Cervical lacerations
Vulval hematoma
Broad ligament hematoma
Placenta accreta and other abnormal placentation
Uterine inversion
Uterine rupture
Coagulopathy
Secondary to hemorrhage or obstetric causes
Inherited or acquired bleeding disorders
Anticoagulant drugs

Primary postpartum hemorrhage

Primary postpartum hemorrhage is traditionally defined as blood loss of more than 500 mL within the first 24 hours of delivery [5]. However, in the 1960s, studies by Pritchard involving ^{51}Cr-labeled red cells demonstrated an average blood loss of 505 mL at vaginal delivery and 930 mL at elective repeat cesarean section [48]. Some clinicians therefore consider as clinically significant only blood loss greater than 500 mL at vaginal and 1000 mL at cesarean delivery, as major obstetric hemorrhage, with a reported incidence of 1.3% [5]. However, visual estimates of blood loss are commonly inaccurate, with frequent underestimation by at least 30–50% [49–51]. Delay in recognizing significant postpartum hemorrhage and therefore in instituting management contributes to maternal mortality from this condition; additionally, the presence of concealed hemorrhage may not be appreciated. A more objective, although retrospective, definition of postpartum hemorrhage is of a 10% change in hematocrit or a need for red blood cell transfusion. On this basis, the incidence of postpartum hemorrhage is 3.9% following vaginal delivery and 6.4% following cesarean section [52,53].

Most major hemorrhage occurs within the first hour post partum. The blood volume expansion of 1.5–2.0 L in healthy pregnant women provides a physiologic reserve for blood loss at delivery [54]. However, women with a below average increase in blood volume (pre-eclampsia, low prepregnancy Body Mass Index) tolerate postpartum hemorrhage less readily and are therefore more at risk of hemorrhagic shock.

Etiology of primary postpartum hemorrhage

Causes of primary postpartum hemorrhage can be divided into four major categories (Table 22.1). Prolonged or severe hemorrhage is the most common cause of coagulopathy post partum and exacerbates bleeding due to other causes [22].

Uterine atony is the most common cause of primary postpartum hemorrhage, accounting for 80% of all cases. At term, the uteroplacental circulation has a blood supply of 600–800 mL per minute. Rapid cessation of blood flow at the placental site is therefore essential, occurring via myometrial contraction causing compression of uterine vasculature. If this fails to occur, life-threatening hemorrhage may rapidly ensue. Many risk factors for uterine atony have been identified. These include high parity, chorioamnionitis, uterine fibroids, overdistension of the uterus (multiple gestation, fetal macrosomia, polyhydramnios), labor-related factors (precipitate labor, prolonged labor, oxytocin use) and uterine-relaxing drugs (magnesium sulfate, halogenated anesthetic agents, nitroglycerin) [49]. Antepartum hemorrhage due to both abruption and placenta previa carries an increased risk for postpartum hemorrhage. Previous postpartum hemorrhage confers a 10% risk of recurrence. Management of uterine atony is outlined in the next section.

Uterine atony unresponsive to medical treatment may be due to retained placental fragments. Visual examination of the placenta following removal cannot always exclude this diagnosis; a placenta appearing complete may be missing an entire or partial cotyledon or there may be a retained succinturiate lobe. In cases where the placenta is not easily removed or appears fragmented or incomplete upon manual extraction, placenta accreta should be suspected. This condition is not uncommonly associated with blood loss often greater than 2500 mL [55]. Examination under anesthesia and evacuation of retained placental tissue are necessary. Care is required with curettage since a postpartum uterus is easily perforated [56].

Genital tract trauma is commonly associated with instrumental delivery. Other risk factors include shoulder dystocia and precipitate delivery. Lacerations may occur throughout the urogenital system, including perineum, vagina, bladder, cervix, uterus, and anorectal tissues. Hemodynamic compromise may occur if diagnosis and repair are not carried out promptly.

Genital tract hematomas may result in postpartum cardiovascular collapse due to concealed blood loss. Vulvovaginal hematomas that lie below the levator ani may contain 1.5–2.0 L of blood [57]. They probably result from contusion or avulsion of the vascular supply due to radial stretching of vaginal tissues during delivery. Spread is usually limited by Colles' fascia and fascia lata. They do not cross the mid-line secondary to the central tendon. Supralevator hematomas can dissect paravaginally and extend into the retroperitoneal space [58]. Supralevator hematomas may present with hemorrhagic shock and can be associated with uterine dehiscense in women with prior cesarean delivery. Usually, laparotomy is required. Infralevator hematomas present with pain although other signs and symptoms include fever, ileus, leg edema and thigh pain. Hematoma formation may also occur in association with inadequate hemostasis during repair of episiotomy or vaginal tears. Evacuation is required for larger hematomas, (>3 cm) [59], best performed by incision through the vaginal wall to minimize scarring. In vulvar hematomas, bleeding vessels usually arise from the pudendal artery. In vaginal hematomas, the descending branch of the uterine artery may be involved. When attempting evacuation, the bleeding vessels should be identified and ligated. Frequently vessels may retract and the source of bleeding cannot be identified. Figure-of-eight sutures may be applied; alternatively, tight packing of the hematoma cavity may be necessary. If bleeding continues despite these measures, arterial ligation or angoigraphic embolization may be necessary (see below).

Broad ligament hematomas may result from uterine tears due to rupture or traumatic extension of a lower segment cesarean hysterotomy. Alternatively, deep cervical tears during spontaneous or operative vaginal delivery may involve the uterine artery at the base of the broad ligament [60]. Conservative management is possible if the patient is hemodynamically stable after vaginal delivery; however, bleeding may be ongoing, and diagnosis may only occur following postpartum collapse. Broad ligament hematomas may be apparent clinically by the presence of a tender, boggy mass suprapubically, with a firmly contracted uterus deviated past the mid-line. By the time a mass is clinically apparent, it may contain several liters of blood, and continued arterial bleeding may result in broad ligament rupture. Conservative surgery may be possible, but hysterectomy may be necessary (see below).

Leiomyoma may increase the risk of postpartum hemorrhage. A recent study demonstrated a 2.5-fold increased risk of postpartum hemorrhage in women with at least one leiomyoma diagnosed during pregnancy [61].

Uterine inversion

Uterine inversion often presents with profound shock, both neurogenic (due to traction on the uterine ligaments) and hemorrhagic (if the placenta is separated and uterus is atonic) in origin. Greater than 90% of patients will present with hemorrhage with typical blood loss approaching 2 L [62]. In complete inversion, clinical diagnosis may be obvious, with the uterus not palpable abdominally and the fundus visible as a mass protruding through the introitus [63]. Partial inversion may not be apparent without vaginal examination, leading to delayed diagnosis. Risk factors relate to the management of the third stage of labor. Predisposing factors include fundal insertion of the placenta and uterine atony, together with cord traction or fundal pressure.

The placenta should not be removed prior to uterine replacement; this exacerbates blood loss [64]. Manual replacement should take place without delay, by placing a hand vaginally with the fingers placed circumferentially and the fundus cupped in the palm. Replacement is such that the region of the uterus that inverted last is the first to be replaced, so avoiding multiple layers of uterine wall within the cervical ring. Uterine relaxation may be necessary, with β-sympathomimetic agents, magnesium sulfate or low-dose nitroglycerine [65]. Caution should be exercised with the use of nitroglycerin secondary to its vasodilatory effect, further potentiating hypotension and tachycardia. Recruitment of anesthesia services for rapid intubation provides full uterine relaxation along with the benefits of a controlled operating room environment, and patient, so that resuscitation/transfusion can be accomplished expeditiously. Intravaginal hydrostatic replacement is an alternative technique [66]. The vaginal introitus is occluded and warm saline infused into the posterior fornix from a meter or more above the patient. Ensuring an adequate vaginal seal may be difficult; a silastic Ventouse cup connected to the infusion and then inserted into the vagina has been successfully employed [67]. In the presence of a cervical ring prohibiting vaginal replacement of the fundus, options include incising the ring through a vaginal approach. An anterior or posterior vaginal incision has been described with subsequent repair once the fundus has been replaced [63]. If these measures fail, laparotomy is required. Two procedures are described. The first involves stepwise traction on the funnel of the inverted uterus or the round ligaments, using ring or Allis forceps reapplied progressively as the fundus emerges (Huntingdon procedure). If this fails, a longitudinal incision is made posteriorly through the cervix, relieving cervical constriction and allowing stepwise replacement (Haultain procedure). This can also be accomplished vaginally as described above. Once the uterus is replaced, all relaxants should be stopped and manual removal of the placenta should follow.

With early diagnosis and prompt replacement of the fundus, most often laparotomy and hysterectomy can be avoided [62,68]. It is delay which leads to increased edema, blood loss and associated morbidities.

Treatment of uterine atony

Emergency procedures

Fundal massage is the simplest treatment for uterine atony, is effective and can be performed while initial resuscitation and administration of uterotonic drugs are in progress. If this fails to rapidly control hemorrhage, bimanual compression may be successful. A fist or hand is placed within the vagina such that the uterus elevated; stretching of the uterine arteries reduces blood flow. The abdominal hand continues fundal massage, whilst also compressing the uterus. A urinary catheter may be inserted; this not only aids assessment of fluid status, but a distended bladder may interfere with uterine contractility. Controlled cord traction, early cord clamping and prophylactic oxytocic administration reduce postpartum hemorrhage by 500–1000 mL.

Aortic compression is a temporizing procedure that can be used in life-threatening hemorrhage, particularly at cesarean section. A closed fist compresses the aorta against the vertebral column just above the umbilicus [69]. Sufficient force is required to exceed systolic blood pressure; this can be assessed by absence of the femoral pulses. Intermittent release of pressure to allow peripheral perfusion then enables bleeding intra-abdominal vessels to be identified.

Following vaginal delivery, external aortic compression may be possible, due to lax abdominal musculature [70]. A study of the hemodynamic effects of aortic compression on healthy non-bleeding women within 4 hours of vaginal delivery found that leg blood pressure was obliterated in 55%, with a substantial reduction in a further 10%. No significant elevation in systemic blood pressure was noted, and the authors concluded that this procedure is safe, and a potentially useful maneuver for patient stabilization and transport. However, there have been no studies addressing the feasibility and efficacy of external aortic compression in patients with uterine atony following vaginal delivery; a high fundus may mean that adequate compression is impossible in this situation.

Medical treatment of uterine atony

The prophylactic use of uterotonic drugs is an effective means of preventing postpartum hemorrhage from uterine atony. Either oxytocin alone (5 IU or 10 IU intramuscularly) or with Syntometrine (5 IU of oxytocin plus 0.5 mg ergometrine: not available in the USA) may be used. The combination drug is more effective, but has more side effects [71]. These drugs are also first-line treatment for postpartum hemorrhage due to atony.

Oxytocin

Oxytocin binds to specific uterine receptors and intravenous administration (dose 5–10 IU) has an almost immediate onset of action [72]. The mean plasma half-life is 3 minutes, so to ensure a sustained contraction, a continuous intravenous infusion is necessary. The usual dose is 20–40 units per liter of crystalloid, with the dose rate adjusted according to response. Plateau concentration is reached after 30 minutes. Intramuscular injection has a time of onset of 3–7 minutes, and the clinical effect is longer lasting, at 30–60 minutes. Most studies find oxytocin alone reduces the need for further medication and is associated with fewer adverse side effects [73]. Compared with other agents, oxytocin has been found to reduce the need for manual placenta removal in some studies, regardless of route of administration (intramuscular versus dilute solution), and is safe [73].

Oxytocin is metabolized by both the liver and kidneys. It has approximately 5% of the antidiuretic effect of vasopressin, and if given in large volumes of electrolyte-free solution, can cause water overload (headache, vomiting, drowsiness, and convulsions), symptoms that may be mistakenly attributed to other causes. Rapid administration of an intravenous bolus of oxytocin results in relaxation of vascular smooth muscle. Hypotension with a reflex tachycardia may occur, followed by a small but sustained increase in blood pressure. Oxytocin is stable at temperatures up to 25°C, but refrigeration may prolong shelf-life.

Methylergonovine/ergometrine

Methylergonovine (methylergometrine) and its parent compound ergometrine result in a sustained tonic contraction of uterine smooth muscle via stimulation of α-adrenergic myometrial receptors [72]. The dose of methylergonovine is 0.2 mg and of ergometrine is 0.2–0.5 mg, repeated after 2–4 hours if necessary. Time to onset of action is 2–5 minutes when given intramuscularly. These agents are extensively metabolized in the liver and the mean plasma half-life is approximately 30 minutes. However, plasma levels do not seem to correlate with uterine effect, since the clinical action of ergometrine is sustained for 3 hours or more. When oxytocin and ergometrine derivatives are used simultaneously, postpartum hemorrhage is therefore controlled by two different mechanisms, oxytocin producing an immediate response, and ergometrine a more sustained action. In a recent large meta-analysis comparing ergometrine-oxytocin with oxytocin alone, a small but statistically significant reduction in postpartum hemorrhage was found with blood loss greater than 500 mL. However, there were no differences between the two groups with greater degrees (>1000 mL) of blood loss [74].

Nausea and vomiting are common side effects. Vasoconstriction of vascular smooth muscle also occurs as a consequence of their α-adrenergic action. This can result in elevation of central venous pressure and systemic blood pressure and therefore pulmonary edema, stroke, and myocardial infarction. Contraindications include heart disease, autoimmune conditions associated with Raynaud's phenomenon, peripheral vascular disease, arteriovenous shunts even if surgically corrected, and hypertension. Women with pre-eclampsia/eclampsia are particularly at risk of severe and sustained hypertension.

Intravenous administration is associated with more severe side effects, but onset of action is almost immediate. This route may be indicated for patients in whom delayed intramuscular absorption may occur (e.g. shock patients). The drug should be given over at least 60 seconds with careful monitoring of blood pressure and pulse. Initial reports suggested that methylergonovine resulted in hypertension less frequently than ergometrine, but no difference has since been reported in randomized controlled trials. Ergometrine and its derivatives are both heat and light sensitive, and should be stored at temperatures below 8°C and away from light.

Prostaglandins

Prostaglandin F-2α results in contraction of smooth muscle cells [72]. Carboprost/hemabate (15-methyl prostaglandin F-2α) is an established second-line treatment for postpartum hemorrhage unresponsive to oxytocic agents. It is available in single-dose vials of 0.25 mg. It may be given by deep intramuscular injection or by direct injection into the myometrium, either under direct vision at cesarean section or transabdominally/transvaginally after vaginal delivery. It is not licensed for the latter route and there is concern about direct injection into a uterine sinus, although it is commonly used in this way [75]. Additionally, it may be more efficacious in shock patients, when tissue hypoperfusion may compromise absorption following intramuscular injection [76]. A second dose may be given after 90 minutes or, if atony and hemorrhage continue, repeat doses may be given every 15–20 minutes to a maximum of eight doses (2 mg), with ongoing bimanual compression and fundal massage.

Small case series have reported an efficacy of 85% or more in refractory postpartum hemorrhage [76,77]. The largest case series to date has involved a multicenter surveillance study of 237 cases of postpartum hemorrhage refractory to oxytocics and found that it was effective in 88% [78]. The majority of women received a single dose. When further oxytocics were given to treatment failures, the overall success rate was 95%. The remaining patients required surgery and many of these had a cause for postpartum hemorrhage other than atony, including laceration and retained products of conception.

F-class prostaglandins cause bronchoconstriction, venoconstriction and constriction of gastrointestinal smooth muscle. Associated side effects include nausea, vomiting, diarrhea, pyrexia, and bronchospasm. There are case reports of hypotension and intrapulmonary shunting with arterial oxygen desaturation, so it is therefore contraindicated in patients with cardiac or pulmonary disease. Studies have demonstrated no significant difference between injectable carboprost compared to ergot compound injections in rates of postpartum hemorrhage [73]. Carboprost is expensive and therefore unaffordable in many developing countries. Dinoprost (prostaglandin F-2α) is more readily available; intramyometrial injection of 0.5–1.0 mg is effective for uterine atony. In randomized controlled trials comparing intramuscular prostaglandin F-2a with ergometrine and combinations of oxytocin and ergometrine, no difference between interventions in measures of blood loss or need for transfusion was found. Low-dose intrauterine infusion via a Foley catheter has also been described, consisting of 20 mg dinoprost in 500 mL saline at 3–4 mL/min for 10 minutes, then 1 mL/min [79]. Intravenous infusion of dinoprost has not been shown to be effective.

Prostaglandin E-2 (dinoprostone) is generally a vasodilatory prostaglandin; however, it causes contraction of smooth muscle in the pregnant uterus [72]. Dinoprostone is widely available on labor wards as an intravaginal pessary for cervical ripening. Rectal administration (2 mg given 2 hourly) has been successful as a treatment for uterine atony, vaginal administration probably being ineffective in the presence of ongoing uterine hemorrhage. Due to its vasodilatory effect, this drug should be avoided in hypotensive and hypovolemic patients. However, it may be useful in women with heart or lung disease in whom carboprost is contraindicated [49]. Case reports also document the use of gemeprost pessaries, a prostaglandin E-1 analog, but with actions resembling PGF-2α rather than its parent compound. Both rectal and intrauterine administration have been reported [80,81].

Misoprostol

Misoprostol is a synthetic analog of prostaglandin E-1 and is metabolized in the liver. The tablet(s) can be given orally, vaginally or rectally. As prophylaxis for postpartum hemorrhage, an international multicenter randomized trial reported that oral misoprostol is less successful than parenteral oxytocin administration [82]. Misoprostol may, however, be of benefit in treating postpartum hemorrhage. In a recent meta-analysis, oral or sublingual misoprostol at a dose of 600 μg was found to be useful in postpartum hemorrhage but did not demonstrate a benefit over other uterotonics [83].

Two small case series have reported an apparently rapid response in postpartum hemorrhage refractory to oxytocin and syntometrine, with rectal doses of 600–1000 μg. Sustained uterine contraction was reported in almost all women within 3 minutes of its administration [84,85]. A single-blinded randomized trial of misoprostol 800 μg rectally versus syntometrine intramuscularly plus oxytocin by intravenous infusion found that misoprostol resulted in cessation of bleeding within 20 minutes in 30/32 cases (93%) compared to 21/32 (66%) [86]. There was no difference in need for blood transfusion or onset of coagulopathy. In a recent meta-analysis comparing the evidence for rectal misprostol, no difference was found with interventions between rectal misoprostol and placebo or combinations of ergometrine and oxytocin, although there was a small decrease in blood loss greater than 500 mL [73,87]. Adverse effects include maternal pyrexia and shivering. Of note, misoprostol is cheap, heat and light stable, and does not require sterile needles and syringes for administration. It may therefore be of particular benefit in developing countries.

Surgical management of postpartum hemorrhage

The majority of the surgical techniques described here aim to arrest hemorrhage due to uterine atony. Many have been utilized for bleeding resulting from placenta accreta and placenta previa or for severe genital tract trauma when simple repair is unable to control hemorrhage.

Surgical intervention for uterine atony is necessary when uterotonic agents have failed to control bleeding, and there is no evidence of retained products of conception or concurrent genital tract trauma. An examination under anesthesia is generally necessary to exclude the latter. An extensive range of surgical techniques has been advocated. Case reports and audit studies constitute the major clinical evidence. Comparison between published reports is difficult – factors such as the severity of hemorrhage, time lapse from delivery to effective surgery, hemodynamic and coagulation status, available surgical expertise, and the presence of other obstetric and medical problems all contribute to differences in outcome.

Uterine tamponade

Uterine packing is a procedure long abandoned by many units but more recently revived, with case reports detailing new techniques for tamponade of the bleeding placental bed. Historically, uterine packing was performed using sterile gauze, with up to 5 m of 5–10 cm gauze introduced into the uterus, either using a specific packing instrument or long forceps [88]. Gauze is applied in layers from side to side, to give maximum pressure on the uterine wall, with the lower segment packed as tightly as possible. Indications for uterine packing include atony, placenta previa, and placenta accreta. Packs are generally left *in situ* for 24–36 hours, and prophylactic antibiotics given.

Uterine packing fell out of use due to concerns about concealed bleeding, infection, trauma, and problems in performing adequate packing. However, there is little documented evidence to support these concerns, and it has been suggested that the risks have been overstated [88,89]. Small studies have demonstrated that uterine packing is effective for controlling hemorrhage refractory to other medical treatment [90,91]. In a case series involving 20 women with postpartum hemorrhage, failure of the uterine packing to control bleeding was demonstrated in three women [92].

The pelvic pressure pack, also known as the "mushroom," "umbrella" or "Logothetopoulos" pack, has been successfully used for control of posthysterectomy hemorrhage in both gynecologic and obstetric patients. Although studies are limited, the success rate of the pelvic pressure pack in controlling posthysterectomy bleeding in obstetrics has approached 86% after other therapies were attempted [93]. Several inflatable mechanical devices have more recently been employed as alternative means of uterine tamponade. Proponents of these devices state that their advantages are that they are rapid and easy procedures to perform, and that their efficacy can readily be evaluated.

A Sengstaken–Blakemore tube has been utilized in this context [89,94]. The first report inflated the gastric balloon with normal saline, and the second inflated only the esophageal balloon. Balloon tamponade has also been performed with a Rusch urologic hydrostatic balloon catheter inflated with 400–500 mL of saline. This was effective in two women with hemorrhage due to morbidly adherent placentae [95]. In a more recent study, the Rusch hydrostatic balloon was effective in controlling postpartum hemorrhage in seven out of eight women when inflated with 1000 mL of normal saline [96]. Balloon tamponade has also been accomplished with the use of a sterile condom inflated with up to 500 mL of solution tied to a Foley catheter [97]. Several case reports have demonstrated similar results with a Foley catheter inflated with 300 mL [98,99]. These temporizing agents may allow for correction of coagulopathy in anticipation of surgical intervention. Often they lead to cessation of hemorrhage altogether and should be attempted in cases where future fertility is a consideration or in low-resource areas. A continuous oxytocin infusion and prophylactic antibiotic cover are advised for these procedures.

Uterine brace suture

The B-Lynch suture is a uterine brace suture designed to vertically compress the uterine body in cases of diffuse bleeding due to uterine atony [100]. In order to assess whether the suture will be effective, bimanual compression is applied to the uterus. If bleeding stops, compression with a brace suture should be equally successful. Single or multiple stitches may be inserted at the same time and, according to the shape, they may be called brace sutures [100], simple brace [101] or square sutures [102]. The patient is placed in the Lloyd-Davies position on the operating table to enable assessment of vaginal bleeding. If delivery occurred via lower segment cesarean section, the incision is reopened. If delivery was vaginal and retained products have been excluded via manual exploration, hysterotomy is not necessary. The uterus is exteriorized and response to bimanual compression assessed. If vaginal bleeding is controlled, the "pair of braces" suture is inserted using a 70 mm round-bodied needle with number 2 chromic catgut suture (Figure 22.1). The two ends are tied while an assistant performs bimanual compression and the lower segment incision is closed as normal. The authors describe five cases in which the procedure was attempted, with success in all cases. They included hemorrhage due to uterine atony, coagulopathy and placenta previa. The authors state that the advantages of this method are its surgical simplicity and that adequate hemostasis can be assessed immediately after its completion. Multiple case reports have described similar success with this procedure with and without other interventions, including radiologic procedures or uterotonics [103–105]. Normal uterine anatomy has been demonstrated on follow-up [106]. Resumption of normal menses along with uncomplicated pregnancies following the B-Lynch procedure for postpartum hemorrhage has also been described [107]. Unexpected occlusion of the uterine cavity with subsequent development of infection (pyometra) has been reported with the occlusive square-stitch [108].

A modification of the B-Lynch suture has been described [109]. A less complex procedure is involved, consisting of two individual sutures, tied at the fundus. A lower segment incision is not necessary, and the authors suggest that more tension may be applied with individual sutures than with one continuous suture. They also describe tying the loose ends of the sutures together, to prevent slippage laterally. A summary of published studies is the subject of a review article [110].

Uterine devascularization

Uterine devascularization is a long-practiced technique for postpartum hemorrhage due to atony, placenta, previa, and trauma. These techniques can also be used prophylactically in women with pregnancies complicated with placenta accreta in the operating room at the time of delivery. Ligation of the uterine arteries and internal iliac arteries is described; ovarian artery ligation may also be performed, generally as an adjunctive procedure. Evidence

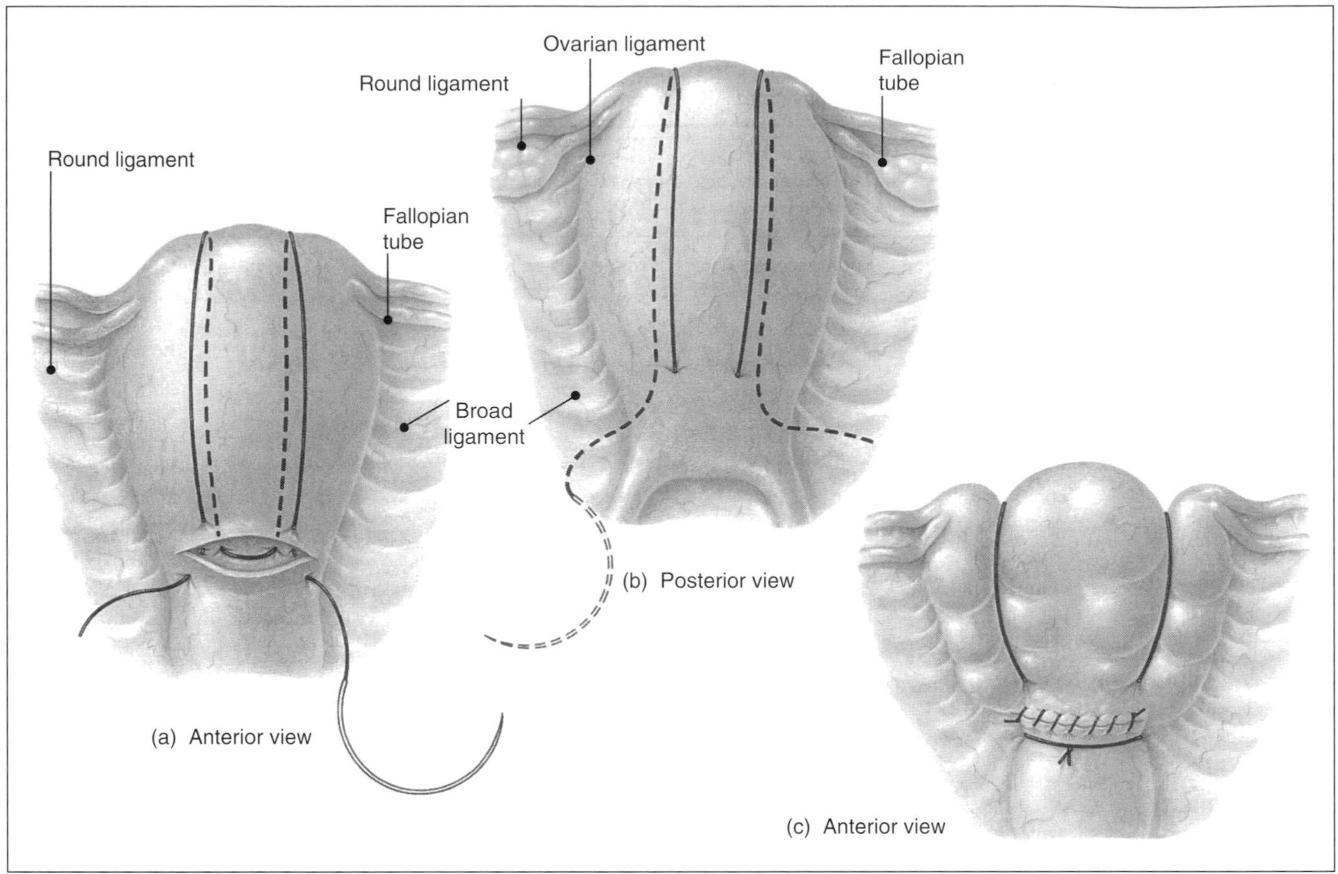

Figure 22.1 The B-Lynch uterine brace suture. (a) Anterior and (b) posterior views are shown during insertion of the suture. (c) After successful insertion. (Reprinted from B-Lynch et al. The B-Lynch surgical technique for the control of massive postpartum haemorrhage: an alternative to hysterectomy? Five cases reported. *Br J Obstet Gynaecol* 1997; 104: 372–375. © 1997 with permission from Elsevier Science.)

for the efficacy of these techniques is based on published case series. The expertise and experience of individual units are important determinants of the surgical approach to postpartum hemorrhage.

Bilateral uterine artery ligation

The pregnant uterus receives 90% of its blood supply from the uterine arteries. Bilateral ligation of the ascending branches of the uterine artery is considered by its practitioners to be a simple, safe, and efficacious alternative to hysterectomy [111]. This procedure was originally utilized to control postpartum hemorrhage at cesarean section. Mass ligation of the uterine artery branches and veins is performed 2–3 cm below the lower segment incision. The suture is placed laterally through an avascular window in the broad ligament, and medially through almost the full thickness of the uterine wall, to include the uterine vessels and 2–3 cm of myometrium. The vessels are not divided, and inclusion of myometrium avoids vascular damage and obliterates intramyometrial ascending arterial branches. An absorbable suture such as number 1 chromic catgut on an atraumatic needle is used. Non-absorbable and figure-of-eight sutures are avoided as they are considered to increase the risk of arteriovenous sinus formation. If vaginal delivery has occurred, the bladder may need to be adequately mobilized prior to suture insertion to avoid ureteric injury.

The largest case series was published in 1995 [112]. This was a 30-year study involving 265 patients with postcesarean postpartum hemorrhage of >1000 mL, refractory to oxytocics, methylergonovine and carboprost. Bilateral uterine artery ligation failed to control hemorrhage in only 10 women, giving a 96% success rate. An immediate effect was reported, with visible uterine blanching; myometrial contractions sometimes occurred, but even if the uterus remained atonic, hemorrhage was usually controlled [111]. No long-term effects on menstrual patterns or fertility have been reported [112,113]. In women who have subsequently undergone repeat caesaran section, the uterine vessels appeared to have recanalized.

Failure of this procedure is most commonly associated with placenta previa with or without accreta. More recently, low bilateral uterine artery ligation has been described for ongoing bleeding from the lower segment in these cases. A series of 103 patients involving stepwise uterine devascularization reported a 75% success rate with conventional uterine artery ligation [113].

Success was highest with uterine atony and abruption. Of seven cases of placenta previa with/without accreta, hemorrhage continued in four women. A further bilateral ligation was performed 3–5 cm below the first sutures, following further mobilization of the bladder. Ligation therefore includes the ascending branches of the cervicovaginal artery and the uterine artery branches supplying the lower segment and upper cervix. This procedure was effective in all cases. A vaginal route for uterine artery ligation has also been described, with moderate success [114]. This intervention includes incising the anterior cervix near the cervicovaginal fold with the bladder retracted. The uterus is then gently pulled to the contralateral side of the intended suture placement. A single absorbable suture is then placed around the vessels while including myometrial tissue. Although this technique may be quick and minimally invasive, more studies are required to prove its utility in postpartum hemorrhage.

Unilateral or bilateral ligation of the ovarian artery may be performed as an adjunct to ligation of uterine arteries. The ligature is tied medial to the ovary to preserve ovarian blood supply. This was the final phase of the stepwise uterine devascularization approach described above [113]. Following uterine artery ligation, 13/96 cases that did not involve placenta previa/accreta had ongoing bleeding. Of these, seven responded to unilateral ovarian artery and six to bilateral ovarian artery ligation. All patients in this case series therefore avoided hysterectomy.

Bilateral internal iliac artery ligation

Internal iliac artery ligation was first performed as a gynecologic procedure by Kelly in 1894 [115]. He termed this "the boldest procedure possible for checking bleeding" and assumed that the blood supply to the pelvis would be completely arrested. From the 1950s, internal iliac ligation was increasingly performed for gynecologic indications, mostly for carcinoma of the cervix. Ligation was still considered to shut off arterial flow, despite the fact that necrosis of pelvic tissues had not been observed.

In the 1960s, Burchell reported cutting a uterine artery following bilateral internal iliac ligation in order to demonstrate the absence of flow. However, to the surprise of those present, blood still flowed freely. This observation led to extensive studies of the hemodynamic effects of internal iliac ligation. These were performed on gynecologic patients, but are quoted widely in the obstetric literature [116,117]. Aortograms performed between 5 minutes and 37 months post ligation demonstrated an extensive collateral circulation, with blood flow throughout the internal iliac artery and its branches. Three collateral circulations were identified: the lumbar and iliolumbar arteries; the middle sacral and lateral sacral arteries; and the superior rectal and middle rectal arteries. Ligation above the posterior division resulted in collateral and therefore reversed flow in its iliolumbar and middle sacral branches (Figure 22.2). Ligation below the posterior division caused collateral flow only in the middle hemorrhoidal artery, again in a retrograde direction. Flow to more distal branches of the internal iliac artery was normal.

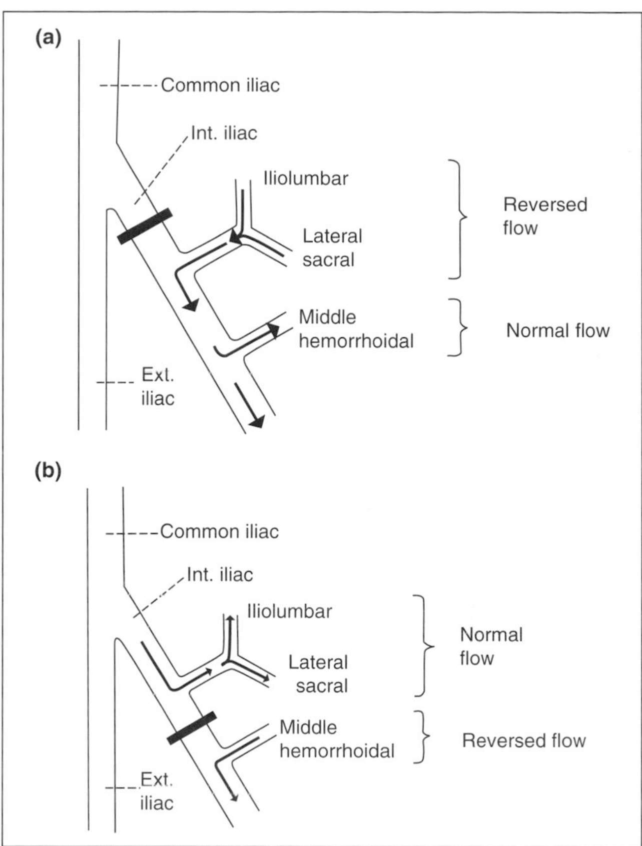

Figure 22.2 Internal iliac artery ligation. (a) Ligation above the posterior diversion; collateral pathways result in reversed flow in the iliolumbar and lateral sacral arteries. (b) Ligation below the posterior diversion; collateral pathways result in reversed flow in the middle hemorrhoidal (middle rectal) artery. (Reprinted from Burchell RC. Arterial physiology of the human pelvis. *Obstet Gynecol* 1968; 31: 855–860, with permission from the American College of Obstetricians and Gynecologists.)

A second study involved intra-arterial pressure recordings before and after ligation [116]. Following bilateral ligation, distal arterial pulse pressure decreased by 85%, with a 24% reduction in mean arterial pressure. In addition, a 48% reduction in blood flow resulted following ipsilateral ligation. The authors concluded that internal iliac ligation controls pelvic hemorrhage mainly by decreasing arterial pulse pressure. The smaller diameter of the anastomoses of the collateral circulation was proposed to explain this phenomenon. The arterial system was considered transformed into a venous-like circulation, with clot formation able to arrest bleeding at the site of injury. These studies have been extensively quoted, but similar studies have not been performed in postpartum women. A single case report found no change in uterine artery Doppler waveform velocity before and 2 days after bilateral internal artery ligation performed to control hemorrhage due to uterine atony [118].

Internal iliac artery ligation is a more complex procedure than uterine artery ligation. The bifurcation of the common iliac artery is identified at the pelvic brim, and the peritoneum opened and reflected medially along with the ureter [109]. The internal iliac artery is identified, freed of areolar tissue, and a right-angled clamp passed under the artery. Two ligatures are tied 1–2 cm apart. The artery is not divided. Both the uterine and vaginal arteries are branches of the anterior division, and ligation should if possible be distal to the origin of the posterior division. This is more efficacious and does not compromise blood supply to the buttocks and gluteal muscles. A retroperitoneal approach may be used when hemorrhage has followed vaginal delivery. Complications of this procedure include damage to the internal iliac vein and ureter. Tissue edema, ongoing hemorrhage, and the presence of a large atonic uterus may make identification of anatomy difficult and prolong operating time. Incorrect identification of the internal iliac artery may result in accidental ligation of the external or common iliac artery, resulting in lower limb and pelvic ischemia. Femoral pulses should therefore be checked after the procedure. Recanalization of ligated vessels may occur, and successful pregnancy has been reported whether or not recanalization has taken place.

Demonstration of the extensive collateral circulation explains why the efficacy of internal iliac ligation is less than for uterine artery ligation. Success rates are generally reported to be approximately 40% [109]. A 1985 study reported a success rate of 42% in a series of 19 patients, with hysterectomy necessary in the remainder [119]. Morbidity was higher than for a group of patients in whom hysterectomy was performed as a primary procedure; mean blood loss was 5125 mL for patients with unsuccessful internal iliac artery ligation followed by hysterectomy, and 3209 mL for those undergoing hysterectomy alone. Complications associated with unsuccessful arterial ligation in this series were associated with delay in instituting definitive treatment (hysterectomy) rather than as a consequence of arterial ligation. These authors consider that there is only a limited role for this procedure in the treatment of postpartum hemorrhage, being restricted to hemodynamically stable patients of low parity in whom future fertility is of paramount concern.

Arterial embolization

Uterine devascularization by selective arterial embolization has recently gained popularity in centers with expertise in interventional radiology. Access is via the femoral artery and the site of arterial bleeding is located by injection of contrast into the aorta. The bleeding vessel is selectively catheterized, and pledgets of absorbable gelatine sponge injected [120]. These effect only a temporary blockade and are resorbed within approximately 10 days. If the site of bleeding cannot be identified, embolization of the anterior branch of the internal iliac artery or the uterine artery is performed.

In published studies, uterine atony and pelvic trauma are the major indications for embolization, and overall success rates of 85–100% are reported [121]. Higher failure rates are associated with placenta accreta and procedures performed following failed bilateral internal iliac artery ligation [122]. Subsequent successful pregnancies have been documented.

Compared to surgical devascularization, embolization has several advantages. It is less invasive and generally results in visualization of the bleeding vessel. Occlusion of distal arteries close to the bleeding site is possible, thereby reducing the risk of ongoing bleeding from a collateral circulation [120]. The efficacy of embolization can immediately be assessed, and repeated embolization of the same or different arteries can be performed. Disadvantages are the necessity of rapid availability of specialist equipment and personnel, and the need for transfer of a hemorrhaging patient to the radiology suite. Embolization may also be a time-consuming procedure, generally requiring between 1 and 3 hours, but with hemostasis of the major bleeding vessel frequently established in 30–60 minutes. Pelage and colleagues evaluated the role of selective arterial embolization in 35 patients with unanticipated postpartum hemorrhage [123]. Bleeding was controlled in all except one who required hysterectomy for rebleeding 5 days later. All women in this series who had successful embolization resumed normal menstruation. These findings have been reported in other studies [124,125]. Patients with life-threatening hemorrhage have also been successfully treated with arterial embolization. A 1998 case series included 27 women with life-threatening bleeding, 12 of whom were intubated and ventilated, and four were successfully resuscitated following cardiac arrest [122]. Fever, contrast media renal toxicity, and leg ischemia are rare but reported complications of this procedure.

A variation on this theme is the prophylactic placement of inflatable balloon catheters in internal iliac arteries of patients who are expected to bleed excessively at the time of surgery, for example elective cesarean delivery in a patient with placenta percreta. In this situation the patient is taken to the interventional radiology suite prior to surgery and the balloon catheters are placed but not inflated. Following delivery of the baby, the catheters can be immediately inflated. Such catheters can be deflated at the completion of surgery and left *in situ* during the next 24–48 hours, to be reinflated if required. The use of prophylactic occlusion balloons in the internal iliac arteries before selective embolization has shown a greater than 80% success rate for control of postpartum hemorrhage [121,124]. Various reports have confirmed these findings with normal resumption of menses within 3–6 months and subsequent uncomplicated pregnancies [126–129]. In a recent study comparing outcomes of over 65 women with placenta accreta who underwent cesarean hysterectomy with and without prophylactic balloon catheters, no differences were found in operative time, blood loss, number of hospital days or transfused products [130].

Hysterectomy

Peripartum hysterectomy is frequently considered the definitive procedure for obstetric hemorrhage, but is not without complications. In the long term, the loss of fertility may be devastating to the patient. In the emergency situation, the major concern is that peripartum hysterectomy can be a complex procedure, due to ongoing blood loss and grossly distorted pelvic anatomy due to edema, hematoma formation, and trauma. Pritchard showed an average blood loss of 1435 mL when hysterectomy was performed at the time of elective repeat cesarean section [48]. At emergency hysterectomy for postpartum bleeding, mean blood loss attributed to the procedure was 2183 mL, with a mean loss of 2125 mL by the time of decision for hysterectomy [131]. Adequate hemostasis is not always achieved, and further procedures may be necessary. Uterine artery embolization has been performed for ongoing bleeding following hysterectomy, both with and without success [122,132]. Re-look laparotomy may also be required; this has been reported in up to 13% of patients [133]. The incidence of febrile morbidity is high, with rates of 5–85% in different series.

Hysterectomy is indicated if conservative procedures such as embolization or uterine devascularization fail to control bleeding. The time lapse between delivery and successful surgery is the most important prognostic factor. If the primary procedure fails, it is recommended that hysterectomy is performed promptly, without attempts at another conservative measure [132]. In severely shocked patients with life-threatening hemorrhage, hysterectomy is in most circumstances the first-line treatment [109]. Hysterectomy may therefore be associated with a higher mortality than other surgical procedures [132].

Uterine atony is the major indication for peripartum hysterectomy, although other factors such as placenta accreta and abruption are frequently present [132]. Many studies have described the profound hemorrhage associated with placenta previa, with a recent analysis [134] revealing blood loss greater than 3000 mL in 23% of patients with this condition. In this series, approximately 10% of patients required greater than five units of blood products and hysterectomy [134]. Surgical re-exploration secondary to postoperative bleeding is needed in up to 7% of patients with placental invasion [135,136]. Other indications for peripartum hysterectomy include placenta previa, uterine rupture, and other genital tract lacerations. Trauma sustained at vaginal delivery may result in concealed bleeding and is therefore associated with a worse outcome; hemorrhage at cesarean section is more readily recognized and more promptly remedied.

A subtotal hysterectomy can generally be performed if bleeding is from the uterine body. It is generally simpler than a total hysterectomy – the cervix and vaginal angles can be difficult to identify in women who have labored to full dilation. There is also less risk of injury to the ureter and bladder. One study reported the incidence of urinary tract injury to be 13% for subtotal hysterectomy, compared to 25% for total hysterectomy [133]. If placenta accreta is suspected, the use of prophylactic ureteral stents may help determine the location of the ureters and assist with difficult dissection planes. In addition, perioperative intentional cystotomy may improve visualization of bladder invasion. If bleeding is from the lower segment (placenta previa, trauma), the cervical branch of the uterine artery must be ligated, and a total hysterectomy will be necessary. Anesthetic considerations include the need for general endotracheal anesthesia in anticipation of prolonged surgical time, placement of a lumbothoracic epidural catheter for postpartum pain relief, and readiness for massive blood transfusion. Prophylaxis for thromboembolism should also be considered and initiated before surgery. Compression stockings placed before induction of anesthesia, prophylactic low molecular weight heparin or unfractionated heparin are also acceptable [137].

The importance of close postpartum observation cannot be overemphasized, and in most cases these patients should be recovered in an ICU setting. Frequently, because of prolonged operative time combined with massive transfusion, there is a risk for laryngeal edema, pulmonary edema, delayed extubation and prolonged ventilation. Continuous vital sign determination and pulse oximetry along with hourly urine output measurement are warranted after significant hemorrhage and blood or product replacement. Patients with periods of prolonged hypotension during surgery should also be followed postoperatively for evidence of the full Sheehan's syndrome or forme fruste of this syndrome.

Bleeding disorders

Consumptive and dilutional coagulopathies secondary to extensive blood loss and crystalloid replacement are the most common bleeding disorders associated with postpartum hemorrhage. Other obstetric causes of disseminated intravascular coagulopathy (acute fatty liver of pregnancy, abruption, anaphylactoid syndrome of pregnancy) or thrombocytopenia (HELLP syndrome, TTP) may cause or contribute to major hemorrhage. Inherited and acquired bleeding disorders unrelated to pregnancy must also be considered. These include abnormalities of the coagulation system and qualitative or quantitative platelet disorders. The most common disorders are discussed below.

Idiopathic thrombocytopenia purpura (ITP)

The differential diagnosis of thrombocytopenia in the gravid patient includes gestational thrombocytopenia, autoimmune disorders such as systemic lupus erythematosus or antiphospholipid syndrome, HELLP syndrome (hemolysis, elevated liver enzymes and low plateletes), folate deficiency, and viral illnesses including human immunodeficiency virus. The most common cause in pregnancy is gestational thrombocytopenia which accounts for 70% of cases when low platelets are discovered [138]. Heparin-induced thrombocytopenia should also be considered in chronically anticoagulated patients.

Idiopathic thrombocytopenia purpura is an autoimmune disorder resulting in increased platelet destruction. The incidence of ITP is 1–2 per 1000 deliveries and accounts for 3% of cases of thrombocytopenia at delivery [139]. The fetal risk of severe thrombocytopenia is 5–10%, and the neonatal nadir occurs between days 2 and 5 after delivery [140]. With ITP, the average platelet lifespan is greatly reduced, being a tenth of the normal 7–10 days. Circulating platelets are therefore younger, larger, and functionally superior compared to normal platelets. Platelet counts are generally between 50 and 75 × 10^9/L, but may fall to exceedingly low levels, particularly following viral infections. Exacerbations of ITP may occur at any time during pregnancy. In non-pregnant patients, spontaneous severe bleeding is rare with platelet counts greater than 10 × 10^9/L, and significant bleeding following trauma unusual with platelet counts above 50 × 10^9/L.

Case series from the 1950s and 1960s reported no increased incidence of postpartum hemorrhage or placental abruption in patients presenting with spontaneous bleeding from other sites [141]. Cesarean section and genital tract lacerations are associated with increased blood loss and an increased need for blood transfusion. Platelet counts should be monitored regularly. Antenatally, treatment is generally recommended with platelet counts of less than 30 × 10^9/L or at any level if there is clinically significant bleeding. The minimal safe platelet count for delivery is unknown. US guidelines demonstrate a diversity of expert opinion [142]; a minimum count between 10 and 50 × 10^9/L (mean 27 × 10^9/L) was recommended for vaginal delivery and 30–50 × 10^9/L (mean 44 × 10^9/L) for cesarean section. A lower limit of 80 × 10^9/L is generally agreed for regional analgesia.

The most common medical treatments for ITP are corticosteroids and intravenous immunoglobulin. High-dose steroids are associated with an increased risk of hypertension in pregnancy and immunoglobulin is extremely expensive. Intravenous anti-D antibodies (WinRho) were introduced in 1995 for the treatment of ITP in non-pregnant patients. The first study evaluating anti-D immunoglobulin in pregnant women occurred in 1993 with a pilot study of eight Rh-positive women with ITP in the second and third trimester. A 75% response rate was demonstrated and no adverse fetal effects were noted [143]. In cases of ITP resistant to conventional therapy, anti-D immunoglobulin should be considered. Platelet levels increase approximately 3–5 days after therapy has been initiated, with peak levels on day 8 [144]. Side effects are rare, with a small risk of hemolysis in the mother and fetus along with a 4% risk of fever, chills and body aches. Platelet transfusions should only be given for life-threatening bleeding or essential surgery; transfused platelets are rapidly destroyed in patients with ITP. Splenectomy remains the definitive treatment. In pregnancy, this may be technically difficult, but is indicated in women who are resistant to medical treatment.

Von Willebrand's disease

Von Willebrand's disease (vWD) is the most common inherited bleeding disorder [145]. The prevalence of vWD has been reported to be as high as 1.3%, with menorrhagia presenting as the most common symptom in the majority of women with this disorder. Pregnant women with this disorder have no increased risk of antepartum hemorrhage; however, the reported incidence of primary postpartum hemorrhage ranges between 22% and 59% [146,147], with an incidence of 20–28% for secondary postpartum hemorrhage [148]. There is also an increased risk of perineal hematoma in women with vWD. In small studies, the rate of perineal hematoma in this group was found to be 7% compared to 2.2 per 1000 in the general population [149,150].

This disorder is characterized by quantitative or qualitative deficiency in the production of von Willebrand factor (vWF), which has a central role in hemostasis [151]. First, it stabilizes the coagulation factor VIIIc, which otherwise is rapidly metabolized. Second, it mediates platelet adhesion following vascular injury. If there is a lack of functional vWF, the plasma level of factor VIIIc is low (normal range 50–150 IU/dL), and the bleeding time is prolonged. Bleeding problems are usually mild (epistaxis, menorrhagia) and the underlying problem may go undetected. However, life-threatening hemorrhage may occur post partum.

There are three types of vWD. Types 1 and 3 are quantitative deficiencies. Type 1 is found in approximately 70% of affected individuals, and is autosomal dominant. It is a partial deficiency state of vWF, and factor VIII levels are usually in the range 5–40 IU/dL. Type 3 is rare and autosomal recessive; there is almost a complete lack of vWF leading to very low levels of factor VIII with severe bleeding problems. Type 2 consists of qualitative differences, with several different subtypes which are inherited as autosomal dominant mutations. Thrombocytopenia may occur in type 2 disease in pregnancy; increased synthesis of abnormal multimers of vWF may cause increased platelet aggregation.

In normal pregnant women and those with type 1 disease, vWF and factor VIII levels rise significantly in the second half of pregnancy. Therefore it is rare that women with mild vWD need treatment in pregnancy. However, women with other types of vWD and low factor levels have an inadequate response. Factor VIII levels should be checked at the initial prenatal care visit and again in the third trimester. Following delivery, there is a rapid fall-off in factor VIII levels, resulting in a high rate of secondary postpartum hemorrhage.

Postpartum hemorrhage in women with vWD generally occurs if the factor VIII level is <50 IU/dL. Prophylactic treatment is therefore required during labor and in the early postpartum period to maintain concentrations above this threshold. Although there is no consensus on levels that are safe for regional anesthesia, if the coagulation profile is normal and factor VIII level is greater than 50 IU/dL, regional anesthesia can be safely administered [148]. The aim is to maintain higher levels for 3–4 days after vaginal delivery and 4–5 days after cesarean section. There are two options for treatment. The first is intravenous infusion of desmopressin (DDAVP; 1-deamino-8-arginine vasopressin), which acts by increasing factor VIII and vWF release into the plasma from storage sites, raising plasma concentrations by 3–5 times within 30 minutes. These levels are usually maintained for 8–10 hours and infusions therefore need to be given 1–2 times daily. Patients with type 1 disease generally respond well, but response is variable in type 3. DDAVP is contraindicated in some subtypes of type 2 because transient thrombocytopenia may result. DDAVP does not appear to cross the placenta in detectable amounts [152]. Caution should be exercised when administering DDAVP during the third stages of labor. In most cases, fluid bolus with the addition of oxytocin is used immediately after delivery. With the addition of DDAVP, synergistic action from both agents can cause fluid retention and hyponatremia [153].

The second treatment option consists of factor VIII and vWF replacement. Fresh frozen plasma contains both factors, but large volumes are required to stop or prevent bleeding. Cryoprecipitate contains 5–10 times higher concentration of both factors. Factor VIII preparations for use in vWD must also contain some vWF, otherwise the half-life of factor VIII is 1 hour or less. Recombinant factor VIII therefore cannot be given, but commercial preparations containing both factors are available. Tranexamic acid may also be useful in women with non-life-threatening postpartum hemorrhage. This agent exerts its effect by competitevely inhibiting the conversion of plasminogen to plasmin, therefore inhibiting the degredation of fibrin This agent does cross the placenta but has not been associated with adverse fetal effects [154,155].

The average time of presentation of postpartum hemorrhage in women with vWD is 15+/−5 days and hemorrhage may occur despite prophylaxis. These women benefit from frequent visits for the first weeks after delivery and may require additional therapy at these times [156].

Hemophilia

Hemophilia A (factor VIII deficiency) and hemophilia B (factor IX deficiency) are X-linked disorders [157]. Some women have levels that are within the normal range (>50 IU/dL), but inactivation of the normal chromosome (lyonization) may result in low factor levels [145]. The overall frequency for these disorders is approximately 1 in 100,000 births [158]. There is also an increased risk of primary and secondary postpartum hemorrhage in hemophilia carriers, with reported rates of 19% and 11% respectively, occurring mostly when factor levels are <50 IU/dL. Although hemorrhage is rare in women with factor levels >50%, severe bleeding may occur with levels between 5% and 30% after surgery or delivery [159]. In small reports, hemophilia A and B were noted to have higher postpartum hemorrhage rates compared to women with other bleeding disorders and required up to 4 days of factor replacement [160].

Carriers of hemophilia A generally experience a pregnancy-induced rise in factor VIII levels. However, factor IX levels are unaffected by pregnancy. Treatment is indicated for labor when factor levels are <50 IU/dL for both types of hemophilia. DDAVP may be used or appropriate factor concentrates. If the diagnosis is not known in the face of hemorrhage, fresh frozen plasma can be used pending test results. Hemophilia A carriers synthesize normal amounts of vWF, and therefore recombinant factor VIII is effective in these patients. Affected fetuses are at risk for extra- and intracranial hemorrhage, but cesarean delivery does not reduce this risk. Fetal scalp electrodes and operative delivery should be used cautiously.

Acquired hemophilia

Acquired hemophilia is caused by the presence of autoantibodies to factor VIII in people with previously normal factor VIII activity [161]. These antibodies are inhibitory, and partially or completely suppress factor VIII procoagulant activity. It is a rare disorder, and bleeding is generally severe with high morbidity and mortality. The incidence is reported as 1.48 per million per year [162]. This disease affects approximately 1 in 350,000 pregnant women [163]. In pregnant women, the time to achieve remission is longer than for non-pregnant patients but there are higher rates of spontaneous remission [164]. The risk of death from hemorrhage is higher in patients with this disorder than in hemophiliacs with factor VIII inhibitors.

Between 7% and 11% of cases are related to pregnancy, and most occur after the first delivery [165]. Presentation is with major bleeding, generally within the first 3 months post partum. Hemorrhage may be apparent at several different sites, including multiple soft tissue hematomas, large ecchymoses, excessive vaginal loss, and postoperative bleeding. Investigations show a prolonged aPTT, together with a normal prothrombin time, bleeding time, and platelet count. In the majority of patients, inhibitors spontaneously disappear and there is complete remission within a few months; however, sometimes these antibodies may persist for years. Until their disappearance, patients are at high risk for further bleeding episodes.

Hemorrhage is controlled by raising the plasma level of factor VIII, to overpower the inhibitory action. Inhibitors bind less readily to porcine factor VIII than human factor VIII, so the former is generally first-line management. Porcine factor VIII has been shown to have excellent efficacy, with a greater than 85% rate of hemostatic control in these patients [166].

Other treatment options include bypassing agents. In a large cohort study evaluating the efficacy of factor VIII inhibitor bypassing activty (FEIBA), complete response was achieved in 76% of severe and 100% of moderate bleeding episodes in these patients [167]. The other bypassing agent used for aquired hemophilia is recombinant factor VIIa. Used as a first-line agent, this demonstrated efficacy within 8 hours in the majority of cases [168]. Several doses may be required. Both agents are associated with thrombotic events and should be administered according to the manufacturer's recommendations based on individual case-by-case situations. There is no validated laboratory monitoring technique for these agents. DDAVP may also be used to increase endogenous factor VIII release from cellular stores. This agent is best used in patients with low inhibitory anti-factor VIII titers and measurable factor VIII levels. The response is unpredictable and it is best used for minor bleeds [169]. Plasmapheresis may be necessary if inhibitor levels are high. Disappearance of inhibitors can be enhanced by treatment with immunosuppressive agents such as corticosteroids, cyclophosphamide, rutiximab and azathioprine. In patients with complete remission, there has been no recurrence in subsequent pregnancies. However, as this is a rare disorder, few cases have as yet been documented.

Secondary postpartum hemorrhage

Secondary or delayed postpartum hemorrhage is defined as blood loss of 500 mL or more from the genital tract occurring more than

24 hours after delivery and up to 6 weeks post partum. The potential severity of this condition should not be underestimated; secondary postpartum hemorrhage may result in the rapid onset of hemorrhagic shock [123]. The peak time for presentation is the second postpartum week, with the third postpartum week the next most common. The great majority of women therefore present with this complication as outpatients.

The reported incidence is 0.5–1.3% of deliveries [170]. Common causes include retained placental tissue, endometritis, and genital tract tears. Rare causes include arteriovenous fistulae and false aneurysms, possibly resulting from surgical trauma and healing at the site of cesarean section incision [123]. Scar dehiscence has also been described. Genital tract malignancy, including choriocarcinoma, may also cause excessive bleeding during the postpartum period. Bleeding disorders may also present in this way, as discussed above. Acquired hemophilia is a rare but potentially lethal cause of secondary postpartum hemorrhage.

Initial acute management of excessive bleeding from the placental bed involves medical treatment. As for primary postpartum hemorrhage, the first-line agents are intramuscular ergometrine/ergotamine and intravenous infusion of oxytocin. Prostaglandins E-2, F-2α, and misoprostol have been used and good responses have been reported. Antibiotics are commonly given, although positive microbial cultures are not frequently found.

Uterine curettage is commonly performed. However, this is not without risk; uterine perforation is reported in 3% of women with secondary postpartum hemorrhage, and has occurred in patients up to 28 days after delivery. Histologic confirmation of products of conception occurs only in about a third of cases; however, an apparent therapeutic benefit may be achieved even in its absence. Ultrasound is no more accurate in the diagnosis of retained placental tissue than clinical assessment.

If bleeding is not controlled by these means, further surgical intervention is necessary. As for primary hemorrhage, ligation of the uterine vasculature, hysterectomy, and arterial embolization have all been successfully performed, although there is little evidence to show which is the optimum procedure. Women with genital tract trauma may also undergo these procedures if primary suturing is unsuccessful or not feasible. Angiography performed prior to embolization may also result in the diagnosis of vascular causes of secondary hemorrhage where otherwise no underlying cause could be identified [123]. A case series of 14 patients revealed a false aneurysm of the uterine artery in two women and an arteriovenous fistula in one woman.

Conclusion

Hemorrhage is a common complication of pregnancy and remains one of the most frequent causes of maternal morbidity and mortality. Early recognition with attention to estimating blood loss, vigilant monitoring of vital signs, prompt intervention to correct the underlying cause of hemorrhage, and in some cases blood component therapy, will minimize serious sequelae of hemorrhage.

References

1 Chang J, Elam-Evans, LD, Berg CJ, et al. Pregnancy-related mortality surveillance – United States. 1991–1997. *MMWR* 2003; 52(2): 1–8.

2 Berg CJ, Chang J, Callaghan WM, et al. Pregnancy related mortality in the United States, 1991–1997. *Obstet Gynecol* 2003; 101(2): 289–296.

3 Clark SL, Belfort MA, Dildy GA, Herbst MA, Meyers JA, Hankins GD. Maternal death in the 21st century: causes, prevention, and relationship to cesarean delivery. *Am J Obstet Gynecol* 2008; 199(1): 36; discussion 91–92.

4 AbouZahr C. Global burden of maternal death and disability. *Br Med Bull* 2003; 67: 1–11.

5 Bonnar J. Massive obstetric haemorrhage. *Baillière's Best Pract Res Clin Obstet Gynaecol* 2000; 14: 1–18.

6 Ananth CV, Savitz DA, Bowes WA, et al. Influence of hypertensive disorders and cigarette smoking on placental abruption and uterine bleeding during pregnancy. *Br J Obstet Gynaecol* 1997; 104: 572–578.

7 Domissee J, Tiltman AJ. Placental bed biopsies in placental abruption. *Br J Obstet Gynaecol* 1992; 99: 651–654.

8 Rana A, Sawhney H, Gopalan S, et al. Abruptio placentae and chorioamnionitis, Microbiologic and histologic correlation. *Acta Obstet Gynecol* 1999; 78: 363–369.

9 Baron F, Hill WC. Placenta previa, placenta abruptio. *Clin Obstet Gynecol* 1998; 41: 527–532.

10 Ananth CV, Smulian JC, Dimissie K, et al. Placental abruption among singleton and twin births in the U.S.: risk factors. *Am J Epidemiol* 2001; 153: 771–778.

11 Lowe TW, Cunningham FG. Placental abruption. *Clin Obstet Gynecol* 1990; 33: 406–413.

12 Ananth CV, Wilcox AJ. Placental abruption and perinatal mortality in the United States. *Am J Epidemiol* 2001; 153: 332–337.

13 Pritchard JA, Cunningham FG, Pritchard SA, Mason RA. On reducing the frequency of severe abruptio placentae. *Am J Obstet Gynecol* 1991; 165: 1345–1351.

14 Ananth CV, Oyelese Y, Prasad V, Getahun D, Smulian JC. Evidence of placental abruption as a chronic process: associations with vaginal bleeding early in pregnancy and placental lesions. *Eur J Obstet Gynecol Reprod Biol* 2006; 128(1–2): 15–21.

15 Goddijn-Wessel TA, Wouters MG, van de Molen EF, Spujbroek MD, Steegers-Theunssen RP. Hyperhomocystenemia – a risk factor for placental abruption or infarction. *Eur J Obstet Gynecol Reprod Biol* 1996; 66: 23–29.

16 Ananth CV, Berkowitz GS, Savitz DA, et al. Plaental abruption and adverse perinatal outcomes. *JAMA* 1999; 282: 1646–1651.

17 Gibbs JM, Weindling AM. Neonatal intracranial lesions following placental abruption. *Eur J Pediatr* 1994; 153: 195–197.

18 Nyberg DA, Cyr DR, Mack LA, Wilson DA, Shuman WP. Sonographic spectrum of placental abruption. *AJR* 1987; 148: 161–164.

19 Dhanraj D, Lambers D. The incidences of Kleihauer–Betke test in low risk pregnancies and maternal trauma patients. *Am J Obstet Gynecol* 2004; 190: 1461–1463.

20 Pritchard JA, Brekken AL. Clinical and laboratory studies on severe abruptio placentae. *Am J Obstet Gynecol* 1967; 97(5): 681–700.

21 Anthony J, Johanson R, Dommisse J. Critical care management of severe preeclampsia. *Fetal Mat Med Rev* 1994; 6: 219–229.

22 Letsky EA. Disseminated intravascular coagulation. *Baillière's Best Pract Res Clin Obstet Gynaecol* 2001; 15: 623–644.

23 Towers CV, Pircon RA, Heppard M. Is tocolysis safe in the management of third trimester bleeding? *Am J Obstet Gynecol* 1999; 180: 1572–1578.

24 Phelan JP. Uterine rupture. *Clin Obstet Gynecol* 1990; 33: 432–437.

25 Plauché WC, von Almen W, Muller R. Catastrophic uterine rupture. *Obstet Gynecol* 1984; 64(6): 792–797.

26 Guise JM, McDonagh M, Osterweil P, et al. Systematic review of the incidence and consequences of uterine rupture in women with prior caesarean section. *BMJ* 2004; 329: 19–23.

27 Devoe LD, Croom CS, Youssef AA, Murray C. The prediction of "controlled" uterine rupture by the use of intrauterine pressure catheters. *Obstet Gynecol* 1992; 80: 626–629.

28 Rodriguez RH, Masaki DI, Phelan JP, Diaz FG. Uterine rupture: are intrauterine pressure catheters useful in the diagnosis? *Am J Obstet Gynecol* 1989; 161: 666–669.

29 McMahon MJ. Vaginal birth after cesarean. *Clin Obstet Gynecol* 1998; 2: 369–381.

30 Endres LK, Barnhart K. Spontaneous second trimester uterine rupture after classical cesarean. *Obstet Gynecol* 2000; 96: 806–808.

31 Lydon-Rochelle M, Holt VL, Easterling TR, Martin DP. Risk of uterine rupture during labor among women with a prior cesarean delivery. *N Engl J Med* 2001; 345: 3–8.

32 Colin A, Baxi LV. Rupture of the primigravid uterus: a review of the literature. *Obstet Gynecol Surv* 2007; 62(5): 327–334.

33 Schrinsky DC, Benson RC. Rupture of the pregnant uterus: a review. *Obstet Gynecol Surv* 1978; 33: 217–232.

34 Senthiles L, Sergent F, Roman H, et al. Late complications of uterine hysteroscopy. Predicting patients at risk of uterine rupture during subsequent pregnancy. *Eur J Obstet Gynecol Reprod Biol* 2005; 120: 134–138.

35 DeRoux SJ, Prendergast NC, Adsay NV. Spontaneous uterine rupture with fatal hemoperitoneum due to placenta percreta/accreta: a case report and revew of the literature. *Int J Gynecol Pathol* 1999; 18; 82–86.

36 Kazandi M. Placenta percreta: report of two cases and a review of the literature. *Clin Exp Obstet Gynecol* 2003; 30; 70–72.

37 Bujold E, Mehta SH, Bujold C, Gauthier RJ. Interdelivery interval and uterine rupture. *Am J Obstet Gynecol* 2002; 187: 1199–1202.

38 Guise JM, Hashima J, Osterweil P. Evidence-based vaginal birth after caesarean section. *Best Pract Res Clin Obstet Gynaecol* 2005; 19: 117–130.

39 Chapman J, Owen J, Hauth JC. One- versus two-layer closure of a low transverse cesarean: the next pregnancy. *Obstet Gynecol* 1997; 89: 16–18.

40 Durnwald C, Mercer B. Uterine rupture, perioperative and perinatal morbidity after single-layer and double-layer closure at cesarean delivery. *Am J Obstet Gynecol* 2003; 189: 925–929.

41 Shipp TD, Zelop C, Cohen A, et al. Post-cesarean delivery fever and uterine rupture in a subsequent trial of labor. *Obstet Gynecol* 2003; 101: 136–139.

42 Phelan P, Eglinton GS, Horenstein JM, et al. Previous cesarean birth: trial of labor in women with macrosomic infants. *J Reprod Med* 1984; 29: 36–40.

43 Flamm BL, Goings JR. Vaginal birth after cesarean section: is suspected fetal macrosomia a contraindication? *Obstet Gynecol* 1989; 74: 694–697.

44 Zelop CM, Shipp TD, Repke JT, et al. Outcomes of trial of labor following previous cesarean delivery among women with fetuses weighing >4000 g. *Am J Obstet Gynecol* 2001; 18: 903–905.

45 Eden RD, Parker RT, Gall SA. Rupture of the pregnant uterus: a 53 year review. *Obstet Gynecol* 1986; 68: 671–674.

46 Thakur A, Heer MS, Thakur V, et al. Subtotal hysterectomy for uterine rupture. *Int J Gynecol Obstet* 2001; 74; 29–33.

47 Ritchie EH. Pregnancy after rupture of the pregnant uterus. *J Obstet Gynaecol Br Commw* 1971; 78: 642–648.

48 Pritchard JA, Baldwin RM, Dickey JC, Wiggins KM. Blood volume changes in pregnancy and the puerperium. II. Red blood cell loss and changes in apparent blood volume during and following vaginal delivery, cesarean section, and cesarean section plus total hysterectomy. *Am J Obstet Gynecol* 1962; 84: 1271–1282.

49 American College of Obstetricians and Gynecologists. Educational Bulletin No. 243. Postpartum haemorrhage. *Int J Gynecol Obstet* 1998; 61: 79–86.

50 Dildy GA, Paine AR, George NC, Velasco C. Estimating blood loss: can teaching significantly improve visual estimation? *Obstet Gynecol* 2004; 104(3): 601–606.

51 Stafford I, Dildy GA, Clark SL, Belfort MA. Visually estimated and calculated blood loss in vaginal and cesarean delivery. *Am J Obstet Gynecol* 2008; 199(5): 519.

52 Combs CA, Murphy EL, Laros RK Jr. Factors associated with hemorrhage in cesarean deliveries. *Obstet Gynecol* 1991; 77(1): 77–82.

53 Combs CA, Murphy EL, Laros RK Jr. Factors associated with postpartum hemorrhage with vaginal birth. *Obstet Gynecol* 1991; 77(1): 69–76.

54 Pritchard JA. Changes in the blood volume during pregnancy and delivery. *Anesthesiology* 1965; 26: 393–399.

55 Read JA, Cotton DB, Miller FC. Placenta accreta: changing clinical aspects and outcome. *Obstet Gynecol* 1980; 56: 31–34.

56 Cruikshank SH. Management of postpartum and pelvic hemorrhage. *Clin Obstet Gynecol* 1986; 29: 213–219.

57 Morgans D, Chan N, Clark CA. Vulval perineal haematomas in the immediate postpartum period and their management. *Aust NZ J Obstet Gynaecol* 1999; 39: 223–227.

58 You WB, Zahn CM. Postpartum hemorrhage: abnormally adherent placenta, uterine inversion, and puerperal hematomas. *Clin Obstet Gynecol* 2006 Mar; 49(1): 184–97.

59 Sotto LS, Collins RJ. Perigenital hematomas; analysis of 47 consecutive cases. *Obstet Gynecol* 1958; 12: 259–263.

60 Maxwell C, Gawler D, Green J. An unusual case of acute postpartum broad ligament haematoma. *Aust NZ J Obstet Gynaecol* 1997; 37: 239–241.

61 Qidwai, GI, Caughey AB, Jacoby AF. Obstetric outcomes in women with sonographically identified uterine leiomyoma. *Obstet Gynecol* 2006; 107: 376–382.

62 Platt LD, Druzin ML. Acute puerperal inversion of the uterus. *Am J Obstet Gynecol* 1981; 141: 187–190.

63 Kitchin JD III, Thiagarajah S, May HV Jr, Thornton WN Jr. Puerperal inversion of the uterus. *Am J Obstet Gynecol* 1975; 123: 51–58.

64 Brar HS, Greenspoon JS, Platt LD, Paul RH. Acute puerperal uterine inversion. New approaches to management. *J Reprod Med* 1989; 34: 173–177.

65 Dayan SS, Schwalbe SS. The use of small-dose intravenous nitroglycerin in a case of uterine inversion. *Anesth Analg* 1996; 82: 1091–1093.
66 O'Sullivan JV. A simple method of correcting puerperal uterine inversion. *BMJ* 1945; 2: 282–284.
67 Ogueh O, Ayida G. Acute uterine inversion: a new technique of hydrostatic replacement. *Br J Obstet Gynaecol* 1997; 104: 951–952.
68 Watson P, Besch N, Bowes WA Jr. Management of acute and subacute puerperal inversion of the uterus. *Obstet Gynecol* 1980; 55: 12–16.
69 Keogh J, Tsokos N. Aortic compression in massive postpartum haemorrhage – an old but lifesaving technique. *Aust NZ J Obstet Gynaecol* 1997; 37: 237–238.
70 Riley DP, Burgess RW. External abdominal aortic compression: a study of a resuscitation manoeuvre for postpartum haemorrhage. *Anesth Intens Care* 1994; 22: 571–575.
71 McDonald S, Prendiville WJ, Elbourne D. Prophylactic syntometrine versus oxytocin for delivery of the placenta. *Cochrane Database Syst Rev* 2000; 2: CD000201.
72 Dollery C, ed. *Therapeutic Drugs*, 2nd edn. Edinburgh: Churchill Livingstone, 1999.
73 Chelmow D, O'Brien B. Postpartum haemorrhage: prevention. *Clin Evid* 2006; 15: 1932–1950.
74 McDonald S, Abbott JM, Higgins SP. Prophylactic ergometrine-oxytocin versus oxytocin for the third stage of labour. *Cochrane Database Syst Rev* 2007; 3: CD000201.pub2.
75 Bigrigg A, Chiu D, Chissell S, Read MD. Use of intramyometrial 15-methyl prostaglandin F2α to control atonic postpartum haemorrhage following vaginal delivery and failure of conventional therapy. *Br J Obstet Gynaecol* 1991; 98: 734–736.
76 Hayashi RH, Castillo MS, Noah ML. Management of severe postpartum hemorrhage with a prostaglandin F2α analogue. *Obstet Gynecol* 1984; 63: 806–808.
77 Toppozada M, El-Bossaty M, El-Rahman HA, El-Din AH. Control of intractable atonic postpartum hemorrhage by 5-methyl prostaglandin F2α *Obstet Gynecol* 1981; 58: 327–330.
78 Oleen MA, Mariano JP. Controlling refractory atonic postpartum haemorrhage with Hemabate sterile solution. *Am J Obstet Gynecol* 1990; 162: 205–208.
79 Kupferminc MJ, Gull I, Bar-Am A, et al. Intrauterine irrigation with prostaglandin F2α for management of severe postpartum haemorrhage. *Acta Obstet Gynaecol Scand* 1998; 77: 548–550.
80 Craig S, Chau H, Cho H. Treatment of severe postpartum hemorrhage by rectally administered gemeprost pessaries. *J Perinat Med* 1999; 27: 231–235.
81 Barrington JW, Roberts A. The use of gemeprost pessaries to arrest postpartum haemorrhage. *Br J Obstet Gynaecol* 1993; 100: 691–692.
82 Gulmezoglu AM, Villar J, Ngoc NT, et al. WHO mulitcentre randomised trial of misoprostol in the management of the third stage of labour. *Lancet* 2001; 358: 689–695.
83 Gülmezoglu AM, Forna F, Villar J, Hofmeyr GJ. Prostaglandins for preventing postpartum haemorrhage. *Cochrane Database Syst Rev* 2007; 3: CD000494.pub3.
84 Abdel-Aleem H, EI-Nashar I, Abdel-Aleem A. Management of severe postpartum hemorrhage with misoprostol. *Int J Gynecol Obstet* 2001; 72: 75–76.
85 O'Brien P, El-Refaey H, Gordon A, Geary M, Rodeck CH. Rectally administered misoprostol for the treatment of postpartum haemorrhage unresponsive to oxytocin and ergometrine: a descriptive study. *Obstet Gynecol* 1998; 92: 212–214.
86 Lokugamage AU, Sullivan KR, Niculescu I, et al. A randomized study comparing rectally administered misoprostol versus syntometrine combined with an oxytocin infusion for the cessation of primary postpartum hemorrhage. *Acta Obstet Gynecol Scand* 2001; 80: 835–839.
87 Mousa HA, Alfirevic Z. Treatment for primary postpartum haemorrhage. *Cochrane Database Syst Rev* 2007; 1: CD003249.
88 Maier RC. Control of postpartum hemorrhage with uterine packing. *Am J Obstet Gynecol* 1993; 169: 317–323.
89 Katesmark M, Brown R, Raju KS. Successful use of a Sengstaken–Blakemore tube to control massive postpartum haemorrhage. *Br J Obstet Gynaecol* 1994; 101: 259–260.
90 Bagga R, Jain V, Kalra J, Chopra S, Gopalan S. Uterovaginal packing with rolled gauze in postpartum hemorrhage. *MedGenMed* 2004; 6(1): 50.
91 Naqvi S, Makhdoom T. Conservative management of primary postpartum haemorrhage. *J Coll Physicians Surg Pak* 2004; 14(5): 296–297.
92 Hag G, Tayyab S. Control of postpartum and post abortal haemorrhage with uterine packing. *J Pak Med Assoc* 2005; 55(9): 369–371.
93 Dildy GA, Scott JR, Saffer CS, Belfort M. An effective pressure pack for severe pelvic hemorrhage. *Obstet Gynecol* 2006; 108: 1222–1226.
94 Chan C, Razvi K, Tham KF, Arulkumaran S. The use of a Sengstaken–Blakemore tube to control post-partum hemorrhage. *Int J Gynecol Obstet* 1997; 58: 251–252.
95 Johanson R, Kumar M, Obhrai M, Young P. Management of massive postpartum haemorrhage: use of a hydrostatic balloon catheter to avoid laparotomy. *Br J Obstet Gynaecol* 2001; 108: 420–422.
96 Keriakos R, Mukhopadhyay A. The use of the Rusch balloon for management of severe postpartum haemorrhage *J Obstet Gynaecol* 2006; 26(4): 335–338.
97 Akhter S, Begum MR, Kabir Z, Rashid M, Laila TR, Zabeen F Use of a condom to control massive postpartum hemorrhage. *MedGenMed* 2003; 5(3): 38.
98 Bowen LW, Beeson JH. Use of a large Foley catheter balloon to control postpartum hemorrhage resulting from a low placental implantation. A report of two cases. *J Reprod Med* 1985; 30(8): 623–625.
99 Ferrazzani S, Guariglia L, Caruso A. Therapy and prevention of obstetric hemorrhage by tamponade using a balloon catheter. *Minerva Ginecol* 2004; 56(5): 481–484.
100 B-Lynch C, Coker A, Lawal AH, Abu J, Cowen MJ. The B-Lynch surgical technique for the control of massive postpartum haemorrhage: an alternative to hysterectomy? Five cases reported. *Br J Obstet Gynaecol* 1997; 104: 372–375.
101 Hayman RG, Arulkumaran S, Steer PJ. Uterine compression sutures: surgical management of postpartum hemorrhage. *Obstet Gynecol* 2002; 99(3): 502–506.
102 Cho JH, Jun HS, Lee CN. Hemostatic suturing technique for uterine bleeding during cesarean delivery. *Obstet Gynecol* 2000; 96(1): 129–131.
103 Smith KL, Baskett TF. Uterine compression sutures as an alternative to hysterectomy for severe postpartum hemorrhage. *J Obstet Gynaecol Can* 2003; 25: 197–200.
104 Holtsema H, Nijland R, Huisman A, Dony J, van den Berg PP. The B-Lynch technique for postpartum haemorrhage: an option for

every gynaecologist. *Eur J Obstet Gynecol Reprod Biol* 2004; 115: 39–42.

105 Pal M, Biswas AK, Bhattacharya SM. B-Lynch brace suturing in primary post-partum hemorrhage during caesarean section. *J Obstet Gynaecol Res* 2003; 29: 317–320.

106 Ferguson JE II, Bourgeois FJ, Underwood PB Jr. B-Lynch suture for postpartum hemorrhage. *Obstet Gynecol* 2000; 95: 1020–1022.

107 Habek D, Kulas T, Bobi-Vukovi M, Selthofer R, Vuji B, Ugljarevi M. Successful of the B-Lynch compression suture in the management of massive postpartum hemorrhage: case reports and review. *Arch Gynecol Obstet* 2006; 273(5): 307–309.

108 Ochoa M, Allaire AD, Stitely ML. Pyometria after hemostatic square suture technique. *Obstet Gynecol* 2002; 99(3): 506–509.

109 Tamizian O, Arulkumaran S. The surgical management of postpartum haemorrhage. *Curr Opin Obstet Gynecol* 2001; 13: 127–131.

110 Dildy GA 3rd. Postpartum hemorrhage: new management options. *Clin Obstet Gynecol* 2002; 45(2): 330–344.

111 O'Leary JL, O'Leary JA. Uterine artery ligation for control of postcesarean section hemorrhage. *Obstet Gynecol* 1974; 43: 849–853.

112 O'Leary JA. Uterine artery ligation in the control of postcesarean hemorrhage. *J Reprod Med* 1995; 40: 1899–1893.

113 AbdRabbo SA. Stepwise uterine devascularisation: a novel technique for management of uncontrollable postpartum hemorrhage with preservation of the uterus. *Am J Obstet Gynecol* 1994; 171: 694–700.

114 Hebisch G, Huch A. Vaginal uterine artery ligation avoids high blood loss and puerperal hysterectomy in postpartum hemorrhage. *Obstet Gynecol* 2002; 100: 574–578.

115 Burchell RC. Arterial physiology of the human pelvis. *Obstet Gynecol* 1968; 31: 855–860.

116 Burchell RC. Internal iliac artery ligation: hemodynamics. *Obstet Gynecol* 1964; 24: 737–739.

117 Burchell RC, Olson G. Internal iliac artery ligation: aortograms. *Am J Obstet Gynecol* 1966; 94: 117–124.

118 Chitrit Y, Guillaumin D, Caubel P, Herrero R. Absence of flow velocity waveform changes in uterine arteries after bilateral internal iliac ligation. *Am J Obstet Gynecol* 2000; 182: 727–728.

119 Clark SL, Phelan JP, Yeh S-Y, Bruce SR, Paul RH. Hypogastric artery ligation for obstetric haemorrhage. *Obstet Gynecol* 1985; 66: 353–356.

120 Vedantham S, Goodwin SC, McLucas B, Mohr G. Uterine artery embolization: an underused method of controlling pelvic hemorrhage. *Am J Obstet Gynecol* 1997; 176: 938–948.

121 Hansch E, Chitkara U, McAlpine J, El-Sayed Y, Dake MD, Razavi MK. Pelvic arterial embolisation for control of obstetric hemorrhage: a five year experience. *Am J Obstet Gynecol* 1999; 180: 1454–1460.

122 Pelage JP, Le Dref O, Mateo J, et al. Life-threatening primary postpartum hemorrhage: treatment with emergency selective arterial embolization. *Radiology* 1998; 208: 359–362.

123 Pelage JP, Soyer P, Repiquet D, et al. Secondary postpartum haemorrhage: treatment with selective arterial embolisation. *Radiology* 1999; 212: 385–389.

124 Alanis M, Hurst BS, Marshburn PB, Matthews ML. Conservative management of placenta increta with selective arterial embolization preserves future fertility and results in a favorable outcome in subsequent pregnancies. *Fertil Steril* 2006; 86(5): 1514.

125 Soncini E, Pelicelli A, Larini P, Marcato C, Monaco D, Grignaffini A. Uterine artery embolization in the treatment and prevention of postpartum hemorrhage. *Int J Gynaecol Obstet* 2007; 96(3): 181–185.

126 Kayem G, Pannier E, Goffinet F, Grangé G, Cabrol D. Fertility after conservative treatment of placenta accreta. *Fertil Steril* 2002; 78(3): 637–638.

127 Clement D, Kayem G, Cabrol D. Conservative treatment of placenta percreta: a safe alternative. *Eur J Obstet Gynecol Reprod Biol* 2004; 114: 108–109.

128 Clark SL, Koonings PP, Phelan JP. Placenta previa/accreta and prior cesarean section. *Obstet Gynecol* 1985; 66: 89–92.

129 Ornan D, White R, Pollak J, Tal M. Pelvic embolization for intractable post partum hemorrhage: long term follow up and implications for fertility. *Obstet Gynecol* 2003; 102: 904 910.

130 Shrivastava V, Nageotte M, Major C, Hayden M, Wing D. Case control comparison of cesarean hysterectomy with and without prophylactic placement of intravascular balloon catheters for placenta accreta. *Am J Obstet Gynecol* 2007; 197(4): 402.

131 Clark SL, Yeh S-Y, Phelan JP, Bruce S, Paul RH. Emergency hysterectomy for obstetric hemorrhage. *Obstet Gynecol* 1984; 64: 376–380.

132 Ledee N, Ville Y, Musset D, Mercier F, Frydman R, Fernandez H. Management in intractable obstetric haemorrhage: an audit study on 61 cases. *Eur J Obstet Gynecol Rep Biol* 2001; 94: 189–196.

133 Lau WC, Fung HYM, Rogers MS. Ten years experience of caesarean and postpartum hysterectomy in a teaching hospital in Hong Kong. *Eur J Obstet Gynecol Reprod Biol* 1997; 74: 133–137.

134 Ihab M, Usta EM, Hobeika AA, et al. Placenta previa-accreta: risk factors and complications. *Int J Gynaecol Obstet* 2006; 93(2): 160–163.

135 Catanzarite VA, Mehalek KE, Wachtel T, Westbrook C. 1996) Sonographic diagnosis of traumatic and later recurrent uterine rupture. *Am J Perinatol* 1996 Apr; 13(3): 177–180.

136 Hoffman-Tretin JC, Koenigsberg M, Rabin A, Anyaegbunam A. Placenta accreta. Additional sonographic observations. *J Ultrasound Med* 1992; 11(1): 29–34.

137 Hudon L, Belfort MA, Broome DR. Diagnosis and management of placenta percreta: a review. *Obstet Gynecol Surv* 1998; 53(8): 509–517.

138 Burrows RF, Kelton JG. Thrombocytopenia at delivery: a prospective survey of 6715 deliveries. *Am J Obstet Gynecol* 1990; 162: 731–734.

139 Crowther MA, Burrows RF, Ginsberg J, Kelton JG. Thrombocytopenia in pregnancy: diagnosis, pathogenesis and management. *Blood Rev* 1996; 10: 8–16.

140 Burrows RF, Kelton JG. Pregnancy in patients with idiopathic thrombocytopenic purpura: assessing the risks for the infant at delivery. *Obstet Gynecol Surv* 1993; 48: 781–788.

141 Silver RM. Management of idiopathic thrombocytopenic purpura in pregnancy. *Clin Obstet Gynecol* 1998; 41: 436–448.

142 George JN, Woolf SH, Raskob GE, et al. Idiopathic thrombocytopenic purpura: a practice guideline developed by explicit methods for The American Society of Hematology. *Blood* 1996; 88: 3–40.

143 Michel M, Novoa M, Bussel J. Intravenous anti-D as a treatment for immune thrombocytopenic purpura (ITP) during pregnancy. *Br J Haematol* 2003; 123: 142–146.

144 Sieunarine K, Shapiro S, Al Obaidi MJ, Girling J. Intravenous anti-D immunoglobulin in the treatment of resistant immune thrombocytopenic purpura in pregnancy. *Br J Obstet Gynaecol* 2007; 114(4): 505–507.

145 Economides DL, Kadir RA, Lee CA. Inherited bleeding disorders in obstetrics and gynaecology. *Br J Obstet Gynaecol* 1999; 106: 5–13.

146 Kouides PA, Phatak PD, Burkart P, et al. Gynaecological and obstetrical morbidity in women with type I von Willebrand disease: results of a patient survey. *Haemophilia* 2000; 6: 643–648.

147 Kirtava A, Drews C, Lally C, et al. Medical, reproductive and psychosocial experiences of women diagnosed with von Willebrand's disease receiving care in haemophilia treatment centres: a case–control study. *Haemophilia* 2003; 9: 292–297.

148 Kadir RA, Lee CA, Sabin CA, Pollard D, Economides DL. Pregnancy in women with von Willebrand's disease or factor XI deficiency. *Br J Obstet Gynaecol* 1998; 105: 314–321.

149 Kadir RA. Women and inherited bleeding disorders: pregnancy and delivery. *Semin Hematol* 1999; 36: 28–35.

150 Gardella C, Taylor M, Benedetti T, et al. The effect of sequential use of vacuum and forceps for assisted vaginal delivery on neonatal and maternal outcomes. *Am J Obstet Gynecol* 2001; 185: 896–902.

151 Mannucci PM. How I treat patients with von Willebrand disease. *Blood* 2001; 97: 1915–1919.

152 Ray JG. DDAVP use during pregnancy: an analysis of its safety for mother and child. *Obstet Gynecol Surv* 1998; 53: 450–455.

153 Chediak JR, Alban GM, Maxey B. von Willebrand's disease and pregnancy: management during delivery and outcome of offspring. *Am J Obstet Gynecol* 1986; 155: 618–624.

154 Walzman M, Bonnar J. Effects of tranexamic acid on the coagulation and fibrinolytic systems in pregnancy complicated by placental bleeding. *Arch Toxicol* 1982; 5(suppl): 214–220.

155 Lindoff C, Rybo G, Astedt B. Treatment with tranexamic acid during pregnancy, and the risk of thrombo-embolic complications. *Thromb Haemost* 1993; 70: 238–240.

156 Roque H, Funai E, Lockwood CJ. von Willebrand disease and pregnancy. *J Matern Fetal Med* 2000; 9: 257–266.

157 Kadir RA, Economides DL, Braithewaite J, Goldman E, Lee CA. The obstetric experience of carriers of haemophilia. *Br J Obstet Gynaecol* 1997; 104: 803–810.

158 Mannucci PM, Tuddenham EGDF. Medical progress: the hemophilias – from royal genes to gene therapy. *N Engl J Med* 2001; 344: 1773–1779.

159 Kulkarni R, Lusher JM. Intracranial and extracranial hemorrhages in newborns with hemophilia: a review of the literature. *J Pediatr Hematol Oncol* 1999; 21: 289–295.

160 Yang MY, Ragni MV. Clinical manifestations and management of labor and delivery in women with factor IX deficiency. *Haemophilia* 2004; 10(5): 483–490.

161 Shobeiri SA, West EC, Kahn MJ, Nolan TE. Postpartum acquired hemophilia (factor VIII inhibitors): a case report and review of the literature. *Obstet Gynecol Surv* 2000; 55: 729–737.

162 Collins P, Macartney N, Davies R, Lees S, Giddings J, Majer R. A population based, unselected, consecutive cohort of patients with acquired haemophilia A. *Br J Haematol* 2004; 124: 86–90.

163 Collins PW. Treatment of acquired hemophilia A. *J Thromb Haemost* 2007; 5(5): 893–900.

164 Solymoss S. Postpartum acquired factor VIII inhibitors: results of a survey. *Am J Hematol* 1998; 59: 1–4.

165 Kadir RA, Koh MB, Lee SA, Pasi KJ. Acquired haemophilia, an unusual cause of severe postpartum haemorrhage. *Br J Obstet Gynaecol* 1997; 104: 854–856.

166 Morrison AE, Ludlam CA, Kessler C. Use of porcine factor VIII in the treatment of patients with acquired hemophilia. *Blood* 1993; 81: 1513–1520.

167 Collins PW, Hirsch S, Baglin TP, et al., for the UK Haemophilia Centre Doctors' Organisation. Acquired haemophilia A in the UK: a two year national surveillance study by UK Haemophilia Centre Doctors Organisation. *Blood* 2007; 109: 1870–1877.

168 Hay CR, Negrier C, Ludlam CA. The treatment of bleeding in acquired haemophilia with recombinant factor VIIa: a multicentre study. *Thromb Haemost* 1997; 78: 1463–1467.

169 Mudad R, Kane WH. DDAVP in acquired hemophilia A: case report and review of the literature. *Am J Hematol* 1993; 43: 295–299.

170 Hoveyda F, MacKenzie IZ. Secondary postpartum haemorrhage: incidence, morbidity and current management. *Br J Obstet Gynaecol* 2001; 108: 927–930.

23 Severe Acute Asthma

Michael A. Belfort[1] & Melissa Herbst[2]

[1]Department of Obstetrics and Gynecology, Division of Maternal-Fetal Medicine, University of Utah School of Medicine, Salt Lake City, UT *and* HCA Healthcare, Nashville, TN, USA
[2]Maternal-Fetal Services of Utah, St. Mark's Hospital, Salt Lake City, UT, USA

Introduction

Asthma is one of the most frequent chronic illnesses encountered in pregnant patients. A recent report found that 9% of the US population reported a diagnosis of asthma at some point in their lifetime [1]. Four to eight per cent of pregnant women have a diagnosis of asthma [2,3]. The prevalence appears to be increasing as demonstrated by the 3% rise reported in the 1997–2001 US survey when compared to the previous survey [3]. With the continuing increase in the number of pregnant patients with asthma, it is important that providers understand the issues surrounding the care of these women during pregnancy.

Asthma is a chronic inflammatory disease of the airways that is manifested as a hyperresponsiveness of the airway to a wide variety of stimuli resulting in airway obstruction that is partially or completely reversible [4]. Most patients with asthma have the classic triad of symptoms: the simultaneous occurrence of cough, shortness of breath, and wheezing [5]. The pathophysiology of asthma is still not fully understood. However, it is known that asthma is a chronic inflammatory disorder of the airways resulting from inflammation causing episodes of wheezing, breathlessness, chest tightness, and cough [6]. A number of different cells are involved and include mast cells, eosinophils, and T lymphocytes. These all interact to increase airway sensitivity leading to inflammation and variable airflow limitation that is generally reversible with treatment [6].

Diagnosis

The diagnosis of asthma is considered in patients who present with episodic, reversible, occurrences of cough, wheeze, dyspnea, hyperventilation or combination of the above [5,7]. As the symptoms are often non-specific in nature, the role of a history, physical, and laboratory evaluation are important to confirm the diagnosis. Patients often give a history of episodic events or symptoms which can be related to exposure to specific triggers. These triggers include allergens, upper respiratory tract infections, medications (such as aspirin and β–blockers), environmental pollutants, occupational exposures (chlorine-based cleaning products), exercise, cold air, emotional stress, and gastroesophageal reflux [8,9]. On physical exam during these events, widespread high-pitched, musical wheezes occurring at various points in the respiratory cycle are characteristic but not specific [5]. These wheezes are often quickly resolved with the use of β-agonists. While the history and physical examination can identify patients with asthma in the majority of cases, it remains important that pulmonary function testing is performed so as to confirm the diagnosis and assist in the determination of management [5].

The mainstay of pulmonary function testing is spirometry. Spirometry allows the measurement of forced expiratory volume in one second (FEV_1) and forced vital capacity (FVC). FEV_1 is the most important in the assessment of airflow obstruction and its severity. This value is constructed based upon the percentage of the predicted forced expiration for that patient as determined by her demographic characteristics. While such testing is important in the initial evaluation, it is impractical for continued management due to logistic constraints. Peak expiratory flow rate (PEFR) however can easily be obtained through a peak flow meter. It is measured during a maximal exhalation that has immediately followed a maximal inhalation [5]. This measurement correlates well with FEV_1. The peak flow meter is easy to use, inexpensive, disposable and portable making it ideal for the determination of severity, therapy response, and for monitoring disease course [10]. It is important to note however that PEFR does have limitations. These include its dependence upon effort and proper technique, making consistent observation and monitoring of technique essential [11–13]. A chest X-ray should be considered to exclude other causes of respiratory difficulty [5]. Once the diagnosis of asthma is made, the same information used to determine the diagnosis can be utilized to determine severity.

Critical Care Obstetrics, 5th edition. Edited by M. Belfort, G. Saade, M. Foley, J. Phelan and G. Dildy.

Table 23.1 Definition of asthma severity.*

Severity classification	Symptoms (A: daytime/B: night-time)	Exacerbations	Lung function testing
Mild intermittent	A: ≤Two times per week B: ≤Two times a month	Brief (lasting 1 hour to a few days) Intensity varies	FEV_1 or PEFR ≥80% predicted PEFR day-to-day variability <20%
Mild persistent	A: ≥Two times per week but not daily B: >Two times per month	Brief (lasting 1 hour to a few days) May affect activity	FEV_1 or PEFR ≥80% predicted PEFR day-to-day variability 20–30%
Moderate persistent	A: Daily B: >Once/week	≥Two times/week and may last days Affects activity	FEV_1 or PEFR >60 but <80% predicted PEFR day-to-day variability >30%
Severe persistent	A/B: Continual	Frequent Limits physical activity	FEV_1 or PEFR ≤60% predicted PEFR day-to-day variability >30%

* From the National Institutes of Health [14].
FEV_1, forced expiratory volume in one second.
PEFR, peak expiratory flow rate.

The classification of asthma severity is important for the choice of therapy as well as for patient monitoring. The classification is based upon diagnostic criteria: symptoms, occurrences, and FEV_1/PEFR. In their 2004 report the National Asthma Education and Prevention Program (NAEPP) Working Group on Asthma in Pregnancy proposed the following classification for asthma in pregnancy: mild intermittent, mild persistent, moderate persistent, and severe persistent [14] (Table 23.1). Patients can be reclassified up or down based upon repeat evaluation and their therapy can be modified accordingly.

Respiratory changes in pregnancy

Pregnancy causes both physical and functional changes which can affect symptoms and influence therapy. Physical changes occur at the macroscopic and microscopic level. Starting in the first trimester, the subcostal angle changes from 68° to as much as 108° [15,16]. The diaphragm may rise up to 4 cm and there may be an increase in chest diameter of 2 cm or more as pregnancy progresses [17]. Diaphragmatic excursion increases up to 2 cm which results in a more barrel-chested appearance [17]. Histologic examination performed by Toppozado et al. showed that the upper respiratory mucosa of pregnant patients demonstrated hyperemia, glandular hyperactivity, increased phagocytic activity and increased mucopolysaccharide content [18]. Such changes are likely due to the increase in estrogen levels and lead to symptomatic nasal stuffiness and more common epistaxis [19]. These physical changes, along with other pregnancy adaptations, lead to many functional respiratory changes. With diaphragmatic elevation, there is a progressive 20% decrease in functional residual capacity along with decreases in expiratory reserve, residual volume, and functional reserve capacity [7,20,21] (Figure 23.1). However, because diaphragmatic function is unchanged, there is no change in forced vital capacity [10] (Figure 23.1). There is a 20% increase in oxygen consumption, and a 15% increase in metabolic rate achieved through a 40–50% increase is resting minute ventilation. This increase in minute ventilation is due to an increase in tidal volume rather than a change in respiratory rate which is unchanged. This hyperventilation increases arterial oxygen tension and decreases carbon dioxide tension. This mild respiratory alkalosis leads to a compensatory decrease in sodium bicarbonate as the kidneys maintain acid–base balance [7]. The normal values of an arterial blood gas are altered in pregnancy (see Table 23.2). Normal values for FEV_1 and PEFR remain unchanged in pregnancy since there are no changes in airway mechanics; therefore most people accept that the standard ranges used outside of pregnancy can be used during pregnancy for management decisions [22,10]. One study did suggest that PEFR and FEV_1 are lower in pregnancy in the supine position as compared to seated, and therefore, it is recommended that patients are positioned in as close to a seated position as possible during acute attacks [23]. Others have found that hypoxemia may be exacerbated during an acute attack due to the decrease in functional residual capacity [24]. Lastly, evaluation of arterial blood gases during an acute asthma attack must be done bearing in mind the underlying respiratory alkalosis.

Table 23.2 Arterial blood gas values in pregnant and non-pregnant patients.

	Non-pregnant	Pregnant
pH	7.38–7.42	7.40–7.45
PaO_2 (mmHg)	90–100	104–108
$PaCO_2$ (mmHg)	35–45	27–32
HCO_3 (mEq/L)	22–26	18–31

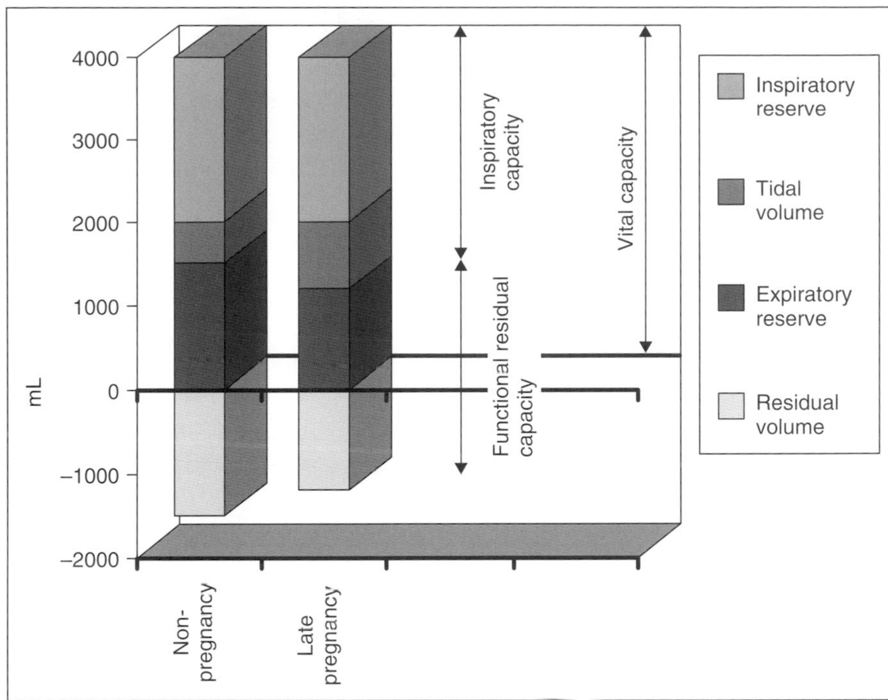

Figure 23.1 Lung volumes.

Table 23.3 Exacerbation and hospitalization rates in pregnancy based upon severity in a large prospective observation cohort study.*

	Mild asthma	Moderate asthma	Severe asthma
Asthma exacerbation rate (%)	12.6	25.7	51.9
Asthma hospitalization rate (%)	2.3	6.8	26.9

* From Dombrowski MP et al. [1].

Effect of pregnancy on asthma

The classic statement in regards to the impact of pregnancy on asthma is the one-third rule: one-third improve, one-third worsen, and one-third remain unchanged. This generality is supported by several recent studies [25,1]. Dombrowski et al. have the most detailed information in their recent prospective study where the asthma group was subdivided by severity [1]. They found that in general 23% improved, 30.3% worsened and 46.7% remained unchanged [1]. It was also noted that as severity increased so did the rate of exacerbation and need for hospitalization [1] (Table 23.3). Exacerbations are most frequent from 17–24 weeks, and appear to be less severe during the last 4 weeks of pregnancy [26–31].

Effect of asthma on pregnancy

The effect of asthma on pregnancy is an area of ongoing debate with some studies showing little to no impact, and others suggesting significant risk.

Early studies evaluating the impact of asthma on pregnancy outcome showed significant adverse effect. The majority of these papers were retrospective, and were based on birth certificate data [32,33]. Patients were classified according to the presence or absence of the diagnostic code for asthma and not on the severity of the asthma. These studies showed an increased risk of preterm birth, low birth weight, pregnancy-induced hypertension, pre-eclampsia, hemorrhage, perinatal mortality and congenital malformations in patients with asthma [2,27,32,34,35]. The findings were supported by Liu et al [36]. in a retrospective cohort study which employed an administrative database with over 2000 asthma patients and 8000 controls. These authors also found an increased risk of preterm labor, pregnancy-induced hypertension, small for gestational age, abruption, chorioamniotis, and cesarean delivery in patients with asthma [36]. Demissie et al. [33] in their case–control study, controlled for confounding factors such as age, education, parity, race, diabetes, hypertension, cigarette use, alcohol and drug use. They also showed an increase in the risk of preterm birth, small for gestation, pregnancy-induced hypertension, previa, congenital anomalies, and cesarean delivery in patients with asthma [33]. While these studies all demonstrated increased risk of perinatal complications in patients with asthma, none controlled for the severity of asthma or possible impact of the medications used as treatment.

More recently, several studies have been specifically designed to address the impact of asthma severity and medication use on pregnancy outcome. In Kallen's population study [37], patients were subdivided into those without asthma, those with asthma of any severity, and those with severe asthma. Patients with asthma

Table 23.4 Odds ration (95% CI) for pregnancy outcomes in patients with asthma versus control in a large population-based study.*

Outcome	All subjects with asthma (n = 36 985)	Severe asthma (n = 1396)
Perinatal mortality	1.21 (1.08–1.35)	1.28 (0.76–2.17)
Pre-eclampsia	1.15 (1.08–1.23)	1.42 (1.09–1.86)
Preterm birth (<37 weeks)	1.15 (1.09–1.21)	1.56 (1.27–1.90)
Low birth weight (<2500 g)	1.21 (1.14–1.29)	1.98 (1.52–2.59)
Congenital malformations	1.05 (0.99–1.10)	1.08 (0.83–1.4)

* From Kallen B, Rydhstroem H, Aberg A [37].

of any severity showed an increase in risk of 15–20% for pre-eclampsia, preterm delivery and low birth weight. This risk was higher (30–100% increase) in those with severe disease [37] (Table 23.4). This study is limited by its retrospective nature and the impact of medication use was not addressed. Perlow et al. [38] addressed the impact of steroid use in a retrospective case–control study. Patients with asthma were subdivided based upon the use of long-term steroids. All patients with asthma were found to have an increased risk of cesarean delivery for fetal distress, and for preterm delivery <37 weeks when compared with controls [38]. Among oral steroid-dependent asthmatics, there was a significant increase in the risk of gestational diabetes and low birth weight [38]. Dombrowski et al. published a prospective observational cohort study in 2004 in which they used the NAEEP Working group on Asthma in Pregnancy definitions for mild, moderate and severe asthma. Over 800 patients were included in each of the groups (control, mild, and moderate to severe asthma) and the patients were followed through pregnancy with monthly visits. No difference was found in antepartum, delivery, or postpartum outcomes including preterm delivery less than 32 or less than 37 weeks in patients with any form of asthma [1]. There was an increase in cesarean delivery in patients with moderate to severe asthma [1]. When only severe asthmatics were evaluated, an increased risk of gestational diabetes and preterm delivery prior to 37 weeks was found. However, the study was not designed to control for steroid use [1].

Thus, despite multiple studies and a tremendous amount of published information, there continues to be controversy regarding the extent of the impact of asthma on pregnancy. There are data suggesting that asthma can be associated with increased risk of pre-eclampsia, pregnancy induced hypertension and preterm birth [27]. and asthma severity has clearly been shown to have an impact on the complication risk in pregnancy [28,30,33,34,38–41]. However, in those studies where asthma was prospectively managed and controlled, such risks were minimized [4,39,41–47]. It remains unclear as to whether these risks are the result of maternal hypoxia and hypocapnia secondary to medication use, or whether they are the result of a fundamental abnormality of smooth muscle in asthmatics which manifests as increased tone in the uterus, airways, and vasculature [48]. While asthma may be associated with significant risk in some (but not all) cases, it does appear that close observation and aggressive management of moderate to severe asthma can result in improved pregnancy outcome.

Management

Prepregnancy

As asthma severity and degree of control clearly impact pregnancy outcome, the optimization of care prior to pregnancy is of great importance. In this regard, given the importance of home monitoring in the management of these cases, review of the appropriate operation of a peak flow meter and the recording of peak expiratory flow rates will be of benefit to the patient. This information should be evaluated regularly and therapy optimized prior to conception. Patients need to be educated on the importance of continuing all medications once pregnancy is achieved to avoid exacerbation of their asthma.

Pregnancy

As discussed above, it is important to maintain tight asthma control to decrease the risk of pregnancy complications. To this end, some discussion of the patient's asthma control should be documented at each prenatal visit. It is important to educate the pregnant patient at the first visit that well controlled asthmatics have little increased risk, yet poor control may significantly increase risk to both mother and fetus [49]. Hence, more critical evaluation of symptoms and reliable objective measurement of pulmonary function by PEFR assessment are vital. As PEFR does not change in pregnancy (typically 380–550 L/min), it can continue to be used to monitor lung function, and to separate asthma-associated dyspnea from pregnancy-associated dyspnea (which does not alter the PEFR). Patients should be asked to perform twice daily (on awakening and at midday) PEFR measurements and record these values for review at each prenatal visit. During these visits, it is recommended that providers verify proper peak flow meter and inhaler use, as well as review asthma management plans with a flexible approach to making adjustments when necessary. Due to the risk of growth restriction, especially in those requiring oral steroids, routine ultrasound should be performed, and antenatal testing should be considered at all levels of severity, but especially in those with severe asthma or recent exacerbation. The NAEEP Working group on Asthma in Pregnancy emphasizes the following five aspects of care:

1 objective evaluation of maternal/fetal condition
2 avoidance/control of triggers such as smoke, dust and pollutants
3 pharmacological treatment
4 educational support, especially with regard to early recognition of symptoms
5 psychological support.

Medications

Prior to discussing therapy recommendations, it may be useful to review the potential impact of asthma medications on pregnancy. In general, it is recommended that patients remain on the same drugs and dosages that are used outside of pregnancy. Inhaled agents are preferred over oral agents to reduce systemic effects and minimize any possible fetal effects [32,50,51].

Medications for asthma are divided into two types: (i) rescue (those used to treat acute bronchospasm and give symptomatic relief without treating the underlying cause of the bronchospasm) and (ii) maintenance (those that help control airway hyperreactivity and treat the underlying inflammation).

Rescue medications

Short-acting β-agonists

These drugs are key to asthma management. Short-acting β-agonists include metaproteronol (Alupent®), terbutaline (Brethine®), and albuterol (Ventolin®, Proventil®). These inhalation agents are good for acute and mild intermittent asthma, as they have a rapid onset resulting in maximum bronchodilation with minimal side effects [52,53]. Side effects of these drugs include tremulousness, palpitations and/or anxiety. However, such side effects can be minimized by the use of a spacer and mouth rinsing after inhalation [54]. Studies have shown no association between short-acting β-agonist use and increased risk of congenital malformations or adverse pregnancy outcome [34,55,56].

Long-acting β–agonists

While much has been published on the short-acting β-agonists, less is known with regard to long-acting β-agonists. These agents include salmeterol (Screvent discus®) and formoterol (Foradil®). Long-acting β-agonists are commonly used as add-on therapy for those not controlled with inhaled steroids [39]. There are currently few data addressing safety in humans, and animal studies have not been particularly reasurring [39]. Of the two drugs, salmeterol appears more promising than formoterol [39]. Currently, consensus recommendations support the use of long-acting β-agonists in patients with moderate to severe asthma who demonstrate a good response to these agents in their prepregnancy state, or as an add-on therapy in patients already using inhaled steroids and who need additional therapy [39].

Anticholinergics

The main anticholinergic drug used in asthma therapy is ipratropium (Atrovent®) which, in its nebulized form, has shown synergistic bronchodilator effect when added to inhaled β-agonists [57,58]. Despite the facts that both animal and human studies have shown negligible adverse effects on the fetus, and that these drugs are felt to be safe, they are not being used widely [59,60]. Anticholinergic use may be appropriate as additional therapy in cases of acute asthma that do not improve significantly after an initial β-agonist treatment [39]. Atropine, a well known anticholinergic, is known to cause significant fetal tachycardia when used systemically and is therefore not recommended [59,60].

Maintenance

Methylxanthines

The most commonly used methylxanthine in pregnant women is theophylline, which is traditionally employed as an add-on therapy to inhaled steroids in patients with moderate persistent asthma [39]. A number of studies have confirmed that this agent is not associated with an increased risk of congenital malformations or poor perinatal outcomes [34,39]. However, theophylline has a narrow range between the therapeutic and toxic concentrations and use of this drug requires close monitoring of serum levels. This situation is made more compelling in pregnancy due to the decreased albumin binding noted in pregnant women and this increases the proportion of free drug in the circulation. With more drug available for metabolism, the total level (free plus bound) falls [61]. To complicate matters more, the clearance of theophylline is reduced by 20% in the third trimester [34,39,62]. Taking the physiologic changes of pregnancy into account, it is recommended that target levels be adjusted in pregnant women to 8–12 mcg/mL instead of the 10–15 used outside of pregnancy [61]. Monitoring of maternal blood levels is not only important for the mother's health, but is similarly important for fetal health. Theophylline crosses the placenta and leads to fetal tachycardia, as well as neonatal irritability, jitteriness, and vomiting if the level is elevated [63,64].

Cromolyn sodium

Cromolyn sodium is a mast cell stabilizer/inhaled non-steroidal agent. It blocks both early- and late-phase pulmonary responses to an allergen challenge, and also prevents the development of airway hyperresponsiveness [65]. It is effective when taken prior to exposure but does not relieve symptoms once they have occurred [39]. Cromolyn sodium is effective in mild intermittent asthma in combination with short-acting β-agonists [54]. There is no increased risk of fetal malformation or poor pregnancy outcome, and this drug should be continued during pregnancy if it has been shown to be effective outside of pregnancy [34,39]. However, since it is not as effective as steroid therapy, cromolyn sodium should not be a first-line agent for managing asthma in pregnancy [34].

Inhaled corticosteroids

Inhaled corticosteroids are considered the mainstay of treatment for persistent asthma [34,54]. Budesonide (Pulmicort®) and beclomethasone (Qvar®) are the two agents with the most data available regarding use during pregnancy [34,60]. Studies have shown that the use of these inhaled steroids in standard doses is not associated with malformations, fetal growth restriction, stillbirth, or fetal mortality [34,39]. However when used in high doses, greater than 1000–1500 mcg/day, systemic effects such as increased intraocular pressure, cataracts, bone loss, growth restriction, and hypothalamic–pituitary–adrenal (HPA) suppression have been reported [54]. Other medications in this group, including triamcinolone (Azmacort®), glunisolide, or fluticasone (Flovent®), are less well studied regarding safety of use in pregnancy. Despite this, most agree that it is not unreasonable to continue their use in patients who are well controlled on the medication prior to becoming pregnant [34,39]. Regardless of the medication used, oral candidiasis (thrush) is a recognized side effect which can be significantly decreased by oral rinsing after inhalation or by using a spacer which maximizes the delivery to the bronchi while minimizing oropharyngeal deposition.

Systemic corticosteroids

In contrast to the low incidence of risk with inhaled corticosteroids, systemic corticosteroid use is associated with definite pregnancy complications. Studies have consistently shown that systemic steroids increases the risk of low birth weight, preterm delivery, pregnancy-induced hypertension, pre-eclampsia, and gestational diabetes [31,37–39,56,66–71]. Some, but not all, studies have reported an association with antepartum and postpartum hemorrhage, and an increased rate of infection [31,34]. One of the most controversial findings is that of the impact of systemic steroid use on the rate of fetal malformation. Early studies found a significantly increased risk of cleft lip and palate when these drugs were taken during pregnancy [69]. However, this study did not classify the outcomes according to the trimester of exposure. In large case control trials stratified by trimester of exposure, a 0.2–0.3-fold increase (20–30%) risk of oral clefting was seen in patients who had experienced first-trimester exposure [39,69,72,73]. This was not confirmed however in a large case control trial [74] in which exposure was stratified by gestational month of exposure. In this study, there was no association with increased risk when steroids were taken during the second and third months of pregnancy [74]. Despite the potential for a small increase in fetal risk, it has been the recommendation of at least two working groups (ACOG and NAEPP) that if oral steroids are needed to control severe asthma, the benefits of using these medications during pregnancy may outweigh the risks. The same two Working Groups also recommend the use of oral steroids for long-term management of patients with severe asthma and in those women with severe asthma who experience exacerbations during pregnancy [14,39].

Leukotriene modifiers

Leukotrienes are potent chemical mediators of the allergic response in asthma. They stimulate bronchoconstriction and mucus hypersecretion, and promote microvascular leakage, edema formation, and eosinophil chemoattraction. Medications which modify and diminish the effects of leukotrienes have been found to allow better asthma control. This class of drugs (leaukotriene modifiers) includes zileuton (Zylfo®), zafirlukast (Accolade®), and montelukast (Singulair®). While few data are available regarding their use in pregnancy, the Human Merck Registry has not shown any increased risk of malformation [39,75]. There are animal studies on zileuton which have suggested a teratologic effect, but zafirlukast showed no teratogenicity at oral doses 160 times greater than the maximum human dose [39,60]. Current ACOG guidelines suggest that any leukotriene modifier except zileuton can be used in pregnant patients who require this class of drug because of resistance to other medications [34].

Combination drugs

These include Advair Discus® and Combivent®. Advair® is a combination of salmeterol, a long-acting β-agonist, and fluticasone, an inhaled steroid. Combivent® is composed of albuterol, a short-acting β-agonist, and ipratropium, an anticholinergic agent. The individual drugs have been discussed in detail above. Current recommendations are for these medications to be continued in patients who are well controlled on them. However, since each combination medication contains at least one component for which few pregnancy data are available, such drugs should only be initiated in pregnancy if benefits outweigh the risk.

Immunotherapy

Allergen immunotherapy can be helpful in those patients whose specific allergy triggers are known, and whose symptoms persist despite optimal avoidance of triggers, and appropriate drug therapy. While there has never been a direct association seen between immunotherapy and poor pregnancy outcome, the risk of a systemic reaction with first-time exposure remains a significant risk [76]. Thus, for those who began therapy prior to pregnancy, who clearly benefit from such treatment, and who have no reaction on a maintenance dose, most authorities would support continuance of the therapy [59,76]. Some authors have recommended that doses should be significantly reduced to avoid a systemic reaction, but this advice is not uniformly supported [77]. It is not currently recommended for patients to initiate immunotherapy during pregnancy because of the above-mentioned potential for systemic reaction [78].

Other medications

The influenza vaccination is recommended for all pregnant patients and especially so in those with respiratory disease. All patients who will be pregnant between October through May should received the inactivated injectable influenza vaccine. The intranasal form is a live virus form and therefore should not be administered in pregnancy [14].

Allergic rhinitis is a common upper respiratory disorder and can induce an asthma exacerbation. Intranasal steroids such as loratadine (Claritin®) and cetirizine (Zyrtec®) are effective treatment for this and have no known impact on pregnancy. While decongestant use is common in pregnancy secondary to nasal hyperemia, inhaled decongestants and steroids are recommended over the oral forms of decongestant since the latter have been associated with gastroschisis when used in the first trimester [74].

Pregnancy-induced hypertension is commonly seen in pregnancy and the incidence appears to be slightly increased in patients with asthma. In many cases the drug of choice for treat-

Table 23.5 Asthma treatment in pregnancy.[±]

Asthma severity	Recommended therapy*	Alternative therapy
Mild intermittent	No daily therapy needed β_2 agonist for symptoms	–
Mild persistent	Low-dose inhaled corticosteroid (budesonide preferred)	Cromolyn Leukotriene receptor antagonist Theophylline
Moderate persistent	Either: Low-dose inhaled corticosteroid and long-acting inhaled β_2 agonist or Medium-dose inhaled corticosteroid with or without long-acting β_2 agonist	Low-dose inhaled corticosteroid and theophylline or leukotriene receptor antagonist
Severe persistent	High-dose inhaled corticosteroid and long-acting inhaled β_2 agonist and oral steroid if needed	High-dose inhaled corticosteroid and theophylline

* Short-acting bronchodilator for all types: 2–4 puffs short-acting inhaled β_2 agonist as needed for symptoms q4–6°.
[±]From the National Institutes of Health [14].

ment is a β–blocker such as labetolol. While such a medication would ordinarily be contraindicated in patients with asthma, if this class of antihypertensive is deemed essential to control the hypertension, a risk/benefit evaluation should be undertaken.

Treatment

Treatment plans are essential in the care of asthmatic patients. They allow for patients to become more involved in their own care and assist in the formation of an action plan for use in the event of an asthma attack. Treatment recommendations are given for each type of asthma in Table 23.5. Initiation of care can either start at the level appropriate to the patient's severity and move up if not controlled, or start at a level above that suggested by severity in order to gain rapid control of the attack and then move down when stable for several weeks [59]. Action plans are based on the best PEFR that a patient has ever obtained. A commonly used action plan for an acute asthma attack is shown in Figure 23.2.

Patients with acute asthma who present to the emergency department require expeditious evaluation and care. Initial care is no different than in non-pregnant patients and includes oxygen, nebulized β-agonists, nebulized anticholiniergic drugs such as ipratropium, as well as oral and/or intravenous steroids as needed. Fetal evaluation should be performed if the baby is beyond 23–24 weeks and in those at lesser gestational age confirmation of heart beat should be documented. There should be a low threshold for admission, and guidelines for admission include a PEFR< 60% of their baseline, PO_2 <70 mmHg at sea level, PCO_2 >35 mmHg, heart rate >120 bpm, or a respiratory rate >22/min. It is important to remember that a PCO_2 > 40 mmHg in pregnancy suggests impending respiratory failure as normal levels are 27–32 mmHg, and thus such patients should be admitted to an ICU where immediate airway management and ventilation options are available. For those who do not respond to initial β-agonist therapy, an oral steroid burst is indicated regardless of severity. This is done by administrating 40–60 mg of oral prednisone per day for 1 week followed by a taper over 7–14 days.

Patients who require admission secondary to concern about potential respiratory failure(P_aCO_2 > 40 or PEFR < 25% of predicted) should be admitted to an intensive care unit and an intensivist should be consulted. When the fetus is beyond 23–24 weeks, continuous fetal heart rate monitoring is recommended. It is important to note that maternal hypercapnia could result in fetal respiratory acidosis and a shift in the fetal hemoglobin dissociation curve to the right. This limits the ability of fetal hemoglobin to bind oxygen. Because of this, the NAEPP Working Group recommends that patients should be intubated and ventilated if any of the following criteria are fulfilled:

1 Inability to maintain a P_aO_2 > 60 mmHg with 90% saturation despite supplemental oxygen.
2 Inability to maintain a P_aCO_2 < 40 mmHg.
3 Maternal exhaustion.
4 Worsening acidosis despite bronchodilator therapy (pH7.2–7.25).
5 Altered maternal consciousness.

An approach to the care of a pregnant patient presenting to an emergency room for an acute asthma attack is shown in Figure 23.3.

Delivery

Women with asthma do not require any alterations in the management of labor or mode of delivery based simply on their affliction. However, additional care is needed in order to avoid specific complications that can occur at the time of delivery. These patients should continue the same inhalation therapy during labor as they have been taking in the preceeding weeks [78,79]. Only patients who used oral corticosteroids in the 4 weeks prior to delivery require additional rescue dose steroid therapy, because

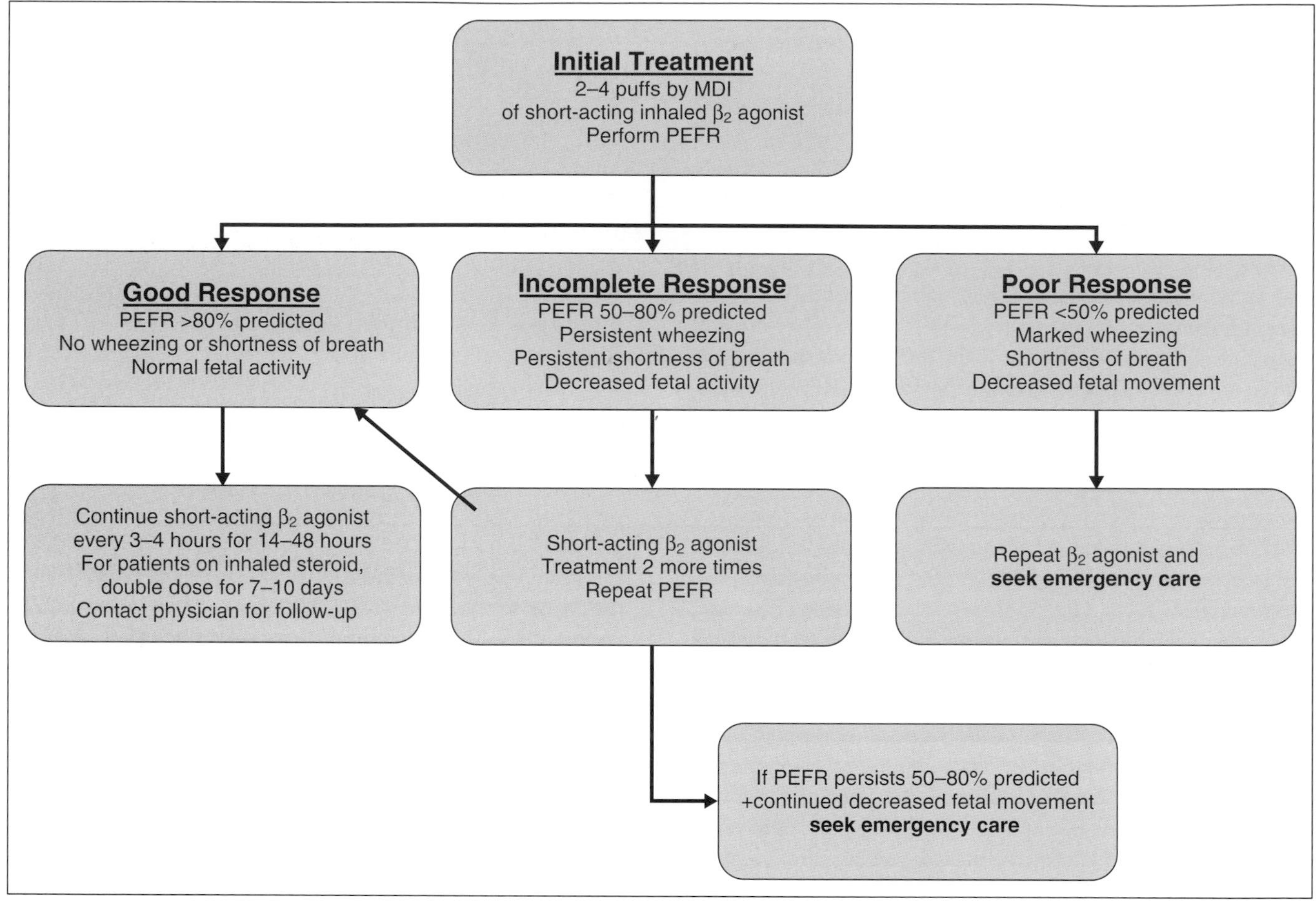

Figure 23.2 Home action plan in the management of acute asthma exacerbations. Reproduced from National Institutes of Health [14].

of potential hypothalamic–pituitary–adrenal axis (HPA) suppression. These patients should receive intravenous hydrocortisone (100 mg every 6–8 hours) during labor until either 24 hours after delivery or until oral medications are tolerated [80]. For labor induction and augmentation oxytocin and prostaglandin E_2 are safe [60,81]. While prostaglandin E_2 is a bronchodilator, prostaglandin $F_{2\alpha}$ is a bronchoconstrictor and therefore should not be used in these patients, even for severe postpartum hemorrhage unless the risk of death from bleeding outweighs the potential risk of precipitating a severe asthma attack [60,81–84]. Ergonovine and other ergots also cause bronchospasm and should also not be used if at all possible [81]. In the management of asthmatic patients with preterm labor, magnesium sulfate is safe (since it has bronchodilator effects). Indomethacin (Indocin®) can induce bronchospasm in aspirin-sensitive patients and therefore should be used with caution [10]. While pain management is strongly encouraged there are some drugs that should be avoided since they cause histamine release (morphine and meperidine). More appropriate alternatives include butorphanol and fentanyl [59,81]. For those who require general anesthesia, ketamine and halogenated anesthetics are preferred due to their bronchodilatory effect [59,81].

Anesthesia consultation is recommended at the time of admission for women with a history of moderate to severe asthma.

Postpartum

Following delivery, patients should continue their inhaled medications in the same dosage and route as they previously used. Those on oral steroids may require intravenous dosing as described above until oral medications are tolerated. Breastfeeding is not contraindicated in the presence of any of the medications used for the treatment of asthma since only small amounts of these drugs enter the breast milk [85]. However, in patients who use theophylline, there is the possibility that sensitive neonates can experience vomiting, jitteriness, tachycardia, and feeding difficulties, and the neonatologist should be aware of the maternal medication exposure history.

Summary

Patients with asthma can expect an uneventful pregnancy for the most part. It is important, however, for each patient to understand the impact of poorly controlled asthma on her pregnancy

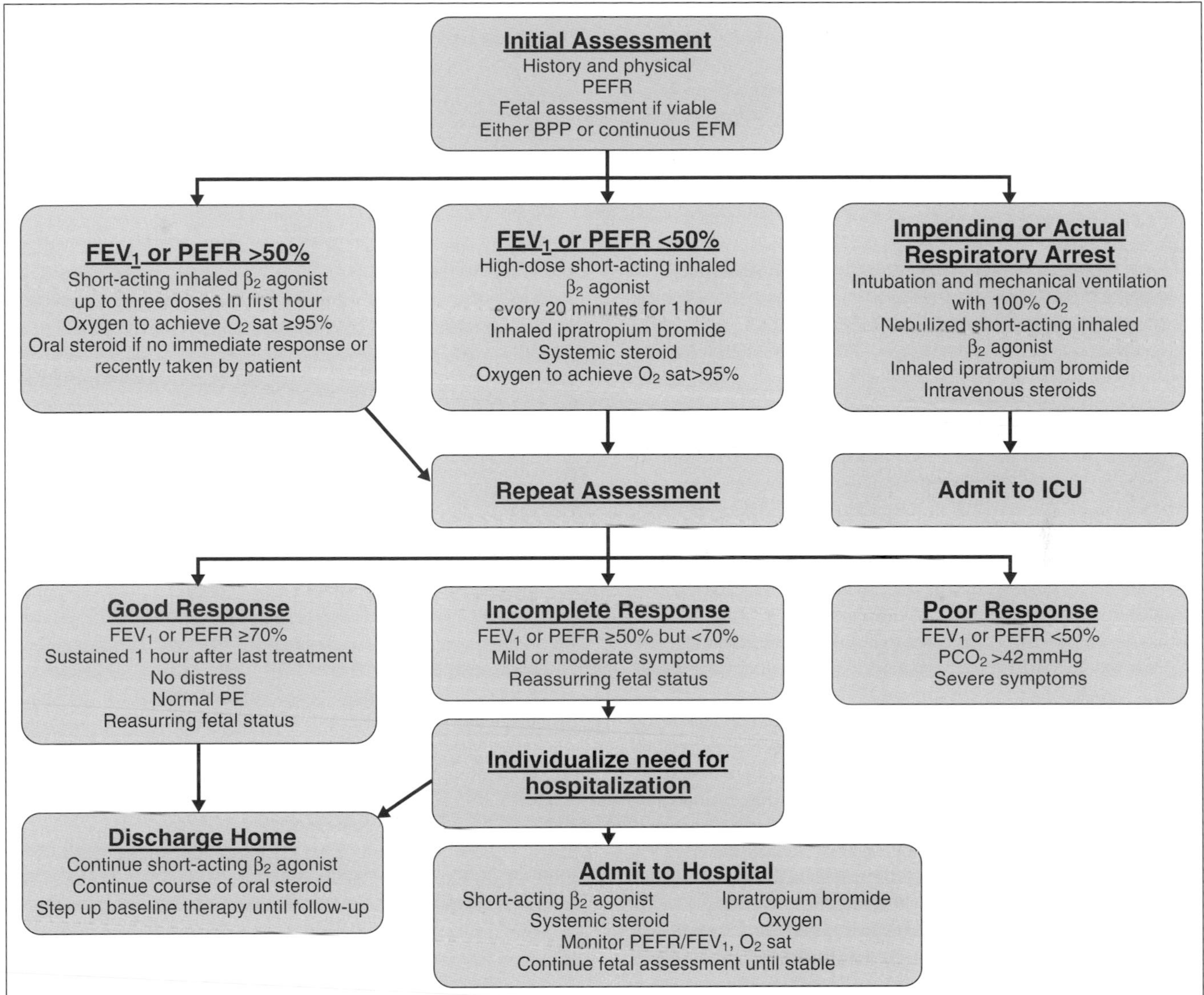

Figure 23.3 Emergency room care of a pregnant patient with acute asthma. Reproduced from National Institutes of Health [14].

(increased risk of complications including preterm birth, pregnancy-induced hypertension, pre-eclampsia and growth restriction). To avoid such outcomes frequent prenatal visits with close attention to asthma symptoms are essential along with regular ultrasound evaluation of fetal growth. Patients should be encouraged to closely monitor their symptoms by the routine use of peak expiratory flow measurements and to seek attention early if worsening symptoms do not respond to initial β-agonist treatment. Through this close observation and early intervention successful pregnancy outcomes are not only possible but routine.

References

1 Dombrowski MP, Schatz M, Wise R, et al. Asthma during pregnancy. *Obstet Gynecol* 2004; 103: 5–12.

2 Alexander S, Dodds L, Armson BA. Perinatal outcomes in women with asthma during pregnancy. *Obstet Gynecol* 1998; 92: 435–440.

3 Kwon HL, Belanger K, Bracken M. Asthma prevalence among pregnant and childbearing-aged women in the United States: estimates from national health surveys. *Ann Epidemiol* 2003; 13: 317–324.

4 Schatz M, Zeiger RS, Hoffman CP. Intrauterine growth is related to gestational pulmonary function in pregnant asthmatic women. Kaiser-Permanente Asthma and Pregnancy Study Group. *Chest* 1990; 98: 389–392.

5 Fanta CH, Fletcher SW. Diagnosis of asthma. In: Rose BD, ed. *UpToDate*. Wellesley, MA: UpToDate, 2006.

6 Global Initiative for Asthma Management and Prevention. NHLBI/WHO Workshop Report. Bethesda, MD: US Department of Health and Human Services. National Institutes of Health, 1995.

7 Weinberger SE, Schatz M. Physiology and clinical course of asthma in pregnancy. In: Rose BD, ed. *UpToDate*. Wellesley, MA: UpToDate, 2006.

8 Bailey WC, Manzella BA. *Learn Asthma Control in Seven Days*. Birmingham, AL: Board of Trustees of the University of Alabama, 1989.
9 Harding SM. Recent clinical investigations examining the association of asthma and gastroesophageal reflux. *Am J Med* 2003; 115(Suppl 3A): 39S.
10 Dombrowski MP. Asthma and pregnancy. *Obstet Gynecol* 2006; 108: 667–681.
11 Enright PL, Lebowitz MD, Cockcroft DW. Physiologic measures: pulmonary function test. *Am J Respir Crit Care Med* 1994; 149: S9.
12 Irvin CG, Eidelman D. Airways mechanics in asthma. In: Holgate S, Busse W, eds. *Rhinitis and Asthma*. Boston: Blackwell Scientific Publications, 1995.
13 Fergusson DM, Horwood LJ, Shannon FT. Parental asthma, parental eczema and asthma and eczema in early childhood. *J Chronic Dis* 1983; 36: 517.
14 National Institutes of Health, National Heart, Lung and Blood Institute, National Asthma Education and Prevention Program. *Working Group Report on Managing Asthma During Pregnancy: Recommendations for Pharmacologic Treatment, Update 2004*. Available at: www.nhlbi.nih.gov?health/prof/lung/asthma/astpreg.htm.
15 Turner AF. The chest radiograph in pregnancy. *Clin Obstet Gynecol* 1975; 18: 65.
16 Thomson K, Cohen M. Studies on the circulation in normal pregnancy: II. Vital capacity observations in normal pregnant women. *Surg Gynecol Obstet* 1938; 66: 591.
17 Gilroy RJ, Mangura BT, Lavietes MH. Rib cage and abdominal volume displacements during breathing in pregnancy. *Am Rev Respir Dis* 1988; 137: 668.
18 Toppozada H, Michaels L, Toppozada M, et al. The human respiratory nasal mucosa in pregnancy. An electron microscopic and histochemical study. *J Laryngol Otol* 1982; 96: 613.
19 Bende M, Hallgarde M, Sjogren U, Uvnas-Moberg K. Nasal congestion during pregnancy. *Clin Otolaryngol* 1989; 14: 385.
20 Bonica J. *Principles and Practice of Obstetric Analgesia and Anesthesia*. Philadelphia: FA Davis, 1962.
21 Bonica JJ. Maternal respiratory changes during pregnancy and parturition. *Clin Anesth* 1974; 10: 1.
22 Weinberger SE,Weiss ST, Cohen WR, et al. Pregnancy and the lung. *Am Rev Respir Dis* 1980; 121: 559.
23 Norregaard O, Schultz P, Ostergaard A, Dahl R. Lung function and postural changes during pregnancy. *Respir Med* 1989; 83: 467.
24 Stenius-Aarniala B. Pulmonary function during pregnancy in health and in asthma. In: Schatz M, Zeiger RS, eds. *Asthma and Allergy in Pregnancy and Early Infancy*. New York: Marcel Dekker, 1993: 53–62.
25 Gluck JC, Gluck PA. The effects of pregnancy on asthma: a prospective study. *Ann Allergy* 1976; 37: 164–168.
26 Stenius-Aarniala B, Hedman J, Teramo K. Acute asthma during pregnancy. *Thorax* 1996; 51: 411.
27 Murphy VE, Gibson PG, Smith R, Clifton VL. Asthma during pregnancy: mechanisms and treatment implications. *Eur Respir J* 2005; 25: 731.
28 Gluck JC. The change of asthma course during pregnancy. *Clin Rev Allergy Immunol* 2004; 26: 171.
29 Kwon HL, Belanger K, Bracken MB. Effect of pregnancy and stage of pregnancy on asthma severity: a systematic review. *Am J Obstet Gynecol* 2004; 190: 1201.
30 Schatz M, Dombrowski MP, Wise R, et al. Asthma morbidity during pregnancy can be predicted by severity classification. *J Allergy Clin Immunol* 2003; 112: 283.
31 Nelson-Piercy C. Asthma in pregnancy. *Thorax* 2001; 56: 325.
32 Bahna SL, Bjerkedal T. The course and outcome of pregnancy in women with bronchial asthma. *Acta Allergol* 1972; 27: 397–406.
33 Demissie K, Breckenridge MB, Rhoads GG. Infant and maternal outcomes in the pregnancies of asthmatic women. *Am J Respir Crit Care Med* 1998; 158: 1091–1095.
34 Tan KS, Thomson NC. Asthma in pregnancy. *Am J Med* 2000; 209: 727.
35 Schatz M, Dombrowski M. Outcomes of pregnancy in asthmatic women. *Immunol Allergy Clin North Am* 2000; 20: 715–727.
36 Liu S, Wen S, Demissie K, et al. Maternal asthma and pregnancy outcomes: a retrospective cohort study. *Am J Obstet Gynecol* 2001; 184: 90–96.
37 Kallen B, Rydhstroem H, Aberg A. Asthma during pregnancy – a population based study. *Eur J Epidemiol* 2000; 16: 167.
38 Perlow JH, Montgomery D, Morgan MA, et al. Severity of asthma and perinatal outcome. *Am J Obstet Gynecol* 1992; 167: 963–967.
39 Namazy JA, Schatz M. Update in the treatment of asthma during pregnancy. *Clin Rev Allergy Immunol* 2004; 26: 139–148.
40 Sorensen TK, Dempsey JC, Xiao R, et al. Maternal asthma and risk of preterm delivery. *Ann Epidemiol* 2003; 13: 267–272.
41 Greenberger PA, Patterson R. The outcome of pregnancy complicated by severe asthma. *Allergy Proc* 1988; 9: 539–543.
42 Schatz M. Interrelationships between asthma and pregnancy: a literature review. *J Allergy Clin Immunol* 1999; 103: S330–336.
43 Jana N, Vasishta K, Saha SC, Khunnu B. Effect of bronchial asthma on the course of pregnancy,labour and perinatal outcome. *J Obstet Gynaecol* 1995; 3: 227–232.
44 Schatz M, Zeiger RS, Hoffman GP, et al. Perinatal outcomes in the pregnancies of asthmatic women: a prospective controlled analysis. *Am J Respir Crit Care Med* 1995; 151: 1170–1174.
45 Stenius-Aarniala B, Piirila P, Teramo K. Asthma and pregnancy: a prospective study of 198 pregnancies. *Thorax* 1988; 43: 12–18.
46 Lao T, Huengsburg M. Labour and delivery in mothers with asthma. *Eur J Obstet Gynecol Reprod Biol* 1990; 35: 183–190.
47 Doucette JT, Bracken MB. Possible role of asthma in the risk of preterm labor and delivery. *Epidemiology* 1993; 2: 143–150.
48 Landau R, Xie HG, Dishy V, Stein CM. β2-Adrenergic receptor genotype and preterm delivery. *Am J Obstet Gynecol* 2002; 187: 1294.
49 National Asthma Education and Prevention Program: Expert Panel Report 2. *Guidelines for the Diagnosis and Management of Asthma*. NIH Publication No. 97-4051. Bethesda, MD: National Institutes of Health, National Heart, Lung, and Blood Institute, 1997.
50 Clark SL. Asthma in pregnancy. National Asthma Education Program Working Group on Asthma and Pregnancy. National Institutes of Health, National Heart, Lung, and Blood Institute. *Obstet Gynecol* 1993; 82: 1036–1040.
51 Schatz M, Patterson R, Zeitz S. Corticosteroid therapy for the pregnant asthmatic patient. *JAMA* 1975; 233: 804–807.
52 Shim C, Williams MH. Bronchial response to oral versus aerosol metaproterenol in asthma. *Ann Intern Med* 1981; 93: 428.
53 Shim C, Williams MH. Comparison of oral aminophylline and aerosol metaproterenol in asthma. *Am J Med* 1981; 71: 452.
54 Fanta CH, Fletcher SW. Overview of asthma management. In: Rose BD, ed. *UpToDate*. Wellesley, MA: UpToDate, 2006.

55 Michigan Medicaid Study, Briggs GG, Freeman RA, Yaffe SJ. *Drugs in Pregnancy and Lactation*, 4th edn. Baltimore, MD: Williams and Wilkins, 1994.

56 Schatz M, Zeiger RS, Harden K, et al. The safety of asthma and allergy medications during pregnancy. *J Allergy Clin Immunol* 1997; 100: 301–306.

57 Schuh S, Johnson DW, Callahan S, et al. Efficacy of frequent nebulized ipratropium bromide added to frequent high-dose albuterol therapy in severe childhood asthma. *J Pediatr* 1995; 126: 639–645.

58 Lin RY, Pesola GR, Bakalchuk L, et al. Superiority of ipratropium plus albuterol over albuterol alone in the emergency department management of adult asthma: a randomized clinical trial. *Ann Emerg Med* 1998; 31: 208–213.

59 National Asthma Education and Prevention Program Expert Panel Executive Summary Report. *Guidelines for the Diagnosis and Management of Asthma, Update on Selected Topics 2002*. Publication No. 02-5075. Bethesda, MD: National Institutes of Health, National Heart, Lung, and Blood Institute, 2002.

60 Busse WW. NAEPP Expert Panel Report. *J Allergy Clin Immunol* 2005; 115: 34.

61 Connelly TJ, Ruo TI, Frederiksen MC, Atkinson AJ. Characterization of theophylline binding to serum proteins in pregnant and nonpregnant women. *Clin Pharmacol Ther* 1990; 47: 68.

62 Schatz M, Dombrowski MP, Wise R, et al. The relationship of asthma medication use to perinatal outcomes. *J Allergy Clin Immunol* 2004; 113: 1040.

63 Labovitz E, Spector S. Placental theophylline transfer in pregnant asthmatics. *JAMA* 1982; 247: 786–788.

64 Arwood LL, Dasta JF, Friedman C. Placental transfer of theophylline: two case reports. *Pediatrics* 1979; 63: 844–846.

65 Cockcroft DW, Murdock KY. Comparative effects of inhaled salbutamol, sodium cromoglycate, and beclomethasone dipropionate on allergen-induced early asthmatic responses, late asthmatic responses, and increased bronchial responsiveness to histamine. *J Allergy Clin Immunol* 1987; 79: 734–740.

66 Namazy JA, Schatz M, Long L, et al. Use of inhaled steroids by pregnant asthmatic women does not reduce intrauterine growth. *J Allergy Clin Immunol* 2004; 113: 427.

67 Bakhireva LN, Jones KL, Schatz M, et al. Asthma medication use in pregnancy and fetal growth. *J Allergy Clin Immunol* 2005; 166: 503.

68 Fitzsimons R, Greenberger PA, Patterson R. Outcome of pregnancy in women requiring corticosteroids for severe asthma. *J Allergy Clin Immunol* 1986; 78: 349.

69 Park-Wyllie L, Mazzotta P, Pastuszak A, et al. Birth defects after maternal exposure to corticosteroids: prospective cohort study and meta-analysis of epidemiological studies. *Teratology* 2000; 62: 385.

70 Bracken MB, Triche EW, Belanger K, et al. Asthma symptoms, severity, and drug therapy: a prospective study of 2205 pregnancies. *Obstet Gynecol* 2003; 102: 739.

71 Reinisch JM, Simon NG, Karow WG, Gandelman R. Prenatal exposure to prednisone in humans and animals retards intrauterine growth. *Science* 1978; 202: 436.

72 Robert E, Vollset SE, Botto L, et al. Malformation surveillance and maternal drug exposure: the Madre Project. *Int J Risk Safety Med* 1994; 6: 75–118.

73 Carmichael SL, Shaw GM. Maternal corticosteroid use and risk of selected congenital anomalies. *Am J Med Genet* 1999; 86: 242–244.

74 Czeizel AE, Rockenbauer M. Population-based case-control study of teratogenic potential of corticosteroids. *Teratology* 1997; 56: 335–340.

75 Schatz M. Asthma during pregnancy: interrelationships and management. *Ann Allergy* 1992; 68: 123–133.

76 Metzer MJ, Turner E, Patterson R. The safety of immunotherapy during pregnancy. *J Allergy Clin Immunol* 1978; 61: 268–272.

77 Metzger MJ. Indications for allergen immunotherapy during pregnancy. *Compr Ther* 1990; 16: 17–26.

78 Liccardi G, Cazzola M, Canonica GW, et al. General strategy for the management of bronchial asthma in pregnancy. *Respir Med* 2003; 97: 778–789.

79 Juniper EF, Daniel EE, Roberts RS, et al. Improvement in airway responsiveness and asthma severity during pregnancy. A prospective study. *Am Rev Respir Dis* 1989; 140: 924.

80 Nelson-Piercy C. Respiratory disease. In: Nelson-Piercy C. *Handbook of Obstetric Medicine*. Oxford: Isis Medical Media, 1997: 45–65.

81 Schatz M, Weinberger S. Management of asthma during pregnancy. In: Rose BD, ed. *UpToDate*. Wellesley, MA: UpToDate, 2006.

82 Nelson-Piercy C, DeSwiet M. Asthma during pregnancy. *Fetal Maternal Med Rev* 1994; 6: 181–189.

83 Smith AP. The effects of intravenous infusion of graded doses of prostaglandin F2α and E2 on lung resistance in patients undergoing termination of pregnancy. *Clin Sci* 1973; 44: 17–25.

84 Crawford JS. Bronchospasm following ergometrine. *Anesthesiology* 1980; 35: 397–398.

85 American Academy of Pediatrics Committee on Drugs. Transfer of drugs and other chemicals into human milk. *Pediatrics* 1989; 84: 924–936.

24 Acute Lung Injury and Acute Respiratory Distress Syndrome (ARDS) During Pregnancy

Antara Mallampalli, Nicola A. Hanania & Kalpalatha K. Guntupalli
Section of Pulmonary, Critical Care, and Sleep Medicine, Baylor College of Medicine, Houston, TX, USA

Introduction

Acute lung injury (ALI) and acute respiratory distress syndrome (ARDS) are uncommon but important causes of acute hypoxemic respiratory failure during pregnancy. Current literature regarding these complications in pregnancy is limited largely to case series, and most of our current approach to the management of ALI/ARDS during pregnancy is based on data from studies performed in non-pregnant patients. This chapter reviews the current understanding of these syndromes, focusing on the definition, clinical presentation, etiologies, and impact of ALI and ARDS, as well as on treatment approaches during pregnancy.

Definitions

The first cohesive description of the acute respiratory distress syndrome was published in 1967 by Ashbaugh and colleagues [1], who used the term ARDS in describing a series of 12 patients with acute onset of hypoxemic respiratory failure characterized by diffuse pulmonary infiltrates on CXR, severe hypoxemia not responsive to supplemental oxygen, and reduced lung compliance. Although initially termed "adult respiratory distress syndrome" in the literature (to distinguish it from the neonatal respiratory distress syndrome seen in prematurity), the condition was later renamed "acute" respiratory distress syndrome when it became clear that the same clinical and pathophysiological process can occur in children as well as adults. Early literature on the syndrome used a variety of criteria to make the diagnosis, but these were not well standardized. In 1994, the findings of the American-European Consensus Conference on ARDS were published and laid out the criteria currently in use to define ARDS (see Table 24.1): (i) acute onset of respiratory distress, (ii) a P_aO_2/F_iO_2 ratio of ≤200 (regardless of PEEP), (iii) bilateral pulmonary infiltrates on chest X-ray, and (iv) a pulmonary artery occlusion (wedge) pressure ≤18 mmHg *or* absence of clinical evidence of left atrial hypertension [2]. The consensus conference also defined the term "acute lung injury" (ALI) to refer to the same clinical syndrome when associated with a milder degree of gas exchange abnormality, i.e. a P_aO_2/F_iO_2 ≤300 [2]. It is important to note that a pulmonary artery catheter is not required to make the diagnosis in the absence of clinical suspicion of left heart dysfunction. However, cardiogenic pulmonary edema and volume overload are always important considerations in the differential diagnosis of ALI and ARDS, and may be especially an issue in pregnancy because of the greater predisposition of these patients for developing volume overload and/or concomitant peripartum cardiomyopathy.

Epidemiology of ALI and ARDS

The reported incidences of ALI and ARDS have varied over the years due in part to changes in the accepted definitions of the syndromes. Several epidemiologic studies have since been published utilizing the now accepted American-European Consensus Conference definitions, allowing more uniform comparisons. One early study from Sweden, Denmark, and Iceland reported an incidence of 17.9 per 100 000 person-years for ALI and 13.5 per 100 000 person-years for ARDS [3]. In the United States, a recent study using the screening data from the ARDS Network clinical trials found an estimated incidence of 64.2 per 100 000 person-years for ALI [4]. There is only limited data on the incidence of ALI and ARDS in pregnancy. Catanzarite and colleagues reported an incidence of 1 per 6227 deliveries based on their series of 28 patients [5]. Other studies in the obstetric population also have reported similar numbers for ALI/ARDS incidence [6,7].

Clinical presentation and pathophysiology of ALI/ARDS

Patients with ALI and ARDS typically present with acute hypoxemic respiratory failure, with symptoms including dyspnea,

Critical Care Obstetrics, 5th edition. Edited by M. Belfort, G. Saade, M. Foley, J. Phelan and G. Dildy.

Table 24.1 Diagnostic criteria for acute lung injury (ALI) and adult respiratory distress syndrome (ARDS).

Acute onset of respiratory distress
Bilateral pulmonary infiltrates on chest X-ray
PAOP ≤18 mmHg *or* absence of clinical evidence of left atrial hypertension
P_aO_2/F_iO_2 ratio of ≤200 for ARDS or ≤300 for ALI, regardless of PEEP

PAOP, pulmonary artery occlusion (wedge) pressure; PEEP, positive end-expiratory pressure.

tachypnea, and tachycardia, and physical examination signs of pulmonary edema (bilateral crackles and/or wheezes on chest auscultation) without signs of left-sided heart failure (e.g. *absent* S3, elevated jugular venous pressure, and peripheral edema). Chest radiography will show diffuse bilateral alveolar and/or interstitial infiltrates, typically without cardiomegaly. Although plain chest radiographs in ALI/ARDS suggest a diffuse process, studies utilizing computed tomography of the chest (CT scans) have shown that in fact lung involvement in ALI and ARDS is inhomogeneous, with alveolar infiltrates, consolidation, and atelectasis that are worst in the dependent lung zones while other areas of the lung may appear to be spared [8,9]. Figure 24.1 shows examples of typical findings on plain chest radiography and CT scan of the chest in ARDS. It should be noted that studies of bronchoalveolar lavage fluid from patients with ARDS have shown that even areas of the lung that appear relatively clear on radiographic examinations may have signs of significant inflammation [10].

A detailed review of the pathogenesis of ALI and ARDS has been published recently by Ware and Matthay [9]. ALI and ARDS are characterized by three distinct stages, although not all patients will progress through all stages. The initial stage is an *acute exudative phase*, which again presents clinically as acute onset of respiratory distress and hypoxemia refractory to supplemental oxygen, most often resulting in respiratory failure requiring mechanical ventilation. The term "non-cardiogenic pulmonary edema" has also been applied to this clinical picture, and the radiographic findings may be indistinguishable from those of congestive heart failure. This acute phase is characterized by increased permeability of the alveolar–capillary barrier leading to leakage of protein-rich edema fluid into the alveolar spaces, accompanied by a pattern of diffuse alveolar damage with increased numbers of neutrophils, macrophages, and erythrocytes, and varying degrees of hyaline membrane formation [9,11,12]. Injury to the alveolar epithelium is a key step in the pathogenesis of ALI and ARDS, and a greater degree of alveolar epithelial injury has been correlated with worse outcomes. Injury to type I alveolar epithelial cells (which make up the majority of alveolar surface area) contributes to alveolar flooding following endothelial injury and increased vascular permeability. Alveolar type II epithelial cells normally function to produce surfactant, transport ions, and differentiate into type I cells as part of recovery from any injury. Injury to type

(a)

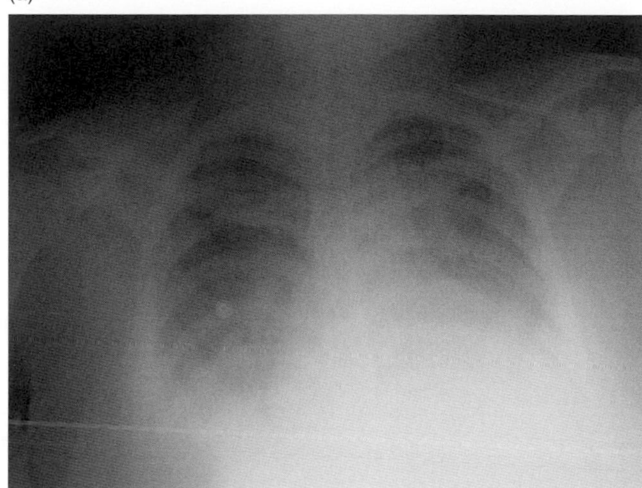

(b)

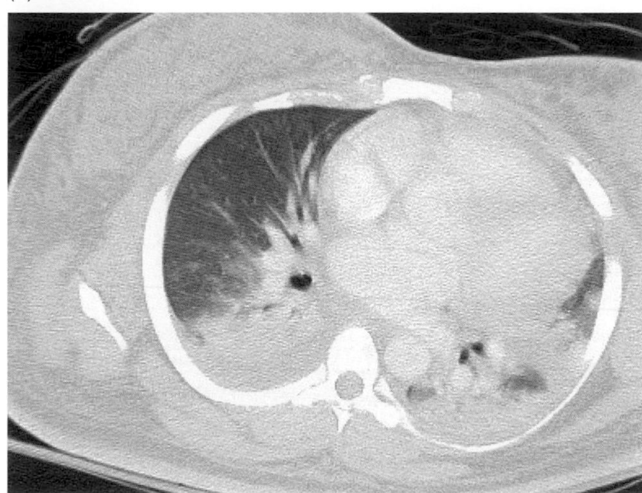

Figure 24.1 (a) Chest radiograph of a woman at 26 weeks gestation with pre-eclampsia and acute non-cardiogenic pulmonary edema (ALI), showing the typical findings of bilateral alveolar and interstitial infiltrates in a perihilar distribution as well as bilateral pleural effusions. (b) Chest CT scan image from the same patient demonstrating the atelectasis/consolidation and small pleural effusions in a predominantly dependent lung zone distribution bilaterally, with areas of relatively normal-appearing lung above. Note that many of the same radiographic findings may be seen with primarily cardiogenic pulmonary edema (see text).

II cells in ALI/ARDS can disrupt removal of alveolar fluid and impair normal surfactant production and turnover, contributing to the alveolar collapse, gas exchange abnormalities, and loss of lung compliance characteristic of this syndrome [9,13–15].

A number of human and animal studies have implicated the neutrophil as one of the key cellular mediators of this early phase of acute lung injury. Histological examinations and analysis of bronchoalveolar lavage fluid from lungs of patients with ARDS have demonstrated increased numbers of neutrophils. Neutrophils are thought to contribute to lung injury through release of proteases, reactive oxygen species, leukotrienes, platelet-activating factor, and other proinflammatory molecules in the pulmonary capillary bed and alveolar spaces. On the other hand, ALI and ARDS can develop in severely neutropenic patients, and neutrophil-independent animal models of ALI also have been developed; thus, whether neutrophils are truly a cause of lung injury in ALI/ARDS or in fact part of the host response is not entirely clear [9].

Other mechanisms implicated in the development of ALI/ARDS include a number of proinflammatory cytokines (such as interleukin-8 and tumor necrosis factor α) that may be produced locally in the lung and also may be regulated by extrapulmonary factors [9]. Disruption of the balance between proinflammatory and anti-inflammatory mediators is likely also important in the development of acute lung injury. Some of the important endogenous inhibitors of these proinflammatory molecules include IL-1 receptor antagonist, autoantibodies against IL-8, and the anti-inflammatory cytokines IL-10 and IL-11 [9]. Other pathways which may be important in the propagation of acute lung injury include secondary abnormalities of the coagulation system which can result in formation of platelet–fibrin thrombi in small vessels and impaired fibrinolysis, leading to further disruption of the pulmonary capillary bed and contributing to the gas exchange abnormalities seen clinically [9,16].

In many patients, the acute phase of ALI/ARDS resolves completely, but in a subset of cases it progresses into a so-called *fibroproliferative phase* (also described as *fibrosing alveolitis* by some authors), typically beginning 5–7 days after the initial insult. This phase may be characterized by persistent hypoxemia, further increase in physiologic dead space, and worsening lung compliance, often associated with pulmonary hypertension secondary to obliteration of the pulmonary capillary bed. Histopathology in this stage may reveal interstitial fibrosis with acute and chronic inflammation [9,11,12,17]. Patients who survive this phase typically go on to a *recovery phase*, which is perhaps the least well-characterized of the phases of ALI/ARDS [9]. In this phase, there is gradual recovery of lung function, with improvements in lung compliance and hypoxemia. Radiographic abnormalities often resolve completely in survivors, although data on the degree of histologic resolution is limited. Some studies of pulmonary function tests in survivors of ARDS have found return to near-normal pulmonary function after 6–12 months [18], but other investigators have shown that the majority has residual abnormalities of diffusing capacity, while 20% have restrictive ventilatory defects and 20% signs of airflow obstruction [19,20].

Etiology

A number of conditions can result in the injury to the alveolar–capillary interface that is characteristic of ALI and ARDS. These are frequently divided into direct, or pulmonary, and indirect, or extrapulmonary, causes of lung injury. Examples of pulmonary causes of ALI/ARDS include pneumonia, lung contusion, gastric aspiration, drowning, or inhalation exposures of smoke or irritant chemicals, all of which may cause direct injury to the lung. In contrast, the extrapulmonary causes trigger a systemic inflammatory cascade that in turn mediates the lung injury; some common extrapulmonary causes include sepsis, acute pancreatitis, massive trauma, burns, and shock of any cause. Some clinical and radiographical differences have been noted between ARDS due to direct versus indirect lung injury, including differences in responsiveness to PEEP and the presence of more lung consolidation on CT scans of the chest in ARDS due to direct lung injury versus a more diffuse pattern of ground glass opacification and pulmonary edema in ARDS due to indirect lung injury. The most common cause of ARDS is sepsis (from pulmonary or extrapulmonary sources), accounting for up to 50% of all cases [9,21]. The risk of developing ARDS has been shown to increase with the presence of multiple risk factors, as well as with concomitant chronic alcohol abuse and chronic lung disease [22,23].

The same conditions mentioned above that predispose to the development of ALI and ARDS in non-pregnant patients can also lead to these complications in the obstetric population, but there are also several conditions unique to pregnancy that have been associated with the development of ALI/ARDS. Among the more frequently reported causes of respiratory distress during pregnancy are sepsis-induced ARDS, pre-eclampsia and eclampsia, pulmonary edema associated with tocolytic therapy, gastric aspiration, and amniotic fluid embolism (Table 24.2).

Severe sepsis, particularly septic shock, is the most common cause of ARDS described in obstetric patients [24]. Acute pyelonephritis seems to be an especially important cause of sepsis-related ARDS in pregnancy, perhaps because this is one of the more common infections that may complicate pregnancy [25,26]. Acute respiratory failure has been reported as a complication in up to 7% of pregnant women with pyelonephritis [24–26].

Table 24.2 Causes of acute lung injury and adult respiratory distress syndrome in pregnancy.

Independent of pregnancy	Specific to pregnancy
Sepsis	Pre-eclampsia and eclampsia
Pneumonia	Tocolytic-induced pulmonary edema
Aspiration of gastric contents	Aspiration pneumonitis (Mendelson's syndrome)
Lung contusion	Amniotic fluid embolism
Acute pancreatitis	Placental abruption
Inhalational injury	Chorioamnionitis
Fat embolism	Endometritis
Severe trauma	Retained placental products
Transfusion-related acute lung injury (TRALI)	Other infections more frequent or more severe in pregnancy (e.g. pyelonephritis, varicella pneumonia, malaria)
Drug overdoses	
Burns	

Pregnancy-associated dilatation of the ureters and increased collecting system volume have been suggested as reasons for the increased frequency of acute pyelonephritis resulting from untreated bacteruria during pregnancy [24]. Besides pyelonephritis, other infections linked to development of ALI and ARDS during pregnancy include viral and bacterial pneumonias, listeriosis, fungal infections with blastomycosis and coccidioidmycosis, and malaria [21]. Chorioamnionitis is another important pregnancy-specific infectious complication to consider in the differential diagnosis of the obstetric patient with ALI/ARDS and clinical suspicion of sepsis without a clear source. Clinical indications of chorioamnionitis include fever, fetal tachycardia, uterine tenderness, and foul-smelling amniotic fluid, but the presentation may be more subtle, and diagnostic amniocentesis should be considered in pregnant patients with ALI/ARDS without a clear cause [21,24].

Preeclampsia, characterized by hypertension, proteinuria, and edema, occurs in up to 8% of pregnancies [24]. Pulmonary edema has been reported to occur in about 3% of patients with severe pre-eclampsia, with most cases (70%) occurring in the immediate postpartum period [27]. Risk factors include older age, multiple prior pregnancies, pre-existing chronic hypertension, and infusion of excessive volumes of crystalloid or colloid [21,27]. A combination of reduced plasma oncotic pressure, altered permeability of pulmonary capillary membranes, and elevated pulmonary vascular hydrostatic pressure have been implicated as factors contributing to the development of pulmonary edema complicating pre-eclampsia/eclampsia [28,29]. Details on the management of pre-eclampsia and eclampsia are discussed in a separate chapter. However, when pulmonary edema complicates these conditions, management is similar to that for pulmonary edema due to other causes, and includes supplemental oxygen, mechanical ventilation when needed, and judicious use of diuretics. Invasive hemodynamic monitoring using a pulmonary artery catheter may be helpful in distinguishing fluid overload and cardiogenic pulmonary edema from ALI/ARDS, but does not seem to impact the outcome of these patients. Therefore, the decision to place these catheters must be individualized.

Tocolytic-induced pulmonary edema is another important pregnancy-specific cause of non-cardiogenic pulmonary edema. The β_2-adrenoceptor agonists terbutaline and ritodrine were until recently used frequently for tocolysis, and their use has been associated with various adverse effects including hyperglycemia, hypokalemia, sodium and water retention, tachycardia, and arrhythmias. In addition, acute pulmonary edema can complicate up to approximately 10% of cases where a β_2-adrenoceptor agonist is used for inhibition of premature labor. This complication can occur during the infusion of these agents or up to 12 hours after their discontinuation [21,24]. The mechanism of tocolysis-related pulmonary edema is not fully understood, but several contributing factors have been suggested, including a combination of medication-induced increases in heart rate and cardiac output (on top of pregnancy-related cardiovascular changes), myocardial dysfunction due to prolonged exposure to catecholamines, increased capillary permeability due to occult infection, and aggressive volume resuscitation in response to maternal tachycardia or hypotension. Possible risk factors for the development of tocolytic-induced acute pulmonary edema include multiple gestation, maternal infection, and corticosteroid therapy [30–32]. In part due to this complication of β_2-adrenoceptor agonist use, magnesium sulfate has increasingly been used in place of these agents for tocolysis. Management of tocolytic-induced pulmonary edema includes immediately stopping the drug, followed by supportive care and diuresis. Most cases resolve rapidly, usually within 12 hours; however, in cases of delayed resolution consideration must be given to possible alternate causes of acute pulmonary edema.

Aspiration of gastric contents is another important cause of ARDS during pregnancy. While this complication is not unique to pregnancy, pregnant patients are at increased risk of pulmonary aspiration of gastric contents because of some of the physiologic and anatomic changes occurring during pregnancy and immediately postpartum. Reduced gastroesophageal sphincter tone, increased intragastric pressure due to the enlarged uterus, reduced gastric motility, and reduced gastric emptying during labor all predispose to aspiration. When it occurs during obstetric anesthesia, aspiration of gastric acid resulting in acute lung injury has been termed Mendelson's syndrome, after the classic description of 66 cases published in 1946 [33]. Mendelson reported an incidence of 1 case per 668 deliveries, with only two fatalities attributed to pulmonary aspiration. A more recent study of perioperative aspiration pneumonitis in pregnant patients reported an incidence of 0.11% for cesarean deliveries and 0.01% for vaginal deliveries [34]. The diagnosis of acid aspiration-induced acute lung injury may be straightforward in cases of witnessed aspiration, but it is important to remember that aspiration may also occur unwitnessed. Occasionally, the only clue for aspiration may be the visualization of gastric contents in the pharynx during laryngoscopy at the time of endotracheal intubation. The degree of lung injury due to aspiration is positively correlated with higher volume and lower pH of aspirated material, and with more particulate matter aspirated.

Amniotic fluid embolism (AFE) is a pregnancy-specific cause of ALI/ARDS which carries a high mortality rate. This condition is discussed in detail in another chapter, and thus will be only mentioned briefly here. The mechanisms underlying AFE are still not fully understood, but it is thought to occur when elements from amniotic fluid enter the maternal circulation, most often at the time of labor or delivery. This can lead to mechanical disruption of pulmonary blood flow as a result of the embolic events and can also trigger release of proinflammatory cytokines that lead to disruption of the alveolar–capillary interface and produce a systemic inflammatory response. The classic clinical presentation of AFE includes acute hypoxemic respiratory distress, hemodynamic collapse (often resulting in cardiac arrest), and disseminated intravascular coagulation, occurring most often during labor or delivery. Reported mortality rates with AFE are generally very high (up to 80%), although more recent reports have disputed this [24].

Management of ALI and ARDS

Mechanical ventilation

The management of patients with acute lung injury and ARDS is largely supportive, in combination with specific therapies directed toward the underlying cause whenever possible. Especially important is identifying infections when present, and treating them expeditiously with appropriate antimicrobials and, if necessary, surgical intervention (e.g. abscess drainage). The mainstay in supportive care for patients with ALI/ARDS is positive-pressure ventilation. Soon after the initial descriptions of ARDS, investigators made the observation that application of positive end-expiratory pressure (PEEP) could produce dramatic improvements in oxygenation [35]. More recently, the application of ventilatory support in ALI and ARDS has evolved further with increased understanding of the potential adverse effects of alveolar overdistention due to the use of excessively high tidal volumes. Ample evidence from animal models has shown that mechanical ventilation using large tidal volumes and high airway pressures can produce lung injury characterized by increased capillary permeability and non-cardiogenic pulmonary edema, even in previously normal lungs [36,37]. This type of lung injury has been termed *ventilator-induced lung injury (VILI)*. In addition to alveolar overdistention, evidence suggests that repetitive opening and closing of surfactant-depleted atelectatic alveoli during mechanical ventilation can itself contribute to VILI, and furthermore can initiate the release of a cascade of proinflammatory cytokines that contributes to a systemic inflammatory response and resulting multiorgan failure [38–40]. A "lung protective" ventilation strategy which aims to avoid both overdistention of alveoli and the repetitive opening and closing of atelectatic lung units has been associated with reductions in this pulmonary and systemic cytokine response [41].

A number of early trials in small numbers of patients using either low tidal volume ventilation or pressure control modes with low target airway pressures in ARDS produced conflicting results as to effect on clinical outcomes. However, the benefit of a low tidal volume approach was clearly demonstrated in the landmark NIH-sponsored ARDS Network randomized trial using volume-controlled mechanical ventilation with 12 mL/kg tidal volumes as compared with 6 mL/kg tidal volumes in 861 patients with ALI and ARDS. This study demonstrated a 22% relative risk reduction in mortality rate in the low tidal volume group (absolute mortality rates 39.8% versus 31.0%, $p = 0.007$) [42]. In this study a detailed algorithm was used to titrate F_iO_2 and PEEP, and plateau pressures were maintained below 30 cmH_2O, with use of sodium bicarbonate infusions if needed to manage severe respiratory acidosis resulting from the controlled hypoventilation caused by low tidal volume ventilation. The ARDS Network trial of low tidal volume ventilation was the first randomized study of a specific strategy of mechanical ventilation to demonstrate convincingly an improvement in mortality in ARDS, and this method of ventilation has now become the standard against which all new ventilatory modes for ALI/ARDS must be compared.

Unfortunately, there are no randomized trials in obstetric patients with ALI/ARDS to guide our approach to mechanical ventilation (or other aspects of management) in this population; indeed, pregnancy has been an exclusion criterion in almost all the clinical trials of therapies for ALI/ARDS. Since maintaining the best environment for the fetus generally requires optimizing intrauterine conditions by supporting the hemodynamic and other organ function of the mother until delivery is feasible, the overall approach to management of ARDS in pregnancy closely parallels the management in non-pregnant patients [24]. There are, however, some important aspects of maternal physiology that may dictate modifications of the targets of mechanical ventilation in this group. During pregnancy, driven in part by progesterone production by the placenta, maternal minute ventilation increases by 50% compared with the non-pregnant state due to increased tidal volume and to a lesser extent increased respiratory rate. The result is mild chronic (compensated) respiratory alkalosis, with P_aCO_2 dropping from 35–45 mmHg at baseline to the 27–34 mmHg range during pregnancy. The renal compensatory response is to increase bicarbonate excretion to maintain normal pH, resulting in normal serum bicarbonate levels in the 18–21 mEq/L range during pregnancy. Lung volumes are also affected by pregnancy, with total lung capacity, functional residual capacity, expiratory reserve volume, and residual volume all decreasing by 4% to 20% from baseline, or non-pregnant values [43,44].

The general approach to mechanical ventilation in the obstetric patient with ARDS is the same as in the general population, aiming to optimize blood gas parameters while preventing ventilator-induced lung injury. However, although volume-controlled mechanical ventilation using the low-tidal volume (target 6 mL/kg ideal body weight) approach should be the goal given the proven mortality benefit in non-pregnant populations, the degree of respiratory acidosis that may be tolerated during pregnancy may be lower as compared with the general population. In fact, the effect of maternal hypercapnia on uteroplacental blood flow is not well understood. Animal studies suggest that with maternal $P_aCO_2 > 60$ mmHg, uterine vascular resistance increases and uterine blood flow decreases. However, these animal models generally examined the impact of acute increases in maternal P_aCO_2, whereas with the controlled hypoventilation strategy in ALI/ARDS the effect on P_aCO_2 is usually more gradual. In ventilating obstetric patients with ALI/ARDS, maintaining maternal P_aCO_2 <45–50 mmHg has been suggested as a general rule [24]. Excessive maternal hyperventilation and hypocapnia also should be avoided when managing mechanical ventilation in pregnancy, as these have been associated with uteroplacental vasoconstriction, decreased uteroplacental blood flow, and fetal hypoxia and acidosis [45–47]. Thus, respiratory alkalosis beyond what is normal in pregnancy also should be avoided.

For the most part, providing positive-pressure ventilatory support in pregnant patients with ALI/ARDS will require establishing an artificial airway first (i.e. endotracheal intubation). Non-invasive positive-pressure ventilation (NIPPV), where ventilatory support is provided by means of a tight-fitting nasal or full-face mask, has only a limited role in the management of carefully selected hemodynamically stable patients with ALI/ARDS [48,49]. Studies in other forms of respiratory failure have shown reduced complications with NIPPV as compared with invasive positive-pressure ventilation (principally reduced nosocomial pneumonias, and also reduced mortality rates in patients with hypercarbic respiratory failure due to COPD). However, NIPPV should not be used in hemodynamically unstable patients or in those with impaired respiratory drive or in patients at increased risk of aspiration, and there are no studies evaluating NIPPV in the management of hypoxemic respiratory failure during pregnancy. In the obstetric population, a trial of NIPPV may be *considered* in carefully selected patients with a rapidly reversible cause for the pulmonary edema, but close monitoring is always warranted due to the increased risk of gastric aspiration during pregnancy. In general, early endotracheal intubation by a clinician experienced in the management of the obstetric airway will be preferable in most cases, especially given the increased risk of encountering a difficult airway in this population.

Fluid management

Optimal fluid management in patients with ALI/ARDS has been another area of controversy over the years, with advocates of fluid restriction pointing to improvements in pulmonary edema and oxygenation with this approach and opponents emphasizing the potential detrimental effects of fluid restriction on cardiac output, renal and other organ perfusion [50,51]. The role of invasive hemodynamic monitoring using pulmonary arterial catheters in this population also has been debated extensively. In an attempt to answer these questions, the NIH ARDS Network undertook the Fluid and Catheter Treatment Trial (FACTT), a randomized multicenter trial involving 1000 patients with ALI and ARDS, which compared a conservative versus liberal fluid management strategy and hemodynamic monitoring with a pulmonary artery catheter (PAC; using primarily the pulmonary artery occlusion pressure, or PAOP, and cardiac index, or CI) versus monitoring with a central venous catheter (CVC; measuring central venous pressure, or CVP) [52,53]. This trial demonstrated that PAC-guided therapy was not associated with any improvements in survival or organ function as compared with CVC-guided therapy, but rather with more catheter-related complications than seen with CVC-guided therapy [53]. In addition, the comparison of fluid management strategies revealed no significant difference in 60-day mortality (the primary outcome), but the conservative fluid strategy was associated with improvement in oxygenation and reduction in ventilator-free days as compared with the liberal fluid strategy without any adverse effect on non-pulmonary organ function [52]. These results lend support to a conservative strategy of fluid management in patients with ALI/ARDS; in the FACTT protocol, the conservative fluid strategy targeted a CVP < 4 mmHg or a PAOP < 8 mmHg, *as long as* the patient was not in shock and maintained adequate renal perfusion and effective circulation (defined for the protocol as mean arterial pressure >60 mmHg without vasopressors, urine output ≥0.5 mL/kg/h, and cardiac index ≥2.5 L/min/m^2 *or* capillary refill time <2 s and the absence of cold, mottled skin). While this study excluded pregnant patients with ALI/ARDS, it suggests that avoidance of volume overload, together with judicious diuresis and fluid restriction, should be the approach to fluid management in this population as well. At the same time, avoidance of maternal hypotension and careful attention to end-organ perfusion parameters as suggested by the FACTT protocol is critical to avoid compromising uteroplacental blood flow.

Prone positioning

Studies have shown improved oxygenation in as many as 70–80% of patients with ALI when ventilated in the prone position [54]. Several factors may be involved in producing the improvement in gas exchange, which interestingly may be sustained for several hours even after return to the supine position. Reduced ventro-dorsal pleural pressure gradient and removal of the effects of compression by heart and mediastinum on dorsal lung units leading to increased recruitment of these previously atelectatic areas of lung, increased functional residual capacity due to the unsupported abdomen in the prone position, and better mobilization of secretions are among the proposed mechanisms for the improvement in oxygenation described with prone positioning [55,56]. However, no randomized trials have demonstrated an impact on mortality or other clinically important outcomes with this approach. Special beds and other devices have been developed to aid in prone positioning of patients, but extreme caution is warranted in order to avoid inadvertent loss of the artificial airway or other support catheters or monitoring equipment, and to prevent the development of pressure ulcers [21]. For obvious reasons, prone positioning is not likely to be a very practical option in the obstetric patient with ARDS, at least not in later stages of pregnancy. In cases where the mother is close to term, maintaining the patient in the left lateral decubitus position will be more important in order to limit the hemodynamic consequences of vena caval compression by the gravid uterus.

Inhaled nitric oxide

Inhaled nitric oxide (NO) has been used in several studies in patients with ARDS and shown to produce improvements in oxygenation. NO is a potent vasodilator, and when administered via the inhaled route produces fairly selective pulmonary vasodilation with minimal effects on systemic blood pressure. Improvement in oxygenation in ALI/ARDS following inhaled NO administration results from improvements in ventilation–perfusion matching through greater vasodilation in the well-ventilated areas of lung [57]. Unfortunately, randomized multicenter trials in adults with ALI and ARDS have failed to show any improvement in mortality or other clinically important outcomes with inhaled NO use despite short-term improvements in oxygenation [58–60]. Thus, there is no evidence to support its use in the routine management of patients with ALI/ARDS [61].

Surfactant therapy

Surfactant therapy has been another potential intervention of great interest in the management of ALI and ARDS. Pulmonary surfactant contains a combination of phospholipids and apoproteins and is produced by alveolar type II epithelial cells. It normally lines the alveoli and respiratory bronchioles and serves to reduce surface tension and stabilize the alveoli, preventing alveolar collapse at low lung volumes. As discussed earlier, loss of surfactant in ALI and ARDS contributes to the atelectasis, gas exchange abnormalities, and reduced lung compliance seen in this syndrome. Exogenous surfactant is routinely used in managing respiratory distress syndrome (RDS) in premature infants, having been shown to improve outcomes in this population. However, a large multicenter randomized trial of exogenous surfactant administered by aerosolization in adults with ARDS failed to show any improvement in outcomes [62]. More recently, small studies suggesting benefits when surfactant preparations were instilled directly into the lower airways using bronchoscopy have revived interest in this therapy for acute lung injury [63,64]. However, larger randomized trials using newer preparations of surfactant and bronchoscopic delivery are still ongoing [21].

Systemic corticosteroids

Because of the prominent role of acute inflammation in the pathology of acute lung injury and ARDS, there was also early interest in potential benefit of anti-inflammatory therapies, in particular corticosteroids. Several studies of high-dose corticosteroids given early in acute-phase ARDS showed no improvement in outcomes including survival, with some suggesting increased rates of infection following early high-dose corticosteroid use [65,66]. However, recent small clinical trials focusing on the administration of corticosteroids in late-phase ARDS (the so-called fibroproliferative phase) reported favorable results, including one small randomized trial which showed improved survival in the steroid-treated group [67]. The ARDS Network recently published results of a multicenter double-blind, placebo-controlled, randomized trial of corticosteroids (methyprednisolone) in persistent ARDS, defined in this study as at least 7 days after the onset of ARDS. The mean duration of ARDS prior to enrolment in this study was 11 days. There was no significant difference in the primary endpoint of 60-day mortality between the placebo and corticosteroid-treated groups, and when begun more than 14 days after onset of ARDS, methylprednisone was associated with significantly increased 60- and 180-day mortality. No significant difference in infectious complications was seen, but rates of neuromuscular weakness were higher in the corticosteroid-treated group [68]. Thus, the routine use of corticosteroids in the treatment of late-phase ARDS is no longer recommended.

Fetal monitoring and potential effects of maternal ARDS on pregnancy

The potential effects of maternal ARDS on a pregnancy include: (i) fetal distress due to maternal hypoxemia, (ii) premature labor triggered by the stress of the maternal condition, (iii) fetal exposure to medications used in management of ARDS, and (iv) interference with assessment of fetal well-being by therapies used to treat the mother [21]. Fetal assessment should be part of the management of any pregnant woman with ALI/ARDS. If the fetus is not yet at the gestational age of viability (at least 24–26 weeks in most centers), assessment may be limited to periodic Doppler auscultation or ultrasonography to determine if the fetal heart tones are still present. However, later in pregnancy, more frequent fetal assessment is needed to help guide decisions regarding the possible need for delivery, especially in the event of changes in the maternal condition such as worsening maternal hypoxemia or acidosis or addition of therapies which may adversely affect the fetus such as use of high doses of vasopressors. Typically such ongoing fetal assessment will be done using continuous fetal heart rate monitoring and periodic ultrasonography with biophysical profile scoring [21,24]. It is important to remember that fetal movements may be affected by sedatives and other medications given to the mother. Furthermore, the mother's critical illness may trigger premature labor, and uterine contractions may in turn worsen maternal hypoxia due to the resulting increased maternal oxygen consumption; in this case, pharmacologic suppression of contractions may be necessary. In cases of maternal ARDS where the fetus is potentially viable, decisions regarding optimal timing of delivery and mode of delivery must be individualized based on the condition of the mother and fetus, and in general the indications for delivery will be the usual obstetric indications [24].

Prognosis of ALI and ARDS

Most epidemiologic studies suggest improvements in survival of patients with ALI/ARDS since the syndrome was first recognized. This is thought to be due to improvements in supportive critical care. Stapleton and colleagues, in a retrospective single-institution study of mortality in patients with ARDS using a uniform definition, describe an overall reduction in mortality rate from 68% in 1981–1982 to a low of 29% in 1996 [69]. Sepsis with multiple organ failure was the most common cause of death (30–50%) and respiratory failure accounted for a smaller proportion (13–19%) of deaths. The ARDS network low tidal volume trial found an overall mortality rate of 31% in the intervention group, and multiple other studies have shown reductions in mortality rates from 50–60% up until the 1980s, down to the 30–40% range since the 1990s [42,70,71]. Several investigators have shown that the mortality for sepsis-related ARDS is higher than that from ARDS associated with trauma and other non-sepsis risk factors [69,72]. Older age (>65), higher elevations in dead space ventilation, and presence of other comorbidities are also important independent risk factors for death in patients with ARDS [3,73,74].

While there are no established registries or studies involving large numbers of cases of ALI and ARDS in pregnancy, data from published series suggest outcomes in obstetric patients with this complication can be expected to be similar or perhaps slightly more favorable than outcomes in the general population. In one of the more recent published series, Catanzarite and colleagues reported a mortality rate of 39% in a cohort of 28 pregnant patients with ARDS, but other investigators reported mortality rates ranging from a low of 24% up to 44% [5–7,75]. The most common cause of death in pregnancy-associated ALI/ARDS cases has been multiple organ system failure [5].

Summary

Acute lung injury (ALI) and ARDS can complicate the course of pregnancy and may result from a number of different causes, which may be unrelated to the pregnancy (such as sepsis, trauma, severe pancreatitis, or inhalation injury, to name only a few) or may be unique to pregnancy (such as pre-eclampsia or amniotic fluid embolism). Management of these complications is directed to the prompt treatment of the underlying precipitating cause, and to supportive care in an intensive care unit. In the absence of pregnancy-specific data to guide supportive care, the existing recommendations are based on evidence from studies in non-obstetric populations with ALI and ARDS. Mechanical ventilation is the mainstay of supportive management in severe ALI/ARDS, and a low tidal volume approach with attention to maternal P_aCO_2 and acid–base status to avoid both excessive hypercarbia and excessive hyperventilation should be utilized. Fluid management, appropriate hemodynamic support, and implementing measures to avoid nosocomial infections also should be part of the routine critical care management of these patients. Unfortunately, none of the specific therapies which have been studied (such as inhaled NO, surfactant, and corticosteroids) have proven to be beneficial in improving outcomes of ALI and ARDS in adults.

References

1 Ashbaugh DG, Bigelow DB, Petty TL, Levine BE. Acute respiratory distress in adults. *Lancet* 1967; 2(7511): 319–323.

2 Bernard GR, Artigas A, Brigham KL, Carlet J, Falke K, Hudson L, et al. The American-European Consensus Conference on ARDS. Definitions, mechanisms, relevant outcomes, and clinical trial coordination. *Am J Respir Crit Care Med* 1994; 149(3 Pt 1): 818–824.

3 Luhr OR, Antonsen K, Karlsson M, Aardal S, Thorsteinsson A, Frostell CG, et al. Incidence and mortality after acute respiratory failure and acute respiratory distress syndrome in Sweden, Denmark, and Iceland. The ARF Study Group. *Am J Respir Crit Care Med* 1999; 159(6): 1849–1861.

4 Goss CH, Brower RG, Hudson LD, Rubenfeld GD. Incidence of acute lung injury in the United States. *Crit Care Med* 2003; 31(6): 1607–1611.

5 Catanzarite V, Willms D, Wong D, Landers C, Cousins L, Schrimmer D. Acute respiratory distress syndrome in pregnancy and the puerperium: causes, courses, and outcomes. *Obstet Gynecol* 2001; 97(5): 760–764.

6 Smith JL, Thomas F, Orme JF Jr, Clemmer TP. Adult respiratory distress syndrome during pregnancy and immediately postpartum. *West J Med* 1990; 153(5): 508–510.

7 Mabie WC, Barton JR, Sibai BM. Adult respiratory distress syndrome in pregnancy. *Am J Obstet Gynecol* 1992; 167(4 Pt 1): 950–957.

8 Gattinoni L, Bombino M, Pelosi P, Lissoni A, Pesenti A, Fumagalli R, et al. Lung structure and function in different stages of severe adult respiratory distress syndrome. *JAMA* 1994; 271(22): 1772–1779.

9 Ware LB, Matthay MA. The acute respiratory distress syndrome. *N Engl J Med* 2000; 342(18): 1334–1349.

10 Pittet JF, Mackersie RC, Martin TR, Matthay MA. Biological markers of acute lung injury: prognostic and pathogenetic significance. *Am J Respir Crit Care Med* 1997; 155(4): 1187–1205.

11 Pratt PC, Vollmer RT, Shelburne JD, Crapo JD. Pulmonary morphology in a multihospital collaborative extracorporeal membrane oxygenation project. I. Light microscopy. *Am J Pathol* 1979; 95(1): 191–214.

12 Bachofen M, Weibel ER. Structural alterations of lung parenchyma in the adult respiratory distress syndrome. *Clin Chest Med* 1982; 3(1): 35–56.

13 Sznajder JI. Strategies to increase alveolar epithelial fluid removal in the injured lung. *Am J Respir Crit Care Med* 1999; 160(5 Pt 1): 1441–1442.

14 Greene KE, Wright JR, Steinberg KP, Ruzinski JT, Caldwell E, Wong WB, et al. Serial changes in surfactant-associated proteins in lung and serum before and after onset of ARDS. *Am J Respir Crit Care Med* 1999; 160(6): 1843–1850.

15 Lewis JF, Jobe AH. Surfactant and the adult respiratory distress syndrome. *Am Rev Respir Dis* 1993; 147(1): 218–233.

16 Gunther A, Mosavi P, Heinemann S, Ruppert C, Muth H, Markart P, et al. Alveolar fibrin formation caused by enhanced procoagulant and depressed fibrinolytic capacities in severe pneumonia. Comparison with the acute respiratory distress syndrome. *Am J Respir Crit Care Med* 2000; 161(2 Pt 1): 454–462.

17 Anderson WR, Thielen K. Correlative study of adult respiratory distress syndrome by light, scanning, and transmission electron microscopy. *Ultrastruct Pathol* 1992; 16(6): 615–628.

18 McHugh LG, Milberg JA, Whitcomb ME, Schoene RB, Maunder RJ, Hudson LD. Recovery of function in survivors of the acute respiratory distress syndrome. *Am J Respir Crit Care Med* 1994; 150(1): 90–94.

19 Orme J Jr, Romney JS, Hopkins RO, Pope D, Chan KJ, Thomsen G, et al. Pulmonary function and health-related quality of life in survivors of acute respiratory distress syndrome. *Am J Respir Crit Care Med* 2003; 167(5): 690–694.

20 Neff TA, Stocker R, Frey HR, Stein S, Russi EW. Long-term assessment of lung function in survivors of severe ARDS. *Chest* 2003; 123(3): 845–853.

21 Bandi VD, Munnur U, Matthay MA. Acute lung injury and acute respiratory distress syndrome in pregnancy. *Crit Care Clin* 2004; 20(4): 577–607.

22 Pepe PE, Potkin RT, Reus DH, Hudson LD, Carrico CJ. Clinical predictors of the adult respiratory distress syndrome. *Am J Surg* 1982; 144(1): 124–130.

23 Hudson LD, Milberg JA, Anardi D, Maunder RJ. Clinical risks for development of the acute respiratory distress syndrome. *Am J Respir Crit Care Med* 1995; 151(2 Pt 1): 293–301.

24 Cole DE, Taylor TL, McCullough DM, Shoff CT, Derdak S. Acute respiratory distress syndrome in pregnancy. *Crit Care Med* 2005; 33(10 Suppl): S269-S278.

25 Cunningham FG, Lucas MJ, Hankins GD. Pulmonary injury complicating antepartum pyelonephritis. *Am J Obstet Gynecol* 1987; 156(4): 797–807.

26 Hill JB, Sheffield JS, McIntire DD, Wendel GD Jr. Acute pyelonephritis in pregnancy. *Obstet Gynecol* 2005; 105(1): 18–23.

27 Sibai BM, Mabie BC, Harvey CJ, Gonzalez AR. Pulmonary edema in severe preeclampsia-eclampsia: analysis of thirty-seven consecutive cases. *Am J Obstet Gynecol* 1987; 156(5): 1174–1179.

28 Gottlieb JE, Darby MJ, Gee MH, Fish JE. Recurrent noncardiac pulmonary edema accompanying pregnancy-induced hypertension. *Chest* 1991; 100(6): 1730–1732.

29 Benedetti TJ, Kates R, Williams V. Hemodynamic observations in severe preeclampsia complicated by pulmonary edema. *Am J Obstet Gynecol* 1985; 152(3): 330–334.

30 Bader AM, Boudier E, Martinez C, Langer B, Sacrez J, Cherif Y, et al. Etiology and prevention of pulmonary complications following betamimetic mediated tocolysis. *Eur J Obstet Gynecol Reprod Biol* 1998; 80(2): 133–137.

31 DiFederico EM, Burlingame JM, Kilpatrick SJ, Harrison M, Matthay MA. Pulmonary edema in obstetric patients is rapidly resolved except in the presence of infection or of nitroglycerin tocolysis after open fetal surgery. *Am J Obstet Gynecol* 1998; 179(4): 925–933.

32 Hatjis CG, Swain M. Systemic tocolysis for premature labor is associated with an increased incidence of pulmonary edema in the presence of maternal infection. *Am J Obstet Gynecol* 1988; 159(3): 723–728.

33 Mendelson C. The aspiration of stomach contents into the lungs during obstetric anesthesia. *Am J Obstet Gynecol* 1946; 52: 191–205.

34 Soreide E, Bjornestad E, Steen PA. An audit of perioperative aspiration pneumonitis in gynaecological and obstetric patients. *Acta Anaesthesiol Scand* 1996; 40(1): 14–19.

35 Petty TL. In the cards was ARDS: how we discovered the acute respiratory distress syndrome. *Am J Respir Crit Care Med* 2001; 163(3 Pt 1): 602–603.

36 Dreyfuss D, Soler P, Basset G, Saumon G. High inflation pressure pulmonary edema. Respective effects of high airway pressure, high tidal volume, and positive end-expiratory pressure. *Am Rev Respir Dis* 1988; 137(5): 1159–1164.

37 Corbridge TC, Wood LD, Crawford GP, Chudoba MJ, Yanos J, Sznajder JI. Adverse effects of large tidal volume and low PEEP in canine acid aspiration. *Am Rev Respir Dis* 1990; 142(2): 311–315.

38 Murphy DB, Cregg N, Tremblay L, Engelberts D, Laffey JG, Slutsky AS, et al. Adverse ventilatory strategy causes pulmonary-to-systemic translocation of endotoxin. *Am J Respir Crit Care Med* 2000; 162(1): 27–33.

39 Verbrugge SJ, Sorm V, van 't Veen A, Mouton JW, Gommers D, Lachmann B. Lung overinflation without positive end-expiratory pressure promotes bacteremia after experimental Klebsiella pneumoniae inoculation. *Intens Care Med* 1998; 24(2): 172–177.

40 Slutsky AS, Tremblay LN. Multiple system organ failure. Is mechanical ventilation a contributing factor? *Am J Respir Crit Care Med* 1998; 157(6 Pt 1): 1721–1725.

41 Ranieri VM, Suter PM, Tortorella C, de Tullio R, Dayer JM, Brienza A, et al. Effect of mechanical ventilation on inflammatory mediators in patients with acute respiratory distress syndrome: a randomized controlled trial. *JAMA* 1999; 282(1): 54–61.

42 Ventilation with lower tidal volumes as compared with traditional tidal volumes for acute lung injury and the acute respiratory distress syndrome. The Acute Respiratory Distress Syndrome Network. *N Engl J Med* 2000; 342(18): 1301–1308.

43 Crapo RO. Normal cardiopulmonary physiology during pregnancy. *Clin Obstet Gynecol* 1996; 39(1): 3–16.

44 Chesnutt AN. Physiology of normal pregnancy. *Crit Care Clin* 2004; 20(4): 609–615.

45 Motoyama EK, Rivard G, Acheson F, Cook CD. Adverse effect of maternal hyperventilation on the foetus. *Lancet* 1966; 1(7432): 286–288.

46 Lumley J, Wood C. Effect of changes in maternal oxygen and carbon dioxide tensions on the fetus. *Clin Anesth* 1974; 10(2): 121–137.

47 Behrman RE, Parer JT, Novy MJ. Acute maternal respiratory alkalosis (hyperventilation) in the pregnant rhesus monkey. *Pediatr Res* 1967; 1(5): 354–363.

48 Rocker GM, Mackenzie MG, Williams B, Logan PM. Non-invasive positive pressure ventilation: successful outcome in patients with acute lung injury/ARDS. *Chest* 1999; 115(1): 173–177.

49 Hilbert G, Gruson D, Vargas F, Valentino R, Chene G, Boiron JM, et al. Non-invasive continuous positive airway pressure in neutropenic patients with acute respiratory failure requiring intensive care unit admission. *Crit Care Med* 2000; 28(9): 3185–3190.

50 Simmons RS, Berdine GG, Seidenfeld JJ, Prihoda TJ, Harris GD, Smith JD, et al. Fluid balance and the adult respiratory distress syndrome. *Am Rev Respir Dis* 1987; 135(4): 924–929.

51 Humphrey H, Hall J, Sznajder I, Silverstein M, Wood L. Improved survival in ARDS patients associated with a reduction in pulmonary capillary wedge pressure. *Chest* 1990; 97(5): 1176–1180.

52 Wiedemann HP, Wheeler AP, Bernard GR, Thompson BT, Hayden D, deBoisblanc B, et al. Comparison of two fluid-management strategies in acute lung injury. *N Engl J Med* 2006; 354(24): 2564–2575.

53 Wheeler AP, Bernard GR, Thompson BT, Schoenfeld D, Wiedemann HP, deBoisblanc B, et al. Pulmonary-artery versus central venous catheter to guide treatment of acute lung injury. *N Engl J Med* 2006; 354(21): 2213–2224.

54 Pelosi P, Brazzi L, Gattinoni L. Prone position in acute respiratory distress syndrome. *Eur Respir J* 2002; 20(4): 1017–1028.

55 Pelosi P, Caironi P, Taccone P, Brazzi L. Pathophysiology of prone positioning in the healthy lung and in ALI/ARDS. *Minerva Anestesiol* 2001; 67(4): 238–247.

56 Albert RK, Hubmayr RD. The prone position eliminates compression of the lungs by the heart. *Am J Respir Crit Care Med* 2000; 161(5): 1660–1665.

57 Rossaint R, Falke KJ, Lopez F, Slama K, Pison U, Zapol WM. Inhaled nitric oxide for the adult respiratory distress syndrome. *N Engl J Med* 1993; 328(6): 399–405.

58 Dellinger RP, Zimmerman JL, Taylor RW, Straube RC, Hauser DL, Criner GJ, et al. Effects of inhaled nitric oxide in patients with acute respiratory distress syndrome: results of a randomized phase II trial. Inhaled Nitric Oxide in ARDS Study Group. *Crit Care Med* 1998; 26(1): 15–23.

59 Lundin S, Mang H, Smithies M, Stenqvist O, Frostell C. Inhalation of nitric oxide in acute lung injury: results of a European multicentre study. The European Study Group of Inhaled Nitric Oxide. *Intens Care Med* 1999; 25(9): 911–919.

60 Taylor RW, Zimmerman JL, Dellinger RP, Straube RC, Criner GJ, Davis K Jr, et al. Low-dose inhaled nitric oxide in patients with acute lung injury: a randomized controlled trial. *JAMA* 2004; 291(13): 1603–1609.

61 Matthay MA, Pittet JF, Jayr C. Just say NO to inhaled nitric oxide for the acute respiratory distress syndrome. *Crit Care Med* 1998; 26(1): 1–2.

62 Anzueto A, Baughman RP, Guntupalli KK, Weg JG, Wiedemann HP, Raventos AA, et al. Aerosolized surfactant in adults with sepsis-induced acute respiratory distress syndrome. Exosurf Acute Respiratory Distress Syndrome Sepsis Study Group. *N Engl J Med* 1996; 334(22): 1417–1421.

63 Walmrath D, Gunther A, Ghofrani HA, Schermuly R, Schneider T, Grimminger F, et al. Bronchoscopic surfactant administration in patients with severe adult respiratory distress syndrome and sepsis. *Am J Respir Crit Care Med* 1996; 154(1): 57–62.

64 Wiswell TE, Smith RM, Katz LB, Mastroianni L, Wong DY, Willms D, et al. Bronchopulmonary segmental lavage with Surfaxin (KL(4)-surfactant) for acute respiratory distress syndrome. *Am J Respir Crit Care Med* 1999; 160(4): 1188–1195.

65 Bernard GR, Luce JM, Sprung CL, Rinaldo JE, Tate RM, Sibbald WJ, et al. High-dose corticosteroids in patients with the adult respiratory distress syndrome. *N Engl J Med* 1987; 317(25): 1565–1570.

66 Luce JM, Montgomery AB, Marks JD, Turner J, Metz CA, Murray JF. Ineffectiveness of high-dose methylprednisolone in preventing parenchymal lung injury and improving mortality in patients with septic shock. *Am Rev Respir Dis* 1988; 138(1): 62–68.

67 Meduri GU, Headley AS, Golden E, Carson SJ, Umberger RA, Kelso T, et al. Effect of prolonged methylprednisolone therapy in unresolving acute respiratory distress syndrome: a randomized controlled trial. *JAMA* 1998; 280(2): 159–165.

68 Steinberg KP, Hudson LD, Goodman RB, Hough CL, Lanken PN, Hyzy R, et al. Efficacy and safety of corticosteroids for persistent acute respiratory distress syndrome. *N Engl J Med* 2006; 354(16): 1671–1684.

69 Stapleton RD, Wang BM, Hudson LD, Rubenfeld GD, Caldwell ES, Steinberg KP. Causes and timing of death in patients with ARDS. *Chest* 2005; 128(2): 525–532.

70 Milberg JA, Davis DR, Steinberg KP, Hudson LD. Improved survival of patients with acute respiratory distress syndrome (ARDS): 1983–1993. *JAMA* 1995; 273(4): 306–309.

71 Abel SJ, Finney SJ, Brett SJ, Keogh BF, Morgan CJ, Evans TW. Reduced mortality in association with the acute respiratory distress syndrome (ARDS). *Thorax* 1998; 53(4): 292–294.

72 Eisner MD, Thompson T, Hudson LD, Luce JM, Hayden D, Schoenfeld D, et al. Efficacy of low tidal volume ventilation in patients with different clinical risk factors for acute lung injury and the acute respiratory distress syndrome. *Am J Respir Crit Care Med* 2001; 164(2): 231–236.

73 Zilberberg MD, Epstein SK. Acute lung injury in the medical ICU: comorbid conditions, age, etiology, and hospital outcome. *Am J Respir Crit Care Med* 1998; 157(4 Pt 1): 1159–1164.

74 Nuckton TJ, Alonso JA, Kallet RH, Daniel BM, Pittet JF, Eisner MD, et al. Pulmonary dead-space fraction as a risk factor for death in the acute respiratory distress syndrome. *N Engl J Med* 2002; 346(17): 1281–1286.

75 Perry KG Jr, Martin RW, Blake PG, Roberts WE, Martin JN Jr. Maternal mortality associated with adult respiratory distress syndrome. *South Med J* 1998; 91(5): 441–444.

25 Pulmonary Edema

William C. Mabie
University of South Carolina, Greenville, SC, USA

Introduction

The clinical circumstances in which pulmonary edema is seen during pregnancy are summarized in Table 25.1. The pathophysiologic mechanism of the pulmonary edema may sometimes be gleaned from the history, physical examination, laboratory data, and chest radiograph. For example, pulmonary edema occurring in the setting of acute pyelonephritis suggests non-cardiogenic or permeability edema. On the other hand, even using echocardiography and pulmonary artery catheterization; we have been unable to fully understand the mechanisms involved in tocolytic-induced pulmonary edema or that associated with pre-eclampsia, two of the more common causes of pulmonary edema in pregnancy.

Two stages in the formation of pulmonary edema are recognized: interstitial and alveolar. The physiology of lung fluid clearance will be reviewed briefly. The lung is divided into alveoli, interstitium, and vessels. Fluid enters the lung interstitium and is pumped out by the lymphatics to the thoracic duct at about 20 mL/h at rest. With strenuous exercise, interstitial edema may be cleared at a rate up to 200 mL/h. In patients with mitral stenosis or chronic congestive heart failure, compensatory hypertrophy of the pulmonary lymphatics and vasculature prevents alveolar flooding even with elevated hydrostatic pressure (e.g. pulmonary artery wedge pressure [PAWP] >18 mmHg) and interstitial edema formation rates.

If the fluid clearance mechanisms are exceeded and alveolar edema results, type I and type II alveolar epithelial cells actively transport fluid back into the interstitium. Fluid enters the cells via the apical sodium channel and is extruded at the base of the cells via the Na,K-ATPase pump with water following isosmotically (Figure 25.1).

There are also water channels called aquaporins within cells and between cells. Aquaporins presumably have a role in water homeostasis as evidenced by their increased expression in the neonatal period during rapid fluid absorption following the initiation of alveolar respiration [1].

Critical Care Obstetrics, 5th edition. Edited by M. Belfort, G. Saade, M. Foley, J. Phelan and G. Dildy.

Pathophysiology

Nearly all cases of pulmonary edema may be classified under one of four mechanisms: hydrostatic, permeability, lymphatic insufficiency, and unknown or poorly understood (see Table 25.2) [2]. In perhaps 10% of cases, more than one mechanism may be operating (e.g. fluid overload in a septic patient with permeability edema) [3].

Hydrostatic pulmonary edema

Hydrostatic pulmonary edema includes cardiogenic causes, colloid osmotic pressure (COP) problems, and rare states resulting in negative interstitial pressure such as rapid reexpansion of a pneumothorax or acute airway obstruction (e.g. blocked endotracheal tube). Excessive intravenous infusions of saline, plasma, or blood can lead to a rise in PAWP and pulmonary edema.

Cardiogenic pulmonary edema can be further divided into disease resulting from systolic dysfunction (decreased myocardial squeeze, ejection fraction <45%), diastolic dysfunction (impaired ventricular muscle relaxation resulting in high filling pressures), or valvular disease (either stenosis or insufficiency). Systolic dysfunction is one of the major causes of pulmonary edema in pregnancy (e.g. peripartum cardiomyopathy) and is the classic pathophysiologic mechanism of congestive heart failure [4,5]. Congestive heart failure may be thought of from different points of view – backward failure versus forward failure, or left heart failure versus right heart failure. Discussing these viewpoints illustrates pathophysiologic mechanisms for the development of the signs and symptoms of heart failure.

With backward failure there is accumulation of excess fluid behind the failing ventricle. In backward failure of the left heart, the ventricle does not empty normally. Left ventricular end-diastolic pressure, wedge pressure, and pulmonary artery

Table 25.1 Clinical setting of pulmonary edema in pregnancy.

Tocolytic therapy
Pre-eclampsia/eclampsia
Cardiac disease
Obesity, chronic hypertension, diastolic dysfunction
Sepsis/acute lung injury
Thyroid storm
Renal failure
Profound anemia
Acute myocardial infarction
Intravenous heroin
Intracranial hemorrhage
Amniotic fluid embolism
Multifactorial

pressure increase. There is a redistribution of intravascular volume from the systemic circulation to the pulmonary circulation resulting in alveolar flooding. With backward failure of the right heart, there is decreased emptying of the right ventricle and elevated central venous pressure (CVP) resulting in peripheral edema, neck vein distension, hepatojugular reflux, hepatic congestion, and jaundice.

Clinical manifestations of forward failure result from an inadequate discharge of blood into the arterial system. If left ventricular forward output is decreased, blood pressure falls. The kidneys sense decreased effective blood volume and increase renin, angiotensin, and aldosterone production resulting in salt and water retention and increased systemic vascular resistance (SVR). With forward failure of the right heart, there is an interventricular septal shift to the left compromising the left ventricular cavity and decreasing stroke volume. This results in increased left ventricular filling pressure, decreased blood flow through the lungs

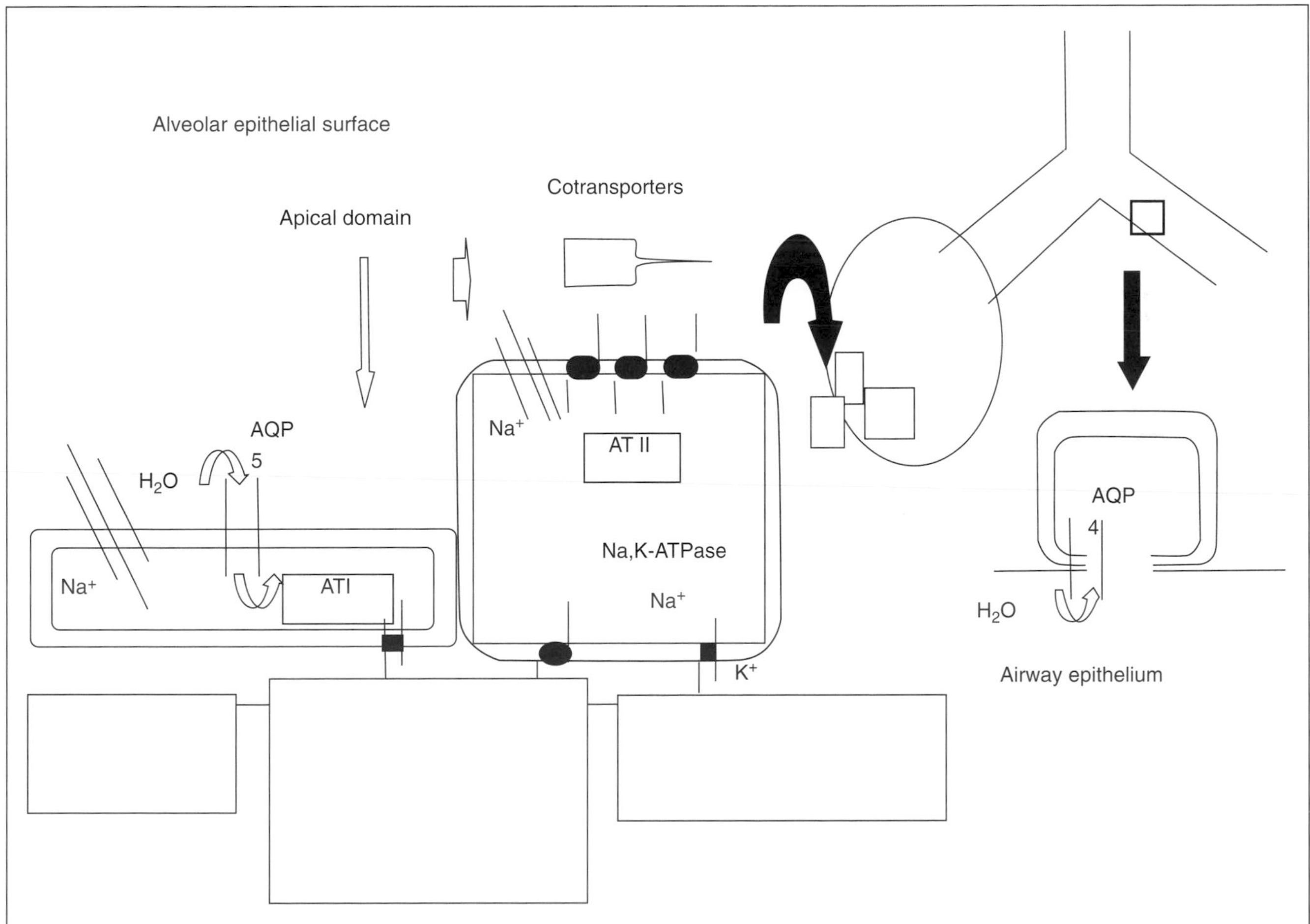

Figure 25.1 Schematic representation of alveolar epithelial cells types I and II, depicting the apical Na^+ channels, the basolaterally located Na,K-ATPase, the aquaporins (AQPs) and some of the cotransporters. Sodium enters through the apical membrane via Na^+ channels and is extruded by the Na,K-ATPase with water following isosmotically. Also shown is an airway epithelial cell with associated basolateral aquaporins. (Reproduced by permission of the publisher, Springer-Verlag, from Dematte JE, Sznajder JI. Mechanisms of pulmonary edema clearance: from basic research to clinical implication. *Intensive Care Med* 2000; 26: 477–480.)

Table 25.2 Mechanisms of pulmonary edema.

Hydrostatic
Cardiogenic
Systolic dysfunction (e.g. peripartum cardiomyopathy)
Diastolic dysfunction (e.g. chronic hypertension)
Valvular disease (e.g. mitral stenosis)
Decreased COP
Hypoalbuminemia secondary to pre-eclampsia, renal, liver, intestinal disease or malnutrition
Increased negative interstitial pressure
Rapid expansion of pneumothorax
Acute airway obstruction
Permeability (ARDS)
Pneumonia (bacterial or viral)
Severe sepsis (e.g. pyelonephritis, ruptured appendix)
Aspiration
Inhaled toxins (e.g. "crack" cocaine, smoke, chlorine gas)
Burns
Non-thoracic trauma
Pancreatitis
Lymphatic insufficiency
Lymphangitic carcinomatosis
Fibrosing lymphangitis (e.g. silicosis)
Post lung transplant
Unknown or incompletely understood
Tocolytic induced
Pre-eclampsia
Narcotic overdose (e.g. intravenous heroin)
Neurogenic (e.g. head trauma)
High altitude

returning to the left atrium, and decreased left ventricular output and systemic blood pressure [2]. Despite the usefulness of these concepts, the ventricles are interdependent. If one ventricle fails, the other will fail.

One of the most interesting developments in cardiology during the last 25 years has been the discovery of congestive heart failure in the absence of systolic dysfunction. Largely based on echocardiographic findings, it is now recognized that, depending on the population studied, about half of patients with heart failure have normal systolic function and presumed diastolic dysfunction [6]. This is particularly common in patients with chronic hypertension and left ventricular hypertrophy. Diastolic relaxation is an active energy-requiring process. The echocardiographic diagnosis of diastolic dysfunction is complex, still evolving, and beyond the scope of this discussion. Some of the parameters measured echocardiographically are the E wave to A wave peak velocity ratio of transmitral filling, the rate of left ventricular posterior wall thinning, and tissue Doppler imaging to calculate myocardial velocity. Many obstetric patients have been found to have diastolic dysfunction as a cause of pulmonary edema, particularly those with both exogenous obesity and chronic hypertension in which the heart has undergone dimorphic adaptation. Obesity results in chamber dilatation while hypertension results in concentric hypertrophy [7,8].

During pregnancy, the valvular heart disease which commonly results in pulmonary edema is rheumatic mitral stenosis. Pregnancy complicates mitral stenosis in two ways: (i) an increase in blood volume; and (ii) an increase in heart rate, shortening diastolic filling time. The pregnant patient with mitral stenosis has a shorter time interval to get an increased amount of blood across a stenotic valve than a non-pregnant patient with mitral stenosis. This results in increased left atrial pressure and, since there are no valves in the pulmonary circulation, increased pressure in the entire pulmonary circuit manifested by elevated pulmonary artery pressure and right ventricular afterload. Thus, the pregnant patient with mitral stenosis is closer to being in pulmonary edema when she is pregnant than when she is not pregnant. These women are apt to go into pulmonary edema postpartum after autotransfusion from the contracting uterus. This autotransfusion is associated with an approximately 10 mmHg increase in the PAWP. Heart rate control with β-blockers and judicious diuresis using Swan–Ganz catheter measurements for guidance has been discussed in an original paper by Clark et al. in 1985 [9].

Colloid osmotic pressure (COP) refers to the pressure resulting from the effect of albumin and globulins that hold water in the vascular space. Intravascular COP opposes hydrostatic pressure and interstitial COP which tend to pull water from the vasculature into the interstitium. The normal intravascular COP in the non-pregnant state is 25 mmHg. Normal PAWP is 6–12 mmHg. Therefore, the normal COP-wedge gradient is about 12 mmHg. Low albumin can occur with liver disease, renal losses, and malnutrition. In normal pregnancy at term, because of increased plasma volume and dilution of albumin, intravascular COP falls to 22 mmHg. With blood loss and crystalloid replacement postpartum, COP falls to 15 mmHg [10]. In patients with pre-eclampsia and hypoalbuminemia, COP may fall from 18 antepartum to 13 mmHg postpartum [11]. Pulmonary edema has been shown to occur when the COP-wedge gradient is less than 4 mmHg. This narrowing of the COP-wedge gradient reflects predisposition to pulmonary edema. The situation is not so simple, however. When COP falls, the intravascular and interstitial COP decrease in parallel, so that the next flux across the membrane should be zero. In addition, patients with nephrotic syndrome and low COP are not more prone to pulmonary edema. Decreased COP is rarely responsible for pulmonary edema on its own, but it can exaggerate the edema that occurs when some other precipitating factor is present [12].

Permeability edema

In permeability pulmonary edema (the second mechanism outlined in Table 25.2), the tight junctions between the endothelial cells open up allowing water, proteins, and cells into the interstitial and alveolar space. The spectrum of severity for permeability edema ranges from acute lung injury (ALI) to the acute respiratory distress syndrome (ARDS). The recommended criteria for ALI are acute onset, bilateral infiltrates on chest radiograph, PAWP of 18 mmHg or less or no clinical evidence of left atrial hypertension, and a ratio of partial pressure of oxygen in arterial blood to fraction of inspired oxygen ($Pa0_2/F_10_2$) of 300 mmHg or less. The criteria for ARDS are the same for timing, chest radiograph, and PAWP, but ARDS requires a $Pa0_2/F_10_2$ of 200 mmHg or less [13].

The mechanisms for this edema formation are numerous. Bacterial or viral pneumonia cause release of prostaglandins, cytokines, and complement components. Septic shock acts similarly by releasing a myriad of mediators including myocardial depressant factor. Aspiration causes a chemical acid injury to the lung as well as bacterial and obstructive components of injury. Inhaled toxins cause direct injury to the alveoli and vasculature (e.g.chlorine gas, smoke). Finally, burns, nonthoracic trauma, and pancreatitis act by systemic transport of a locally-initiated cytokine cascade.

Permeability edema can be substantiated by obtaining edema fluid (e.g. suctioned from an endotracheal tube) and measuring the edema fluid to plasma protein ratio. In hydrostatic pulmonary edema, there should be a low protein content in the edema fluid; whereas, in permeability pulmonary edema, there should be a high protein content. Thus, the edema fluid protein to plasma protein ratio is ≥0.6 in permeability pulmonary edema.

Another way to look at the difference between hydrostatic pulmonary edema and permeability edema is to consider the histologic picture of the lung. In hydrostatic pulmonary edema, one sees nice, lacy alveoli filled with salt water. In permeability edema (particularly in ARDS), one sees "chopped chicken liver." Distorted alveoli are filled with inflammatory cells, protein, blood, hyaline membranes due to fibrin deposition, and collagen.

Hydrostatic pulmonary edema clears in a few hours with aggressive diuresis, whereas permeability edema takes days or weeks to clear, because polymorphonuclear leukocytes have to ingest and eliminate the protein and debris in the lung.

One may also use a pulmonary artery catheter to differentiate hydrostatic from permeability edema. Hydrostatic pulmonary edema is accompanied by a PAWP > 18 mmHg. Permeability edema is thus associated with a normal PAWP (6–12 mmHg) or at least a PAWP < 18 mmHg. There are problems with trying to document an elevated wedge pressure. There may be "flash" pulmonary edema where the wedge pressure goes to 35 mmHg and then falls because of decompression of the pulmonary vasculature with alveolar flooding, delay in inserting the pulmonary artery catheter, or partial treatment with diuretics. Table 25.3 summarizes the differences between cardiogenic and non-cardiogenic pulmonary edema.

Lymphatic insufficiency

The third mechanism of pulmonary edema in Table 25.2 is lymphatic insufficiency. This is rarely seen in pregnancy and will not be discussed further.

Table 25.3 Cardiogenic versus non-cardiogenic pulmonary edema.

Cardiogenic	Non-cardiogenic
Hydrostatic	Permeability related
Left ventricular systolic or diastolic dysfunction, interstitial fluid overwhelms lymphatics, alveolar flooding, interference with gas exchange	Injury to semipermeable alveolar-capillary membrane, leakage of proteinaceous fluid into interstitium even at normal hydrostatic pressures, alveolar flooding, disrupted gas exchange
Decreased compliance	Decreased compliance
Clears rapidly	Clears slowly
	Recovery – nearly normal lung function or fibrosis, inability to wean, eventual death

Unknown or poorly understood mechanisms of pulmonary edema

The fourth category (Table 25.2) includes diseases in which the mechanisms of pulmonary edema are incompletely understood. Tocolytic-induced pulmonary edema is associated with open fetal surgery, twin gestation, maternal anemia, low maternal weight, use of intravenous ritodrine or terbutaline for more than 24 hours, simultaneous use of two or three tocolytic agents, and corticosteroid therapy to accelerate fetal lung maturity. Several mechanisms have been proposed for the development of tocolytic-induced pulmonary edema. These include antidiuretic hormone release, underlying heart disease, fluid overload, occult chorioamnionitis, hypokalemia, myocardial ischemia, mineralocorticoid effect of corticosteroids, catecholamine injury to the myocardium, and permeability edema. The most plausible explanation is that catecholamine tocolytics increase antidiuretic hormone release from the posterior pituitary causing oliguria. This has been confirmed clinically by finding an hematocrit fall of 6–8 points after a 24-hour infusion of β-agonist tocolytics. Many times occult abruption has been suspected because of this hematocrit fall. The mineralocorticoid effect of steroid therapy is now thought to be too small to be contributing to pulmonary edema. With the switch from catecholamine tocolytics to magnesium sulfate as the first agent of choice for tocolysis and the limitation of intravenous therapy to 24 hours, the incidence of tocolytic-induced pulmonary edema has decreased [14–16].

Preeclampsia should also be considered in the unknown or incompletely understood category. Preeclamptic patients frequently have multiple abnormalities including increased capillary permeability due to endothelial cell injury, hypoalbuminemia, afterload-induced left ventricular dysfunction, and increased hydrostatic pressure due to delayed postpartum mobilization of extravascular fluid [17–20].

Narcotic overdose pulmonary edema has been thought to be due to contaminants. Neurogenic pulmonary edema, as seen in head trauma or intracranial hemorrhage, has been thought to be due to a massive sympathetic discharge with an acute rise in PAWP. High altitude pulmonary edema is thought to be caused by hypoxic pulmonary vasoconstriction. The wedge pressure is normal, but pulmonary artery pressures are high. The pulmonary edema fluid has a high protein content, however, suggesting capillary leak [12].

Several physiologic changes of pregnancy may predispose to the development of pulmonary edema. These include increased cardiac output, increased blood volume, decreased plasma colloid osmotic pressure, increased heart rate, and decreased functional residual capacity in the lung [21].

A chronological review of some of the advancements in our knowledge of pulmonary edema in pregnancy is found in Table 25.4 [7,17–20,22–27].

Lung mechanics and gas exchange

Pulmonary edema reduces the distensibility of the lung and edematous alveoli shrink in size. Perfusion of partially fluid-filled or flooded alveoli results in ventilation–perfusion mismatching or an absolute shunt. Hypoxic pulmonary vasoconstriction reduces the ventilation-perfusion mismatch, but pulmonary vascular resistance rises thereby increasing the right ventricular work load. Airway resistance is increased, especially if the large airways are filled with fluid. Rapid, shallow breathing occurs early in the course of pulmonary edema because of stimulation of J receptors in the alveolar walls. This breathing pattern minimizes the high elastic work of breathing. Arterial hypoxemia is an additional stimulus to breathing [12].

Diagnosis

The diagnosis of pulmonary edema is summarized in Table 25.5. In the history, one seeks the onset and duration of symptoms, precipitating factors, comorbidity (e.g. anemia, underlying heart, lung, kidney, or liver disease), and any medication the patient is taking. Symptoms of pulmonary edema include dyspnea, orthopnea, paroxysmal nocturnal dyspnea, Cheyne–Stokes or periodic respiration, and decreased exercise tolerance. Signs include tachypnea, upright posture, air hunger, sweating, rales, use of accessory muscles of respiration, resting tachycardia, displaced point of maximal impulse, third heart sound, neck vein distension, hepatojugular reflux, hepatomegaly, jaundice, and peripheral edema.

The chest X-ray usually shows bilateral air space disease more prominent in the bases (Figure 25.2). Chest radiography cannot reliably distinguish hydrostatic from permeability edema, although claims to the contrary have been made. Features suggesting cardiogenic or hydrostatic pulmonary edema are increased heart size, "bat-wing" or perihilar distribution of edema, prominence of the upper lobe veins, pleural effusions, and septal lines or B-lines of Kerley. On the other hand, non-cardiogenic pulmonary edema is more likely if the radiograph shows normal heart size, peripheral distribution of edema, normal central vasculature, and air bronchograms.

Arterial blood gases are measured less frequently now, because non-invasive pulse oximetry allows continuous oxygen saturation measurement. If the patient is critically ill or has comorbid conditions such as renal disease, chronic obstructive pulmonary disease, or sepsis, an arterial blood gas measurement may be needed to check for acidosis or carbon dioxide retention. Typical blood gases in pulmonary edema reveal hypoxemia with low or normal P_aCO_2. With florid pulmonary edema, carbon dioxide retention and respiratory acidosis may develop.

A 12-lead electrocardiogram should be performed to detect chamber hypertrophy, ischemia, infarction, conduction defects, or arrhythmias.

A recent development in the diagnosis of congestive heart failure has been the measurement of plasma brain natriuretic peptide (BNP) in patients who present with acute dyspnea. BNP was initially identified in the brain, but it is also synthesized by the cardiac ventricles in response to increased wall stress. Like atrial natriuretic peptide which is released by atrial myocardial cells, BNP has diuretic, natriuretic, and hypotensive effects. Both hormones inhibit the renin–angiotensin system, endothelin secretion, and systemic and renal sympathetic activity. The BNP level is most useful if the value is below 100 pg/mL, a level at which congestive heart failure is unlikely. Concentrations higher than 500 pg/mL are likely to be associated with heart failure. BNP levels cannot be used to distinguish between systolic and diastolic heart failure [28].

In pregnancy, median BNP values are less than 20 pg/mL and do not change significantly between trimesters. In severe preeclampsia, however, median BNP levels are elevated to around 100 pg/mL, possibly reflecting increased ventricular wall stress due to hypertension [29]. The role of BNP levels in the diagnosis of heart failure in pregnancy has not been adequately studied.

An extremely useful diagnostic test in pulmonary edema is the echocardiogram. This allows non-invasive evaluation of cardiac structure and function. In a prospective study of pregnant women with pulmonary edema, Mabie et al. used echocardiography to differentiate between cardiogenic and non-cardiogenic forms of pulmonary edema, determine the type of cardiac dysfunction (systolic, diastolic, or valvular), and plan long-term therapy [25]. It is important to recognize that the echocardiogram does not have to be done acutely while the patient is in pulmonary edema. The underlying cardiac abnormalities do not change rapidly despite therapy.

A pulmonary artery catheter (PAC) may be needed for diagnosis and/or management of patients with pulmonary edema. The PAC can be used to diagnose hypovolemia; hydrostatic pulmonary edema (PAWP > 18 mmHg); severe mitral regurgitation (V wave); pulmonary hypertension; low, normal, or high cardiac output state; cardiac tamponade (equalization of pressures PAWP, CVP, pulmonary artery diastolic), and ventricular septal rupture (step-up in oxygenation). Many of these diagnostic uses have been replaced by echocardiography. The PAC is primarily

Table 25.4 Selective literature review of pulmonary edema in obstetrics.

Year	Authors	Cardiac monitoring	Significant findings
1980	Berkowitz, Rafferty [22]	Swan–Ganz	Used in 20 obstetric patients over 3 years. Differentiated cardiogenic from non-cardiogenic pulmonary edema. Followed patients with multiple organ system failure. Early detection of loss of cardiac reserve and effectiveness of therapeutic manipulations.
1980	Strauss et al. [17]	Swan–Ganz	Three cases of pre-eclampsia with pulmonary edema. Elevated PAWP (22–33 mmHg). Simultaneous CVP normal. Isolated left ventricular dysfunction was primarily the result of increased afterload and responded to vasodilators (sodium nitroprusside, hydralazine). Cardiac output nearly doubled without a significant change in heart rate or blood pressure. Limit nitroprusside therapy to 30 minutes if fetus still *in utero*.
1981	Keefer et al. [18]	Swan–Ganz	Four cases of non-cardiogenic pulmonary edema treated with supportive care with mechanical ventilation and positive end-expiratory pressure. Pulmonary artery catheter allowed documentation of normal wedge pressure.
1984	Hankins et al. [19]	Swan–Ganz	Eight primigravid women with eclampsia. Initial hemodynamic findings: low CVP and PAWP, high cardiac output, and elevated SVR. Postpartum, women without spontaneous diuresis had elevated PAWP and cardiac output. Proposed concept of delayed mobilization of extravascular fluid occurring 24–72 hours postpartum.
1985	Benedetti et al. [20]	Swan–Ganz	Ten pre-eclamptic patients with pulmonary edema. Eight of 10 developed pulmonary edema postpartum. Five patients had COP-wedge gradient ≤4. Three had findings consistent with pulmonary capillary leak. Two had left ventricular failure. CVP did not correlate with PAWP. Eight of 10 received colloidal fluid before onset of pulmonary edema, raising the possibility that colloid was contributory.
1986	Cotton et al. [23]	Swan–Ganz	Used intravenous nitroglycerin to drop mean arterial pressure by 20% in three pre-eclamptic women with pulmonary edema. Mean PAWP decreased from 27 ± 4 to 14 ± 6 mmHg, resulting in a COP-wedge gradient change from −10 to 2 mmHg. There was no change in heart rate, CVP or cardiac output.
1987	Sibai et al. [24]	None	Retrospective chart review of 37 patients. Incidence of pulmonary edema 2.9% among 1290 severe pre-eclampsia/eclampsia patients. Incidence was higher in older, multiparas with chronic hypertension. Seventy per cent of cases occurred postpartum. Four maternal deaths. Perinatal mortality 530/1000. Sick patients with much comorbidity: 18 had disseminated intravascular coagulation, 17 sepsis, 12 abruptio placentae, 10 acute renal failure, 6 hypertensive crisis, 5 cardiopulmonary arrest, 2 liver rupture, and 2 ischemic cerebral damage.
1988	Mabie et al. [7]	Echocardiography	Used the concept of diastolic dysfunction to explain pulmonary edema in four obese, chronically hypertensive pregnant women.
1993	Mabie et al. [25]	Echocardiography	Prospective study of 45 obstetric patients with pulmonary edema. Three therapeutically and prognostically distinct groups were identified: (i) systolic dysfunction (n = 19); (ii) diastolic dysfunction (n = 17); and (iii) normal heart (n = 9). Two patients with systolic dysfunction died and one underwent cardiac transplantation. Patients with systolic dysfunction required short- and long-term treatment with digoxin, diuretics, and angiotensin-converting enzyme inhibitors. Those with diastolic dysfunction received diuretics and long-term antihypertensive therapy. Women with normal hearts required acute therapy only. Because clinical and roentgenographic findings do not accurately differentiate patients with respect to the presence and type of cardiac dysfunction, echocardiography was recommended to evaluate all pregnant women with pulmonary edema.
1998	DiFederico et al. [26]	None	Retrospective chart review of pulmonary edema in obstetric patients(1985–1995). Eighty-six cases out of 16 810 deliveries (prevalence about 1/200 deliveries). Associated clinical conditions were pre-eclampsia 28%, preterm labor 24%, fetal surgery 17%, and infection 14%. Forty-five per cent of patients required intensive care unit admission; 15% required mechanical ventilation. Sixty-nine patients (80%) received tocolysis; 37 patients (41%) received multiple, simultaneous tocolytics. An interesting subgroup was found. Fifteen of 65 patients (23%) undergoing open fetal surgery developed pulmonary edema. Most received intravenous nitroglycerin as a tocolytic. The increased severity and delayed resolution of pulmonary edema in the open fetal surgery group suggested permeability edema.
2003	Sciscione et al. [27]	None	Ten-year retrospective chart review of acute pulmonary edema in pregnancy (1989–99). The main causes were tocolytic agents, underlying heart disease, fluid overload, and pre-eclampsia. Fifty-one cases among 62 917 consecutive deliveries (prevalence 8/10 000 deliveries).

Table 25.5 Diagnosis and treatment.

Diagnosis
History
Physical
Pulse oximetry ± blood gas
Chest radiograph
Electrocardiogram
Brain natriuretic peptide
Echocardiogram
Initial management
Sit patient upright
Oxygen
Furosemide
Morphine

useful for management to obtain CVP, PAWP, intermittent or continuous cardiac output, mixed venous oxygen saturation, and right ventricular ejection fraction – depending on the type of catheter used. The author has found the PAC most useful in treating pregnant patients with tight mitral stenosis (valve area <1 cm^2), a "white out" on chest X-ray, and those patients who do not respond to aggressive diuresis with furosemide.

The PAC provides information that one could not obtain by history, physical examination, and chest X-ray [30]. Nevertheless, it has become highly controversial with calls for a moratorium on its use [31]. Problems are lack of physician ability to interpret hemodynamic waveforms and non-randomized trials showing increased length of stay with increased cost and mortality in patients undergoing Swan–Ganz monitoring [32,33]. It has been suggested that use of the right heart catheter is a marker for a more aggressive and morbid style of care [30]. This controversy has stimulated recent prospective, randomized trials which have shown that use of the PAC is relatively safe, but it does not improve outcome [34,35]. Therefore, its role in critical care is diminishing.

Treatment

The treatment of acute pulmonary edema in pregnancy depends on whether the excessive accumulation of extravascular lung water is due to increased hydrostatic pressures (e.g. left ventricular failure, mitral stenosis, volume overload); to increased capillary permeability (e.g. sepsis-induced ARDS, pneumonia, trauma); or to one of the poorly understood causes such as tocolytic-induced pulmonary edema or pre-eclampsia. Although the algorithm for diagnosis is stepwise, providing care is a dynamic process requiring simultaneous diagnosis and treatment. In the absence of contraindications, initial management can proceed as outlined in Table 25.5 for suspected hydrostatic pulmonary edema [3].

Initial treatment includes sitting the patient upright and administering oxygen, furosemide, and morphine. Oxygen may be given by nasal cannula at rates of up to 4 L/min. Flow rates above this do not increase the inhaled oxygen fraction and cause nasal irritation. Face-mask oxygen can be given with a non-rebreathing mask using flow rates up to 15 L/min. Non-invasive positive-pressure ventilation may be given with a nasal mask or the better tolerated oronasal mask. Either a portable pressure-limited or a standard mechanical ventilator may be used. This increases intra-alveolar pressure, reduces transudation of fluid from alveolar capillaries, and impedes venous return to the thorax. It is most useful as a temporizing measure to maintain oxygenation until furosemide-induced diuresis clears the lungs. Intubation and mechanical ventilation may be required for patient exhaustion or refractory hypoxemia. Mechanical ventilation decreases the work of breathing, allows delivery of increased inhaled oxygen fractions, and permits the use of positive end-expiratory pressure to recruit atelectatic alveoli or to maintain partially expanded alveoli. The route of oxygen administration depends on the severity of the pulmonary edema and the response to initial therapy. The goal is to maintain the arterial partial pressure of oxygen >60 mmHg and the oxygen saturation >90%.

Furosemide may be given in a dose of 40 mg intravenously. This causes venodilation, decreasing preload, and blockage of chloride and sodium reabsorption in the ascending limb of the loop of Henle. The aim should be to obtain roughly a 2000 mL diuresis over a few hours. This is often associated with radiographic clearing of the pulmonary edema.

Morphine (2–5 mg intravenously) is also a venodilator and will decrease the patient's anxiety. Frequently in obstetrics, these mainstays of therapy are all that are needed.

Further management will depend on the cause of the pulmonary edema. If it is tocolytic-induced, consideration should be given to stopping tocolysis and allowing delivery to occur. A recent review of pulmonary edema associated with magnesium sulfate tocolysis advocated continuing the tocolytic once pulmonary edema has been treated [36]. The present author disagrees with this advice for several reasons: (i) pulmonary edema may be a life-threatening complication; (ii) frequently labor does not progress even after tocolysis is stopped; (iii) actual fetal weight may exceed 1800 g; (iv) occult chorioamnionitis or placental abruption may be present; (v) there may be a maternal contraindication to tocolysis such as pre-eclampsia, appendicitis, or hyperthyroidism; and (vi) there may be a fetal contraindication to tocolysis such as an anomaly or intrauterine growth restriction.

If pulmonary edema occurs antepartum in a patient with pre-eclampsia, delivery will usually be indicated. When pulmonary edema is associated with severe hypertension, antihypertensive therapy with intravenous hydralazine, labetalol, or nicardipine will reduce afterload and improve cardiac performance. Oral short-acting nifedipine is also efficacious for severe hypertension, but may produce overshoot hypotension. Sodium nitroprusside, a balanced arterial and venular vasodilator, can be used for minute-to-minute titration of blood pressure; however, it is rarely used in pregnancy because of the risk of fetal cyanide and thiocyanate toxicity. Nitroglycerin is primarily a venular vasodilator

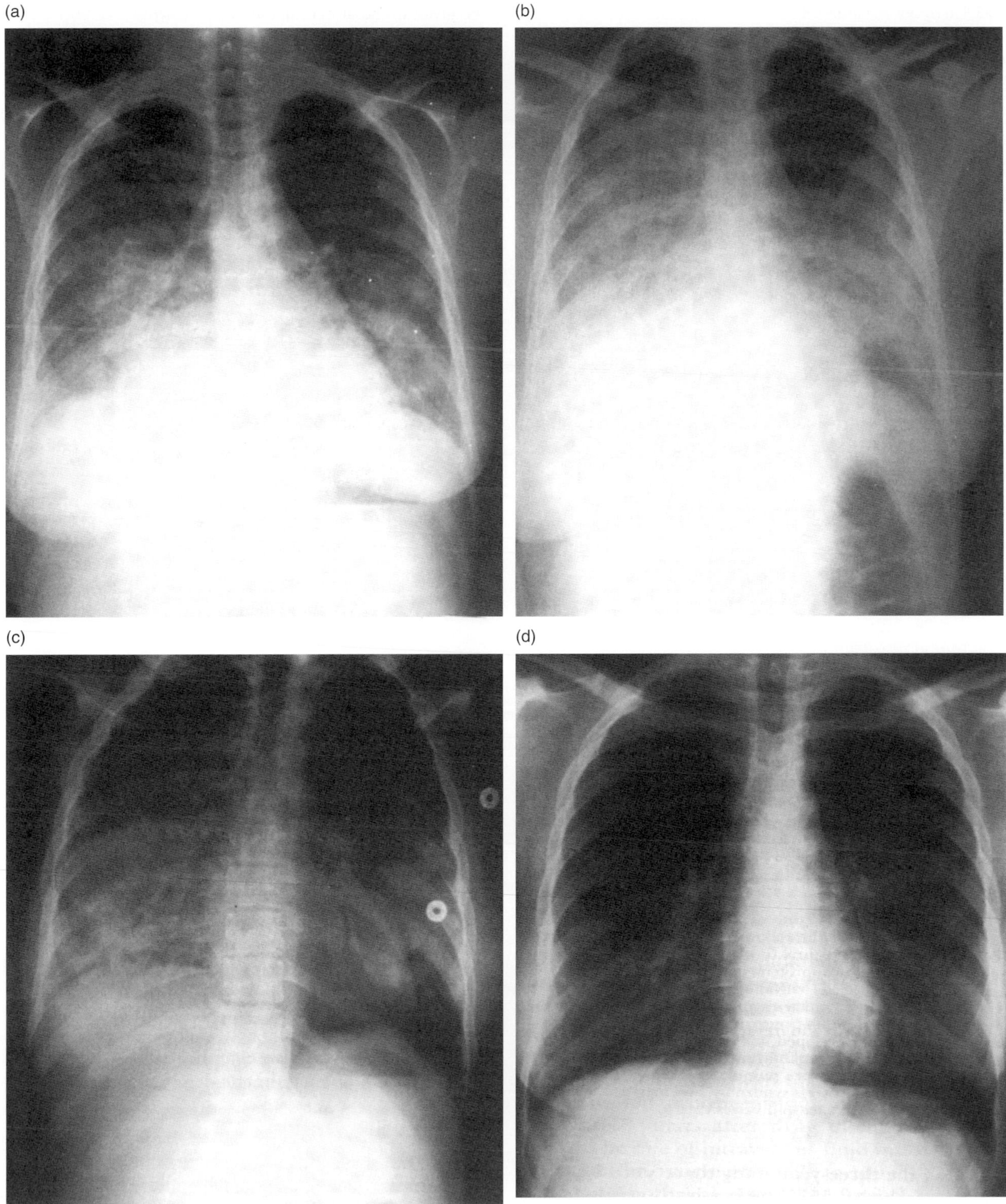

Figure 25.2 Pulmonary edema induced by 48 hours of tocolysis with intravenous and then oral ritodrine. (a) Roentgenogram of the chest taken at the onset of pulmonary edema showing bilateral perihilar and basilar infiltrates. (b) Postpartum film taken 22 hours after (a) shows worsening infiltrates despite fluid restriction and furosemide-induced diuresis. (c) Portable AP film taken 50 hours after the onset of pulmonary edema demonstrating some resolution of the infiltrates. Notice air bronchograms and normal pulmonary vasculature. (d) Standard PA film taken 30 days after the onset of pulmonary edema demonstrating a normal cardiac silhouette and clear lungs. (Adapted from: Mabie WC, Pernoll ML, Witty JB, and Biswas MK. Pulmonary edema induced by betamimetic drugs. *S Med J.* 1983;76:1354–60.)

Table 25.6 Treatment of systolic heart failure.

Treatment
Angiotensin-converting enzyme inhibitors
Angiotensin receptor blockers
Other vasodilators
Diuretics
Aldosterone blockers
β-blockers
Digoxin
Amiodarone
Calcium channel blockers
Inotropic agents
Nesiritide
Acute hemodialysis and ultrafiltration
Anticoagulants
Implantable cardioverter-defibrillators
Biventricular pacemakers (cardiac resynchronization therapy)
Ventricular assist devices
Cardiac transplantation

that has arterial vasodilator effects when given in higher intravenous doses. Although it crosses the placenta, nitroglycerin is safe for the fetus. It is the drug of choice in hypertension associated with acute coronary syndromes such as myocardial infarction or unstable angina; however, symptomatic coronary artery disease is uncommon in pregnancy.

The treatment of cardiogenic or non-cardiogenic pulmonary edema is complex and may be thought of in terms of how cardiologists or pulmonary/critical care physicians handle their specialty patients. Table 25.6 summarizes the cardiologist's options for the treatment of systolic heart failure [37]. The indications and details of this treatment are beyond the scope of this chapter. Angiotensin-converting enzyme inhibitors, angiotensin receptor blockers, amiodarone, and coumadin are contraindicated in pregnancy. Hydralazine and isosorbide dinitrate may be substituted for angiotensin-converting enzyme inhibitors or angiotensin receptor blockers in the treatment of systolic heart failure during pregnancy. Treatment for diastolic heart failure consists of diuretics, treating the underlying etiology by controlling hypertension, and rate control with β-blockers to allow time for diastolic filling.

The pulmonary/critical care approach to permeability edema includes supportive care until the lung can heal and a lung-protective strategy for mechanical ventilation (tidal volume 6 mL/kg) [38]. Management of severe sepsis and septic shock includes early goal-directed therapy, antibiotics and source control, activated protein C, replacement-dose hydrocortisone, and tight glucose control [39].

Prevention

Tocolytic-induced pulmonary edema is the etiology most amenable to prevention by the obstetrician. A strategy for prevention includes: (i) attention to contraindications to tocolytic therapy (e.g. pre-eclampsia, infection); (ii) careful intake and output with total fluid administration limited to 2500 mL/day; (iii) recognition of predisposing factors (e.g. twins, anemia, low maternal weight); and (iv) use of magnesium sulfate as the tocolytic agent of first choice.

Other strategies to prevent pulmonary edema include: (i) invasive hemodynamic monitoring in patients with New York Heart Association class III or IV cardiac disease, particularly mitral stenosis with a valve area less than 1.0 cm^2; and (ii) close monitoring of the patient undergoing "conservative" management of severe pre-eclampsia.

References

1 Dematte JE, Sznajder JI. Mechanisms of pulmonary edema clearance: from basic research to clinical implication. *Intens Care Med* 2000; 26(4): 477–480.

2 Ingram RH Jr, Braunwald E. Dyspnea and pulmonary edema. In: Kasper DL, Braunwald E, Fauci AS, et al., eds. *Harrison's Principles of Internal Medicine*, 16th edn. New York: McGraw-Hill, 2005: 201–205.

3 Ware LB, Matthay MA. Acute pulmonary edema. *N Engl J Med* 2005; 353: 2788–2796.

4 Heider AL, Kuller JA, Strauss RA, Wells SR. Peripartum cardiomyopathy: a review of the literature. *Obstet Gynecol Surv* 1999; 54(1): 526–531.

5 Pearson GD, Veille JC, Rahimtoola S, et al. Peripartum cardiomyopathy: National Heart, Lung, and Blood Institute and Office of Rare Diseases (National Institute of Health) workshop recommendations and review. *JAMA* 2000; 283(9): 1183–1188.

6 Gandhi SK, Powers JC, Nomeir AM, et al. The pathogenesis of acute pulmonary edema associated with hypertension. *N Engl J Med* 2001; 344(1): 17–22.

7 Mabie WC, Ratts TE, Ramanathan KB, Sibai BM. Circulatory congestion in obese hypertensive women: a subset of pulmonary edema in pregnancy. *Obstet Gynecol* 1988; 72(4): 553–558.

8 Desai DK, Moodley J, Naidoo DP, Bhorat I. Cardiac abnormalities in pulmonary edema associated with hypertensive crises in pregnancy. *Br J Obstet Gynaecol* 1996; 103(6): 523–528.

9 Clark SL, Phelan JP, Greenspoon J, Aldahl D, Horenstein J. Labor and delivery in the presence of mitral stenosis: central hemodynamic observations. *Am J Obstet Gynecol* 1985; 152(8): 984–988.

10 Cotton DB, Gonik B, Spillman T, Dorman KF. Intrapartum to postpartum changes in colloid osmotic pressure. *Am J Obstet Gynecol* 1984; 149(2): 174–177.

11 Benedetti TJ, Carlson RW. Studies of colloid osmotic pressure in pregnancy-induced hypertension. *Am J Obstet Gynecol* 1979; 135(3): 308–311.

12 West JB. Pulmonary edema. In: *Pulmonary Physiology and Pathophysiology*, 2nd edn. Philadelphia, PA: Wolters Kluwer Lippincott, Williams and Wilkins, 2007: 94–104.

13 Bernard GR, Artigas A, Brigham KL, et al. and the Consensus Committee. The American-European Consensus Conference on ARDS: definitions, mechanisms, relevant outcomes, and clinical trial coordination. *Am J Respir Crit Care Med* 1994; 149: 818–824.

14 Pisani RJ, Rosenow EC 3rd. Pulmonary edema associated with tocolytic therapy. *Ann Intern Med* 1989; 110(9): 814–818.

15 Lampert MB, Hibbard J, Weinert L, Briller J, Lindheimer M, Lang RM. Peripartum heart failure associated with prolonged tocolytic therapy. *Am J Obstet Gynecol* 1993; 168(2): 493–495.

16 Leduc D, Naeije K, Leeman M, Homans C, Kahn RJ. Severe pulmonary edema associated with tocolytic therapy: case report with hemodynamic study. *Intens Care Med* 1996; 22(11): 1280–1281.

17 Strauss RG, Keefer JR, Burke T, Civetta JM. Hemodynamic monitoring of cardiogenic pulmonary edema complicating toxemia of pregnancy. *Obstet Gynecol* 1980; 55(2): 170–174.

18 Keefer JR, Strauss RG, Civetta JM, Burke T. Non-cardiogenic pulmonary edema and invasive cardiovascular monitoring. *Obstet Gynecol* 1981; 58(1): 46–51.

19 Hankins GDV, Wendel GD, Cunningham FG, Leveno KJ. Longitudinal evaluation of hemodynamic changes in eclampsia. *Am J Obstet Gynecol* 1984; 150(5pt1): 506–512.

20 Benedetti TJ, Kates R, Williams V. Hemodynamic observations in severe preeclampsia complicated by pulmonary edema. *Am J Obstet Gynecol* 1985; 152(3): 330–334.

21 Zlatnik MG. Pulmonary edema: etiology and treatment. *Semin Perinatol* 1997; 21(4): 298–306.

22 Berkowitz RL, Rafferty TD. Invasive hemodynamic monitoring in critically ill pregnant patients: role of Swan–Ganz catheterization. *Am J Obstet Gynecol* 1980; 137(1): 127–134.

23 Cotton DB, Jones MM, Longmire S, Dorman KF, Tessem J, Joyce TH 3rd. Role of intravenous nitroglycerin in the treatment of severe pregnancy-induced hypertension complicated by pulmonary edema. *Am J Obstet Gynecol* 1986; 154(1): 91–93.

24 Sibai BM, Mabie BC, Harvey CJ, Gonzales AR. Pulmonary edema in severe preeclampsia-eclampsia: analysis of 37 consecutive cases. *Am J Obstet Gynecol* 1987; 156(4): 1174–1179.

25 Mabie WC, Hackman BB, Sibai BM. Pulmonary edema associated with pregnancy: echocardiographic insights and implications for treatment. *Obstet Gynecol* 1993; 81(2): 227–234.

26 DiFederico EM, Burlingame JM, Kilpatrick SJ, Harrison M, Matthay MA. Pulmonary edema in obstetric patients is rapidly resolved except in the presence of infection or of nitroglycerin tocolysis after open fetal surgery. *Am J Obstet Gynecol* 1998; 179: 925–933.

27 Sciscione AC, Ivester T, Largoza M, Manley J, Schlossman P, Colmorgen GHC. Acute pulmonary edema in pregnancy. *Obstet Gynecol* 2003; 101: 511–515.

28 Mueller C, Scholer A, Laule-Kilian K, et al. Use of B-type natriuretic peptide in the evaluation and management of acute dyspnea. *N Engl J Med* 2004; 350: 647–654.

29 Resnik, JL, Hoag C, Resnik R, et al. Evaluation of B-type natriuretic peptide (BNP) levels in normal and preeclamptic women. *Am J Obstet Gynecol* 2005; 193: 450–454.

30 Connors AF, Speroff T, Dawson NV, et al. for the SUPPORT (Study to Understand Prognoses and Preferences for Outcomes and Risks of Treatments) Investigators. The effectiveness of right heart catheterization in the initial care of critically ill patients. *JAMA* 1996; 276(11): 889–897.

31 Dahlen JE, Bone RC. Is it time to pull the pulmonary artery catheter? *JAMA* 1996; 276(11): 916–918.

32 Iberti TJ, Fischer EP, Leibowitz AB, Panacek EA, Silverstein JH, Albertson TE, and the Pulmonary Artery Catheter Study Group. A multicenter study of physicians' knowledge of the pulmonary artery catheter. *JAMA* 1990; 264(22): 2928–2932.

33 Dahlen JE. The pulmonary artery catheter – friend, foe, or accomplice? *JAMA* 2001; 286(3): 348–350.

34 Richard C, Warszawski J, Anguel N, et al. Early use of the pulmonary artery catheter and outcomes in patients with shock and acute respiratory distress syndrome: a randomized trial. *JAMA* 2003; 290: 2713–2720.

35 National Heart, Lung, and Blood Institute Acute Respiratory Distress Syndrome (ARDS) Clinical Trials Network. Pulmonary-artery versus central venous catheter to guide treatment of acute lung injury. *N Engl J Med* 2006; 354: 2213–2224.

36 Samol JM, Lambers DS. Magnesium sulfate tocolysis and pulmonary edema: the drug or the vehicle? *Am J Obstet Gynecol* 2005; 192: 1430–1432.

37 Hunt SA, Abraham WT, Chin MH, et al. ACC/AHA 2005 guideline update for the diagnosis and management of chronic heart failure in the adult – summary article. *J Am Coll Cardiol* 2005; 46: 1116–1143.

38 Acute Respiratory Distress Syndrome Network. Ventilation with lower tidal volumes as compared with traditional tidal volumes for acute lung injury and the acute respiratory distress syndrome. *N Engl J Med* 2000; 342: 1301–1318.

39 Dellinger RP, Carlet JM, Masur H, et al. Surviving sepsis campaign guidelines for management of severe sepsis and septic shock. *Crit Care Med* 2004; 32: 858–873.

26 The Acute Abdomen During Pregnancy

Howard T. Sharp
Department of Obstetrics and Gynecology, University of Utah School of Medicine, Salt Lake City, UT, USA

Introduction

Effective communication between physicians and medical services is critically important in the treatment of the pregnant patient with an acute abdomen.

Caring for two patients, both with unique vulnerabilities, is optimally performed with the coordination of appropriate obstetric, surgical, radiological, and in later gestational ages, neonatal services. Proper communication with radiologists can help to minimize exposure to ionizing radiation, while maternal and fetal recommendations to the surgical team can help maximize intraoperative safety if surgery is necessary.

Timely communication can also help avoid treatment delay, which can ultimately be the greatest risk for maternal and fetal morbidity and mortality. As a general rule, the acute abdomen during pregnancy should be treated as it would in the non-pregnant state. It is important for physicians caring for obstetric patients with acute surgical issues to be aware of the unique circumstances associated with each trimester of pregnancy, in particular organogenesis in the first trimester and preterm labor issues in the later part of the second and the third trimesters. Lastly, with the popularization of laparoscopy, surgical approaches are evolving, the limits of which are currently being investigated for safety and efficacy.

This chapter will review contemporary diagnostic and surgical modalities available for patients with the acute abdomen in pregnancy. The morbidity and mortality associated with these surgical conditions will also be reviewed. The vast majority of data regarding the acute abdomen in pregnancy are based upon case reports and case series, and are therefore considered level III data as outlined by the US Preventive Services Task Force.

Critical Care Obstetrics, 5th edition. Edited by M. Belfort, G. Saade, M. Foley, J. Phelan and G. Dildy. © 2010 Blackwell Publishing Ltd.

Laparoscopy during pregnancy

The refinement of operative laparoscopy has allowed for a significant shift in the way many surgeries are performed during pregnancy. There remain questions about the potential for decreased maternal uterine blood flow due to increased intra-abdominal pressures from insufflation, and possible fetal carbon dioxide absorption. Some data from animal models suggest that the risk of fetal acidosis may be higher than expected [1]. Other possible drawbacks of laparoscopic surgery during pregnancy include injury to the pregnant uterus, and the technical difficulty of laparoscopic surgery due to the growing mass of the gravid uterus.

The most commonly performed laparoscopic surgeries during pregnancy are cholecystectomy and appendectomy. Laparoscopy is routinely performed during the second trimester at most hospitals, and is becoming more common during the first and third trimesters [2]. In a review of appendectomy and cholecystectomy during pregnancy at a tertiary care hospital, one group reported an increase in the use of laparoscopy from 54% in 1998 to 97% in 2002 with no significant differences in preterm delivery rates, birth weights, or 5-minute Apgar scores compared to a control group of pregnant women who underwent laparotomy [3].

Most evidence for the use of laparoscopy during pregnancy comes from case series demonstrating feasibility and reporting favorable outcomes from surgeons with significant interest and skill in laparoscopy [4,5]. Therefore, their results may not accurately reflect complication rates at other centers. Some groups are less enthusiastic about the use of laparoscopy during pregnancy and caution that the broad application and acceptance of laparoscopy in pregnancy should follow favorable outcomes from high-quality evidence [6]. Due to the limited amount of high-quality studies, data on laparoscopic surgery during pregnancy are insufficient to draw firm conclusions on its safety and complication rate [7]. However, the trend of the cumulative experience over the past 10 years suggests that laparoscopic surgery is becoming more widely used and may be performed safely during pregnancy in most cases. Though preliminary evidence on short-term as well as long-term [8] outcomes is promising, higher-quality studies (level I) are eagerly awaited.

If laparoscopic surgery is to be performed after the first trimester, open laparoscopy is recommended to best avoid trocar or Veress needle injury to the gravid uterus. The use of a uterine manipulator is contraindicated in pregnancy.

Diagnostic imaging during pregnancy

There is often concern over the use of diagnostic imaging during pregnancy. Organogenesis occurs predominately during days 31 through 71 from the last menstrual period. According to the American College of Radiology, no single diagnostic X-ray procedure results in enough radiation exposure to threaten the well-being of the developing pre-embryo, embryo, or fetus. Radiation exposure of less than 5 rad is not associated with an increased risk of teratogenesis. However, carcinogenesis is thought to be associated with ionizing radiation at higher doses (>5 rad), and the avoidance of unnecessary radiological testing is a valid concern.

Ultrasound uses sound waves rather than ionizing radiation and is considered safe during pregnancy. At the time of this writing, there are no reports of adverse fetal effects from its use. Therefore, it should be considered a first-line diagnostic procedure if appropriate for the suspected condition.

All diagnostic X-ray procedures result in fetal exposure of less than 5 rad (Table 26.1). These range from approximately 100 mrad for a single view abdominal film to 2–4 rad for a barium enema or small bowel series. The amount of radiation exposure is largely dependent upon the number of exposures. Consultation with a radiologist can assist in estimating the amount of ionizing radiation to the fetus before tests are performed.

The dose of ionizing radiation from a computed tomography (CT) study of the maternal pelvis using standard parameters varies, but is usually associated with a fetal exposure of between 2.4 rad and 4.6 rad, and is therefore below the 5-rad threshold of potential teratogenesis risk. The 5-rad dose range has been associated with an up to two times increased risk of childhood cancer [9]. Spiral or helical CT scans, also called multidetector CT scans, are now able to perform imaging much faster with less radiation exposure.

Table 26.1 Estimated fetal exposure from radiologic procedures.

Procedure	Fetal exposure
Abdominal film	100 mrad
Helical CT of abdomen	300 mrad
Barium enema	2–4 rads
Small bowel series	2–4 rads
CT of abdomen	3.5 rads
Intravenous pyelogram	>1 rad

Magnetic resonance imaging (MRI) uses magnets that alter the energy state of hydrogen protons instead of using ionizing radiation. Though there has been no reported adverse fetal effect from its use, current FDA labeling of MRI devices states that fetal safety "has not been established." Although the elective use of MRI during pregnancy should be avoided, its use is preferable to CT.

Appendicitis during pregnancy

The most common cause of the acute abdomen in pregnancy is appendicitis, which occurs with a rate of approximately 1 in 1500 deliveries [10,11]. The diagnosis of appendicitis in pregnancy can be difficult to make because of the blunted signs and symptoms during pregnancy, along with the changing location of the appendix as pregnancy advances. When appendicitis is suspected during pregnancy, the physician must balance the risks associated with delaying surgery with the effects of surgery on the mother and fetus. Ultimately, as in the non-pregnant state, the decision to operate should be made on clinical grounds, accepting that there is an inherent chance of a negative exploration. Most larger series of appendectomy during pregnancy quote a negative exploration rate of approximately 20–35%. If the appendix appears normal at surgery, it is important to look for other non-obstetric causes (Table 26.2) as well as obstetric causes (Table 26.3).

Presentation

It is important to realize the changes that the uterus undergoes throughout the 9 months of gestation. In 1932, Baer et al. demonstrated the migration of the appendix based on serial radiographs in pregnant women [12]. They described a progressive upward displacement of the appendix after the third month, reaching the level of the iliac crest at the end of the sixth month. The appendix was noted to return to its normal position by the 10th postpartum day. These observations were recently confirmed in a study using MRI in pregnant women [13].

Table 26.2 Non-obstetric conditions mimicking appendicitis.

Acute intermittent porphyria
Acute mesenteric adenitis
Bowel obstruction
Carcinoma of large bowel
Cholecystitis/cholelithiasis
Crohn's disease
Diverticulitis (including meckel's)
Gastroenteritis
Hernia
Ischemic mesentaric necrosis
Pancreatitis
Perforated duodenal ulcer
Pyelonephritis
Rectus hematoma
Urinary calculi

Table 26.3 Obstetric conditions mimicking appendicitis.

Abruptio placenta
Adnexal torsion
Chorioamnionitis
Ectopic / heterotopic pregnancy
Myomatous red degeneration
Pelvic inflammatory disease
Preterm labor
Round ligament pain
Rupture of uterine avm
Uterine rupture
(placenta percreta)
(rudimentary uterine horn)
Uterine torsion
Utero-ovarian vein rupture

The most typical presentation of appendicitis is colicky epigastric or periumbilical pain (referred from the appendiceal viscera), which eventually localizes to the right side of the abdomen. Anorexia and vomiting, though common in pregnant women with appendicitis, are not necessarily specific or sensitive indicators; likewise, fever is often not present. The single most reliable symptom in pregnant patients with appendicitis is right lower quadrant pain [14]. Rebound tenderness and guarding are not particularly specific.

Due to the natural physiology of pregnancy, laboratory values are not reliably predictive of appendicitis during pregnancy. In the first and second trimesters, the white blood cell count may normally range from 6000 to 16,000 cells/mm^3. During labor, it may rise to 20,000–30,000 cells/mm^3. Therefore, leukocytosis may not be helpful in diagnosing appendicitis in pregnancy; however, a persistent white blood cell count in the normal range provides reassurance. Larger case series have questioned the usefulness of relying on laboratory data to confirm or dismiss a diagnosis of appendicitis in pregnancy [15].

Diagnostic imaging

In the non-pregnant state, graded compression ultrasound (GCU) has been used to diagnose acute appendicitis with a sensitivity of 86%. Because of its accuracy and favorable safety profile, it is the initial diagnostic imaging test of choice for evaluating pregnant women. In pregnancy, GCU has been shown to be accurate in the first and second trimesters, but technically difficult in the third. In a series of 42 women with suspected appendicitis during pregnancy, GCU was found to be 100% sensitive, 96% specific, and 98% accurate in diagnosing appendicitis [16]. Three patients were unable to be adequately evaluated due to the technical difficulties associated with gestational ages over 35 weeks. Though ultrasound is the preferred imaging modality for suspected acute appendicitis during pregnancy, in the late third trimester, or if ultrasound is otherwise inconclusive, MRI or CT may be necessary. Consultation with a radiologist is recommended if MRI or CT is to be used.

MRI has the advantage over CT of using no ionizing radiation and has been shown to be accurate in its ability to demonstrate abdominal and pelvic disease in pregnant patients [17]. It has been reported to have an overall sensitivity and specificity of 100% and 93.6% respectively for appendicitis in pregnancy [18].

Helical CT is a technology that has the advantage of being performed rapidly, with less exposure to ionizing radiation compared to standard CT. In a prospective comparison with standard CT in non-pregnant patients with acute abdominal pain, simple agreement among radiologists was obtained in 79% of cases [19]. Though the initial results in pregnant patients are promising, only one case series has been reported which included seven patients [20]. Helical CT of the pregnant abdomen can be accomplished in 15 minutes with an exposure of approximately 300 mrad to the fetus. Larger studies are needed to validate the initial favorable results of this case series.

Mortality and morbidity

Babler wrote in 1908, "The mortality of appendicitis complicating pregnancy and the puerperium is the mortality of delay" [21]. Though the fetal mortality rate associated with appendicitis has improved over the past 50 years, when appendiceal perforation occurs, the fetal loss rate may be as high as 36% [10]. In contrast, in the absence of appendiceal perforation, the incidence of fetal loss is 1.5% or less [10]. Appendiceal rupture has been reported to occur twice as often in the third trimester (69%) as in the first and second trimesters (31%) [22].

Preterm labor is a concern due to peritoneal irritation and its inflammatory response. Though preterm contractions are common after appendectomy in pregnancy (83%), they rarely result in preterm labor and delivery (5–14%) [12,15]. Therefore tocolytic agents are not routinely recommended.

Over the past several decades, maternal mortality rates associated with appendicitis have dropped. This is likely due to the development of improved surgical techniques and antibiotics. Maternal death from appendicitis, which was not uncommon in the early 20th century (25% mortality rate), is now a rarity and is usually associated with significant surgical delay.

Prompt surgical intervention has been shown to decrease the morbidity and mortality associated with appendicitis during pregnancy in several case series. Horowitz reported on a series of 12 patients with a preoperative diagnosis of appendicitis, 10 of which were documented to have appendicitis [23]. Surgery was delayed more than 24 hours in 7 of the 12 patients. Six of the 7 patients had appendiceal perforation resulting in two fetal deaths, one preterm delivery, and one maternal death. A larger series by Tamir reported appendiceal perforation in 66% of patients when surgical delay occurred for greater than 24 hours (n = 35), yet no cases of perforation in patients taken to surgery within 24 hours of presentation [24].

Preparing for surgery

When preparing for surgery in the pregnant patient, it is useful for care to be coordinated between consulting services in a timely fashion. Obstetrics, general surgery, anesthesia, and neonatology services each may have important details to convey to optimize the team approach.

If laparotomy is to be performed, the patient should be placed in the supine position with a right hip roll, rotating the patient 30° to the left to optimize blood flow to the fetus. Uterine manipulation should be avoided as much as possible to decrease the risk of uterine irritability and preterm labor. Intraopterative external fetal monitoring should be considered if the gestational age is in the range of fetal viability. This can be done by wrapping a sterile plastic bag around the fetal heart rate monitor and displacing it from the skin incision. The main argument for performing intraoperative fetal monitoring is in case appendiceal perforation has occurred, wherein there is a greater risk of fetal mortality. If perforation has occurred, an important part of therapy is the use of copious irrigation and broad-spectrum antibiotics, including anerobic coverage. The use of an intraperitoneal drain has been advocated in such cases.

Various incisions have been recommended. The most popular is a muscle-splitting incision over the point of maximum tenderness, which is particularly useful in the second and third trimesters. The paramedian and midline vertical incisions should be used if there is significant doubt about the diagnosis, for improved access to the left adnexa if necessary.

In a case–control study of 22 laparoscopic appendectomies, compared to 18 open appendectomies, all were performed without birth defects, fetal loss or uterine injury. Preterm delivery rates in the both groups were similar. Neither birth weights nor Apgar scores were significantly different across groups [25]. In a prospective series, maternal and fetal outcomes in pregnant women undergoing laparoscopic appendectomy was compared with a control group of pregnant women who underwent open appendectomy [26]. There was no significant difference in the length of procedure (60 vs 46 min) or complications rate. There was no conversion to laparotomy in the laparoscopic group, and the length of postoperative stay was shorter in the laparoscopic group (3.6 vs 5.2 days; $p = 0.05$). There was no fetal loss or other adverse outcome of pregnancy in either group, and all the women in both groups had normal full-term delivery. The infants' development was normal in both groups for a mean follow-up period of 30 months (see section on laparoscopy in pregnancy).

Cholecystitis during pregnancy

Cholecystitis is the second most common surgical condition in pregnancy, occurring in approximately 1 in 1600 to 10,000 pregnancies. During pregnancy, there is an increase in maternal cholesterol synthesis with an increased concentration of cholesterol in the gallbladder, yet stasis of bile in the gallbladder. Cholelithiasis is the cause of cholecystitis in pregnancy in over 90% of cases. The incidence of cholelithiasis in pregnant women undergoing routine obstetric ultrasound examinations is 3.5%; however, it is unclear whether pregnancy predisposes women to cholecystitis, as statistically fewer cholecystectomies are performed on pregnant women than on non-pregnant women [27]. This lower rate may be due to physicians' reluctance to perform surgery on pregnant patients.

Table 26.4 Differential diagnosis of cholecystitis during pregnancy.

Appendicitis
Acute hepatitis
Herpes zoster
Myocardial infarction
Pancreatitis
Peptic ulcer disease
Pneumonia
Preeclampsia
Pyelonephritis

Presentation

The presentation of cholecystitis in pregnancy is essentially the same as in as in the non-pregnant state. Nausea, vomiting, and an acute onset of a colicky or stabbing pain that begins over the midepigastrium or right upper abdominal quadrant with radiation to the back, is common. Biliary colic, usually sudden in onset, may persist for approximately 3 hours after a meal. Symptoms also may be localized to the flank, right scapula, or shoulder. Murphy's sign (tenderness under the right costal margin upon deep inspiration) is less common in pregnant women with cholecystitis. Fever, tachycardia, and tachypnea may be present. When upper abdominal pain presents during pregnancy, the differential diagnosis should include potentially life-threatening processes such as myocardial infarction, acute fatty liver in pregnancy, and HELLP syndrome. Other less serious but significant conditions should also be considered in the differential diagnosis (Table 26.4).

Diagnosis

Leukocytosis and hyperamylasemia are common, the later usually resolving upon hydration. Serum transaminases and direct bilirubin levels may also be elevated. Jaundice is rare, but if present, may be associated with common bile duct stones. Alkaline phosphatase is less helpful in diagnosing cholecystitis in pregnancy because estrogen secretion causes these levels to be elevated.

Ultrasound imaging of the gallbladder is indicated when there is significant right upper quadrant pain in pregnancy. It is the diagnostic test of choice in pregnancy because it is non-invasive, readily available, and accurate. The diagnostic accuracy of ultrasound for detecting gallstones is approximately 95% [27]. Good views of the gallbladder can usually be obtained during pregnancy without fasting.

Clinical management

The treatment for cholecystitis in pregnancy has typically been supportive, especially in the third trimester. Surgery has generally been reserved for those cases in which supportive medical treatment failed after several days, or in patients who experienced repeated attacks of biliary colic. Surgery has also typically been performed outright in patients with suspected perforation, sepsis, or peritonitis. This traditional approach is now being challenged by some investigators in favor of a more aggressive surgical approach, managed by laparoscopy [23] or laparotomy regardless of trimester.

Medical management

The medical treatment of cholecystitis in pregnancy consists of supportive intravenous hydration, enteric rest with nasogastric suction, and judicious use of narcotics. Morphine is avoided because it can exacerbate biliary colic. Broad-spectrum antibiotics are probably helpful in most cases, but clearly indicated for signs of sepsis.

Active surgical management

In 1987, Dixon made an argument for a more aggressive approach during the second trimester. He reported a retrospective study of 44 pregnant women with biliary colic, 26 who received supportive medical management and 18 who underwent primary open cholecystectomy in the second trimester [28]. In the group receiving medical management, 58% suffered recurrent episodes. Total parenteral nutrition was necessary in 8% of patients for an average of 29 days, and one patient developed pancreatitis. The mean length of hospital admission was 14 days which did not including hospital days for subsequent cholecystectomy. In the group of women treated primarily by surgery the mean length of hospital stay was 6 days. Larger subsequent studies have also demonstrated improved pregnancy outcomes in terms of both reduced hospitalization and a reduction of preterm delivery rates in women who underwent surgical management [29,30].

Laparoscopic cholecystectomy in pregnancy has been compared favorably to open cholecystectomy [31], wherein investigators have reported a decreased risk of spontaneous abortion in the first trimester, and a lower rate of preterm labor in the third trimester in women undergoing laparoscopic cholecystectomy. In a series of 16 women who underwent laparoscopic cholecystectomy during pregnancy, nine of 11 women who underwent cholecystectomy more than 5 weeks after onset of symptoms, experienced recurrent symptoms. These symptoms necessitated 15 hospital admissions and four emergency room visits [32]. Moreover, four women who experienced symptoms in the first and second trimesters, had surgery delayed to the third trimester, resulting in 11 hospital admissions and four emergency room visits. Cholecystectomy was completed laparoscopically in 14 women. There was no hospital infant or maternal mortality or morbidity. As a result, the authors recommend that prompt laparoscopic cholecystectomy in pregnant women with symptomatic biliary disease be considered as a means of reducing hospital admissions and the frequency of premature labor.

Bowel obstruction during pregnancy

Bowel obstruction in pregnancy occurs 1 in 2500 to 3500 deliveries, adhesions being the cause in the majority of cases. The incidence of intestinal obstruction caused by adhesions during stages in pregnancy were found to be 6% in the first trimester, 27% in the second trimester, 44% in the third trimester, and 21% postpartum [33]. In the first trimester this is probably caused by the uterus becoming a suprapubic organ, and later due to rapid uterine size changes that take place during delivery and the puerperium. Volvulus is the second most common cause of bowel obstruction in pregnancy, occurring in approximately 25% of cases [34]. Other causes such as intussusception, hernia, and cancer are rare. The incidence of bowel obstruction has been climbing since the 1940s, likely because of an increase in the number of surgeries performed. As with appendicitis, the morbidity and mortality of bowel obstruction is related to diagnostic and therapeutic delay [35]. Beware of the diagnosis of hyperemesis gravidarum in the second and third trimesters in patients who have had abdominal surgery, as this is a common misdiagnosis.

Bowel obstruction can result in significant maternal and fetal morbidity and mortality. Perdue et al. reviewed the literature written between 1966 and 1991 and found four maternal deaths in 66 reported cases of bowel obstruction in pregnancy [36]. The fetal mortality rate was 26%. Bowel strangulation requiring resection occurred in 23% of cases. The mean length of time from admission to surgery in these cases was 48 hours.

Presentation

The symptoms associated with bowel obstruction in pregnancy are crampy abdominal pain, obstipation, and vomiting. In the case of a high obstruction, the period between attacks is usually short, 4 or 5 minutes, and is frequently characterized by diffuse, poorly localized upper abdominal pain. Colonic obstruction may manifest as low abdominal or perineal pain with a longer pain attack interval of 15–20 min. The abdomen is frequently distended and tender. Fever, leukocytosis, and electrolyte abnormalities increase the likelihood of finding intestinal strangulation.

Diagnosis

Upright and flat-plate abdominal films should be obtained if intestinal obstruction is suspected. It is often helpful to compare serial radiographic findings to identify the presence of air–fluid levels or progressive bowel dilatation, in order to assess whether conservative management is effective. In one series, flat and upright radiographs showed typical patterns of obstruction in 75% of cases [34]. Radiologic studies following the administration of oral contrast media should be performed if bowel obstruction still is suspected in the absence of typical findings on flat and upright abdominal images.

Clinical management

The clinical management of bowel obstruction during pregnancy is essentially no different from treatment in the non-pregnant state. Treatment consists of fluid and electrolyte replacement, bowel decompression via nasogastric tube, and timely surgery for failed medical management. Fluid is lost by way of vomiting, nasogastric suctioning, intralumenal losses, bowel wall edema, and free peritoneal fluid. A Foley catheter should be placed to monitor urine output. The amount of fluid loss is often underestimated and may result in renal insufficiency, hypovolemia, shock, and death.

If the decision is made to take the patient to surgery, a midline vertical incision is recommended. Exposure is often a challenge, and depending on the gestational age in the third trimester, cesarean delivery may be necessary. The entire bowel should be examined, as there may be more than one area of obstruction. Bowel viability should be assessed carefully by a surgeon experienced in the management of necrotic bowel. Segmental resection with or without anastomosis may be needed.

Adnexal torsion during pregnancy

Adnexal torsion is one of the few causes of the acute abdomen that is more common in pregnancy than in the non-pregnant state. The typical presentation is lateralized lower quadrant pain, often sudden in onset. Though nausea, vomiting, fever, and leukocytosis may be present, none of these are reliable findings during pregnancy. On physical examination, the abdomen is tender, often with peritoneal signs. If it occurs in the first trimester, the adnexum is usually enlarged and exquisitely tender on bimanual exam.

Ultrasonography is the diagnostic modality of choice, as the presence of an adnexal mass is usually detectable. Doppler studies may assist to document the presence or absence of ovarian blood flow. However, the diagnosis of ovarian and adnexal torsion cannot be based solely on the absence or presence of flow on color Doppler sonography, because the presence of arterial or venous flow does not exclude the diagnosis of adnexal torsion [37]. Doppler studies of the ovarian vessels in pregnancy have not been investigated at the time of this writing.

If adnexal torsion is suspected, surgery should not be delayed, as the viability of the ovary may be compromised. If a laparotomy is to be performed, a midline vertical incision is recommended. This gives the surgeon excellent access to the adnexa and allows for enough room to properly explore the upper abdomen, as is standard for the presence of an adnexal mass. The laparoscopic approach to adnexal torsion in pregnancy has been reported with favorable outcomes [38,39]. If ovarian cystectomy is performed prior to 12 weeks gestation, supplemental progesterone should be provided if the mass was the corpus luteum.

There has been a common misconception that the untwisting of an ovary that has undergone torsion may cause venous embolism. A review of the literature failed to document any cases of venous embolic phenomena associated with this practice. Growing evidence supports ovarian-sparing surgery in the non-pregnant state, even in the case of persistently black-blue ovaries after untwisting [40,41]. In a series of 54 non-pregnant women with ovarian torsion resulting in black-bluish ovaries, all underwent adnexal or ovarian untwisting with sparing of the affected ovary. On follow-up, 93% were documented to have normal ovarian size with follicular development [42]. The authors conclude that ovaries that have undergone torsion should be untwisted regardless of color and that cystectomy should be performed instead of oophorectomy.

Summary

Maternal mortality is rare in cases of appendicitis during pregnancy. However, fetal mortality can be as high as 33% in cases associated with appendiceal perforation. During pregnancy, laboratory tests are often unreliable, and diagnostic radiologic tests such as ultrasound, MRI, and helical CT are understudied. Therefore, a clinical diagnosis based on the patient's history and physical examination is essential. Due to the low incidence of maternal and fetal complications in patients surgically explored early, pregnant patients with suspected appendicitis should be treated with a similar decision-making process as non-pregnant patients. Though ultrasound is the preferred imaging modality for suspected acute appendicitis during pregnancy, in the late third trimester, or if ultrasound is otherwise inconclusive, MRI or CT may be necessary. Consultation with a radiologist is recommended if MRI or CT is to be used.

For patients with cholecystitis in pregnancy, individualization of treatment is recommended. Current data favors primary surgical management as a treatment option. Laparoscopic cholecystectomy is gaining popularity, as surgeons experienced in this technique have had favorable preliminary results in all trimesters. Outcomes associated with laparoscopic surgery in pregnancy need further study, especially in terms of complication rates.

References

1 Amos JD, Schorr SJ, Norman PF, et al. Laparoscopic surgery during pregnancy. *Am J Surg* 1997; 174: 22.

2 Barnes SL, Shane MD, Schoemann MB, et al. Laparoscopy appendectomy after 30 weeks pregnancy: report of two cases and description of technique. *Am Surg* 2004; 70: 733–736.

3 Rollins MD, Chan KJ, Price RR. Laparoscopy for appendicitis and cholelithiasis during pregnancy: a new standard of care. *Surg Endosc* 2004; 18: 237–241.

4 Ueberrueck T, Kock A, Meyer L, et al. Ninety-four appendectomies for suspected acute appendicitis during pregnancy. *World J Surg* 2004; 28: 508–551.

5 Wu JM, Chen KH, Lin HF, et al. Laparoscopic appendectomy in pregnancy. *J Laparoendosc Adv Surg Tech A* 2005; 15: 447–450.

6 Carver TW, Antevil J, Egan JC, et al. Appendectomy during early pregnancy: what is the preferred surgical approach? *Am Surg* 2005; 71: 809–812.

7 Fatum M, Rojansky N. Laparoscopic surgery during pregnancy. *Obstet Gynecol Surv* 2001; 56: 50–59.

8 Rizzo AG. Laparoscopic surgery in pregnancy: long-term follow-up. *J Laparoendosc Adv Surg Tech A.* 2003; 13: 11–15.

9 Damilakis J, Perisinakis K, Voloudaki A, et al. Estimation of fetal radiation dose from computed tomography scanning late in pregnancy: depth-dose data from routine examinations. *Invest Radiol* 2000; 35: 527–533.

10 Babaknia A, Parsa H, Woodruff JD. Appendicitis during pregnancy. *Obstet Gynecol* 1977; 50: 40–44.

11 Black WP. Acute appendicitis in pregnancy. *BMJ* 1960; 1: 1938–1941.

12 Baer JL, Reis RA, Arens RA. Appendicitis in pregnancy with changes in position and axis of the normal appendix in pregnancy. *JAMA* 1932; 52: 1359–1364.

13 Oto A, Srinivasan PN, Ernst RD, et al. Revisiting MRI for appendix location during pregnancy. *AJR* 2006; 186: 883–887.

14 Mourad J, Elliott JP, Erickson L, Lisboa L. Appendicitis in pregnancy: new information that contradicts long-held clinical beliefs. *Am J Obstet Gynecol* 2000; 182: 1027–1029.

15 Andersen B, Nielsen TF. Appendicitis in pregnancy: diagnosis, management and complications. *Acta Obstet Gynecol Scand* 1999; 78: 758–762.

16 Lim HK, Bae SH, Seo GS. Diagnosis of acute appendicitis in pregnant women: value of sonography. *AJR* 1992; 159: 539–442.

17 Birchard KR, Brown MA, Hyslop WB. MRI of the acute abdominal and pelvic pain in pregnant patients. *AJR* 2005; 184: 452–458.

18 Pedosa I, Levine D, Eyvazzadeh AD, et al. MR imaging evaluation of acute appendicitis in pregnancy. *Radiology* 2006; 238: 891–899.

19 Lee SY, Coughlin B, Wolfe JM, et al. Prospective comparison of helical CT of the abdomen and pelvis with and without oral contrast in assessing acute abdominal pain in adult Emergency Department patients. *Emerg Radiol* 2006; 12: 150–157.

20 Castro MA, Shipp TD, Castro EE, Ouzounian J, Rao P. The use of helical computed tomography in pregnancy for the diagnosis of acute appendicitis. *Am J Obstet Gynecol* 2001; 184: 954–957.

21 Babler EA. Perforative appendicitis complicating pregnancy. *JAMA* 1908; 51: 1313.

22 Weingold AB. Appendicitis in pregnancy. *Clin Obstet Gynecol* 1983; 26: 801–809.

23 Horowitz MD, Gomez GA, Santiesteban R, Burkett G. Acute appendicitis during pregnancy. *Arch Surg* 1995; 120: 1362–1367.

24 Tamir IL, Bongard FS, Klein SR. Acute appendicitis in the pregnant patient. *Am J Surg* 1990; 160: 571–576.

25 Affleck DG, Handrahan DL, Egger MJ, Price RR. The laparoscopic management of appendicitis and cholelithiasis during pregnancy. *Am J Surg* 1999; 178: 523–529.

26 Lyass S, Pikarsky A, Eisenberg VH, Elchalal U, Schenker JG, Reissman P. Is laparoscopic appendectomy safe in pregnant women? *Surg Endosc* 2001; 15: 377–379.

27 Stauffer RA, Adams A, Wygal J, Lavery PJ. Gallbladder disease in pregnancy. *Am J Obstet Gynecol* 1982; 6: 661–664.

28 Dixon NP, Faddis DM, Silberman H. Aggressive management of cholecystitis during pregnancy. *Am J Surg* 1987; 154: 292–294.

29 Lee S, Bradley JP, Mele MM, Sehdev HM, Ludmir J. Cholelithiasis in pregnancy: surgical versus medical management. *Obstet Gynecol* 2000; 95: S70–S71.

30 Lu EJ, Curet MJ, El-Sayed YY, et al. Medical versus surgical management of biliary tract disease in pregnancy. *Am J Surg* 2004; 188: 755–759.

31 Graham G, Baxi L, Tharakan T. Laparoscopic cholecystectomy during pregnancy: a case series and review of the literature. *Obstet Gynecol Surv* 1998; 53: 566–574.

32 Muench J, Albrink M, Serafini F, Rosemurgy A, Carey L, Murr MM. Delay in treatment of biliary disease during pregnancy increases morbidity and can be avoided with safe laparoscopic cholecystectomy. *Am Surg* 2001; 67: 539–542.

33 Connolly MM, Unit JA, Nora PF. Bowel obstruction in pregnancy. *Surg Clin North Am* 1995; 75: 101–113.

34 Wenetick LH, Roschen FP, Dunn JM. Volvulus of the small bowel complicating pregnancy. *J Reprod Med* 1973; 14: 82–83.

35 Kalu E, Sherriff E, Alsibai MA, et al. Gestational intestinal obstruction: a case report and review of the literature. *Arch Gynecol Obstet* 2006; 274: 60–62.

36 Perdue PW, Johnson HW, Stafford PW. Intestinal obstruction complicating pregnancy. *Am J Surg* 1992; 164: 384–388.

37 Albayram F, Hamper UM. Ovarian and adnexal torsion: a spectrum of sonographic findings with pathologic correlation. *J Ultrasound Med* 2001; 20: 1083–1089.

38 Morice P, Louis-Sylvestre C, Chapron C, Dubuisson JB. Laparoscopy for adnexal torsion in pregnant women. *J Reprod Med* 1997; 42: 435–439.

39 Abu-Musa A, Nassar A, Usta I, Khalil A, Hussein M. Laparoscopic unwinding and cystectomy of twisted dermoid cyst during second trimester of pregnancy. *J Am Assoc Gynecol Laparosc* 2001; 8: 456–460.

40 Oelsner G, Bider D, Goldenberg M, et al. Long-term follow-up of the twisted ischemic adnexal managed by detorsion. *Fertil Steril* 1993; 60: 976–979.

41 Cohen SB, Wattiez A, Seidman DS, et al. Laparoscopy versus laparotomy for detorsion and sparing of twisted ischemic adnexa. *JSLS* 2003; 7: 295–299.

42 Cohen SB, Oelsner G, Seidman DS, Admon D, Mashiach S, Goldenberg M. Laparoscopic detorsion allows sparing of the twisted ischemic adnexa. *J Am Assoc Gynecol Laparosc* 1999; 6: 139–1343.

27 Acute Pancreatitis

Shailen S. Shah[1] & Jeffrey P. Phelan[2]

[1]Maternal-Fetal Medicine, Virtua Health, Voorhees, NJ *and* Thomas Jefferson University Hospital, Philadelphia, PA, USA
[2]Department of Obstetrics and Gynecology, Citrus Valley Medical Center, West Covina *and* Clinical Research, Childbirth Injury Prevention Foundation, City of Industry, Pasadena, CA, USA

Introduction

Pancreatitis is uncommon in pregnancy [1] and is most commonly due to cholelithiasis [1]. Pregnancy-associated pancreatitis, however, may have a significant impact on maternal and fetal well-being. A clearer understanding of the natural history of this disease as it exists in the gravid woman has evolved over the past three decades. While the clinical presentation of pancreatitis is not significantly altered by pregnancy, the diagnosis of pancreatitis during pregnancy, as with all abdominal processes, may be challenging. Maternal outcome, however, does not appear to be altered by the concurrent state of pregnancy.

Pancreatitis spans the clinical spectrum from mild disease to multisystem organ failure. Reports of maternal mortality range from 0% to 3.4% and compare favorably with an overall mortality of 9% in the general population [1–6]. Fetal and neonatal outcomes, however, are often adversely affected by this disease, with prematurity accounting for a portion of morbidity [1]. However, earlier reports of perinatal mortality as high as 35% have been tempered by studies demonstrating fetal loss directly attributable to pancreatitis of 0–11% [1,3,5,7,8]. This chapter focuses on the epidemiology, clinical course, diagnosis, prognostic indicators, and management of pancreatitis occurring in pregnancy.

Epidemiology

The reported incidence of pancreatitis complicating pregnancy varies widely, with studies demonstrating rates as frequent as 1 in 459 and as uncommon as 1 in 6790 [9,10,11]. Many retrospective studies have been generated from tertiary care hospitals evaluating the frequency of pancreatitis within individual institutions. A more contemporary view found that the incidence of pancreatitis is approximately 1 case per 3333 pregnancies [1]. In a review of cholecystectomies performed for gallstone pancreatitis, Block and Kelly [3] found that among 152 female patients, 21 (13.8%) were either pregnant at the time of surgery or within 6 weeks postpartum.

Many studies have shown an increasing incidence of pancreatitis with advancing gestational age, although first-trimester pancreatitis is well described [1]. While pancreatitis may occur throughout pregnancy and the puerperium, as many as 35–50% of cases occur during the third trimester [1]. Approximately 70–80% of patients are multigravidas [1], correlating with the overall distribution within the general obstetric population. Parity, therefore, does not appear to influence the development of pancreatitis. Increased risk among ethnic groups has not been demonstrated within the obstetric population. Incidence rates, however, do correlate with the prevalence of etiologic factors such as cholelithiasis [1] and alcohol abuse, which are known to vary among populations.

Early reports of phenomenally high maternal mortality led to a long-held belief that pancreatitis in pregnancy gravely endangered maternal well-being. It is now accepted that previous maternal mortality figures approaching 35–50% considerably overestimated the lethality of the disease [7]. Klein [2] collected data from five single institution series and found only three maternal deaths among 87 cases of pancreatitis, a mortality rate of 3.4%. However, contemporary investigations have demonstrated no maternal deaths occurring among 94 cumulative cases [1,3,5]. Biased reporting of more severe cases, as well as confounding concurrent disease, such as fatty liver of pregnancy, may have contributed to the higher mortality reported in earlier studies. Commonly used pharmacologic agents, including methyldopa, may produce unpredictable idiosyncratic or hypersensitivity reactions, including hepatitis and pancreatitis [12,13]. Additionally, two drugs previously used liberally in pregnancy, thiazide diuretics and tetracycline, have been linked to pancreatitis but are rarely used today [4,14,15]. The course of pancreatitis associated with these drugs may have incited a more frequently

Critical Care Obstetrics, 5th edition. Edited by M. Belfort, G. Saade, M. Foley, J. Phelan and G. Dildy.

fulminant disease process. Conversely, improvements in laboratory assays and radiologic modalities may now enable detection of a greater number of mild cases. Regardless of the underlying cause of this discrepancy, current maternal mortality from pancreatitis is only a tenth of previously reported rates.

Etiology

Acute pancreatitis is caused by many different factors. While the list of etiologies is extensive (Table 27.1), approximately 80% of cases are attributable to either biliary tract disease or alcohol abuse in the general population [4,16]. Gallstones are the most common cause of pancreatitis in the United States, Western Europe, and Asia, accounting for 45% of cases [4]. Alcoholism accounts for another 35%, roughly 10% are idiopathic, and the remainder is divided among miscellaneous causes.

Among pregnant patients, causes of pancreatitis parallel those of the general population. Physiologic changes in biliary function, however, appear to influence the incidence of cholelithiasis, although not necessarily gallstone pancreatitis, during pregnancy. Behavioral changes secondary to teratogenic concerns also may decrease the relative proportion of alcohol-induced pancreatitis. This section focuses on those causes most commonly seen in pregnancy: gallstones, hypertriglyceridemia, and drug-associated pancreatitis. It should also be noted that pancreatitis in pregnancy has been associated with pre-eclampsia, HELLP syndrome, and acute fatty liver of pregnancy (AFLP). It is a potentially lethal complication of AFLP and some have suggested that all patients with this diagnosis be screened [17].

Biliary disease in pregnancy

Cholelithiasis is the most common etiology of pancreatitis in pregnancy, representing a larger percentage of cases than in the non-pregnant population. Biliary disease has been identified in 68–100% of pregnant patients with pancreatitis [1,3,5]. The increased proportion of gallstone-induced pancreatitis may be attributable to the direct effects of pregnancy on gallstone formation, rather than a decreased incidence of other etiologies, and remains an area of active investigation.

Table 27.1 Potential causes of acute pancreatitis in pregnancy.

Acute fatty liver of pregnancy
Pre-eclampsia
Obstruction (cholelithiasis)
Drugs (ethanol, thiazides, azathioprine, valproic acid)
Hyperlipidemia
Abdominal trauma
Hypercalcemia
Infection (viral, parasitic)
Vascular disease (systemic lupus erythematosus)
Miscellaneous (Crohn's disease, perforating ulcer, cystic fibrosis)

Physiology of the biliary system during gestation appears to promote the incidence of gallstone formation through changes in both gallbladder function and bile composition. Using direct observation, intravenous contrast, and, most recently, serial ultrasound evaluation, residual gallbladder volume has been shown to increase throughout pregnancy [18]. Braverman et al. [18] also demonstrated a slower rate of gallbladder emptying in the latter part of pregnancy. It is felt that these functional changes result in bile stasis, thereby facilitating gallstone formation. Furthermore, studies of bile composition have demonstrated an increase in the lithogenic index of bile, as well as increased bile acid pool size, increased cholesterol secretion, and decreased enterohepatic circulation [19]. The functional changes that contribute to bile stasis act in concert with physiologic changes that increase the lithogenicity of bile constituents, leading to gallstone formation during pregnancy. This is demonstrated in a study of gallstones in Chilean women, by Valdivieso and associates [19] who demonstrated the effect of pregnancy on the incidence of gallstone formation, noting gallstones in 12.2% of puerperal women, compared with 1.3% in age-matched controls.

The mechanism by which gallstones initiate pancreatitis remains incompletely understood. In 1901, Opie [20] proposed the "common channel theory," by which stone impaction at the ampulla of Vater occludes the biliopancreatic duct, creating a channel that allows bile to reflux into the pancreatic duct. Another theory suggests that the pancreatic duct itself becomes blocked, obstructing the outflow of pancreatic secretions, which, in turn, damage the pancreatic acini. While further investigations have challenged these theories, the actual sequence of events remains elusive. Regardless of the mechanism by which stone passage initiates pancreatitis, it is clear that passage is temporally related to the onset of symptoms. Recovery of stones from stool collections has been reported to be as high as 85% [15].

Hypertriglyceridemia

Elevation of plasma triglycerides is a well-established cause of pancreatitis. While this type of pancreatitis is rare during pregnancy with a reported incidence of 1 in 25 000 births [21], the physiologic changes of pregnancy can exacerbate and unmask an underlying familial disorder and can compound the effects of other etiologies of hypertriglyceridemia. The mechanism by which hyperlipidemia causes pancreatitis is not fully understood. Local injury to the pancreatic acini, however, is felt to occur through the release of free fatty acids by the action of lipases on the excessive triglycerides [2,21,22]. Patients with triglyceride levels exceeding 1000 mg/dL are at greatest risk for pancreatitis, especially those with type V hyperlipidemia [2,21].

Pregnancy alters lipid metabolism by several mechanisms. An increase in triglyceride production and very low density lipoprotein (VLDL) secretion, as well as a decrease in lipolysis, result in a 50% increase in cholesterol and a threefold increase in triglycerides, with the peak effect observed in the third trimester

[2,22,23]. Superimposed on a familial hyperlipidemia, the metabolic changes of pregnancy can lead to markedly elevated serum levels and greatly increase the risk of pancreatitis. Postpartum total cholesterol and VLDL fall to baseline by 6 weeks [23].

Several features of a patient's medical and family history may suggest an underlying lipid disorder. A history of pancreatitis, recurrent (unexplained) abdominal pain, and known familial disorders can suggest the presence of inherited hyperlipidemia. Chronic renal failure, poorly controlled diabetes mellitus, hypothyroidism, alcohol use, and drugs such as glucocorticoids and β-blockers can lead to elevated lipid levels [24]. In the presence of such conditions in a patient with a familial lipid disorder, the superimposition of pregnancy may result in fulminant pancreatitis [21,24]. Intravenous fat emulsions administered to patients receiving parenteral nutrition are also a rare cause of pancreatitis.

Drugs

Numerous drugs have the potential to occasionally cause pancreatitis. One review classified the following drugs as toxic to the pancreas: azathioprine, estrogens, furosemide, methyldopa, pentamidine, procainamide, sulfonamides, and thiazide diuretics [25]. The immunosuppressants 6-mercaptopurine and azathioprine and the common HIV therapies pentamidine and 2′,3′-dideoxyinosine have been strongly associated with this condition [15]. Antibiotics, including erythromycin and sulfonamides, also have been implicated.

More pertinent to the pregnant population, thiazide diuretics and tetracycline historically accounted for a significant portion of pancreatitis during pregnancy. When these agents were used more commonly in the treatment of pre-eclampsia, thiazides were associated with 8% of cases of pancreatitis in pregnancy [7]. In the same review, tetracycline accounted for nearly 28% of cases and was also commonly associated with acute fatty liver of pregnancy. With subsequent elucidation of the teratogenic effects of tetracycline, this agent should no longer cause pancreatitis in pregnancy. Similarly, use of thiazide diuretics has little or no role in the modern management of pre-eclampsia.

Pathology and pathophysiology

The pancreas secretes approximately 20 enzymes in 2000–3000 mL of alkaline fluid each day. The fluid is rich in bicarbonate, which serves to neutralize gastric acid and provide the correct pH within the intestinal tract for activation of the pancreatic enzymes. Under hormonal and neural control, amylolytic, lipolytic, and proteolytic enzymes are released into the duodenum. The pancreas is normally protected from autodigestion by the presence of protease inhibitors and storage of proteases as precursors (zymogens).

Pancreatitis can be classified based on its chronicity and severity. Acute pancreatitis implies return of normal pancreatic function, while chronic disease represents residual damage to the gland. The acute form can be further classified as either mild (interstitial or edematous) or severe (necrotizing or hemorrhagic) pancreatitis. Edematous pancreatitis represents roughly 75–90% of cases and is typically self-limiting in its course [4,26]. Morphologically, pancreatic interstitial edema and fat necrosis are present, but pancreatic necrosis is absent. In severe cases, the parenchyma of the gland undergoes necrosis and can lead to parenchymal and extrapancreatic hemorrhage.

Multiple diverse etiologies appear to trigger a sequence of events that ultimately leads to parenchymal inflammation and premature activation of pancreatic enzymes. Zymogen activation results in local damage by direct action on the acinar cells and pancreatic blood vessels. Systemic effects occur when complement and kallikrein activation induce disseminated intravascular coagulation and cardiovascular compromise. Degradation of surfactant by activated phospholipase A2 has been implicated as a possible mechanism of pulmonary injury in acute pancreatitis [27].

Clinical manifestations

Pregnancy does not significantly alter the clinical presentation of pancreatitis, but can certainly confound it. Symptoms of acute pancreatitis may develop abruptly or intensify over several hours. Present in nearly 100% of patients, epigastric or umbilical pain is constant and non-colicky in nature and often radiates to the back [5]. The pain is variable in severity, often peaking in a matter of hours but frequently continuing for many days, and can be exacerbated by meals. In some patients, the pain is worse in the supine position and relieved partially by sitting and leaning forward. Nausea and vomiting affect 80% of patients, but vomiting does not usually relieve the pain [5,15].

Physical examination generally reveals anxious and restless behavior as the patient strives to attain a comfortable position. Fever is present in as many as 60% of patients. Tachycardia and hypotension may result from hemorrhage, vasodilation, increased vascular permeability, or sequestration of fluids in the retroperitoneum or peritoneal cavity (ascites). Pulmonary findings are present in a minority of patients, ranging from decreased breath sounds secondary to effusions (more often left-sided) to severe respiratory distress. Evaluation of the abdomen reveals areas of tenderness, both epigastric and generalized. Voluntary and involuntary guarding is frequently present. Pancreatic pseudocysts may be palpable. The abdomen is commonly distended, and bowel sounds are diminished or absent. Bluish discoloration around the umbilicus (Cullen's sign) or at the flanks (Grey Turner's sign) occurs in less than 1% of patients but represents the ominous development of hemorrhagic pancreatitis with retroperitoneal dissection.

While pregnancy complicates diagnosis, and other disorders can have similar presentations, deep epigastric pain particularly when radiating to the back or associated with nausea and vomiting should be evaluated for pancreatitis.

Table 27.2 Complications of acute pancreatitis in pregnancy.

Hypovolemic shock (third-space sequestration)
Disseminated intravascular coagulation
Acute respiratory distress syndrome
Acute tubular necrosis
Hypocalcemia, hyperglycemia
Pseudocyst formation
Pancreatic abscess
Upper gastrointestinal hemorrhage
Premature labor and delivery

Complications

Most cases of pancreatitis during pregnancy are mild and self-limited, but it can progress to multisystem disease [28] (Table 27.2). Locally, pancreatic necrosis and infection may occur early in the course of disease, often within the first 2 weeks. Necrosis of greater than 50% of the pancreas is associated with high rates of infection. Increased abdominal tenderness, fever, and leukocytosis signal the onset of infection. Late complications include pseudocyst and abscess formation. Pseudocysts are collections of pancreatic secretions that lack epithelial linings and develop in 1–8% of cases of acute pancreatitis [4,15]. They usually occur 2–3 weeks after the onset of illness. Patients frequently complain of upper abdominal pain and may develop symptoms related to growth and pressure on adjacent structures. Abscesses differ from pseudocysts by the presence of a capsule surrounding a purulent fluid collection. Abscesses complicate 1–4% of cases and are most often diagnosed 3–4 weeks after the onset of pancreatitis [4].

Systemic complications arising in severe cases of pancreatitis are often manifest within the first week of illness and are potentially life-threatening. Multisystem organ failure may involve the pulmonary, cardiovascular, and renal systems, contributing to a mortality rate of nearly 9% [4,6]. Pulmonary involvement ranges from pleural effusions and pneumonia to acute respiratory distress syndrome (ARDS). The frequency of ARDS as a cause of death has previously been underestimated. In a review of 405 autopsy cases, 60% of deaths occurred in the first week of illness; and among these patients, pulmonary failure was the most common cause [29]. The exact mechanism of pulmonary injury has not been elucidated. As mentioned earlier, however, patients with pancreatitis-associated pulmonary complications have been noted to have higher phospholipase A and phospholipase A2 catalytic activity [27].

Various other organ systems are vulnerable in severe pancreatitis. Cardiovascular compromise may occur secondary to several mechanisms. Hemorrhage (intra- or retroperitoneal), fluid sequestration, and activation of vasoactive substances can lead to profound, refractory hypotension. Renal failure may develop following hypotensive episodes and acute tubular necrosis. Overwhelming sepsis is the most common cause of death after the first week of illness [5].

Uncommon complications also may occur during severe cases of pancreatitis. Stress ulcers leading to gastrointestinal hemorrhage, pancreatic pseudoaneurysms, or colonic obstruction or fistulas may develop. Rarely, sudden blindness has been reported (Purtscher's angiopathic retinopathy), with fundoscopy revealing cotton-wool spots and flame-shaped hemorrhages found solely at the optic disk and macula.

Diagnosis

Laboratory evaluation

While elevated serum amylase has been the cornerstone of diagnosis for many decades, a variety of biochemical indicators have been identified as markers of pancreatitis. Amylase isoenzymes, serum lipase, and more recently, trypsinogen-2 may increase the diagnostic accuracy of more standard serum assays. Several factors influence the accuracy of these tests. For example, amylase levels may be falsely elevated by non-pancreatic production, impaired renal clearance, or acidemia, as in diabetic ketoacidosis. Furthermore, concurrent conditions, such as hypertriglyceridemia, can falsely lower measured values.

Serum amylase is a rapidly performed, readily available serum marker of pancreatic enzyme levels. Many organs contribute to total amylase values. The pancreas contributes roughly 40%, while salivary glands contribute 60%, as measured by the P-isoenzyme and S-isoenzyme levels, respectively. Other tissues, such as the lung and fallopian tubes, also produce S-isoamylase. Isoenzyme measurement can improve the sensitivity of amylase testing. However, it is not as widely available. Amylase rises in the first few hours of disease onset and falls rapidly, returning to normal in 24–72 hours. It is, therefore, not an accurate test for patients presenting more than several days after the onset of symptoms. Overall, serum amylase has a sensitivity of 95–100% and a specificity of 70% [30].

In contrast, serum lipase rises in a fashion parallel to amylase but remains elevated for a longer period of time (as many as 7–14 days). Serum lipase, therefore, has greater sensitivity in the subset of patients with late presentation. It is also unaffected by diabetic ketoacidosis. Lipase is produced mainly by the pancreas but is produced by other gastrointestinal sources as well, namely, liver, intestine, biliary tract, and salivary glands. The effect of non-pancreatic production on serum lipase levels, however, is unclear. It is generally regarded that lipase is more specific (99%) and as sensitive (99–100%) as serum amylase and merits wider use in the evaluation of pancreatitis [30].

The effect of pregnancy on amylase and lipase levels has been investigated. Strickland et al. [31] studied 413 asymptomatic women of varying gestational ages. In contrast to earlier studies reporting higher levels in pregnancy that vary through gestation, they concluded that mean amylase activities did not significantly differ among gestational age groups, nor compared with women 6 weeks postpartum [31,32]. Amylase levels measured as high as 150 IU/L. Ordorica et al. [33] and Karsenti et al. [34] corrobo-

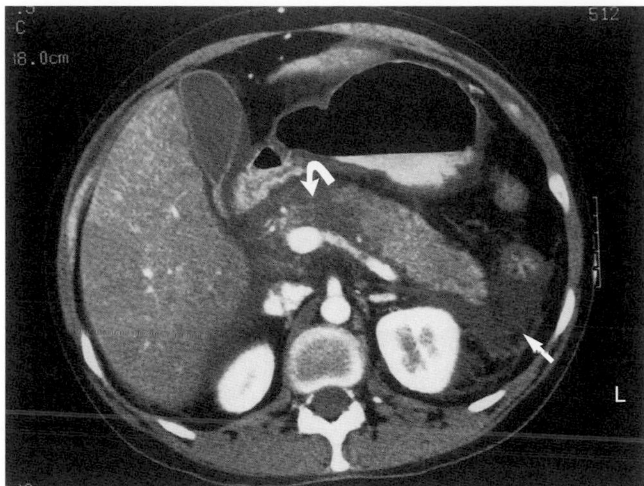

Figure 27.1 Computed tomography scan demonstrating necrosis in the head of the pancreas (curved arrow) and free fluid in the anterior pararenal space (straight arrow). (Courtesy of Dr Paula Woodward.)

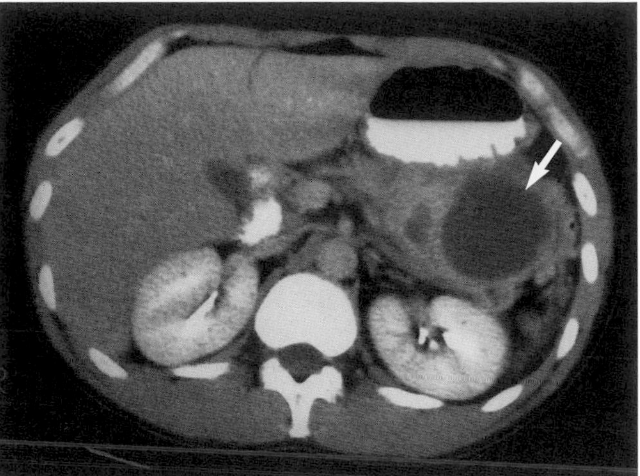

Figure 27.2 Computed tomography scan demonstrating pseudocyst in the tail of the pancreas (arrow). (Courtesy of Dr Paula Woodward.)

rated these findings, noting no difference in amylase activity related to pregnancy. Lipase levels were also studied, and no significant difference was found between the second and third trimesters or compared with non-pregnant controls, although one study noted a lower lipase level in the first trimester [34]. Mean values of lipase in 175 women were approximately 12 IU/L, with none exceeding 30 IU/L.

As a screening tool for acute pancreatitis, urinary trypsinogen-2 has also been evaluated in the general population. Using a dipstick test for urinary trypsinogen-2, Kemppainen et al. [35] evaluated 500 consecutive patients presenting to the emergency room with abdominal pain. The authors found 94% sensitivity and 95% specificity in detecting acute pancreatitis. While requiring further study, the 99% negative predictive value achieved with this urinary dipstick test may prove a useful adjunctive test to standard serum evaluation of amylase and lipase.

Leukocytosis, hyperglycemia, hyperbilirubinemia, abnormal coagulation tests, and elevated liver enzymes may also be present. Although other diseases can result in abnormal values, amylase and lipase remain the cornerstone of diagnosis. These values are typically elevated more than threefold over normal.

Radiologic evaluation

While the diagnosis of acute pancreatitis is based on clinical suspicion, physical examination, and elevated amylase and lipase, radiologic tests aid in the confirmation of acute pancreatitis and can be used to monitor the development and progression of complications. A plain film of the abdomen may show dilation of an isolated loop of intestine (sentinel loop) adjacent to the pancreas. Pleural effusions may be detected on chest X-ray.

Computed tomography (CT) is considered the radiographic procedure of choice for determining the extent or the severity of the pancreatitis [36]. Since CT is unhindered by bowel gas patterns, CT scans can demonstrate pancreatic necrosis, pseudocysts, hemorrhage, thrombophlebitis, and abcess formation [36] and provide guidance for directed sampling of abscess cavities (Figures 27.1 & 27.2). CT is also useful in differentiating pancreatitis from other intra-abdominal pathologies.

The role of ultrasound is typically quite limited in the initial evaluation of patients who have pancreatitis, because the pancreas often is obscured by bowel gas. Additionally, the pancreas may have an entirely normal sonographic appearance in the acute phase. In patients suspected of having acute pancreatitis, the primary role of ultrasound is to assess for gallstones and biliary obstruction [36].

Table 27.3 Differential diagnosis of acute pancreatitis

Non-obstetric conditions
Acute cholecystitis
Appendicitis
Biliary colic
Intestinal obstruction
Duodenal ulcer
Splenic rupture
Mesenteric vascular occlusion
Perinephric abscess
Pneumonia
Pulmonary embolus
Myocardial infarction
Diabetic ketoacidosis
Obstetric conditions
Pre-eclampsia
Ruptured ectopic pregnancy
Hyperemesis gravidarum

Differential diagnosis

Abdominal complaints in pregnancy present unique diagnostic challenges (Table 27.3). Non-obstetric conditions include acute cholecystitis, duodenal ulcer (including perforation), appendicitis, splenic rupture, perinephric abscess, mesenteric vascular occlusion, pneumonia, diabetic ketoacidosis, biliary colic, and intestinal obstruction. In the pregnant patient, pre-eclampsia, hyperemesis gravidarum, and ruptured ectopic pregnancy must be added to the differential diagnosis.

Preeclampsia may mimic pancreatitis with upper abdominal pain, nausea, and vomiting. Concomitant hypertension, proteinuria, and edema, however, will usually be present. Hyperemesis gravidarum most often affects patients in the first trimester, without a significant component of pain. Ruptured ectopic pregnancy may produce symptoms similar to those seen in acute pancreatitis. Hemoperitoneum can occur with either and may require laparotomy for diagnosis. But ruptured ectopics are not typically associated with an elevated lipase.

Table 27.4 Clinical indicators of poor prognosis: Ranson's criteria [36–38].

Non-gallstone pancreatitis	
On admission	
Age	>55 y
WBC	>16 000/mm^3
Glucose	>200 mg/dL
LDH	>350 IU/L
AST	>250 IU/L
Within 48 h	
Decrease in hematocrit	>10%
Increase in BUN	>5 mg/dL
Calcium	<8 mg/dL
P_aO_2	<60 mmHg
Base deficit	>4 mmol/L
Fluid deficit	>6 L
Gallstone pancreatitis	
On admission	
Age	>70 y
WBC	>18 000/mm^3
Glucose	>220 mg/dL
LDH	>400 IU/L
AST	>250 IU/L
Within 48 h	
Decrease in hematocrit	>10%
Increase in BUN	>2 mg/dL
Calcium	<8 mg/dL
Base deficit	>5 mmol/L
Fluid deficit	>4 L

AST, aspartate amino transferase; BUN, blood urea nitrogen; LDH, lactic dehydrogenase.

Prognostic indicators

Several methods utilizing clinical and laboratory data have been developed to indicate the severity of acute pancreatitis and allow refinement of prognosis [37–39]. The most widely used criteria were developed by Ranson (Table 27.4). The number of criteria met correlates with the mortality risk for the individual. For non-gallstone pancreatitis, patients with fewer than three signs have rates of mortality less than 3% and morbidity less than 5%. Patients with three or more positive signs carry a 62% mortality rate and a 90% morbidity rate. Utilizing a modified set of criteria for gallstone pancreatitis, individuals with fewer than three signs have a 1.5% mortality rate, while those with three or more signs demonstrate a 29% mortality rate. Critics of this system cite poor sensitivity, specificity, delayed assessment (due to the labs required at 48 hours), and inability to perform repeated assessments as major deterrents to its usefulness.

Another method of clinically evaluating the severity of several types of critical illnesses, including pancreatitis, is the Acute Physiology and Chronic Health Evaluation (APACHE) III criteria [40]. Unlike Ranson's criteria [37–39], the APACHE assessment [40] can be updated and the patient's course monitored on a continuing basis. This system evaluates several variables, both biochemical and physiologic, and calculates scores based on deviation from normal values. A 5-point increase in score is independently associated with a statistically significant increase in the relative risk of hospital death within a specific disease category. Within 24 hours of admission, 95% of patients admitted to the intensive care unit could be given a risk estimate for death within 3% of that actually observed [40]. Although more complex and computer dependent, the APACHE scoring system appears more accurate than Ranson's criteria in predicting morbidity [41]. The addition of body mass index seems to improve prediction as obesity predicts severity [42]. Several single prognostic indicators have been investigated in order to achieve early identification of pancreatic necrosis. Paracentesis can be performed; return of dark, prune-colored fluid is characteristic of necrotizing pancreatitis. Utilizing color charts, Mayer and McMahon [43] identified 90% of the patients who subsequently died and 72% of patients with severe morbidity.

Biochemical indicators that have been evaluated as predictors of severity of disease include C-reactive protein [44–46], trypsinogen activation peptide [47–49], procalcitonin [50,51], thrombomodulin [45], and serum amyloid A [46]. Only C-reactive protein is currently used clinically, but is limited in that it is predictive only after 48–72 hours following onset of symptoms. While interleukin-6, trypsinogen activation peptide and granulocyte nuclear elastase all show promise in acutely identifying patients destined for a severe clinical course, they await confirmatory trials and widespread acceptance into routine clinical use.

Compared with scoring systems and laboratory markers, contrast-enhanced CT scans offer broader information regarding intra-abdominal anatomy. Location and extent of necrosis are identified and can be serially evaluated (see Figure 27.1). Infection within pseudocysts is suggested by evidence of gas production. This test, however, may be limited in its availability and is difficult to obtain in severely ill patients.

Management

Treatment of acute pancreatitis in pregnancy is similar to that of non-pregnant individuals. The initial treatment of acute pancreatitis is supportive medical management. Because most cases are mild and self-limiting, this approach is largely successful. Correction of any underlying predisposing factors, such as avoidance or cessation of exacerbating factors like alcohol or drugs, early endoscopic retrograde cholangiopancreatography (ERCP) with obstructive jaundice, and reversal of hypercalcemia, is a basic principle to be observed. Assessment of prognostic indicators, as discussed earlier, permits appropriate surveillance. Patients with more severe disease should be transferred to an intensive care unit for continuous monitoring, because shock and pulmonary failure can present early in the course of disease and require prompt recognition and management.

Medical therapy is comprised of fluid and electrolyte management, adequate analgesia, and elimination of oral intake. Intravenous fluid resuscitation is a vital component of treatment in both mild and severe cases. Restoration of intravascular volume and avoidance of hypotension is important for cardiovascular stability and renal perfusion. Electrolyte abnormalities are common, including hypokalemia and metabolic alkalosis from severe vomiting and hypocalcemia from fat saponification. Serial assessment of electrolytes and appropriate replacement are essential. Parenteral analgesia is frequently necessary; morphine compounds, however, should be avoided secondary to their actions on the sphincter of Oddi. Oral intake is withheld for the duration of illness. Most patients with mild pancreatitis can be managed with intravenous fluids. In contrast, nutrition should be implemented early in the hospital course of patients with severe disease. Enteral feeding may have advantages over parenteral. It has the potential benefit of maintaining the intestinal barrier (it is felt that bacterial translocation is probably the major source of infection). Enteral nutrition also avoids catheter-related complications of parenteral nutrition such as line sepsis [52,53].

Nasogastric suction may be appropriate in a subset of patients with acute pancreatitis. Nasogastric suction, however, does not appear to influence duration of disease or its symptoms. Several studies have investigated the role of nasogastric suction in mild to moderate pancreatitis and found no difference in duration of abdominal pain, tenderness, nausea, and elevated pancreatic enzymes or time to resumption of oral feeding [54–56]. Therefore, nasogastric suction should be utilized on an elective basis for symptomatic relief for those patients with severe emesis or ileus.

Prophylactic antibiotics also have been advocated in an effort to prevent the development of infectious complications. Mild cases of pancreatitis do not appear to benefit from antibiotic prophylaxis, although studies are few [57,58]. In contrast, severe cases with pancreatic necrosis have a high rate (40%) of bacterial contamination and represent a subset of patients that may benefit from antibiotic administration [59]. A study of 74 patients with acute necrotizing pancreatitis treated with prophylactic imipenem demonstrated a significantly decreased incidence of pancreatic sepsis (12% vs 30%) [60]. Similar results were observed by Sainio and colleagues [61]. While further studies are needed to better define both patient and antibiotic selection, antibiotic prophylaxis appears to be indicated in patients at high risk for septic complications such as pancreatic necrosis.

Antienzyme and hormonal therapies have been designed to reduce the severity of disease by halting the production of pancreatic enzymes and the subsequent cascade activation of the complement, kallikrein–kinin, fibrinolytic, and coagulation systems. Studies evaluating atropine, calcitonin, glucagon, somatostatin, and the enzyme inhibitors, aprotinin and gabexate, however, have not shown improved morbidity or mortality in severe acute pancreatitis [4,26]. Octreotide, a somatostatin analogue, has received considerable attention as a means to improve the course of acute pancreatitis. Five randomized trials have been performed [62–66] which failed to demonstrate a clinical benefit.

Surgical therapy

Although supportive measures are the mainstay of therapy, surgical intervention also has a place in the management of acute pancreatitis. The exact role, timing, and form of surgery remain a matter of debate. The one clear indication for surgery is for diagnosis of an acute abdomen. An uncertain diagnosis mandates exploration for possible surgically correctable conditions. Two other situations also may require surgery: gallstone pancreatitis and select anatomic or infectious complications.

The goals of biliary surgery in cases of gallstone pancreatitis are to prevent recurrence and to decrease morbidity and mortality by removing the instigating agent. Cholecystectomy and bile duct exploration are not performed, however, during the acute episode. Because nearly 95% of stones pass during the first week of illness, the utility of surgery early in the illness does not weigh heavily against the high mortality rates that have been reported for early biliary surgery [67]. While not indicated in the acute phase of illness, biliary surgery should be performed after the acute pancreatitis subsides, prior to discharge from the hospital.

An alternative to open surgical removal of bile duct stones has been developed utilizing ERCP. Combined with endoscopic sphincterotomy, ERCP offers both diagnostic and therapeutic advantages in the critically ill patient [68,69]. If performed within the first 72 hours of illness, this procedure has been shown to decrease morbidity and length of hospital stay in patients with severe pancreatitis [69,70].

ERCP has been used in a number of pregnant patients without complications and has been found advantageous in the avoidance of the potential risks of major surgery during pregnancy [71–76]. ERCP during pregnancy is used to treat choledocholithiasis [69]. Choledocholithiasis that causes cholangitis and pancreatitis during pregnancy increases the risk of morbidity and mortality for both the fetus and mother. ERCP is safe during pregnancy and may be performed with modified techniques to reduce radiation exposure to the fetus and without fluoroscopy [75,76]. If there is radiation exposure during ERCP, the dosimetry should be routinely recorded.

Surgery for early and late complications of pancreatitis has also been the subject of controversy. A few situations appear to be clear indications for surgical intervention, such as acute, life-threatening hemorrhage. However, the timing and type of surgical procedures for later complications, such as sterile necrosis, pseudocyst, and abscess, are less straightforward. Using the development or persistence of organ failure despite 72 hours of intensive medical therapy as indications for surgery, Gotzinger and colleagues [77] reported on 340 patients who underwent surgical exploration for acute pancreatitis. Control of pancreatic necrosis (total removal of necrotic tissue) was accomplished in 73% of patients, requiring an average of 2.1 operations. Mortality was 100% in patients in whom surgical control of necrosis could not be accomplished versus 19% in those patients who did achieve surgical control of necrosis.

Arterial hemorrhage occurs in 2% of patients with severe pancreatitis. Necrosis and erosion into surrounding arteries of the gastrointestinal tract result in massive intra-abdominal or retroperitoneal hemorrhage. Arteriographic embolization followed by surgical debridement and artery ligation improved survival from 0% to 40% [78]. In contrast, the development of sterile pancreatic necrosis is not an automatic indication for surgery, because up to 70% of cases will resolve spontaneously. While few studies have been performed, no benefit for early debridement has been demonstrated [79,80].

The formation of pseudocysts may mandate surgical debridement based on clinical characteristics. Occurring in as many as 10–20% of patients with severe acute pancreatitis, pseudocysts resolve in approximately 50% of cases [26]. Surgery is performed if symptoms of hemorrhage, infection, or compression develop or if the pseudocyst exceeds 5–6 cm or persists longer than 6 weeks. Internal drainage represents the superior surgical approach, although percutaneous drainage may temporize a critically ill patient. Fluid should be collected for culture to rule out infection.

Finally, pancreatic abscess formation occurs in 2–4% of patients with severe pancreatitis and is 100% lethal if left undrained. Although percutaneous drainage may be temporizing, the catheter often becomes occluded secondary to the thick purulent effluent. With early and aggressive surgical debridement, mortality is reduced to 5% [81]. Either transperitoneal or retroperitoneal approaches may be appropriate. Postoperatively, 20% will require reoperation for incomplete drainage, ongoing infection, fistulas, or hemorrhage [81].

Considerations in pregnancy

Treatment of pancreatitis does not differ in the pregnant patient. Supportive measures are identical to those of the non-pregnant patient, and severe complications are managed aggressively. Two situations, however, merit special consideration in pregnancy: the treatment of biliary disease and hypertriglyceridemia.

The management of biliary disease in pregnancy raises the issue of timing of surgery. On resolution of acute pancreatitis, cholecystectomy is typically performed in a non-pregnant patient prior to discharge from the hospital. Some advocate continued conservative management in pregnancy to avoid operative complications and fetal morbidity. A high relapse rate (72%), however, is often encountered [5,82]. For patients presenting in the first trimester, this may be as high as 88%. Surgical intervention decreases the incidence of relapse and the risk of systemic complications.

Several studies support the use of second-trimester cholecystectomy for cholecystitis or pancreatitis [1,3,5,83,84]. The second trimester appears optimal in order to avoid medication effect on organogenesis and a possible increased rate of spontaneous abortion in the first trimester [1,3,5,83,84]. Third-trimester patients are best managed conservatively because they are close to the postpartum period when operative risks are reduced. Cholecystectomy may be performed by laparotomy or open laparoscopy. The open technique for the laparoscopic approach is often best, in order to avoid puncture of the gravid uterus with blind trocar insertion.

Fetal loss following cholecystectomy was once reported to be as high as 15% [85]. Many earlier reports, however, included patients undergoing surgery in the first trimester suffering spontaneous abortion many weeks postoperatively. Because at least 15% of all pregnancies are now known to end in spontaneous abortion, and preterm labor is seen in up to 10% of all continuing pregnancies, it would appear that the actual rate of complications related to surgery probably approaches nil, a figure confirmed by several recent studies [5,86,87]. A review of studies from 1963 to 1987, evaluating fetal loss in patients undergoing cholecystectomy, revealed an 8% spontaneous abortion rate and an 8% rate of premature labor [86]. In a similar manner, laparoscopic cholecystectomy in the second trimester has been reported in a small number of patients, with no increase in fetal or maternal morbidity or mortality [88,89].

Treatment of hypertriglyceridemia in pregnancy is aimed primarily at prevention of pancreatitis. Fats should be limited to fewer than 20 g/day. This restrictive diet, however, is not palatable and is difficult for patients to maintain. Sanderson and associates [90] reported successful management of hypertrigliceridemia during an episode of pancreatitis and the remainder of gestation by utilizing intravenous fluid therapy to provide calories in the form of 5% dextrose and restricting oral intake to clear liquids. Total parenteral nutrition offers another therapeutic approach when dietary adjustments are inadequate to prevent excessive triglyceride elevations. Plasma exchange and immunospecific apheresis also have been investigated and have suggested that long-term extracorporeal elimination of lipoproteins may offer a safe and effective method of prevention and treatment of hypertriglyceridemic pancreatitis in pregnancy [91]. Fish oil supplement (>3 g/day) can also be quite effective in lowering triglycerides [92,93].

References

1 Ramin KD, Ramin SM, Richey SD, Cunningham FG. Acute pancreatitis in pregnancy. *Am J Obstet Gynecol* 1995; 173: 187–191.

2 Klein KB. Pancreatitis in pregnancy. In: Rustgi VK, Cooper JN, eds. *Gastrointestinal and Hepatic Complications in Pregnancy*. New York: Wiley, 1986.

3 Block P, Kelly TR. Management of gallstone pancreatitis. *Surg Gynecol Obstet* 1989; 168: 426–428.

4 Steinberg W, Tenner S. Acute pancreatitis. *N Engl J Med* 1994; 330: 1198–1210.

5 Swisher SG, Hunt KK, Schmit PJ, et al. Management of pancreatitis complicating pregnancy. *Am Surg* 1994; 60: 759–762.

6 Gullo L, Migliori M, Olah A, et al. Acute pancreatitis in five European countries: etiology and mortality. *Pancreas* 2002; 24(3): 223–227.

7 Wilkinson EJ. Acute pancreatitis in pregnancy: a review of 98 cases and a report of 8 new cases. *Obstet Gynecol Surv* 1973; 28: 281–303.

8 Jouppila P, Mokka R, Larmi TK. Acute pancreatitis in pregnancy. *Surg Gynecol Obstet* 1974; 139: 879–882.

9 Langmade CF, Edmondson HA. Acute pancreatitis during pregnancy and the postpartum period: a report of nine cases. *Surg Gynecol Obstet* 1951; 92: 43–46.

10 Herfort K, Fialova V, Srp B. Acute pancreatitis in pregnancy. *Mater Med Pol* 1981; 13: 15–17.

11 Chang CC, Hsieh YY, Tsai HD, Yang TC, Yeh LS, Hsu TY. Acute pancreatitis in pregnancy. *Chinese Med J* 1998; 61(2): 85–92.

12 Underwood TW, Frye CB. Drug-induced pancreatitis. *Clin Pharmacol* 1993; 12(6): 440–448.

13 Eland IA, van Puijenbroek EP, Sturkenboom MJ, Wilson JH, Stricker BH. Drug-associated acute pancreatitis: twenty-one years of spontaneous reporting in The Netherlands. *Am J Gastroenterol* 1999; 94(9): 2417–2422.

14 Greenberger NJ, Toskes PP, Isselbacher KJ. Acute and chronic pancreatitis. In: Wilson JD, Isselbacher KJ, Fauci A, et al. eds. *Harrison's Principles of Internal Medicine*, 12th edn. New York: McGraw-Hill, 1991: 1372–1378.

15 Gorelick FS. Acute pancreatitis. In: Yamada T, Alpers DH, Kalloo AN, et al. eds. *Textbook of Gastroenterology*, 2nd edn. Philadelphia: JB Lippincott, 1995: 2064–2091.

16 Steer ML. Acute pancreatitis. In: Ayres SM, Gronvik A, Holbrook PR, Shoemaker WC, eds. *Textbook of Critical Care*, 3rd edn. Philadelphia: WB Saunders, 1995.

17 Moldenhauer JS, O'brien JM, Barton JR, Sibai B. Acute fatty liver of pregnancy: a life-threatening complication. *Am J Obstet Gynecol* 2004; 190(2): 502–505.

18 Braverman DZ, Johnson ML, Kern F Jr. Effects of pregnancy and contraceptive steroids on gallbladder function. *N Engl J Med* 1980; 302: 362–364.

19 Valdivieso V, Covarrubias C, Siegel F, Cruz F. Pregnancy and cholelithiasis: pathogenesis and natural course of gallstones diagnosed in early puerperium. *Hepatology* 1993; 17: 1–4.

20 Opie EL. The relation of cholelithiasis to disease of the pancreas and to fat necrosis. *Am J Med Surg* 1901; 12: 27–43.

21 Crisan L, Steidl E, Rivera-Alsina M. Acute hyperlipidemic pancreatitis in pregnancy. *Am J Obstet Gynecol* 2008; 198(5): e57–59.

22 DeChalain TMB, Michell WL, Berger GMB. Hyperlipidemia, pregnancy and pancreatitis. *Surg Gynecol Obstet* 1988; 167: 469–473.

23 Montes A, Walden CE, Knopp RH, et al. Physiologic and supraphysiologic increases in lipoprotein lipids and apoproteins in late pregnancy and postpartum. *Arteriosclerosis* 1984; 4: 407–417.

24 Stone NJ. Secondary causes of hyperlipidemia. *Med Clin North Am* 1994; 78: 117–141.

25 Scarpelli DG. Toxicology of the pancreas. *Toxicol Appl Pharmacol* 1989; 101(3): 543–554.

26 Reynaert MS, Dugernier T, Kestens PJ. Current therapeutic strategies in severe acute pancreatitis. *Intens Care Med* 1990; 16: 352–362.

27 Buchler M, Malfertheiner P, Schadlich H, et al. Role of phospholipase A2 in human acute pancreatitis. *Gastroenterology* 1989; 97: 1521–1526.

28 Boakye M, Macfoy D, Rice C. Alcoholic pancreatitis. *Obstet Gynecol* 2006; 26: 814–817.

29 Renner IG, Savage WT, Pantoja JL, Renner VJ. Death due to acute pancreatitis. *Dig Dis Sci* 1985; 30: 1005–1018.

30 Agarwal N, Pitchumoni CS, Sivaprasad AV. Evaluating tests for acute pancreatitis. *Am J Gastroenterol* 1990; 85: 356–366.

31 Strickland DM, Hauth JC, Widish J, et al. Amylase and isoamylase activities in serum of pregnant women. *Obstet Gynecol* 1984; 64: 389–391.

32 Kaiser R, Berk JE, Fridhandler L. Serum amylase changes during pregnancy. *Am J Obstet Gynecol* 1975; 122: 283–286.

33 Ordorica SA, Frieden FJ, Marks F, et al. Pancreatic enzyme activity in pregnancy. *J Reprod Med* 1991; 36: 359–362.

34 Karsenti D, Bacq Y, Brechot JF, Mariotte N, Vol S, Tichet J. Serum amylase and lipase activities in normal pregnancy: a prospective case-control study. *Am J Gastroenterol* 2001; 96(3): 697–699.

35 Kemppainen EA, Hedstrom JI, Puolakkainen PA, et al. Rapid measurement of urinary trypsinogen-2 as a screening test for acute pancreatitis. *N Engl J Med* 1997; 336(25): 1788–1793.

36 Scout L, Sawyers S, Bokhari J, Hamper U. Ultrasound evaluation of the acute abdomen. *Ultrasound Clin* 2007; 2: 493–523.

37 Ranson JHC, Rifkind KM, Roses DF, et al. Prognostic signs and the role of operative management in acute pancreatitis. *Surg Gynecol Obstet* 1974; 139: 69–81.

38 Ranson JC. The timing of biliary surgery in acute pancreatitis. *Ann Surg* 1979; 189: 654–663.

39 Imrie CW, Benjamin IS, Ferguson JC. A single-centre double-blind trial of Trasylol therapy in primary acute pancreatitis. *Br J Surg* 1978; 65: 337–341.

40 Knaus WA, Wagner DP, Draper EA, et al. The APACHE III prognostic system. Risk prediction of hospital mortality for critically ill hospitalized adults. *Chest* 1991; 100: 1619–1636.

41 Larvin M, McMahon MJ. APACHE-II score for assessment and monitoring of acute pancreatitis. *Lancet* 1989; 2: 201–205.

42 Johnson CD, Toh SH, Campbell MJ. Combination of APACHE-II Score and an obesity score (APACHE-O) for the prediction of severe acute pancreatitis. *Pancreatology* 2004; 4: 1–6.

43 Mayer DA, McMahon MJ. The diagnostic and prognostic value of peritoneal lavage in patients with acute pancreatitis. *Surg Gynecol Obstet* 1985; 160: 507–512.

44 Buchler M, Malfertheiner P, Schoetensack C, Uhl W, Beger HG. Sensitivity of antiproteases, complement factors and C-reactive protein in detecting pancreatic necrosis. Results of a prospective clinical study. *Int J Pancreatol* 1986; 1(3–4): 227–235.

45 Mantke R, Pross M, Kunz D, et al. Soluble thrombomodulin plasma levels are an early indication of a lethal course in human acute pancreatitis. *Surgery* 2002; 131(4): 424–432.

46 Mayer JM, Raraty M, Slavin J, et al. Serum amyloid A is a better early predictor of severity than C-reactive protein in acute pancreatitis. *Br J Surg* 2002; 89(2): 163–171.
47 Tenner S, Fernandez-del Castillo C, Warshaw A, et al. Urinary trypsinogen activation peptide (TAP) predicts severity in patients with acute pancreatitis. *Int J Pancreatol* 1997; 21(2): 105–110.
48 Neoptolemos JP, Kemppainen EA, Mayer JM, et al. Early prediction of severity in acute pancreatitis by urinary trypsinogen activation peptide: a multicentre study. *Lancet* 2000; 355(9219): 1955–1960.
49 Lempinen M, Kylanpaa-Back ML, Stenman UH, et al. Predicting the severity of acute pancreatitis by rapid measurement of trypsinogen-2 in urine. *Clin Chem* 2001; 47(12): 2103–2107.
50 Kylanpaa-Back ML, Takala A, Kemppainen EA, et al. Procalcitonin, soluble interleukin-2 receptor, and soluble E-selectin in predicting the severity of acute pancreatitis. *Crit Care Med* 2001; 29: 63–69.
51 Kylanpaa-Back ML, Takala A, Kemppainen EA, et al. Procalcitonin strip test in the early detection of severe acute pancreatitis. *Br J Surg* 2001; 88: 222–227.
52 Marik PE, Zaloga GP. Meta-analysis of parenteral nutrition versus enteral nutrition in patients with acute pancreatitis. *BMJ* 2004; 328: 1407.
53 McClave SA, Chang WK, Dhaliwal R, Heyland DK. Nutrition support in acute pancreatitis: a systematic review of the literature. *J Parenter Enteral Nutr* 2006; 30: 143.
54 Levant JA, Secrist DM, Resin HR, et al. Nasogastric suction in the treatment of alcoholic pancreatitis. *JAMA* 1974; 229: 51–52.
55 Loiudice TA, Lang J, Mehta H, Banta L. Treatment of acute alcoholic pancreatitis: the roles of cimetidine and nasogastric suction. *Am J Gastroenterol* 1984; 79: 553–558.
56 Naeije R, Salingret E, Clumeck N, et al. Is nasogastric suction necessary in acute pancreatitis? *BMJ* 1978; 2: 659–660.
57 Howes R, Zuidema GD, Cameron JL. Evaluation of prophylactic antibiotics in acute pancreatitis. *J Surg Res* 1975; 18: 197–200.
58 Finch WT, Sawyers JL, Schenker S. A prospective study to determine the efficacy of antibiotics in acute pancreatitis. *Ann Surg* 1976; 183: 667–671.
59 Berger HG, Bittner R, Block S, Buchler M. Bacterial contamination of pancreatic necrosis: a prospective clinical study. *Gastroenterology* 1986; 91: 433–438.
60 Pederzoli P, Bassi C, Vesentini S, Campedelli A. A randomized multicenter clinical trial of antibiotic prophylaxis of septic complications in acute necrotizing pancreatitis with imipenem. *Surg Gynecol Obstet* 1993; 176: 480–483.
61 Sainio V, Kemppainen E, Puolakkainen P, et al. Early antibiotic treatment in acute necrotizing pancreatitis. *Lancet* 1995; 346: 663.
62 Beechey-Newman N. Controlled trial of high-dose octreotide in treatment of acute pancreatitis. *Dig Dis Sci* 1993; 38: 644–647.
63 Paran H, Neufeld D, May A, et al. Preliminary report of a prospective randomized study of octreotide in the treatment of severe acute pancreatitis. *J Am Coll Surg* 1995; 181: 121–124.
64 McKay C, Baxter J, Imrie C. A randomized, controlled trial of octreotide in the management of patients with acute pancreatitis. *Int J Pancreatol* 1997; 21: 13–19.
65 Karakoyunlar O, Sivrel E, Tani N, Denecli AG. High-dose octreotide in the management of acute pancreatitis. *Hepatogastroenterology* 1999; 46: 1968–1972.
66 Uhl W, Buchler MW, Malfertheiner P, et al. A randomized, double-blind, multicentre trial of octreotide in moderate to severe acute pancreatitis. *Gut* 1999; 45: 97–104.
67 Osborne DH, Imrie CW, Carter DC. Biliary surgery in the same admission for gallstone-associated acute pancreatitis. *Br J Surg* 1981; 68: 758–761.
68 Venu RP, Brown RD, Halline AG. The role of endoscopic retrograde cholangiopancreatography in acute and chronic pancreatitis. *J Clin Gastroenterol* 2002; 34(5): 560–568.
69 Adler DG, Baron TH, Davila RE, et al. ASGE guidelines: the role of ERCP in diseases of the biliary tract and the pancreas. *Gastrointest Endosc* 2005; 62: 1–8.
70 Neoptolemos JP, Carr-Locke DL, London NJ, et al. Controlled trial of urgent endoscopic retrograde cholangiopancreatography and endoscopic sphincterotomy versus conservative treatment for acute pancreatitis due to gallstones. *Lancet* 1988; 2: 979–983.
71 Buchner WF, Stoltenberg PH, Kirtley DW. Endoscopic management of severe gallstone pancreatitis during pregnancy. *Am J Gastroenterol* 1988; 83: 1073.
72 Baillie J, Cairns SR, Putnam WS, Cotton PB. Endoscopic management of choledocholithiasis during pregnancy. *Surg Gynecol Obstet* 1990; 171: 1–4.
73 Uomo G, Manes G, Picciotto FO, Rabitti PG. Endoscopic treatment of acute biliary pancreatitis in pregnancy. *J Clin Gastroenterol* 1994; 18: 250–252.
74 Nesbitt TH, Kay HH, McCoy MC, Herbert WN. Endoscopic management of biliary disease during pregnancy. *Obstet Gynecol* 1996; 87: 806–809.
75 Kahaleh M, Hartwell G, Arseneau K, et al. Safety and efficacy of ERCP in pregnancy. *Gastrointest Endosc* 2004; 60: 287–292.
76 Simmons D, Tarnasky P, Rivera-Alsin M, Lopez J, Edman C. Endoscopic retrograde cholangiopancreatography (ERCP) in pregnancy without radiation. *Am J Obstet Gynecol* 2004; 190: 1467–1469.
77 Gotzinger P, Sautner T, Kriwanek S, et al. Surgical treatment for severe acute pancreatitis: extent and surgical control of necrosis determine outcome. *World J Surg* 2002; 26(4): 474–478.
78 Waltman AC, Luers PR, Athanasoulis CA, Warshaw AL. Massive arterial hemorrhage in patients with pancreatitis. *Arch Surg* 1986; 121: 439–443.
79 Bradley EL, Allen K. A prospective longitudinal study of observation versus surgical intervention in the management of necrotizing pancreatitis. *Am J Surg* 1991; 16: 19–25.
80 Karimigani I, Porter KA, Langevin RE, Banks P. Prognostic factors in sterile pancreatic necrosis. *Gastroenterology* 1992; 103: 1636–1640.
81 Warshaw AL, Gongliang J. Improved survival in 45 patients with pancreatic abscess. *Ann Surg* 1985; 202: 408–417.
82 Hernandez A, Petrov MS, Brooks DC, Banks PA, Ashley SW, Tavakkolizadeh A. Acute pancreatitis and pregnancy: a 10-year single center experience. *J Gastrointest Surg* 2007; 11: 1623–1627.
83 Martin IG, Dexter SP, McMahon MJ. Laparoscopic cholecystectomy in pregnancy. A safe option during the second trimester? *Surg Endosc* 1996; 10: 508–510.
84 Cosenza CA, Saffari B, Jabbour N, et al. Surgical management of biliary gallstone disease during pregnancy. *Am J Surg* 1990; 178: 545–548.
85 Green J, Rogers A, Rubin L. Fetal loss after cholecystectomy during pregnancy. *Can Med Assoc J* 1963; 88: 576–577.
86 McKellar DP, Anderson CT, Boynton CJ. Cholecystectomy during pregnancy without fetal loss. *Surg Gynecol Obstet* 1992; 174: 465–468.

87 Kort B, Katz VL, Watson WJ. The effect of nonobstetric operation during pregnancy. *Surg Gynecol Obstet* 1993; 177: 371–376.

88 Morrell DG, Mullins JR, Harrison PB. Laparoscopic cholecystectomy during pregnancy in symptomatic patients. *Surgery* 1992; 112: 856–859.

89 Elerding SC. Laparoscopic cholecystectomy in pregnancy. *Am J Surg* 1993; 165: 625–627.

90 Sanderson SL, Iverius P, Wilson DE. Successful hyperlipemic pregnancy. *JAMA* 1991; 265: 1858–1860.

91 Swoboda K, Derfler K, Koppensteiner R, et al. Extracorporeal lipid elimination for treatment of gestational hyperlipidemic pancreatitis. *Gastroenterology* 1993; 104: 1527–1531.

92 Nestel P, Connor WE, Reardon MF, et al. Suppression by diets rich in fish oil of very low density lipoprotein production in man. *J Clin Invest* 1984; 74: 72.

93 Harris WS, Connor WE, Illingworth DR, et al. Effects of fish oil on VLDL triglyceride kinetics in humans. *J Lipid Res* 1990; 31: 1549.

28 Acute Renal Failure

Shad H. Deering[1] & Gail L. Seiken[2]
[1]Department of Obstetrics and Gynecology, Uniformed Services University of Health Sciences, Old Madigan Army Medical Center, Tacoma, WA, USA
[2]Washington Nephrology Associates, Bethesda, MD, USA

Introduction

Renal failure is now an uncommon complication of pregnancy in developed countries, occurring in less than 1% of all pregnancies in developing countries, although specific diagnostic criteria have not always been well defined in the literature [1,2]. In fact, the incidence of acute renal failure (ARF) requiring dialysis is now not significantly different in pregnant women in Western countries compared with the worldwide population. One large analysis reported that the incidence of ARF in pregnancy fell from 1 in 3000 to 1 in 18 000 between the years 1958 and 1994 [3]. In previous decades, rates of ARF as high as 20–40% were reported in pregnancy, largely attributed to the high incidence of septic abortion [4–6]. When ARF does occur in underdeveloped parts of the world, it is often secondary to limited prenatal/delivery care and illegal abortion.

As the incidence of pregnancy-related ARF in developed countries has sharply declined and treatment has improved, so have maternal mortality rates reported in most studies. This improvement is related to both earlier recognition and intervention, as well as availability of dialytic support. Stratta et al. reported no deaths over the last 7 years of their experience, as compared with previously reported rates as high as 31% [3]. This is in sharp contrast, however, to another study at an inner city hospital in Georgia from 1986 to 1996 which documented 15% maternal and 43% perinatal mortality rates, respectively, as well as data from India that suggest ARF in pregnancy may have a mortality rate as high as 50% [7]. These studies suggest that ARF in pregnancy remains a potentially devastating complication.

Etiologies of acute renal failure

The approach to the pregnant patient with ARF is similar to that of the non-pregnant patient, although diseases unique to pregnancy (Table 28.1) must be considered in the differential diagnosis [8]. Disorders causing ARF in pregnancy include prerenal azotemia, intrinsic renal disease, urinary obstruction, as well as pre-eclampsia, HELLP syndrome (*h*emolysis, *e*levated *l*iver enzymes, *l*ow *p*latelets), acute fatty liver of pregnancy (AFLP), and postpartum renal failure, also known as postpartum hemolytic uremic syndrome (HUS). Bilateral renal cortical necrosis (BRCN) is another consideration in the evaluation of the pregnant women with ARF, which, though not unique to the pregnant state, is seen overwhelmingly in pregnancy.

In the past, a bimodal incidence of ARF was seen in pregnancy, with a peak in the first trimester corresponding to the high incidence of septic abortion, and a second peak in the third trimester corresponding to a number of other disorders seen uniquely in pregnancy. Currently, with the decrease in the number of septic abortions, the majority of ARF is now seen in the latter part of gestation. Additionally, accelerated loss of renal function, along with more difficult to control hypertension and increased proteinuria, is seen in 10% of women entering pregnancy with underlying moderate to severe renal insufficiency due to a variety of causes [9]. Although less common, significant deterioration in renal function may also occur during pregnancy in women with underlying diabetic nephropathy [10].

Renal biopsy is infrequently performed during pregnancy as the clinical presentation and timing of renal failure is usually adequate to establish a diagnosis. A renal biopsy may be indicated in pregnancy if there is a sudden deterioration of renal function without a definite cause before 32 weeks of gestation, especially if a diagnosis of pre-eclampsia is in doubt and a premature delivery may be avoided by the information obtained. A large retrospective study of over 1000 percutaneous renal biopsies performed during pregnancy between 1970 and 1996 reported a complication rate of 2.4% [11]. Another recent but smaller study of 18 renal biopsies performed in pregnancy and the early postpartum period reported a 38% incidence of renal hematoma, with nearly one-third of those affected requiring a blood transfusion [12]. Because of advances in neonatal intensive care and the favorable long-term prognosis for infants born after 32 weeks of gestation, renal biopsy is generally not

Critical Care Obstetrics, 5th edition. Edited by M. Belfort, G. Saade, M. Foley, J. Phelan and G. Dildy.

Table 28.1 Differential diagnosis of acute renal failure in pregnancy.

Prerenal azotemia
Acute tubular necrosis
Acute interstitial nephritis
Acute glomerulonephritis
Obstruction
Pre-eclampsia*
HELLP syndrome*
Acute fatty liver of pregnancy*
Postpartum renal failure
Pyelonephritis
Bilateral renal cortical necrosis

*These occur almost exclusively after 20 weeks gestation, and mostly in the third trimester of pregnancy.

Table 28.2 Laboratory evaluation of acute renal failure.

	Prerenal azotemia	Acute tubular necrosis
BUN: creatinine ratio	>20:1	10:1
Urine Na^+ (mEq/L)	<20	>40
Fractional excretion of Na^+ ($FENa^+$)	<1%	>2%
Urine osmolality (mosm/kg H_2O)	>500	<350
Urine sp gr	>1.020	1.010
Urine sediment	Bland	Granular casts, renal tubular epithelial cells

performed after this gestational age as prolongation of pregnancy is less of a concern.

Prerenal azotemia

Prerenal azotemia is the result of decreased renal perfusion, due to either true intravascular volume depletion, decreased cardiac output, or altered renal perfusion. The latter can be seen with cirrhosis, nephrotic syndrome, renal artery stenosis, or the use of non-steroidal anti-inflammatory agents. By definition, prerenal azotemia is readily reversible with restoration of renal perfusion.

Early in pregnancy, hyperemesis gravidarum is one of the more common causes of ARF secondary to profound volume depletion resulting from poor oral intake and vomiting. Similarly, any gastrointestinal illness with vomiting or diarrhea, excessive use of cathartics or laxatives, or bulimia may result in prerenal azotemia. Generally, these disorders are readily apparent on the basis of history and laboratory findings. However, eating disorders, which occur in up to 1% of pregnancies, are often difficult to diagnose and require a high index of suspicion [13]. To prevent the development of fixed renal tubular injury, prerenal azotemia, due to hemorrhage or other causes, must be treated aggressively with blood product support and fluid resuscitation.

Laboratory studies that may be of benefit in establishing the diagnosis of prerenal azotemia include urinary electrolytes and osmolality (Table 28.2). The urine sodium is typically low, as is the fractional excretion of sodium [(urine Na^+/serum Na^+)/(urine creatinine/serum creatinine) × 100%], reflecting a sodium-avid state, and urine osmolality is high, indicating intact urine concentrating ability. A low urine chloride may also provide a clue to surreptitious vomiting.

Uterine hemorrhage is an important cause of hypovolemia and subsequent prerenal azotemia late in pregnancy. Although usually presenting as profuse vaginal bleeding, hemorrhage from placental abruption may be concealed or may occur in the postpartum period secondary to lacerations, uterine atony, or retained products of conception. Hemorrhage with resultant hypotension was a major cause of pregnancy-associated ARF in 7% of patients studied at the Necker Hospital, and was a contributing factor in as many as 79% of cases in other studies [1]. A more recent study implicated postpartum hemorrhage in nearly 10% of ARF cases, and placental abruption in another 4% [7].

Patients with pre-eclampsia may be particularly susceptible to ARF associated with hemorrhage due to pre-existing alterations in maternal physiology, including decreased intravascular volume, heightened vascular responsiveness to catecholamines and angiotensin II, and altered prostaglandin synthesis [14]. In a study of 31 patients with pre-eclampsia and acute renal failure, Sibai and colleagues reported that 90% had experienced some form of significant hemorrhage [15].

Intrinsic renal disease

Acute renal failure may result from a variety of intrinsic renal diseases similar to those in the non-pregnant patient. Involvement of the glomeruli may predominate in one of the many primary or secondary glomerulonephritides. The renal tubules and interstitium are the primary areas of injury in acute tubular necrosis (ATN) and acute interstitial nephritis (AIN). Both clinical presentation and examination of the urinary sediment can provide valuable clues to the diagnosis, although renal biopsy may eventually be required to distinguish among the many glomerular diseases and to predict prognosis (Table 28.3).

Acute glomerulonephritis

The numerous causes of acute glomerulonephritis (GN) include primary glomerular disease such as poststreptococcal GN, membranoproliferative GN, idiopathic rapidly progressive (or crescentic) GN (RPGN), as well as secondary glomerular diseases such as lupus nephritis, systemic vasculitis, and bacterial endocarditis (Table 28.4).

The classic presentation of acute GN is that of hypertension, edema and volume overload, nephrotic range proteinuria, and an active urinary sediment with red blood cell casts (Table 28.3). In

Table 28.3 Acute renal failure: evaluation of intrinsic renal disease.

	Acute tubular necrosis	Acute interstitial nephritis	Acute glomerulonephritis
Urine sediment	Brown granular casts	Hematuria, pyuria, eosinophils, WBC casts	Hematuria, renal tubular cells RBC casts, oval fat bodies
Proteinuria	<2 g/day	<2 g/day	>2 g/day, possible nephrotic syndrome
FENa+	>2%	>2%	<1%
Hypertension	Uncommon	Uncommon	Common
Systemic manifestations	Hypotension, sepsis, hemorrhage	Fever, skin rash, new medication	Collagen-vascular disease, infection

Table 28.4 Causes of glomerulonephritis.

Primary
Minimal change disease
Focal segmental glomerulosclerosis
IgA nephropathy
Membranoproliferative glomerulonephritis
Membranous nephropathy
Poststreptococcal glomerulonephritis

Secondary
SLE
Henoch–Schönlein purpura
Cryoglobulinemia
Polyarteritis nodosa
Wegener's granulomatosis
Hypersensitivity vasculitis
Goodpasture's syndrome
Infection-related (i.e. shunt nephritis, endocarditis)

Table 28.5 Causes of acute interstitial nephritis.

Drug-induced
Infection
  Viral: cytomegalovirus, infectious mononucleosis, hemorrhagic fever
  Bacterial: streptococcal infections, diphtheria, Legionnaires' disease
  Parasitic: malaria, leptospirosis, toxoplasmosis
Systemic disease
  Sarcoidosis
  Systemic lupus erythematosus
  Sjögren's syndrome
  Transplant rejection
  Leukemic or lymphomatous infiltration
Idiopathic

those women with pre-existing renal disease, these features are often noted in the first two trimesters of gestation, although systemic lupus erythematosus (SLE) may manifest at any time during pregnancy. Laboratory analysis including serum complement levels, antinuclear antibodies, antistreptolysin-O titers, antineutrophil cytoplasmic antibodies, and other autoantibodies may be helpful in establishing a diagnosis, although in most cases renal biopsy is eventually necessary. Pre-eclampsia may mimic acute glomerulonephritis in presentation, although serologic evaluation should be negative. It is important to attempt to differentiate between the two in order to avoid delivery at a very early gestational age as may be required for severe pre-eclampsia. Treatment of acute GN is largely supportive, including diuretics, antihypertensive agents, and occasionally dialysis. Depending on the underlying disease, corticosteroids or cytotoxic agents may be employed as well.

Acute interstitial nephritis (AIN)

The most common cause of AIN is drug exposure and an extensive list of agents have been implicated. Among those more commonly noted are the β-lactam antibiotics such as the semisynthetic penicillins, sulfa-based drugs, histamine H_2 blockers, and nonsteroidal anti-inflammatory agents (NSAIDs). While NSAID use is usually avoided in pregnancy, it may be encountered in the case of an intentional overdose. Antibiotics such as the penicillins and β-lactam antibiotics, and H_2 blockers are, however, used routinely in pregnancy.

Acute interstitial nephritis may also occur in association with viral infections, including cytomegalovirus and infectious mononucleosis, direct bacterial invasion, parasitic infections such as malaria and leptospirosis, and systemic diseases such as SLE and sarcoidosis (Table 28.5). Unlike acute GN, acute interstitial nephritis typically presents with modest proteinuria (<2 g/day), pyuria, eosinophiluria, hematuria, and white blood cell casts on urinalysis. Systemic manifestations may include fever, rash, arthralgias, and other signs of a hypersensitivity reaction in those patients with drug-induced interstitial nephritis. Hypertension and edema are infrequently seen with AIN, except in those cases of severe renal failure. Withdrawal of the offending agent or treatment of the underlying infection or disease usually results in improvement of renal function. In some cases of drug-induced or idiopathic AIN, steroids have been used with varying degrees of success. When history, physical examination, and laboratory evaluation are inadequate to establish a diagnosis, renal biopsy may be necessary.

Acute tubular necrosis

Acute tubular necrosis may result from a variety of toxic exposures, including aminoglycosides, radiographic contrast, heavy metals, and several chemotherapeutic agents. Pigment-induced

ATN may occur in cases of rhabdomyolysis or massive hemolysis. More commonly in pregnancy, however, ATN is ischemic in nature, as a result of a hemodynamic insult with hypotension and impaired renal perfusion. This is commonly due to a hemorrhage during pregnancy, which may be the result of either placental abruption or a postpartum hemorrhage which complicates approximately 1% and 4–6% of pregnancies respectively [16].

In those patients with pre-eclampsia who develop renal failure, ATN appears to be the underlying renal lesion. Clinically, it may be difficult to distinguish between severe prerenal azotemia and ATN, although urinary indices and urinalysis may be helpful (Table 28.2). Urinalysis typically reveals muddy brown granular casts and renal tubular epithelial cells. In light of impaired renal tubular function, laboratory evaluation reveals a high urinary sodium excretion as well as urine that is neither concentrated nor dilute. Acute tubular necrosis may be either oliguric (urine output <400 mL/day) or non-oliguric (>400 mL/day), depending on the mechanism of injury and the severity. Treatment of ATN is supportive and necessitates optimization of hemodynamics, avoidance of potential nephrotoxin exposure, nutritional support with careful monitoring of fluids and electrolytes and, occasionally, dialysis. Renal function typically recovers in 7–14 days with appropriate treatment.

Urinary obstruction

Although urinary obstruction is a relatively uncommon cause of ARF in pregnancy, it is readily reversible and, therefore, must be considered in the differential. Obstruction may occur at any level of the urinary tract due to a wide variety of causes, many of which are not unique to pregnancy (Table 28.6). Additionally, gravidas with an abnormally configured or overdistended uterus, such as those with uterine leiomyomata, polyhydramnios, or multiple gestations, may be particularly susceptible. Ureteral compression by the gravid uterus, with resultant ARF and hypertension, has been reported [17] and large leiomyomata have even been reported to cause ureteral obstruction in the first trimester [18]. Another cause unique to pregnancy is an incarcerated uterus, which may cause urinary retention as the gravid uterus enlarges but becomes trapped in the pelvis secondary to significant retroflexion and then compresses the bladder [19,20]. Other risk factors for urinary obstruction in pregnancy include pyelonephritis, renal calculi, ureteral narrowing, and low abdominal wall compliance [21].

Table 28.6 Causes of urinary obstruction.

Upper tract	Lower tract
Stones	Stones
Blood clots	Blood clots
Tumor	Tumor
Sloughed papillae	Neuropathic bladder
Ureteral stricture or ligation	Urethral stricture
Retroperitoneal fibrosis	
Extrinsic compression by tumor, gravid uterus	

Renal ultrasound is the first step in the evaluation of possible urinary tract obstruction, although results may be inconclusive due to the physiologic dilation of the collecting system often seen in pregnancy due to both the effects of progesterone and the mechanical pressure of the gravid uterus. Thus, anterograde or retrograde pyelography may be necessary for definitive diagnosis. Relief of the obstruction may be accomplished by ureteral stent placement, percutaneous nephrostomy, manual reduction of an incarcerated uterus, or amnioreduction in the case of polyhydramnios. If the fetus is significantly premature, correcting the obstruction should allow for a substantial delay in delivery as well as recovery of renal function. If the patient is near term, however, delivery may be indicated to remove both the mechanical and hormonal causes of the obstruction. It should be noted that the fetal mortality rate for reversible obstructive uropathy with associated renal failure has been reported to be as high as 33% [22].

Pyelonephritis

Pyelonephritis is an important cause of ARF during pregnancy. As a result of the normal physiologic changes that accompany pregnancy, the urinary collecting system is prone to dilation and urinary stasis. In addition, there is an increased sensitivity to bacterial endotoxin-induced tissue damage. These normal changes result in an increased incidence in both upper and lower tract infections. The incidence of pyelonephritis in pregnancy is approximately 2% and it is one of the most common causes of sepsis during pregnancy [23]. Presenting symptoms generally include fever, flank pain, nausea, vomiting, and possibly urinary frequency, dysuria, and urgency. The most common causative organism is *E. coli*, which accounts for nearly 75% of cases [24]. Other potential pathogens include *Proteus mirabilis*, *Klebsiella pneumoniae*, group B streptococci, enterococci, and *Pseudomonas aeruginosa*. Prompt and appropriate antibiotic treatment is generally very effective in treating pyelonephritis during pregnancy, with improvement seen in the first 24–48 hours. After resolution of the initial infection, suppressive antibiotic treatment throughout pregnancy should be considered as the recurrence rate is as high as 20%.

Although pyelonephritis rarely results in a significant decline in renal function in non-pregnant patients, Gilstrap and colleagues demonstrated a substantial decrease in creatinine clearance among gravidas with pyelonephritis, with a return to normal or near-normal renal function in the majority of women re-evaluated following antibiotic therapy [25,26]. As mentioned previously, it has been postulated that this decline in renal function is related to an increased vascular sensitivity to bacterial endotoxins and vasoactive mediator release in pregnancy [1]. It is this sensitivity to endotoxin that may account for the greater incidence of septic shock and adult respiratory distress syndrome from pyelonephritis during pregnancy.

Pre-eclampsia

Among those causes of ARF unique to pregnancy, pre-eclampsia/eclampsia accounts for the majority. One study of ARF in pregnancy performed in Uruguay, which included patients from 1976 to 1994, reported that pre-eclampsia was the cause of ARF in approximately 47% of cases [27]. Another retrospective study conducted at an inner-city hospital in Georgia described pre-eclampsia in more than one-third of 21 cases of ARF diagnosed at their institution from 1986 to 1996 [7].

Classically, pre-eclampsia is defined as the development of hypertension, proteinuria, and edema after the 20th week of gestation. (It should be noted, however, that severe pre-eclampsia may occur earlier than 20 weeks in the presence of gestational trophoblastic disease, also called a molar pregnancy.) Elevated liver enzymes, coagulation abnormalities, and microangiopathic hemolytic anemia may be seen in severe pre-eclampsia as well. The diagnosis is established clinically and rarely confirmed by renal biopsy.

Pathologically, pre-eclampsia is characterized by swollen glomerular capillary endothelial cells or glomerular endotheliosis, with resultant capillary obstruction and glomerular ischemia [28]. Importantly, the extent of the morphologic lesion does not necessarily correspond to the degree of renal functional impairment [4]. In addition, the presence of subtle volume depletion and enhanced sensitivity of the renal vasculature to vasoconstriction may contribute to superimposed ATN, which many believe to be the lesion associated with significant ARF in pre-eclampsia.

Treatment of severe pre-eclampsia and the associated renal failure ultimately depends on delivery of the infant and seizure prophylaxis with magnesium sulfate during the delivery and for at least 24 hours postpartum. This is accomplished regardless of the gestational age of the fetus, though consultation with a maternal-fetal medicine specialist is recommended with a premature fetus to determine if it is possible to delay delivery long enough to administer corticosteroids in an attempt to improve fetal lung maturity. It is important to monitor fluid administration closely while magnesium sulfate is given as patients with impaired renal function will not clear the medication as well and dose reductions may be necessary.

Recovery of renal function is usually seen within days to weeks after delivery with isolated pre-eclampsia, although up to 20% may have some degree of residual impairment [29]. In contrast, when patients with chronic hypertension and underlying renal disease experience ARF in pregnancy, approximately 80% will require long-term renal replacement therapy [15]. Histologic evaluation in those patients with persistent renal impairment, proteinuria, or hypertension postpartum has revealed evidence of underlying chronic renal disease, presumably unmasked by pregnancy and/or pre-eclampsia [5].

HELLP syndrome

HELLP is an acronym used to describe a constellation of findings, including *h*emolysis, *e*levated *l*iver enzymes, and *l*ow *p*latelets. Nausea, epigastric or right upper quadrant pain, and tenderness may be present at the time of diagnosis, as well as proteinuria and renal dysfunction. Coagulation studies including fibrinogen, prothrombin time, and partial thromboplastin time may be useful in distinguishing this disorder from others associated with disseminated intravascular coagulation (DIC), in that they are often normal in patients with HELLP syndrome in the absence of placental abruption.

HELLP syndrome has been described in 4–12% of patients with severe pre-eclampsia [30] and is considered to represent a variant of severe pre-eclampsia. However, in a small study by Krane, in which patients with HELLP syndrome underwent renal biopsy, less than half had the glomerular endotheliosis classic for pre-eclampsia [31]. Sibai et al. observed acute renal failure in 7.4% (32/435) of patients with HELLP syndrome, and approximately one-third of these patients required hemodialysis [32]. Evidence of disseminated intravascular coagulation was present in 84% of these patients, and 44% had abruptio placentae. HELLP syndrome associated with acute renal failure in this study carried a maternal mortality rate of 13% and perinatal mortality rate of 34%. The poor prognoses described by Sibai likely reflect the severity of disease seen in his patient population.

Generally, treatment of HELLP syndrome consists of expeditious delivery once the diagnosis is established, as well as magnesium sulfate for seizure prophylaxis as discussed earlier, with rapid recovery of renal function expected. In a group of 23 patients with HELLP syndrome who were normotensive prior to pregnancy, no residual renal impairment was observed following delivery. However, 40% of patients with chronic hypertension and subsequent HELLP syndrome eventually required chronic dialysis [32,33].

Acute fatty liver of pregnancy

Acute fatty liver of pregnancy is another uncommon cause of ARF in pregnancy, with an incidence reported as between 1 in 6700 and 1 in 13000 deliveries [34,35]. The disease exhibits a slight predominance in nulliparas; it has been diagnosed as early as 24 weeks of gestation and as late at 7 days postpartum [4,35], but usually occurs in the last few weeks of gestation. Initial manifestations are non-specific, including nausea, vomiting, headache, malaise, and abdominal pain. Laboratory evaluation reveals mild elevation of serum transaminase levels, hyperbilirubinemia, and leukocytosis as well as hypoglycemia. Renal failure develops in the majority of cases and, left untreated, patients may progress to fulminant hepatic failure with jaundice, encephalopathy, disseminated intravascular coagulopathy, gastrointestinal hemorrhage, and death. Maternal and fetal mortality rates as high as 85% were seen in the past, although with earlier diagnosis and treatment a recent analysis of 28 consecutive cases reported no maternal deaths [35].

Diagnosis of fatty liver may be established by liver biopsy revealing microvesicular fatty infiltration. Computed tomography (CT) may reveal decreased hepatic attenuation. A report by Usta and colleagues described their experience with 13 patients (14 cases) of AFLP over an 8-year period, all of whom had ARF on presentation [36]. They reported 100% maternal survival, with 13% perinatal mortality. Although nine of 14 cases were initially diagnosed as pre-eclampsia, the diagnosis of AFLP was subsequently confirmed either by liver biopsy (10/14), CT of the liver (2/14), or clinically. One patient experienced a recurrence of AFLP in a subsequent pregnancy. Although CT revealing hepatic density below the normal range of 50–70 Hounsfield units has been reported as suggestive of AFLP, Usta's study demonstrated a high false-negative rate with only two of 10 abnormal scans, including nine biopsy-proven cases [36]. Contributing to the diagnostic dilemma in these women is the frequent occurrence of hypertension, edema, and proteinuria suggestive of pre-eclampsia, although renal pathology has failed to reveal evidence of glomerular endotheliosis. As is the case with severe pre-eclampsia, expeditious delivery is warranted, with prompt improvement in both hepatic and renal failure noted in nearly all cases [34,35].

Thrombotic thrombocytopenic purpura/hemolytic uremic syndrome

Thrombotic thrombocytopenic purpura/hemolytic uremic syndrome (TTP/HUS) is an uncommon disorder during pregnancy with an incidence of approximately 1 in 25 000 births [37]. It is characterized by the classic pentad of thrombocytopenia, hemolytic anemia, fever, neurologic abnormalities, and some degree of renal dysfunction. During pregnancy, the disorder tends to present earlier than pre-eclampsia, with a median gestational age of onset of 23 weeks [38]. The underlying pathophysiology of the disorder is apparently due to intravascular thrombi that result in fragmentation of red blood cells, platelet consumption, and varying degrees of systemic ischemia.

Although treatment guidelines are not well established, plasma exchange is recommended due to an apparent benefit in survival in a small number of patients. Due to the continuum of disease, both HUS and TTP have been considered together in most clinical trials. The Canadian Apheresis Study Group and a group at Johns Hopkins University examined therapeutic outcomes in TTP and TTP/HUS, respectively [39,40]. Both reported the superiority of plasma exchange therapy in terms of clinical response and survival, with mortality rates of 22% and 9% respectively, in those receiving such treatment. Additional therapeutic interventions varied, including aspirin, dipyridamole, and corticosteroids. Greater than 50% of all patients had evidence of renal dysfunction, although those with severe ARF or anuria were excluded from the Canadian multicenter trial.

Delivery in cases of TTP/HUS is not necessarily indicated, especially at very early gestational ages, which is why care must be taken to differentiate this disease from severe pre-eclampsia.

Nine of the 76 women seen at Johns Hopkins presented in their third trimester of pregnancy, although there was no comment as to the degree of renal impairment in this subset of patients. A recent report of three patients with postpartum HUS at the Rhode Island hospital who were treated with frequent plasma exchange and prednisone reported survival in all three patients [41]. Additionally, Hayward and colleagues described nine pregnant women presenting between the first trimester of gestation and 1 month postpartum with TTP-HUS [42]. Of these 21 women from three institutions, all but one survived, and none required renal replacement therapy. With respect to future pregnancies, one recent report cites only an 18% recurrence risk in subsequent pregnancies in patients with a history of postpartum TTP/HUS [43].

Postpartum renal failure

Idiopathic postpartum renal failure, also referred to as postpartum HUS, is a unique cause of pregnancy-associated ARF that typically develops in the puerperium following an uncomplicated pregnancy and delivery. Women may present up to several months following delivery with severe hypertension, microangiopathic hemolytic anemia, and oliguric renal failure, often with congestive heart failure and CNS manifestations. A prodromal flu-like illness or initiation of oral contraceptives may be associated with postpartum renal failure as well as with idiopathic HUS, suggesting a toxic or hormonal influence.

Pathologically, the disease is often indistinguishable from the thrombotic microangiopathies, idiopathic HUS and TTP, with arteriolar injury, fibrin deposition, and microvascular (arteriolar and glomerular capillary) thrombosis. The major pathologic involvement is renal, as opposed to CNS involvement seen in TTP. The pathogenesis of the thrombotic microangiopathies remains unclear, although intravascular coagulation, disordered platelet aggregation, endothelial damage, and alterations in prostaglandins have been suggested [44]. Therapies have been chosen in an attempt to intervene in one or more of these processes, including plasma exchange, plasma infusion, antiplatelet agents, and anticoagulation. In addition, acute and long-term dialytic support is often necessary, with approximately 12–15% of patients developing end-stage renal disease. The maternal mortality rate was estimated at between 46% and 55% in the 1980s [45,46] but appears to be improving with the use of plasma exchange and other treatments.

Bilateral renal cortical necrosis

Acute, bilateral renal cortical necrosis is a pathologic entity consisting of partial or complete destruction of the renal cortex, with sparing of the medulla. While not unique to pregnancy, this rare and catastrophic form of ARF occurs most commonly in pregnancy, with obstetric causes accounting for 50–70% of cases [47]. Although BRCN represents less than 2% of cases of ARF in the non-pregnant population, it has been reported to account for 10–38% of obstetric cases of renal failure, perhaps secondary to the hypercoagulable state and altered vascular sensitivity of pregnancy [31,48]. Patients typically present between 30 and 35 weeks of gestation in association with profound shock and renal hypoperfusion, such as that seen with abruptio placentae, placenta previa, and other causes of obstetric hemorrhage. Acute BRCN has also been observed early in pregnancy associated with septic abortion. Abruption placentae, with either overt or concealed hemorrhage, appears to be the most common antecedent event [47].

Patients with BRCN present with severe and prolonged oliguria or anuria (urine output <50 mL/day), flank pain, gross hematuria, and urinalysis demonstrating RBC and granular casts. Diagnosis is established by renal arteriogram demonstrating virtual absence of cortical blood flow (interlobular arteries), despite patency of the renal arteries. Diagnosis may also be established by ultrasonography, contrast-enhanced CT demonstrating areas of cortical lucency, and MRI [49]. The prognosis for patients with BRCN is extremely poor, again likely related to the severity of illness, with one study of 15 cases during pregnancy reporting a mortality rate of 93% [48].

Management of acute renal failure

Management of ARF in pregnancy is similar to that in the non-pregnant patient, including supportive therapy as well as dialysis. General principles include treating the underlying cause, prevention of further renal injury, and supportive care until renal function recovers. Close attention to fluid balance is critical because either superimposed volume depletion or fluid overload may exacerbate ARF or necessitate earlier dialytic intervention. In addition, magnesium sulfate administration in cases of pre-eclampsia may also increase the patient's risk for fluid overload or toxicity from the medication and should be monitored closely. Correction of the metabolic acidosis seen with ARF may require bicarbonate therapy or dialysis, if it remains refractory to medical therapy or occurs in the setting of congestive heart failure. Prevention of hyperphosphatemia includes dietary phosphate restriction and non-absorbable or calcium-containing phosphate binders given with meals. Dietary potassium restriction also is imperative to avoid potentially life-threatening hyperkalemia. A cation-exchange resin, such as kayexalate, can be used for mild hyperkalemia or until dialysis is available. For hyperkalemia with associated electrocardiographic changes, acute therapy includes intravenous calcium gluconate to stabilize the cardiac membrane, infusion of glucose and insulin or inhaled β-agonists to transiently shift potassium intracellularly, and acute dialysis. Additional conservative measures include avoiding further nephrotoxic exposure and hypotension, control of hypertension, and medication dose adjustment according to the degree of renal impairment.

In patients with severe metabolic abnormalities that are unresponsive to conservative medical management, volume overload and pulmonary congestion that cannot be corrected with diuretics, or signs and symptoms of uremia including pericarditis and encephalopathy, dialysis is indicated.

As discussed previously, if the underlying etiology is determined to be severe pre-eclampsia, then delivery may be indicated, even at very early gestational ages as there is no other way to prevent progression of the disease.

Prognosis

The prognosis for return of renal function depends on multiple variables, including baseline renal status, duration of renal failure,

Table 28.7 Classification of pregnancy-associated acute renal failure.

Pre-eclampsia	HELLP syndrome	Acute fatty liver of pregnancy	Postpartum (HUS) renal failure	Pyelonephritis	Bilateral renal cortical necrosis
Proteinuria	RUQ pain	Elevated LFTs	Occurring postpartum	Positive urine culture	Hemorrhage
Hypertension	Proteinuria	Hyperbilirubinemia	MAHA	Fever	Hypotension/shock
Edema	Hemolysis Elevated LFTs Thrombocytopenia Normal coags	Coagulopathy Oliguria Nausea Abdominal pain Leukocytosis	Oliguria Severe HTN Prodromal illness Thrombocytopenia CNS involvement		Oliguria/anuria Flank pain Gross hematuria

HTN, hypertension; LFTs, liver function tests; MAHA, microangiopathic hemolytic anemia; RUQ, right upper quadrant.

and the etiology of the ARF. For instance, if the patient had normal renal function before ARF from an acute obstructive process that is relieved in a timely manner, then a full recovery should be expected. On the other hand, as previously discussed, studies have demonstrated that, of patients with compromised renal function who develop pre-eclampsia with ARF, up to 80% may require long-term dialysis [15].

Summary

Evaluation of the pregnant patient with ARF encompasses a broad range of disorders, some of which are unique to pregnancy. Prerenal azotemia, intrinsic renal disease, including ATN, GN, and interstitial nephritis, and urinary obstruction should be considered based on clinical presentation. Evaluation of ARF during pregnancy is similar to that in the non-pregnant patient, including urinalysis and urinary diagnostic indices, and in some cases, renal biopsy. In addition, diseases unique to pregnancy and those more common during pregnancy must be considered, including pre-eclampsia, HELLP syndrome, AFLP, postpartum renal failure, and BRCN (Table 28.7). Treatment may necessitate prompt delivery of the infant, even at early gestational ages when issues of prematurity may exist.

References

1 Pertuiset N, Ganeval D, Grunfeld JP. Acute renal failure in pregnancy: an update. *Semin Nephrol* 1984; 3: 232–239.

2 Gammill HS, Jeyabalan A. Acute renal failure in pregnancy. *Crit Care Med* 2005; 33(Suppl): S372–S384.

3 Stratta P, Besso L, Canavese C, et al. Is pregnancy-related acute renal failure a disappearing clinical entity? *Ren Fail* 1996; 18(4): 575–584.

4 Lindheimer MD, Katz AI, Ganeval D, et al. Acute renal failure in pregnancy. In: Brenner BN, Lazarus JM, eds. *Acute Renal Failure*. New York: Churchill Livingstone, 1988: 597–620.

5 Stratta P, Canavese C, Dogliani M, et al. Pregnancy-related renal failure. *Clin Nephrol* 1989; 32: 14–20.

6 Turney JH, Ellis CM, Parsons FM. Obstetric acute renal failure 1956–1987. *Br J Obstet Gynaecol* 1989; 96: 679–687.

7 Nzerue CM, Hewan-Lowe K, Nwawka C. Acute renal failure in pregnancy: a review of clinical outcomes at an inner-city hospital from 1986–1996. *J Natl Med Assoc* 1998; 90: 486–490.

8 Thadhani R, Pascual M, Bonventre JV. Acute renal failure. *N Engl J Med* 1996; 334: 1448–1460.

9 Jones DC, Hayslett JP. Outcome of pregnancy in women with moderate or severe renal insufficiency. *N Engl J Med* 1996; 335: 226–232.

10 Gordon M, Landon MB, Samuels P, et al. Perinatal outcome and long-term follow-up associated with modern management of diabetic nephropathy. *Obstet Gynecol* 1996; 87: 401–409.

11 Gonzalez M, Chew W, Soltero L, Gamba G, Correa R. Percutaneous kidney biopsy, analysis of 26 years: complication rate and risk factors. *Rev Invest Clin* 2000; 52: 125–131.

12 Kuller JA, D'Andrea NM, McMahon MJ. Renal biopsy and pregnancy. *Am J Obstet Gynecol* 2001; 184(6): 1093–1096.

13 Turton P, Hughes P, Bolton H, Sedgwick P. Incidence and demographic correlates of eating disorder symptoms in a pregnant population. *Int J Eat Disord* 1999; 26: 448–452.

14 Grunfeld JP, Ganeval D, Bournerias F. Acute renal failure in pregnancy. *Kidney Int* 1980; 18: 179–191.

15 Sibai BM, Villar MA, Mabie BC. Acute renal failure in hypertensive disorders of pregnancy. Pregnancy outcome and remote prognosis in thirty-one consecutive cases. *Am J Obstet Gynecol* 1990; 162(3): 777–783.

16 Ovelese Y, Ananth CV. Placental abruption. *Obstet Gynecol* 2006; 108: 1005–1016.

17 Satin AJ, Seiken GL, Cunningham FG. Reversible hypertension in pregnancy caused by obstructive obstetric uropathy. *Obstet Gynecol* 1993; 81: 823–825.

18 Courban D, Blank S, Harris MA, Bracy J, August P. Acute renal failure in the first trimester resulting from uterine leiomyomas. *Am J Obstet Gynecol* 1997; 177(2): 472–473.

19 Myers DL, Scotti RJ. Acute urinary retention and the incarcerated, retroverted, gravid uterus. A case report. *J Reprod Med* 1995; 40(6): 487–490.

20 Nelson MS. Acute urinary retention secondary to an increased gravid uterus. *Am J Emerg Med* 1986; 4(3): 231–232.

21 Brandes JC, Fritsche C. Obstructive acute renal failure by a gravid uterus: a case report and review. *Am J Kidney Dis* 1991; 18: 398–401.

22 Khanna N, Nguyen H. Reversible acute renal failure in association with bilateral ureteral obstruction and hydronephrosis in pregnancy. *Am J Obstet Gynecol* 2001; 184(2): 239–240.

23 Cunningham FG, Lucas MJ. Urinary tract infections complicating pregnancy. *Baillière's Clin Obstet Gynaecol* 1994; 8: 353–373.

24 Davison JM, Lindheimer MD. Renal disorders. In: Creasy RK, Resnick R, eds. *Maternal Fetal Medicine*, 4th edn. Philadelphia: WB Saunders, 1999: 873–894.

25 Whalley PJ, Cunningham FG, Martin FG. Transient renal dysfunction associated with acute pyelonephritis of pregnancy. *Obstet Gynecol* 1975; 46: 174–177.

26 Gilstrap LC, Cunningham FG, Whalley PJ. Acute pyelonephritis during pregnancy: an anterospective study. *Obstet Gynecol* 1981; 57: 409–413.

27 Ventura JE, Villa M, Mizraji R, Ferreiros R. Acute renal failure in pregnancy. *Ren Fail* 1997; 19(2): 217–220.

28 Antonovych TT, Mostofi FK. *Atlas of Kidney Biopsies*. Washington, DC: Armed Forces Institute of Pathology, 1981: 266–275.

29 Suzuki S, Gejyo F, Ogino S. Post-partum renal lesions in women with pre-eclampsia. *Nephrol Dial Transplant* 1997; 12: 2488–2493.

30 Martin JN, Blake PG, Perry KG, et al. The natural history of HELLP syndrome: patterns of disease progression and regression. *Am J Obstet Gynecol* 1991; 164: 1500–1513.

31 Krane NK. Acute renal failure in pregnancy. *Arch Intern Med* 1988; 148: 2347–2357.

32 Sibai BM, Ramadan MK. Acute renal failure in pregnancies complicated by hemolysis, elevated liver enzymes, and low platelets. *Am J Obstet Gynecol* 1993; 168: 1682–1690.

33 Nakabayashi M, Adachi T, Itoh S, Kobayashi M, Mishina J, Nishida H. Perinatal and infant outcome of pregnant patients undergoing chronic hemodialysis. *Nephron* 1999; 82: 27–31.

34 Kaplan MM. Acute fatty liver of pregnancy. *N Engl J Med* 1985; 313: 367–370.

35 Castro MA, Fassett MJ, Reynolds TB, Shaw KJ, Goodwin TM. Reversible peripartum liver failure: a new perspective on the diagnosis, treatment, and cause of acute fatty liver of pregnancy, based on 28 consecutive cases. *Am J Obstet Gynecol* 1999; 181(2): 389–395.
36 Usta IM, Barton JR, Amon EA, et al. Acute fatty liver of pregnancy: an experience in the diagnosis and management of fourteen cases. *Am J Obstet Gynecol* 1994; 171(5): 1342–1347.
37 Dasche JS, Ramin SM, Cunningham FG. The long-term consequences of thrombotic microangiopathy (thrombotic thrombocytopenic purpura and hemolytic uremic syndrome) in pregnancy. *Obstet Gynecol* 1998; 91: 662–668.
38 Elliott MA, Nichols WL. Thrombotic thrombocytopenic purpura and hemolytic uremic syndrome. *Mayo Clin Proc* 2001; 76: 1154–1162.
39 Bell WR, Braine HG, Ness PM, Kickler TS. Improved survival in thrombotic thrombocytopenic purpura-hemolytic uremic syndrome. *N Engl J Med* 1991; 325: 398–403.
40 Rock GH, Shumak KH, Buskard NA, et al. Comparison of plasma exchange with plasma infusion in the treatment of thrombotic thrombocytopenic purpura. *N Engl J Med* 1991; 325: 393–397.
41 Shemin D, Dworkin LD. Clinical outcome in three patients with postpartum hemolytic uremic syndrome treated with frequent plasma exchange. *Ther Apher* 1998; 2(1): 43–48.
42 Hayward CPM, Sutton DMC, Carter WH, et al. Treatment outcomes in patients with adult thrombotic thrombocytopenic purpura-hemolytic uremic syndrome. *Arch Intern Med* 1994; 154: 982–987.
43 Vesely SK, Li X, McMinn JR, Terrell DR, George JN. Pregnancy outcomes after recovery from thrombotic thrombocytopenic purpura-hemolytic uremic syndrome. *Transfusion* 2004; 44(8): 1149–1158.
44 Hayslett JP. Postpartum renal failure. *N Engl J Med* 1985; 312: 1556–1559.
45 Weiner CP. Thrombotic microangiopathy in pregnancy and the postpartum period. *Semin Hematol* 1987; 24: 119–129.
46 Li PK, Lai FM, Tam JS, Lai KN. Acute renal failure due to postpartum hemolytic uremic syndrome. *Aust NZ J Obstet Gynaecol* 1988; 28(3): 228–230.
47 Donohoe JF. Acute bilateral cortical necrosis. In: Brenner BM, Lazarus JM, eds. *Acute Renal Failure*. Philadelphia: WB Saunders, 1983: 252–269.
48 Prakash J, Tripathi K, Pandey LK, Gadela SR. Renal cortical necrosis in pregnancy-related acute renal failure. *J Indian Med Assoc* 1996; 94(6): 227–229.
49 Francois M, Tostivint I, Mercadal L, Bellin M, Izzedine H, Deray G. MR imaging features of acute bilateral renal cortical necrosis. *Am J Kidney Dis* 2000; 35(4): 745–748.

29 Acute Fatty Liver of Pregnancy

T. Flint Porter

Department of Obstetrics and Gynecology, University of Utah Health Science UT, *and* Maternal-Fetal Medicine, Urban Central Region, Intermountain Healthcare, Salt Lake City, UT, USA

Introduction

Acute fatty liver of pregnancy (AFLP) is a rare, yet potentially fatal complication of late pregnancy. Also known as acute fatty metamorphosis or acute yellow atrophy, the incidence ranges between 1 in 7000 and 1 in 15 000 depending on the population studied [1–3]. Older published series reported maternal and perinatal mortality rates as high as 75 and 85%, respectively [4]. However, more recent experience suggests that both morbidity and mortality can be reduced by early recognition and prompt treatment [1,2,5].

Epidemiology

The majority of cases of AFLP occur during the third trimester [1,5,6], usually between 30 and 38 weeks of gestation [3]; some do not become clinically evident until after delivery [7]. Rare mid-trimester cases have also been reported [8,9]. There are no clear epidemiologically distinct risk factors for AFLP. Neither maternal age nor ethnicity appears to affect risk. Most affected women are in their first pregnancy [7] though AFLP has been diagnosed in multiparous women with otherwise normal obstetric histories. Recurrence in subsequent pregnancy has also been reported [10,12]. Additional suggested risk factors include the presence of a male fetus [13], and multiple gestation [7,14].

Pathogenesis

The pathogenesis of AFLP has not been fully elucidated but abnormalities in mitochondrial fatty acid oxidation likely play an important role. Fatty acid oxidation (FAO) is the major source of energy for skeletal and heart muscle, a process that occurs primarily in the liver during conditions of prolonged fasting, illness, and increased muscular activity [3]. Hepatic FAO also plays an essential role in intermediary liver metabolism and synthesizes alternative sources of energy for the brain when blood glucose levels are low [13].

Mitochondrial FAO functions via a protein complex known as mitochondrial trifunction protein (MTP). It is composed of three enzymes, one of which is long-chain 3-hydroxyacyl-CoA dehydrogenase (LCHAD). Human defects in MTP have emerged as an important group of metabolic errors because of their serious clinical implications (Figure 29.1). They are recessively inherited and result in either isolated LCHAD deficiency or dramatically reduced functionality of all three of the MTP enzymes. Most reported cases involve children with isolated LCHAD deficiency who present within the first few hours to months of life with non-ketotic hypoglycemia and hepatic encephalopathy, which progresses to coma and death if untreated [15,16]. Cardiomyopathy, slowly progressing peripheral neuropathy, skeletal myopathy, or sudden, unexpected death are also reported [17,18].

Schoeman [11] and colleagues were the first group to suggest an association between recurrent maternal AFLP and a fetal fatty acid oxidation disorder in two siblings, both whom died at 6 months of age [16]. Other reports of a potential causative relationship followed [15,19–22]. In one series of 12 affected pregnancies, several offspring delivered of mothers with AFLP were diagnosed postnatally with a homozygous form of LCHAD [19,23]. Parental heterozygosity was subsequently confirmed. LCHAD deficiency was later reported in three families in association with pregnancies complicated by AFLP [20]. Ibdah [15] reported that 80% of mothers who delivered babies with confirmed MTP defects developed either AFLP or HELLP during their pregnancy. Three of them had a history of AFLP in a previous pregnancy. In a subsequent prospective study, the same group [24,25] found that in approximately 1 in 5 pregnancies complicated by AFLP, the fetus is LCHAD-deficient. These findings support the potentially life-saving role of screening for MTP defects in children born to women with AFLP. Prenatal diagnosis

Critical Care Obstetrics, 5th edition. Edited by M. Belfort, G. Saade, M. Foley, J. Phelan and G. Dildy.

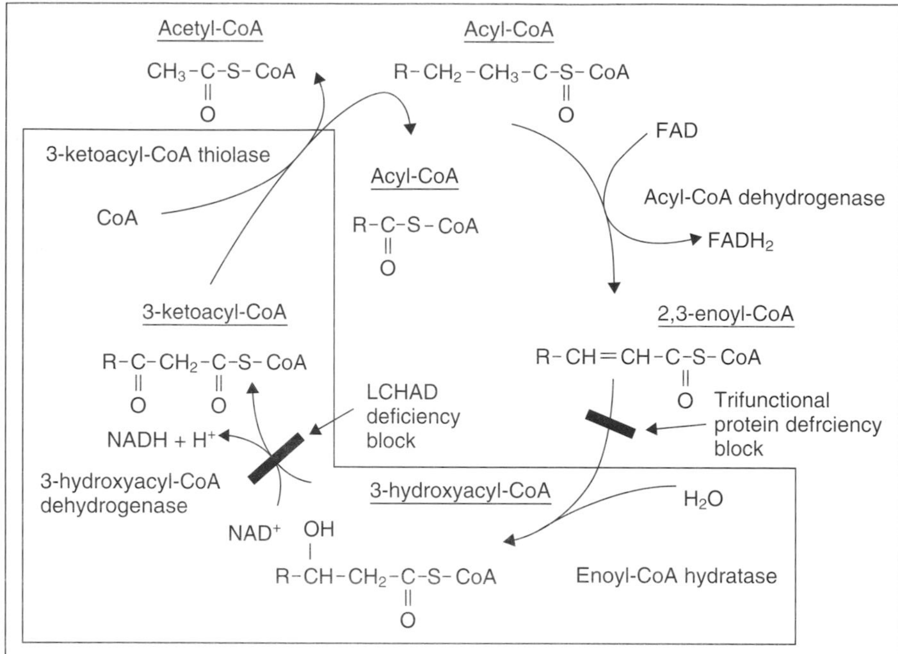

Figure 29.1 The biochemistry of mitochondrial trifunctional protein (MTP) deficiencies. Mitochondrial fatty acid β-oxidation spiral where the MTP catalyzes long chain fatty acids substrates (see box). In isolated LCHAD deficiency, the pathway is blocked after the enoyl Co-A hydratase reaction and before the 3-hydroxyacyl Co-A dehydrogenase reaction, causing the accumulation of medium- and long-chain 3-hydroxy fatty acids and their metabolites. In complete MTP deficiency, the pathway is blocked after the acyl Co-A dehydrogenase reaction and before the enoyl Co-A dehydrogenase reaction causing the accumulation of straight-chain fatty acids and their metabolites. Adapted from Ibdah JA. Acute fatty liver of pregnancy: an update on pathogenesis and clinical implications. *World J Gastroenterol* 2006; 12(46): 7397–7404 [2].

in subsequent pregnancies has also been performed using chorionic villus sampling in an effort to identify at-risk pregnancies [26].

Clinical presentation

The clinical presentation of AFLP is non-specific and most commonly includes nausea, vomiting, anorexia, tachycardia, and abdominal pain (Table 29.1) [1,3,5,7]. Symptoms may develop suddenly or over a 2–3 week period. Though liver size is usually normal or small, 50% of women with AFLP are jaundiced and complain of right upper quadrant or epigastric pain. Fever, headache, and pruritus are not uncommon [1,3]. Symptoms of preeclampsia are present in 50% of women with AFLP including hypertension, proteinuria, and edema [7]. Some women present with isolated obstetric complaints including contractions, decreased fetal movement, and vaginal bleeding [1].

Systemic complications of AFLP are due to fulminant hepatic failure and include encephalopathy, acute renal failure, infection, pancreatitis, gastrointestinal hemorrhage, coagulopathy, and at least mild hypoglycemia. Neurological dysfunction begins early and should immediately alert the physician to the possibility of AFLP. Symptoms may rapidly progress from restlessness, confusion, and disorientation, to asterixis, seizures, psychosis, and ultimately coma [1,3,5]. Other systemic effects include respiratory failure, sometimes requiring assisted ventilation [5], ascites [7], and gastrointestinal bleeding from gastric ulceration and Mallory–Weiss syndrome [2,7].

Renal insufficiency associated with AFLP is due to fatty infiltration of the kidneys [1]. Hepatorenal syndrome eventually develops and leads to oliguria and acute tubular necrosis [1]. In turn, damage to the proximal renal tubules results in decreased sensitivity to vasopressin and transient diabetes insipidus [27,28]. Laboratory evidence of renal dysfunction is evident early in the disease with increased serum creatinine levels. Uric acid and blood urea nitrogen concentrations are also elevated, and with the onset of jaundice, urobilinogen appears in the urine. Serum electrolytes may reflect metabolic acidosis and plasma glucose is often below 60 mg/dL suggesting reduced hepatic glycogenolysis [29]. It is not uncommon for mild hypoglycemia to be masked

Table 29.1 Signs and symptoms of acute fatty liver of pregnancy.

Symptoms	
Nausea, vomiting	Almost always
Malaise	Always
Abdominal pain	Almost always, may be variable in position and severity
Physical signs	
Hypertension	Almost always
Edema	Almost always
Proteinuria	Variable
Jaundice	Always
Elevated liver transaminases	Always
Hypoglycemia	Always, may be masked by administration of glucose-containing intravenous fluids
Coagulopathy	Common
Diabetes insipidus	Common
Encephalopathy	Common, may correlate with ammonia levels

by the administration of dextrose solutions which often routinely occurs at the time of admission.

Virtually all women with AFLP have laboratory evidence of coagulopathy and at least 50% require replacement of blood components [1,2,5,30]. Impaired hepatic synthesis of coagulation factors leads to prolongation of prothrombin time (PT) and activated partial thromboplastin time (aPTT). Hypofibrinogenemia, profound antithrombin III deficiency, and thrombocytopenia are common. Factor VIII levels most accurately reflect the extent of coagulopathy and their return toward normal signals recovery. Coagulopathy may worsen in the postpartum period, most likely secondary to low antithrombin III levels [31].

Serum transaminase concentrations are typically mildly increased, usually between 100 and 1000 U/L. Bilirubin levels are variable but generally exceed 5 mg/dL. Alkaline phosphatase is elevated but is not helpful in making the diagnosis because of placental production. Serum albumin is usually low. Ammonia levels are elevated, due to decreased utilization by urea cycle liver enzymes and may predict the degree of altered sensorium. Elevated amylase and lipase should raise suspicions of concomitant pancreatitis [32]. Liver function tests usually return to normal 4–8 weeks after delivery [4].

The gold standard used for confirmation of AFLP remains the liver biopsy. However, it is rarely necessary when other clinical and laboratory parameters are consistent with the diagnosis. Microscopic examination of fresh specimens stained with special fat stains, most commonly oil red, demonstrate hepatocellular cytoplasm distended by numerous fine vacuoles giving the cells a distinct foamy appearance (Figure 29.2). The myriad of tiny vacuoles are separated from each other by thin eosinophilic cytoplasmic strands and do not coalesce to form a single large vacuole. In contrast to the cytoplasm, the cell nucleus is located centrally and is normal in size and appearance.

Histologic changes are most prominent in the central portion of the lobule with a thin rim of normal hepatocytes at the periphery. The lobular architecture is usually preserved and, with rare exceptions, necrosis and inflammation are absent [33]. This is distinct from the periportal fibrin deposition and hemorrhagic necrosis reported in pre-eclampsia (Figure 29.3). Characteristic histologic changes may be present up to 3 weeks after the onset of jaundice.

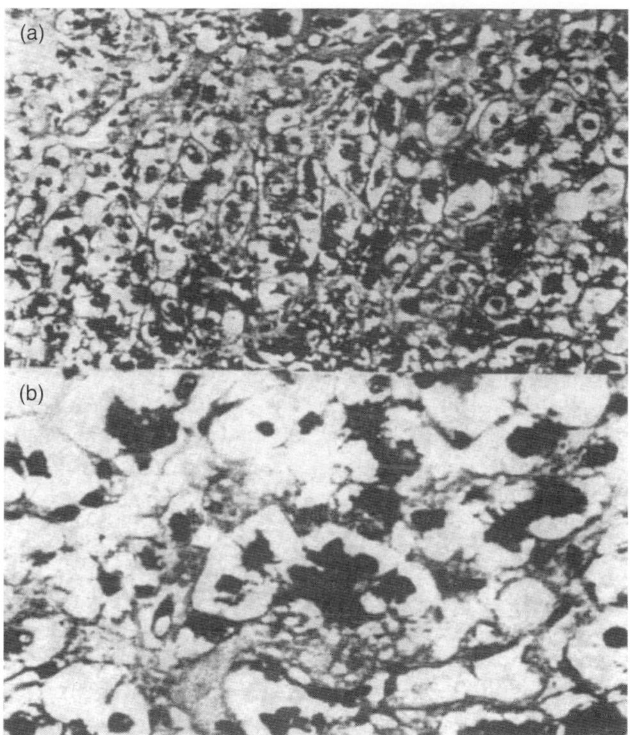

Figure 29.2 (a) Acute fatty liver of pregnancy (H&E stain; magnification 200×). Note diffuse fatty infiltration and absence of necrosis and inflammation. (b) Higher magnification demonstrates the fine cytoplasmic vacuoles and centrally placed nuclei (H&E stain; magnification 1000×). (Courtesy of Dr Patricia Latham, University of Maryland Hospital.)

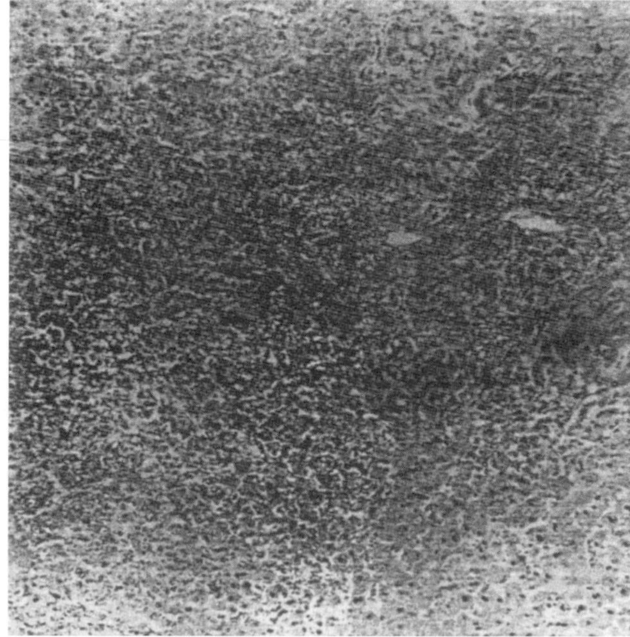

Figure 29.3 Liver section from a patient who died of complications of pre-eclampsia (H&E stain; magnification 40×). Note extensive hepatocellular inflammation and necrosis. (Courtesy of Dr James Kelley, Madigan AMC.)

Diagnosis

A high index of suspicion based on clinical presentation correlated with correct interpretation of laboratory testing is usually sufficient to make the diagnosis of AFLP [1,7]. Liver biopsy is usually not necessary or even possible because of coagulopathy. Most common among the differential diagnoses are pre-eclampsia/HELLP syndrome, viral hepatitis, and cholestasis (Table 29.2). Women with AFLP or pre-eclampsia/HELLP may have elevated serum transaminases, thrombocytopenia or coagulation defects. However, liver failure and jaundice are rare in

Table 29.2 Differential diagnosis of acute fatty liver of pregnancy.

	Acute fatty liver of pregnancy	Acute hepatitis	Cholestasis of pregnancy	Severe pre-eclampsia
Trimester	Third	Variable	Third	Third
Clinical manifestations	Nausea, vomiting, malaise, encephalopathy, abdominal pain, coagulopathy	Malaise, nausea, vomiting, jaundice, anorexia, encephalopathy	Pruritus, jaundice	Hypertension, edema, proteinuria, oliguria, CNS hyperexcitability
Bilirubin	Elevated	Elevated	Elevated	Normal or minimally elevated
Transaminases	Minimally elevated	Markedly elevated	Minimally elevated	Normal or minimal to moderate increase
Alkaline phosphatase	Usually normal for pregnancy	Minimally elevated	Moderately elevated	Normal for pregnancy
Histology	Fatty infiltration, no inflammation or necrosis	Marked inflammation and necrosis	Biliary stasis, no inflammation	Inflammation, necrosis, fibrin deposition
Recurrence	Reported	No	Yes	Yes

pre-eclampsia/HELLP. Some authorities believe that AFLP and pre-eclampsia may occur concomitantly [1]. The diagnosis of viral hepatitis can be established quickly and with reasonable certainty via specific serologic testing. In addition, serum transaminase levels in women with hepatitis are usually elevated well beyond those typically seen in AFLP. Women with cholestasis of pregnancy are usually not as ill-appearing as those with AFLP, pre-eclampsia, or viral hepatitis. While liver function tests are abnormal in cholestasis of pregnancy, concentrations of bilirubin and transaminase are usually much lower compared to those of AFLP or viral hepatitis and signs and symptoms typical of pre-eclampsia are rarely present.

Ultrasonography, CT, and MRI are often performed as part of the diagnostic work-up for jaundice during pregnancy. Ultrasound demonstrates echogenicities within the liver of women with AFLP [7]. While non-specific, ultrasound may also identify subcapsular hematoma, cholecystitis, and/or cholangitis. Both CT and MRI may suggest AFLP based on lower density that occurs with fatty infiltration of the liver [34,35]. However, both have high false-negative rates that limit their usefulness [30]. In clinical practice, imaging studies are complementary but not necessary to make the diagnosis of AFLP and their performance should not delay appropriate treatment. Moreover, a normal study does not exclude AFLP.

Treatment

Women suspected of having AFLP should be hospitalized in an intensive care setting where comprehensive supportive care can be given and preparations for delivery can be made. All published series have reported improved maternal and perinatal outcome when prompt delivery is accomplished [1,3–5,7]. Most women begin to show clinical improvement and resolution of laboratory abnormalities by the second day postpartum [5]. There are no reported cases of AFLP resolving prior to delivery; Therefore, once the diagnosis is established, expectant management is absolutely contraindicated. AFLP should not be considered an indication for cesarean, even though expeditious delivery is recommended. Indeed, most hemorrhagic complications in women with AFLP occur as a result of surgical trauma [1]. Attempts at induction of labor and vaginal delivery are appropriate as long as adequate maternal supportive care and fetal surveillance are possible. Even so, fetal compromise during labor is common and cesarean delivery is often necessary [1]. Women who are critically ill should not be subjected to long arduous induction of labor. The ultimate decision regarding route of delivery should be individualized, based on the maternal and fetal conditions as well as the favorability of the cervical exam.

Anesthetic options in patients with AFLP are limited. General anesthesia can further damage an already compromised liver and regional anesthetic poses a risk of hemorrhage when coagulopathy is present. If general anesthesia must be used, inhalation agents with potential hepatotoxicity (e.g. halothane) should be avoided. Isoflurane is a logical choice since it has little or no hepatotoxicity and may preserve liver blood flow [36,37]. Epidural anesthesia is probably the best option under most circumstances because it preserves hepatic blood flow without hepatotoxic effects [37,38]. Recognition and treatment of thrombocytopenia and coagulopathy is essential prior to neuraxial techniques.

Supportive care

Supportive care of patients with AFLP should include careful monitoring for evidence of progressive hepatic failure, hypoglycemia, and coagulopathy. This should occur in an intensive care setting and in consultation with physicians well-versed in the care of critically ill patients. Prevention of worsening hypoglycemia and reduction of endogenous production of nitrogenous wastes can be accomplished by providing approximately 2000–2500 calories per day, primarily in the form of glucose. Most patients require solutions containing more than 5% dextrose, sometimes as high as 25%, administered intravenously or through a nasogastric tube. Nitrogenous waste production can be reduced further by exclusion of protein intake during the acute phase of the illness. Once clinical improvement is evident, protein intake should gradually be restored. With rare exceptions, any drug that requires hepatic metabolism should be withheld from the patient. Colonic emptying should be facilitated through the use of enemas and/or magnesium citrate; ammonia production by intestinal bacteria may be diminished by the administration of neomycin, 6–12 g orally per day.

Exchange transfusion, hemodialysis, plasmapheresis, extracorporeal perfusion, and corticosteroids have all been used to treat fulminant hepatic failure [39] and should be considered in cases unresponsive to traditional management. Successful liver transplantation has also been reported in women with AFLP who continue to deteriorate in spite of delivery and appropriate supportive care [40–42]. However, because the pathophysiologic changes associated with AFLP are reversible, transplantation is inappropriate in all but the most extreme cases [1,43]. Successful temporary auxiliary liver transplant has also been reported [41].

Mild coagulation abnormalities need not be corrected if delivery can be accomplished atraumatically and there is no evidence of clinical bleeding. However, in the presence of hemorrhagic complications or if surgery is contemplated, the coagulation abnormalities should be corrected with platelet, fresh frozen plasma, or cryoprecipitate transfusion based on the results of laboratory evaluation. The successful use of antithrombin [1,43] and factor VII [44] concentrations have also been reported.

Morbidity from other potential complications may be prevented by prophylactic treatment and careful surveillance. The liberal use of broad-spectrum antibiotics may decrease the incidence of concomitant infection [1]. Prophylactic administration of antacid solutions and H_2 blocking agents may decrease the risk of gastrointestinal bleeding.

Summary

Acute fatty liver of pregnancy is fortunately uncommon but when it occurs, results in serious morbidity and even mortality in the worst cases. Early diagnosis and prompt treatment remain the best strategy for managing patients with AFLP. Defects in long-chain fatty acid oxidation play a role in the development of AFLP and genetic testing may useful in preventing neonatal morbidity as well as future pregnancy morbidity. Delivery is the treatment of choice and supportive care and treatment of systemic manifestations of AFLP improve both maternal and perinatal survival.

References

1 Castro MA, Fassett MJ, Reynolds TB, Shaw KJ, Goodwin TM. Reversible peripartum liver failure: a new perspective on the diagnosis, treatment, and cause of acute fatty liver of pregnancy, based on 28 consecutive cases. *Am J Obstet Gynecol* 1999; 181(2): 389–395.

2 Ibdah JA. Acute fatty liver of pregnancy: an update on pathogenesis and clinical implications. *World J Gastroenterol* 2006; 12(46): 7397–7404.

3 Reyes H, Sandoval L, Wainstein A, et al. Acute fatty liver of pregnancy: a clinical study of 12 episodes in 11 patients. *Gut* 1994; 35: 101–106.

4 Kaplan MM. Acute fatty liver of pregnancy. *N Engl J Med* 1985; 313: 367.

5 Usta IM, Barton JR, Amon EA, Gonzalez A, Sibai BM. Acute fatty live of pregnancy: an experience in the diagnosis and management of fourteen cases. *Am J Obstet Gynecol* 1994; 171: 1342–1347.

6 Pockros PJ, Peters RL, Reynolds TB. Idiopathic fatty liver of pregnancy: findings in ten cases. *Medicine* 1984; 63: 1.

7 Bacq Y. Acute fatty liver of pregnancy. *Semin Perinatol* 1998; 22(2): 134–140.

8 Monga M, Katz AR. Acute fatty liver in the second trimester. *Obstet Gynecol* 1999; 93(5 Pt 2): 811–813.

9 Suzuki S, Watanabe S, Araki T. Acute fatty liver of pregnancy at 23 weeks of gestation. *Br J Obstet Gynaecol* 2001; 108: 223–224.

10 Barton JR, Sibai BM, Mabie WC, Shanklin DR. Recurrent acute fatty liver of pregnancy. *Am J Obstet Gynecol* 1990; 163: 534–538.

11 Schoeman MN, Batey RG, Wilcken B. Recurrent acute fatty liver of pregnancy associated with a fatty-acid oxidation defect in the offspring. *Gastroenterology* 1991; 100: 544–548.

12 Wilcken B, Leung KC, Hammond J, Kamath R, Leonard JV. Pregnancy and fetal long-chain 3-hydroxyacyl coenzyme A dehydrogenase deficiency. *Lancet* 1993; 341: 407–408.

13 Burroughs AK, Seong NGJ, Dojcinov DM, et al. Idiopathic acute fatty liver of pregnancy in twelve patients. *Q J Med* 1982; 204: 481.

14 Davidson KM, Simpson LL, Knox TA, d'Alton ME. Acute fatty liver of pregnancy in triplet gestation. *Obstet Gynecol* 1998; 91(5 Pt 2): 806–808.

15 Ibdah JA, Bennett MJ, Rinaldo P, et al. A fetal fatty-acid oxidation disorder as a cause of liver disease in pregnant women. *N Engl J Med* 1999; 340(22): 1723–1731.

16 Rinaldo P, Raymond K, al-Odaib A, Bennett MJ. Clinical and biochemical features of fatty acid oxidation disorders. *Curr Opin Pediatr* 1998; 10: 615–621.

17 Pons R, Roig M, Riudor E, et al. The clinical spectrum of long-chain 3-hydroxyacyl-CoA dehydrogenase deficiency. *Pediatr Neurol* 1996; 14: 236–243.

18 Ibdah JA, Tein I, Dionisi-Vici C, et al. Mild trifunctional protein deficiency is associated with progressive neuropathy and myopathy and suggests a novel genotype-phenotype correlation. *J Clin Invest* 1998; 102: 1193–1199.

19 Treem WR, Rinaldo P, Hale DE, et al. Acute fatty liver of pregnancy and long-chain 3-hydroxyacyl-coenzyme A dehydrogenase deficiency. *Hepatology* 1994; 19: 339–345.

20 Sims HF, Brackett JC, Powell CK, et al. The molecular basis of pediatric long chain 3-hydroxyacyl-CoA dehydrogenase deficiency associated with maternal acute fatty liver of pregnancy. *Proc Natl Acad Sci USA* 1995; 92: 841–845.

21 Isaacs JD Jr, Sims HF, Powell CK, et al. Maternal acute fatty liver of pregnancy associated with fetal trifunctional protein deficiency: molecular characterization of a novel maternal mutant allele. *Pediatr Res* 1996; 40: 393–398.

22 Matern D, Hart P, Murtha AP, et al. Acute fatty liver of pregnancy associated with short-chain acyl-coenzyme A dehydrogenase deficiency. *J Pediatr* 2001; 138(4): 585–588.

23 Treem WR. Mitochondrial fatty acid oxidation and acute fatty liver of pregnancy. *Semin Gastrointest Dis* 2002; 13: 55–66.

24 Yang Z, Zhao Y, Bennett MJ, Strauss AW, Ibdah JA. Fetal genotypes and pregnancy outcomes in 35 families with mitochondrial trifunctional protein mutations. *Am J Obstet Gynecol* 2002; 187: 715–720.

25 Yang Z, Yamada J, Zhao Y, Strauss AW, Ibdah JA. Prospective screening for pediatric mitochondrial trifunctional protein defects in pregnancies complicated by liver disease. *JAMA* 2002; 288: 2163–2166.

26 Ibdah JA, Zhao Y, Viola J, Gibson B, Bennett MJ, Strauss AW. Molecular prenatal diagnosis in families with fetal mitochondrial trifunctional protein mutations. *J Pediatr* 2001; 138: 396–399.

27 Kennedy SK, Hall PM, Seymore AE, Hague WM. Transient diabetes insipidus and acute fatty liver of pregnancy. *Br J Obstet Gynaecol* 1994; 101: 387–391.

28 Tucker ED, Calhoun BC, Thorneycroft IH, Edwards MS. Diabetes insipidus and acute fatty liver: a case report. *J Reprod Med* 1993; 38: 835–838.

29 Purdie JM, Waters BNJ. Acute fatty liver of pregnancy. Clinical features and diagnosis. *Aust NZ J Obstet Gynaecol* 1988; 28: 62–67.

30 Castro MA, Ouzounian JG, Colletti PM, Shaw KJ, Stein SM, Goodwin TM. Radiologic studies in acute fatty liver of pregnancy. A review of the literature and 19 new cases. *J Reprod Med* 1996; 41(11): 839–843.

31 Liebman HA, McGhee WG, Patch MJ, Feinstein DI. Severe depression of antithrombin III associated with disseminated intravascular coagulation in women with fatty liver of pregnancy. *Ann Intern Med* 1983; 98: 330–333.

32 Lauersen B, Frost B, Mortensen JZ. Acute fatty liver of pregnancy with complicating disseminated intravascular coagulation. *Acta Obstet Gynecol Scand* 1983; 62: 403.

33 Duma RJ, Dowling EA, Alexander HC, et al. Acute fatty liver of pregnancy: report of a surviving patient with serial liver biopsies. *Ann Intern Med* 1965; 63: 851.

34 Clements D, Young WT, Thornton JG, Rhodes J, Howard C, Hibbard B. Imaging in acute fatty liver of pregnancy. Case report. *Br J Obstet Gynaecol* 1990; 97: 631–633.

35 Farine D, Newhouse J, Owen J, Fox HE. Magnetic resonance imaging and computed tomography scan for the diagnosis of acute fatty liver of pregnancy. *Am J Perinatol* 1990; 7: 316–318.

36 Goldfarb G, Debaene B, Ang ET, Roulot D, Jolis P, Lebrec D. Hepatic blood flow in humans during isoflurane N_2O and halothane-N_2O anesthesia. *Anesth Analg* 1990; 71: 349–353.

37 Holzman RS, Riley LE, Aron E, Fetherston J. Perioperative care of a patient with acute fatty liver of pregnancy. *Anesth Analg* 2001; 92(5): 1268–1270.

38 Antognini JF, Andrews S. Anaesthesia for caesarean section in a patient with acute fatty liver of pregnancy. *Can J Anaesth* 1991; 38: 904–907.

39 Katelaris PH, Jones DB. Fulminant hepatic failure. *Med Clin North Am* 1989; 73: 955–970.

40 Amon E, Allen SR, Petrie RH, Belew JE. Acute fatty liver or pregnancy associated with pre-eclampsia: management of hepatic failure with postpartum live transplantation. *Am J Perinatol* 1991; 8: 278–279.

41 Franco J, Newcomer J, Adams M, Saeian K. Auxiliary liver transplant in acute fatty liver of pregnancy. *Obstet Gynecol* 2000; 95(6 Pt 2): 1042.

42 Ockner SA, Brunt E, Cohn SM, Krul ES, Hanto DW, Peters MG. Fulminant hepatic failure caused by acute fatty liver of pregnancy by orthotopic liver transplantation. *Hepatology* 1990; 11: 59–64.

43 Doepel M, Backas HN, Taskinen EI, Isoniemi HM, Hockerstedt KA. Spontaneous recovery of post partus liver necrosis in a patient listed for transplantation. *Hepatogastroenterology* 1996; 43(10): 1084–1087.

44 Gowers CJ, Parr MJ. Recombinant activated factor VIIa use in massive transfusion and coagulopathy unresponsive to conventional therapy. *Anaesth Intens Care* 2005; 33(2): 196–120.

30 Sickle Cell Crisis

Michelle Y. Owens & James N. Martin

Department of Obstetrics and Gynecology, Division of Maternal-Fetal Medicine, University of Mississippi Medical Center, Jackson, MS, USA

Introduction

Sickle cell disease represents a spectrum of heritable disorders of hemoglobin synthesis that result in the production of abnormal hemoglobin molecules (hemoglobin S). Included in this group are sickle cell anemia (Hgb $\beta^S\beta^S$), SC disease (Hgb $\beta^S\beta^C$), and sickle β-thalassemia (Hgb $\beta^+\beta^0$). In sickle cell trait (Hgb $\beta^A\beta^S$) only one β-chain is abnormal. As such, sickle trait is considered to be an essentially benign disease, except under extremely stressful physiologic conditions. In sickle cell disease, the production of abnormal hemoglobin causes deformities of the red cell membrane which result in hemolytic anemia, tissue ischemia, organ failure, and episodic vaso-occlusive pain crises. Other sequelae include chronic pain from long-term or repeated ischemic events, and altered immunity leading to an increased susceptibility to infections. When compared with unaffected pregnancies, sickle cell disease in pregnancy is associated with an increased incidence of pre-eclampsia, preterm labor, spontaneous abortion, and stillbirth compared to unaffected pregnancies [1,2].

Over the past few decades, much has been learned about this particular class of hemoglobinopathies. In one generation, survival for individuals with sickle cell disease has increased from 14 years to almost 50 years, and 50% survive beyond the fourth decade [3]. With the advent of widespread screening, prophylactic antibiotic therapy, vaccine use, and the application of novel technologies such as transcranial Doppler, morbidity and mortality from sickle cell disease have diminished greatly and significant increases in quality of life have occurred.

Epidemiology

The sickle cell mutation arose, independently, in five geographic locations worldwide [4]. The mutations are identified by their association with different β-globin gene haplotypes (Tables 30.1 & 30.2). Four occurred in Africa (Senegal, Bantu, Benin, and Cameroon types), and one originated in Southern India (Indian/Saudi Arabian type). The high prevalence of such a deleterious gene among some ethnic groups has been attributed to selective pressure from falciparum malaria. Heterozygotes (sickle cell trait) are usually asymptomatic and have partial protection against the malarial parasite.

Sickle cell anemia is the most common heritable hemoglobinopathy. It is the most common single gene disorder in the United States, with 1 in 400 African Americans affected and 1 in 12 being carriers of the trait. The disorder is also common among other ethnic groups around the world, including Asian Indians, those of Mediterranean descent, and inhabitants of the Arabian Peninsula. Hemoglobin SC disease has an approximate frequency of 1 in 1250 and the sickle β-thalassemias occur in approximately 1 in 24 000 African Americans [5]. However, because American society is made up of immigrants from many countries, it is useful to be aware that the sickle hemoglobin gene has a prevalence of 25% in some parts of Saudi Arabia and 30% among some Indian populations. The gene has also been identified in parts of the former Soviet Union, in Arabs living in Israel, in Central and South America, and in the Mediterranean countries of Greece, Italy, and Spain [4,6].

Similarly, the β-thalassemia mutations are common in Africa, some parts of India and around the Mediterranean and in Southeast Asia.

Fertility is not impaired in women with sickle cell disease. Although no statistics are available on the number of births to affected women, the high prevalence of the disease makes it very likely that a clinician will at some time be responsible for the care of a pregnant sickle cell patient.

Molecular basis of the sickle hemoglobinopathies

The sickle hemoglobinopathies are inherited as autosomal recessive traits. Individuals with sickle cell disease possess at least one

Critical Care Obstetrics, 5th edition. Edited by M. Belfort, G. Saade, M. Foley, J. Phelan and G. Dildy.

Table 30.1 Mutations that cause sickle cell disease.

$\beta^{6glu\rightarrow val}\beta^{6glu\rightarrow val}$	Sickle cell anemia
$\beta^{6glu\rightarrow val}\beta^{6glu\rightarrow lys}$	SC disease
$\beta^{6glu\rightarrow val}\beta^{0}$ or β^{+}	Sickle β-thalassemia
$\beta^{6glu\rightarrow val}\beta^{A}$	Sickle trait

Table 30.2 Known double mutations.

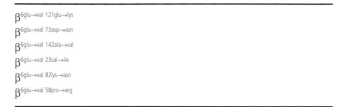

$\beta^{6glu\rightarrow val\ 121glu\rightarrow lys}$
$\beta^{6glu\rightarrow val\ 73asp\rightarrow asn}$
$\beta^{6glu\rightarrow val\ 142ala\rightarrow val}$
$\beta^{6glu\rightarrow val\ 23val\rightarrow ile}$
$\beta^{6glu\rightarrow val\ 82lys\rightarrow asn}$
$\beta^{6glu\rightarrow val\ 58pro\rightarrow arg}$

gene for sickle hemoglobin in addition to another abnormal hemoglobin gene. Those with sickle cell trait possess one gene for sickle hemoglobin and another for normal adult hemoglobin. The offspring of parents with sickle cell trait have a 25% chance of being homozygous for sickle cell anemia, a 25% chance of having normal hemoglobin, and a 50% chance of being a carrier. Clinical manifestations of sickle cell disease vary according to the type of abnormal hemoglobin produced as well as the amount of abnormal hemoglobin present.

The β-globin chain is coded on the short arm of chromosome 11. Sickle cell anemia was the first disease determined to have a molecular basis [7]. Though the first clinical description of sickle cell anemia was published by Herrick in 1910 [8], it was not until 1949 that Pauling and colleagues [7] discovered the underlying mechanism of disease. They determined that sickle cell anemia was the result of a point mutation in the gene coding for the β-chain of the hemoglobin molecule which resulted in the substitution of a single amino acid (valine for glutamic acid) in the sixth position of the β-globin chain. When present on both chromosomes in a patient, the result was sickle cell hemoglobin (Hgb S) [7]. It was later discovered that another abnormal hemoglobin, hemoglobin C, was also the result of a missense mutation at the sixth position causing lysine to replace glutamic acid.

In addition to the more common point mutations, double mutations also sometimes occur. These resultant hemoglobin variants still exhibit the characteristic sickling tendencies, but when electrophoresed, they demonstrate different migration patterns. There are six known double mutation variants, which result in abnormalities of the tertiary structure of the resulting globin chain [4].

Unlike the sickle gene which is responsible for the production of a dysfunctional globin chain, the thalassemia genes result in an abnormal amount of globin produced. The β-thalassemia mutations are subdivided into two categories, β^{+} and β^{0}, based on globin gene production. In β^{+}, there is reduced production of β-chains, while β^{0} is the result of a gene deletion or abnormal gene which precludes any production of β-chains. Sickle β^{+}-thalassemia is the mildest variant of sickle cell disease, followed in order of increasing severity by doubly heterozygous sickle hemoglobin C (SC), sickle β^{0}-thalassemia, and homozygous sickle cell disease.

Diagnosis

The diagnosis of sickle cell disease cannot and must not be made from either a sickle cell preparation or a solubility test. While these are adequate screening tools, neither of these tests will reliably distinguish sickle cell trait from sickle cell disease. Cellulose acetate electrophoresis or an isoelectric focusing test can be used for diagnostic purposes [9]. Preimplantation genetic diagnosis is also available for use with assisted reproductive technologies.

Pathophysiology

Under conditions of normal oxygenation, sickle hemoglobin has normal form and function. Under conditions that cause reduced oxygen concentrations, the sickle β-globin demonstrates a high affinity for other Hgb S chains. This process is facilitated by the neutrally charged valine which is substituted for glutamic acid. Tetramers of deoxyhemoglobin polymerize to form longer deoxyhemoglobin strands within the erythrocyte [10,11]. These rigid polymers deform the erythrocyte membrane, causing occlusion of the smaller-caliber blood vessels. Fully oxygenated hemoglobin is sterically prevented from polymerization. Additionally, sickled cells adhere to the vascular endothelium and precipitate intimal hyperplasia and the release of inflammatory cytokines which accelerate endothelial injury. Most importantly, there is a delay between the deoxygenation and the formation of the hemoglobin polymer that is inversely dependent upon the concentration of sickle hemoglobin [12]. Thus, the higher the intracellular hemoglobin concentration, the more readily polymerization will occur. It is this polymerization that is responsible for the distortion of the red cell membrane. This process remains cyclical throughout the life of the red blood cell, and is also responsible for alterations in cellular membrane permeability leading to the overall egress of water from the erythrocyte [13]. While polymerization is a reversible process, the dehydration process is not. Over time, the net effect of multiple episodes of polymerization and dehydration is an irreversibly sickled cell.

It has been shown that the presence of fetal hemoglobin (Hgb F) decreases the severity of sickle cell anemia. Fetal hemoglobin has a higher affinity for oxygen and does not polymerize. Individuals with higher percentages (20–30%) of hemoglobin F rarely experience crises because the speed of the sickling is reduced and the presence of the alternate globin chain inhibits the polymerization process [6].

Sickling can be precipitated by a number of physiologic and environmental factors. Among the more common aggravating factors are acidosis, dehydration, extremes of temperature (hot or cold), hypoxia, elevation, and infection. In the initial stages, the sickling process is reversible with oxygenation. However, with repeated episodes of deoxygenation, the red blood cell membrane becomes rigid and irreversibly sickled [10]. The alterations in the molecular structure of sickled cells significantly reduce the lifespan of the erythrocyte. While the lifespan of a normal red blood cell is approximately 120 days, the life span of a sickled cell ranges from 10 to 20 days. These damaged cells are cleared by the reticuloendothelial system (largely the spleen and liver) where the majority of the hemolysis occurs, with approximately one-third of hemolysis occurring intravascularly. A chronic compensated anemia results via the bone marrow and extramedullary hematopoiesis.

Vaso-occlusive crises occur first as a result of occlusion of the microvasculature. Unlike the more pliable normal red blood cells, sickled cells lack the flexibility to maneuver through the smaller diameters of the microcapillary beds. These rigid cells become entrapped within the capillaries, producing a vicious cycle of local hypoxia, deoxygenation, and more sickling.

Secondary organ system effects

Sickle cell disease effects may be seen in multiple organ systems. As a result of the wide variety of systemic effects, the pregnant sickle cell patient is at increased risk for more frequent pain crises, hypertensive disorders of pregnancy, intrauterine growth restriction, preterm labor, and infections. Maternal mortality is reported to be 1% in this population, but is continuing to decline [14]. Though the effects of chronic sickling may be numerous, we have decided to focus on those organ systems most commonly affected in the gravid adult with sickle cell disease.

Cardiovascular

Cardiac abnormalities are almost ubiquitous in this patient population. Cardiac output is increased to compensate for the reduced oxygen-carrying capacity of the blood caused by anemia. This increase in output occurs without an elevation in heart rate and thus must be accomplished by increasing stroke volume. Cardiomegaly is found in 80–100% of adults with sickle cell disease. The right and left ventricles and left atrium are usually enlarged and the interventricular septum is thickened, though contractility appears to remain normal [15,16]. On an ECG, 10% of sicklers have prolongation of PR interval and 50% have some evidence of left ventricular hypertrophy [17]. Fortunately, despite the known effects of sickle cell disease on the cardiovascular system, it is uncommon for women with sickle cell anemia to die of cardiac disease. However, the physiologic adaptations to chronic anemia combined with the volume changes of pregnancy put the pregnant sickle cell patient at an increased risk of heart failure should volume overload occur.

Additionally, parturients with sickle cell disease are at increased risk for gestational hypertension, pre-eclampsia, and growth restriction. The reasons why this occurs is unknown. The authors recommend screening for hypertensive disorders at the time of registration which includes a 24- or 12-hour urine collection for urine protein and creatinine, liver function tests, uric acid, and a complete blood count to establish a baseline from which to evaluate these patients if and when symptoms occur. Furthermore, close monitoring of maternal weight, blood pressure, clinical symptoms, and urine protein is essential. In sickle cell disease, blood pressures tend to be lower than that with normal hemoglobin. Part of our routine care also includes serial ultrasonography to evaluate the fetal rate of growth. The authors typically follow these patients serially (4–6 weeks) if fetal growth rate is normal and every 3 weeks in the presence of growth restriction. However, alterations in the timing of such examinations may be necessary as clinical indications arise.

Respiratory

Another common site for sickle cell involvement is the lung. The degree of involvement is variable, and comprises both acute and chronic processes. Pulmonary complications are the second leading cause of hospitalization, and represent the leading cause of death in the patient with sickle cell disease [18]. Pulmonary mortality has declined with the initiation of penicillin prophylaxis and widespread vaccination protocols in childhood sicklers, but pneumonia remains a serious complication of sickle cell anemia. Pneumonia is the third leading cause of death in pregnancy complicated by sickle cell disease. Though *Streptococcus pneumoniae* is most common, atypical organisms such as *Chlamydia* species should also be considered in this population [9]. It is also recommended that these patients receive the influenza vaccine annually and the polyvalent pneumococcal vaccine. In cases of asplenia, vaccination against *Haemophilus influenzae* type B and the meningococcus is also recommended [19].

Acute chest syndrome (ACS) is an acute life-threatening illness that can occur in sickle cell disease. It will be discussed in further detail later in this chapter.

Chronic pulmonary changes such as pulmonary hypertension and pulmonary fibrosis are the respiratory sequelae of recurrent episodes of ACS and the widespread endothelial injury that occurs in sickle cell disease. In one study, 90% of adults with sickle cell disease were found to have abnormal pulmonary function tests, the majority of which demonstrated a restrictive physiology (76%) [20]. It is estimated that approximately one-third of patients with sickle cell disease will develop pulmonary hypertension. The maternal mortality rate associated with pregnancy and pulmonary hypertension ranges from 30 to 50%, and in severe cases, termination of pregnancy is recommended for maternal benefit. In the event that pregnancy is continued, management should include frequent visits, serial cardiopulmonary evaluation (including transthoracic Doppler echocardiography), and a multidisciplinary approach to care. Successful medical management has been reported in some cases with the utilization of sildenafil, inhaled nitric oxide, and L-arginine therapy [21–24]. Though data are limited regarding pulmonary fibrosis in pregnancy, scattered case reports demonstrate that successful outcomes are possible with close follow-up [25,26].

Renal

Sickle cell anemia is also associated with alterations in renal morphology and function. Light microscopy has demonstrated sickled blood cells in glomerular capillaries and afferent arterioles. The glomerulus is prone to glomerulosclerosis, which may lead to proteinuria, nephritic syndrome, or renal failure [27]. In sickle cell disease, destruction of the vasa recta through exposure to the hypertonic interstitium of the medulla leads to hyposthenuria, the inability to maximally concentrate the urine, further potentiating sickling and dehydration. Hemorrhage from surrounding medullary veins is thought to be responsible for occasional self-limited bouts of hematuria which are commonly seen in patients with sickle cell disease [28].

As pregnant patients with sickle cell disease are at an increased risk for urinary tract infections, it is recommended that they undergo routine urinary screening. The authors use urine dipsticks at each visit, with serial urine cultures at least every trimester.

Sickle cell disease affects almost every organ system. From cerebrovascular accidents, Moya-Moya disease (chronic cerebrovascular disease characterized by severe bilateral stenosis or occlusion of the arteries around the circle of Willis with prominent collateral circulation), and sensorineural hearing loss, to proliferative retinopathy and acute retinal artery occlusion with resultant vision loss, the complications are many. A high index of suspicion and a low threshold for further investigation is imperative.

Sickle crisis management (Figure 30.1)

Uncomplicated acute pain crisis

Pain crises without major organ involvement are the most common types of crises during pregnancy. Clinical features of acute pain crises vary with age and sex and frequently recur in a pattern, which is stereotypical for each individual. Pregnancy and the puerperium are associated with an increased frequency of painful episodes.

Musculoskeletal pain, limited motion and swollen tender joints with effusions may be present. Dark urine is a common complaint reflecting excretion of urinary porphyrin.

The diagnosis of pain crisis is a diagnosis of exclusion because objective laboratory and physical findings are lacking. Approximately 50% of patients with pain crises have alterations in vital signs including mild to moderate fever (37.8°C or higher), elevations of blood pressure, tachycardia and tachypnea. Fever can occur in the absence of infection due to release of endogenous pyrogens by ischemic tissue. Nonetheless, when fever is encountered, an infectious cause should be sought. Moderate leukocytosis (12–17 000 cells/μL) usually occurs even in the absence of infection and is most likely a reaction to tissue ischemia. In the presence of infection the white blood cell count can exceed 20 000 with an associated bandemia. Serum lactate dehydrogenase values (LDH), especially isoenzymes 1 and 2, are elevated in sickle pain crises most likely due to marrow infarction [17]. Levels of LDH rise in proportion to the severity of systemic vaso-occlusion. C-reactive protein is elevated within 1–2 days of onset of a crisis and the erythrocyte sedimentation rate is decreased. Approximately, one-third of pain crises are associated with infection. The most common infections during pregnancy are pneumonia, urinary tract infections, endomyometritis and osteomyelitis.

Standard management of sickle pain crises is supportive: rest, hydration, oxygenation, and pain control. The majority of patients will be dehydrated due to an inability to concentrate urine. Fluid resuscitation should be initiated with normal saline. Fluid therapy probably has no effect on irreversibly sickled cells but euvolemia will decrease blood viscosity and thereby decrease the predisposition to ongoing vaso-occlusion. Input and output should be followed closely to limit the occurrence of pulmonary edema, though Foley catheterization should be avoided, if possible, to decrease the risk of infection. If infection is suspected, blood and urine cultures and a chest radiograph should be taken and broad-spectrum antibiotic coverage should be started empirically.

Fetal assessment

During and immediately after a vaso-occlusive crisis, there is significant risk for fetal distress, premature labor, and fetal loss. Continuous electronic fetal monitoring should be initiated for fetuses at the age of viability, and continued until the patient is stable. A non-reactive fetal heart tracing is common during vaso-occlusive crises. One-third of fetuses will have a biophysical profile score of 6 or less [29]. Fetal assessments typically improve as the sickle crisis resolves. The maternal condition should be stabilized and intrauterine resuscitation initiated before emergent operative delivery is considered. Once the patient is well hydrated, oxygenation optimized, her vital signs stabilized, there is no evidence of major organ involvement or severe infection, and her pain is well controlled, continuous fetal monitoring can be replaced by intermittent fetal assessments such as daily or twice weekly non-stress testing or biophysical profiles for fetuses 26 weeks and older. As with most pregnancy complications, antenatal assessments should be individualized to the patient and her clinical situation.

Chest syndrome

Acute chest syndrome (ACS) or pulmonary crisis is a potentially fatal complication of sickle cell disease characterized by fever, pleuritic chest pain, tachypnea and pulmonary infiltrates. If a cough is present it is usually non-productive.

The syndrome results from infarction of the pulmonary vasculature or pulmonary infection or a combination of these. The

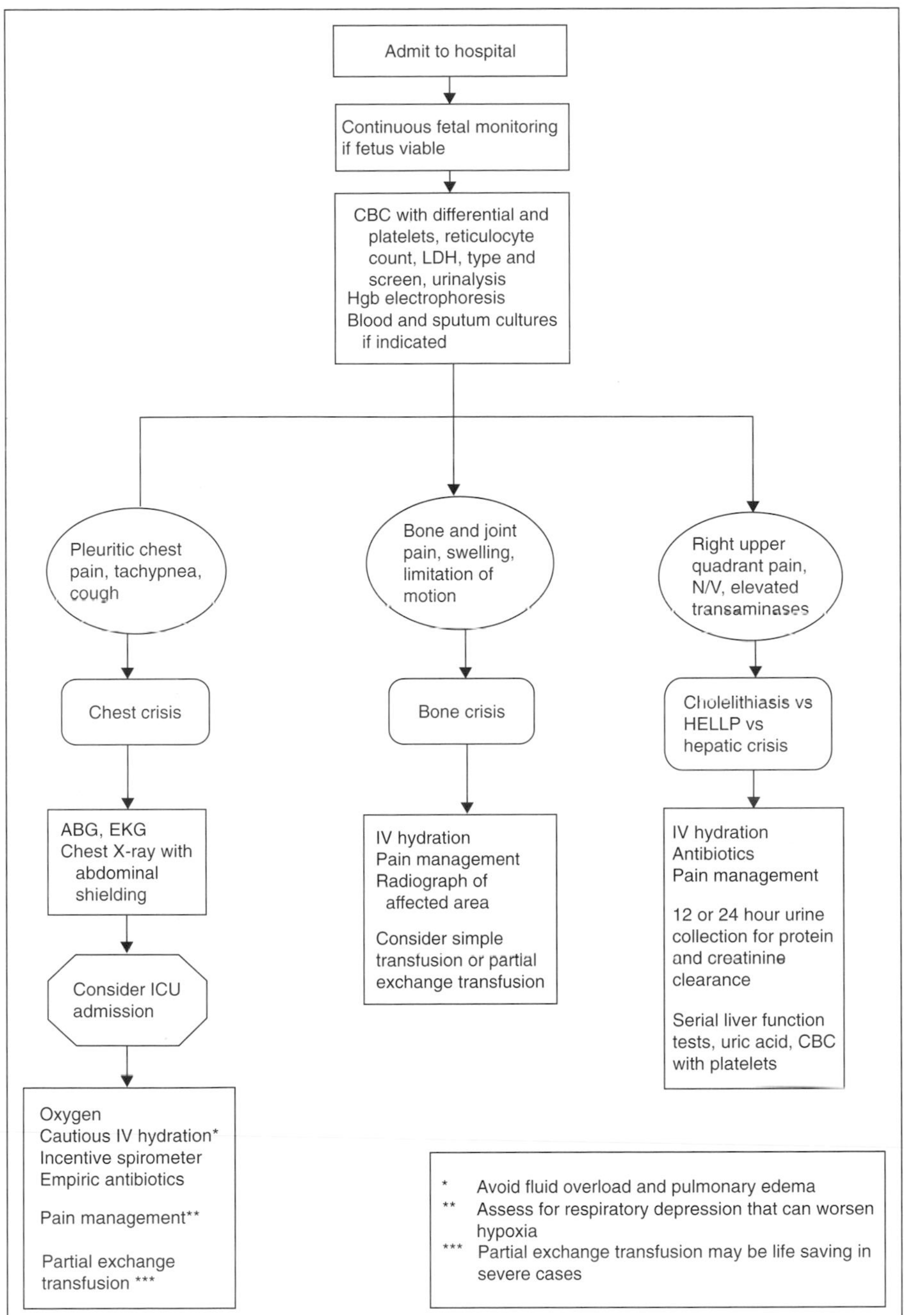

Figure 30.1 Proposed clinical management approach for the patient in sickle cell crisis.

differential diagnosis of chest syndrome includes pulmonary embolus, fat embolus from bone marrow infarction, and amniotic fluid embolus [30]. The ventilation–perfusion scan may be abnormal due to recurrent episodes of pulmonary infarction. It is important to realize that chest syndrome is often a secondary diagnosis, developing in hospitalized sicklers or in the immediate postoperative period.

Treatment is supportive. The goals of therapy are adequate oxygenation, hydration, treatment of infection, and pain relief. An arterial blood gas should be obtained and oxygen provided to keep arterial oxygen tension above 70 mmHg. Hypoventilation due to pleuritic chest pain can worsen hypoxia. Likewise, narcotics should be used cautiously to prevent respiratory depression. Use of an incentive spirometer may minimize atelectasis and infiltrates [31]. Empiric antibiotic coverage for community-acquired pneumonia should be started. In a multicenter trial with 538 patients, the most frequent organisms identified in sputum were *Chlamydia pneumoniae*, *Mycoplasma pneumoniae*, and respiratory syncytial virus [30]. Transfusion to increase the level of hemoglobin A to 30–50% without exceeding a hematocrit of

30% has been shown to reverse acute respiratory distress during pulmonary crisis [30,32].

Davies [33] recommended exchange transfusion for worsening hypoxia, continuing fever and tachycardia, or worsening chest radiograph. Atz [34] reported the successful use of inhaled nitric oxide in two patients with chest syndrome. Inhaled nitric oxide selectively dilates the pulmonary vasculature, increases oxygenation, and potentially alleviates the vaso-occlusive process.

Hepatic crisis

Hepatic crisis due to disseminated vaso-occlusion of the hepatic microvasculature with sickled red cells simulates acute cholecystitis with fever, right upper quadrant pain, leukocytosis, and elevations in transaminases and bilirubin. Differentiating this syndrome from cholecystitis or the syndrome of hemolysis, elevated liver enzymes and low platelets (HELLP) can be a diagnostic challenge. It is reasonable to manage such patients with parenteral hydration, broad-spectrum antibiotics, pain control, and serial laboratory assessments of liver function, uric acid, and complete blood count with platelets.

Pain management

The management of pain (Figure 30.2) in the sickle cell population presents difficulties to the clinician for multiple reasons. Sickle cell patients are often economically disadvantaged and sometimes non-compliant. There are no objective criteria for identifying a pain crisis or for quantifying the pain. The patient's self-report of her level of pain is the only assessment tool available. Factitious disorder and Munchausen's syndrome are well documented among sickle patients. On the other hand, patients who require large doses of narcotics to control their pain may be incorrectly labeled as drug seeking. In an effort to optimize the management of pain associated with sickle cell, the American Pain Society released the first evidence-based guideline for acute and chronic pain management in sickle cell disease. This guideline includes a comprehensive initial pain assessment which includes the patient's treatment history, physical factors, demographic and psychosocial factors, dimensions of pain, and the impact of pain on functioning [35].

The initial dose of pain medicine should be individualized based on the patient's prior use of analgesia, including the type, route and frequency of dosage. Traditional therapy includes non-opioid and opioid analgesics with analgesic adjuvants.

For mild pain, peripherally acting oral analgesia, such as acetaminophen, may be sufficient, combined with aggressive oral hydration. Acetaminophen provides analgesia and antipyresis. The recommended adult dosage should not exceed 6g in a 24-hour period. Mild to moderate pain can be managed by the addition of codeine.

Hospitalization is recommended for greater than mild to moderate pain, as severe pain should be considered a medical emergency, with timely and aggressive management provided until the pain becomes tolerable [35]. Opioids combined with non-opioids and adjuvant analgesics are the mainstay of treatment. Though morphine is the preferred opioid, the type of opioid used should be based on the type and expected duration of the pain. Demerol should be avoided if possible, because of the increased potential for dependency and abuse.

Morphine should be given in a loading dose to provide pain relief. The loading dose should be based on the patient's previous use of narcotics. A possible starting dose is 4 mg of morphine sulfate IV or 8–10 mg IM. After the loading dose, subsequent doses are titrated with the goal of providing quick and sustained relief of the pain. The patient should be reassessed frequently for amount of pain and sedation. One-fourth of the initial loading dose should be given at each reassessment until the pain is relieved or there is concern about sedation. Once relief of pain is achieved, maintenance dosing should be started either at scheduled intervals or by patient-controlled pump. Sickle cell patients with pain crises who are given patient-controlled analgesia use less medication, develop less respiratory depression, and report better pain control than those receiving bolus injections on demand [36]. The maintenance dose can be calculated as the medication required during the titration phase divided by the number of hours over which it was given.

An alternative to morphine, for those patients who report morphine allergies, is butorphanol. An intramuscular injection of 2 mg of butorphanol has equivalent analgesic effect to 10 mg of IM morphine or 80 mg of IM meperidine. It is a mixed agonist–antagonist and can precipitate withdrawal in addicted patients. In a study comparing butorphanol to morphine for the control of pain due to sickle cell crisis, no difference was found in pain relief or level of alertness [37]. Butorphanol can be given as 2 mg IM or 1 mg IV with assessment of the patient in 30 minutes and repeated doses until pain is relieved. Maintenance dosing should be the initial dose given at schedule times every 2–4 hours.

Adjuvant analgesics are often added to improve the effect of the opioids and minimize side effects. The most commonly used adjuvants are antihistamines [12]. They counteract the opioid-induced release of histamines that cause pruritus, reduce nausea, and have a mild sedative effect. In the event that sedatives and anxiolytics are needed, they should always be used in combination with analgesics and not alone in the management of pain, as they may mask the behavioral response to pain without providing analgesia [35].

Once consistent pain control has been achieved, the parenteral opioids should be tapered over several days while maintaining pain control with oral opioids. Once pain control is achieved, the patient may be followed in the outpatient setting, with oral analgesia for home use. Of note, long-term opioid use produces opioid tolerance and physical dependence. This should be expected to develop over time, and should not be confused with psychologic dependence [35]. The authors have also experienced great success in the outpatient population with fentanyl patches, which provide a more steady level of analgesia over time, and may also be utilized in patients who suffer from chronic pain as a result of their disease process.

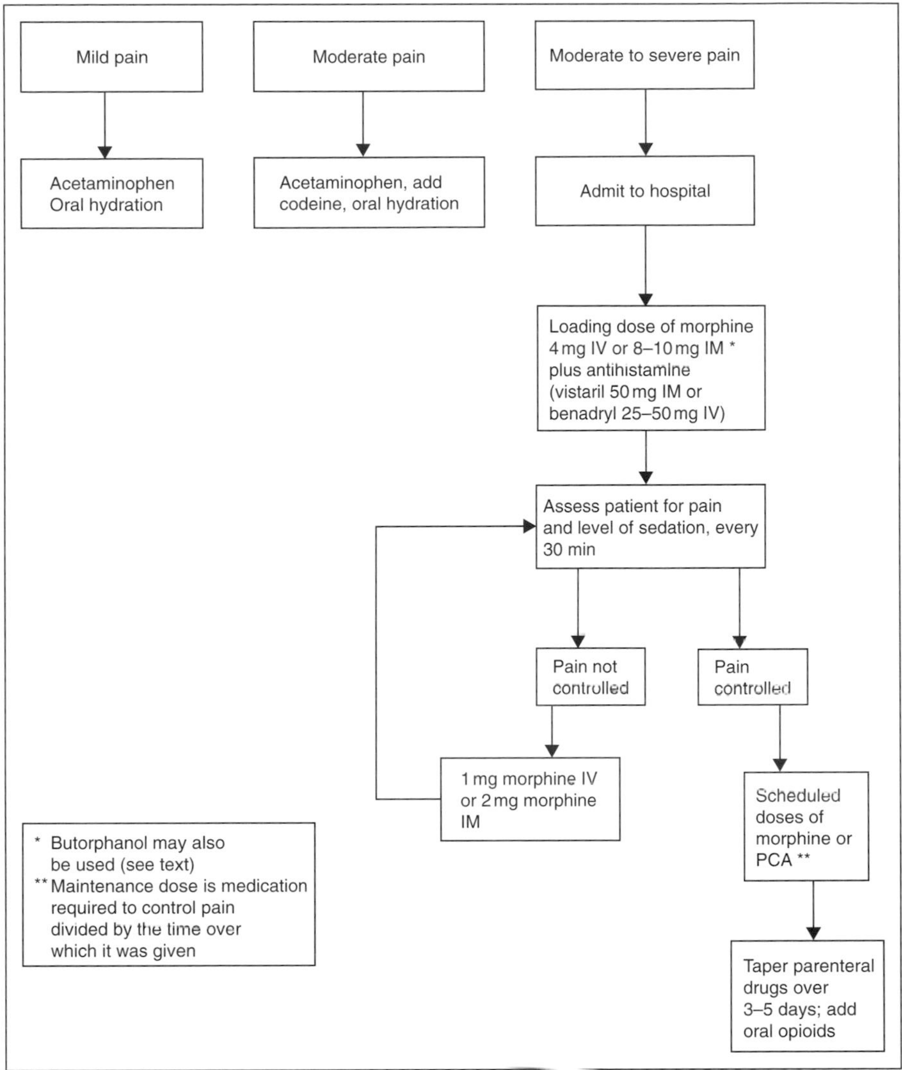

Figure 30.2 Pain management approach for patients with sickle cell crisis.

Therapeutic options

Oxygen therapy

The benefit of oxygen therapy in non-hypoxic patients is uncertain. Although oxygen has been shown to reduce the number of reversibly sickled cells *in vitro*, clinical trials of such therapy have not produced a reduction in the duration of pain, analgesic administration, or length of hospitalization [38]. The therapeutic goal is to maintain a normal P_aO_2.

If oxygen therapy is needed, 3 L supplied by nasal cannula is usually sufficient. In severe oxygenation failure refractory to supplemental oxygen, continuous positive airway pressure or positive end-expiratory pressure may be necessary.

Exchange transfusion

Prophylactic partial exchange transfusion during pregnancy, before the onset of a vaso-occlusive crisis, is controversial. It has been shown to improve both maternal and fetal outcomes in one study [39]. In contrast, no improvement in pregnancy outcome was found in a retrospective review of matched patients who received prophylactic exchange during pregnancy compared to those who did not [40]. The major disadvantage is the potential for isosensitization. Patients can become so severely sensitized that cross-matching becomes nearly impossible. During an emergency requiring transfusion, inability to find compatible blood can be fatal. During pain crises, exchange transfusion has been shown to provide symptomatic relief within 1 hour of initiation of the procedure [41]. This procedure rapidly decreases the amount of hemoglobin S and increases hemoglobin A, thereby improving oxygenation and decreasing the risk of sickling and associated complications. The goal is to achieve a hemoglobin A concentration of at least 60–70% with a hematocrit of 30–35%.

Tables are available to calculate the required volume of transfusion given a target percentage of hemoglobin A, the hematocrit of the transfused blood, and the patient's weight in kilograms.

Patients usually require placement of a double-lumen central catheter before the procedure and should be premedicated as for any blood transfusion. We have found that a standard exchange of 6 units of washed packed red blood cells results in approximately 70% of hemoglobin A.

Simple transfusion

Simple transfusion of packed red cells is indicated for hematocrit less than 15% or hemoglobin less than 6 g/dL. A hematocrit of 30–35% is considered optimal. This should not be exceeded due to the increased viscosity of sickled cells which can precipitate a crisis when the hematocrit is elevated.

Hydroxyurea

Hydroxyurea is an antineoplastic agent that has been shown to induce production of hemoglobin F. It is commonly used in non-pregnant sicklers and has been shown to decrease the frequency of pain crises, acute chest syndrome, and the necessity of transfusions [42–44]. Hydroxyurea works by selectively killing cells in the bone marrow thus increasing the number of erythroblasts producing hemoglobin F [43,44]. Because it is cytotoxic, the risk of teratogenesis when used during the first trimester, its long-term effect, and the risk of carcinogenesis are a concern. No randomized studies exist on its use in pregnancy. There are case reports reporting favorable outcomes even in the first trimester of pregnancy. Diav-Citrin [45] reported a case of hydroxyurea use during the first 9 weeks of pregnancy and additionally reviewed case reports of 15 other exposures to the drug during pregnancy. Nine cases had first-trimester exposure. All of those pregnancies had phenotypically normal children. However, there is no long-term follow-up on those children. Though the available data suggest that use of hydroxyurea during pregnancy is not commonly associated with adverse short-term outcomes, at this time, use of hydroxyurea in pregnancy cannot be advocated [46]. However, for patients with unplanned exposure to the drug during pregnancy, the prognosis may not be as grim as expected. There are no human data available regarding reproductive toxicity of hydroxyurea in the female patient.

Erythropoietin

Erythropoietin is a hormone that stimulates red blood cell production. It has been shown to increase the number of reticulocytes containing fetal hemoglobin in humans [47]. It has been used alone and in alternating doses with hydroxyurea to increase the amount of hemoglobin F [43,47]. Studies have produced conflicting results about its efficacy in either augmenting the effect of hydroxyurea or of enhancing production of fetal hemoglobin [47,48]. Erythropoietin is currently not used for induction of fetal hemoglobin in sickle cell patients, but may be useful in sickle patients with renal insufficiency.

Bone marrow transplant

Bone marrow transplantation has emerged as the only cure for the patient with sickle cell disease. Two large trials in Europe [49] and the United States [50] have reported on a total of 116 patients with sickle cell disease. Though cure rates are reported at 80–85% in both studies, the mortality ranges from 5 to 10%. Complications are high, with 25% neurologic morbidity (including intracranial hemorrhage) and 10% incidence of graft-versus-host disease. The transplants have been predominantly performed in children and young adults [49,50]. There are no reports of bone marrow transplantation during pregnancy, and the procedure remains unproven in adults. Due to concerns over safety, bone marrow transplantation has been reserved for only the most severe cases of sickle cell disease. It is hoped that further advances may someday make bone marrow transplantation a more plausible treatment option for a greater majority of patients.

References

1 Seoud MAF, Cantwell C, Nobles G, Lerry DL. Outcome of pregnancies complicated by sickle cell and sickle-C hemoglobinopathies. *Am J Perinatol* 1994; 11: 187.

2 Sun PM, Wilburn W, Raynor BD, Jamieson D. Sickle cell disease in pregnancy: twenty years of experience at Grady Memorial Hospital, Atlanta, Georgia. *Am J Obstet Gynecol* 2001; 184(6): 1127–1130.

3 Mehta SR, Afenyi-Annan A, Byrns P, Lottenberg R. Opportunities to improve outcomes in sickle cell disease. *J Am Fam Pract* 2006; 74(2): 303–310.

4 Bain BJ. *Haemoglobinopathy Diagnosis*. London: Blackwell Science, 2001: 113–117.

5 Whitten CF, Whitten-Shurney W. Sickle cell. *Clin Perinatol* 2001; 28(2): 435–448.

6 Sergeant GR, Sergeant BE. *Sickle Cell Disease*, 3rd edn. Oxford: Oxford University Press, 2001.

7 Pauling L, Itano HA, Singer SJ, Wells IC. Sickle cell anemia: a molecular disease. *Science* 1949; 110: 543–549.

8 Herrick JB. Peculiar elongated and sickle-shaped red blood corpuscles in a case of severe anemia. *Arch Intern Med* 1910; 6: 517–521.

9 Dauphin-McKenzie N, Gilles JM, Jacques E, Harrington T. Sickle cell anemia and the female patient. *Obstet Gynecol Surv* 2006; 61(5): 343–352.

10 Bunn HF. Pathogenesis and treatment of sickle cell disease. *N Engl J Med* 1997; 337(11): 762–769.

11 Rust OA, Perry KG Jr. Pregnancy complicated by sickle hemoglobinopathy. *Clin Obstet Gynecol* 1995; 38(3): 472–484.

12 Steinberg MH, Rodgers GP. Pathophysiology of sickle cell disease: role of cellular and genetic modifiers. *Semin Hematol* 2001; 38(4): 299–306.

13 Lonergan GJ, Cline DB, Abbondanzo SL. Sickle cell anemia. *Radiographics* 2001; 21(4): 971–994.

14 Howard RJ, Tuck SM. Sickle cell disease and pregnancy. *Curr Obstet Gynaecol* 1995; 5(1): 36–40.

15 Covitz W, Espeland M, Gallagher D, Hellenbrand W, Leff S, Talner N. The heart in sickle cell anemia: the Cooperative Study of Sickle Cell Disease (CSSCD). *Chest* 1995; 108: 1214–1219.

16 James TN, Riddick L, Massing GK. Sickle cells and sudden death: morphologic abnormalities of the cardiac conduction system. *J Lab Clin Med* 1994; 124: 507–520.

17 Mentzer WC Jr, Wang WC. Sickle-cell disease: pathophysiology and diagnosis. *Pediatr Ann* 1980; 9(8): 287–296.

18 Stark P, Pfeiffer WR. Intrathoracic manifestations of sickle cell disease. *Radiology* 1985; 25: 33–35.

19 Cunningham FG, Hauth JC, Leveno KJ, et al. *Williams' Obstetrics.* Stamford, CT: McGraw-Hill, 2005.

20 Klings ES, Wyszynski DF, Nolan VG, Steinberg MH. Abnormal pulmonary function in adults with sickle cell anemia. *Am J Respir Care Med* 2006;173: 1264–1269.

21 Castro O, Gladwin M. Pulmonary hypertension in sickle cell disease: mechanisms, diagnosis, and management. *Hematol Oncol Clin North Am* 2005; 19(5): 881–896.

22 Derchi G, Formi GL, Formisano F, et al. Efficacy and safety of sildenafil in the treatment of severe pulmonary hypertension in patients with hemoglobinopathies. *Haematologica* 2005; 90: 452–458.

23 Morris CR, Morris SM Jr, Hagar W, et al. Arginine therapy: a new treatment for pulmonary hypertension in sickle cell disease? *Am J Respir Crit Care Med* 2003; 168: 63–69.

24 Reiter CD, Gladwin MT. An emerging role for nitric oxide in sickle cell disease vascular homeostasis and therapy. Erythroid system and its diseases. *Curr Opin Haematol* 2003; 10(2): 99–107.

25 Ratto D, Balmes J, Boylen T, Sharma OP. Pregnancy in a woman with severe pulmonary fibrosis secondary to hard metal disease. *Chest* 1988; 93: 663–665.

26 Sharma CP, Aggarwal AN, Vashisht K, Jindal SK. Successful outcome of pregnancy in idiopathic pulmonary fibrosis. *J Assoc Physicians India* 2002; 50: 1446–1448.

27 Schmitt F, Martinez F, Brillet G, et al. Early glomerular dysfunction in patients with sickle cell anemia. *Am J Kidney Dis* 1998; 32: 208–214.

28 Pham PT, Pham PC, Wilkinson AH, Lew SQ. Renal abnormalities in sickle cell disease. *Kidney Int* 2000; 57: 1–8.

29 Anyaegbunum A, Morel M, Merkatz IR. Antepartum fetal surveillance tests during sickle cell crisis. *Am J Obstet Gynecol* 1991; 165(4Pt1): 1081–1083.

30 Vichinsky EP, Neumayr LD, Earles AN, et al. Causes and outcomes of the acute chest syndrome in sickle cell disease. *N Engl J Med* 2000; 25(342): 1855–1865.

31 Bellet PS, Kalinyak KA, Shukla R, Gelfand JM, Rucknagel DL. Incentive spirometry to prevent acute pulmonary complications in sickle cell disease. *N Engl J Med* 1995; 333(11): 699–703.

32 Mallouh AA, Asha MA. Beneficial effect of blood transfusion in children with sickle cell chest syndrome. *Am J Dis Child* 1988; 142(2): 178–182.

33 Davies SC, Win AA, Luce PJ, Riordan JF. Acute chest syndrome in sickle cell disease. *Lancet* 1984; 1(8367): 36–38.

34 Atz AM, Wessel DL. Inhaled nitric oxide in sickle cell disease with acute chest syndrome. *Anesthesiology* 1997; 87(4): 988–990.

35 Benjamin LJ, Dampier CD, Jacox AK, et al. *Guideline for the Management of Acute and Chronic Pain in Sickle Cell Disease.* APS Clinical Practice Guidelines Series No. 1. Glenview, IL: American Pain Society, 1999: 12–13.

36 Shapiro BS, Cohen DE, Howe CJ. Patient-controlled analgesia for sickle-cell-related pain. *J Pain Symptom Manage* 1993; 8(1): 22–28.

37 Gonzalez ER, Ornato JP, Ware D, Bull D, Evens RP. Comparison of intramuscular analgesic activity of butorphanol and morphine in patients with sickle cell disease. *Ann Emerg Med* 1988; 17(8): 788–791.

38 Zipursky A, Robieux IC, Brown EJ, et al. Oxygen therapy in sickle cell disease. *Am J Pediatr Hematol Oncol* 1992; 14(3): 222–228.

39 Morrison JC, Wiser WL. The use of prophylactic partial exchange transfusions in pregnancies associated with sickle cell hemoglobinopathies. *Obstet Gynecol* 1976; 48(5): 516–520.

40 Miller JM, Horger EO, Key TC, Walker EM. Management of sickle hemoglobinopathies in pregnant patients. *Am J Obstet Gynecol* 1981; 141(3): 237–241.

41 Martin JN Jr, Martin RW, Morrison JC. Acute management of sickle cell crisis in pregnancy. *Clin Perinatol* 1986; 13(4): 853–869.

42 Charache TS, Moore RD, Dover GJ, et al. Effect of hydroxyurea on the frequency of painful crisis in sickle cell anemia. *N Engl J Med* 1995; 332: 1317–1322.

43 Steinberg MH. Management of sickle cell disease. *N Engl J Med* 1999; 13(340): 1021–1030.

44 Steinberg MH, Barton F, Castro O, et al. Effect of hydroxyurea on mortality and morbidity in adult sickle cell anemia. Risks and benefits up to 9 years of treatment. *JAMA* 2003; 289: 1645–1651.

45 Diav-Citrin O, Hunnisett L, Sher GD, Koren G. Hydroxyurea use during pregnancy: a case report in sickle cell disease and review of the literature. *Am J Hematol* 1999; 60: 148–150.

46 Liebelt EL, Balk, SJ, Faber W, et al. NTP-CERHR Expert Panel Report on the Reproductive and Developmental Toxicity of Hydroxyurea. *Birth Defects Res B* 2007; 80: 259–366.

47 Rodgers GP, Dover GJ, Uyesaka N, Noguchi CT, Schecter AN, Nienhuis AW. Augmentation by erythropoietin of the fetal-hemoglobin response to hydroxyurea in sickle cell disease. *N Engl J Med* 1993; 328(2): 73–80.

48 Goldberg MA, Brugnara C, Dover GJ, Schapira L, Charache S, Bunn HF. Treatment of sickle cell anemia with hydroxyurea and erythropoietin. *N Engl J Med* 1990; 323(6): 366–372.

49 Vermylen C, Cornu G. Bone marrow transplantation for sickle cell disease. The European experience. *Am J Pediatr Hematol Oncol* 1994; 16(1): 18–21.

50 Walters MC, Patience M, Leisenring W, et al. Bone marrow transplantation for sickle cell disease. *N Engl J Med* 1996; 335: 369–376.

31 Disseminated Intravascular Coagulopathy

Nazli Hossain[1] & Michael J. Paidas[2]

[1]Department of Obstetrics and Gynaecology Unit-III, Dow University of Health Sciences, Civil Hospital, Karachi, Pakistan
[2]Yale Women & Children's Center for Blood Disorders, Department of Obstetrics, Gynecology and Reproductive Sciences, Yale School of Medicine, New Haven, CT, USA

Normal coagulation during pregnancy

Pregnancy brings about changes in the circulating levels of coagulation factors. The hemostatic system is dependent upon an intricate balance between platelets, procoagulants and endogenous anticoagulant pathways. Table 31.1 indicates the changes, if any, in the coagulation factors during each trimester of pregnancy. Levels of vWF increase as much as 400% near term. Except for factors V and II, the rest of the factors show a 20–1000% increase in circulating levels [1]. Serum markers of hypercoagulation in normal pregnancy include increased levels of D-dimer, thrombin–antithrombin (TAT) complexes, and prothrombin fragments 1+2 (F1+2). The anticoagulant pathway includes tissue factor pathway inhibitor (TFPI), activated protein C resistance (APC) and the protein Z-dependent protease inhibitor (ZPI). The ZPI causes inactivation of factor Xa, and this inhibition is enhanced 1000-fold in the presence of protein Z. There is a fall in the levels of anticoagulant activity, especially protein S, both free and circulating level [2]. Free protein S levels decline significantly as much as 55% during pregnancy. In addition 40% of the women may develop an acquired resistance to activated protein C, unrelated to factor V Leiden mutation. This may be due to increase in factor VIII activity, or a decrease in protein S activity or other as yet undefined mechanisms. Fibrinolytic activity is reduced in pregnancy by the secretion of plasminogen activator inhibitor type 2 (PAI-2) by the placenta, and plasminogen activator inhibitor type 1 (PAI-1) produced by the liver and endothelium. Levels of both PAI-1 and PAI-2 are increased in pregnancy. Plasmin is directly and indirectly inhibited by α2 plasmin inhibitor and by thrombin-activatable fibrinolysis inhibitor (TAFI). Levels of TAFI are increased in the third trimester.

Critical Care Obstetrics, 5th edition. Edited by M. Belfort, G. Saade, M. Foley, J. Phelan and G. Dildy. © 2010 Blackwell Publishing Ltd.

Pathophysiology

General principles

Disseminated intravascular coagulation (DIC) in obstetrics is typically due to one of three etiologies: (i) a release of thromboplastin-like substances that causes activation of both intrinsic and extrinsic pathways; (ii) endothelial damage that may cause activation of intrinsic pathway; or (iii) cytokine release in conditions like Gram-negative sepsis. Any of the above mechanisms may activate both thrombin and plasmin in the circulation. Thrombin causes conversion of fibrinogen into fibrin. During this process, there is formation of fibrin monomers. These monomers then polymerize to form fibrin, which in turn cause occlusion of the microvessels. This may involve multiple organs or peripheral vasculature. This vessel occlusion results in multiple organ damage seen in DIC. The deposition of fibrin, leads to trapping of platelets, leading to thrombocytopenia. Activation of plasmin also causes release of fibrin degradation products from the fibrinogen, recognized as X, Y, D and E. These degradation products (FDPs) combine with fibrin monomers before polymerization to form soluble fibrin monomer. This further impairs hemostasis and leads to hemorrhage. FDPs also interfere with myometrial and myocardial contraction, thus leading to hemorrhage and hypotension. Thrombin also induces monocyte release of IL-1, IL-6 and tumor necrosis factor (TNF), along with endothelial release of thrombomodulin, endothelin and selectin. Endothelin causes intense vasospasm and vasoconstriction, followed by thrombus formation and vascular occlusion. The selectin E (ELAM-1), binds to monocytes, lymphocytes, and granulocytes causing more release of cytokines. These degradation products cause synthesis and release of monocyte- or macrophage-derived interleukins IL-1 and IL-6, and PAI-1. Interleukins induce additional endothelial damage, whereas PAI-1 inhibits fibrinolysis, causing further thrombosis. Free plasmin in the circulation also causes the activation of complement system. This leads to further destruction of platelets and thrombocytopenia. Complement activation also leads to increased vascular permeability, leading

Table 31.1 Normal clotting values in pregnancy.

Variables (mean ± SD)	First trimester	Second trimester	Third trimester	Normal range
Platelets	275 ± 64	256 ± 49	244 ± 52	150–400
Fibrinogen (g/L)	3.7 ± 0.6	4.4 ± 1.2	5.4 ± 0.8	2.1–4.2
Prothrombin complex (%)	120 ± 27	140 ± 27	130 ± 27	70–30
Antithrombin (U/mL)	1.02 ± 0.10	1.07 ± 0.14	1.07 ± 0.11	0.85–1.25
Protein C (U/mL)	0.92 ± 0.13	1.06 ± 0.17	.94 ± 0.2	0.68–1.25
Protein S, total (U/mL)	0.83 ± 0.11	0.73 ± 0.11	0.77 ± 0.10	0.70–1.70
Protein S, free (U/mL)	0.26 ± 0.07	0.17 ± 0.04	0.14 ± 0.04	0.20–0.50
Soluble fibrin (nmol/L)	9.2 ± 8.6	11.8 ± 7.7	13.4 ± 5.2	<15
Thrombin-antithrombin(μg/L)	3.1 ± 1.4	5.9 ± 2.6	7.1 ± 2.4	<2.7
D-dimers (ug/L)	91 ± 24	128 ± 49	198 ± 59	<80
Plasminogen activator inhibitor-1 (AU/mL)	7.4 ± 4.9	14.9 ± 5.2	37.8 ± 19.4	<15
Plasminogen activator inhibitor-2 (ug/L)	31 ± 14	84 ± 16	160 ± 31	<5
Protein Z (ug/mL)	2.01 ± 0.76	1.47 ± 0.45	1.55 ± 0.48	

to hypotension. The diffuse endothelial damage leads to activation of factor XII. Activated XII induces the conversion of prekallikrien to kallikrein, which in turn causes activation of kinins. This further increases vascular permeability.

In summary, a triggering event leads to activation of thrombin and plasmin in circulation. Once activated a vicious cycle ensues, leading to generation of FDPs, release of IL-1, IL-6, TNF-α and complement activation. Subsequent endothelial activation further aggravates the situation. Inflammatory cytokines such as IL-6 and TNF-α have been shown to be prothrombotic by increasing endothelial tissue factor production and affecting protein C activation by changes in the endothelial protein C receptor and thrombomodulin [3]. Cytokines also cause increased platelet formation, and these new platelets are more sensitive to thrombin activation and increased procoagulant activity [4]. This cycle is further aggravated by a decrease in the circulating anticoagulants, namely antithrombin (AT), and protein C and S. This decrease is markedly seen in pre-eclampsia and sepsis. The decreased levels correlate directly with the severity of the disease as well [5]. There is consumption of coagulation factors and platelets, leading to hemorrhage. Both coagulation and hemorrhage coexist, but mostly it is the hemorrhage that seeks obstetrician attention.

Etiological factors for DIC

There are number of clinical scenarios in obstetrics that can lead to DIC (Table 31.2).

Table 31.2 Clinical scenarios in obstetrics associated with disseminated intravascular coagulation (DIC).

Amniotic fluid embolus syndrome
Placental abruption
Gram-positive and Gram-negative septicemia
Massive blood loss leading to DIC
Massive transfusions secondary to blood loss
Severe pre-eclampsia and eclampsia
Intrauterine fetal death
Acute fatty liver of pregnancy

Amniotic fluid embolism and DIC

Mechanism

Amniotic fluid is rich in both procoagulant and fibrinolytic substances. All the procoagulant activity is dependent upon the presence of tissue factor, whose concentration increases with gestational age [6]. Amniotic fluid embolus syndrome (AFE) has been found to be associated with multiple pregnancies, older maternal age, cesarean or instrumental vaginal deliveries, polyhdramnios, eclampsia, abruption, uterine rupture and fetal distress [7]. Pathophysiologically, AFE results from a simultaneous tear in the fetal membranes and uterine vessel, through which amniotic fluid can pass into uterine venous circulation, and then into maternal pulmonary arterial circulation [8]. The presence of amniotic fluid debris in the maternal circulation causes the release of thromboplastin-like material, which in turn causes activation of factor X. Activated factor X is the most potent activator of thrombin. This results in the occlusion of small microvasculature with platelet-rich fibrin microthrombi. The end result is fulminant DIC. Amniotic fluid also causes release of complement, and platelet factor III, hence causing platelet-rich fibrin microthrombi [9]. Coagulopathy is seen in 83% of cases of amniotic fluid embolism, and may appear as early as within 4 hours of a triggering event [8]. The laboratory diagnosis of DIC is based on levels of ATIII, fibrinopeptide levels, D dimers, and platelet counts. Hemodynamic stabilization, oxygen inhalation, and use of vasopressor drugs are the mainstay of treatment. AFE is the only condition where heparin can be used in DIC to clear the microvascular occlusion [10,11].

Eclampsia and DIC

Coagulation abnormalities and intravascular coagulation do occur in hypertensive disorders of pregnancy, but are not clinically significant. Laboratory assessments like prothrombin time, activated partial thromboplastin time and plasma fibrinogen levels are usually not affected in hypertensive disorders of pregnancy. Severe pre-eclampsia and eclampsia lead to low-grade DIC in circulation. It is usually seen in 10% of cases of severe pre-eclampsia and eclampsia. The basic mechanism is the damage to the endothelial cells resulting in activation of both extrinsic and intrinsic pathways. This results in the disappearance of procoagulants, the appearance of fibrin degradation products and end-organ damage secondary to the formation of microthrombi. Significantly higher levels of thrombin–antithrombin complex, soluble fibrin, fibrin degradation product and plasmin-α_2 antiplasmin are found in pre-eclamptic women [12]. This has been established in peripheral as well as in uteroplacental circulation [5]. Platelet counts are decreased, and low platelet counts correlate well with the severity of disease. The occurrence of HELLP syndrome in severe pre-eclampsia is reported at between 13% to 17%. Activation of endothelial cells causes increased release of VWF, which in turn leads to consumptive thrombocytopenia and thrombotic microangiopathy [13]. In severe cases, decrease of procoagulants like fibrinogen and platelets may produce spontaneous hemorrhage.

Placental abruption and DIC

Advanced maternal age, hypertension, cocaine use, trauma and multiparity can be associated with abruptio placentae. Thrombophilic mutations have also identified as a risk factor for abruptio. Factor V Leiden mutation, protein S deficiency and prothrombin gene mutations have been identified in the etiology of abruptio placentae [14]. Placental abruption has been graded into the following categories, first introduced in 1978 [15].

Grade 0: refers to a retrospective diagnosis of abruptio placentae.

Grade 1: vaginal bleeding.

Grade 2: vaginal bleeding, concealed hemorrhage, uterine tenderness, non-reassuring FHR.

Grade 3: vaginal bleeding, shock, extensive concealed hemorrhage, uterine tenderness, fetal death, and sometimes coagulopathy. Grade 3 is further subdivided based on the presence or absence of a coagulopathy.

Coagulopathy as seen in grade 3 placental abruption causes a release of procoagulant substances and thromboplastin-like material into the circulation. This causes the activation of extrinsic coagulation pathway. This, if left unattended for an excessive period of time, will lead to consumption of coagulation factors and fulminant DIC. Only 10% of patients show significant coagulopathy with abruption [10]. In the event of massive separation, coagulopathy is seen in 20–30% of cases. The risk of developing DIC in abruptio placentae depends upon the degree of abruption, the time interval between placental abruption and delivery, and the prognosis of fetus as well. In abruption of a lesser degree it is assumed that silent placental infarcts will cause consumption of coagulation factors like factor VIII, along with release of degradation products, whereas in massive abruption, placental thromboplastin and activated coagulation factors enter into the systemic circulation through uterine veins and cause DIC. Clinical features are the same as described below, along with the laboratory evidence. Recently elevated levels of thrombomodulin (TM) have been identified in acute phases of abruption [16]. TM is not only found in endothelial cells, but is also present in the syncytiotrophoblast. Elevated TM has been identified in TTP, pre-eclampsia and SLE. The efficacy of TM as a marker of DIC in acute phases of abruptio placentae requires confirmation in larger studies.

Intrauterine death and DIC

Intrauterine death causes release of necrotic tissue material and enzymes into maternal circulation. This happens when the fetus has been dead for more than 5 weeks. In such cases coagulopathy is seen in around 25% of cases. The pathway is same as for placental abruption, by the release of thromboplastin into the circulation, but consumption of coagulation factors take place slowly, over weeks. Serum fibrinogen levels are decreased, and fibrinogen degradation products are increased in circulation. This clinical scenario is also seen in cases of single fetal demise in twin pregnancy. Hemostatic failure is of concern for the surviving fetus and not for the mother.

Intrauterine infections and DIC

Antepartum and postpartum uterine infections and septic abortion can trigger DIC. Endothelial injury, caused by TNF-α, results in release of tissue factor. Tissue factor leads to the production of thrombin, which combines with thrombomodulin to activate protein C. This leads to inhibition of factors Va and VIIIa. This procoagulant effect results in fibrin deposition in microvasculature. In sepsis there is a decrease in the activity of protein C and S, EPCR expression. TNF-α also leads to increased PAI-1 levels, and hence decreased fibrinolysis [17]. Thus sepsis leads to alteration in procoagulant–anticoagulant balance, with an increase in procoagulant factors and decrease in anticoagulant factors.

Evacuation of uterus under antibiotic cover helps in stopping further progression of the disease. The choice of antibiotic depends upon prevalence and susceptibility patterns in the facility. Both laboratory parameters and clinical signs should be taken into account when diagnosing DIC.

Acute fatty liver of pregnancy

Acute fatty liver of pregnancy (AFLP) is a rare, potentially fatal complication of pregnancy, usually seen in the third trimester. There are case reports of earlier appearance in the second trimester as well. It has been found associated with DIC, which is seen in a majority of patients (>50%). Castro et al. in a series of 28 patients, found DIC in all of their patients [18]. The coagulation abnormalities include a marked decrease in AT levels, which precede the onset of clinical symptoms, thrombocytopenia and consumptive coagulopathy leading to a decrease in the circulating coagulation factors. These coagulation abnormalities persist for many days after delivery [19]. Maternal and fetal mortality are high in AFLP. Apart from supportive treatment, investigators have looked at the potential role of AT concentrate in the treatment. Empirical therapy with AT did not show any improvement in the clinical outcome [12].

Clinical diagnosis

The clinical presentation of DIC may be hemorrhagic or thrombotic. Commonly, it is the hemorrhagic variety which is seen in obstetric practice. Hemorrhagic DIC denotes an acute condition, whereas thrombotic DIC indicates chronic activation of the coagulation cascade. Hemorrhagic DIC involves skin or mucous membranes, resulting in ecchymosis, petechiae, bleeding from venepuncture sites, bleeding from gums, hematuria and gastrointestinal bleeding. Thrombotic DIC may involve the neurologic, renal and pulmonary systems. It is usually seen in chronic compensated DIC, as in malignancy and intrauterine fetal demise. It usually involves deposition of fibrin microthrombi, resulting in organ dysfunction. Microvascular cerebral thrombosis causes cortical dysfunction, which is manifested clinically as an altered state of conciousness. Similarly, renal involvement results in acute tubular necrosis and renal failure, seen in DIC. Involvement of peripheral veins and arteries may result in phlebitis and peripheral gangrene. Here, DIC is characterized by skin hemorrhagic necrosis and gangrene in the extremities of the digits as a consequence of arterial fibrin microthrombi. This is usually seen in patients with Gram-negative bacterial sepsis [20] and is also seen in patients with protein C and S deficiencies [21].

Laboratory diagnosis

Laboratory tests in a bleeding obstetric patient are of value, but prompt treatment should not be withheld while awaiting results. Unnecessary delay in starting the treatment further aggravates the situation. Table 31.3 illustrates the common laboratory tests to obtain in suspected DIC.

Table 31.3 The common laboratory tests to obtain in suspected DIC.

1	Prothrombin time
2	Partial thromboplastin time
3	Thrombin time
4	Platelet count
5	Fibrinogen levels
6	FDP
7	D-dimer assay
8	Antithrombin levels

Prothrombin time (PT) tests the extrinsic system of coagulation. This test may be abnormal in 50% of patients and may be normal or short in 50% of cases, thus making it less reliable in establishing a diagnosis of DIC. It may be normal or short because of circulating activated clotting factors like factor Xa, which accelerates the formation of fibrin, thus giving a normal or short PT time.

Partial thromboplastin time (APTT) is less important. It may also be prolonged in 50–60% of patients and normal or short in 50% of patients.

The thrombin time is more reliable than either PT or APTT. A fibrin clot not dissolving within 10 minutes signifies that fibrinolysis is an unlikely event. If the clot begins to lyse within 10 minutes, it shows significant plasmin activity. Prolonged thrombin time is seen with hypofibrinogenemia and also with increased fibrin degradation products.

Platelets counts are low in DIC, as explained previously. In cases of thrombocytopenia (<100 000) counts should be repeated at 4-hourly intervals. A repeat low count indicates increased consumption by the generated thrombin. Low platelet counts are not characteristic of DIC, as they may also be seen in the presence of underlying disorders leading to DIC. Hence a low platelet count is not diagnostic of DIC.

Serum fibrinogen levels fall below 100 mg/dL before the clinical manifestation of DIC. Measurement of FDPs will be raised, due to the increased plasmin activity. FDPs are raised in 85–100% of cases of DIC, but they do not predict the clinical course of DIC [21]. An elevated FDP acts as an indirect test for fibrinolysis. It signifies the presence of acute or chronic DIC. In acute situations it only confirms the presence of DIC, but is not diagnostic. FDP may be found elevated in conditions like pulmonary embolism, myocardial infarction or surgical trauma, in women taking oral contraceptive pills and in patients with arterial or venous thromboembolism.

The D-dimer test is specific for fibrin degradation products, and is more specific for DIC, though elevated levels of D-dimer may also be found in deep venous thrombosis and pulmonary embolism. D-dimer is a neo-antigen formed as a result of digestion of cross-linked fibrin by plasmin. The use of D-dimer along with FDP and AT levels has been found to be more sensitive in the diagnosis of DIC in clinical practice [22].

Antithrombin levels are found to be low in DIC. This is due to the formation of complexes of thrombin and coagulation factors with antithrombin, leading to considerable decrease in the level of circulating antithrombin. Thus antithrombin testing helps not only in diagnosis, but also for monitoring therapy in ongoing DIC.

PF 1+2 assay is a reliable molecular marker which shows the generation of factor Xa and thrombin. ELISA assays are now available to quantitate the levels of circulating PF1+2 and TAT complexes in the circulation [23].

While most of the above tests are available in a routine laboratory, the last two tests require a specialty laboratory. There is no single definitive test for the diagnosis of DIC. The practicing clinician may benefit from routine global tests, AT levels and FDP. In many cases, serial laboratory studies may be clinically necessary.

Management of DIC

Fluid balance, adequate tissue perfusion, avoidance of tissue hypoxia and removal of underlying etiologic agent are the mainstays of treatment of DIC. The guidelines for management of a bleeding obstetric patient are the same whether bleeding is caused by or is augmented by a coagulation failure. Blood may be drawn for laboratory work, but availability of results should not delay the start of treatment. Identification of etiologic factors and their removal are the cornerstone of treatment for DIC in obstetrics. Delivery of the fetus and placenta should be the first aim in the management of DIC. This results in return of plasma factors to normal levels within 24 hours of cessation of DIC. Platelets return to normal within 7–9 days, the time period required for maturation and release from bone marrow.

Fluid choices

Initially fluids may be required to maintain hemodynamic balance until blood and blood products are available for transfusion. Crystalloid solutions like Ringer's lactate and Hartmann's solution are the first choices for intravenous fluid replacement. The volume infused should be two to three times more than the estimated blood loss. Infusion of crystalloid also helps in maintaining renal function. Plasma substitutes like dextran, gelatin, and starch solution may be used as well. Dextran is associated with allergic reactions, and interferes with subsequent blood grouping and cross-matching tests. Gelatin is also an important substitute, with minimal immunologic reactions, that improves renal function in the presence of hypovolemia [9].

Blood and blood products

Although transfusion support may be needed, there is no consensus regarding optimal treatment. In a bleeding patient, a combination of fresh frozen plasma (FFP) and cryoprecipitate is indicated. However, if there is no bleeding, blood products are not indicated, irrespective of laboratory tests. There is no evidence supporting prophylaxis with platelets or plasma.

Whole blood may be the treatment of choice for correction of coagulation failure, but is not readily available, because it requires at least 18–24 hours for screening. Transfusion of packed red blood cells is necessary to increase the oxygen-carrying capacity. In case the same blood group is not available, non-cross-matched O-negative blood should be available for transfusion. It should be noted that stored bank blood is deficient in labile clotting factors V, VIII and platelets. It is advisable to transfuse 2 units of FFP for every 4–6 units of bank red cells administered. Fresh frozen plasma (FFP) contains all the clotting factors present in whole blood and is readily available. FFP is obtained from fresh whole blood within 6 hours of donation and immediately stored at −30°C, and if stored properly, can be used over a period of 1 year. Though there are no randomized trials on the use of FFP in DIC, it is generally understood that FFP is beneficial in patients with active DIC and consumptive coagulopathy who are treated for underlying disorders prior to any invasive procedure. Use of FFP in such circumstances is well indicated, compared to patients with low-grade DIC without bleeding. There is no role of FFP as prophylactic agent, in situations where bleeding is anticipated [24]. Cryoprecipitate contain more fibrinogen than FFP, but carries more risk of transmissible infections. It lacks antithrombin which is depleted in bleeding obstetric patients.

There is no evidence for the prophylactic use of platelets in patients with DIC who are not bleeding, or are not at high risk for bleeding. The need for platelet transfusion depends upon the platelet count. If the platelet count is below 50 000/cu mm, and operative intervention is required, platelet transfusions are required. Platelet transfusions may also be required in bleeding patients with low platelet counts. Thus, the clinical scenario and not the laboratory reports should guide the clinician with regard to further treatment.

Use of heparin

Heparin may be required in the thrombotic variety of DIC involving the renal system and peripheral gangrene. Heparin itself has no anticoagulant activity, but combines with AT and enhances the reactivity of AT with serine proteases. Decreased levels of AT in DIC makes heparin ineffective. It is initially given as a loading dose, followed by continuous intravenous infusion at a rate of 500–1000 units per hour. Platelet transfusions may be required in the event of thrombocytopenia. Laboratory control of heparin therapy is difficult. In obstetrics, heparin is required in cases of AFE and in intrauterine fetal death [10,11]. Heparin in these circumstances blocks the further conversion of fibrinogen and other clotting factors. Heparin should only be used in women with an intact circulation. Active bleeding and vascular disruption are contraindications to treatment with heparin.

Use of activated protein C

Use of recombinant activated protein C (APC) has been shown to have a beneficial effect in DIC due to sepsis. It has anti-inflammatory and antithrombotic effects and has also been found to have profibrinolytic properties. Side effects include increased risk of bleeding with its use. A large double-blind, placebo-controlled, multicenter trial, evaluating the use of recombinant activated protein C, found a significant reduction of 6.1% in mortality as compared to the placebo [25]. There are few published case reports of its use in pregnancy. Kobayashi et al. used APC in 16 cases of placental abruption with DIC. They found administration of APC was associated with a decrease in FDP and TAT complexes, and a significant increase in the fibrinogen level [26]. Use of APC has also been found useful in the treatment of coagulopathy due to AFLP [27].

Role of antithrombin III in DIC

Antithrombin is a major serine protease inhibitor. It inhibits the activities of thrombin and factors Xa, IXa, VIIa, and XIIa. A double-blind, placebo-controlled, multicenter trial in patients with severe sepsis did not find any beneficial effect on overall survival and mortality with the use of high-dose AT [28]. The investigators did find some beneficial effect when it was not used concomitantly with heparin in follow-up substudies. There is increased risk of hemorrhage when combined with heparin. It is recommended before surgery or delivery in patients with DIC, as decreased AT levels may induce severe bleeding in a deficient patient.

Use of rVIIa in DIC

There have been numerous case reports and case series about the successful off-label use of rFVIIa in DIC in postpartum hemorrhage [29–32]. The mechanism of action of activated recombinant factor VII is by formation of complexes with exposed tissue factor (TF) in the absence of factors VII and X. This leads to generation of a thrombin burst. *In vitro* studies have shown that the clots formed in the presence of rVIIa are firmer, stronger and more resistant to digestion by fibrinolytic enzymes. Concerns about the use of rVIIa use in DIC are that by raising the levels of factor rFVIIa by more than 1000-fold by the drug can potentially cause widespread thrombosis. *In vitro* studies have not supported this idea. Moreover, the reported incidence of thromboembolism in more than 700 000 doses administered to hemophiliac individuals is as low as 1%. In other series covering its use in trauma and massive bleeding, the incidence varied between 5 and 7% [33]. These patients had other comorbid factors such as obesity, diabetes mellitus, malignancy and advanced age. A literature search did not show any link with thromboembolism in pregnant patients who were given the drug. In our series of 18 patients [34], we also did not find any adverse side effects related to the use of drug. Though it has proved to be a life-saving medicine in bleeding obstetric patients, further studies are needed to define its use. There are anecdotal reports about its use in DIC due to various obstetric conditions [35,36].

References

1 Lockwood CJ. Pregnancy-associated changes in the hemostatic system. *Clin Obstet Gynecol* 2006; 49(4): 836–843.

2 Paidas MJ, Ku DH, Lee MJ, et al. Protein Z, protein S levels are lower in patients with thrombophilia and subsequent pregnancy complications. *J Thromb Haemost* 2005; 3(3): 497–501.

3 Ku DH, Arkel YS, Paidas MP, Lockwood CJ. Circulating levels of inflammatory cytokines (IL-1 beta and TNF-alpha), resistance to activated protein C, thrombin and fibrin generation in uncomplicated pregnancies. *Thromb Haemost* 2003; 90(6): 1074–1079.

4 Esmon CT. Possible involvement of cytokines in diffuse intravascular coagulation and thrombosis. *Baillière's Best Pract Res Clin Haematol* 1999; 12(3): 343–359.

5 Higgins JR, Walshe JJ, Darling MR, Norris L, Bonnar J. Hemostasis in the uteroplacental and peripheral circulations in normotensive and pre-eclamptic pregnancies. *Am J Obstet Gynecol* 1998; 179(2): 520–526.

6 Lockwood CJ, Bach R, Guha A, Zhou XD, Miller WA, Nemerson Y. Amniotic fluid contains tissue factor, a potent initiator of coagulation. *Am J Obstet Gynecol* 1991; 165(5Pt 1): 1335–1341.

7 Villar J, Carroli G, Wojdyla D, et al. Preeclampsia, gestational hypertension and intrauterine growth restriction, related or independent conditions? *Am J Obstet Gynecol* 2006; 194(4): 921–931.

8 Moore J, Baldisseri MR. Amniotic fluid embolism. *Crit Care Med* 2005; 33(10 Suppl): S279–285.

9 Green BT, Umana E. Amniotic fluid embolism. *South Med J* 2000; 93(7): 721–723.

10 Letsky EA. Disseminated intravascular coagulation. *Best Pract Res Clin Obstet Gynaecol* 2001; 15(4): 623–644.

11 Richey ME, Gilstrap LC, Ramin SM. Management of disseminated intravascular coagulation. *Clin Obstet Gynecol* 1995; 38(3): 514–520.

12 Levi M, de Jonge E, van der Poll T. New treatment strategies for disseminated intravascular coagulation based on current understanding of the pathophysiology. *Ann Med* 2004; 36(1): 41–49.

13 Hulstein JJ, van Runnard Heimel PJ, Franx A, et al. Acute activation of the endothelium results in increased levels of active von Willebrand factor in hemolysis, elevated liver enzymes, and low platelets (HELLP) syndrome. *J Thromb Haemost* 2006; 4(12): 2569–2575.

14 Facchinetti F, Marozio L, Grandone E, Pizzi C, Volpe A, Benedetto C. Thrombophilic mutations are a main risk factor for placental abruption. *Haematologica* 2003; 88(7): 785–788.

15 Sher G. A rational basis for the management of abruptio placentae. *J Reprod Med* 1978; 21(3): 123–129.

16 Magriples U, Chan DW, Bruzek D, Copel JA, Hsu CD. Thrombomodulin: a new marker for placental abruption. *Thromb Haemost* 1999; 81(1): 32–34.

17 Dempfle CE. Coagulopathy of sepsis. *Thromb Haemost* 2004; 91(2): 213–224.

18 Castro MA, Goodwin TM, Shaw KJ, Ouzounian JG, McGehee WG. Disseminated intravascular coagulation and antithrombin III depression in acute fatty liver of pregnancy. *Am J Obstet Gynecol* 1996; 174(1 Pt 1): 211–216.

19 Castro MA, Fassett MJ, Reynolds TB, Shaw KJ, Goodwin TM. Reversible peripartum liver failure: a new perspective on the diagnosis, treatment, and cause of acute fatty liver of pregnancy, based on 28 consecutive cases. *Am J Obstet Gynecol* 1999; 181(2): 389–395.

20 Powars DR, Rogers ZR, Patch MJ, McGehee WG, Francis RB Jr. Purpura fulminans in meningococcemia: association with acquired deficiencies of proteins C and S. *N Engl J Med* 1987; 317(9): 571–572.

21 Molos MA, Hall JC. Symmetrical peripheral gangrene and disseminated intravascular coagulation. *Arch Dermatol* 1985; 121(8): 1057–1061.

22 Yu M, Nardella A, Pechet L. Screening tests of disseminated intravascular coagulation: guidelines for rapid and specific laboratory diagnosis. *Crit Care Med* 2000; 28(6): 1777–1780.

23 Wada H, Gabazza E, Nakasaki T, et al. Diagnosis of disseminated intravascular coagulation by hemostatic molecular markers. *Semin Thromb Hemost* 2000; 26(1): 17–21.

24 Mueller MM, Bomke B, Seifried E. Fresh frozen plasma in patients with disseminated intravascular coagulation or in patients with liver diseases. *Thromb Res* 2002; 107(Suppl 1): S9–17.

25 Bernard GR, Vincent JL, Laterre PF, et al. Efficacy and safety of recombinant human activated protein C for severe sepsis. *N Engl J Med* 2001; 344(10): 699–709.

26 Kobayashi T, Terao T, Maki M, Ikenoue T. Activated protein C is effective for disseminated intravascular coagulation associated with placental abruption. *Thromb Haemost* 1999; 82(4): 1363.

27 MacLean AA, Almeida Z, Lopez P. Complications of acute fatty liver of pregnancy treated with activated protein C. *Arch Gynecol Obstet* 2005; 273(2): 119–121.

28 Hoffmann JN, Wiedermann CJ, Juers M, et al. Benefit/risk profile of high-dose antithrombin in patients with severe sepsis treated with and without concomitant heparin. *Thromb Haemost* 2006; 95(5): 850–856.

29 Pepas LP, Arif-Adib M, Kadir RA. Factor VIIa in puerperal hemorrhage with disseminated intravascular coagulation. *Obstet Gynecol* 2006; 108(3 Pt 2): 757–761.

30 Shamsi TS, Hossain N, Soomro N, et al. Use of recombinant factor VIIa for massive postpartum haemhorrage: case series and review of literature. *J Pak Med Assoc* 2005; 55(11): 512–515.

31 Michalska-Krzanowska G, Czuprynska M. Recombinant factor VII (activated) for haemorrhagic complications of severe sepsis treated with recombinant protein C (activated). *Acta Haematol* 2006; 116(2): 126–130.

32 Moscardo F, Perez F, de la Rubia J, et al. Successful treatment of severe intra-abdominal bleeding associated with disseminated intravascular coagulation using recombinant activated factor VII. *Br J Haematol* 2001; 114(1): 174–176.

33 Scarpelini S, Rizoli S. Recombinant factor VIIa and the surgical patient. *Curr Opin Crit Care* 2006; 12(4): 351–356.

34 Hossain N, Shamsi T, Haider S, Paidas M. Use of activated recombinant factor VII for massive postpartum hemorrhage. *Acta Obstet Gynecol Scand* 2007; 86(10): 1200–1206.

35 Gowers CJ, Parr MJ. Recombinant activated factor VIIa use in massive transfusion and coagulopathy unresponsive to conventional therapy. *Anaesth Intens Care* 2005; 33(2): 196–200.

36 Baudo F, Caimi TM, Mostarda G, de Cataldo F, Morra E. Critical bleeding in pregnancy: a novel therapeutic approach to bleeding. *Minerva Anestesiol* 2006; 72(6): 389–393.

32 Thrombotic Thrombocytopenic Purpura, Hemolytic–Uremic Syndrome, and HELLP

Joel Moake[1] & Kelty R. Baker[2]

[1]Rice University, Houston, TX, USA

[2]Department of Internal Medicine, Hematology-Oncology Section and Baylor College of Medicine, Houston, TX, USA

Thrombotic thrombocytopenic purpura (TTP)

Dr Eli Moschcowitz of New York City initially recognized and reported the first patient with thrombotic thrombocytopenic purpura (TTP) in 1923 [1,2]. Terminal arterioles and capillaries were occluded by hyaline thrombi, later determined to be composed mostly of platelets, without perivascular inflammation or endothelial desquamation.

TTP is now considered to be the most extensive and dangerous microvascular (arteriolar/capillary) platelet clumping disorder. From about 1970–80 on, for unknown reasons, the incidence of this once rare disease has increased considerably.

Clinical features

Severe thrombocytopenia and hemolytic anemia with one to several fragmented red cells (schistocytes) in many oil fields of the blood smear (i.e. more than 1% of total red cells) [3], along with neurological symptoms and signs, constitute the characteristic clinical triad. Neurological disorders may range in severity from transient bizarre thought and behavior to sensory motor deficits, aphasia, seizures, or coma. The peripheral blood smear typically shows increased reticulocytes (polychromatic large erythrocytes) and often nucleated red blood cells, in response to the intense hemolysis. Fever and/or renal dysfunction occur in a minority of patients. Renal abnormalities may include proteinuria and hematuria, as well as azotemia. Symptoms and signs of ischemia in the retinal (visual defects), coronary (conduction abnormalities), and abdominal circulation (abdominal pain) may be present. Microvascular occlusions that cause ischemia of the sinoatrial or atrioventricular node, or of the bundle of His or Purkinje conduction system, may cause sudden death [4–6]. Abdominal presentations, sometimes resembling pancreatitis, have become more commonly recognized during the past few years (about 5–10% of TTP episodes may present with abdominal symptoms) [7].

Critical Care Obstetrics, 5th edition. Edited by M. Belfort, G. Saade, M. Foley, J. Phelan and G. Dildy.

Laboratory findings

The degree of thrombocytopenia in TTP reflects the extent of intravascular platelet clumping. Platelet counts are often less than 20 000/mL during acute episodes of TTP. Erythrocyte fragmentation occurs as red cells attempt to bypass, at high flow rates, the partially occlusive microvascular platelet aggregates, producing the characteristic schistocytes on peripheral blood films (Figure 32.1). Hemolysis is predominantly intravascular and, along with tissue damage, contributes to the increased serum levels of lactate dehydrogenase (LDH) [7].

Coagulation studies are characteristically normal in the early stages of a TTP episode [7]. If there is considerable tissue necrosis, however, secondary disseminated intravascular coagulation (DIC) may occur as a result of overactivation of the coagulation pathway that follows the binding of factor VIIa to exposed tissue factor molecules on injured tissue cells. The ominous development of secondary DIC is indicated by the appearance of elevated levels of D-dimers (or fibrin degradation products), prolongation of the prothrombin or activated partial thromboplastin times, and a decreasing fibrinogen level.

Types

Since the general application of plasma therapy, many patients have survived episodes of TTP. It has become apparent that there are several conditions associated with the disorder, and more than one etiology [7] (Table 32.1). About two-thirds of adult patients with the relatively common acquired idiopathic TTP ('out-of-the-blue' TTP) have a single episode that never recurs (presuming successful treatment). About one-third of adult patients who recover from an initial TTP episode will have recurrences at irregular intervals, often commencing within the first year after the initial episode.

In the rarest type of the disease, familial (or congenital) TTP, frequent episodes may occur at regular (approximately 3–4 week) intervals. This entity has also been called chronic relapsing TTP,

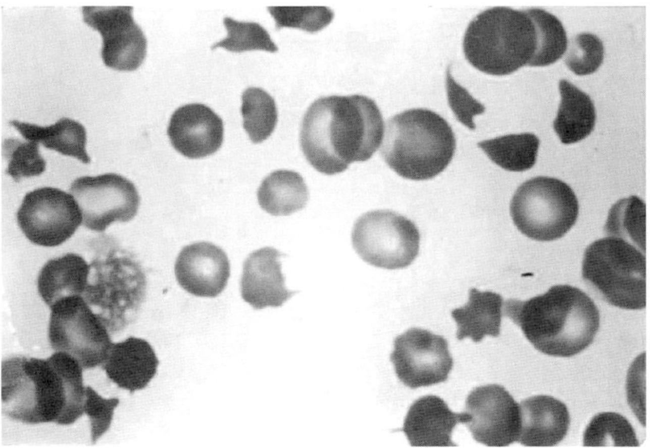

Figure 32.1 Schistocytes or "split" red blood cells, are inevitably present on the peripheral blood smear of patients with TTP.

Table 32.1 Clinical types of TTP.

Familial (congenital; recurrent)
Acquired idiopathic (recurrent in ~1/3)
Drugs: thienopyridine-associated
ticlopidine (Ticlid)
clopidogrel (Plavix)
Thrombotic microangiopathies that resemble TTP (or HUS)
Drugs:
mitomycin
cyclosporine; tacrolimus
quinine
combination chemotherapy; gemcitamine
Total-body irradiation
Bone marrow/stem cell tansplantation
Solid organ transplantation

and is usually seen initially in infants and children [8–10]. A subgroup of familial TTP patients have only occasional episodes, beginning later in life.

During the past few years, the structurally similar platelet function inhibitors ticlopidine (Ticlid) [11,12] and clopidogrel (Plavix) [13] have been associated with the induction of TTP in a fraction of exposed patients. These two drugs, which differ only by a single carboxymethyl group, inhibit a platelet adenosine diphosphate (ADP) receptor site and are used to suppress arterial platelet thrombosis. A fraction of patients with human immunodeficiency virus-1 (HIV-1) infection also develop TTP.

Mitomycin C, quinine, cyclosporine, FK506 (tacrolimus), che motherapeutic agents in combination, gemcitabine and total-body irradiation have been associated with the subsequent development of thrombotic microangiopathy [14–23]. The syndrome often more closely resembles the hemolytic–uremic syndrome (HUS, discussed later in this chapter) than TTP, and usually develops weeks to months after exposure [20]. Patients who have been treated for various illnesses with bone marrow/stem cell transplantation make up a relatively large subgroup [20]. Thrombotic microangiopathy has also been reported after solid organ transplantation (kidney, liver, heart, and lung) [22]. (Transplantation of all types is often managed with immunosuppression using cyclosporine and/or tacrolimus.)

Although TTP may occur at any stage of pregnancy, episodes most frequently occur during the last trimester [24–26]. In contrast, if HUS occurs it is usually during the postpartum period [27–31]. HUS during pregnancy is likely to be associated with diarrhea [32] caused by Shiga toxin-producing enterohemorrhagic *E. coli* [33].

Causes and pathophysiology

Early vascular lesions in TTP consist almost exclusively of platelet thrombi without evidence of perivascular inflammation or other overt vessel wall pathology [34,35]. Microvascular occlusions are seen in most organs. Most frequently involved are the brain, heart, spleen, kidneys, pancreas, and adrenals; however, even the lungs and eyes are affected in some patients.

The histopathological and clinical findings in TTP suggest that organ ischemia and thrombocytopenia are caused by potentially reversible platelet adhesion/aggregation in the microcirculation of multiple organs concurrently. Immunohistochemical studies of TTP thrombi reported in 1985 by Asada and coworkers [34] revealed an abundance of von Willebrand factor (VWF) with little fibrinogen/fibrin, supporting the initial 1982 suggestion [9] that VWF is involved in the microvascular platelet adhesion/aggregation that characterizes some types of the disorder.

von Willebrand factor and ADAMTS-13

Monomers of VWF (280000 daltons) are linked by disulfide bonds into multimers with varying molecular masses that range into the millions of daltons [36]. Multimers of VWF are constructed within megakaryocytes and endothelial cells, and stored within platelet α-granules and endothelial cell Weibel–Palade bodies. Most plasma VWF multimers are derived from endothelial cells. Both endothelial cells and platelets produce VWF multimers larger than the multimers in normal plasma [36]. These ULVWF (ultralarge VWF) multimers bind more efficiently than the largest plasma VWF multimers to the glycoprotein (GP) Iba components of platelet GPIb-IX-V receptors [37,38]. The initial attachment of ULVWF multimers to GPIba receptors [37], and subsequently to activated platelet integrin aIIbb3 (GPIIb-IIIa complexes), induces platelet adhesion and aggregation *in vitro* in the presence of elevated levels of fluid shear stress [38,39]. After retrograde secretion by endothelial cells, ULVWF multimers become entangled in subendothelial collagen, thereby maximizing the VWF-mediated adhesion of blood platelets to any subendothelium exposed by vascular damage and endothelial cell desquamation. An efficient "processing activity" [9,40] in normal plasma prevents the highly adhesive, ULVWF multimers, that are also secreted antegrade into the vessel lumen, from persisting in the bloodstream.

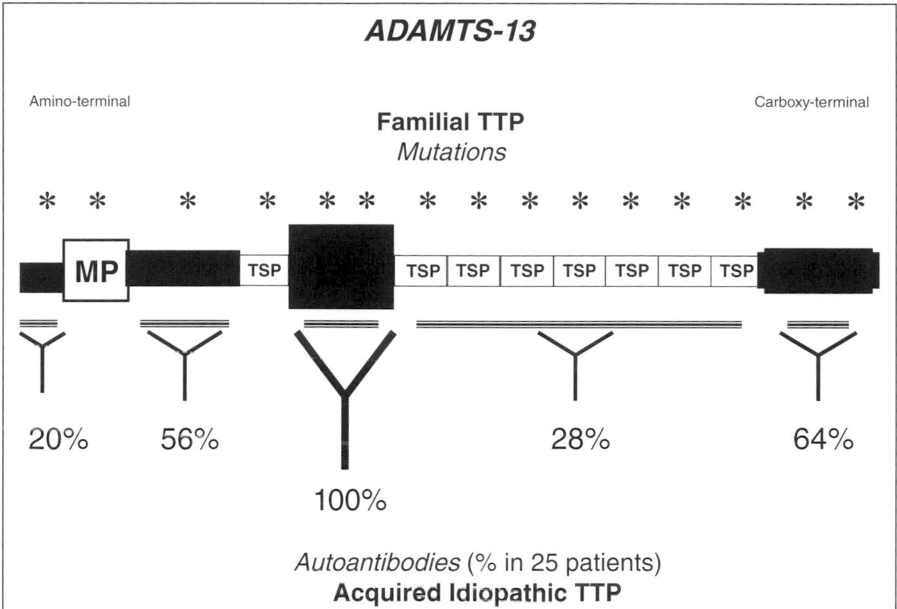

Figure 32.2 Domain structure of ADAMTS-13 (the plasma VWF-cleaving metalloprotease). P, propeptide; MP, metalloprotease (proteolytic) domain; TSP, thrombospondin-1-like domain (eight are present); CUB, two non-identical domains containing peptide segments similar to *c*omplement components, C1r/C1s, a sea *u*rchin protein, and a *b*one morphogenic protein. *Indicates the location of mutations in familial TTP patients that affect secretion or function of ADAMTS-13 (above enzyme structure). The percentages of polyclonal autoantibodies directed against specific domains of ADAMTS-13 in 25 patients with acquired idiopathic TTP are indicated below the enzyme structure [79].

This VWF "processing activity," initially described in 1982 [9], is now known to be a specific VWF-cleaving metalloprotease in normal plasma that prevents the persistence in the circulation of ULVWF multimers [8,41,42]. The enzyme degrades ULVWF multimers by cleaving 842Tyr–843Met peptide bonds in susceptible A2 domains of VWF monomeric subunits [43–45]. The VWF-cleaving metalloprotease is number 13 in a family of 18 distinct ADAMTS-type enzymes identified to date that share structural similarities [46,47]. "ADAMTS-13" is *a d*isintegrin *a*nd *m*etalloprotease with eight *t*hrombo*s*pondin-1-like domains. More precisely, plasma ADAMTS-13 is composed of an amino-terminal reprolysin-type metalloprotease domain followed by: a disintegrin domain; a thrombospondin-1-like domain; a cysteine-rich domain containing an arginine-glycine-aspartate (RGD) sequence; a spacer domain; seven additional thrombospondin-1-like domains; and two non-identical CUB-type domains at the carboxyl-terminal end of the molecule (Figure 32.2). CUB domains contain peptide sequences similar to: *c*omplement sub-components C1r/C1s; embryonic sea *u*rchin protein egf; and *b*one morphogenic protein-1 [48].

ADAMTS-13 is a Zn^{2+}- and Ca^{2+}-requiring 190 000-Da glycosylated protein that is encoded on chromosome 9q34. It is produced (predominantly) by endothelial cells [49,50], and by hepatic stellate cells [51–53]. Plasma ADAMTS-13 activity is inhibited by the strong divalent cation-chelating agent, EDTA. Functional assays of the enzyme *in vitro* are usually performed in plasma anticoagulated using citrate, a weak divalent cation chelator [8,41–47,54,55].

ULVWF multimers are cleaved by ADAMTS-13 as they are secreted as long "strings" from stimulated endothelial cells (Figure 32.3) [56,57]. The ULVWF multimeric strings may be anchored in the endothelial cell membrane to P-selectin molecules that are secreted concurrently with the ULVWF multimers from Weibel–Palade bodies [58]. Included among the agents that stimulate endothelial cells to secrete ULVWF multimers are the proinflammatory cytokines, tumor necrosis factor (TNF)-α, interleukin (IL)-8 and IL-6 (in complex with the IL-6 receptor), [59] and the Shiga toxins (discussed in the section below on HUS). One of the repeated CUB domains at the carboxyl-terminal end of each ADAMTS-13 enzyme, as well as one or more of the thrombospondin-1-like domains along the length of the molecule, may modulate the binding of ADAMTS-13 to ULVWF multimers as they are secreted by endothelial cells [60–62]. Specifically, ADAMTS 13 enzymes may attach under flowing conditions to accessible A3 domains in the monomeric subunits of ULVWF multimers, [56] and then cleave Tyr842–843Met peptide bonds in adjacent A2 domains (Figure 32.4). Partial unfolding of emerging ULVWF multimers by fluid shear stress may increase the efficiency of ADAMTS-13 attachment to ULVWF multimers, as well as ULVWF cleavage [45,57]. Platelet GPIba binding to the VWF A1 domain pulls the adjacent VWF A2 domain into a position that is susceptible to proteolysis by ADAMTS-13 [63]. This may explain why ADAMTS-13, secreted by endothelial cells along with ULVWF multimeric strings, does not cleave the ULVWF strings until platelet–ULVWF adhering begins.

Failure to degrade ULVWF multimers has been suspected since the 1980s to cause familial and acquired idiopathic types of TTP, or to predispose an individual to these disorders (Figures 32.3 & 32.4) [9,64]. Critical experiments verifying this concept were reported in 1997–8. In 1997, four patients were described with chronic relapsing TTP who had a deficiency of VWF-cleaving protease activity (ADAMTS-13) in plasma [8]. No inhibitor of the enzyme was detected, and so the deficiency was ascribed to

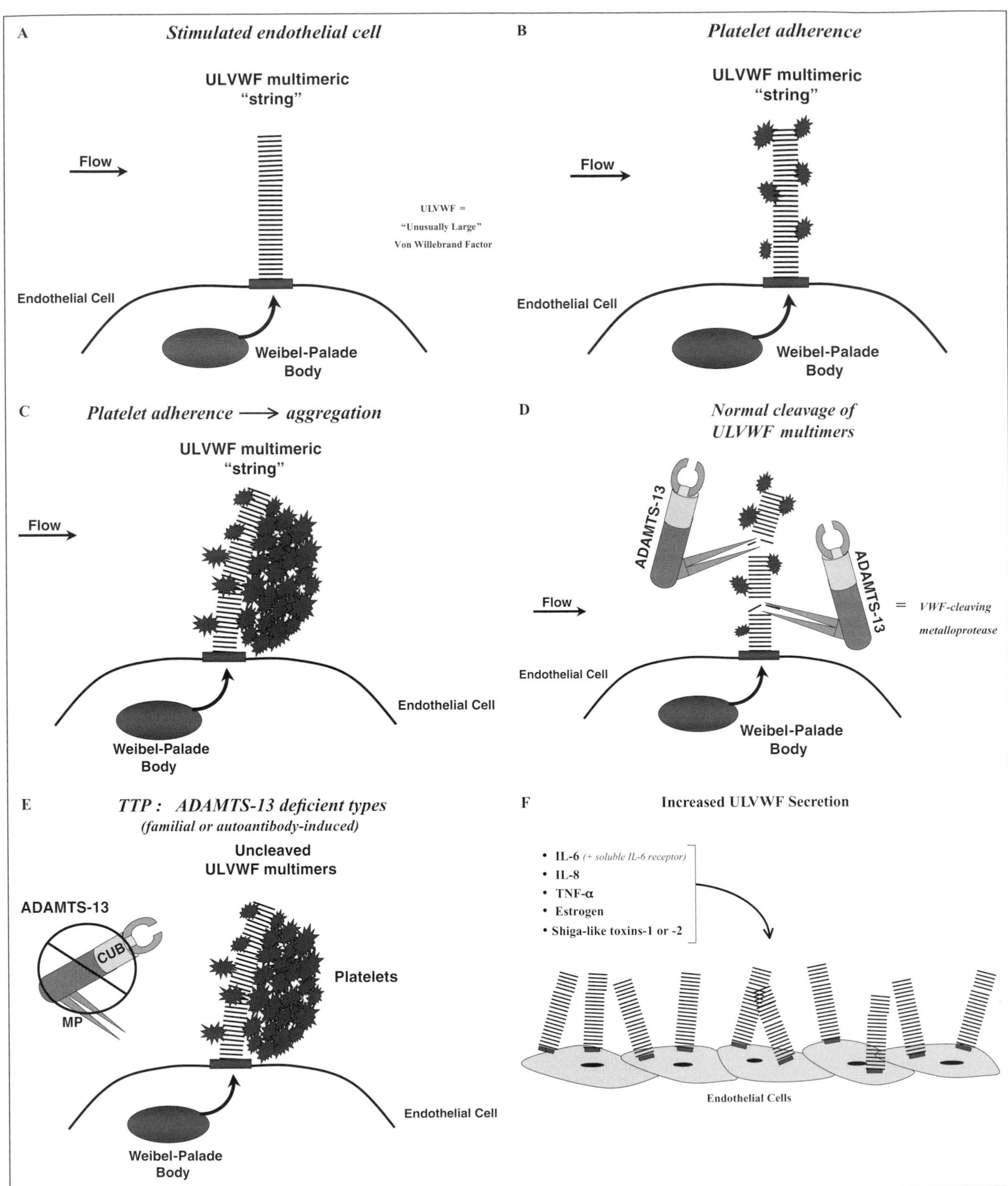

Figure 32.3 Proposed mechanism for the cleavage of unusually large von Willebrand factor (ULVWF) multimeric strings by ADAMTS-13. (a) Stimulation of endothelial cells causes secretion of long ULVWF multimeric strings. (b) Platelets from flowing blood adhere to the long ULVWF multimeric strings immediately after string secretion. (c) Additional blood platelets then cohere (aggregeate) onto those initially adherent to the ULVWF multimeric strings. (d) Adequate quantities of ADAMTS-13 enzymes are present in the plasma of normal individuals to cleave quickly the ULVWF–platelet strings. (e) Absent or severely reduced activity of ADAMTS-13 in the plasma of patients with TTP prevents the timely cleavage of ULVWF multimeric strings as they are secreted from endothelial cells. Uncleaved ULVWF multimers induce the adhesion and subsequent aggregation of platelets in flowing blood. TTP can be caused by familial deficiencies of ADAMTS-13 secretion or activity caused by ADAMTA-13 gene mutations, or by acquired autoantibody-induced defects of ADAMTS-13 activity (or survival). (f) Stimulation of ULVWF multimeric secretion by cytokines or toxins may precipitate TTP episodes in individuals who have marginal levels of plasma ADAMTS-13 activity. Stx, Shiga toxin (Stx-1 and -2 are from enterohemorrhagic *E. coli*); TNF, tumor necrosis factor; IL, interleukin.

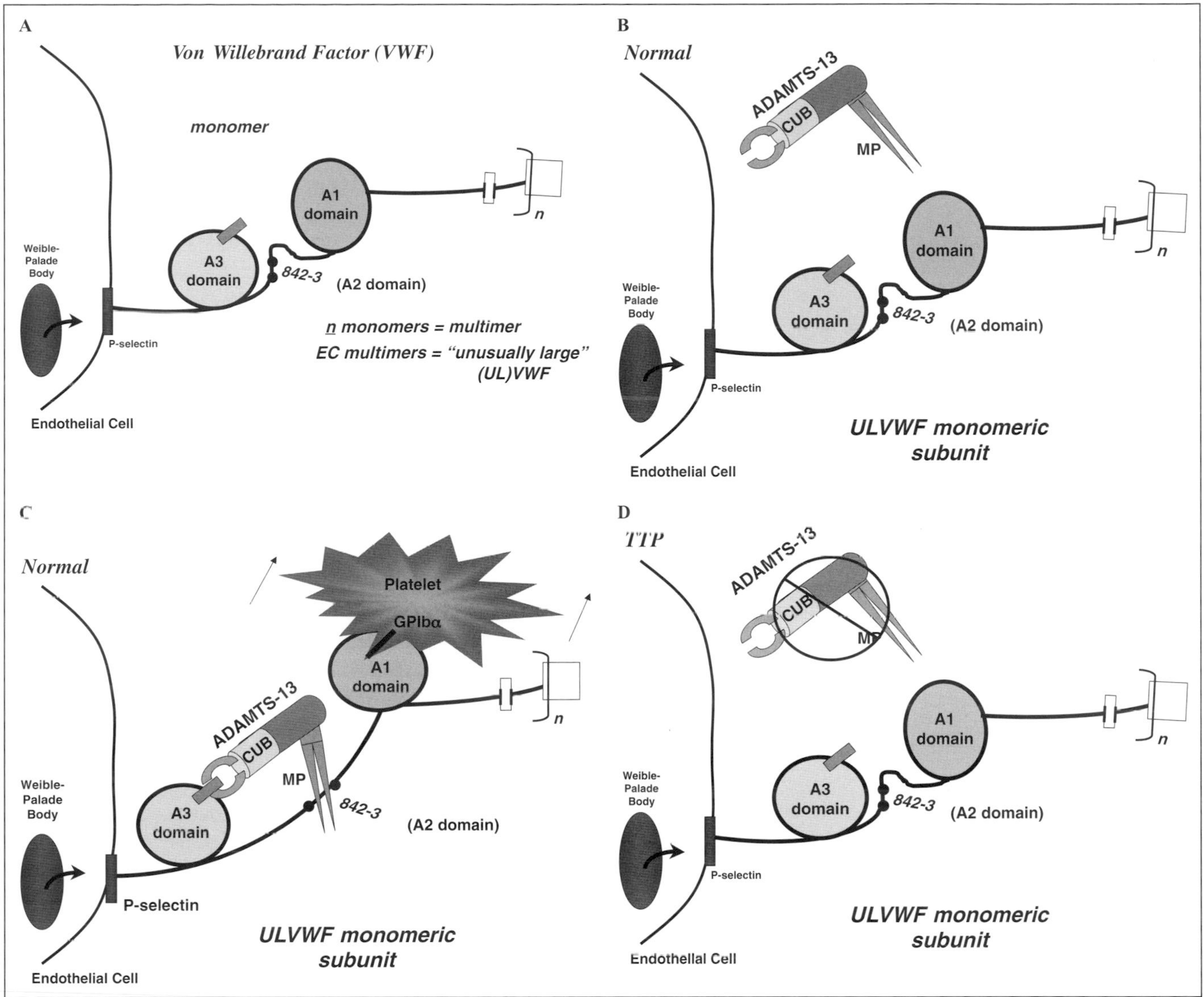

Figure 32.4 Proposed mechanism of ULVWF multimeric string cleavage by ADAMTS-13. (A) One of the many monomeric subunits that comprise an ULVWF multimeric string secreted by stimulated endothelial cells. The ULVWF multimeric strings may be anchored in the endothelial cell membrane to P-selectin molecules that are secreted concurrently with the ULVWF multimers from Weibel-Palade bodies. The A1, A2 (with the tyr842-843met ADAMTS-13 proteolytic cleavage site), and A3 domains are shown. (B) Adequate quantities of ADAMTS-13 enzymes are present in the plasma of normal individuals. The carboxy-terminal CUB domain is indicated, and the metalloprotease domain (MP) is drawn as a pincer-like structure on the amino-terminal portion of the enzyme. (C) Platelets from flowing blood adhere to the long ULVWF multimeric strings immediately after string secretion. Platelet adherence (via platelet GPIbα) to the A1 domain of ULVWF monomeric subunits increases the exposure of neighboring A2 tyr842-843met peptide bonds in ULVWF multimeric strings. ADAMTS-13 molecules may attach via one of their CUB domains (and possibly the spacer domain) to the A3 domain of ULVWF monomeric subunits, and cleave the adjacent (and now-exposed) tyr842-843met bond. ADAMTS-13 cleavage by this mechanism occurs in various monomers along the length of ULVWF multimeric strings. The smaller VWF forms that circulate after cleavage do not induce the adhesion and aggregation of platelets during normal blood flow. (D) Absent or severely reduced activity of ADAMTS-13 in the plasma of patients with TTP prevents the timely cleavage of ULVWF-multimeric strings.

an abnormality in the production, survival or function of the protease. The following year, the pathogenesis of the more common acquired idiopathic type of TTP was elucidated [41,42,65]. Acquired idiopathic TTP patients have little or no plasma VWF-cleaving protease activity during acute episodes; however, the activity often returns towards normal upon recovery. The plasma assays used in the 1997–8 studies were "non-physiologic;" they were, however, innovative and informative. IgG autoantibodies against components of the enzyme probably accounted for the lack of protease activity in most of the acquired idiopathic TTP patients reported in 1998 [41,42,65]. The explanation for the transient immune dysregulation, as well as for the selective antigenic targeting of the VWF-cleaving protease, is not yet known.

Most patients with familial TTP have less than about 5–10% of normal ADAMTS-13 activity in their plasma, regardless of whether the sample is obtained during or after acute episodes (provided that they have not recently received plasma infusions). Most patients with acquired idiopathic types of TTP have less than 5–10% of normal activity of ADAMTS-13 in their plasma, but this is only during (or for a variable period following) acute TTP episodes [7,41,42,65,66]. Severe deficiency of ADAMTS-13 activity in TTP patient plasma correlates with a failure to cleave ULVWF multimeric strings as they emerge from the surface of endothelial cells (Figures 32.3 & 32.4) [57]. As a consequence, ULVWF multimers secreted by endothelial cells remain anchored to the cells in long strings [57]. The anchoring may be via P-selectin molecules, which have transmembrane domains and are secreted along with ULVWF multimers from the Weibel–Palade bodies of endothelial cells [58]. (P-selectin molecules are predominantly retained in the cell membrane as the Weibel–Palade contents are secreted.) Passing platelets adhere via their GPIba receptors to these long uncleaved ULVWF multimeric strings [57]. (Platelets do not adhere to the smaller VWF forms that circulate after cleavage of ULVWF multimers [36].) Many additional platelets subsequently aggregate under flowing conditions, probably via their activated membrane integrin aIIbb3 (GP IIb–IIIa) complexes, onto the ULVWF multimeric strings to form large, potentially occlusive, platelet thrombi [57,67] (Figure 32.3).

Plasma ADAMTS-13 activity is almost always absent or severely reduced in familial TTP patients, [8,68,69] as a consequence of homozygous (or doubly heterozygous) mutations in each of the two ADAMTS-13 9q34 genes (Table 32.2) [7,25,66,70,71]. Mutations in familial TTP have been detected all along the gene structure, in regions encoding different domains (Figure 32.2) [7,25,66,70,71]. In severe familial deficiencies of ADAMTS-13 activity, episodes of TTP usually commence in infancy or childhood. In some of these patients, however, overt TTP episodes may not develop for years (e.g. during a first pregnancy) [25,72]. This latter observation suggests that *in vivo* ADAMTS-13 activity on ULVWF multimers emerging from stimulated endothelial cells may exceed the plasma enzyme activity measured by *in vitro* (non-physiologic) assays. Additionally, or alternatively, accentuated secretion of ULVWF multimers by endothelial cells induced by estrogen or proinflammatory cytokines [59] may be required to provoke TTP episodes in some patients with severe plasma ADAMTS-13 deficiency (Figure 32.3).

Table 32.2 TTP: inadequate cleavage of ULVWF multimers secreted by endothelial cells.

VWF-cleaving metalloprotease (ADAMTS-13) plasma activity "absent (or <5–10 %)"

Familial (congenital) TTP (often "chronic relapsing"):
- Severe defect of ADAMTS-13 production, function or survival
- Doubly heterozygous or homozygous mutations

Acquired idiopathic TTP ("out of the blue"):
- Severe defect of ADAMTS-13 function or survival
- Autoantibodies (often IgG) detectable in 44–94% of patients who are ADAMTS-13 deficient

Types
- Transient single episode
- Recurrent (irregular intervals)
- Ticlopidine/clopidogrel

HIV/AIDS

Pregnancy

ULVWF, unusually large von Willebrand factor.

In some infants with less than 5–10% ADAMTS-13 and neonatal onset of familial chronic relapsing TTP, transient or progressive renal failure is a prominent component of the disorder [73]. These patients clinically resemble two children described in 1960 by Schulman et al. [9,74] and in 1978 by Upshaw [9,75] and so this pediatric subgroup is sometimes said to have "Upshaw–Schulman syndrome."

Many patients with acquired idiopathic TTP have absent or severely reduced plasma ADAMTS-13 activity during an initial episode, as well as during any later recurrence [41,42,65] (Table 32.2). ADAMTS-13 activity usually increases in these patients following recovery from either a single, or recurrent, episode. IgG antibodies (presumably autoantibodies) that inhibit plasma ADAMTS-13 activity can be detected in 44–94% of patients using the non-physiologic techniques currently available [25,41,42,65,76,77]. These results suggest a transient, or intermittently recurrent, defect of immune regulation in many patients who have acquired idiopathic TTP associated with transient, or recurrent, ADAMTS-13 deficiency. Antibodies that inhibit plasma ADAMTS-13 have also been demonstrated in a few patients with ticlopidine- or clopidogrel-associated TTP [13,78].

It is not yet known if there is a transient, severe defect of ADAMTS-13 production or survival in patients with acquired TTP who do not have detectable autoantibodies against the enzyme. Alternatively, failure to detect autoantibodies in some patients may reflect the limited sensitivity of the test systems in current use.

In one recent study [79] of polyclonal autoantibodies against ADAMTS-13 in 25 acquired TTP patients, the epitope targets of autoantibodies always included the cysteine-rich/spacer domain sequence. The CUB domains were additional antigenic targets of other autoantibodies in about two-thirds of the patients in this study (Figure 32.2).

Autoantibodies either inhibit the activity of ADAMTS-13 or decrease its survival. Relapses occur in 23–44% of patients with acquired idiopathic TTP, [25,76,80,81], often in the first year after the initial episode [25]. These relapsing patients usually have acquired idiopathic TTP with severe plasma ADAMTS-13 deficiency that is often due to the presence of detectable autoantibodies against ADAMTS-13 [25].

In a few instances, pregnancy-related TTP episodes have been demonstrated to be caused by autoantibodies against ADAMTS-

13 [25]. The risk of recurrent TTP during any subsequent pregnancies is controversial, with estimates of possible recurrence (per woman) ranging from 26 to 73% [25].

Plasma ADAMTS-13 activity in healthy adults ranges from approximately 50 to 178% using currently available static, nonphysiologic assays. Activity is often reduced below normal in liver disease, disseminated malignancies, [82] chronic metabolic and inflammatory conditions and pregnancy, and in newborns [83]. With the exception of those peripartum women who develop overt TTP, [25,76] the ADAMTS-13 activity in these conditions is not reduced to the extremely low values (<5–10% of normal) found in most patients with familial or acquired idiopathic TTP.

Other observations

About twice as many women as men develop acquired idiopathic TTP. Most patients are 20–60 years old, no racial or seasonal predisposition is obvious, and case clustering is rare. The majority of patients who develop acute idiopathic TTP have no identifiable associated risk factor. TTP during pregnancy or the postpartum period accounts for a small percentage of total TTP cases [24–26]. Neame [84] suggested that abnormal immune modulation might contribute to the etiology in these circumstances. Indeed, a specific defect in immune regulation is likely to be the basis for the "escape" of autoantibody production against ADAMTS-13 in most acute idiopathic TTP patients.

The possibility that immunologic events are involved in acute idiopathic TTP is supported by studies that suggest macrophage/lymphocyte activation in some patients [85,86]. Elevated levels of IL-1, IL-6, the soluble IL-2 receptor, TNF-α, and transforming growth factor-β (TGF-β) have all been reported in the disorder. There is also one report that patients lacking the class II HLA antigen, DR53, may be more susceptible to thrombotic microangiopathy [87].

Acquired idiopathic TTP has been associated occasionally with diseases characterized by autoimmune or other types of abnormal immune responses, including systemic lupus erythromatosus (SLE) [88], autoimmune "idiopathic" thrombocytopenic purpura (ITP), [89] and the acquired immunodeficiency syndrome (AIDS) [90–92].

Treatment

The demonstration by Byrnes and Khurana in 1977 [93] that TTP relapses could be prevented or reversed by the infusion of fresh frozen plasma or cryosupernatant (plasma depleted of VWF-rich cryoprecipitate, fibrinogen, fibronectin and IgM) was followed in 1985 by the observation that the processing of ULVWF multimers was restored in patients with familial, chronic relapsing TTP by transfusing fresh frozen plasma, cryosupernatant [40,94] or (in 1994) solvent/detergent-treated plasma [10]. These plasma products contain functionally active ADAMTS-13, and are effective alone (in quantities varying from one to several units), without the need for concurrent plasmapheresis [41,42], in patients with familial TTP who produce inadequate quantities or functionally defective forms of ADAMTS-13 (Table 32.3) [7,8,41,42,69].

Table 32.3 TTP: ADAMTS-13-deficient types.

Familial TTP (ADAMTS-13 <u>mutations</u>; often chronic relapsing):
Plasma (or cryosupernatant) infusion alone (~ every 2–4 weeks)
Acquired idiopathic TTP (ADAMTS-13 <u>autoantibodies</u>):
Plasma (or cryosupernatant) exchange (plasma infusion with plasmapheresis) (daily)
Other therapy for acquired idiopathic TTP:
Glucocorticoids
Transfusion: RBC (as needed)
Platelets only for emergency bleeding, surgery or invasive procedures
No aspirin
Rituximab (anti-CD20 on B-lymphocytes)
Splenectomy
Cytoxan; vincristine; cyclosporine?
Future: recombinant ADAMTS-13?

The reason why the infusion of normal ADAMTS-13 only about every 3 weeks prevents TTP episodes in some of these patients is not known. The plasma $t_{1/2}$ of the infused ADAMTS-13 activity is relatively long (about 2 days) [69]. The functional $t_{1/2}$ of the enzyme may be even longer, as a result of ADAMTS-13 docking and cleaving on one ULVWF multimeric string after another as each string is secreted from endothelial cells [56,62].

Adults and some older children with acquired idiopathic TTP episodes associated with ADAMTS-13 deficiency require daily plasma exchange (Table 32.3). Plasma exchange combines plasmapheresis (which may remove circulating ULVWF–platelet strings; cytokines, hormones or agents that stimulate endothelial cells to secrete ULVWF multimers; and autoantibodies against ADAMTS-13) and the infusion of FFP or cryosupernatant (containing uninhibited ADAMTS-13). Skipping even 1 day before complete remission may lead to rapid relapse. More than one exchange (or multiple plasma volumes) per day has not been demonstrated to be beneficial.

Infusion of normal FFP at the rate of about 30 mL/kg/day can be used initially until plasma exchanges are arranged. This should be as quickly as practical, but often requires from a few to many hours. Plasma infusion alone is less effective in acquired idiopathic TTP than plasma exchange [95] and may result in volume overload. TTP patients with coma, cardiac failure, or severe renal dysfunction should receive plasma exchange commencing as soon as possible. Plasma exchange with FFP or cryosupernatant allows about 80% ± 10% of acquired, "out-of-the-blue" idiopathic TTP patients who have severe ADAMTS-13 deficiency to survive an episode [25,95,96].

Lower titers of plasma ADAMTS-13 autoantibodies may be associated with better responses to plasma exchange procedures than higher levels of ADAMTS-13 autoantibodies produced for longer periods [81,97,98]. Autoantibodies are, however, difficult to quantify precisely using currently available assay procedures. In association with plasma exchange, production of ADAMTS-13 autoantibodies may be suppressed by high-dose glucocorticoids [96], 4–8 weekly doses of rituximab (monoclonal antibody against CD20 on B-lymphocytes) [99–102] rituximab combined with cyclophosphamide [25,103], (possibly) cyclosporine [31,104], or (most radically) splenectomy to remove a major organ comprised of immunologic cells (Table 32.3) [105–107].

Recovery from TTP is not usually associated with persistent, overt organ damage [95,96]; however, some compromise of cognitive function may be detectable subsequently by careful testing [25]. Almost all TTP recurrences can be recognized quickly by blood counts/smears and LDH measurements.

If a patient with a TTP episode is taking either ticlopidine or clopidogrel, or any other suspicious drug (e.g. mitomycin, cyclosporin, quinine), then this medicine should be stopped immediately.

Although adult patients have recovered from TTP episodes without receiving glucocorticoids, in one large series a subset of TTP patients recovered in association with glucocorticoid therapy alone [96]. On the basis of this study by Bell and colleagues [96], it is probably prudent to institute glucocorticoid therapy – in association with plasma exchange – in all adult patients with initial or recurrent TTP episodes, unless there is a strong contraindication. The usefulness of glucocorticoids may reflect the proposed autoimmune pathogenesis in many adult patients (e.g. glucocorticoids may suppress the production of autoantibodies against ADAMTS-13). Bell and coworkers [96] administered prednisolone intravenously immediately following diagnosis in a dosage of about 200 mg/day, and continued it until the patient recovered.

Depending on the hemoglobin level and intensity of hemolysis, red blood cell transfusions may be required. Transfusion of platelets is likely to be necessary if the platelet count is very low and (i) bleeding (e.g. GI hemorrhage) is a primary problem; (ii) serious bleeding is anticipated in association with an operative or invasive diagnostic procedure); or (iii) intracranial bleeding is demonstrated by computed tomography or magnetic resonance imaging. Otherwise, it may be better to withhold platelet transfusions because they have been temporally associated too frequently with exacerbation of the microcirculatory thrombotic process in the central nervous system [35,108].

The study by Bell, et al. also suggests that plasma exchange should be continued for *more than 3 days* [96] after patients attain complete remission (i.e. a normal neurologic status, a platelet count of 150 000–200 000/mL, a rising hemoglobin value, and a normal serum LDH level) in order to prevent incomplete response with rapid relapse. This is more aggressive than recommendations by blood bank organizations [109]. Plasma exchange should then be stopped, and the glucocorticoid dosage tapered and discontinued over a period of several weeks. Schistocytes in declining numbers often persist for many days on peripheral blood films, and so cannot be used as a reliable marker for remission [110]. Either tapered or intermittent plasma exchanges over days or weeks has not been demonstrated to provide additional benefit in most patients. Platelet counts should be monitored regularly in order to detect incipient relapse. If TTP does recur, the same treatment program (i.e. glucocorticoids and plasma exchanges) that has previously induced remission should be repeated.

In some adult patients with acquired idiopathic TTP who turn out to have recurrent episodes, many will have their first recurrence during the year following their initial episode [25]. In others, episodes do not recur for months to years after an initial episode. A small study of a few patients suggests that frequent relapses *may* be controlled by splenectomy [105].

In patients who achieve only a partial response, or worsen during therapy, plasma exchanges should be continued for a period of a few to many additional days in an effort to achieve a complete remission. In these patients, concomitant heparin-associated thrombocytopenia (HIT) or bacterial infection (e.g. from the plasma exchange catheter) should be suspected. HIT is especially likely if platelets begin to decrease without a concomitant increase in the LDH values that have been decreasing progressively toward normal during therapy. In the latter situation, all exposure of the patient to heparin should be eliminated (including via keep-open intravenous lines or indwelling catheters, during dialysis, or on the tips of Swan–Ganz catheters). It is not known if any additional treatment for HIT, other than heparin removal, is required (e.g. hirudin or argatroban) in patients who are also undergoing plasma exchange for TTP. In the absence of evidence to the contrary, the addition or hirudin or argatroban during therapy for TTP is probably too dangerous.

First-line treatment does not work in some patients with acquired idiopathic TTP episodes. Other forms of therapy can be added if plasma exchanges with FFP or cryosupernatant, glucocorticoids, and rituximab are unsuccessful or incompletely successful. (Table 32.3). These other options include: addition of vincristine [111], which depolymerizes platelet microtubules and may alter the availability of GPIb-IX-V or GPIIb/IIIa receptors for VWF on platelet surfaces; splenectomy [107]; and addition of other immunosuppressive agents in an attempt to suppress production of ADAMTS-13 autoantibodies (e.g. azathioprine [Imuran] [40], cyclophasphamide [Cytoxan] [103], or even cyclosporine [104]. Aspirin may exacerbate hemorrhagic complications in these severely thrombocytopenic patients [112].

If the differential diagnosis in an adult patient includes TTP as a serious possibility, then plasma infusion/exchange should commence immediately and be continued until the precise diagnosis is clarified.

Possible future treatment

The sequence of the 190 000-Da ADAMTS-13 has been determined, and the enzyme has been partially purified from normal human plasma fractions [43,46,47]. Recombinant, active ADAMTS-13 has also been prepared [113], and may soon be produced in therapeutic quantities using insect, mammalian or bacterial cells. As a consequence, purified or recombinant ADAMTS-13 may soon be developed for therapeutic use in TTP. It may also be possible to produce active, truncated forms of recombinant ADAMTS-13 that have less binding affinity for

ADAMTS-13 autoantibodies. This type of ADAMTS-13 might be useful in the treatment of acquired idiopathic TTP [53].

Specific obstetric issues

The plasma levels of VWF increase throughout normal pregnancy, probably in response to estrogen. Concurrently, plasma ADAMTS-13 levels steadily decline, possibly because of compensatory attachment of plasma ADAMTS-13 to the increased secretion ULVWF strings by estrogen-stimulated endothelial cells. It is anticipated, therefore, that pregnancy is likely to provoke episodes of TTP in women who have congenital defects in ADAMTS-13 production, function or survival. Occasionally, the *initial* TTP episode may occur during a first pregnancy in these susceptible women with familial defects of ADAMTS-13. Recurrences of TTP are likely during subsequent pregnancies in familial TTP. Regular infusions of FFP (containing ADAMTS-13) are probably necessary to prevent relapses.

More commonly, TTP episodes during pregnancy (usually, but not inevitably, around the time of delivery) may be caused by maternal production of autoantibodies against ADAMTS-13. This escape from immune regulatory control of a specific autoantibody against ADAMTS-13 may be an uncommon and anomalous consequence of the immune alterations associated with pregnancy. Only a small number of patients with apparently acquired TTP episodes during pregnancy have had plasma ADAMTS-13 activity/inhibitor titers determined. In several, ADAMTS-13 was severely reduced or absent and, in a few, inhibitors (presumably autoantibodies) were detectable using the imperfect testing systems currently in use.

Fortunately, infants delivered successfully from mothers with pregnancy-related, presumably ADAMTS-13 autoantibody-mediated, TTP usually do not have the disorder. This indicates that maternal ADAMTS-13 autoantibodies do not cross the placenta into the fetal circulation in sufficient quantities to cause neonatal TTP.

The risk of a recurrent TTP episode during a subsequent pregnancy after an episode of acquired idiopathic (ADAMTS-13 autoantibody) TTP, either "out of the blue" or during a previous pregnancy, varies widely in the modest number of individuals reported in several studies [24–26]. It is not possible on the basis of the observations available to make decisions with a high level of confidence on the danger of TTP recurrence during a subsequent pregnancy in women who have previously had episodes of acquired idiopathic TTP. The following are management suggestions to consider until the matter is resolved with additional clinical and laboratory observations.

Option 1

Most women have a progressive decline in plasma ADAMTS-13 level as pregnancy proceeds; consequently, a subsequent pregnancy after a previous TTP episode (especially an episode provoked by pregnancy) is too dangerous and should be discouraged. Estrogen-containing birth control pills should also be avoided because these promote ULVWF secretion by endothelial cells. Exogenous estrogen should especially be avoided in a woman who has already had an episode of TTP during the estrogen "flood" (and ADAMTS-13 decline) of pregnancy. Option 1 is safer, and definitely preferable, if the woman had a complicated therapeutic course during a previous TTP episode (e.g. a prolonged number of plasma exchange procedures required for remission; hypotensive allergic reaction to plasma components [114,115]; venous access infection; HITT; or any other life-threatening condition associated with therapy).

Option 2

If the patient who has a previous episode of TTP becomes pregnant (especially if the previous episode was provoked by pregnancy), then blood counts/smear and serum LDH level should be determined at baseline, about every other week through the second trimester, and every week thereafter. It would also be helpful to obtain plasma ADAMTS-13 values at baseline, about monthly through the second trimester, and weekly thereafter. Rapid and reliable laboratory testing and turnaround are, however, currently unavailable generally. (This may change soon.) Access to the services of a major medical center also is prudent. If platelets progressively fall, schistocytes appear, LDH increases, or ADAMTS-13 values drop toward 10% of normal, plasma infusion or exchange (especially in the presence a detectable ADAMTS-13 inhibitor) should commence. The baby should be delivered as soon as possible using induction via the vaginal route or by Caesarean section, depending on fetal age and maternal condition.

Other thrombotic microangiopathies

Some patients develop the characteristic clinical manifestations of thrombotic microangiopathy without either overt associated conditions or plasma ADAMTS-13 deficiency (at least as measured by techniques currently available) [76,80,81,116,117]. The etiology of the disorder in this subgroup of patients, who have a higher mortality rate than patients with severe ADAMTS-13 deficiency, is unknown. In some of these patients, any possible relationship with ADAMTS-13 deficiency is clouded by the transfusion of normal blood products containing ADAMTS-13 before the testing of patient plasma for enzyme activity [25].

Neither bone marrow/stem cell transplantation-associated thrombotic microangiopathy nor diarrhea-associated HUS (caused by Shiga toxin-producing enterohemorrhagic *E. coli)* is usually associated with an absence or severely reduced level of plasma ADAMTS-13 activity [12,41,80,118,119]. The explanation for VWF abnormalities in the plasma of some chemotherapy/transplant-associated thrombotic microangiopathy patients [15] is not known.

Differential diagnosis

The initial diagnostic algorithm should include a review of the blood counts and peripheral blood smear, and ordering of additional laboratory studies (LDH, creatinine, prothrombin time and activated partial thromboplastin time, D-dimer and fibrinogen levels, and direct Coombs' test). The constellation of thrombocytopenia, hemolysis with schistocytosis, and LDH elevation also occurs (to an extent that is usually less extreme than in TTP) in HUS, disseminated intravascular coagulation (DIC), pre-eclampsia/eclampsia, the HELLP syndrome (pre-eclampsia-associated hemolytic anemia with elevated liver enzymes and low platelets), malignant hypertension, severe vasculitis, scleroderma with associated hypertension and renal failure, Evans' syndrome (concurrent autoantibody-mediated thrombocytopenia and hemolysis with positive direct Coombs' test), malfunctioning prosthetic cardiac valve, and, occasionally, after cocaine use [7,120]. Heparin-induced thrombocytopenia/thrombosis (HITT), which causes progressive thrombocytopenia and thrombosis, is not usually accompanied by schistocytes.

Among all of the above entities, only familial and acquired idiopathic types of TTP are associated with absent or severely reduced plasma ADAMTS-13 levels.

Hemolytic–uremic syndrome (HUS)

Platelet adhesion/aggregations on uncleaved ULVWF multimeric strings in the microcirculation in TTP produce fluctuating ischemia or infarction in various organs, including the brain in 50–71% of episodes [95,96]. In the closely related hemolytic–uremic syndrome (HUS), initially reported by Gasser and colleagues in 1955 [121], the ischemia is predominantly renal as a consequence of platelet adhesion/aggregation and fibrin polymer formation atop glomerular endothelial cells. Thrombocytopenia, erythrocyte fragmentation, and increased serum levels of LDH are often less extreme in HUS. However, the variability of organ dysfunction in TTP (including minor to modest renal abnormalities in 50–75% of episodes) [95] and the extrarenal manifestations that may complicate HUS can make the two syndromes difficult to distinguish [7,57,95,96,122]. Furthermore, clinical presentations resembling either TTP or HUS are sometimes associated with similar underlying conditions (e.g. transplantation, chemotherapy/total-body irradiation).

Clinical features, laboratory findings, causes and pathophysiology

HUS is a triad of thrombocytopenia, acute renal failure, and intravascular hemolytic anemia with schistocytosis and elevated serum LDH. Renal dysfunction is severe in HUS, in contrast to most cases of TTP, and often requires dialysis. Oliguria, anuria, chronic renal failure, and hypertension may complicate HUS, whereas this is uncommon in patients who recover from episodes of TTP. Although the microvascular thrombi in HUS are usually predominantly renal, other organs are sometimes involved [7,122,123]. Especially in children, HUS is frequently preceded by hemorrhagic enterocolitis caused by cytotoxin-producing serotypes of *Escherichia coli* (e.g. O157:H7) or *Shigella* species [7,122,124,125]. Shiga toxin (Stx)-1 and Stx-2 produced by enterohemorrhagic *E. coli* usually cause diarrhea-associated HUS. This relatively common disorder is characterized by obstruction of the glomerular microvasculature by platelet–fibrin thrombi, acute renal failure, thrombocytopenia, intravascular hemolytic anemia, elevated plasma VWF antigen, and plasma levels of ADAMTS-13 activity that are within a broad normal range. This latter finding may partially explain the poor response of these patients to plasma infusion or exchange [7,12,41].

It was recently demonstrated [126] that Stx-1 and Stx-2 stimulate the rapid and profuse secretion of unusually large ULVWF multimeric strings from human endothelial cells, including glomerular microvascular endothelial cells. Perfused normal human platelets immediately adhere to the secreted ULVWF multimeric strings, and the rate of ULVWF–platelet string cleavage by ADAMTS-13 is delayed in the presence of Stx-1 or Stx-2. These studies suggest that Stx-induced formation of ULVWF strings, along with impairment of ULVWF–platelet string cleavage by ADAMTS-13, explain the initial platelet adhesion atop Stx-stimulated glomerular endothelial cells in diarrhea-associated HUS. The findings may explain glomerular microvascular occlusion and acute renal failure, associated with consumptive thrombocytopenia, in diarrhea-associated HUS [126].

Recurrent episodes are common in familial TTP. Truly recurrent TTP episodes (i.e. not a single protracted episode with brief intervening periods of incomplete remission) [96] occur in about one-third of acquired idiopathic TTP patients. In contrast, diarrhea-associated HUS usually occurs as a single episode.

Some patients, however, have a familial and recurrent type of the disease. In these latter patients (often children), the level of the plasma complement control protein, factor H, may be abnormally low. The result is excessive activation of complement component 3 (C3) whenever the alternative complement pathway is stimulated [127,128]. A similar clinical syndrome results from deficiency in another alternative complement pathway C3 control substance, membrane cofactor protein (MCP) [127,128], or from deficiency of C3b-cleaving protease (C3 inactivator, or factor I) [129].

In adults, a thrombotic microangiopathy that clinically more often resembles HUS than TTP may follow (sometimes after weeks to months) the administration of mitomycin, cyclosporin, bone marrow or solid organ transplantation, total-body irradiation, gemcitabine or multiple chemotherapeutic agents [20,130,131]. More recent exposure to quinine also induces a similar syndrome. Plasma ADAMTS-13 levels are within a broad normal range, and the pathophysiology of these entities is currently unknown [7,119].

If excessive microvascular platelet adhesion/aggregation is systemic and extensive, and especially if the central nervous system is involved, the disorder is usually called "TTP." If platelet adhesion/aggregation (and secondary fibrin formation) predominantly involves the kidneys, the patient is considered to have "HUS". Severe renal involvement in a "TTP" patient, or extrarenal manifestations in a patient with "HUS," can cloud clinical boundaries between the two syndromes. This situation will persist until there are rapid, trustworthy and accessible clinical laboratory tests available for plasma ADAMTS-13 activity. Furlan and colleagues initially reported in 1998 that patients diagnosed with TTP usually have little or no plasma ADAMTS-13 activity, in contrast to the normal (or nearly normal) levels in patients considered to have acquired idiopathic HUS [12,65,66]. This may eventually provide the laboratory basis for more rapid and precise differentiation of the two entities.

Treatment

Neither plasma infusion nor exchange is consistently useful in Shiga toxin-induced HUS [7]. Discontinuation of any putative disease-inducing drug should occur immediately. Patients in the "pathogenesis-unknown" category of thrombotic microangiopathies often also respond poorly to plasma exchange [7,20]. It has been demonstrated recently, however, that some of these latter patients may improve in association with exchange [76]. It is, therefore, appropriate to commence daily plasma exchange procedures and continue for a sufficient period to determine effectiveness.

Several patients with HUS-like thrombotic microangiopathy following solid organ transplantation have been reported to respond to plasma exchange plus intravenous IgG [132,133]. Plasma adsorption over staphylococcal protein A columns was reported in one 1986 study to be useful in thrombotic microangiopathy associated with mitomycin C exposure [134].

HELLP syndrome

The constellation of severe eclampsia, hemolysis and thrombocytopenia was initially described by Stahnke in 1922 [135]. Pritchard et al. [136] subsequently described three other cases and suggested that an immunologic process might account for both the pre-eclampsia/eclampsia and the hematologic abnormalities. Although initially known as edema–proteinuria–hypertension gestosis type B [137], the more enduring "HELLP syndrome" (*h*emolysis, *el*evated *l*iver enzymes in serum, and *l*ow *p*latelets) was applied to this life-threatening pre-eclampsia/eclampsia complication by Weinstein in 1982 [138].

Clinical features

HELLP syndrome occurs in approximately 5 per 1000 pregnancies [139], in 4–12% of pregnancies complicated by pre-eclampsia, and in 30–50% of pregnancies complicated by eclampsia. About 15% of women ultimately diagnosed with HELLP syndrome do not have either hypertension or proteinuria [140]. Two-thirds of HELLP diagnoses are made antepartum, frequently between 27 and 37 weeks, and more often in white, multiparous women over 34 years of age. HELLP is diagnosed in the remaining third within hours to 6 days following delivery (the majority within 48 hours [141–143]). Although the homozygous cytidine to thymidine polymorphism at position 677 of the methylenetetrahydrofolate reductase gene may be a modest risk factor for pre-eclampsia, this is not true for HELLP syndrome [144]. Whether or not either the factor V Leiden or the prothrombin 20210 gene mutations is a risk factor for HELLP is controversial [145–147].

Most (90%) HELLP patients have malaise and right upper quadrant or epigastric pain; 45–86% have nausea or vomiting; 55–67% have edema; 31–50% have headache; and a few report visual changes. Fever is atypical. Hypertension is found in 85% [140].

Laboratory features

Schistocytes, consistent with microangiopathic hemolytic anemia, are seen on the peripheral blood films of 54–86% of patients [140]. Reticulocytosis can be present. Absent haptoglobin levels indicate intravascular hemolysis [148,149]. Haptoglobin often returns to normal within 24–48 hours postpartum [149].

The serum LDH level is increased considerably above normal. The ratio of LDH 5 (LDH isoenzyme found specifically in the liver) to total LDH has been reported to be elevated in proportion to the severity of pre-eclampsia [150]. The elevated LDH value is, therefore, more likely due to liver damage than intravascular hemolysis [149]. Serum levels of aspartic acid transaminase (AST) and alanine transaminase (ALT) can be increased by 100-fold; in contrast, elevations of alkaline phosphatase and total bilirubin are usually less extreme. In most patients, liver enzymes return to baseline values within 3–5 days postpartum [140]

The severity of thrombocytopenia has been utilized to predict maternal morbidity and mortality, rapidity of postpartum recovery, risk of disease recurrence, perinatal outcome, and the need for plasmapheresis. In this "Mississippi triple class system," patients with platelet counts below 50 000/μL are "class 1" (13% incidence of bleeding); those with platelets of 50 000–100 000/μL are "class 2" (8% incidence of bleeding); and those with platelets over 100 000/μL are "class 3" (no increased bleeding) [142,143]. Patients with "class 1" HELLP syndrome have the highest incidence of perinatal morbidity and mortality, and the most protracted recovery postpartum [143]. Thiagarajah et al. [151] also found a direct correlation between the severity of thrombocytopenia and liver enzyme abnormalities; however, this association was not observed when the underlying hepatic histopathologic abnormalities were reviewed [152].

Abundant megakaryocytes are found bone by bone marrow aspiration/biopsy, consistent with a consumptive thrombocytopenia (platelet life span reduced from ~ 10 to 3–5 days [143]). The platelet count nadir usually occurs 23–29 hours postpartum, with subsequent normalization within 6–11 days [142,143].

The prothrombin time (PT) is usually within normal limits, and the activated partial thromboplastin time (APTT) can be either normal or prolonged. Although low fibrinogen levels are inconsistently found, other indicators of increased coagulation and secondary fibrinolysis may be positive. These include decreased protein C and antithrombin III (AT III) levels, and increased D-dimer and thrombin-ATIII values [153].

In some patients, hepatic ultrasonography reveals large, irregular, well-demarcated areas of increased echogenicity [154]. Biopsy samples may show periportal or focal necrosis, fibrin deposits in the sinusoids, and vascular microthrombi. As the disease progresses, large areas of necrosis can coalesce and dissect into the liver capsule, producing subcapsular hematomas or hepatic rupture [139].

Causes and pathogenesis

Trophoblastic invasion into the decidua during normal pregnancy occurs at 10–12 days, and again at 16–22 weeks. These specialized placental epithelial cells replace the endothelium of uterine spiral arteries and intercalate within the arterial muscular tunica, thereby increasing vessel diameter (and decreasing resistance). As a result, the spiral arteries are remodeled into hybrid vessels composed of fetal and maternal cells with a high flow/low resistance design that is protective against the effects of vasoconstrictors circulating in the maternal bloodstream [155]. In a pre-eclamptic pregnancy, the second wave of trophoblastic invasion fails to penetrate the spiral arteries of the uterus completely, possibly because of inadequate placental expression of syncytin-mediated cell fusion processes during placentogenesis [156]. As a consequence, the poorly perfused placenta may release factors that include soluble fms-like tyrosine kinase 1 (sFlt-1), an anti-angiogenic protein that binds placental growth factor and vascular endothelial growth factor (VEGF) and prevents their interaction with endothelial cell receptors. The result may be endothelial dysfunction [157] with increased vascular tone, alteration of prostacyclin/thromboxane ratios, and enhanced platelet adhesion/aggregation. Excessive thrombin generation may occur, and this potentiates further activation of the coagulation cascade, systemic platelet and fibrin polymer deposition in capillaries, additional platelet aggregation and thrombocytopenia, and multiorgan microvascular obstruction. The microvascular obstruction is the likely cause of the microangiopathic hemolytic anemia and the enzyme release from ischemic, injured or necrotic hepatic cells [139].

In one study [158], all women with HELLP syndrome had modestly lower plasma levels of ADAMTS-13 activity (median, 31% of normal) than healthy pregnant (71%) or non-pregnant women (101%). These lower plasma ADAMTS-13 values, which are distinct from the absent or severely reduced plasma levels in many patients with TTP, normalized (to 115%) as the HELLP patients recovered. Inactivating autoantibodies against ADAMTS-13 were not detected in HELLP plasma, in contrast to patients with acquired idiopathic TTP. The levels of VWF antigen in this HELLP study were higher than the (elevated) levels associated with normal pregnancy, perhaps because of endothelial cell injury or excessive stimulation in HELLP. ULVWF multimers have not been found to be circulating in HELLP plasma [158,159], in contrast to the plasma of patients with congenital TTP (and sometimes acquired idiopathic TTP).

Treatment

Therapy for HELLP includes intravenous magnesium sulfate to prevent eclamptic seizures, control of hypertension, management of fluids and electrolytes, transfusion of red cells and/or platelets, as needed, possible stimulation of fetal lung maturation with betamethasone if less than 34 weeks and delivery is to be delayed, and consideration of rapid delivery [143]. Indications for immediate delivery include maternal or fetal distress, worsening symptoms and signs of HELLP syndrome, and under most circumstances a gestational age of greater than 32 weeks [140]. Cesarean section under general anesthesia is used in 60–97% of cases; however, induction of labor and vaginal delivery is a consideration if the maternal and fetal condition are favorable. Whether or not postpartum curettage is helpful in lowering the mean arterial pressure and increasing urinary output and platelet count is not resolved [143,160].

Adjunctive antepartum and postpartum therapy for HELLP with dexamethasone and plasma exchange have been reported [142,161,162]. Dexamethasone (10 mg intravenously every 12 hours) is believed by some to increase urinary output and platelet count, decrease AST and LDH levels and decrease time to delivery, and may reduce neonatal morbidity/mortality [142], without affecting the rate of infection or maternal recovery postpartum. Those who support steroid use have recommended continued use for at least 2 days following delivery, in order to prevent a recurrence of liver enzyme elevation (including LDH), thrombocytopenia and oliguria [143]. Not all studies have been positive, however, and Fonseca et al. [161] reported no benefit in the resolution of HELLP syndrome with dexamethasone in a prospective, double-blind, placebo-controlled, clinical trial in 132 women. The patients in the steroid group received 10-mg doses of dexamethasone intravenously every 12 hours until delivery and three additional doses after delivery. Puerperal women received three 10-mg doses of dexamethasone after delivery. The same schedule was used in the placebo group. Although the main outcome variable was the duration of hospitalization, other parameters evaluated were time to recovery of laboratory and clinical parameters, as well as frequency of complications. The mean duration of hospitalization was not significantly affected by the dexamethasone treatment (6.5 vs 8.2 days; $p = 0.37$) and there were no significant differences between the two groups in terms of the time to recovery of the platelet count (hazard ratio [HR] 1.2; 95% CI 0.8–1.8), lactate dehydrogenase (HR 0.9; 95% CI 0.5–1.5), aspartate aminotransferase (HR 0.6; 95% CI 0.4–1.1), or development of complications. These results were similar in both pregnant and puerperal women. Matchaba and Moodley [162] published a review on the subject in 2004 in the Cochrane Library. They reviewed five studies ($n = 170$), of which three were antepartum and two postpartum. In four of the studies patients were randomised to standard therapy or dexamethasone. One study compared dexamethasone with betamethasone. There were no significant differences in the primary outcomes of maternal mortality and morbidity due to placental abruption, pulmonary edema, or liver hematoma and rupture. Analysis of the secondary maternal outcomes demonstrated a tendency to a greater platelet count increase over 48 hours, statistically significantly shorter hospital stay (weighted mean difference (WMD) –4.50 days; 95%

CI −7.13 to −1.87), mean interval (hours) to delivery (41 ± 15) versus (15 ± 4.5) ($p = 0.0068$) in favor of women randomised to dexamethasone.

There were no significant differences in perinatal mortality or morbidity due to respiratory distress syndrome, need for ventilatory support, intracerebral hemorrhage, necrotizing enterocolitis and a 5-min Apgar less than 7. The mean birthweight was significantly greater in the group allocated to dexamethasone (WMD 247.00; 95% CI 65.41–428.59). These authors concluded that based on these five studies there was insufficient evidence to determine whether adjunctive steroid use in HELLP syndrome decreases maternal and perinatal mortality, or major maternal and perinatal morbidity.

Antepartum plasma exchanges do not arrest or reverse HELLP syndrome; however, peripartum exchanges may minimize hemorrhage and morbidity. Plasma exchanges should probably be employed in women who fail to improve within 72–96 hours after delivery. This is a subgroup of about 5% of HELLP patients who are usually either nulliparous or younger than 20 years of age [142,143]. Liver transplantation may eventually be necessary in cases complicated by large destructive hematomas or total hepatic necrosis [163]

Although the condition of most HELLP patients stabilizes within 24–48 hours following delivery, death occurs in 3–5%. Maternal mortality rates as high as 25% were reported prior to 1980, usually because of cerebral hemorrhage, cardiopulmonary arrest, DIC, adult respiratory distress syndrome, or hypoxic ischemic encephalopathy [139]. Other complications can include infection, abruptio placentae, postpartum hemorrhage, intra-abdominal bleeding, pulmonary edema, retinal detachment, postictal cortical blindness, hypoglycemic coma, and subcapsular liver hematoma with subsequent rupture (mortality about 50%) [140,164]. Patients with the latter complication may complain of right-sided shoulder pain, and may develop shock with ascites and/or pleural effusions. Hepatic hematomas are usually in the anterior superior right lobe. Deep and repeated abdominal palpation, seizures, or vomiting makes rupture and catastrophic hemorrhage more likely. The safest therapy for hepatic rupture in HELLP syndrome is to pack the liver and abdomen, place a large-bore drain to monitor continued bleeding, close the abdomen and continue supportive therapy with blood and blood product (including activated factor VIIa) transfusion [165,166]. Emergent hepatic artery embolization or ligation, and lobectomy, have been attempted but are associated with significantly worse outcome than the "pack and support" approach. In some cases where total liver shutdown has occurred following massive necrosis, liver transplantation may be necessary [139,143].

Renal complications of HELLP may include transient elevation of serum creatinine, hyponatremia, nephrogenic diabetes insipidus, or acute renal failure. Nephrogenic diabetes insipidus may result in HELLP syndrome from the impaired hepatic metabolism of placental-produced vasopressinase. This inadequately metabolized vasopressinase is postulated to cause excessive breakdown of antidiuretic hormone (vasopressin) produced by the posterior pituitary gland, and "resistance to vasopressin" [164,167]. The small subset of patients with progressive deterioration of renal function after delivery may require either temporary or permanent hemodialysis.

Fetal morbidity and mortality, once estimated to be anywhere from 5 to 100%, has now decreased to between 9 and 24% [140]. Fetal complications are usually due to prematurity, placental abruption, and intrauterine hypoxia or asphyxia. Some infants (39%) of HELLP syndrome mothers have intrauterine growth restriction (IUGR), and about one-third have thrombocytopenia. Intraventricular hemorrhage occurs in 4% of infants with severe thrombocytopenia [168].

HELLP syndrome itself has been reported to recur in up to 27% of women during subsequent pregnancies [139] and the incidence of any hypertensive disorder of pregnancy (eclampsia, pre-eclampsia, or gestational hypertension) is of the order of 30% in women with previous preterm HELLP syndrome who have another pregnancy [169].

Differential diagnosis

Complications of pregnancy that may be confused with HELLP include TTP, HUS, DIC, sepsis, connective tissue disorders, antiphospholipid antibody syndrome, and acute fatty liver of pregnancy. This latter entity is also seen in the last trimester or postpartum, and presents with thrombocytopenia and right upper quadrant pain; however, the serum levels of AST and ALT increase more modestly (up to about fivefold) and the PT and APTT are both consistently prolonged. Liver biopsy samples reveal inflammation and patchy hepatocellular necrosis, and specific staining demonstrates fat in the cytoplasm of centrilobular hepatocytes.

Because it can cause right upper quadrant pain and nausea, HELLP has been misdiagnosed as viral hepatitis, biliary colic, esophageal reflux, cholecystitis, and gastric ulcer. Conversely, other conditions misdiagnosed as HELLP syndrome have included cardiomyopathy, dissecting aortic aneurysm, acute cocaine intoxication, essential hypertension with renal disease, and alcoholic liver dysfunction [143].

References

1 Moschcowitz E. Hyaline thrombosis of the terminal arterioles and capillaries: a hitherto undescribed disease. *Proc NY Pathol Soc* 1924; 24: 21–24.

2 Moschcowitz E. An acute febrile pleiochromic anamia with hyaline thrombosis of the terminal arterioles and capillaries. *Arch Intern Med* 1925; 36: 89–93.

3 Burns ER, Lou Y, Pathak A. Morphologic diagnosis of thrombotic thrombocytopenic purpura. *Am J Hematol* 2004; 75: 18–21.

4 James T, Monto R. Pathology of the cardiac conduction system in thrombotic thrombocytopenic purpura. *Ann Intern Med* 1966; 65: 37–43.

5 Bell M, Barnhart J, Martin JM. Thrombotic throbocytopenic purpura causing sudden unexpected death – a series of eight patients. *J Forens Sci* 1990; 35: 601–613.
6 Ridolfi R, Hutchins G, Bell WR. The heart and cardiac conduction system in thrombotic thrombocytopenic purpura. A clinicopathologic study of 17 autopsied patients. *Ann Intern Med* 1979; 91: 357–363.
7 Moake JL. Thrombotic microangiopathies. *N Engl J Med* 2002; 347: 589–600.
8 Furlan M, Robles R, Solenthaler M, et al. Deficient activity of von Willebrand factor-cleaving protease in chronic relapsing thrombotic thrombocytopenic purpura. *Blood* 1997; 89: 3097–3103.
9 Moake J, Rudy CK, Troll J, et al. Unusually large plasma factor VIII: von Willebrand factor multimers in chronic relapsing thrombotic thrombocytopenic purpura. *N Engl J Med* 1982; 307: 1432–1435.
10 Moake J, Chintagumpala M, Turner N, et al. Solvent/detergent-treated plasma suppresses shear-induced platelet aggregation and prevents episodes of thrombotic thrombocytopenic purpura. *Blood* 1994; 84: 490–497.
11 Bennett C, Davidson CS, Raisch DW, et al. Thrombotic thrombocytopenic purpura associated with ticlopidine: a review of 60 cases. *Ann Intern Med* 1998; 128: 541–544.
12 Tsai HM, Chandler WL, Sarode R, et al. von Willebrand factor and von Willebrand factor-cleaving metalloprotease activity in Escherichia coli 0157:H7-associated hemolytic uremic syndrome. *Pediatr Res* 2001;49: 653–659.
13 Bennett C, Connors JM, Carwile JM, et al. Thrombotic thrombocytopenic purpura associated with clopidogrel. *N Engl J Med* 2000; 342: 1773–1777.
14 Atkinson K, Biggs J, Hayes J, et al. Cyclosporin A associated nephrotoxicity in the first 100 days after allogeneic bone marrow transplantation: three distinct syndromes. *Br J Haematol* 1983; 54: 59–67.
15 Charba D, Moake J, Harris M, Hester JP. Abnormalities of von Willebrand factor multimers in drug- associated thrombotic microangiopathies. *Am J Hematol* 1993; 42: 268–277.
16 Gottschall J, et al. Quinine-induced immune thrombocytopenia associated with hemolytic-uremic syndrome: a new clinical entity. *Blood* 1991; 77: 306–310.
17 Humphreys B, Sharman JP, Henderson JM, et al. Gemcitabine-associated thrombotic microangiopathy. *Cancer* 2004; 100: 2664–2670.
18 Kojouri K, Vesely SK, George JN. Quinine-associated thrombotic thrombocytopenic-hemolytic uremic syndrome: frequency, clinical features, and long-term outcomes. *Ann Intern Med* 2001; 135: 1047–1051.
19 Mach-Pascual S, Samii K, Beris P. Microangiopathic hemolytic anemia complicating FK506 (tacrolimus) therapy. *Am J Hematol* 1996; 52: 310–312.
20 Moake JL, Byrnes JJ. Thrombotic microangiopathies associated with drugs and bone marrow transplantation. *Hematol/Oncol Clin North Am* 1996; 10: 485–497.
21 Rabadi SJ, Khandekar JD, Miller HJ. Mitomycin-induced hemolytic uremic syndrome: case presentation and review of literature. *Cancer Treat Rep* 1982; 66: 1244–1247.
22 Singh N, Gayowski T, Marino IR. Hemolytic uremic syndrome in solid-organ transplant recipients. *Transplant Int* 1996; 9: 68–75.
23 Venat-Bouvet L, Ly K, Szelag JC, et al. Thrombotic microangiopathy and digital necrosis: two unrecognized toxicities of gemcitabine. *Anticancer Drugs* 2003; 14: 829–832.
24 George JN. The association of pregnancy with thrombotic thrombocytopenic purpura-hemolytic uremic syndrome. *Curr Opin Hematol* 2003; 10: 339–344.
25 Sadler JE, Moake JL, Miyata T, George JN. Recent advances in thrombotic thrombocytopenic purpura. *Hematology (Am Soc Hematol Educ Program)* 2004; 407–423.
26 Vesely SK, Li X, McMinn JR, Terrell DR, George JN. Pregnancy outcomes after recovery from thrombotic thrombocytopenic purpura-hemolytic uremic syndrome. *Transfusion* 2004; 44: 1149–1158.
27 Anacleto FE, Cifra CL, Elises JS. Postpartum hemolytic uremic syndrome in a 17-year-old Filipina primigravid. *Pediatr Nephrol* 2003; 18: 1283–1285.
28 Dashe JS, Ramin SM, Cunningham FG. The long-term consequences of thrombotic microangiopathy (thrombotic thrombocytopenic purpura and hemolytic uremic syndrome) in pregnancy. *Obstet Gynecol* 1998; 91: 662–668.
29 Robson JS, Ruckley VA, MacDonald MK. Irreversible post partum renal failure. A new syndrome. *QJ Med* 1968; 37: 423.
30 Martinez-Roman S, Gratacos E, Torné A, et al. Successful pregnancy in a patient with hemolytic-uremic syndrome during the second trimester of pregnancy. *J Reprod Med* 1996; 41: 211–214.
31 Iannuzzi M, Siconolfi P, d'Angelilo A, et al. A post-partum hemolytic-uremic-like-syndrome in a patient with pre-eclampsia: description of a clinical case. *Transfus Apher Sci* 2006; 34: 11–14.
32 Ribeiro FM, Rocha E, Maccariello E, et al. Early gestational hemolytic uremic syndrome: case report and review of literature. *Ren Fail* 1997; 19: 475–479.
33 Banatvala N, Griffin PM, Greene KD, et al. The United States National Progressive Hemolytic Uremic Syndrome Study: microbiologic, serologic, clinical. and epidemiologic findings. *J Infect Dis* 2001; 183: 1063–1070.
34 Asada Y, Sumiyoshi A, Hayashi T, Suzumiya J, Kaketani K. Immunochemistry of vascular lesions in thrombotic thromocytopenic purpura, with special reference to factor VIII related antigen. *Throm Res* 1985; 38: 469–479.
35 Harkness DR, Byrnes JJ, Lian E, Williams W, Hensley GT. Hazard of platelet transfusion in thrombotic thrombocytopenic purpura. *JAMA* 1981; 246: 1931–1933.
36 Ruggeri ZM. Developing basic and clinical research on von Willebrand factor and von Willebrand disease. *Thromb Haemost* 2000; 84: 147–149.
37 Arya M, Anvari B, Romo GM, et al. Ultra-large multimers of von Willebrand factor form spontaneous high-strength bonds with the platelet GP Ib-IX complex: studies using optical tweezers. *Blood* 2002; 99: 3971–3977.
38 Moake JL, Turner NA, Stathopoulos NA, Nolasco LH, Hellums JD. Involvement of large plasma von Willebrand factor (vWF) multimers and unusually large vWF forms derived from endothelial cells in shear stress-induced platelet aggregation. *J Clin Invest* 1986; 78: 1456–1461.
39 Moake JL, Turner NA, Stathopoulos NA, Nolasco L, Hellums JD. Shear-induced platelet aggregation can be mediated by vWF released from platelets, as well as by exogenous large or unusually large vWF multimers, requires adenosine diphosphate, and is resistant to aspirin. *Blood* 1988; 71: 1366–1374.

40 Moake JL, Rudy CK, Troll JH, et al. Therapy of chronic relapsing thrombotic thrombocytopenic purpura with prednisone and azathioprine. *Am J Hematol* 1985; 20: 73–79.

41 Furlan M, Robles R, Galbusera M, et al. von Willebrand factor-cleaving protease in thrombotic thrombocytopenic purpura and hemolytic-uremic syndrome. *N Engl J Med* 1998; 339: 1578–1584.

42 Tsai HM, Lian E. Antibodies of von Willebrand factor cleaving protease in acute thrombotic thrombocytopenic purpura. *N Engl J Med* 1998; 339: 1585–1594.

43 Furlan M, Robles R, Lammle B. Partial purification and characterization of a protease from human plasma cleaving von Willebrand factor to fragments produced by in vivo proteolysis. *Blood* 1996; 87: 4223–4234.

44 Tsai HM. Physiologic cleavage of von Willebrand factor by a plasma protease is dependent on its confirmation and requires calcium ion. *Blood* 1996; 87: 4235–4244.

45 Tsai HM, Sussman II, Nagel RL. Shear stress enhances the proteolysis of von Willebrand factor in normal plasma. *Blood* 1994; 83: 2171–2179.

46 Fujikawa K, Suzuki H, McMullen B, Chung D. Purification of von Willebrand factor-cleaving protease and its identification as a new member of the metalloproteinase family. *Blood* 2001; 98: 1662–1666.

47 Zheng X, Chung D, Takayama TK, et al. Structure of von Willebrand factor-cleaving protease (ADAMTS13), a metalloprotease involved in thrombotic thrombocytopenic purpura. *J Biol Chem* 2001; 276: 41059–41063.

48 Bork P, Beckmann G. The CUB domain – a widespread module in developmentally regulated proteins. *J Molec Biol* 1993; 231: 530–545.

49 Shang D, Zheng XW, Niiya M, Zheng XL. Apical sorting of ADAMTS13 in vascular endothelial cells and Madin-Darby canine kidney cells depends on the CUB domains and their association with lipid rafts. *Blood* 2006; 108(7): 2207–2215.

50 Turner N, Nolasco L, Tao Z, Dong JF, Moake J. Human endothelial cells synthesize and release ADAMTS-13. *J Thromb Haemost* 2006; 4: 1396–1404.

51 Niiya M, Uemura M, Zheng XW, et al. Increased ADAMTS-13 proteolytic activity in rat hepatic stellate cells upon activation in vitro and in vivo. *J Thromb Haemost* 2006; 4: 1063–1070.

52 Uemura M, Tatsumi K, Matsumoto M, et al. Localization of ADAMTS13 to the stellate cells of human liver. *Blood* 2005; 106: 922–924.

53 Zhou W, Inada M, Lee TP, et al. ADAMTS13 is expressed in hepatic stellate cells. *Lab Invest* 2005; 85: 780–788.

54 Barbot J, Costa E, Guerra M, et al. Ten years of prophylactic treatment with fresh-frozen plasma in a child with chronic relapsing thrombotic thrombocytopenic purpura as a result of a congenital deficiency of von Willebrand factor-cleaving protease. *Br J Haematol* 2001; 113: 649–651.

55 Chung DW, Fujikawa K. Processing of von Willebrand factor by ADAMTS-13. *Biochemistry* 2002; 41: 11065–11070.

56 Dong JF, Moake JL, Bernardo A, et al. ADAMTS-13 metalloprotease interacts with the endothelial cell-derived ultra-large von Willebrand factor. *J Biol Chem* 2003; 278: 29633–29639.

57 Dong JF, Moake JL, Nolasco L, et al. ADAMTS-13 rapidly cleaves newly secreted ultralarge von Willebrand factor multimers on the endothelial surface under flowing conditions. *Blood* 2002; 100: 4033–4039.

58 Padilla A, Moake JL, Bernardo A, et al. P-selectin anchors newly released ultralarge von Willebrand factor multimers to the endothelial cell surface. *Blood* 2004; 103: 2150–2156.

59 Bernardo A, Ball C, Nolasco L, Moake JL, Dong JF. Effects of inflammatory cytokines on the release and cleavage of the endothelial cell-derived ultralarge von Willebrand factor multimers under flow. *Blood* 2004; 104: 100–106.

60 Tao Z, Wang Y, Choi H, et al. Peptides from the C-terminal regions of ADAMTS-13 specifically block cleavage of ultra-large von Willebrand factor multimers on the endothelial surface under flow. *J Thromb Haemost* 2003; 1 July, Abstract #OC405 (2003).

61 Majerus EM, Anderson PJ, Sadler JE. Binding of ADAMTS13 to von Willebrand factor. *J Biol Chem* 2005; 280: 21773–21778.

62 Tao Z, Peng Y, Nolasco L, et al. Recombinant CUB-1 domain polypeptide inhibits the cleavage of ULVWF strings by ADAMTS13 under flow conditions. *Blood* 2005; 106: 4139–4145.

63 Nishio K, Anderson PJ, Zheng XL, Sadler JE. Binding of platelet glycoprotein Ibalpha to von Willebrand factor domain A1 stimulates the cleavage of the adjacent domain A2 by ADAMTS13. *Proc Natl Acad Sci USA* 2004; 101: 10578–10583.

64 Moake JL, McPherson PD. Abnormalities of von Willebrand factor multimers in thrombotic thrombocytopenic purpura and hemolytic-uremic syndrome. *Am J Med* 1989; 87: 9N–15N.

65 Furlan M, Robles R, Solenthaler M, Lammle B. Acquired deficiency of von Willebrand factor-cleaving protease in a patient with thrombotic thrombocytopenic purpura. *Blood* 1998; 91: 2839–2846.

66 Bianchi V, Robles R, Alberio L, Furlan M, Lammle B. Von Willebrand factor-cleaving protease (ADAMTS13) in thrombotic thrombocytopenic disorders: a severely deficient activity is specific for thrombotic thrombocytopenic purpura. *Blood* 2002; 100: 710–713.

67 Bernardo A, Ball C, Nolasco L, et al. Platelets adhered to endothelial cell-bound ultra-large von Willebrand factor strings support leukocyte tethering and rolling under high shear stress. *J Thromb Haemost* 2005; 3: 562–570.

68 Allford SL, Harrison P, Lawrie AS, et al. Von Willebrand factor-cleaving protease in congenital thrombotic thrombocytopenic purpura. *Br J Haematol* 2000; 111: 1215–1222.

69 Furlan M, Robles R, Morselli B, Sandoz P, Lammle B. Recovery and half-life of von Willebrand factor-cleaving protease after plasma therapy in patients with thrombotic thrombocytopenic purpura. *Thromb Haemost* 1999; 81: 8–13.

70 Levy GA, Nichols WC, Lian EC, et al. Mutations in a member of the ADAMTS gene family cause thrombotic thrombocytopenic purpura. *Nature* 2001; 413: 488–494.

71 Pimanda JE, Maekawa A, Wind T, et al. Congenital thrombotic thrombocytopenic purpura in association with a mutation in the second CUB domain of ADAMTS13. *Blood* 2004; 103: 627–629.

72 Furlan M, Lammle B. Aetiology and pathogenesis of thrombotic thrombocytopenic purpura and the haemolytic syndrome: the role of von Willebrand factor-cleaving protease. *Best Pract Res Clin Haematol* 2001; 14: 437–454.

73 Veyradier A, Obert B, Haddad E, et al. Severe deficiency of the specific von Willebrand factor-cleaving protease (ADAMTS 13) activity in a subgroup of children with atypical hemolytic uremic syndrome. *J Pediatr* 2003; 142: 310–317.

74 Schulman I, Pierce M, Lukens A, Currimbhoy Z. Studies on thrombopoiesis. I. A factor in normal human plasma required for platelet production; chronic thrombocytopenia due to its deficiency. *Blood* 1960; 16: 943–957.

75 Upshaw JD Jr. Congenital deficiency of a factor in normal plasma that reverses microangiopathic hemolysis and thrombocytopenia. *N Engl J Med* 1978; 298: 1350–1352.

76 Vesely SK, George JN, Lammle B, et al. ADAMTS13 activity in thrombotic thrombocytopenic purpura-hemolytic uremic syndrome: relation to presenting features and clinical outcomes in a prospective cohort of 142 patients. *Blood* 2003; 102: 60–68.

77 Veyradier A, Girma JP. Assays of ADAMTS-13 activity. *Semin Hematol* 2004; 41: 41–47.

78 Tsai HM, Rice L, Sarode R, Chow TW, Moake JL. Antibody inhibitors to von Willebrand factor metalloproteinase and increased von Willebrand factor-platelet binding in ticlopidine-associated thrombotic thrombocytopenic purpura. *Ann Intern Med* 2000; 132: 794–799.

79 Klaus C, Plaimauer B, Studt J, et al. Epitope mapping of ADAMTS13 autoantibodies in acquired thrombotic thrombocytopenic purpura. *Blood* 2004; 103(12): 4514–4519.

80 Veyradier A, Obert B, Houllier A, Meyer D, Girma JP. Specific von Willebrand factor-cleaving protease in thrombotic microangiopathies: a study of 111 cases. *Blood* 2001; 98: 1765–1762.

81 Zheng XL, Kaufman RM, Goodnough LT, Sadler JE. Effect of plasma exchange on plasma ADAMTS13 metalloprotease activity, inhibitor level, and clinical outcome in patients with idiopathic and non-idiopathic thrombotic thrombocytopenic purpura. *Blood* 2004; 103(11): 4043–4049.

82 Oleksowicz L, Bhagwati N, DeLeon-Fernandez M. Deficient activity of von Willebrand's factor-cleaving protease in patients with disseminated malignancies. *Cancer Res* 1999; 59: 2244–2250.

83 Mannucci PM, Canciani MT, Forza I, et al. Changes in health and disease of the metalloprotease that cleaves von Willebrand factor. *Blood* 2001; 98: 2730–2735.

84 Neame PD. Immunologic and other factors in thrombotic thrombocytopenic purpura (TTP). *Semin Thromb Hemost* 1980; 6: 416–429.

85 Wada H, Kaneko T, Ohiwa M, et al. Plasma cytokine levels in thrombotic thrombocytopenic purpura. *Am J Hematol* 1992; 40: 167–170.

86 Zauli G, Gugliotta L, Catani L, et al. Increased serum levels of transforming growth factor beta-1 in patients affected by thrombotic thrombocytopenic purpura (TTP): its implications on bone marrow haematopoiesis. *Br J Haematol* 1993; 84: 381–386.

87 Joseph G, Smith KJ, Hadley TJ, et al. HLA-DR53 protects against thrombotic thrombocytopenic purpura/adult hemolytic uremic syndrome. *Am J Hematol* 1994; 47: 189–193.

88 Nesher G, Hanna VE, Moore TL, Hersh M, Osborn TG. Thrombotic microangiographic hemolytic anemia in systemic lupus erythematosus. *Semin Arthritis Rheum* 1994; 24: 165–172.

89 Zacharski LR, Lusted D, Glick JL. Thrombotic thrombocytopenic purpura in a previously splenectomized patient. *Am J Med* 1976; 60: 1061–1063.

90 Leaf AN, Laubenstein LJ, Raphael B, et al. Thrombotic thrombocytopenic purpura associated with human immunodeficiency virus type 1 (HIV-1) infection. *Ann Intern Med* 1988; 109: 194–197.

91 Nair JM, Bellevue R, Bertoni M, Dosik H. Thrombotic thrombocytopenic purpura in patients with the acquired immunodeficiency syndrome (AIDS)-related complex. A report of two cases. *Ann Intern Med* 1988; 109: 209–212.

92 Yospur LS, Sun NC, Figueroa P, Niihara Y. Concurrent thrombotic thrombocytopenic purpura and immune thrombocytopenic purpura in an HIV-positive patient: case report and review of the literature. *Am J Hematol* 1996; 51: 73–78.

93 Byrnes JJ, Khurana M. Treatment of thrombotic thrombocytopenic purpura with plasma. *N Engl J Med* 1977; 297: 1386–1389.

94 Frangos JA, Moake JL, Nolasco L, Phillips MD, McIntireL V. Cryosupernatant regulates accumulation of unusually large vWF multimers from endothelial cells. *Am J Physiol* 1989; 256: H1635–44.

95 Rock GA, Shumak KH, Buskard NA, et al. Comparison of plasma exchange with plasma infusion in the treatment of thrombotic thrombocytopenic purpura. *N Engl J Med* 1991; 325: 393–397.

96 Bell WR, Braine HG, Ness PM, Kickler TS. Improved survival in thrombotic thrombocytopenic purpura-hemolytic-uremic syndrome clinical experience in 108 patients. *N Engl J Med* 1991; 325: 398–403.

97 Tsai HM. High titers of inhibitors of von Willebrand factor-cleaving metalloproteinase in a fatal case of acute thrombotic thrombocytopenic purpura. *Am J Hematol* 2000; 65: 251–255.

98 Tsai HM, Li A, Rock G. Inhibitors of von Willebrand factor-cleaving protease in thrombotic thrombocytopenic purpura. *Clin Lab* 2001; 47: 387–392.

99 Chemnitz J, Draube A, Scheid C, et al. Successful treatment of severe thrombotic thrombocytopenic purpura with the monoclonal antibody rituximab. *Am J Hematol* 2002; 71: 105.

100 Gutterman LA, Kloster B, Tsai HM. Rituximab therapy for refractory thrombotic thrombocytopenic purpura. *Blood Cells Mol Dis* 2002; 28: 385.

101 Reff M, Carner K, Chambers K, et al. Depletion of B cells in vivo by a chimeric mouse human monoclonal antibody to CD20. *Blood* 1994; 83: 435–445.

102 Tsai HM, Shulman K. Rituximab induces remission of cerebral ischemia caused by thrombotic thrombocytopenic purpura. *Eur J Haematol* 2003; 70: 183–185.

103 Zheng X, Pallera AM, Goodnough LT, Sadler JE, Blinder MA. Remission of chronic thrombotic thrombocytopenic purpura after treatment with cyclophosphamide and rituximab. *Ann Intern Med* 2003; 138: 105–108.

104 Cataland SR, Jin M, Zheng XL, George JN, Wu HM. An evaluation of cyclosporine alone for the treatment of early recurrences of thombotic thrombocytopenic purpura. *J Thromb Haemost* 2006; 4(5): 1162–1164.

105 Crowther MA, Heddle N, Hayward CPM, Warkentin T, Kelton JG. Splenectomy done during hematologic remission to prevent relapse in patients with thrombotic thrombocytopenic purpura. *Ann Intern Med* 1996; 125: 294–296.

106 Kremer Hovinga JA, Studt JD, Demarmels Biasuitti F, et al. Splenectomy in relapsing and plasma-refractory acquired thrombotic thrombocytopenic purpura. *Haematologica* 2004; 89: 320–324.

107 Thompson CE, Damon LE, Ries CA, Linker CA. Thrombotic microangiopathics in the 1980s: clinical features, response to treatment, and the impact of the human immunodeficiency virus epidemic. *Blood* 1992; 80: 1890–1895.

108 Gordon LI, Kwaan HC, Rossi EC. Deleterious effects of platelet transfusions and recovery thrombocytosis in patients with thrombotic microangiopathy. *Semin Hematol* 1987; 24: 194–201.

109 Bandarenko N, Brecher ME. United States Thrombotic Thrombocytopenic Purpura Apheresis Study Group (US TTP ASG):

multicenter survey and retrospective analysis of current efficacy of therapeutic plasma exchange. *J Clin Apher* 1998; 13: 133–141.

110 Egan JA, Hay SN, Brecher ME. Frequency and significance of schistocytes in TTP/HUS patients at the discontinuation of plasma exchange therapy. *J Clin Apher* 2004; 19: 165–167.

111 Gutterman LA, Stevenson TD. Treatment of thrombotic thrombocytopenic purpura with vincristine. *JAMA* 1982; 247: 1433–1436.

112 Rosove MH, Ho WG, Goldfinger D. Ineffectiveness of aspirin and dipyridamole in the treatment of thrombotic thrombocytopenic purpura. *Ann Intern Med* 1982; 96: 27–33.

113 Plaimauer B, Zimmerman K, Volkel D, et al. Cloning, expression, and functional characterization of the von Willebrand factor-cleaving protease (ADAMTS13). *Blood* 2002; 100: 3626–3632.

114 Howard MA, Williams LA, Terrell DR, et al. Complications of plasma exchange in patients treated for clinically suspected thrombotic thrombocytopenic purpura-hemolytic uremic syndrome. *Transfusion* 2006; 46(1): 154–156.

115 Reutter JC, Sanders KF, Brecher ME, Jones HG, Bandarenko N. Incidence of allergic reactions with fresh frozen plasma or cryo-supernatant plasma in the treatment of thrombotic thrombocytopenic purpura. *J Clin Apher* 2001; 16: 134–138.

116 Mori Y, Wada H, Gabazza EC, et al. Predicting response to plasma exchange in patients with thrombotic thrombocytopenic purpura with measurement of vWF-cleaving protease activity. *Transfusion* 2002; 42: 572–580.

117 Raife T, Atkinson B, Montgomery R, Vesely S, Friedman K. Severe deficiency of VWF-cleaving protease (ADAMTS13) activity defines a distinct population of thrombotic microangiopathy patients. *Transfusion* 2004; 44: 146–150.

118 Elliott MA, Nichols WL Jr, Plumhoff EA, et al. Posttransplantation thrombotic thrombocytopenic purpura: a single-center experience and a contemporary review. *Mayo Clin Proc* 2003; 78: 421–430.

119 van der Plas RM, Schiphorst ME, Huizinga EG, et al. von Willebrand factor proteolysis is deficient in classic, but not in bone marrow transplantation-associated thrombotic thrombocytopenic purpura. *Blood* 1999; 93: 3798–3802.

120 Volcy J, Nzerue CM, Oderinde A, Hewan-Iowe K. Cocaine-induced acute renal failure, hemolysis, and thrombocytopenia mimicking thrombotic thrombocytopenic purpura. *Am J Kidney Dis* 2000; 35: E3.

121 Gasser C, Gautier E, Steck A, Siebenmann RE, Oechslin R. [Hemolytic-uremic syndrome: bilateral necrosis of the renal cortex in acute acquired hemolytic anemia.]. *Schweiz Med Wochenschr* 1955; 85: 905–909.

122 Moake JL. Haemolytic-uremic syndrome: basic science. *Lancet* 1994; 343: 393–397.

123 Kaplan BS, Proesmans W. The hemolytic uremic syndrome of childhood and its variants. *Semin Hematol* 1987; 24: 148–160.

124. Karmali MA. Infection by Shiga toxin-producing Escherichia coli: an overview. *Mol Biotechnol* 2004; 26: 117–122.

125 Karmali MA, Petric M, Lim C, et al. The association between idiopathic hemolytic uremic syndrome and infection by verotoxin-producing Escherichia coli. *J Infect Dis* 1985; 151: 775–782.

126 Nolasco L, Turner NA, Bernardo A, et al. Hemolytic uremic syndrome-associated Shiga toxins promote endothelial-cell secretion and impair ADAMTS13 cleavage of unusually large von Willebrand factor multimers. *Blood* 2005; 106: 4199–4209.

127 Bonnardeaux A, Pichette V. Complement dysregulation in haemolytic uraemic syndrome. *Lancet* 2003; 362: 1514–1515.

128 Warwicker P, Goodship TH, Donne RL, et al. Genetic studies into inherited and sporadic hemolytic uremic syndrome. *Kidney Int* 1998; 53: 836–844.

129 Fremeaux-Bacchi V, Dragon-Durey MA, Blouin J, et al. Complement factor I: a susceptibility gene for atypical haemolytic uraemic syndrome. *J Med Genet* 2004; 41: e84.

130 Byrnes JJ, Moake JL. Thrombotic thrombocytopenic purpura and the hemolytic-uremic syndrome: evolving concepts of pathogenesis and therapy. *Clin Haematol* 1986; 15: 413–442.

131 Moake JL. Haemolytic-uraemic syndrome: basic science. *Lancet* 1994; 343: 393–397.

132 Banerjee D, Kupin W, Roth D. Hemolytic uremic syndrome after multivisceral transplantation treated with intravenous immunoglobulin. *J Nephrol* 2003; 16: 733–735.

133 Gatti S, Arru M, Reggiani P, et al. Successful treatment of hemolytic uremic syndrome after liver-kidney transplantation. *J Nephrol* 2003; 16: 586–590.

134 Korec S, Schein PS, Smith FP, et al. Treatment of cancer-associated hemolytic-uremic syndrome with staphylococcal protein A immunoperfusion. *J Clin Oncol* 1986; 4: 210–215.

135 E, S. Über das Verhalten der Blutplättchen bei Eklampsie. *Zentralbl Gynäkol* 1922; 46: 391.

136 Pritchard JA, Weisman RJ, Ratnoff OD, Vosburgh GJ. Intravascular hemolysis, thrombocytopenia and other hematologic abnormalities associated with severe toxemia of pregnancy. *N Engl J Med* 1954; 250: 89–98.

137 Goodlin RC, Cotton DB, Haesslein HC. Severe edema-proteinuria-hypertension gestosis. *Am J Obstet Gynecol* 1978; 132: 595–598.

138 Weinstein L. Syndrome of hemolysis, elevated liver enzymes, and low platelet count: a severe consequence of hypertension in pregnancy. *Am J Obstet Gynecol* 1982; 142: 159–167.

139 Rahman TM, Wendon J. Severe hepatic dysfunction in pregnancy. *QJM* 2002; 95: 343–357.

140 Rath W, Faridi A, Dudenhausen JW. HELLP syndrome. *J Perinat Med* 2000; 28: 249–260.

141 Sibai BM, Ramadan MK, Usta I, et al. Maternal morbidity and mortality in 442 pregnancies with hemolysis, elevated liver enzymes, and low platelets (HELLP syndrome). *Am J Obstet Gynecol* 1993; 169: 1000–1006.

142 Magann EF, Bass D, Chauhan SP, et al. Antepartum corticosteroids: disease stabilization in patients with the syndrome of hemolysis, elevated liver enzymes, and low platelets (HELLP). *Am J Obstet Gynecol* 1994; 171: 1148–1153.

143 Magann EF, Martin JNJ. Twelve steps to optimal management of HELLP syndrome. *Clin Obstet Gynecol* 1999; 42: 532–550.

144 Zusterzeel PL, Visser W, Blom HJ, et al. Methylenetetrahydrofolate reductase polymorphisms in pre-eclampsia and the HELLP syndrome. *Hypertens Pregn* 2000; 19: 299–307.

145 Benedetto C, Marozio L, Salton L, et al. Factor V Leiden and factor II G20210A in preeclampsia and HELLP syndrome. *Acta Obstet Gynecol Scand* 2002; 81: 1095–1100.

146 Bozzo M, Carpani G, Leo L, et al. HELLP syndrome and factor V Leiden. *Eur J Obstet Gynecol Reprod Biol* 2001; 95: 55–58.

147 Krauss T, Augustin HG, Osmers R, et al. Activated protein C resistance and factor V Leiden in patients with hemolysis, elevated liver enzymes, low platelets syndrome. *Obstet Gynecol* 1998; 92: 457–460.

148 Marchand A, Galen RS, van Lente F. The predictive value of serum haptoglobin in hemolytic disease. *JAMA* 1980; 243: 1909–1911.

149 Wilke G, Rath W, Schutz E, Armstrong VW, Kuhn W. Haptoglobin as a sensitive marker of hemolysis in HELLP-syndrome. *Int J Gynaecol Obstet* 1992; 39: 29–34.

150 Shukla PK, Sharma D, Mandal RK. Serum lactate dehydrogenase in detecting liver damage associated with pre-eclampsia. *Br J Obstet Gynaecol* 1978; 85: 40–42.

151 Thiagarajah S, Bourgeois FJ, Harbert G, Caudle MR. Thrombocytopenia in preeclampsia: associated abnormalities and management principles. *Am J Obstet Gynecol* 1984; 150: 1–7.

152 Barton JR, Riely CA, Adamec TA, et al. Hepatic histopathologic condition does not correlate with laboratory abnormalities in HELLP syndrome (hemolysis, elevated liver enzymes, and low platelet count). *Am J Obstet Gynecol* 1992; 167: 1538–1543.

153 de Boer K, Buller HR, ten Cate JW, Treffers PE. Coagulation studies in the syndrome of haemolysis, elevated liver enzymes and low platelets. *Br J Obstet Gynaecol* 1991; 98: 42–47.

154 Thomas EA, Copplestone JA, Dubbins PA, Friend JR. The radiologist cries "HELLP"!. *Br J Radiol* 1991; 64: 964–966.

155 Zhou Y, McMaster M, Woo K, et al. Vascular endothelial growth factor ligands and receptors that regulate human cytotrophoblast survival are dysregulated in severe preeclampsia and hemolysis, elevated liver enzymes, and low platelets syndrome. *Am J Pathol* 2002; 160: 1405–1423.

156 Knerr I, Beinder E, Rascher W. Syncytin, a novel human endogenous retroviral gene in human placenta: evidence for its dysregulation in preeclampsia and HELLP syndrome. *Am J Obstet Gynecol* 2002; 186: 210–213.

157 Levine RJ, Maynard SE, Qian C, et al. Circulating angiogenic factors and the risk of preeclampsia. *N Engl J Med* 2004; 350: 672–683.

158 Lattuada A, Rossi E, Calzarossa C, Candolfi R, Mannucci PM. Mild to moderate reduction of a von Willebrand factor cleaving protease (ADAMTS-13) in pregnant women with HELLP microangiopathic syndrome. *Haematologica* 2003; 88: 1029–1034.

159 Thorp JMJ, White G, Moake JL, Bowes W. von Willebrand factor multimeric levels and patterns in patients with severe preeclampsia. *Obstet Gynecol* 1990; 75: 163–167.

160 Schlenzig C, Maurer S, Goppelt M, Ulm K, Kolben M. Postpartum curettage in patients with HELLP-syndrome does not result in accelerated recovery. *Eur J Obstet Gynecol Reprod Biol* 2000; 91: 25–28.

161 Fonseca JE, Mendez F, Catano C, Arias F. Dexamethasone treatment does not improve the outcome of women with HELLP syndrome: a double-blind, placebo-controlled, randomized clinical trial. *Am J Obstet Gynecol* 2005; 193(5): 1591–1598.

162 Matchaba P, Moodley J. Corticosteroids for HELLP syndrome in pregnancy. *Cochrane Database of Systematic Reviews* 2004, Issue 1. Art. No.: CD002076.

163 Erhard J, Lange R, Niebel W, et al. Acute liver necrosis in the HELLP syndrome: successful outcome after orthotopic liver transplantation. A case report. *Transpl Int* 1993; 6: 179–181.

164 Reubinoff BE, Schenker JG. HELLP syndrome – a syndrome of hemolysis, elevated liver enzymes and low platelet count – complicating preeclampsia-eclampsia. *Int J Gynaecol Obstet* 1991; 36: 95–102.

165 Smith LG Jr, Moise KJ Jr, Dildy GA 3rd, Carpenter RJ Jr. Spontaneous rupture of liver during pregnancy: current therapy. *Obstet Gynecol* 1991; 77(2): 171–175.

166 Merchant SH, Mathew P, Vanderjagt TJ, Howdieshell TR, Crookston KP. Recombinant factor VIIa in management of spontaneous subcapsular liver hematoma associated with pregnancy. *Obstet Gynecol* 2004; 103(5 Pt 2): 1055–1058.

167 Yamanaka Y, Takeuchi K, Konda E, et al. Transient postpartum diabetes insipidus in twin pregnancy associated with HELLP syndrome. *J Perinat Med* 2002; 30: 273–275.

168 Harms K, Rath W, Herting E, Kuhn W. Maternal hemolysis, elevated liver enzymes, low platelet count, and neonatal outcome. *Am J Perinatol* 1995; 12: 1–6.

169 van Pampus MG, Wolf H, Mayruhu G, Treffers PE, Bleker OP. Long-term follow-up in patients with a history of (H)ELLP syndrome. *Hypertens Pregn* 2001; 20: 15–23.

33 Endocrine Emergencies

Carey Winkler & Fred Coleman
Legacy Health Systems, Maternal-Fetal Medicine, Portland, OR, USA

Introduction

Disorders of the endocrine system are not uncommon in women of childbearing age and therefore, are not uncommon during pregnancy. Significant disturbances of many of the endocrine organs can result in dramatic alterations in maternal physiology which in turn, may affect the maternal–placental–fetal unit. Early recognition and rapid correction of these abnormalities will result in improved maternal and fetal outcomes. This chapter reviews the management of the more common (and severe) endocrine emergencies seen in obstetrics: diabetic ketoacidosis, thyroid disorders, pheochromocytoma, adrenal crisis, and altered parathyroid states.

Diabetic ketoacidosis

In recent years, diabetes has accounted for approximately 3–5% of all maternal mortality. Of these, 15% were secondary to diabetic ketoacidosis (DKA) [1]. Because of improvements in care provided to critically ill patients, along with prompt recognition and treatment, the risk of maternal death from an episode of DKA is now 1% or less [2]. Unfortunately, the fetal death rate has not fallen to that level. Despite aggressive treatment of the mother and improvements in perinatal and neonatal care, studies suggest a 10–25% fetal loss rate for a single episode of DKA [3,4].

Factors that predispose pregnant patients to DKA include accelerated starvation, dehydration, decreased caloric intake secondary to pregnancy-related nausea, decreased buffering capacity (compensated respiratory alkalosis), stress, and increased insulin antagonists such as human placental lactogen, prolactin, and cortisol [5]. The most common precipitating events in DKA are infection related (viral or bacterial 30%) and inadequate insulin treatment usually from patient non-compliance (30%). Other less common reasons include insulin pump failure and medications (glucocorticoids with/without β-adrenergic agents) for preterm labor [6–8]. In one series, 7 of 11 patients decreased their insulin dosage because of decreased food intake and lower glucose levels [9]. In addition, Montoro et al. [4] noted that 6 of 20 patients who presented with DKA were newly diagnosed with diabetes.

In a retrospective study by Cullen and associates [9], 11 pregnant patients presented in diabetic ketoacidosis over a 10-year period. Of these 11 patients, four had an initial blood glucose <200 mg/dL. The precipitating event for ketoacidosis in these four cases was maternal nausea and vomiting due to an underlying gastrointestinal disorder such as hyperemesis gravidarum or a viral gastroenteritis. In response to the persistent nausea and vomiting, these patients reduced not only their caloric intake but also their insulin dose. Thus, it is important to remember that when an insulin-dependent diabetic presents with a history of persistent nausea and vomiting, a blood glucose <200 mg/dL does not necessarily eliminate the potential for ketoacidosis. Under these circumstances, an evaluation for the potential of diabetic ketoacidosis should be undertaken.

The underlying cause of DKA is an absolute, or more commonly during pregnancy, a relative deficiency in circulating insulin levels in relationship to an excess of insulin counter-regulatory hormones, specifically catecholamines, glucagon, cortisol, and growth hormone. The sequence of events has been reviewed by Kitabchi et al. [8]. The levels of catecholamines (700–800%), glucagon (400–500%), cortisol (400–500%), and growth hormone (200–300%) are all increased during DKA when compared to baseline levels. The net result is an increase in glucose levels and hyperglycemia. Glucagon increases production of hepatic ketone bodies from fatty acids. Because insulin is also needed for the effective degradation of ketone bodies, the excessive degree of ketonemia is due to both overproduction as well as continued undermetabolization.

The main ketone bodies are β-hydroxybutyric acid, acetic acid, and acetone. These are moderately strong acids and when released

Critical Care Obstetrics, 5th edition. Edited by M. Belfort, G. Saade, M. Foley, J. Phelan and G. Dildy.

into the maternal circulation, exceed the maternal buffering capacity of the serum bicarbonate, resulting in the metabolic acidosis component of DKA. As hydrogen ions move into the intracellular space from the extracellular compartment, potassium ions shift in the opposite direction. As a result, there is a depletion of intracellular potassium stores that may be greater than indicated by plasma levels. Maternal respiratory changes to excrete carbon dioxide include an increase in the rate and depth of inspirations, also known as Kussmaul respirations. This results in a compensatory respiratory alkalosis. As the degree of hyperglycemia and ketonemia increases, there is a rise in serum osmolarity. In addition, the hyperglycemia and ketonuria result in a profound osmotic diuresis and severe dehydration. Hypovolemia and hypotension soon follow, resulting in decreased peripheral perfusion, increased production of lactic acid, and a further decrease in serum pH. This sequence of events sets up a vicious cycle of worsening dehydration, increasing serum osmolarity, increasing release of insulin counter-regulatory hormones from stress and cellular dysfunction, and worsening acidosis.

The loss of free water from osmotic diuresis can be extensive: up to 150 mL/kg body weight. In a typical pregnant patient, this equates to 7–10 L of free water. Along with the loss of urinary water, there is the depletion of many electrolytes, specifically sodium, potassium, and phosphorus. The hypovolemia and hypotension may result in emesis, which can exacerbate dehydration and electrolyte losses. Finally, the increased respiratory rate can cause additional water loss and dehydration.

Usually, the diagnosis is quite obvious from a clinical perspective. The patient will present with feelings of malaise, emesis, weakness/lethargy, polyuria, polydipsia, tachypnea, and signs of dehydration (decreased skin turgor, dry mucous membranes, tachycardia, hypotension). The patient may complain of fever, suggesting infection as a precipitating event. Because of the decreased peripheral perfusion and resultant ischemia, patients may have abdominal pain of such severity that it may mimic an intra-abdominal process such as appendicitis. Acetone is highly volatile and is excreted in the patient's breath, producing a classic fruity smell.

Laboratory evaluation should include serum electrolytes, osmolality, creatinine, blood urea nitrogen, urine leukocyte esterase, and arterial blood gases. Classically, the serum glucose will be elevated to 300 mg/dL or more. An arterial blood gas will confirm an acidotic pH (<7.30) along with a decreased serum bicarbonate level. The anion gap will be increased (>12) suggesting the presence of non-volatile acids. Finally, the serum will test strongly for acetone (1 : 2 dilution or greater). The predominant ketone produced in DKA is β-hydroxybutyric acid. A commonly used test for evaluating the presence of ketones is the nitroprusside reactions. Neither β-hydroxybutyric acid nor acetone reacts as strongly with nitroprusside as acetoacetate. Therefore, the severity of the ketonemia may be severely underestimated by this test. If possible, direct measurement of plasma β-hydroxybutyric acid should be performed. As insulin therapy is begun, there is a preferential fall in the level of β-hydroxybutyric acid and increased conversion to acetoacetate. Paradoxically, the nitroprusside reaction may worsen as the condition of the patient improves. However, there should be an improvement in the patient's pH, a decrease in the anion gap, and an overall improvement in the patient's clinical condition.

In order to optimize maternal/fetal outcome, the diagnosis needs to be made quickly with immediate initiation of treatment [4]. Therapy should consist of rapidly correcting the volume deficits, initiation of insulin, treatment of infection if present, and careful monitoring to aid in correction of the metabolic and electrolyte abnormalities. A transurethral catheter should be placed and urine sent for culture and sensitivity. The initial intravenous solution replacement consists of isotonic saline (0.9% NaCl) solution at 1000mL/h for at least 2 hours. Using a hypotonic intravenous solution such as half-normal saline (0.45% NaCl) solution can lead to rapid decline in serum osmolarity. If this occurs too quickly for intracellular equilibrium to take place, rarely, cellular swelling can occur, leading to cerebral edema [10]. After 2 L of an isotonic solution over 2 hours, the solution should be changed to one more similar to electrolyte losses during osmotic diuresis (0.45% NaCl) given at 250 mL/h, until serum glucose is between 200 and 250 mg/dL. Continuing the use of an isotonic saline solution can result in excessive chloride and metabolic acidosis during the resolution phase. Once glucose levels reach 250 mg/dL, intravenous fluids should be changed to 0.45% NaCl with 5% dextrose to prevent an excessively rapid drop in serum glucose. Approximately 75% of the total fluid replacement should occur during the first 24 hours and the remaining 25% over the next 24–48 hours. Unless there are signs of severe dehydration and cardiovascular collapse, a good estimate of the total fluid loss is 100 mL/kg actual body weight.

Since DKA is precipitated by an absolute or relative deficiency in insulin, it is critical that insulin therapy is started in order to correct the many metabolic abnormalities that have occurred. Treatment should be an initial intravenous bolus followed by continuous infusion. Intramuscular or subcutaneous therapy should be avoided as decreased perfusion may result in inadequate absorption [8]. The initial bolus should be in the neighborhood of 10 units of regular insulin (0.1 units/kg) followed by a continuous infusion of 0.1 units/kg/h. Serum glucose levels should be determined every hour. The decrease in serum glucose levels should be gradual to prevent excessive movement of water into the cells from a rapid drop in serum osmolarity. A reasonable target is a decrease of 50–75 mg/dL every hour. If serum glucose levels fail to decrease by at least 50 mg/dL in the first 2 hours, the rate of insulin infusion should be doubled [8]. The insulin infusion should be maintained until most of the metabolic abnormalities have corrected and the patient is feeling well enough to eat. At that time, subcutaneous insulin can be initiated and the insulin infusion discontinued. A thorough search for and treatment of the precipitating event and continuation of insulin is necessary to limit recurrence.

In DKA, there is a significant loss in total body sodium and potassium. The total body loss of potassium can approach over

300 mEq. As the acidosis is corrected, potassium ions shift intracellularly. The intracellular movement of potassium is accelerated in the presence of insulin and can lead to a precipitous decrease in the serum potassium level. As the patient's volume status improves, potassium levels must be followed closely and immediately corrected when low. It is important to replace potassium slowly and not cause hyperkalemia. Serum potassium levels should be determined every 2–4 hours depending on the levels. Two ways to replace potassium are as follows.

1 Add KCl (40 mEq/L) to each liter of replacement fluids and run at the usual 150–250 mL/h. This will give approximately 5–10 mEq/h replacement.

2 Intermittent intravenous infusion boluses: in an additional intravenous port, give 10 mEq/h infusion for 4–6 hours, check the serum potassium level, and continue the "piggyback" infusion as necessary.

Because of concerns for toxicity/cardiac arrhythmias, potassium supplements should not be given more quickly than 20 mEq/h. After the patient is stable and eating a regular diet, oral supplementation can be given for 1–2 days to completely replenish the total body stores of potassium.

The use of intravenous bicarbonate to increase pH and improve organ function has become a minority view and for most patients, in fact, is becoming discouraged. Sodium bicarbonate treatment has failed to show a difference in outcome in DKA with a pH in the range of 6.8–7.1 [8,11]. However, due to the paucity of patients with a pH 6.9–7.0, it is difficult to state whether bicarbonate replacement was helpful in this subset of cases. Therefore, if the patient has a pH less than 7.0 or the serum bicarbonate levels is <5 mEq/L, administration of one ampule (44 mEq) is prudent. Otherwise, the treatment of choice is correction of the underlying problem with hydration, insulin, and potassium. Rapid administration of sodium bicarbonate has the potential to cause paradoxical central nervous system acidosis, as the blood–brain barrier is freely permeable to carbon dioxide but not bicarbonate. For overall management options, see Figure 33.1.

One final point is evaluation and care of the fetus. Fetal distress may occur due to several mechanisms. Uterine blood flow may decrease due to catecholamine-induced vasoconstriction or dehydration. Secondly, fetal β-hydroxybutyric acid and glucose concentrations parallel maternal levels [12] and fetal hyperglycemia may in itself lead to an osmotic diuresis, fetal intravascular volume depletion, and decreased placental perfusion. Finally, a leftward shift of the oxygen dissociation curve with a decreased 2,3-diphosphoglycerate increases hemoglobin affinity for oxygen and reduces tissue oxygen delivery. In any case, uterine blood

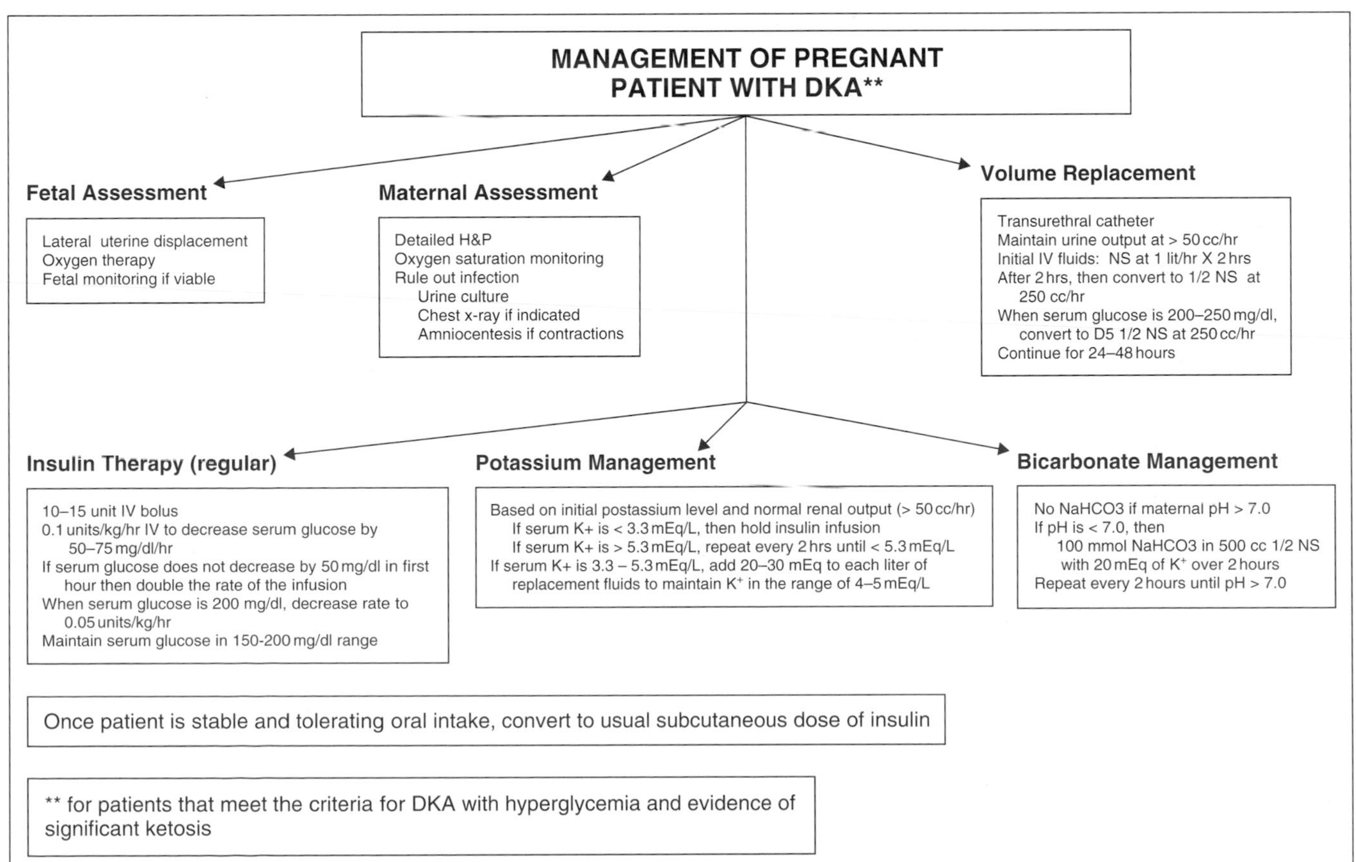

Figure 33.1 Management of pregnant patient with DKA.

flow may be reduced in poorly controlled diabetics [13]. A significant reduction in the maternal pH thus will result in a corresponding fall in fetal pH. This will often be reflected in abnormal fetal heart rate tracings. Unless there are other overriding reasons for prompt delivery, it is usually prudent to correct the underlying DKA, as the abnormal fetal heart rate tracings and Doppler studies seen in maternal ketoacidosis improve with diabetic control [14,15]. In the majority of cases, improving the maternal condition allows for prolongation of the pregnancy.

Thyroid dysfunction

Multiple changes occur in the maternal and fetal thyroid gland during pregnancy. These physiologic changes have been extensively detailed [16,17]. A brief review of changes that affect the interpretation of thyroid tests or thyroid hormone metabolism in relationship to clinical management follows.

Changes in thyroid hormone levels during pregnancy occur both in the maternal circulation and in the developing fetus. Thyroid-binding globulin (TBG) levels increase during pregnancy secondary to an estrogen-stimulated increase in synthesis and a decrease in clearance that is associated with altered sialylation of TBG [18]. Because of the increase in TBG, there is also an increase in the total thyroxine (T4) blood levels in the maternal circulation. Maternal free T4 and free triiodothyronine (T3) blood levels remain within the range of normal values but are minimally decreased in the second and third trimester [16,19]. Sensitive thyroid-stimulating hormone (TSH) and free T4 assays have replaced the free T4 index and have improved the diagnosis of thyroid disorders during pregnancy. The newer TSH assays are extremely sensitive for determining early hypothyroidism. The current upper limits of the normal range is 4.5 mU/L but because 95% of the normal population have a TSH <2.5 mU/L, there is growing support to decrease the normal values [20]. However, currently, there is no compelling evidence that early treatment of these "borderline hypothyroid" pregnant patients compared to close follow-up improves long-term outcomes [21]. In the non-pregnant patient, there are accumulating data suggesting treatment of subclinical hypothyroidism decreases morbidity, especially cardiovascular disease [22–24].

One exception to the interpretation of free T4 and TSH during pregnancy is the increase in maternal free T4 and decrease in TSH at 8–12 weeks of gestation when human chorionic gondatotropin (hCG) levels peak [17]. This is thought, in part, to reflect the weak thyrotropic activity of hCG. Thus, a mild elevation of free T4 and suppressed TSH level in the first trimester, in the absence of clinical signs of thyrotoxicosis, is more likely to reflect a physiologic adjustment and does not suggest hyperthyroidism.

The clinical consequences of T4 metabolism are threefold. The first is that thyroid replacement in the hypothyroid patient is usually initiated at 100 μg/day [25,26] and often increases during pregnancy. Mandel et al. [25] found that to normalize TSH levels in pregnant women, the mean T4 dose increased from 102 to 147 μg/day, or an increase of 45%. Second, in the acute setting of thyroid storm, it is logical to use propylthiouracil instead of methimazole as the former inhibits peripheral conversion of T4 to T3, while the latter does not. Finally, clinical symptomatic improvement in patients with acute hyperthyroidism treated with propylthiouracil (measured in days) precedes normalization of thyroid function tests (which may take 6–8 weeks).

Hyperthyroidism

Hyperthyroidism during pregnancy is rare, complicating less than 0.2% of all births [27,29]. Early treatment and normalization of maternal thyroid function is important because poor metabolic control increases the risk of preterm delivery, fetal wastage, and thyroid crisis [27,28]. By far the most common cause of thyrotoxicosis during pregnancy is Graves' disease, accounting for greater than 90% of cases [30,31]. Less common causes are listed in Table 33.1 and include thyroid adenomas, thyroiditis, or secondary hCG-dependent disorders.

Graves' disease is an autoimmune disorder where maternal antibodies (thyrotropin receptor antibodies or TRAb) attach to the thyroid gland and stimulate the production of thyroid hormone, similar to TSH. Prior to the use of thionamides, it was recognized that some 25% of patients undergo long-term remission without therapy [32]. During pregnancy, the course is variable. As in other autoimmune disorders, some patients appear to improve during pregnancy and relapse postpartum. Amino et al. [33] noted in women with Graves' disease near remission at the

Table 33.1 Causes of hyperthyroidism.

Autoimmune
Graves' disease
Hashimoto's disease
Autonomous
Toxic multinodular goiter
Solitary toxic adenoma
Thyroiditis (transient)
Postpartum thyroiditis
Subacute thyroiditis
Painless thyroiditis
Drug induced
Iodide-induced (Jod–Basedow)
Radiocontrast agents
Thyroxine (factitous or dietary supplements containing thyroid hormones)
Secondary
TSH-secreting tumor
hCG dependent (hyperemesis gravidarum, hydatidiform mole)
Thyroid hormone resistance
Ectopic struma ovarii
Metastatic follicular carcinoma

onset of pregnancy that the free T4 index was increased in the first trimester, fell in the second and third trimester, and was again increased postpartum. A fall in antimicrosomal antibodies during pregnancy and an increase postpartum was also measured in patients with Graves' disease or postpartum thyroiditis [34]. For further information, the reader is referred to a recent review of postpartum thyroiditis, which occurs in 5–7% of patients [35].

The diagnosis of Graves' disease is suggested by the presence of thyrotoxicosis, ophthalmopathy, a diffuse goiter, dermopathy, and thyroid receptor antibodies. The diagnosis is clinical and is supported by thyroid function tests; thyroid receptor antibody tests are often not necessary but levels of the antibodies at 36 weeks correlate with the risk of neonatal thyrotoxicosis [36]. However, pretibial dermopathy is rarely present in pregnant women, and active clinical ophthalmopathy is evident in only half of patients with Graves' disease [37,38]. Exophthalmos, weakness of the extraocular muscles, chemosis, and impairment of convergence are signs of infiltrative ophthalmopathy and may remain despite normalization of thyroid hormone levels.

In pregnancy, the signs and symptoms of hyperthyroidism are slightly more difficult to interpret due to the normal changes that occur during gestation. Heart rate and cardiac output increase, and heat intolerance, nausea, and weight loss are common. Thyrotoxicosis is suggested by clinical findings which include a pulse rate persistently greater than 100 that fails to decrease with Valsalva in the presence of a tremor, previously mentioned signs, thyroid bruit, thyromegaly, and mild systolic hypertension. The cardiac effects of hyperthyroidism are summarized in Table 33.2. An elevated free T4 and low serum TSH confirms the diagnosis. Clinical signs of thyrotoxicosis without elevated total or free T4 should suggest free T3 thyrotoxicosis or deficient TBG states [39] but these are much less common.

"Thyroid receptor antibodies" is a generalized term that may be used to include both thyroid-stimulating immunoglobulins (TSIs) as well as thyrotropin-binding inhibitor immunoglobulins (TBIIs) and may be a useful predictor of neonatal thyroid dysfunction [40]. Consequently, neonatal thyroid effects may occur years after the diagnosis of Graves' disease, when the mother is either euthyroid or hypothyroid after radioactive thyroid ablation. Thyroid disease in pregnancy has recently been reviewed by Glinoer [41].

Table 33.2 Cardiovascular changes in hyper- and hypothyroid states.

	Hyperthyroid	Hypothyroid
Cardiac output	↑	↓
Heart rate	↑	↓
Stroke volume	↑	↓
Cardiac contractility	↑	↓
Systemic vascular resistance	↑	↓
Mean arterial pressure	↑	↓
Blood volume	↑	↓
Other	Atrial fibrillation ↓QT, ↑ PR interval ST elevation ↑conduction abnormalities	Ascites Pleural effusion ↑QT interval

Neonatal thyroid status may be affected transiently by either thionamides therapy or thyroid receptor antibodies. The incidence of neonatal hyperthyroidism or hypothyroidism due to maternal passive transmission of thyroid receptor antibodies appears to be 1–3% [38]. Mitsuda et al. [42] reported overt thyrotoxicosis in six neonates of 230 women with Graves' disease. In four of the mothers, TBII levels were elevated. In addition, transient hypothyroidism was found in five neonates with normal TBII levels and thionamides treatment. Mortimer et al. [43] reported a higher incidence of neonatal thyrotoxicosis in four infants of 44 mothers with Graves' disease; in all four cases, the mothers had TBII levels greater than 70%. These investigators observed that the neonatal free T4 index correlated inversely with maternal thionamides dose. In addition, women who had a free T4 index in the lower half of the reference range on thionamides were more likely to deliver a child with an elevated TSH than women with a free T4 index in the upper half of the reference range. Similarly, Momotani et al. [44] studied 43 women maintained on thionamide therapy until delivery and 27 women in whom thionamides therapy was discontinued due to normalization of thyroid function tests prior to delivery. They found in women who took thionamides until delivery, a greater number had fetuses with increased TSH levels, lower T4 levels, and higher maternal TBII levels. It is important to note that in both of these studies there was only evidence of mild chemical, not clinical, hypothyroidism. However, taken together these data suggest that the minimal dose of thionamides therapy should be used to keep maternal thyroid function at the upper limits of normal. Because TBII antibodies are positive although at lower levels in 50–80% of women with Graves' disease [38,43,44], their utility remains to be further demonstrated. In patients with Graves disease, the fetal heart rate may also be an indicator of fetal thyroid function and should be auscultated for a persistent fetal heart rate tachycardia at each prenatal visit. In 1–5% of cases, TSH receptor-stimulating antibodies may cross the placenta producing fetal/neonatal thyrotoxicosis. Findings suggestive of fetal thyrotoxicosis could include the presence of a persistent fetal heart rate tachycardia [45], fetal goiter, or intrauterine growth impairment.

Wing et al. [28] found that only one infant of 185 women treated with propylthiouracil or methimazole had transient hypothyroidism at birth. Similarly, Davis et al. [27] found one neonate had transient hypothyroidism and a second was euthyroid with an asymptomatic goiter among 43 mothers receiving propylthiouracil. Both were on high doses of propylthiouracil at the time of delivery. This is consistent with a review of the literature by Mandel et al. [46] in which the incidence of neonatal goiter in women exposed to antithyroid medications was 4%. PTU may be concentrated in the fetal compartment since umbilical blood levels were higher than maternal serum samples in five maternal–fetal pairs [47].

In thyroid crisis or storm, an acute increase in the signs and symptoms of thyrotoxicosis may be life-threatening. The overall incidence of thyroid crisis in women who receive thionamides treatment during pregnancy, some of whom remain thyrotoxic, is about 2% [27]. A clinical diagnosis must be established and treatment initiated well before confirmatory thyroid function tests are available. The classic signs of thyroid storm (altered mental status, temperature above 41°C, hypertension, and diarrhea) are not necessarily present. Postpartum congestive heart failure, tachycardia, and severe hypertension should suggest the diagnosis and prompt an evaluation for other signs of thyrotoxicosis [48]. Rarely loss of consciousness following cesarean section [49] or seizures mimicking eclampsia [50] may complicate the presentation of thyrotoxicosis.

The risks appear to be related to metabolic status and to the precipitating cause. Pekonen et al. [51] reported that two of seven untreated thyrotoxic women in labor developed thyroid crisis. Similar results were described in eight untreated women in labor, of whom five developed heart failure, and four had stillbirths [27]. In that series, among 16 other women who had received thionamides but were still thyrotoxic at the time of delivery, two had stillbirths and one developed heart failure whereas there were no complications in 36 women who were euthyroid. In an expanded review, Sheffield and Cunningham [52] found that nearly 10% of thyrotoxic women developed reversible congestive heart failure. Kriplani et al. [29] also reported three patients who developed thyroid storm, including one maternal death, among 32 patients who were hyperthyroid during pregnancy. Although thyroid functions were not specifically detailed, thyroid storm was associated with either emergent operative delivery or infection. Thionamide therapy, even of short duration, is generally effective in preventing storm. Therefore, congestive heart failure that occurs after administration of propylthiouracil should suggest another precipitating event, such as underlying infection, hypertension, or anemia.

The treatment of thyroid storm is somewhat empiric and consists of thionamides, iodide, and β-blockers. Therapy differs from the usual management of hyperthyroidism in the dose and choice of thionamide. Although propylthiouracil and methimazole are equally effective in the treatment of hyperthyroidism in pregnancy [28], in the setting of thyroid storm, propylthiouracil is administrated by mouth and if necessary by nasogastric tube to inhibit peripheral conversion of T4 to T3. Despite inhibition of T4 synthesis, it may take 7–8 weeks of therapy to deplete thyroid colloid stores and normalize thyroid function tests [27,28]. Clinical improvement commonly precedes resolution of the tachycardia due to the long half-life of T4. Iodide inhibits thyroid release rapidly [53,54]. Iodide should be given only after propylthiouracil is administered and should be discontinued when there is clinical improvement to avoid the risk of congenital goiter if the pregnancy continues. Propranolol (1 mg IV every 5 minutes and repeated as necessary) may be used to control autonomic symptoms. The fast-acting/short half-life β-blocker, esmolol, is also a reasonable choice. The loading dose is 250–500 μg/kg followed by a continuous infusion at 50–100 μg/kg/min. Labetalol has also been used successfully [55]. Although β-adrenergic blockade may inhibit peripheral conversion of T4 to T3, this does not alter thyroid release and does not prevent thyroid storm [56,57]. Because large increases in pulmonary diastolic pressure may be precipitated [58] and because congestive heart failure may be a common presentation of thyroid crisis in pregnant women, propranolol and other β-blocking agents should be used with caution.

Corticosteroids have been advocated for inhibiting peripheral conversion of T4 and to prevent adrenal insufficiency, but there are few data to support their use. Fever should be treated with cooling blankets or acetaminophen to decrease cardiovascular demands. A thorough search for underlying infection is necessary because pyelonephritis, endometritis, or sepsis are common precipitating factors. Because of the increased incidence of atrial arrhythmia and central nervous system emboli, thromboembolic disease should be considered in the patient with altered mental status that does not respond to the aforementioned therapy [59].

Complications of propylthiouracil and methimazole include chemical hepatitis, rash or other drug reactions (5%) and rarely agranulocytosis (0.3%) [60]. Because of the seriousness of the latter, patients with fever or sore throat should be instructed to discontinue mediation until a white cell count is checked. Agranulocytosis, as defined by a total leukocyte count of < 1,000/mm^3 or granulocyte count of less than 250/mm^3, is generally seen in older patients and within 2 months of the onset of therapy [60]. Finally lactation may be continued if the total dose of propylthiouracil does not exceed 450 mg/day and if methimazole dosage does not exceed 20 mg/day [61,62]. See Table 33.3 for an overview of thyroid storm management in pregnancy.

Hypothyroidism

Overt hypothyroidism during pregnancy is uncommon as many women with overt hypothyroidism are anovulatory. The most common etiologies are prior surgical thyroidectomy, radioiodine, ablation, and autoimmune thyroiditis. Clinical signs and symptoms include delayed deep tendon reflexes, fatigue, weight gain, cold intolerance, hair loss, dry skin, brawny edema, thickened tongue, hoarse voice, hypertension, and bradycardia, some of which are more difficult to ascertain during pregnancy. The hemodynamic changes of hypothyroidism are summarized in the table. Hyponatremia, ascites, pericardial effusions, or psychosis are not commonly present but may herald myxedema coma. Laboratory confirmation of hypothyroidism can be established by a low free T4 in the presence of an elevated TSH. However, TSH levels may be suppressed in the first trimester with less sensitive tests and undetectable in as many as 13% of women [63]. More sensitive TSH assays are unlikely to return undetectable.

Although earlier studies of hypothyroidism suggested an increase in congenital anomalies, perinatal mortality, and infant neurologic dysfunction, more recent studies report better outcomes with adequate replacement [64]. Leung et al. [65] studied 23 women with overt hypothyroidism and 45 women with sub-

Table 33.3 Treatment of thyroid storm.

Propylthiouracil 800 mg administered orally, then 150–200 mg every 4–6 hours
Starting 1–2 hours after propylthiouracil administration Saturate solution of potassium iodide 2–5 drops orally every 8 hours, or Sodium iodide 0.5–1.0 g IV every 8 hours
Dexametasone 2 mg IV every 6 hours for 4 doses
β-blockade to decrease hypermetabolic state Propranolol 12 mg IV, repeated every 5 min, up to a total of 6 mg for extreme tachycardia or Esmolol 250–500 μg/kg IV loading dose followed by 50–100 μg /kg/min continuous infusion
Treatment of anxiety/restlessness Hydroxyzine 50–100 mg orally every 6 hours or Lorazepam 1–2 mg orally every 6–8 hours or 20–25 μg /kg IV every 6 hours Phenobarbital 30–60 mg every 8 hours as needed for extreme restlessness
Search for precipitating event, in particular infection
Control temperature if hyperthermic Acetaminophen 500–1000 mg every 4–6 hours, not to exceed 4000 mg/day Cooling blanket
Critical tests Free T4, TSH, urine culture Evaluate for other autoimmune disorders Chest X-ray if indicated EKG (atrial fibrillation)

clinical hypothyroidism (elevated TSH level with a normal T4 index). One stillbirth occurred in an untreated overtly hypothyroid patient who was also eclamptic. Other than one infant with clubfeet, neonatal outcomes were satisfactory. Pre-eclampsia, pregnancy-induced hypertension, and eclampsia were common in women who were not yet euthyroid at delivery (9/30 subjects). In another study of 16 pregnancies in overtly hypothyroid women and 12 cases of subclinical hypothyroidism, complications were more common in overtly hypothyroid women including postpartum hemorrhage, anemia, pre-eclampsia, and placental abruption [66]. Two women also had evidence of cardiac dysfunction, one of whom developed congestive heart failure. It is likely that the etiology of the increase in abruption was secondary to the higher incidence of chronic hypertension in hypothyroid patients [67]. Rarely hypothyroid patients may have prolonged bleeding times that normalize with T4 replacement [68].

As previously mentioned, thyroid replacement requirements may increase during pregnancy [64,69]. Mandel et al. [25] found it necessary to increase the mean T4 dose from 102 to 147 μg/day in 9 of 12 patients in order to normalize TSH levels. Another group of investigators studied 35 pregnancies and noted that only 20% of women required an increase in T4 dosage [70]. TSH measurement should be used to guide thyroid replacement therapy because of the advantage of treating subclinical thyroid disease [26,71].

The importance between the maternal and fetal thyroid axis has recently been examined. A study using 25 216 second-trimester maternal serum α-fetoprotein samples [72] selected 62 women with TSH levels greater than the 98th percentile. At 8 years of age, the children of women with elevated TSH levels had a mean IQ that was 4 points less than matched controls ($p = 0.06$). In 48 of the women who did not receive thyroid replacement during pregnancy, the IQ was 7 points less than matched controls ($p = 0.05$) and these children scored lower on 8 of 15 neuropsychological tests. Within 11 years, 64% of the untreated women and 4% of the match-control women had confirmed hypothyroidism. Similar differences have been found by Pop et al. [73]. A recent workshop was held to discuss the many issues surrounding hypothyroidism and pregnancy [74]. Although universal thyroid screening is not currently recommended [21,45], screening of women with a history of thyroid disorders and normalization of TSH levels would appear beneficial in these women.

Pheochromocytoma

Pheochromocytoma is a rare tumor of catecholamine-secreting chromaffin cells. Recent reviews have noted 43 cases associated with pregnancy between 1988 and 1997 [75–77]. Compared to the period of 1980–1987, maternal mortality fell from 16 to 2%, fetal loss decreased from 26 to 11%, and cases diagnosed antenatally increased from 52 to 83%.

The most common signs are hypertension (90%), headache, excessive truncal sweating, and paroxysmal attacks in 40–50% of patients. Pallor, flushing, anxiety, chest pain, nausea, and vomiting are less common. The diagnosis should be considered in the differential with hyperthyroidism and pre-eclampsia as higher maternal mortality is increased with hypertensive crisis when the diagnosis is not established prior to delivery. [75]. Most (90%) pheochromocytomas occur sporadically and some 10% are associated with familial disorder including multiple endocrine neoplasia (MEN) II syndromes, von Recklinghausen's disease, or von Hippel–Lindau syndrome [78]. Hypertension in the setting of café-au-lait spots and neurofibromas should raise the suspicion of pheochromocytoma. Genetic screening may be warranted not only in familial syndromes [79] but also in sporadic cases [80]. MEN 2A is an autosomal dominant syndrome in which medullary thyroid carcinoma is associated with pheochromocytoma and hyperparathyroidism. A more extensive review of pheochromocytoma has been published by Prys-Roberts [78].

Advances in biochemical testing have improved the diagnosis. Table 33.4 summarizes the sensitivity and specificity of plasma and urine tests [79]. If biochemical evaluation and the history suggest a pheochromocytoma, MRI can be safely performed in pregnancy to confirm the presence of an adrenal mass, as 90% of pheochromocytomas arise in the adrenal glands. After delivery,

Table 33.4 Biochemical tests for pheochromocytoma.

Test	Sensitivity (%)	Specificity (%)
Plasma metanephrine	99	89
Plasama catecholamine	85	80
Urinary catecholamine	88	64
Urinary metanephrine	94	53
Urinary vanillymandelic acid	63	94

radioactive iodine-labeled metiodobenzylguanidine scintigraphy offers greater than 95% specificity in the detection [79] of a pheochromocytome.

The most frequently used treatment consists of non-specific α-adrenergic blockade with phenoxybenzamine given by mouth, 10 mg daily, increased by 0.5–1.0 mg/kg/daily [76,79]. Alternatively, the shorter-acting selective α_1-blocker prazosin is less likely to cause tachycardia. The initial dosage is 1 mg three times a day, increased to 2–5 mg three times a day. Beta-blockers should be used in conjunction only after adrenergic blockade is initiated as unopposed α-adrenergic activity may lead to vasoconstriction and a marked increase in blood pressure. Commonly, labetalol is used as it has both α- and β-adrenergic antagonist properties. As hypertension is the most common presenting feature, pre-eclampsia will often be included in the differential diagnosis. Interestingly, magnesium sulfate given as a bolus followed by a 2-g infusion has been used in non-pregnant patients for operative control during surgical removal of pheochromocytoma [81,82]. The use of magnesium sulfate may therefore be advantageous.

Hyperparathyroidism

Primary hyperparathyroidism is more common in women than men (3 : 1 ratio). Since the average age of diagnosis is 55 years, the combination of hyperparathyroidism and pregnancy is uncommon. Approximately 145 cases of primary hyperparathyroidism have been reported during pregnancy, which is proportionately less than the expected incidence of 8 new cases per 100 000 per year in women of childbearing age [83,84]. The discrepancy is in part due to the asymptomatic nature of most cases of hyperparathyroidism. Combining the results of two series [85,86], the majority of patients were diagnosed postpartum following the presentation of neonatal tetany. A recent review summarizes parathyroid disorders [87].

Whether in pregnancy or not, the diagnosis of hyperparathyroidism is suggested by elevated levels of ionized calcium in the presence of inappropriately elevated parathyroid hormone (PTH). The majority of calcium is bound to albumin. The reduced serum albumin levels in pregnancy, acquisition by the fetus of 25–30 g of calcium, increase in glomerular filtration rate, and the expanded extracellular fluid volume result in an overall decrease in total serum calcium levels of 0.5 mg/dL [88]. However, ionized calcium levels are not affected. Pregnant women with primary hyperparathyroidism have biochemical parameters similar to those who are not pregnant [89]. In normal gestation, PTH levels are stable or slightly lower in the second trimester, refuting earlier studies of elevated PTH levels [90–92]. Thus, repeatedly elevated PTH levels in the presence of increase ionized calcium, or total calcium adjusted for albumin, must be considered significant.

When hyperparathyroidism is diagnosed, a search for MEN is indicated [87]. Most non-parathyroid causes of hypercalcemia are associated with suppression of PTH and urinary cAMP levels. Non-parathyroid causes of hypercalcemia include malignancy (breast, melanoma, lymphoma), hypocalcuric hypercalcemia (familial, thiazides, lithium), granulomatous disease (sarcoidosis, tuberculosis), thyrotoxicosis, drug-induced causes (hypervitaminosis D or A, calcium, milk–alkali syndrome), adrenal insufficiency, and immobilization. Hypercalcemia secondary to PTH-related protein produced by breast tissue during pregnancy and lactation with normal PTH levels has also been reported [93]. A history should include the use of over-the-counter vitamin preparations and other medications.

Primary hyperparathyroidism may be due to parathyroid adenomas (89% of cases), parathyroid hyperplasia (9%), or parathyroid cancer (2%) [94]. The majority of patients with primary hyperparathyroidism are thought to be asymptomatic and are found to have elevated serum calcium levels on routine screening. However, on closer questioning, nearly half of these patients may complain of weakness or fatigue [95]. Approximately 20% of patients with hyperparathyroidism will have nephrolithiasis. Other common signs and symptoms include nausea or vomiting, mental disturbances, pancreatitis, and bone pain [83,96,97]. Hypercalcemic crisis is characterized by progressive hypercalcemia with hypovolemia, renal insufficiency, altered mentation, and pancreatitis in the most severe cases. Rarely, seizures from hypercalcemia may mimic eclampsia [98].

The only definitive treatment is surgical removal of the glands. Since only 25% of asymptomatic patients will have progressive disease, which is usually in the form of a decrease in bone mass, the management of asymptomatic hyperparathyroidism is somewhat controversial. In non-pregnant patients with mild to moderate hyperparathyroidism that was left untreated, no increase in mortality was seen. The only increase in mortality occurred in those patients with serum calcium levels in the uppermost quartile [99]. Treatment during pregnancy, however, may be warranted in view of the risk of neonatal tetany as well as the increase in perinatal complications including miscarriage and stillbirth seen in maternal hypercalcemia [100].

There is no satisfactory medical treatment for primary hyperparathyroidism in the pregnant or non-pregnant state. Mithramycin and bisphosphonates are contraindicated during pregnancy. Asymptomatic patients with mild hypercalcemia can be followed closely through pregnancy, with surgery deferred until after delivery [85,101,102]. Occasionally, a patient with significant symptoms due to hypercalcemia but who is not a surgical candidate has been controlled safely and effectively with oral phosphate therapy (1.5 g/day in divided doses) throughout gestation [103]. This therapy is only indicated in patients in whom the initial serum phosphorus level is less than 3 mg/dL; phosphate administration should be adjusted to maintain serum phosphate below 4 mg/dL. Furosemide increases the excretion of calcium in the urine and can be given orally to help lower the serum calcium levels on a chronic basis. In contrast, patients with progressive symptoms, significant hypercalcemia (>12 mg/dL), or deterioration of renal function should be treated surgically by an experienced parathyroid surgeon [83,94]. Neck exploration should not be deferred in the symptomatic woman because of pregnancy, unless delivery is imminent [83].

Medical management for stabilization in hypercalcemic crisis includes hydration with normal saline (2–3 L over 3–6 hours), correction of electrolyte abnormalities, furosemide, which decreases distal tubular calcium reabsorption (10–40 mg IV every 2–4 hours) to maintain urine output at 200 mL/h, and calcium restriction. Hypercalcemia resistant to this regimen may be alleviated with more potent agents, such as calcitonin (100–400 units/day). Although effective initially, tachyphylaxis to calcitonin generally occurs in 4–6 days. Glucocorticoids can be used to decrease gastrointestinal calcium absorption. The reader is referred to a recent review [84] for greater detail.

In hyperparathyroid mothers, neonatal hypocalcemia is predictable and can be prevented. Transient neonatal tetany should not be associated with long-term sequelae. Management of maternal hyperparathyroidism diagnosed during pregnancy should be individualized, taking into consideration the patient's symptoms, the gestational age of the fetus, and the severity of the disease.

Hypoparathyroidism

Hypocalcemia caused by hypoparathyroidism is an extremely rare disorder in pregnancy. The most common cause of hypoparathyroidism is non-production of PTH because of excision of the parathyroid gland, usually following thyroidectomy. Anywhere from 0.5 to 3.5% of thyroid surgeries result in hypoparathyroidism. As mentioned earlier, although total calcium concentration decreases in pregnancy, ionized calcium does not [88,90]. In response to hypocalcemia, PTH normally increases, which in turn augments renal tubular calcium reabsorption and phosphate excretion. PTH also increases 25-hydroxyvitamin D transformation to the active hormone 1,25-dihydroxyvitamin D, which stimulates intestinal calcium and phosphate absorption as well as osteoclastic bone reabsorption [87]. Ineffective PTH syndromes may be caused by failure to respond to increased PTH (pseudohypoparathyroidism), deficient vitamin D from malabsorption, or increased vitamin D metabolism seen with phenytoin or other anticonvulsants [104,105].

Chronic candidiasis, alopecia, vitiligo, and multiple endocrinopathies should suggest the autoimmune polyendocrinopathy–candidiasis–ectodermal dystrophy syndrome [87,106]. Perioral paresthesias, psychiatric disturbances, and Chvostek's or Trousseau's sign may be present. Trousseau's sign, also known as the "obstetrician's hand", or carpal spasm due to ulnar and median nerve ischemia, is elicited by inflating a sphygmomanometer cuff around the arm to 20 mmHg above systolic pressures.. The thumb adducts and the fingers are extended, except at the metacarpophalangeal joints, within minutes, indicating latent tetany. Cardiac changes of hypocalcemia are non-specific but include electrocardiogram Q–T prolongation, hypotension, and reversible congestive cardiomyopathy [104,107]. Hypopharyngeal tetany may present as stridor and seizures and may be life-threatening. Magnesium sulfate rarely has been implicated in hypocalcemia and should be used cautiously when pre-eclampsia is superimposed on hypoparathyroidism [108]. Dilantin may increase vitamin D metabolism. In one case, decreased fetal heart rate variability was reported although there was no evidence of acidosis [109]. Secondary fetal or neonatal hyperparathyroidism, bone demineralization, and skeletal and skull fracture have been reported.

Medical treatment of hypocalcemia can be divided into long-term and acute management. Vitamin D (50 000–100 000 units/day) or 1,25-dihydroxyvitamin D (calcitriol 0.5–3.0 μg/day) and 1–2 g/day of elemental calcium have been used successfully in pregnancy [88]. Vitamin D_2 is the least expensive form of vitamin D, but several weeks may be needed for its full effect. Calcitriol has a faster onset of action (1–2 days) but requires more frequent monitoring to prevent hypercalcemia. Requirements during pregnancy may increase in the latter half of pregnancy, presumably due to increased vitamin D-binding protein. It is often necessary to reduce replacement doses in the postpartum period to avoid hypercalcemia, even in women who are breastfeeding [110]. The latter require closer monitoring of calcium levels, because it may be difficult to predict calcium need during lactation. Of interest, in some species (cattle in particular), the onset of lactation can result in hypocalcemia and parturient paresis [111].

Acute hypocalcemia or impending signs of tetany are treated by 10% calcium gluconate (10 mL diluted in 150 mL of D5W given over 10 minutes), followed by continuous infusion of calcium (0.5–2.0 mg/kg/h). Serial calcium measurements should be measured initially every 2–4 hours to assess the adequacy of the administered dose and adjust the infusion rate accordingly [112]. Laboratory evaluation in addition to ionized calcium should include magnesium, phosphorus, and PTH levels. Hypoparathyroidism is diagnosed by normal serum magnesium concentration, low or inappropriately normal PTH level, and low ionized calcium. High PTH and low phosphorus levels suggest vitamin D deficiency, whereas high PTH and high phosphorus levels are consistent with the diagnosis of pseudohypoparathyroidism or renal insufficiency.

Adrenal crisis

Adrenal insufficiency may be primary or secondary. The most common cause of primary adrenal insufficiency (Addison's disease) is idiopathic or autoimmune adenitis. Less frequently, tuberculosis, sarcoidosis, AIDS, or bilateral hemorrhage (antiphospholipid syndrome or anticoagulation) may be the cause. Autoimmune adenitis may be associated with gonadal failure, hypothyroidism, hyperthyroidism, Hashimoto's thyroiditis, vitiligo, hypoparathyroidism, and pernicious anemia (polyglandular failure type I or II). For further details, the reader is referred to the review of Williams and Dluhy [113]. Except for those patients on corticosteroid therapy for other medical reasons, secondary adrenal insufficiency is rare in pregnancy.

Adrenal insufficiency is more commonly diagnosed during the puerperium than earlier in pregnancy, in part due to the similar symptoms of pregnancy, including nausea, fatigue, diffuse tan or bronze darkening of the elbows or creases of the hands, and bluish-black patches that may appear on the mucous membranes. Axillary and pubic hair may be reduced as adrenal androgens are diminished. The diagnosis may not be suspected until adrenal crisis develops, with potentially serious sequelae. Pregnancy may be well tolerated until stresses such as infection, trauma, surgery, labor, or dehydration from vomiting or diarrhea precipitate adrenal crisis. The clinical features of acute primary adrenocortical insufficiency include hypotension and shock (cardiovascular collapse), weakness, apathy, nausea, vomiting, anorexia, abdominal or flank pain, and hyperthermia. Electrolyte abnormalities include hyponatremia, hyperkalemia, mild azotemia, and metabolic acidosis. Hypoglycemia and mild hypercalcemia may also be seen. Importantly, secondary adrenal insufficiency may present similarly but without electrolyte changes (normal renin–aldosterone response) and should be considered in patients previously on corticosteroids.

Treatment of acute adrenal insufficiency includes hydrocortisone 100 mg IV every 6 hours for 24 hours. This dose can be reduced to 50 mg every 6 hours if the patient is improving, and tapered to an oral maintenance dose in 4–5 days. Doses of hydrocortisone in the range of 100–200 mg maximize mineralocorticoid effects and therefore supplementary mineralocorticoid is not necessary [113]. Additional therapy includes intravenous saline and glucose and correction of precipitating factors (infection) and electrolyte abnormalities. Volume replacement is critical in improving cardiovascular status. Patients with cardiovascular collapse may not respond well to pressor agents until hydrocortisone is given.

Patients on chronic corticosteroid therapy should receive stress doses for infections, surgery, labor, and delivery. Adrenal suppression is unlikely to occur when corticosteroids are used for less than 3 weeks [114]. Following withdrawal of prolonged corticosteroids, approximately 70% of patients will have normal function within a month but in some individuals up to 9 months may be necessary for restoration of normal function [115,116]. However, abnormal ACTH testing measures physiologic reserve and does not necessarily predict whether adrenal crisis will develop following stress. The risk of clinically apparent adrenal insufficiency developing in unsupplemented patients undergoing surgery is well recognized [117]. In obstetric patients, chemical adrenal suppression has been noted in women receiving two courses of betamethasone for fetal lung maturation, yet neither of these patients had clinical signs of adrenal insufficiency during pregnancy [118]. One suggested regimen is to use hydrocortisone 100 mg every 8 hours for 24 hours if the patient has received more than 20 mg of prednisone daily for more than 3 weeks within the previous year [114].

For chronic replacement in patients with primary adrenocortical insufficiency, doses are similar to those in the non-pregnant patient: hydrocortisone 20 mg each morning and 10 mg each evening. Since this dosage of hydrocortisone does not replace the adrenal mineralocorticoid component, mineralocorticoid supplementation is usually needed. This is accomplished by the administration of 0.05–0.2 mg/day fluorocortisone by mouth. Patients should also be instructed to maintain an ample intake of sodium (3–4 g/day). During conditions of increased sweating, exercise, nausea and vomiting, these doses may need to be increased.

References

1 Gabbe SG, Mestman JH, Hibbard LT. Maternal mortality in diabetes mellitus: an 18 year Survey. *Obstet Gynecol* 1976; 48: 549–551.

2 Drury MI, Greene AT, Stronge JM. Pregnancy complicated by clinical diabetes mellitus: a study of 600 pregnancies. *Obstet Gynecol* 1977; 49: 519–522.

3 Kilvert JA, Nicholson HO, Wright AD. Ketoacidosis in diabetic pregnancy. *Diabet Med* 1993; 10: 278–281.

4 Montoro MN, Myers VP, Mestman JH, et al. Outcome of pregnancy in diabetic ketoacidosis. *Am J Perinatol* 1993; 10: 17–20.

5 Chauhan SP, Perry KG. Management of diabetic ketoacidosis in the obstetric patient. *Obstet Gynecol Clin North Am* 1995; 22: 143–155.

6 Bedalov A, Balasubramanyam A. Glucocorticoid induced ketoacidosis in gestational diabetes. *Diabetes Care* 1997; 20: 922–924.

7 Bouhanick B, Biquard F, Hadjadj S, et al. Does treatment with antenatal glucocorticoids for the risk of premature delivery contribute to ketoacidosis in pregnant women with diabetes who receive CSII? *Arch Intern Med* 2000; 160: 242–243.

8 Kitabchi A, Umpierez G, Murphy M, Barret E. Management of hyperglycemic crises in patients with diabetes. *Diabetes Care* 2001; 24: 131–153.

9 Cullen MT, Reece EA, Homko CJ, Sivan E. The changing presentations of diabetic ketoacidosis during pregnancy. *Am J Perinatol* 1996; 13: 449–451.

10 Van der Meulen JA, Klip A, Grinstein S. Possible mechanisms for cerebral oedema in diabetic detoacidosis. *Lancet* 1987; ii: 306–308.

11 Viallon A, Zeni F, Lafond P, et al. Does bicarbonate therapy improve the management of severe diabetic ketoacidosis? *Crit Care Med* 1999; 27: 2690–2693.

12 Miodovnik M, Lavin J, Harrington D, et al. Effect of maternal ketoacidemia on the pregnant ewe and the fetus. *Am J Obstet Gynecol* 1982; 144: 585–593.

13 Nylund L, Lunell N, Lewander R, et al. Uteroplacental blood flow in diabetic pregnancy: measurements with indium 113m and a computer-linked gamma camera. *Am J Obstet Gynecol* 1982; 144: 298–302.

14 Hughes AB. Fetal heart rate changes during diabetic ketosis. *Acta Obstet Gynecol Scand* 1987; 66: 71–73.

15 Takahashi Y, Kawabata I, Shinohara A, Tamaya T. Transient fetal blood flow redistribution induced by maternal diabetic ketoacidosis diagnosed by Doppler ultrasonography. *Prenat Diagn* 2000; 20: 524–525.

16 Burrow GN, Fisher DA, Larsen PR. Maternal and fetal thyroid function. *N Engl J Med* 1994; 331: 1072–1078.

17 Glinoer D, Delange F. The potential repercussions of maternal, fetal and neonatal hypothyroxinemia on the progeny. *Thyroid* 2000; 10: 871–887.

18 Ain KB, Mori Y, Refetoff S. Reduced clearance rate of thyroxine-binding globulin (TBG) with increased sialylation: a mechanism for estrogen-induced elevation of serum TBG concentrations. *J Clin Endocrinol Metab* 1987; 65: 689–696.

19 Berghout A, Endert E, Ross A, et al. Thyroid function and thyroid size in normal pregnant women living in an iodine replete area. *Clin Endocrinol (Oxf)* 1994; 41: 375–379.

20 Wartofsky L, Dickey RA. The evidence for a narrower thyrotropin reference range is compelling. *J Clin Endocrinol Metab* 2005; 90: 5483–5488.

21 Surks MI, Ortiz E, Daniels GH, et al. Subclinical thyroid disease: scientific review and guidelines for diagnosis and management. *JAMA* 2004; 291: 228–238.

22 Hak AE, Pols HAP, Visser TJ, et al. Subclinical hypothyroidism is an independent risk factor for atherosclerosis and myocardial infarction in elderly women: the Rotterdam study. *Ann Intern Med* 2000; 132: 270–278.

23 Imaizumi M, Akahoshi M, Ichimaru S, et al. Risk for ischemic heart disease and all-cause mortality in subclinical hypothyroidism. *J Clin Endocrinol Metab* 2004; 89: 3365–3370.

24 Redondi N, Newman AB, Vittinghoff E, et al. Subclinical hypothyroidism and the risk of heart failure, other cardiovascular events, and death. *Arch Intern Med* 2005; 165: 2460–2466.

25 Mandel SJ, Larsen RP, Seely EW, et al. Increased need for thyroxine during pregnancy in women with primary hypothyroidism. *N Engl J Med* 1990; 323: 91–96.

26 Toft AD. Thyroxine therapy. *N Engl J Med* 1994; 331: 174–180.

27 Davis LE, Lucas MJ, Hankins GD, et al. Thyrotoxicosis complicating pregnancy. *Am J Obstet Gynecol* 1989; 160: 63–70.

28 Wing DA, Miller LK, Koonings PP, et al. A comparison of propylthiouracil versus methimazole in the treatment of hyperthyroidism in pregnancy. *Am J Obstet Gynecol* 1994; 170: 90–95.

29 Kriplani A, Buckshee K, Bhargava VL, et al. Maternal and perinatal outcome in thyrotoxicosis complicating pregnancy. *Eur J Obstet Gynecol Reprod Biol* 1994; 54: 159–163.

30 Neale D, Burrow G. Thyroid disease in pregnancy. *Obstet Gynecol Clin* 2004; 31: 893–905.

31 Nader S. Thyroid disease and other endocrine disorder in pregnancy. *Obstet Gynecol Clin North Am* 2004; 31: 257–285.

32 Volpe R, Ehrlich R, Steriner G, et al. Graves' disease in pregnancy years after hypothyroidism with recurrent passive-transfer neonatal Graves' disease in offspring. Therapeutic considerations. *Am J Med* 1984; 77: 572–578.

33 Amino N, Tanizawa O, Mori H, et al. Aggravation of thyrotoxicosis in early pregnancy and after delivery in Grave's disease. *J Clin Endocrinol Metab* 1982; 55: 108–112.

34 Amino N, Kuro R, Tanizawa O, et al. Changes of serum anti-thyroid antibodies during and after pregnancy in autoimmune thyroid diseases. *Clin Exp Immunol* 1978; 31: 30–37.

35 Muller A, Drexhage H Berghout A. Postpartum thyroiditis and autoimmune thyroiditis in women of childbearing age: recent insights and consequences for antenatal and postnatal care. *Endocrine Rev* 2001; 22: 605–630.

36 Zimmerman D. Fetal and neonatal hyperthyroidism. *Thyroid* 1999; 9: 727–733

37 Epstein RH. Pathogenesis of Graves' ophthalmopathy. *N Engl J Med* 1993; 329: 1468.

38 Weetman AP. Graves' disease. *N Engl J Med* 2000; 343: 1236–1248.

39 Bitton RN, Wexler C. Free triiodothyronine toxicosis: a distinct entity. *Am J Med* 1990; 88: 531–533.

40 Peleg D, Cada S, Peleg A, Ben-Ami M. The relationship between maternal serum thyroid stimulating immunoglobulin and fetal and neonatal thyroitoxicosis. *Obstet Gynecol* 2002; 99: 1040–1043.

41 Glinoer D. Thyroid disease in pregnancy. In: Braverman LE, Utiger RD, eds. *Werner and Ingbar's The Thyroid*, 9th edn. Philadelphia: JB Lippincott, 2004: 1086.

42 Mitsuda N, Tamaki H, Amino N, et al. Risk factors for developmental disorders in infants born to women with Graves disease. *Obstet Gynecol* 1992; 80: 359–364.

43 Mortimer TH, Tyuack SA, Galligan JP, et al. Graves's disease in pregnancy: TSH receptor binding inhibiting immunoglobulins and maternal and neonatal thyroid function. *Clin Endocrinol* 1990; 32: 141–152.

44 Momotani N, Noh J, Oyanagi, Ishikawa N, Ito K. Antithyroid drug therapy for Grave's disease during pregnancy. Optimal regimen for fetal thyroid status. *N Engl J Med* 1986; 315: 24–28.

45 American College of Obstetricians and Gynecologists. *Practice Bulletin No. 32. Thyroid Disease in Pregnancy*. Washington, DC: American College of Obstetricians and Gynecologists, 2001.

46 Mandel SJ, Brent GA, Larsen PR. Review of antithyroid drug use during pregnancy and a report of aplasia cutis. *Thyroid* 1994; 4: 129–133.

47 Gardner DF, Cruishank DP, Hays PM, et al. Pharmacology of propylthiouracil (PTU) in pregnant hyperthyroid women: correlation of maternal PTU concentrations with cord serum thyroid function test. *J Clin Endocrinol Metab* 1986; 62: 217–220.

48 Easterling TR, Schmucker BC, Carlson KL, et al. Maternal hemodynamics in pregnancies complicated by hyperthyroidism. *Obstet Gynecol* 1991; 78: 348–352.

49 Pugh S, Lalwani K, Awal A. Thyroid storm as a cause of loss of consciousness following anaesthesia for emergency caesarean section. *Anaesthesia* 1994; 49: 35–37.

50 Mayer DC, Thorp J, Baucom D, et al. Hyperthyroidism and seizures during pregnancy. *Am J Perinatol* 1995; 12: 192–194.

51 Pekonen F, Lamberg BA, Ikonen E. Thyrotoxicosis and pregnancy: an analysis of 43 pregnancies in 42 thyrotoxic mothers. *Ann Chir Gynaecol* 1978; 67: 1–7.

52 Sheffield J, Cunningham FG. Thyrotoxicosis and heart failure that complicate pregnancy. *Am J Obstet Gynecol* 2004; 190(1): 211–217.

53 Wartofsky L, Ransil B, Ingbar S. Inhibition by iodine of the release of thyroxine from the thyroid gland of patients with thyrotoxicosis. *J Clin Invest* 1970; 49: 78–86.
54 Tan TT, Morat P, Ng ML, et al. Effects of Lugol's solution on thyroid function in normals and patients with untreated thyrotoxicosis. *Clin Endocrinol* 1989; 30: 645–649.
55 Bowman ML, Bergmann M, Smith JF. Intrapartum labetalol for the treatment of maternal and fetal thyrotoxicosis. *Thyroid* 1998; 8: 795–796.
56 Eriksson M, Rubenfeld S, Garber AJ, et al. Propranolol does not prevent thyroid storm. *N Engl J Med* 1977; 296: 263–264.
57 Ashikaga H. Propranolol administration in a patient with thyroid storm. *Ann Intern Med* 2000; 132: 681–682.
58 Ikram H. The nature and prognosis of thyrotoxic heart disease. *Q J Med* 1985; 54: 19–28.
59 Woeber K. Update on the management of hyperthyroidism and hypothyroidism. *Arch Intern Med* 2000; 160: 1067–1071.
60 Cooper DS, Goldminz D, Levin A, et al. Agranulocytosis associated with antithyroid drugs. *Ann Intern Med* 1983; 98: 26–29.
61 Azizi F, Khoshniat M, Bahrainian M, et al. Thyroid function and intellectual development of infants nursed by mothers taking methimazole. *J Clin Endocrinol Metab* 2000; 85: 3233–3238.
62 Mandel SJ, Cooper DS. The use of antithyroid drugs in pregnancy and lactation. *J Clin Endocrinol Metab* 2001; 86: 2354–2359.
63 Glinoer D, de Nayer P, Bourdoux P, et al. Regulation of maternal thyroid during pregnancy. *J Clin Endocrinol Metab* 1990; 71: 276–278.
64 Abalovich M, Gutierrez S, Alcaraz G, et al. Overt and subclinical hypothyroidism complicating pregnancy. *Thyroid* 2002; 12: 63–68.
65 Leung AS, Millar LK, Koonings PP, et al. Perinatal outcome in hypothyroid pregnancies. *Obstet Gynecol* 1993; 81: 349–353.
66 Davis LE, Leveno KJ, Cunningham FG. Hypothyroidism complicating pregnancy. *Obstet Gynecol* 1988; 72: 108–112.
67 Bing RF, Briggs RSJ, Burden AC, et al. Reversible hypertension and hypothyroidism. *Clin Endocrinol (Oxf)* 1980; 12: 339–342.
68 Myrup B, Bregengard C, Faber J. Primary haemostasis in thyroid disease. *J Intern Med* 1995; 238: 59–63.
69 Chopra I, Baber K. Treatment of primary hypothyroidism during pregnancy: is there an increase in thyroxine dose requirement in pregnancy? *Metabolism* 2003; 52: 122–128.
70 Girling JC, de Swiet M. Thyroxine dosage during pregnancy in women with primary hypothyroidism. *Br J Obstet Gynaecol* 1992; 99: 368–370.
71 Monzani F, di Bello V, Caraccion N, et al. Effect of levothyroxine on cardiac function and structure in subclinical hypothyroidism: a double blind, placebo-controlled study. *J Clin Endocrinol Metab* 2001; 86: 1110–1115.
72 Haddow J, Palomaki G, Allan W, et al. Maternal thyroid deficiency during pregnancy and subsequent neurophyschological development of the child. *N Engl J Med* 1999; 341: 549–555.
73 Pop VJ, Brouwers EP, Vader HL, et al. Maternal hypothyroxinaemia during early pregnancy and subsequent child development: a 3 year follow up study. *Clin Endocrinol* 2003; 59: 282–288.
74 LaFranchi SH, Haddow JE, Hollowell JG. Is thyroid inadequacy during gestation a risk factor for adverse pregnancy and developmental outcomes? *Thyroid* 2005; 15(1): 60–71.
75 Ahlawat S, Jain S, Kumari S, et al. Pheochromocytoma associates with pregnancy: case report and review of the literature. *Obstet Gynecol Surv* 1999; 54: 728–737.
76 Hermayer K, Szpiech M. Diagnosis and management of pheochromocytoma during pregnancy: a case report. *Am J Med Sci* 1999; 318: 186–189.
77 Almog B, Kupferminc M, Many A, Lessing J. Pheochromocytoma in pregnancy: a case report and review of the literature. *Acta Obstet Gynecol Scand* 2000; 79: 709–711.
78 Prys-Roberts C. Phaeochromocytoma: recent progress in its management. *Br J Anaesth* 2000; 85: 44–57.
79 Pacak K, Linehan WM, Eisenhofer G, et al. Recent advances in genetics, diagnosis, localization and treatment of pheochromocytoma. *Ann Intern Med* 2001; 134: 315–329.
80 Neumann H, Bausch B, McWhinney SR, et al. Germ-line mutations in nonsyndromic pheochromocytoma. *N Engl J Med* 2002; 346: 1459–1466.
81 James MF, Use of magnesium sulphate in the anaesthetic management of phaeochromocytoma: a review of anaesthetics. *Br J Anaesth* 1989; 62: 616–623.
82 James M. Phaeochromocytoma: recent progress in its management. *Br J Anaesth* 2001; 86; 594–595.
83 Carella MJ, Gossain V. Hyperparathyroidism and pregnancy. *J Gen Intern Med* 1992; 7: 448–453.
84 Schnatz P, Curry S. Primary hyperparathyroidism in pregnancy: evidence based management. *Obstet Gynecol Surv* 2002; 57: 365–376.
85 Gelister JS, Sanderson JD, Chapple CR, et al. Management of hyperparathyroidism in pregnancy. *Br J Surg* 1989; 76: 1207–1208.
86 Kort KC, Schiller HJ, Numann PJ. Hyperparathyroidism and pregnancy. *Am J Surg* 1999; 177: 66–68.
87 Marx SJ. Hyperparathyroid and hypoparathyroid disorders. *N Engl J Med* 2000; 343: 1863–1875.
88 Pitkin RM. Calcium metabolism in pregnancy and the perinatal period. A review. *Am J Obstet Gynecol* 1985; 151: 99–109.
89 Ammann P, Irion O, Gast J, et al. Alterations of calcium and phosphate metabolism in primary hyperparathyroidism during pregnancy. *Acta Obstet Gynecol Scand* 1993; 72: 488–492.
90 Seki K, Makimura N, Mitsui C, et al. Calcium-regulating hormones and osteocalcin levels during pregnancy: a longitudinal study. *Am J Obstet Gynecol* 1991; 164: 1248–1252.
91 Kohlmeier L, Marcus R. Calcium disorder of pregnancy. *Endocrinol Metab Clin North Am* 1995; 24: 15–39.
92 Seely EW, Brown EM, DeMaggio DM, et al. A prospective study of calciotropic hormones in pregnancy and postpartum reciprocal changes in serum intact parathyroid hormone and 1,25-dihydroxyvitamin D. *Am J Obstet Gynecol* 1997; 176: 214–217.
93 Lepre F, Grill V, Ho PW, et al. Hypercalcemia in pregnancy and laction associated with parathyroid hormone-related protein. *N Engl J Med* 1993; 328: 666–667.
94 Kelly TR. Primary hyperparathyroidism during pregnancy. *Surgery* 1991; 110: 1028–1033.
95 Bilezibian JP, Silverbert SJ, Gartenberg F, et al. Clinical presentation of primary hyperparathyroidism. In: Bilezibian JP, Levine MA, Marcu R, eds. *The Parathyroids: Basic and Clinical Concepts*, 2nd edn. San Diego, CA: Academic Press, 2001.
96 Kristoffersson A, Dahlgren S, Lithner F, et al. Primary hyperparathyroidism in pregnancy. *Surgery* 1985; 97: 326–330.
97 Murray J, Newman W, Dacus J. Hyperparathyroidism in pregnancy: diagnostic dilemma? *Obstet Gynecol Surv* 1999; 541: 183.
98 Whalley PJ. Hyperparathyroidism and pregnancy. *Am J Obstet Gynecol* 1963; 86: 517.

99 Silverberg SJ, Shane E, Jacobs TP, Siris E, Bilezikian JP. A 10 year review prospective study of primary hyperparathyroidism with or without parathyroid surgery. *N Engl J Med* 1993; 341: 1249–1255.

100 Shangold MN, Dor N, Welt S, et al. Hyperparathyroidism and pregnancy: a review. *Obstet Gynecol Surv* 1982; 37: 217–228.

101 Croom RD, Thomas CG. Primary hyperparathyroidism during pregnancy. *Surgery* 1984; 96: 1109–1118.

102 Hill NC, Lloyd-Davies SV, Bishop A, et al. Primary hyperparathyroidism and pregnancy. *Int J Gynaecol Obstet* 1989; 29: 253–255.

103 Montoro MN, Collear JV, Mestman JH. Management of hyperparathyroidism in pregnancy with oral phosphate therapy. *Obstet Gynecol* 1980; 55: 431–434.

104 Zalonga GP, Eil C. Diseases of the parathyroid glands and nephrolithiasis during pregnancy. In: Brody SA, Ueland K, Kase N, eds. *Endocrine Disorders in Pregnancy*. Norwalk, CT: Appleton and Lange, 1989: 231.

105 Potts JT. Disease of the parathyroid gland and other hyper and hypocalcemic disorders. In: Braunwald E, Fauci AS, Isselbacher KJ, et al., eds. *Harrison's Principles of Internal Medicine*, 15th edn. New York: McGraw-Hill, 2001.

106 Ahonen P, Myllarniemi S, Sipila I, et al. Clinical variation of autoimmune poly-endocrinopathy-candidiasis-ectodermal dystrophy (APECED) in a series of 68 patients. *N Engl J Med* 1990; 322: 1829–1836.

107 Csanady M, Forster T, Juesz J. Reversible impairment of myocardial function in hypoparathyroidism causing hypocalcaemia. *Br Heart J* 1990; 63: 58–60.

108 Eisenbud E, LoBue C. Hypocalcemia after therapeutic use of magnesium sulfate. *Arch Intern Med* 1976; 136: 688–691.

109 Hagay S, Mazor M, Leiberman J, et al. The effect of maternal hypocalcemia on fetal heart rate baseline variability. *Acta Obstet Gynecol Scand* 1986; 65: 513–515.

110 Caplan RH, Beguin EA. Hypercalcemia in a calcitriol-treated hypoparathyroid women during lactation. *Obstet Gynecol* 1990; 76: 485–489.

111 Goff JP, Reinhardt TA, Horst RL. Recurring hypocalcemia of bovine parturient paresis is associated with failure to produce 1,25-dihydroxyvitamin D. *Endocrinology* 1989; 125: 49–53.

112 Reber PM, Heath H. Hypocalcemic emergencies. *Med Clin North Am* 1995; 79(1): 93–106.

113 Williams G, Dluhy R. Primary adrenocortical deficiency (Addison's disease). In: Braunwald E, Fauci AS, Isselbacher KJ, et al., eds. *Harrison's Principles of Internal Medicine*, 15th edn. New York: McGraw-Hill, 2001.

114 Jabbour S. Steroids and the surgical patient. *Med Clin North Am* 2001; 85: 1311–1317.

115 Graber A, Ney R, Nicholson W, et al. Natural history of pituitary-adrenal function recovery after long-term suppression with corticosteroids. *J Clin Endocrinol* 1965; 25: 11.

116 Aceto T, Beckhorn G, Jorgensen J, et al. Iatrogenic ACTH-cortisol insufficiency. *Pediatr Clin North Am* 1966; 13: 543.

117 Kehlet J, Binder C. Adrenocortical function and clinical course during and after surgery in unsupplemented glucocorticoid-treated patients. *Br J Anaesth* 1973; 45: 1043–1048.

118 Helal K, Gordon MC, Lightner CR, et al. Adrenal suppression induced by betamethasone in women at risk for premature delivery. *Obstet Gynecol* 2000; 96: 287–290.

34 Complications of Pre-eclampsia

Gary A. Dildy III[1] & Michael A. Belfort[2]

[1]Maternal-Fetal Medicine, Mountain Star Division, Hospital Corporation of America, Salt Lake City, UT *and* Department of Obstetrics and Gynecology, LSU Health Sciences Center, School of Medicine in New Orleans, New Orleans, LA, USA
[2]Department of Obstetrics and Gynecology, Division of Maternal-Fetal Medicine, University of Utah School of Medicine, Salt Lake City, UT *and* HCA Healthcare, Nashville, TN, USA

Introduction

Hypertensive disorders complicate 6–8% of pregnancies and remain significant contributors to maternal and perinatal morbidity and mortality [1]. Classification systems of hypertensive diseases during pregnancy tend to be confusing. A National Institutes of Health (NIH) sponsored working group proposed a modified classification system (Table 34.1) for the purpose of providing clinical guidance in managing hypertensive patients during pregnancy. Chronic hypertension is defined as hypertension that is present before pregnancy or diagnosed before the 20th week of gestation. Pre-eclampsia is defined as the appearance of hypertension plus proteinuria, usually occurring after 20 weeks of gestation. Chronic hypertension may be complicated by superimposed pre-eclampsia or eclampsia. In this classification system, gestational hypertension is reassigned retrospectively following the puerperium as transient hypertension of pregnancy or chronic hypertension.

In the United States, pre-eclampsia is one of the top three causes of maternal mortality in advanced gestations [2–5]. Substandard care is often an underlying factor leading to maternal mortality and severe morbidity [6–9].

Pathologic changes commonly affect the maternal cardiovascular, renal, hematologic, neurologic, and hepatic systems (Table 34.2). Equally important are the adverse effects on the uteroplacental unit, resulting in fetal and neonatal complications [10–12]). Our goal is to help guide the clinician in managing potentially severe complications of pre-eclampsia. Therapy for pregnant women with chronic hypertension will not be addressed in this chapter [13,14].

Critical Care Obstetrics, 5th edition. Edited by M. Belfort, G. Saade, M. Foley, J. Phelan and G. Dildy. © 2010 Blackwell Publishing Ltd.

Etiology of pre-eclampsia

Pre-eclampsia has been a recognized pathologic entity since the time of the ancient Greeks [15,16]. The inciting factor remains unknown, however, and an empty shield located on a portico at the Chicago Lying-In Hospital awaits inscription of the name of the person who discovers the etiology of the disease [17]. A significant amount of investigation has been undertaken during recent decades to elucidate the cause and improve the treatment of this disease. During the past 40 years of medical research, the number of published articles has grown in a geometric manner.

Numerous risk factors are associated with the development of pre-eclampsia (Table 34.3), allowing for antenatal recognition of potential problems in some cases. Multiple interrelated pathophysiologic processes have been proposed as etiologic in the development of this disease [18–20], including prostaglandin imbalance [21–25], immunologic mechanisms [26–30], hyperdynamic increase in cardiac output [31], and subclinical blood coagulation changes [32]. Endothelial involvement and the role of tumor necrosis factor, β-carotene, and reduced antithrombin III have also been investigated, but remain incompletely understood [33–38].

Increased vascular reactivity to vasoactive agents was demonstrated by Dieckmann and Michel in 1937 [39]. In 1961, Abdul-Karim and Assali [40] found that normal pregnant women were less responsive to angiotensin II than non-pregnant women. Gant et al. [41] published data that demonstrated an early loss of refractoriness to angiotensin II in those patients who later were to develop pre-eclampsia. Although clinical improvement may follow hospitalization and bed rest, vascular sensitivity to angiotensin II does not decrease until after delivery of the fetus [42].

A molecular variant of the angiotensinogen gene (T235), found to be associated with essential hypertension, also has been associated with pre-eclampsia [43]. It is postulated that increased concentrations of plasma or tissue angiotensinogen could lead to increased baseline or reactive production of angiotensin II,

Table 34.1 Classification of hypertensive diseases during pregnancy.

Chronic hypertension
Hypertension that is present before pregnancy or diagnosed before 20 weeks of gestation

Pre-eclampsia – eclampsia
Hypertension plus proteinuria usually occurring after 20 weeks of gestation or earlier with trophoblastic diseases

Pre-eclampsia superimposed upon chronic hypertension
Chronic hypertension with signs and symptoms of pre-eclampsia such as:
- Blood pressure ≥160/110 mmHg
- Proteinuria ≥2.0 g/24 h
- Serum creatinine >1.2 mg/dL unless previously elevated
- Thrombocytopenia
- Persistent epigastric pain
- Elevated hepatic transaminases
- Persistent neurologic disturbances

Gestational hypertension
These are retrospective diagnoses. If pre-eclampsia is not present at the time of delivery and elevated blood pressure:
- Transient hypertension of pregnancy: returns to normal by 12 weeks post partum
- Chronic hypertension: persists beyond 12 weeks

Modified from the Working Group Report on High Blood Pressure in Pregnancy. National Heart, Lung, and Blood Institute. NIH Publication No. 00-3029, July 2000.

chronically stimulating autoregulatory mechanisms, thus increasing vascular tone and producing vascular hypertrophy. These changes then may impede pregnancy-induced plasma volume expansion, which occurs in normal pregnancies, and result in general circulatory maladaptation.

One of the more striking clinical risk factors for the development of pre-eclampsia is the antiphospholipid syndrome. At the University of Utah, Branch et al. [44] studied 43 women who presented with severe pre-eclampsia prior to 34 weeks of gestation and found 16% to have significant levels of antiphospholipid antibodies. They recommended that women with early-onset severe pre-eclampsia be screened for antiphospholipid antibodies and, if detected, be considered for prophylactic therapy in subsequent pregnancies. The same group [45] found a high incidence of pre-eclampsia (51%) and severe pre-eclampsia (27%) in 70 women with antiphospholipid syndrome whose pregnancies progressed beyond 15 weeks of gestation, despite various medical treatment protocols.

An integrated model of pre-eclampsia pathophysiology has been proposed by Romero et al. [46]. Abnormal placentation is thought to be the first step in the development of the disease, possibly related to immune mechanisms. Trophoblastic prostacyclin, which may be important with respect to trophoblast invasion and prevention of blood clotting in the intervillous space, becomes deficient. A relative decrease in the prostacyclin–thromboxane ratio allows platelet aggregation, thrombin activation, and fibrin deposition in systemic vascular beds. Thrombosis and vasospasm develop and lead to multiorgan involvement, including renal, hepatic, neurologic, hematologic, and uteroplacental dysfunction.

Table 34.2 Complications of severe pregnancy-induced hypertension.

Cardiovascular
Severe hypertension
Pulmonary edema

Renal
Oliguria
Renal failure

Hematologic
Hemolysis
Thrombocytopenia
Disseminated intravascular coagulopathy

Neurologic
Eclampsia
Cerebral edema
Cerebral hemorrhage
Amaurosis

Hepatic
Hepatocellular dysfunction
Hepatic rupture

Uteroplacental
Abruption
Intrauterine growth retardation
Fetal distress
Fetal death

Table 34.3 Risk factors for the development of pregnancy-induced hypertension.

Risk factor	Risk ratio
Nulliparity	3
Age >40 years	3
African-American race	1.5
Family history of pregnancy-induced hypertension	5
Chronic hypertension	10
Chronic renal disease	20
Antiphospholipid syndrome	10
Diabetes mellitus	2
Twin gestation	4
Angiotensinogen gene T235 mutation	
Homozygous	20
Heterozygous	4

Revised from American College of Obstetricians and Gynecologists. *Hypertension in Pregnancy*. ACOG Technical Bulletin 219. Washington, DC: American College of Obstetricians and Gynecologists, 1996.

Women with a previous pregnancy complicated by pre-eclampsia have an increased risk for recurrence in subsequent pregnancies. For severe pre-eclamptic women in an initial pregnancy, recurrence rates for pre-eclampsia are very high, approaching 50% in some studies. Furthermore, significant maternal and fetal complications are more common in recurrent pre-eclampsia compared with an initial episode [47].

All of the preceding theories still do not allow accurate prediction of which gravidas will develop pre-eclampsia, and an ideal screening test is currently not available [19,48]. Furthermore, it is still not clear which process or processes separate mild disease from the development of critical illness and multiorgan dysfunction.

Diagnosis of pre-eclampsia

The diagnosis of pre-eclampsia is often clinically confusing and erroneous [49–52]. Blood pressure (BP) criteria include a systolic BP of at least 140 mmHg or a diastolic BP of at least 90 mmHg. The relative rise from baseline values in systolic pressure of 30 mmHg or diastolic pressure of 15 mmHg appears to be of questionable value [53,54]. Significant proteinuria is defined as at least 300 mg in a 24-hour period. Semiquantitative dipstick analysis of urinary protein is poorly predictive of the actual degree of proteinuria measured by 24-hour urinary collections; thus, classification of pre-eclampsia based on proteinuria should be confirmed with a 24-hour quantitative collection [55]. Edema and weight gain historically have been included in the diagnostic triad (hypertension, proteinuria, edema) of pre-eclampsia, but have been de-emphasized recently due to the ubiquitous nature of edema during pregnancy [1]. These changes usually occur after 20 weeks of gestation, except when there exist hydatidiform changes of the chorionic villi, such as seen with hydatidiform mole or hydrops fetalis.

The signs and symptoms of severe pre-eclampsia are summarized in Table 34.4. The development of these manifestations necessitates careful evaluation, management in a tertiary care facility, and consideration for delivery [3].

Table 34.4 Diagnostic criteria for severe pre-eclampsia.

Blood pressure >160–180 mmHg systolic or >110 mmHg diastolic
Proteinuria >5 g/24 h
Oliguria defined as <500 mL/24 h
Cerebral or visual disturbances
Pulmonary edema
Epigastric or right upper quadrant pain
Impaired liver function of unclear etiology
Thrombocytopenia
Fetal intrauterine growth retardation or oligohydramnios
Elevated serum creatinine
Grand mal seizures (eclampsia)

Revised from American College of Obstetricians and Gynecologists. *Hypertension in Pregnancy.* ACOG Technical Bulletin 219. Washington, DC: American College of Obstetricians and Gynecologists, 1996.

General management principles for pre-eclampsia

On suspecting the diagnosis of pre-eclampsia, several steps are initiated simultaneously to treat and further evaluate the mother and her fetus. A peripheral intravenous line is placed and fluid therapy initiated. These patients are often volume-depleted and benefit from intravenous hydration, but are also susceptible to volume overload, so meticulous monitoring of intake and output is recommended.

Routine laboratory evaluation for pre-eclampsia (Table 34.5) includes complete blood count, platelet count, serum creatinine, and liver enzyme analyses [46,56–59]. If delivery is not felt to be imminent, a 24-hour collection of urine should be started for volume, creatinine clearance, and total protein excretion. The patient should be placed in a lateral recumbent position and fetal assessment (ultrasound, non-stress test, or biophysical profile) performed as indicated [60]. Amniocentesis for fetal lung maturity may be considered in those cases in which fetal maturity is in question and the disease process is not severe enough to mandate delivery.

When severe pre-eclampsia is diagnosed, immediate delivery, regardless of gestational age, has generally been recommended [61]. Conservative management has been proposed in select cases [62–64]). Sibai and colleagues retrospectively reviewed 60 cases of conservatively managed severe pre-eclampsia during the second trimester (18–27 weeks gestation). They found a high maternal morbidity rate, with complications such as abruptio placentae, eclampsia, coagulopathy, renal failure, hypertensive encephalopathy, intracerebral hemorrhage, and ruptured hepatic hematoma. Additionally, an 87% perinatal morality rate was noted [65]. In subsequent prospective studies, Sibai and colleagues reported improved perinatal outcomes with no increased rate of maternal complications in a select group of women with severe pre-eclampsia between 24–27 weeks of gestation and 28–32 weeks of gestation [66] who were managed with intensive fetal and maternal monitoring under strict protocols in a tertiary care center. In another randomized controlled trial, expectant management in selected severe pre-eclamptics between 28 and 34

Table 34.5 Laboratory evaluation for pre-eclampsia.

Complete blood count
Platelet count
Liver function tests (ALT and AST)
Renal function tests (creatinine, blood urea nitrogen, uric acid)
Urinalysis and microscopy
24-hour urine collection for protein and creatinine clearance
Blood type and antibody screen

weeks of gestation was not associated with an increase in maternal complications, but did result in a significant prolongation of the pregnancy, reduction of neonates requiring ventilation, and a reduction in the number of neonatal complications [67].

The presence of pre-eclampsia does not guarantee accelerated lung maturation, and a high incidence of neonatal respiratory complications has been associated with premature delivery for pre-eclampsia [68,69]. In a stable maternal–fetal environment, steroid therapy may be considered if amniocentesis reveals fetal lung immaturity or the clinical situation is consistent with prematurity. Although delivery is generally indicated for severe pre-eclampsia regardless of gestational age, we feel that conservative therapy in a tertiary care center is appropriate in select premature patients with proteinuria exceeding 5 g/24 h, mild elevations of serum transaminase levels, or borderline decreases in platelet count and blood pressure that is controllable.

Fluid therapy for pre-eclampsia

Fluid management in severe pre-eclampsia consists of crystalloid infusions of normal saline or lactated Ringer's solution at 100–125 mL/h. Additional fluid volumes, in the order of 1000–1500 mL, may be required prior to use of epidural anesthesia or vasodilator therapy to prevent maternal hypotension and fetal distress [70].

Epidural anesthesia appears to be safe and is the anesthetic method of choice in severe pre-eclampsia, if preceded by volume preloading to avoid maternal hypotension [71–75]. Likewise, severely hypertensive patients receiving vasodilator therapy may require careful volume preloading to prevent an excessive hypotensive response to vasodilators. Abrupt and profound drops in blood pressure leading to fetal bradycardia and distress may occur in severe pre-eclampsia when vasodilator therapy is not accompanied by volume expansion [76–78].

Intravenous fluids are known to cause a decrease in colloid oncotic pressure (COP) in laboring patients [79]. In addition, baseline COP is decreased in patients with pre-eclampsia and may decrease further postpartum as a result of mobilization of interstitial fluids. This may be clinically relevant with respect to the development of pulmonary edema in pre-eclamptic patients [80]. Therefore, close monitoring of fluid intake and output, hemodynamic parameters, and clinical signs must be undertaken to prevent an imbalance of hydrostatic and oncotic forces that potentiate the occurrence of pulmonary edema.

Kirshon et al. [77] placed systemic and pulmonary artery catheters in 15 primigravid patients with severe pre-eclampsia during labor. A hemodynamic protocol requiring strict control of COP, pulmonary capillary wedge pressure (PCWP), and mean arterial pressure (MAP) throughout labor, delivery, and the postpartum period was followed. Low COP and PCWP were corrected with the administration of albumin. Severe hypertension was treated as needed with intravenous nitroglycerin, nitroprusside, or hydralazine. Furosemide was administered for elevated PCWP. These investigators found that the only benefit of such management was avoidance of sudden profound drops in systemic blood pressure and fetal distress during antihypertensive therapy. The overall incidence of fetal distress in labor was not affected, however. Because of a significant requirement for pharmacologic diuresis to prevent pulmonary edema in the study group, these authors recommended that COP not be corrected with colloid unless markedly decreased (12 mmHg) or a prolonged negative COP–PCWP gradient was identified. While the infusion of colloids has been shown to result in less of a decrease in COP when compared with crystalloids, there is no evidence of any clinical benefit of colloids over crystalloids for the pregnant patient [81]. Thus, in the absence of a firm clinical indication for colloid infusion, carefully controlled crystalloid infusions appear to be the safest mode of fluid therapy in severe pre-eclampsia.

A randomized clinical trial (n = 264) compared the postpartum management of pre-eclampsia with brief furosemide therapy (20 mg oral furosemide daily for 5 days with 20 mEq per day of oral potassium supplementation) versus no furosemide therapy, after spontaneous onset of postpartum diuresis and discontinuation of intravenous magnesium sulfate. Only patients with severe pre-eclampsia appeared to benefit from furosemide therapy, defined by more rapid normalization of blood pressure and reduction in the need for antihypertensive therapy. Shortening of hospitalization and reduction of delayed postpartum complications were not observed.

Seizure prophylaxis for pre-eclampsia

Magnesium sulfate ($MgSO_4 \cdot 7H_2O$ USP) has been used for the prevention of eclamptic seizures since the early 20th century [82–84] and has long been the standard treatment of pre-eclampsia–eclampsia in the United States [85,86]. The mechanism of action of magnesium sulfate remains controversial [87]. Some investigators feel that magnesium acts primarily via neuromuscular blockade, while others believe that magnesium acts centrally [88,89]. Two separate investigations evaluating the effect of parenteral magnesium sulfate on penicillin-induced seizure foci in cats report conflicting data [88,90]. Koontz and Reid [90] postulate that magnesium may be effective as an anticonvulsant only when the blood–brain barrier is disrupted. Human data reveal that abnormal EEG findings are common in pre-eclampsia–eclampsia, and they are not altered by levels of magnesium considered to be therapeutic [91]. In the rat model, Hallak et al. [92] and Hallak [93] proposed that magnesium's anticonvulsant mechanism of action was central, mediated through excitatory amino acid (N-methyl-D-aspartate) receptors. In a randomized placebo-controlled study, Belfort et al. [94] evaluated the effect of magnesium sulfate on maternal retinal blood flow in pre-eclamptics by way of Doppler blood flow measurements of central retinal and posterior ciliary arteries. Their findings suggested that magnesium sulfate vasodilates small vessels in the retina and proposed that this may reflect similar changes occurring in the cerebral circulation. More recently, Belfort et al. [95] showed that magnesium sulfate reduces cerebral perfusion pressure while at the same time maintaining cerebral blood flow. This finding suggests that at least in part, magnesium sulfate acts by preventing or reducing hypertensive encephalopathy and barotrauma of the cerebral microcirculation [96].

Magnesium sulfate regimens are illustrated in Table 34.6. Because a regimen of a 4-g IV loading dose followed by a 1–2-g/h IV maintenance dose failed to prevent eclampsia in a significant number of pre-eclamptic women, Sibai et al. [97] modified this regimen to a 4-g IV loading dose followed by a 2–3-g/h IV maintenance dose. Sibai compared Pritchard's regimen of a 4-g IV and 10-g IM loading dose followed by a 5-g IM maintenance dose every 4 hours, with a 4-g IV loading dose followed by a 1–2-g/h continuous IV maintenance infusion. The IV loading dose with maintenance dose of 1 g/h did not produce adequate serum levels of magnesium (4–7 mEq/L); thus, they recommended a 2–3-g/h maintenance dose [97]. We employ a regimen of a 4–6-g IV loading dose over 20 minutes, followed by a 2–3-g/h continuous IV infusion. The maintenance infusion may be adjusted according to clinical parameters and serum magnesium levels. Pruett et al. [98] found no significant effects on neonatal Apgar scores at these doses.

Until relatively recently there remained considerable controversy regarding the best agent for eclampsia prophylaxis. In the United States, magnesium sulfate has been the agent of choice [61,69,99], whereas in the United Kingdom and in a few US centers, conventional antiepileptic agents have been advocated [100–103]. Recently, several important randomized clinical trials of magnesium sulfate for prevention or control of eclamptic seizures have been published (Table 34.7).

Table 34.6 Magnesium sulfate protocols.

	Loading dose	Maintenance dose
Pritchard [85]		
Eclampsia	4 g IV and 10 g IM	5 g IM every 4 h
Zuspan [323]		
Severe pre-eclampsia	None	1 g/h IV
Eclampsia	4–6 g IV over 5–10 min	1 g/h IV
Sibai et al. [97]		
Pre-eclampsia–eclampsia	6 g IV over 15 min	2 g/h

In a randomized trial comparing magnesium sulfate with phenytoin for the prevention of eclampsia, Lucas et al. [104] found a statistically significant difference ($P = 0.004$) in the development of seizures between the magnesium sulfate group (0/1049) and the phenytoin group (10/1089), with no significant differences in eclampsia risk factors between the two study groups.

The Eclampsia Trial Collaborative Group [105] enrolled 1,687 women with eclampsia in an international multicenter randomized trial comparing standard anticonvulsant regimens of magnesium sulfate, phenytoin, and diazepam. Women allocated magnesium sulfate had a 52% lower risk of recurrent convulsions than those allocated diazepam, and a 67% lower risk of recurrent convulsions than those allocated phenytoin. Women allocated magnesium sulfate were less likely to require mechanical ventilation, to develop pneumonia, and to be admitted to intensive care than those allocated phenytoin. Furthermore, the babies of mothers allocated magnesium sulfate were less likely to be intubated at delivery and less likely to be admitted to the newborn intensive care nursery when compared with babies of mothers treated with phenytoin. The Eclampsia Trial Collaborative Group concluded that magnesium sulfate is the drug of choice for routine anticonvusant management of women with eclampsia, rather than diazepam or phenytoin, and recommended that other anticonvulsants be used only in the context of randomized trials.

Coetzee et al. [106] conducted a blinded, randomized, controlled trial ($n = 822$) of intravenous magnesium sulfate versus placebo in the management of women with severe pre-eclampsia. They found that use of intravenous magnesium sulfate significantly reduced the development of eclampsia (0.3% vs 3.2%, relative risk 0.09; 95% confidence interval 0.01–0.69; $P = 0.003$) compared to placebo.

Thus at present, magnesium sulfate is strongly endorsed as the agent of choice for eclampsia prophylaxis and treatment

Table 34.7 Randomized trials comparing magnesium sulfate ($MgSO_4$) with other agents in prophylaxis (preventing eclampsia in pre-eclamptics) and treatment (preventing recurrent seizures) of eclampsia.

Reference	Study population	*n*	$MgSO_4$	Placebo	Phenytoin	Diazepam	Lytic cocktail	Nimodipine
Bhalla [326]	Eclamptics	91	2.2%	–	–	–	24.4%	–
Lucas et al. [104]	Mixed pre-eclamptics	2138	0%	–	0.9%	–	–	
Eclampsia Trial Collaborative Group [105]	Eclamptics	905	13.2%	–	–	27.9%	–	–
	Eclamptics	775	5.7%	–	17.1%	–	–	–
Coetzee et al. [106]	Severe pre-eclamptics	685	0.3%	3.2%	–	–	–	–
Magpie Trial Collaborative Group [319]	Mixed pre-eclamptics	10,141	0.8%	1.9%	–	–	–	–
Belfort et al. [287]	Severe pre-eclamptics	1650	0.8%	–	–	–	–	2.6%

[1,107–110]. The Cochrane Review of randomized clinical trials found magnesium superior to lytic cocktail (chlorpromazine, promethazine, pethidine), diazepam, and phenytoin for prevention and/or treatment of eclampsia [111–114]. The role of magnesium sulfate seizure prophylaxis for mild pre-eclamptics is still subject to debate.

Plasma magnesium levels maintained at 4–7 mEq/L are felt to be therapeutic in preventing eclamptic seizures [3]. Patellar reflexes usually are lost at 8–10 mEq/L, and respiratory arrest may occur at 13 mEq/L [85,115]. Urine output, patellar reflexes, and respiratory rates should be monitored closely during magnesium sulfate administration. In those patients who have renal dysfunction, serum magnesium levels should be monitored as well. Calcium gluconate, oxygen therapy, and the ability to perform endotracheal intubation should be available in the event of magnesium toxicity [115]. Calcium will reverse the adverse effects of magnesium toxicity. Calcium gluconate is administered as a 1-g dose (10 mL of a 10% solution) IV over a period of 2 minutes [116].

Bohman and Cotton [117] reported a case of supralethal magnesemia (38.7 mg/dL) with patient survival and no adverse sequelae. The essential elements in the resuscitation and prevention of toxic magnesemia are: (i) respiratory support as determined by clinical indicators; (ii) use of continuous cardiac monitoring; (iii) infusion of calcium salts to prevent hypocalcemia and the enhanced cardiotoxicity associated with concurrent hypocalcemia and hypermagnesemia; (iv) use of loop or osmotic diuretics to excrete the magnesium ion more rapidly, as well as careful attention to fluid and electrolyte balances; (v) a consideration that toxic magnesium is neither anesthetic nor amnestic to the patient; and (vi) assurance that all magnesium infusions be administered in a buretrol-type system or by intramuscular injection to prevent toxic magnesemia.

Magnesium sulfate is not an antihypertensive agent [85]. Administration produces a transient decrease in BP in hypertensive, but not normotensive, non-pregnant subjects [118]. Young and Weinstein [119] noted significant respiratory effects and a transient fall in maternal BP in patients who received a 10-g IM loading dose of magnesium sulfate followed by maintenance push doses of 2 g every 1–2 hours, but not in patients who received the 10-g loading dose followed by a 1-g/h continuous infusion [119]. Cotton et al. [76] observed a transient hypotensive effect related to bolus infusion, but not with continuous infusion in severe pre-eclampsia.

Duration of magnesium administration post-delivery for seizure prophylaxis in severe pre-eclampsia has traditionally been 24 hours in many centers. A randomized clinical trial of 98 severe pre-eclamptics compared standard 24-hour treatment with discontinuation of magnesium upon the onset of maternal diuresis, defined as urine output >100 mL/h for 2 consecutive hours [120]. This study showed no untoward outcomes or need for re-initiation of treatment with discontinuation of therapy at diuresis.

Antihypertensive therapy for severe pre-eclampsia

Pre-eclampsia is sometimes manifested by severe systemic hypertension. Careful control of hypertension must be achieved to prevent complications such as maternal cerebral vascular accidents and placental abruption. Medical intervention is usually recommended when the diastolic BP exceeds 110 mmHg [116,121,122]. The degree of systolic hypertension requiring therapy is less certain, but most would treat for a level exceeding 160–180 mmHg, depending on the associated diastolic pressure. In the previously normotensive patient, cerebral autoregulation is lost and the risk of intracranial bleeding increases when MAP exceeds 140–150 mm Hg, as illustrated in Figure 34.1 [123]. Although many different antihypertensive agents are available, we confine our discussion to those agents most commonly used for acute hypertensive crises in pregnancy (Table 34.8).

Hydralazine hydrochloride

Hydralazine hydrochloride (Apresoline) has long been the gold standard of antihypertensive therapy for use by obstetricians in the United States. Hydralazine reduces vascular resistance via direct relaxation of arteriolar smooth muscle, affecting precapillary resistance vessels more than postcapillary capacitance vessels [124]. Assali et al. [125] noted the hypotensive effect to be marked and prolonged in pre-eclamptic patients, moderate in patients with essential hypertension, and slight in normotensive subjects. Using M-mode echocardiography, Kuzniar et al. [126] found an attenuated response to a 12.5-mg IV dose of hydralazine in patients with pre-existing hypertension, compared with those with severe pre-eclampsia. Cotton et al. [127] studied the cardiovascular alterations in six severe pre-eclamptics following intra-

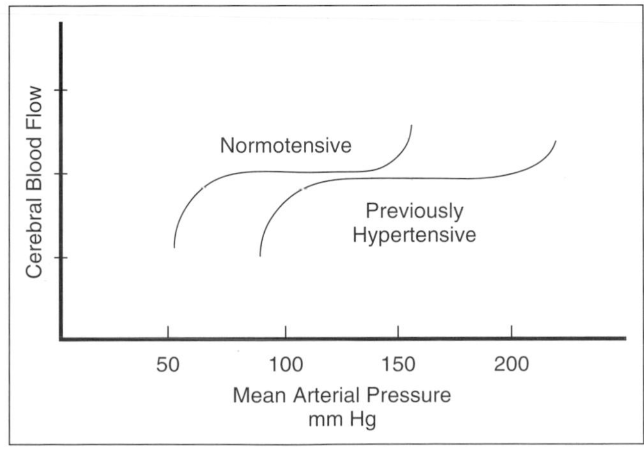

Figure 34.1 Cerebral blood flow remains constant over a wide range of pressures in normotensive individuals. This range is shifted to the right in individuals with chronic hypertension. (Modified from Zimmerman JL. Hypertensive crisis: emergencies and urgencies. In: Ayers SM, ed. *Textbook of Critical Care*. Philadelphia: WB Saunders, 1995.)

Table 34.8 Pharmacologic agents for antihypertensive therapy in pre-eclampsia–eclampsia.

Generic name	Trade name	Mechanism of action	Dosage	Comment
Hydralazine	Apresoline	Arterial vasodilator	5 mg IV, then 5–10 mg IV/20 min up to total dose of 40 mg; titrated IV infusion 5–10 mg/h	Must wait 20 min for response between IV doses; possible maternal hypotension
Labetalol	Normodyne Trandate	Selective α- and non-selective β-antagonist	20 mg IV, then 40–80 mg IV/10 min to 300 mg total dose; titrated IV infusion 1–2 mg/min	Less reflex tachycardia and hypotension than with hydralazine
Nifedipine	Procardia Adalat	Calcium channel blocker	10 mg PO, may repeat after 30 min	Oral route only; possible exaggerated effect if used with $MgSO_4$
Nitroglycerin	Nitrostat IV Tridil Nitro-Bid IV	Relaxation of venous (and arterial) vascular smooth muscle	5 μg/min infusion; double every 5 min	Requires arterial line for continuous blood pressure monitoring; potential methemoglobinemia
Nitroprusside	Nipride Nitropress	Vasodilator	0.25 μg/kg/min infusion; increase by 0.25 μg/kg/min every 5 min	Requires arterial line for continuous blood pressure monitoring; potential cyanide toxicity

Modified from Dildy GA, Cotton DB. Hemodynamic changes in pregnancy and pregnancy complicated by hypertension. *Acute Care* 1988–89; 14–15: 26–46.

venous administration of a 10-mg bolus of hydralazine. They observed a significant increase in maternal heart rate and cardiac index (CI), with a decrease in MAP and systemic vascular resistance (SVR) index. There was a wide range of individual response with respect to peak and duration. Jouppila et al. [128] measured maternal–fetal effects with Doppler in severe pre-eclamptics receiving dihydralazine and demonstrated a fall in maternal BP with no change in intervillous blood flow and an increase in umbilical vein blood flow. Dihydralazine also has been shown to cross the placenta to the fetus [129]. The administration of hydralazine may result in maternal hypotension and fetal distress [130]. For this reason, we recommend an initial dose of 2.5–5.0 mg IV, followed by observation of hemodynamic effects. If appropriate change in BP is not achieved, 5–10 mg IV may be administered at 20-minute intervals to a total acute dose of 30–40 mg. Hypertension refractory to the preceding approach warrants the use of alternative antihypertensive agents [131,132].

Diazoxide

Diazoxide (Hyperstat) is a benzothiadiazine derivative that exerts its antihypertensive effect by reducing peripheral vascular resistance through direct relaxation of arterioles [133]. The commonly used 300-mg bolus injection to treat severe hypertension may induce significant hypotension with resultant morbidity. Minibolus diazoxide titration is clinically effective and relatively free of side effects in non-pregnant, severely hypertensive adults; a suggested dose would be 30–60 mg IV in 5-minute intervals, titrating to desired clinical response. Thien et al. [134] recommended that diazoxide for the treatment of severe pre-eclampsia–eclampsia be administered by the infusion method (15 mg/min; total amount, 5 mg/kg body weight) rather than by bolus injection (300 mg within 10 s), because the infusion method results in a more gradual decline in BP and can be interrupted in cases of exaggerated drop in BP.

Calcium channel blockers

Calcium channel blockers such as nifedipine (Procardia, Adalat) lower BP primarily by relaxing arterial smooth muscle. An initial oral dose of 10 mg is administered, which may be repeated after 30 minutes, if necessary, for the acute management of severe hypertension; 10–20 mg may then be administered orally every 3–6 hours as needed [121]. Principal side effects in severe pre-eclamptics include headache and cutaneous flushing. Care must be given when nifedipine is administered to patients receiving concomitant magnesium sulfate because of the possibility of an exaggerated hypotensive response [135]. In a randomized clinical trial, 49 women with severe pre-eclampsia and severe hypertension between 26 and 36 weeks of gestation were primarily treated with sublingual (then oral) nifedipine or intravenous (then oral) hydralazine [136]. Effective control of BP (values consistently below 160/110 mmHg) was achieved in 96% of the nifedipine group and 68% of the hydralazine group ($P < 0.05$), with acute fetal distress occurring more commonly in the hydralazine group. A beneficial effect may also be seen on urine output in women with severe pre-eclampsia treated with nifedipine [137,138]. Other calcium channel blockers (nimodipine) have been studied in the management of pre-eclampsia [139–142] and are the subject of ongoing investigation.

Labetalol

Labetalol (Normodyne, Trandate) is a combined α- and β-adrenoceptor antagonist that may be used to induce a controlled rapid decrease in BP via decreased SVR in patients with severe hypertension [143]. Reports on the efficacy and safety of labetalol in the treatment of hypertension during pregnancy have been favorable ([144–150]. Mabie et al. [149] compared bolus intravenous labetalol with intravenous hydralazine in the acute treatment of severe hypertension. They found that labetalol had a quicker onset of action and did not result in reflex tachycardia. Labetalol also may exert a positive effect on early fetal lung maturation in patients with severe hypertension who are remote from term [145,151]. An initial dose of 10 mg is given and is followed by progressively increasing doses (20, 40, 80 mg) every 10 minutes, to a total dose of 300 mg. Alternately, constant intravenous infusion may be started at 1–2 mg/min until therapeutic goals are achieved, then decreased to 0.5 mg/min or completely stopped [121]. Lunell et al. [152] studied the effects of labetalol on uteroplacental perfusion in hypertensive pregnant women and noted increased uteroplacental perfusion and decreased uterine vascular resistance. Morgan et al. [153] evaluated the effects of labetalol on uterine blood flow in the hypertensive gravid baboon and found that low doses (0.5 mg/kg) significantly reduced MAP without adversely affecting uterine blood flow. Belfort et al. have shown that labetalol has a favorable profile in terms of its cerebral hemodynamic effects. It reduces elevated cerebral perfusion pressure while maintaining cerebral blood flow [154]. This may be important in its control of cerebral overperfusion and prevention of hypertensive encephalopathy and associated pathology.

Nitroglycerin

Nitroglycerin (Nitrostat IV, Nitro-Bid IV, Tridil) relaxes predominantly venous but also arterial vascular smooth muscle, decreasing preload at low doses and afterload at high doses [155]. It is a rapidly acting potent antihypertensive agent with a very short hemodynamic half-life. Using invasive hemodynamic monitoring, Cotton et al. [131,156] noted that the ability to control BP precisely was dependent on volume status. Although larger doses of nitroglycerin were required following volume expansion, the ability to effect a smoother and more controlled drop in BP required prevasodilator hydration [156]. Nitroglycerin is administered via an infusion pump at an initial rate of 5 μg/min and may be doubled every 5 minutes. Methemoglobinemia may result from high-dose (7 μg/kg/min) intravenous infusion. Patients with normal arterial oxygen saturation who appear cyanotic should be evaluated for toxicity, defined as a methemoglobin level greater than 3% [155].

Sodium nitroprusside

Sodium nitroprusside (Nipride, Nitropress) is another potent antihypertensive agent that may be used to control severe hypertension associated with pre-eclampsia. A dilute solution may be started at 0.25 μg/kg/min and titrated to the desired effect through an infusion pump by increasing the dose by 0.25 μg/kg/min every 5 minutes. The solution is light sensitive and should be covered in foil and changed every 24 hours [157]. Arterial blood gases should be monitored for developing metabolic acidosis, which may be an early sign of cyanide toxicity. In non-pregnant subjects, sodium nitroprusside infusion rates in excess of 4 μg/kg/min led to red blood cell cyanide levels that after 2–3 hours of administration extended into the toxic range (>40 nmol/mL); infusion rates of less than 2 μg/kg/min for several hours remained non-toxic [157]). Treatment time should be limited because of the potential for fetal cyanide toxicity [158]. Correction of hypovolemia prior to initiation of nitroprusside infusion is essential in order to avoid abrupt and often profound drops in BP.

Angiotensin-converting enzyme inhibitors

Angiotensin-converting enzyme (ACE) inhibitors (captopril, enalapril) interrupt the renin–angiotensin–aldosterone system, resulting in a lowering of BP [159]. The risk of inducing neonatal renal failure and other serious complications would contraindicate the use of ACE inhibitors during pregnancy [160–163]. Fetal abortion has been reported in pregnant rabbits [164]. Additionally, the ACE inhibitors as a class do not appear to be useful in acute treatment of severe hypertension because of a 1–4-hour delay in achievement of peak serum levels after ingestion [159].

Severe hypertension

We recommend labetalol for the initial management of severe hypertension in pre-eclampsia (BP 180–160/110 mmHg). Labetalol will be effective in restoring BP to a desired range (160–130/110–80 mmHg) in the majority of cases and has favorable cerebral hemodynamic effects with a minimum of adverse fetal effects. Hydralazine is used if labetalol is ineffective and if maximum doses (up to 40 mg) have not corrected the severe hypertension, we then proceed to nifedipine. Hydralazine in high doses has been associated with diversion of blood from the uteroplacental ciculation and sudden-onset fetal decompensation. In rare cases, these agents are ineffective, and we resort to intravenous infusion of nitroglycerin or nitroprusside, which requires an intensive care setting.

Analgesia–anesthesia for pre-eclampsia

The use of conduction anesthesia in pre-eclampsia was, at one time, controversial. Concerns have been voiced by some authors that the sympathetic blockade and peripheral vasodilation resulting from epidural anesthesia may lead to hypotension and fetal distress in patients who are already volume contracted [3,86,165]. However, induction of general endotracheal anesthesia is not without its own inherent risks. General anesthesia has been shown to result in significant rises in systemic arterial pressure in patients with severe pre-eclampsia. An average increase in systolic arterial BP of 56 mmHg during endotracheal intubation of 20 patients with hypertension was reported by Connell et al. [166].

Hodgkinson et al. [167] evaluated 10 severe pre-eclamptic–eclamptic patients undergoing general anesthesia using the pulmonary artery catheter. They noted severe systemic and pulmonary hypertension during endotracheal intubation and extubation. Ten patients undergoing epidural anesthesia with 0.75% bupivacaine for cesarean section maintained stable systemic and pulmonary arterial pressures, with the exception of one patient who developed systemic hypotension that responded promptly to ephedrine.

Newsome et al. [75] demonstrated a drop in MAP and a slight but insignificant decrease in SVR without change in CI, peripheral vascular resistance (PVR), central venous pressure (CVP), or PCWP in 11 patients with severe pre-eclampsia undergoing lumbar epidural anesthesia. Jouppila et al. [73] measured intervillous blood flow in nine patients with severe pre-eclampsia during labor with lumbar epidural block and found a significant increase in uterine blood flow. Ramos-Santos et al. [168] studied the effects of epidural anesthesia on uterine and umbilical artery blood flow by way of Doppler velocimetry in mild pre-eclamptics, chronic hypertensives, and normal controls during active term labor. In the pre-eclamptic group, the uterine artery systolic/diastolic ratios decreased to levels similar to those of the control group, suggesting a possible beneficial effect in reducing uterine artery vasospasm.

Deleterious hypotension may be avoided by lateral maternal tilt, thus preventing aortocaval occlusion, and preloading with crystalloid solution to compensate for peripheral vasodilation [73]. Contraindications to epidural anesthesia include patient refusal, fetal distress requiring immediate delivery, local infection, septicemia, severe spinal deformities, and coagulopathy [74]. If preceded by volume loading, epidural anesthesia appears beneficial and safe in severe pre-eclampsia [70–75,132]. Clark and Cotton [132] state, "In skilled hands, a cautiously administered epidural anesthetic is, in our opinion, not only justified, but the method of choice for anesthesia in cesarean section or for control of the pain of labor in the patient with severe pre-eclampsia." The safety and efficacy of neuraxial analgesia for severe pre-eclamptics appears to be well supported by recent studies [169,170]). When general anesthesia is necessary, careful control of maternal BP, especially around the time of induction and awakening, is essential. Small doses of nitroglycerin or other similar agents are often useful in this regard.

Hemodynamic monitoring for pre-eclampsia

The pulmonary artery catheter, introduced over 30 years ago, has been very useful in the management of critically ill patients [171]. In cases of severe pre-eclampsia, most clinicians have obtained excellent results without invasive monitoring [69]. Protocols developed to study the central hemodynamic parameters of severe pre-eclampsia have revealed interesting data, which are sometimes confounded by differences in clinical patient management prior to and at the time of catheterization [70]. Hemodynamic changes observed in normal pregnancies and pregnancies complicated by hypertension are summarized by Dildy and Cotton [172,173]. Central hemodynamic findings in severe pre-eclampsia are summarized by Clark and Cotton [132] in Table 34.9. Hemodynamic findings in non-pregnant women, normal third-trimester pregnancy, and severe pre-eclamptics are provided in Table 34.10.

Table 34.9 Hemodynamic findings in severe pregnancy-induced hypertension.

Cardiac output is variable
Mean arterial pressure is elevated; systemic vascular resistance is normal (early) or elevated (late)
Central venous pressure is usually low to normal and does not correlate with pulmonary capillary wedge pressure
Pulmonary hypertension and pulmonary vascular resistance are not present, but low pulmonary artery pressure may occur in the presence of hypovolemia
Pulmonary capillary wedge pressure may be low, normal or high
Oliguria may not reflect volume depletion
Ventricular function is usually hyperdynamic, but may be depressed in the presence of marked elevation in systemic vascular resistance
Colloid oncotic pressure is usually low

Reproduced with permission from Clark SL, Cotton DB. Clinical indications for pulmonary artery catheterization in the patient with severe preeclampsia. *Am J Obstet Gynecol* 1988; 158: 453–458.

Current indications for the use of a pulmonary artery catheter in pre-eclampsia are listed in Table 34.11 [132,174–176]. Routine use of the pulmonary artery catheter in uncomplicated severe pre-eclampsia is not recommended. In these cases, the potential morbidity of pulmonary artery catheterization does not appear to be justified. Known complications of invasive monitoring at the time of insertion include cardiac arrhythmias, pneumothorax, hemothorax, injury to vascular and neurologic structures, pulmonary infarction, and pulmonary hemorrhage. Later complications include balloon rupture, thromboembolism, catheter knotting, pulmonary valve rupture, and catheter migration into the pericardial and pleural spaces, with subsequent cardiac tamponade and hydrothorax [177–179]. It should be noted, however, that Clark et al. [174] observed no significant complications from pulmonary artery catheterization in a series of 90 patients who underwent the procedure on an obstetrics–gynecology service. A retrospective study of 115 pregnant women with severe pre-eclampsia and eclampsia managed by pulmonary artery catheterization concluded that catheterization was subjectively beneficial in 93% of cases with an acceptable complication rate of 4% [180].

An alternate approach to the use of invasive monitoring is the use of echocardiography to determine central hemodynamic parameters [181–183]. In almost all cases of severe pre-eclampsia an initial echocardiogram will allow determination of cardiac function (cardiac output and ejection fraction), and central venous pressure. This is generally all that is needed to make the important clinical decisions regarding fluid management and antihypertensive drug choice. It also allows rapid determination of cardiac function and the potential for hypertensive cardiomyopathy and diastolic dysfunction – two important complications frequently seen in severe hypertension in pre-eclampsia. We have

Table 34.10 Hemodynamic profiles of non-pregnant women, normal women during the late third trimester, and severe pre-eclamptics.

Normal	Normal late non-pregnant (n = 10)* (mean ± SD)	Normal/late third trimester (n = 10)* (mean ± SD)	Severe pre eclampsia (n = 45)† (mean ± SEM)	Severe preeclampsia (n = 41)‡ (mean ± SEM)
Heart rate (beats/min)	71 ± 10	83 ± 10	95 ± 2	94 ± 2
Systolic blood pressure (mmHg)	N/A	N/A	193 ± 3	175 ± 3
Diastolic blood pressure (mmHg)	N/A	N/A	110 ± 2	106 ± 2
Mean arterial blood pressure (mmHg)	86.4 ± 7.5	90.3 ± 5.8	138 ± 3	130 ± 2
Pulse pressure (mmHg)	N/A	N/A	84 ± 2	70 ± 2
Central venous pressure (mmHq)	3.7 ± 2.6	3.6 ± 2.5	4 ± 1	4.8 ± 0.4
Pulmonary capillary wedge pressure (mmHg)	6.3 ± 2.1	7.5 ± 1.8	10 ± 1	8.3 ± 0.3
Pulmonary artery pressure (mmHg)	11.9 ± 2.0§	12.5 ± 2.0§	17 ± 1	15 ± 0.5
Cardiac output (L/min)	4.3 ± 0.9	6.2 ± 1.0	7.5 ± 0.2	8.4 ± 0.2
Stroke volume (mL)	N/A	N/A	79 ± 2	90 ± 2
Systemic vascular resistance (dynes·sec·cm^{-5})	1530 ± 520	1210 ± 266	1496 ± 64	1,226 ± 37
Pulmonary vascular resistance (dynes·sec·cm^{-5})	119 ± 47	78 ± 22	70 ± 5	65 ± 3
Serum colloid osmotic pressure (mmHg)	20.8 ± 1.0	18.0 ± 1.5	19.0 ± 0.5	N/A
Body surface area (m^2)	N/A	N/A	N/A	N/A
Systemic vascular resistance index (dynes·sec·cm^{-5}·m^2)	N/A	N/A	2726 ± 120	2,293 ± 65
Pulmonary vascular resistance index (dynes·sec·cm^{-5}·m^2)	N/A	N/A	127 ± 9	121 ± 7
Right ventricular stroke work index (g·m·M^{-2})	N/A	N/A	8 ± 1	10 ± 0.5
Left ventricular stroke work index (g·m·M^{-2})	41 ± 8	48 ± 6	81 ± 2	84 ± 2
Cardiac index (L·min^{-1}·m^2)	N/A	N/A	4.1 ± 0.1	4.4 ± 0.1
Stroke volume index (mL·beat·m^2)	N/A	N/A	44 ± 1	48 ± 1
COP–PCWP (mmHg)	14.5 ± 2.5	10.5 ± 2.7	N/A	N/A

Data from * Cotton et al. [176], † Clark et al. [195], ‡ Mabie et al. [318]; § Clark et al., unpublished data.
N/A, not available; SD, standard deviation; SEM, standard error of the mean.

Table 34.11 Indications for use of pulmonary artery catheter in pregnancy-induced hypertension.

Complications related to central volume status
Pulmonary edema of uncertain etiology
Pulmonary edema unresponsive to conventional therapy
Persistent oliguria despite aggressive volume expansion
Induction of conduction anesthesia in hemodynamically unstable patients
Medical complication that would otherwise required invasive monitoring

found that this approach is very useful and in all but the most severe cases allows non-invasive management and avoids the need for a pulmonary artery catheter.

Cardiopulmonary complications of pre-eclampsia

During normal pregnancy, plasma volume increases approximately 42% while red blood cell volume increases approximately 24% [184]. Earlier studies of cardiovascular changes in pre-eclampsia revealed increased vascular resistance, decreased circulatory volume, and decreased perfusion of various organ systems, most notably the renal and uteroplacental circulations, when compared with normal non-pregnant subjects [17,185], In pregnancies complicated by pre-eclampsia, a reduction in plasma volume with hemoconcentration occurs in proportion to the severity of the disease [184]. Significant plasma volume depletion and reduction in circulating plasma protein may occur prior to the clinical manifestations of pre-eclampsia [185–187]. In subjects who developed hypertension during pregnancy, various degrees of increased cardiac output (CO) and/or SVR were noted [188].

Although the precise cause of these changes remains unknown, further insight into the exact cardiovascular parameters associated with pregnancy-related disease states evolved around 1980, when obstetric and gynecologic indications for use of the pulmonary artery catheter were described, and measurements of CVP, pulmonary artery pressure (PAP), PCWP, CO, and mixed venous oxygen became available [178].

Rafferty and Berkowitz [189] studied three pre-eclamptic patients with a pulmonary artery catheter and noted an increased left ventricular stroke index (LVSWI) and normal pulmonary artery resistance. At delivery, the CI and PCWP increased in these patients, probably secondary to increased venous return. These investigators noted an increased PCWP postpartum, which also was felt to be secondary to increased circulatory volume. These findings suggest that the pulmonary vasculature is not involved in the vasospastic process and that pulmonary hypertension is not present in severe pre-eclampsia.

Observations made from pulmonary artery catheterization in 10 patients with severe pre-eclampsia during labor showed an increased LVSWI (suggesting hyperdynamic ventricular function), normal PAP, and poor correlation between CVP and PCWP [190]. The poor correlation of PCWP and CVP has been verified by subsequent investigations [127,158].

Hemodynamic studies have consistently demonstrated hyperdynamic left ventricular function in pre-eclamptic patients [76,191,192]. Phelan and Yurth [191] studied 10 severe pre-eclamptics and noted hyperdynamic cardiac function with elevated CO and variable elevation of SVR. Immediately postpartum, a transient fall in left ventricular function with a rise in CVP and PCWP was noted in 6 of 10 patients, possibly secondary to an autotransfusion effect. Hyperdynamic ventricular function returned 1 hour postpartum. One criticism of this study as it related to CO is the fact that several of these patients received intrapartum hydralazine, which could account for the elevated CO.

Groenendijk et al. [193] noted a low CI, low PCWP, and high SVR in pre-eclamptics prior to volume expansion. Volume expansion resulted in an elevation of PCWP and CI to normal pregnant values, a drop in SVR, and no change in BP. Vasodilation using hydralazine then resulted in a further drop in SVR and BP, with a rise in CI, and no change in PCWP.

Eclamptics studied by Hankins et al. [194] initially demonstrated hyperdynamic left ventricular function and elevated SVR, as well as low right and left ventricular filling pressures. Following labor management, consisting of fluid restriction, magnesium sulfate, and hydralazine, the authors observed a postpartum rise in PCWP in patients who did not have an early spontaneous diuresis. This rise in PCWP was thought to be secondary to mobilization of extravascular fluids before the diuresis phase. They concluded that the hemodynamic status was influenced by the severity and duration of the disease, other underlying disease states, and therapeutic interventions such as epidural anesthesia.

Cotton et al. [176] summarized the hemodynamic profile in 45 patients with severe pre-eclampsia or eclampsia. They observed a wide variety of hemodynamic measurements in these patients; however, the majority were found to have an elevated BP, variably elevated SVR, hyperdynamic left ventricular function, normal to increased PCWP, and low CVP. They hypothesized that the elevated PCWP with decreased CVP was secondary to elevated left ventricular afterload, combined with a hypovolemic state. These findings are summarized in Table 34.9.

Clark et al. [195] documented for the first time central hemodynamic parameters in normotensive late third-trimester pregnant patients (see Table 34.10). They demonstrated that most reported patients with severe pre-eclampsia have SVR in the normal range for pregnancy, and that left ventricular function in normal pregnancy as assessed by LVSWI is not hyperdynamic. This supports the model of an initially hyperdynamic hypertension without vasospasm in pre-eclampsia. This may be followed by the development of elevated SVR associated with vasospasm and a secondary decline in CO and LVSWI. Such a phenomenon has been documented in untreated non-pregnant patients with essential hypertension [196].

Pulmonary edema

Sibai et al. [197] reported a 2.9% incidence of pulmonary edema in severe pre-eclampsia–eclampsia; 70% of these 37 cases developed postpartum. In 90% of the cases that developed antepartum, chronic hypertension was identified as an underlying factor. A higher incidence of pulmonary edema was noted in older patients, multigravidas, and patients with underlying chronic hypertension. The development of pulmonary edema was also associated with the administration of excess infusions, either colloids or crystalloids.

Reduction of COP, alteration of capillary membrane permeability, and elevated pulmonary vascular hydrostatic pressures may lead to extravasation of fluids into the interstitial and alveolar spaces, resulting in pulmonary edema [192]. Cotton et al. [127] observed a negative COP–PCWP gradient in five pre-eclamptic patients who developed pulmonary edema. Interestingly, Clark et al. [175] compared the hemodynamic alterations in severe pre-eclamptics and eclamptics and suggested that the occurrence of eclamptic seizures may have also been associated with decreased COP rather than with the intensity of peripheral vasospasm.

The etiology of pulmonary edema in pre-eclamptic patients appears to be multifactorial, as illustrated by Benedetti's work involving 10 pre-eclamptic women with pulmonary edema [198]. Of these patients eight developed pulmonary edema in the postpartum period. Five patients had an abnormal COP–PCWP gradient, three demonstrated increased pulmonary capillary permeability, and two suffered left ventricular failure. Pulmonary edema secondary to capillary leak versus that due to increased hydrostatic pressure was distinguished by evaluating the ratio of edema fluid protein to plasma protein [199]. The diagnosis of capillary leak was made in Benedetti's study when the ratio of protein in pulmonary edema fluid to serum protein was greater than 0.4 [198]. Again, CVP was found not to correlate with PCWP. A decreased COP–PCWP gradient has long been correlated with the development of pulmonary edema in non-pregnant patients [199]. Pregnancy is known to lower COP, and COP is lower in pre-eclamptic patients than in normal pregnant patients. COP decreases further postpartum, secondary to supine positioning, bleeding at the time of delivery, and intrapartum infusion of crystalloid solutions [200]. In 50% of Benedetti's pre-eclamptic patients, a lowered COP–PCWP gradient may have contributed to pulmonary edema [201].

From the foregoing discussion, it is clear that non-hydrostatic factors (pulmonary capillary leak and deceased COP) may cause or contribute to pulmonary edema in patients with pre-eclampsia. In other patients, highly elevated SVR may lead to decreased CO and LVSWI and secondary cardiogenic pulmonary edema. A similar hydrostatic pulmonary edema may have been seen with normal left ventricular function following iatrogenic fluid overload.

The diagnosis of pulmonary edema is made on clinical grounds. Symptoms of dyspnea and chest discomfort are usually elicited. Tachypnea, tachycardia, and pulmonary rales are noted on examination. Chest X-ray and arterial blood gas analysis confirm the diagnosis. Other life-threatening conditions, such as thromboembolism, should be considered and ruled out as quickly as possible.

Initial management of pulmonary edema includes oxygen administration and fluid restriction. A pulse oximeter should be placed so that oxygen saturation may be monitored continuously. A pulmonary artery catheter may be considered for severe pre-eclamptic patients who develop pulmonary edema antepartum, in order to distinguish between fluid overload, left ventricular dysfunction, and non-hydrostatic pulmonary edema, each of which may require different approaches to therapy.

Furosemide (Lasix) 10–40 mg IV over 1–2 minutes represents the first line of conventional therapy for patients with pulmonary edema associated with fluid overload. If adequate diuresis does not commence within 1 hour, an 80-mg dose may be slowly administered to achieve diuresis. In severe cases of pulmonary edema, a diuresis of 2–3 L needs to be achieved before oxygenation begins to improve. Again, the degree of diuresis appropriate for these hemodynamically complex patients may be clarified by complete hemodynamic evaluation, using parameters derived by a pulmonary artery catheter. An alternative approach in patients without evidence of fluid overload, but with congestive failure secondary to intense peripheral vasospasm [158], involves the administration of intravenous nitroprusside. While hydrostatic derangements may be corrected quickly, rapid improvement in arterial oxygenation may not be seen [155,156]. Continuous arterial BP monitoring is often helpful in this setting because of the potent activity of some arteriodilating agents.

When hypoxemia persists despite initial treatment, mechanical ventilation may be required for respiratory support, pending correction of the underlying problem. In all cases, close monitoring of the patient's respiratory status with arterial blood gas analysis should be performed. Fluid balance is maintained by careful monitoring of intake and output. An indwelling catheter with urometer should be placed to follow hourly urine output. Serum electrolytes should also be closely monitored, especially in patients receiving diuretics.

Hypertensive cardiomyopathy

During pregnancy pregnant women show an increase in left ventricular muscle mass index and a decrease in fractional shortening. When studied with echocardiography, many normal pregnant women show a degree of "physiologic" diastolic dysfunction. Schannwell et al. [202] demonstrated affected LV relaxation with a reduction in peak early diastolic flow and an increase of isovolumetric relaxation time at 33 weeks gestation in normal pregnant women. In pregnant patients with mild chronic hypertension they showed definite signs of diastolic dysfunction with delayed relaxation noted as early as the beginning of the gestation. Some patients with pregnancy-associated hypertension developed diastolic dysfunction at midgestation, while others only showed this abnormality at term. They concluded that in healthy pregnant women, the increased preload associated with normal pregnancy results in a reversible physiologic left ventricular hypertrophy, a significant alteration in diastolic left ventricular function (disturbed relaxation pattern) and a temporary decrease in the efficacy of systolic function. In women with chronic hypertension however, there is delayed LV relaxation demonstrable at the beginning of pregnancy and in as many as 50% of cases signs of restrictive cardiomyopathy may develop.

Desai et al. [203] used echocardiography to show that 25% (4/16) of patients they studied with pulmonary edema and hypertensive crisis in pregnancy had impaired left ventricular systolic function. The remaining 75% (12/16) had abnormal left ventricular diastolic filling.

Diastolic dysfunction in patients with severe hypertension from pre-eclampsia needs to be recognized as a potential cause for fulminant pulmonary edema, cardiac failure and sudden death [204] It is important that the obstetrician understand that diastolic dysfunction can occur despite normal left ventricular systolic function, and in the face of an elevated blood pressure. Pulmonary edema from diastolic dysfunction occurs frequently with severe hypertension, and "cardiac failure" is not always associated with hypotension or a diminished ejection fraction. In fact, up to 40% of hypertensive patients presenting with clinical signs of congestive heart failure have normal systolic left ventricular function [204]. The concept that a pre-eclamptic patient with elevated blood pressure cannot be in cardiac failure needs to be discarded. Likewise, the idea that a pre-eclamptic patient who develops severe pulmonary edema always has peripartum cardiomyopathy should be questioned. Peripartum cardiomyopathy is a distinct entity that carries significant implications for long-term therapy and future pregnancies. Pre-eclamptic women who develop pulmonary edema due to diastolic dysfunction and hypertensive cardiomyopathy should not be labeled as having had peripartum cardiomyopathy. The pathophysiology is different, and in most cases of hypertensive cardiomyopathy associated with pre-eclampsia the ejection fraction rapidly returns to normal after treatment of the pre-eclampsia. It is highly unlikely that a pre-eclamptic patient with severely elevated blood pressure who develops pulmonary edema, is then delivered and recovers rapidly within 24–48 hours has peripartum cardiomyopathy. The most likely diagnosis in this scenario is that of hypertensive cardiomyopathy and diastolic dysfunction. Witlin et al. [205] have shown that patients with severe myocardial dysfunction due to peripartum cardiomyopathy are unlikely to regain normal cardiac function on follow-up. In addition, the same group showed that pre-eclampsia and chronic hypertension are likely to unmask underlying cardiac abnormalities [206]. In situations where it is unclear why the patient is in pulmonary edema echocardiography can be very useful. Not only does it allow an assessment of the systolic and diastolic function, as well as cardiac output, but the state of filling of the vasculature can also be evaluated. This is especially important in a severely pre-eclamptic patient who may have intravascular dehydration but pulmonary congestion and increased capillary permeability. Mabie et al. [207] showed that obese women with chronic hypertension are at particular risk of underlying cardiac abnormality and diastolic dysfunction.

Malignant ventricular arrythmias

Ventricular arrhythmias are not a commonly noted feature of severe pre-eclampsia. This is perhaps more due to the fact that we do not monitor for these arrhythmias than that they do not occur. Naidoo et al. [208] studied 24 patients with hypertensive crises during pregnancy with continuous electrocardiographic monitoring over a period of 24 hours to detect the presence of serious ventricular arrhythmias. They excluded three patients from the analysis because of low serum potassium levels. Thirteen of the remaining 21 patients (62%) had ventricular tachycardia on subsequent analysis of the electrocardiogram. These arrhythmias subsided after induction of anesthesia when blood pressure control was optimal. The authors of this paper felt that their finding may explain, in part, the pathogenesis of pulmonary edema and sudden death in some patients with malignant hypertension in pre-eclampsia. The high rate of ventricular arrhythmia in this study may be explained by the fact that many of these patients had little or no prenatal care and were admitted with severe, prolonged hypertensive crises. Hopefully, in an environment where prenatal care is more prevalent we are less likely to see such ventricular dysfunction. Another explanation as to why this complication is less frequently seen in the USA is that β-blocker use is common and we use hydralazine (not dihydralazine) for blood pressure control. Regardless of the potential pathophysiology, this paper underlines the importance of expeditious control of the blood pressure in severely hypertensive pregnant women.

The same group [209] studied the effects of β-adrenergic blockade during the peripartum period on their previously observed high incidence of ventricular arrhythmias in 40 eclamptic postpartum patients. Cardiac rhythm was assessed by blinded analysis of a 24-hour Holter record using the Lown classification of arrhythmias. They showed a significantly higher incidence of serious ventricular arrhythmias in patients receiving dihydralazine (81%) than in those receiving labetalol (17%, $P < 0.0001$). Patients receiving labetalol showed a significant decrease in mean heart rate ($P < 0.0001$), whereas patients receiving dihydralazine showed a significant increase ($P < 0.0001$). They concluded that introduction of β-adrenergic blockade into peripartum hypertensive management of eclampsia significantly reduced the incidence of dangerous ventricular arrhythmias. This may be on the basis of improved myocardial oxygen supply/demand ratio with β-blockade. This paper makes a cogent argument for control of severely elevated blood pressure with labetalol instead of hydralazine or similar agents.

Renal complications of pre-eclampsia

Renal plasma flow and glomerular filtration rate are diminished significantly in pre-eclamptic women [210]. Renal biopsy of pre-eclamptic patients often demonstrates a distinctive glomerular capillary endothelial cell change, termed "glomerular endotheliosis." Damage to the glomerular membrane results in renal dysfunction [211,212]. Urinary sediment changes (granular, hyaline, red-cell, and tubular cell casts) are common in severe pre-eclampsia; they reflect renal parenchymal damage but do not correlate with or predict the clinical course of disease [213,214].

Acute renal failure in pre-eclamptic pregnancies is uncommon [215]. In 245 cases of eclampsia reported by Pritchard et al. [69], none required dialysis for renal failure. Among a group of 435 women with HELLP syndrome, however, 7% developed acute renal failure. Maternal and perinatal complications were extremely high, although subsequent pregnancy outcome and long-term prognosis were usually favorable in the absence of pre-existing chronic hypertension [11]. Acute renal failure secondary to pre-eclampsia is usually the result of acute tubular necrosis but may be secondary to bilateral cortical necrosis [11,12]. Precipitating factors include abruption, coagulopathy, hemorrhage, and severe hypotension [216]. The urine sediment may show granular casts and renal tubular cells [214,215]. Renal cortical necrosis may be associated with pre-eclampsia and may present as anuria or oliguria. Renal failure presenting in association with pre-eclampsia may be secondary to other underlying medical disorders, especially in the older multiparous patient [50]. Should acute renal failure occur, hemodialysis or peritoneal dialysis may be required, pending return of renal function [215].

Oliguria

Severe renal dysfunction in pre-eclampsia is most commonly manifested as oliguria, defined as urinary output less than 25–30 mL/h over 2 consecutive hours. This often parallels a rise in serum creatinine and blood urea nitrogen (BUN) and a fall in creatinine clearance. Reversible hyperuricemia is a common feature of pre-eclampsia and usually precedes the development of uremia and proteinuria [217]. Significant alterations in albumin/creatinine ratio have also been described [218].

Clark et al. [219] have described three different hemodynamic subsets of pre-eclamptic–eclamptic patients with persistent oliguria, based on invasive monitoring parameters. The first group was found to have a low PCWP, hyperdynamic left ventricular function, and mild to moderately increased SVR. These patients responded to further volume replacement. This is the most common clinical scenario, and it is felt to be secondary to intravascular volume depletion.

The second group is characterized by normal or increased PCWP, normal CO, and normal SVR, accompanied by intense uroconcentration. The pathophysiologic basis of oliguria in this group is thought to be secondary to intrinsic renal arterial spasm out of proportion to the degree of generalized systemic vasospasm. Low-dose dopamine (1–5 μg/kg/min) has been shown to produce a significant rise in urine output in severe pre-eclamptic patients in this hemodynamic subgroup [220]. Alternatively, afterload reduction may also improve urine output in this setting.

The third group of oliguric patients has markedly elevated PCWP and SVR, with depressed ventricular function. These patients respond to volume restriction and aggressive afterload reduction. In many cases, a forced oliguria in this subgroup may often be accompanied by incipient pulmonary edema, with fluid accumulation in the pulmonary interstitial space. Such patients would certainly not benefit from further volume infusion, yet they may be clinically indistinguishable from patients in the first group, who do respond to additional fluid infusion. Central hemodynamic assessment will allow the clinician to distinguish the preceding subgroups and tailor therapy accordingly.

Lee et al. [221] studied seven pre-eclamptic women with oliguria, utilizing the pulmonary artery catheter, and also found that oliguria was not a good index of volume status. They determined that urinary diagnostic indices such as urine–plasma ratios of creatinine, urea nitrogen, and osmolality were clinically misleading if applied to fluid management. Five of seven patients were found to have urinary diagnostic indices consistent with prerenal dehydration, but PCWP consistent with euvolemia. Normal PCWPs in pre-eclamptics with oliguria support the hypothesis that oliguria is often secondary to severe regional vasospasm [69,221].

Close monitoring of fluid intake and output is of paramount importance in all patients diagnosed with pre-eclampsia. If urine output falls below 25–30 mL/h over 2 consecutive hours, oliguria is said to be present, and a management plan should be instituted. Given the fact that plasma volume is diminished in pre-eclamptics, the cause of oliguria may be considered prerenal in most instances [184,187,219]. A fluid challenge of 500–1000 mL of normal saline or lactated Ringer's solution may be administered over 30 minutes. If urine output does not respond to an initial fluid challenge, additional challenges should be withheld pending delivery or the institution of pulmonary artery catheterization for a more precise definition of hemodynamic status [219]. If at any time oxygen saturation drops during a volume challenge, pulmonary artery catheterization is indicated if further fluid is contemplated in an effort to resolve the oliguria [132,174,176,219]. Repetitive fluid challenges are to be avoided in the absence of close monitoring of oxygenation status. In the presence of oliguria, delivery is of course indicated.

HELLP syndrome

The HELLP syndrome is a variant of severe pre-eclampsia, affecting up to 12% of patients with pre-eclampsia–eclampsia. In one study, the incidence of HELLP syndrome (442 cases) was 20% among women with severe pre-eclampsia [12]. HELLP syndrome is characterized by hemolysis, elevated liver enzymes, and low platelets [68]. The acronym, HELLP syndrome, was coined by Weinstein in 1982, but the hematologic and hepatic abnormalities of three cases were described by Pritchard et al. in 1954 [222]. Pritchard credited association of thrombocytopenia with severe pre-eclampsia to Stahnke in 1922 [223], and hepatic changes to Sheehan in 1950 [224]. Despite the high maternal and perinatal mortality rates associated with the HELLP syndrome, considerable controversy exists as to the proper management of these patients, who constitute a heterogeneous group with a wide array of clinical and laboratory manifestations. In addition, HELLP syndrome may be the imitator of a variety of non-obstetric medical entities [49,225] and serious medical–surgical pathology may be misdiagnosed as HELLP syndrome [226].

Unlike most forms of pre-eclampsia, HELLP syndrome is not primarily a disease of primigravidas. For example, several studies have found that nearly half of HELLP syndrome patients were multigravidas, the incidence among multigravidas being almost twice that seen in primigravid patients [57,62,227,228].

Clinically, many HELLP syndrome patients do not meet the standard BP criteria for severe pre-eclampsia. In one series of 112 women with severe pre-eclampsia–eclampsia complicated by HELLP syndrome, diastolic BP was less than 110 mmHg in 31% of cases and less than 90 mmHg in 15% at admission [229].

The multisystem nature of pre-eclampsia is often manifested by hepatic dysfunction. Hepatic artery resistance is increased in patients with HELLP syndrome [230]. Liver dysfunction, as defined by an elevated SGOT, was retrospectively identified in 21% of 355 patients with pre-eclampsia [58]. Liver dysfunction has been associated with intrauterine growth retardation (IUGR), prematurity, increased cesarean section rates, and lower Apgar scores [58]. Using immunofluorescent staining, Arias and Mancilla-Jimenez [231] found fibrin deposition in hepatic sinusoids of pre-eclamptic women, thought to be the result of ischemia secondary to vasospasm. Continued prolonged vasospasm may lead to hepatocellular necrosis [231,232].

The clinical signs and symptoms of patients with HELLP syndrome are classically related to the impact of vasospasm on the maternal liver. Thus, the majority of patients present with signs or symptoms of liver compromise. These include malaise, nausea (with or without vomiting), and epigastric pain. In most series, hepatic or right upper quadrant tenderness to palpation is seen consistently in HELLP syndrome patients [57,62,68,229].

Laboratory studies often create the illusion of medical conditions unrelated to pregnancy or pre-eclampsia. Peripheral smears demonstrate burr cells and/or schistocytes with polychromasia, consistent with microangiopathic hemolytic anemia. Hemolysis can also be demonstrated by abnormal haptoglobin or bilirubin levels [233–236]. Scanning electron microscopy demonstrates evidence of microangiopathic hemolysis in patients with HELLP syndrome [236]. The microangiopathic hemolytic anemia is felt to occur secondary to passage of the red cells through thrombosed, damaged vessels [58,234,235,237,238]. Increased red-cell turnover has also been evidenced by increased levels of carboxyhemoglobin and serum iron [238]. Although some degree of hemolysis is noted, anemia is uncommon.

Thrombocytopenia is defined as a platelet count of less than 100,000–150,000/μL. This process is not usually encountered in pregnant patients with essential hypertension [222]. Thrombocytopenia in pre-eclampsia occurs secondary to increased peripheral platelet destruction, as manifested by increased bone marrow megakaryocytes, the presence of circulating megathrombocytes, evidence of reduced platelet lifespan, and platelet adherence to exposed vascular collagen [235,237–239]. Thrombocytopenia has been found in as many as 50% of pre-eclamptic patients studied prospectively for hemostatic and platelet function [237]. Evidence for platelet destruction, impaired platelet function, and elevated platelet-associated IgG has been found in thrombocytopenic pre-eclamptic patients.

In a retrospective review of 353 patients with pre-eclampsia, Romero et al. [59] reported an 11.6% incidence of thrombocytopenia, defined as a platelet count less than 100,000/μL. Patients with thrombocytopenia had an increased risk for cesarean section, blood transfusion, preterm delivery, IUGR, and low Apgar scores. Thrombocytopenia has also been reported to occur in the neonates of pre-eclamptic women [57,68,240], although others have disputed these findings [241].

Clotting parameters, such as the prothrombin time, partial thromboplastin time, fibrinogen, and bleeding time, in the patient with HELLP syndrome are generally normal in the absence of abruptio placentae or fetal demise [229]. Platelet or fresh frozen plasma transfusion is necessary in 8–10% of patients with HELLP syndrome [222,229].

Significant elevation of alkaline phosphatase is seen in normal pregnancy; the elevation of SGOT and/or SGPT, however, indicates hepatic pathology. In HELLP syndrome, SGOT and SGPT are rarely in excess of 1,000 IU/L; values in excess of this level suggest other hepatic disorders, such as hepatitis. However, HELLP syndrome progressing to liver rupture may be associated with markedly elevated hepatic transaminases.

Laboratory abnormalities usually return to normal within a short time after delivery; it is not unusual, however, to see transient worsening of both thrombocytopenia and hepatic function in the first 24–48 hours postpartum [242]. An upward trend in platelet count and a downward trend in lactate dehydrogenase concentration should occur in patients without complications by the fourth postpartum day [243]. Martin et al. [243] evaluated postpartum recovery in 158 women with HELLP syndrome at the University of Mississippi Medical Center. A return to a normal platelet count (100,000/μL) occurred in all women whose platelet nadir was below 50,000/μL by the 11th postpartum day, and in all women whose platelet nadir was 50,000–100,000/μL by the sixth postpartum day.

HELLP syndrome can be a "great masquerader," and both clinical presentation and laboratory findings associated with this syndrome may suggest an array of clinical diagnoses (Table 34.12). Because of the numerous misdiagnoses associated with this syndrome, and because a delay in diagnosis may be life-threatening, a pregnant woman with thrombocytopenia, elevated serum transaminase levels, or epigastric pain should be considered as having HELLP syndrome until proven otherwise. Furthermore, HELLP syndrome occasionally presents before 20 weeks of gestation, usually in conjunction with underlying conditions such as fetal triploidy or antiphospholipid syndrome. However it may rarely present early without identifiable comorbidities [244].

Complications associated with HELLP syndrome include placental abruption, acute renal failure and hepatic hematoma with rupture, and ascites. Placental abruption in HELLP syndrome occurs at a rate 20 times that seen in the general obstetric population; the reported incidence ranges from 7 to 20% [222,229,236,245]. Abruption in the presence of HELLP syndrome is frequently associated with fetal death and/or consumptive coagulopathy.

A review of the literature discloses significantly elevated maternal (Table 34.13) and perinatal (Table 34.14) mortality rates associated with HELLP syndrome. As with other severe pre-eclampsia variants, delivery is ultimately the treatment of choice. The timing of delivery, however, remains controversial. Several investigators recommend immediate delivery, while others reasonably suggest that under certain conditions with marked fetal immaturity, delivery may safely be delayed for a short time [62,63,68,225,246,247]. In support of this latter approach, Clark et al. [248] have demonstrated transient improvement in patients with HELLP syndrome following bed rest and/or corticosteroid administration. Following an initial improvement, however, each patient's clinical condition worsened. Similar observations were seen in 3 of 17 (18%) patients in Sibai's series following steroid administration to enhance fetal pulmonary maturity [229]. Thus, it appears that in the mother with a very premature fetus and borderline disturbances in platelet count or serum transaminase

Table 34.12 Differential diagnoses of HELLP syndrome.

Autoimmune thrombocytopenic purpura
Chronic renal disease
Pyelonephritis
Cholecystitis
Gastroenteritis
Hepatitis
Pancreatitis
Thrombotic thrombocytopenic purpura
Hemolytic–uremic syndrome
Acute fatty liver of pregnancy

Table 34.13 Maternal outcomes in HELLP syndrome.

Reference	Location	Years	Cases (*n*)	Incidence (%)	Maternal mortality (%)	Cesarean rate (%)
MacKenna et al. [62]	Greenville, NC	1978–82	27	12*	0	N/A
Weinstein [57]	Tucson, AZ	1980–84	57	0.67†	3.5	58
Sibai et al. [97]	Memphis, TN	1977–85	112	9.7‡	1.8	63
Romero et al. [58]	New Haven, CT	1981–84	58	21*	N/A	57
Sibai et al. [12]	Memphis, TN	1977–92	442	20§	0.9	42

*Among all pre-eclamptic–eclamptic patients.
†Among all live births.
‡Among severe pre-eclamptic–eclamptic pregnancies.
§Among severe pre-eclamptic women.
N/A, not available.

Table 34.14 Perinatal outcomes in HELLP syndrome.

Reference	Location	Years	Cases (*n*)	Perinatal mortality (%)	Small for gestational age (%)	Respiratory distress syndrome (%)
MacKenna et al. [62]	Greenville, NC	1978–82	27	11	N/A	8
Weinstein [57]	Tucson, AZ	1980–84	57	8	N/A	16
Sibai et al. [97]	Memphis, TN	1977–85	112	33	32	N/A
Romero et al. [58]	New Haven, CT	1981–84	58	7	41	31

N/A, not available.

values, and in the absence of other absolute indications for delivery, careful in-hospital observation may at times be appropriate. Certainly, uncontrollable BP or significantly changing liver enzymes or platelet count would mandate delivery irrespective of gestational age.

The mode of delivery should depend on the state of the cervix and other obstetric indications for cesarean birth. HELLP syndrome, by itself, is not an indication for cesarean delivery. At least half of patients with HELLP syndrome, however, will undergo operative delivery (see Table 34.13). A commonly encountered situation involves a mother with a premature fetus, an unfavorable cervix, and a platelet count less than 100 000/μL. In such patients, cesarean delivery is often preferred in order to avoid the necessity of later operative delivery for failed induction in the face of more significant thrombocytopenia.

Sullivan et al. [249] evaluated 481 women who developed HELLP syndrome at the University of Mississippi Medical Center; 195 subsequent pregnancies occurred in 122 patients. The incidence of recurrent HELLP syndrome was 19–27%, and the recurrence of any form of pre-eclampsia–eclampsia was 42–43%. Sibai et al. [250] reviewed 442 pregnancies complicated by HELLP syndrome at the University of Tennessee in Memphis; follow-up data were available in 341 cases. In 192 subsequent pregnancies, obstetric complications were common, including pre-eclampsia (19%), although only 3% experienced recurrent HELLP syndrome. They attributed the discrepancy in recurrence risk between their study and that of Sullivan et al. [249] to differences in definitions of the syndrome and patient populations.

Schwartz and Brenner [251] reported the use of exchange plasmapheresis with fresh frozen plasma to treat hemolysis and thrombocytopenia that did not resolve following delivery and standard medical treatment. Corticosteroids have been proposed for the treatment of postpartum HELLP syndrome [252]; a recent metanalysis [253] addressing this matter found that women randomised to dexamethasone demonstrated significantly better outcome for several parameters (oliguria, mean arterial pressure, mean increase in platelet count, mean increase in urinary output and liver enzyme elevations), but the authors concluded that there is insufficient evidence to determine whether steroid use decreases maternal perinatal mortality and major maternal morbidity. In addition, Fonseca et al [254] showed in a double-blinded randomized placebo-controlled trial in 132 women that corticosteroid therapy did not decrease hospitalization duration, alter platelet or liver enzyme values significantly, or improve outcomes in women with HELLP syndrome

Liver rupture

Hepatic infarction may lead to intrahepatic hemorrhage and development of a subcapsular hematoma, which may rupture into the peritoneal space and result in shock and death [231,255].

Subcapsular hematomas usually develop on the anterior and superior aspects of the liver [256]. The diagnosis of a liver hematoma may be aided by use of ultrasonography, radionuclide scanning, computed tomography (CT), magnetic resonance imaging (MRI), and selective angiography [256,257].

Henny et al. [257] described a biphasic chronologic sequence of events during rupture of the subcapsular hematoma. The initial presenting symptoms are constant, progressively worsening pain in the epigastrium or right upper quadrant of the abdomen, with or without nausea and vomiting. The second phase is manifested by the development of vascular collapse, shock, and fetal death. The maternal and fetal prognoses of liver rupture are poor. Bis and Waxman [258] reported a 59% maternal and 62% fetal mortality rate.

Significant or persistent elevations of serum transaminase levels in conjunction with pre-eclampsia and right upper quadrant or epigastric tenderness indicate delivery regardless of gestational age. Especially when such dysfunction occurs in the presence of thrombocytopenia, careful clinical observation during the postpartum period is essential. When the diagnosis of liver hematoma is suspected in severe pre-eclampsia prior to delivery of the fetus, immediate exploratory laparotomy and cesarean section should be performed in order to prevent rupture of the hematoma secondary to increased abdominal pressure in the second stage of labor, with vomiting, or during eclamptic convulsions [257]. When the diagnosis of liver hematoma is made in the postpartum period, conservative management with blood transfusion and serial ultrasonography may be reasonable [257,259].

Smith et al. [260] reviewed the medical literature for the period 1976–90 (28 cases) and reported their experience at Baylor College of Medicine for the period 1978–90 (seven new cases) of spontaneous rupture of the liver during pregnancy. The incidence was 1 per 45 145 live births in the Baylor series. A significant improvement in maternal outcome (P = 0.006) was seen among patients who were managed by packing and drainage (82% survival) compared with those managed by hepatic lobectomy (25% survival). This conservative approach is supported by the trauma literature. At Baylor College of Medicine, 1000 consecutive cases of liver injury were evaluated; extensive resection of the liver or lobectomy with selective vascular ligation resulted in a 34% mortality rate, whereas conservative surgery (packing and drainage and/or use of topical hemostatic agents) resulted in a 7% mortality [261]. Smith et al. [260] proposed an algorithm for antepartum and postpartum management of hepatic hemorrhage in their review.

Liver rupture with intraperitoneal hemorrhage, when suspected, requires laparotomy. Hemostasis may be achieved by compression, simple suture, topical coagulant agents, arterial embolization, omental pedicles, ligation of the hepatic artery, or lobectomy, depending on the extent of the hepatic damage [262]. Temporary control of bleeding may be achieved by packing the rupture site or by application of a gravity suit [262,263]. Management by liver transplant has been reported [264,265].

Few cases of pregnancy following hepatic rupture have been reported. There have been several reported cases of non-recurrence in subsequent pregnancies [266] and one case of recurrence with survival in a subsequent pregnancy [267]. Spontaneous splenic rupture associated with pre-eclampsia has been reported [268].

Pancreatitis

Pancreatitis has been observed in association with pre-eclampsia and HELLP syndrome, thought to be secondary to ischemia or possibly diuretics administered for oliguria [269–272]. The association between diuretic use and postpartum pancreatitis is interesting [269]. It is possible that pancreatic ischemia due to generalized vasoconstriction from pre-eclampsia is worsened by the use of loop diuretics in the setting of oliguria with renal failure. The authors suggest that in postpartum women with pregnancy-induced hypertension and acute renal failure, diuretics should be cautiously used because they may increase the risk of pancreatitis. In cases where unrelenting upper abdominal or chest pain is documented, especially where there is radiation to the back, it would be wise to consider pancreatitis and aortic dissection as differential diagnoses. Serum amylase and lipase levels should be checked and appropriate pancreatitis management regimens instituted in those cases where pre-eclampsia and pancreatitis co-exist.

Neurologic complications of pre-eclampsia

Cerebral hemorrhage, cerebral edema, temporary blindness (amaurosis), and eclamptic seizures are separate but related neurologic conditions that may occur in pre-eclampsia. Cerebral hemorrhage and cerebral edema are two major causes of maternal mortality in pre-eclampsia [273]. Intracranial hemorrhage may result from the combination of severe hypertension and hemostatic compromise [46].

Cerebral edema

Cerebral edema is defined as increased water content of one or more of the intracranial fluid compartments of the brain [274]. Signs of diffuse cerebral edema may be found in eclamptic women on CT scan [275] and may develop when the forces affecting the Starling equilibrium are disturbed. The three most important etiologic factors include increased intravascular pressure, damage to the vascular endothelium, and reduced plasma COP [276]. Miller's classification of cerebral edema includes: (i) vasogenic edema with breakdown of the blood–brain barrier, secondary to vascular damage; (ii) cytotoxic edema, secondary to damage to the cellular sodium pump; (iii) hydrostatic edema from increased intravascular pressure; (iv) interstitial edema related to acute obstructive hydrocephalus; and (v) hypo-osmotic edema, in which intravascular free water decreases plasma osmolality [276].

In the general population, vasogenic edema, which predominantly occurs in the cerebral white matter, is the most common type of cerebral edema [277].

In pre-eclampsia, cerebral edema is thought to occur secondary to anoxia associated with eclamptic seizures or secondary to loss of cerebral autoregulation as a result of severe hypertension [278]. Cerebral edema is diagnosed on CT scan by the appearance of areas with low density or a low radiographic absorption coefficient [275,277,279]. MRI has also been useful in providing an index of water content in select areas of the brain [277].

General therapeutic principles in the treatment of cerebral edema include correction of hypoxemia and hypercarbia, avoidance of volatile anesthetic agents, control of body temperature, and control of hypertension [276,277]. Assisted hyperventilation reduces intracranial hypertension and the formation of cerebral edema. The partial pressure of carbon dioxide is maintained between 25 and 30 mmHg [276].

The administration of hypertonic solutions such as mannitol increases serum osmolality and draws water from the brain into the vascular compartment, thus reducing brain tissue water and volume. A 20% solution of mannitol is given as a dose of 0.5–1.0 g/kg over 10 minutes or as a continuous infusion of 5 g/h. The serum osmolality is maintained in a range between 305 and 315 mosmol [276,277]. Steroid therapy (dexamethasone, betamethasone, methylprednisolone) is thought to be most effective in the treatment of focal chronic cerebral edema, which may occur in association with a tumor or abscess. Steroid therapy is less beneficial in cases of diffuse or acute cerebral edema [276]. Other pharmacologic agents that have been used to reduce intracranial pressure and cerebral edema include acetazolamide (Diamox), furosemide (Lasix), spironolactone (Aldactone), and ethacrynic acid (Edecrin).

In pre-eclamptic–eclamptic patients diagnosed with cerebral edema, therapy should be directed at correcting hypoxemia, hypercarbia, hyperthermia, and/or hypertension or hypotension. If assisted ventilation is employed, hyperventilation with controlled hypocapnia should be used. Mannitol may be administered with careful observation of pulmonary, cardiovascular, and renal function. The inciting factor of cerebral edema in pre-eclampsia and eclampsia, albeit unknown, is eliminated by delivery of the products of conception and thus the condition is ultimately treatable in this patient population.

Temporary blindness

Temporary blindness may complicate 1–3% of cases of pre-eclampsia–eclampsia [279–283] and was recently reported in 15% of women with eclampsia at Parkland Hospital [284]. Pregnancy-related blindness has been associated with eclampsia, cavernous sinus thrombosis, and hypertensive encephalopathy [279–282]. Beeson and Duda [279] reported one case associated with eclampsia and occipital lobe edema. Hill et al. [282] noted that recovery of vision correlated with the return of a normal PCWP in severe pre-eclamptics with amaurosis. The injury is usually the result of severe damage to the retinal vasculature or occipital lobe ischemia [280]. Cunningham et al. [284] evaluated the clinical courses of 15 women with severe pre-eclampsia or eclampsia who developed cortical blindness over a 14-year period. Blindness persisted from 4 hours to 8 days but resolved completely in all cases. Based on data from CT imaging and MRI, the Parkland group concluded that cortical blindness resulted from petechial hemorrhages and focal edema in the occipital cortex. Hinchey et al. [285] described a syndrome of reversible posterior leukoencephalopathy, with neuroimaging findings characteristic of subcortical edema without infarction in patients who presented with headache, altered mental functioning, seizures, and loss of vision.

Transient blindness usually resolves spontaneously after delivery of the fetus [279,281,282]. Nevertheless, focal neurologic deficits such as this require ophthalmologic and neurologic consultation and CT or MRI of the brain. Generally, management guidelines are the same as for pre-eclamptics without this complication [284]. Associated conditions, such as cerebral edema, should be treated as indicated. Paralysis of the sixth cranial nerve has been reported as a complication of eclampsia [286].

Eclampsia

The precise cause of seizures in pre-eclampsia remains unknown. Hypertensive encephalopathy, as well as vasospasm, hemorrhage, ischemia, and edema of the cerebral hemispheres, have been proposed as etiologic factors. The weight of the most current data and the general consensus at this time is that eclampsia is the result of cerebral overperfusion and hypertensive encephalopathy [287].

Thrombotic and hemorrhagic lesions have been identified on autopsy of pre-eclamptic women [224,288]. Clark et al. [175] noted lower COP associated with eclamptic patients, as opposed to matched severe pre-eclamptic patients. The importance of low COP in the development of pulmonary dysfunction has been described previously [198].

Douglas and Redman [289] reported that the incidence of eclampsia in the United Kingdom during 1992 was 4.9 per 10 000 maternities. During the period 1979–86, the incidence of eclampsia in the United States was 5.6 per 10 000 births [290]. The eclampsia rate decreased by 36% from 6.8 per 10 000 births during the first half of the series to 4.3 per 10 000 births during the latter half of the series.

Eclamptic seizures usually occur without a preceding aura, although many patients will manifest some form of apprehension, excitability, or hyperreflexia prior to the onset of a seizure. Eclampsia unheralded by hypertension and proteinuria occurred in 38% of cases reported in the United Kingdom [289]. Douglas and Redman conclude that "the term pre-eclampsia is misleading because eclampsia can precede pre-eclampsia." In a study of 179 cases of eclampsia, approximately one-third of patients received obstetric care that met standards for delivery of obstetric services and were thus classified as "unavoidable" cases of eclampsia

[291]. Sibai and colleagues have recommended magnesium prophylaxis in all pre-eclamptics, regardless of degree, because a significant percentage of eclamptics demonstrated only mild signs and symptoms of pre-eclampsia prior to the onset of seizures [291]. Once a seizure occurs, it is usually a forerunner of more convulsions unless anticonvulsant therapy is initiated.

Eclamptic seizures occur prior to delivery in roughly 80% of patients (Table 34.15). In the remainder, convulsions occur postpartum, and have been reported up to 23 days following delivery [292,293]. Douglas and Redman [289] observed that most antepartum convulsions (76%) occurred prior to term, while most intrapartum or postpartum convulsions (75%) occurred at term. Late postpartum eclampsia (convulsions more than 48 hours but less than 4 weeks after delivery) constituted 56% of total postpartum eclampsia and 16% of all cases of eclampsia in a series collected at the University of Tennessee, Memphis, between 1977 and 1992 [294]. Severe headache or visual disturbances were noted in 83% of patients before the onset of convulsions. When seizures occur more than 24 hours postpartum, however, a thorough search for other potential causes is mandatory.

A maternal seizure typically results in fetal bradycardia, and the fetal heart rate pattern usually returns to normal upon resolution of the seizure. Appropriate steps should be taken to enhance maternal–fetal well-being, including maintenance of the maternal airway, oxygen administration, and maternal lateral repositioning. Complete maternal recovery following eclampsia usually is expected.

The standard therapy for the management of eclampsia includes magnesium sulfate and delivery of the fetus. We administer magnesium sulfate 4–6 g IV over 20 minutes, and initiate an intravenous infusion at 2–3 g/h. If control of seizures is not successful after the initial intravenous bolus, a second 2-g bolus of magnesium sulfate may be cautiously administered. No more than a total of 8 g of magnesium sulfate is recommended at the outset of treatment.

Seizures may recur despite apparently appropriate magnesium therapy. The incidence of recurrent seizures ranges from 8 to 13% [291]. Both intramuscular and intravenous magnesium sulfate regimens may be associated with recurrent seizures. Of such patients, half may have subtherapeutic magnesium levels [291]. This underscores the importance of individualized therapy in order to achieve adequate serum magnesium levels and minimize the risk of recurrent seizures. Seizures refractory to standard magnesium sulfate regimens may be treated with a slow 100-mg IV dose of thiopental sodium (Pentothal) or 1–10 mg of diazepam (Valium). Alternatively, sodium amobarbital (up to 250 mg IV) may be administered. In a clinical study, Lucas et al. [295] described a simplified regimen of phenytoin for the treatment of pre-eclampsia. An intravenous infusion rate of 16.7 mg/min over 1 hour provided an initial dose of 1000 mg; an additional 500 mg of phenytoin administered orally 10 hours after treatment initiation maintained therapeutic levels for an additional 14 hours.

Eclamptic patients with repetitive seizures despite therapeutic magnesium levels may warrant CT evaluation of the brain. Dunn et al. [296] found five of seven such patients to have abnormalities including cerebral edema and cerebral venous thrombosis. However, Sibai et al. [297] reported 20 cases of eclampsia with neurologic signs or repetitive seizures who all had normal CT

Table 34.15 Eclampsia: maternal–fetal complications.

Reference	Location	Years	Cases (*n*)	Antepartum eclampsia (%)	Cesarean rate (%)	Maternal mortality (%)	Perinatal mortality (%)
Bryant & Fleming [312]	Cincinnati, OH	1930–40	120	62	0	1.7	29*
Zuspan [323]	Augusta, GA	1956–65	69	88	1.4†	2.9	32*
Harbert et al. [315]	Charlottesville, VA	1939–63	168	78	6†	4.8	22*
Pritchard & Pritchard [86]	Dallas, TX	1955–75	154	82	23	0	15†
Lopez-Llera [300]	Mexico City, Mexico	1963–79	704	83	57†	14	27
Pritchard et al. [69]	Dallas, TX	1975–83	91	91	33†	1.1	16†
Adetoro [324]	Ilorin, Nigeria	1972–87	651	N/A	N/A	14	N/A
Sibai [322]	Memphis, TN	1977–89	254	71	49†	0.4	12*
Douglas & Redman [289]	United Kingdom	1992	383	56	54†	1.8	7*
Majoko & Mujaji [320]	Harare, Zimbabwe	1997–98	151	68	63	26.5	N/A
Onwuhafua et al. [321]	Kaduna Stage, Nigeria	1990–97	45	60	53	42	44
Chen et al. [313]	Singapore	1994–1999	62	81	79	1.6	10
Lee et al. [317]	Nova Scotia, Canada	1981–2000	31	74	79	0	6
Efetie & Okafor [314]	Abuja, Nigeria	2000–2005	46	74	72	28	N/A
Knight [316]	United Kingdom	2005	314	64	N/A	0	6

* All cases.
† Antepartum and intrapartum cases only.
N/A, not available.

findings. Their recommendation regarding CT scan was restricted to patients with late-onset postpartum pre-eclampsia or those patients with focal neurologic deficits.

Eclamptic patients require delivery without respect to gestational age [298]. Cesarean delivery should be reserved for obstetric indications or deteriorating maternal condition. As demonstrated in Table 34.15, vaginal delivery may be achieved in at least half of eclamptic patients. Pritchard et al. [69] reported successful vaginal delivery in 82% of oxytocin-induced patients.

Maternal mortality rates are increased in eclamptics, although the rates have declined dramatically in recent years [69]. According to Chesley [16], the average maternal mortality rate of eclampsia during the mid-19th century (1837–67) was approximately 30%. In the latter half of the 19th century, the average maternal mortality rate was around 24%. During the early 20th century (1911–25), the maternal mortality rate was 11% and 22% among women managed conservatively and delivered operatively, respectively. Lazard [83] reported a 13% gross mortality rate among 225 eclamptics treated in Los Angeles between 1924 and 1932. Eastman and Steptoe [84] reported a 7.6% maternal mortality and 21.7% fetal mortality rate of eclampsia in Baltimore between 1924 and 1943.

Contemporary maternal mortality rates of eclampsia are under 2% in developed countries but are significantly higher in developing nations (see Table 34.15). In Pritchard's series of 245 eclamptics, one maternal death occurred, which was attributed to magnesium intoxication [69]. In Sibai's series of 254 eclamptic women, there was one maternal death in a woman who suffered seizures prior to arrival at the hospital and who arrived in a moribund state [299]. In the United Kingdom during 1992, a 1.8% maternal case mortality rate was reported for eclampsia [289].

At a referral hospital in Mexico City, 704 eclamptic women were managed during a 15-year period [300]. The maternal mortality rate was 14%, a relatively high rate likely secondary to a high proportion of advanced cases of disease. According to Lopez-Llera [300], maternal mortality rates are higher in those women with seizures before (15%) than after (10%) delivery. The most common cause of death in the Mexico City series among 86 fatal cases of antepartum and intrapartum eclampsia was cerebrovascular damage (72%), followed by severe respiratory insufficiency (12%), postpartum hemorrhage (6%), and disseminated intravascular coagulation (4%). Autopsy findings have mirrored these observations [224].

Overall, the contemporary perinatal mortality rate among eclamptics ranges from 7 to 16% in the United States and the United Kingdom (see Table 34.15) and is most commonly secondary to placental abruption, prematurity, and perinatal asphyxia. Antenatal deaths accounted for a significant proportion of the overall perinatal mortality. Depending on the gestational age and the clinical circumstances, it may be prudent to have a person capable of neonatal resuscitation immediately available at delivery.

Eclamptic patients are at increased risk for developing pre-eclampsia–eclampsia in a subsequent pregnancy [227,299]. Remote mortality is not greater for white primiparous eclamptics but is increased from two to five times the expected rate for white multiparous eclamptics and all black eclamptics [301]. Moreover, these women appear to be at a greater risk of developing chronic hypertension and diabetes mellitus [227,301,302]. However, long-term neurologic deficits are rare and long-term anticonvulsant therapy is usually not necessary in the eclamptic woman [297].

Uteroplacental–fetal complications of pre-eclampsia

Uteroplacental blood flow is significantly decreased in pre-eclamptic patients [24,303–305] and may lead to IUGR [325], fetal distress, or fetal death. Hypertensive patients are also at higher risk for abruption. The pathophysiology of placental abruption in pre-eclamptic patients has been proposed to result from thrombotic lesions in the placental vasculature, leading to decidual necrosis, separation, and hemorrhage. A vicious cycle then continues as the decidual hemorrhage results in further separation. This cycle may be aggravated by coexisting hemostatic compromise. Abdella et al. [306] evaluated 265 cases of abruption and estimated an incidence of approximately 1% in the total obstetric population; 27% were complicated by a hypertensive disorder. Pre-eclamptics, chronic hypertensives, and eclamptics were found to have a 2, 10, and 24% incidence of abruption, respectively [306,307]. Severe pre-eclamptic patients with chronic hypertension have a significantly increased perinatal mortality rate, abruption rate, and frequency of growth-retarded infants compared with severe pre-eclamptics without pre-existing hypertension [91]. Fetal growth retardation appears to occur frequently in multiparous women with pre-eclampsia compared with nulliparous women with pre-eclampsia; the cause of this difference, however, is uncertain [308]. Oxygen transport and extraction may be negatively affected by pre-eclampsia. Wheeler et al. [309] demonstrated a strong negative linear correlation between base deficit and oxygen delivery index and suggested that a base deficit exceeding 8.0 mEq/L consistently predicted fetal acidosis, death, and maternal end-organ ischemic injury [310]. The reader is referred to a recent review of antenatal fetal surveillance techniques for hypertensive women [60]. Even near-term (delivery between 35 and 37 weeks of gestation) pregnancies complicated by pre-eclampsia or gestational hypertension have higher rates of neonatal intensive care unit admission, small for gestational age birthweight, and longer neonatal stay than normotensive pregnancies, regardless of the severity of hypertensive disease [311].

Conclusions

Pre-eclampsia and eclampsia have the potential to produce significant maternal and fetal complications. Advances in clinical medicine have provided for improved outcomes for our patients.

While the critically ill pre-eclamptic today is much better off than her predecessors, continued evolution of medical services and technology are needed to reduce these complications to an acceptable level.

References

1 Report of the National High Blood Pressure Education Program Working Group on High Blood Pressure in Pregnancy. *Am J Obstet Gynecol* 2000; 183: S1–S22.

2 Kaunitz AM, Hughes JM, Grimes DA, et al. Causes of maternal mortality in the United States. *Obstet Gynecol* 1985; 65: 605–612.

3 Pritchard JA, MacDonald PC, Grant NF. In: Pritchard JA, MacDonald PC, eds. *Hypertensive Disorders in Pregnancy Williams' Obstetrics*, 17th edn. Norwalk, CT: Appleton-Century-Crofts, 1985: 525.

4 Grimes DA. The morbidity and mortality of pregnancy: still risky business. *Am J Obstet Gynecol* 1994; 170: 1489–1494.

5 Berg CJ, Atrash HK, Koonin LM, Tucker M. Pregnancy-related mortality in the United States, 1987–1990. *Obstet Gynecol* 1996; 88: 161.

6 Berg CJ, Harper MA, Atkinson SM, et al. Preventability of pregnancy-related deaths: results of a state-wide review. *Obstet Gynecol* 2005; 106(6): 1228–1234.

7 Royal College of Obstetricians and Gynaecologists. *Confidential Enquiry into Maternal and Child Health. Why Mothers Die 2000–2002*. London: Royal College of Obstetricians and Gynaecologists, 2004.

8 Schutte JM, Schuitemaker NW, van Roosmalen J, Steegers EA, Dutch Maternal Mortality Committee. Substandard care in maternal mortality due to hypertensive disease in pregnancy in the Netherlands. *Br J Obstet Gynaecol* 2008; 115(6): 732–736.

9 Clark SL, Belfort MA, Dildy GA, Herbst MA, Meyers JA, Hankins GD. Maternal death in the 21st century: causes, prevention, and relationship to cesarean delivery. *Am J Obstet Gynecol* 2008; 199(1): 36.

10 Lin CC, Lindheimer MD, River P, Moawad AH. Fetal outcome in hypertensive disorders of pregnancy. *Am J Obstet Gynecol* 1982; 142: 255–260.

11 Sibai BM, Ramadan MK. Acute renal failure in pregnancies complicated by hemolysis, elevated liver enzymes, and low platelets. *Am J Obstet Gynecol* 1993; 168: 1682–1690.

12 Sibai BM, Ramadan MK, Usta I, et al. Maternal morbidity and mortality in 442 pregnancies with hemolysis, elevated liver enzymes, and low platelets (HELLP syndrome). *Am J Obstet Gynecol* 1993; 169: 1000–1006.

13 Sibai BM. Treatment of hypertension in pregnant women. *N Engl J Med* 1996; 335: 257.

14 American College of Obstetricians and Gynecologists. Chronic hypertension in pregnancy. *Obstet Gynecol* 2001; 98(1, suppl): 177–185.

15 Chesley LC. A short history of eclampsia. *Obstet Gynecol* 1974; 43: 599–602.

16 Chesley LC. History and epidemiology of pre-eclampsia–eclampsia. *Clin Obstet Gynecol* 1984; 27: 801–820.

17 Zuspan FP. Problems encountered in the treatment of pregnancy-induced hypertension. *Am J Obstet Gynecol* 1978; 131: 591–597.

18 Worley RJ. Pathophysiology of pregnancy-induced hypertension. *Clin Obstet Gynecol* 1984; 27: 821–823.

19 Conde-Agudelo A, Lede R, Belizan J. Evaluation of methods used in the prediction of hypertensive disorders of pregnancy. *Obstet Gynecol Surv* 1994; 49: 210–222.

20 Stone JL, Lockwood CJ, Berkowitz GS, et al. Risk factors for severe preeclampsia. *Obstet Gynecol* 1994; 83: 357–361.

21 Lewis PJ, Shepherd GI, Ritter J. Prostacyclin and preeclampsia. *Lancet* 1981; i: 559.

22 Dadek C, Kefalides A, Sinzinger H, Weber G. Reduced umbilical artery prostacyclin formation in complicated pregnancies. *Am J Obstet Gynecol* 1982; 144: 792–795.

23 Downing I, Shepherd GI, Lewis PJ. Kinetics of prostacyclin synthetase in umbilical artery microsomes from normal and preeclamptic pregnancies. *Br J Clin Pharmacol* 1982; 13: 195–198.

24 Friedman SA. Preeclampsia: a review of the role of prostaglandins. *Obstet Gynecol* 1988; 71: 122–137.

25 Sorensen JD, Olsen SF, Pederson AK, et al. Effects of fish oil supplementation in the third trimester of pregnancy on prostacyclin and thromboxane production. *Am J Obstet Gynecol* 1993; 168: 915–922.

26 Balasch J, Mirapeix E, Borche L, et al. Further evidence against preeclampsia as an immune complex disease. *Obstet Gynecol* 1981; 58: 435.

27 Redman CWG. Immunologic factors in the pathogenesis of preeclampsia. *Contrib Nephrol* 1981; 25: 120.

28 Rote NS, Caudle MR. Circulating immune complexes in pregnancy, preeclampsia, and auto-immune diseases: evaluation of Raji cell enzyme-linked immunosorbent assay and polyethylene glycol precipitation methods. *Am J Obstet Gynecol* 1983; 147: 267–273.

29 Massobrio M, Benedetto C, Bertini E, et al. Immune complexes in preeclampsia and normal pregnancy. *Am J Obstet Gynecol* 1985; 152: 578–583.

30 Robillard P, Hulsey TC, Perianin J, et al. Association of pregnancy-induced hypertension with duration of sexual cohabitation before conception. *Lancet* 1994; 344: 973–975.

31 Easterling TR, Benedetti TJ. Preeclampsia: a hyperdynamic disease model. *Am J Obstet Gynecol* 1989; 160: 1447–1453.

32 Savelieva GM, Efimov VS, Grishin VL, et al. Blood coagulation changes in pregnant women at risk of developing preeclampsia. *Int J Gynecol Obstet* 1995; 48: 3–8.

33 Weenink GH, Treffers PE, Vijn P, Smorenberg-Schoorl ME, Ten Cate JW. Antithrombin III levels in preeclampsia correlate with maternal and fetal morbidity. *Am J Obstet Gynecol* 1984; 148: 1092–1097.

34 Weiner CP, Kwaan HC, Xu C, et al. Antithrombin III activity in women with hypertension during pregnancies. *Obstet Gynecol* 1985; 65: 301–306.

35 Rodgers GM, Taylor RN, Roberts JM. Preeclampsia is associated with a serum factor cytotoxic to human endothelial cells. *Am J Obstet Gynecol* 1988; 159: 908–914.

36 Friedman SA, de Groot CJM, Taylor RN, et al. Plasma cellular fibronectin as a measure of endothelial involvement in preeclampsia and intrauterine growth retardation. *Am J Obstet Gynecol* 1994; 170: 838–841.

37 Kupferminc MJ, Peaceman AM, Wigton TR, et al. Tumor necrosis factor-α is elevated in plasma and amniotic fluid of patients with severe preeclampsia. *Am J Obstet Gynecol* 1994; 170: 1752–1759.

38 Mikhail MS, Anyaegbunam A, Garfinkel D, et al. Preeclampsia and antioxidant nutrients: decreased plasma levels of reduced ascorbic

acid, α-tocopherol, and beta-carotene in women with preeclampsia. *Am J Obstet Gynecol* 1994; 171: 150–157.
39 Dieckmann WJ, Michel HL. Vascular–renal effects of posterior pituitary extracts in pregnant women. *Am J Obstet Gynecol* 1937; 33: 131–137.
40 Abdul-Karim R, Assali NS. Pressor response to angiotensin in pregnant and non-pregnant women. *Am J Obstet Gynecol* 1961; 82: 246–251.
41 Gant NF, Daley GL, Chand S, et al. A study of angiotensin II pressor response throughout primigravid pregnancy. *J Clin Invest* 1973; 52: 2682–2689.
42 Whalley PJ, Everett RB, Gant NF, et al. Pressor responsiveness to angiotensin II in hospitalized primigravid women with pregnancy-induced hypertension. *Am J Obstet Gynecol* 1983; 145: 481–483.
43 Ward K, Hata A, Jeunemaitre X, et al. A molecular variant of angiotensinogen associated with preeclampsia. *Nat Genet* 1993; 4: 59–61.
44 Branch DW, Andres R, Digre KB, et al. The association of antiphospholipid antibodies with severe preeclampsia. *Obstet Gynecol* 1989; 73: 541–545.
45 Branch DW, Silver RM, Blackwell JL, et al. Outcome of treated pregnancies in women with antiphospholipid syndrome: an update of the Utah experience. *Obstet Gynecol* 1992; 80: 614–620.
46 Romero R, Lockwood C, Oyarzun E, Hobbins JC. Toxemia: new concepts in an old disease. *Semin Perinatol* 1988; 12: 302–323.
47 Dildy GA, Belfort MA, Smulian JC. Preeclampsia recurrence and prevention. *Semin Perinatol* 2007; 31: 135–41.
48 Masse J, Forest JC, Moutquin JM, et al. A prospective study of several potential biologic markers for early prediction of the development of preeclampsia. *Am J Obstet Gynecol* 1993; 169: 501–508.
49 Goodlin RC. Severe preeclampsia: another great imitator. *Am J Obstet Gynecol* 1976; 125: 747–753.
50 Fisher KA, Luger A, Spargo BH, Lindheimer MD. Hypertension in pregnancy: clinical–pathological correlations and remote prognosis. *Medicine* 1981; 60: 267–276.
51 Chesley LC. Diagnosis of preeclampsia. *Obstet Gynecol* 1985; 65: 423–425.
52 Sibai BM. Pitfalls in diagnosis and management of preeclampsia. *Am J Obstet Gynecol* 1988; 159: 1–5.
53 Villar MA, Sibai BM. Clinical significance of elevated mean arterial blood pressure in second trimester and threshold increase in systolic or diastolic blood pressure during third trimester. *Am J Obstet Gynecol* 1989; 160: 419.
54 Conde-Agudelo A, Belizan JM, Lede R, Bergel EF. What does an elevated mean arterial pressure in the second half of pregnancy predict – gestational hypertension or preeclampsia? *Am J Obstet Gynecol* 1993; 169: 509–514.
55 Meyer NL, Mercer BM, Friedman SA, Sibai BM. Urinary dipstick protein: a poor predictor of absent or severe proteinuria. *Am J Obstet Gynecol* 1994; 170: 137–141.
56 Pritchard JA, Cunningham FG, Mason RA. Coagulation changes in preeclampsia: their frequency and pathogenesis. *Am J Obstet Gynecol* 1976; 124: 855–864.
57 Weinstein L. Preeclampsia/eclampsia with hemolysis, elevated liver enzymes, and thrombocytopenia. *Obstet Gynecol* 1985; 66: 657–660.
58 Romero R, Vizoso J, Emamian M, et al. Clinical significance of liver dysfunction in pregnancy-induced hypertension. *Am J Perinatol* 1988; 5: 146–151.
59 Romero R, Mazor M, Lockwood CJ, et al. Clinical significance, prevalence, and natural history of thrombocytopenia in pregnancy-induced hypertension. *Am J Perinatol* 1989; 6: 32–38.
60 Dildy GA. Antenatal surveillance in preeclampsia and chronic hypertension. In: Belfort MA, Thornton S, Saade GR, eds. *Hypertension in Pregnancy*. New York: Marcel Dekker, 2003.
61 National High Blood Pressure Education Program Working Group. Report on high blood pressure in pregnancy. *Am J Obstet Gynecol* 1990; 163: 1689–1712.
62 MacKenna J, Dover NL, Brame RG. Preeclampsia associated with hemolysis, elevated liver enzymes, and low platelets: an obstetric emergency? *Obstet Gynecol* 1983; 62: 751–754.
63 Thiagarajah S, Bourgeois FJ, Harbert GM, Caudle MR. Thrombocytopenia in preeclampsia: associated abnormalities and management principles. *Am J Obstet Gynecol* 1984; 150: 1–7.
64 Van Dam PA, Reiner M, Baekelandt M, et al. Disseminated intravascular coagulation and the syndrome of hemolysis, elevated liver enzymes, and low platelets in severe preeclampsia. *Obstet Gynecol* 1989; 73: 97–102.
65 Sibai BM, Saslimi M, Abdella TN, et al. Maternal and perinatal outcome of conservative management of severe preeclampsia in midtrimester. *Am J Obstet Gynecol* 1985; 152: 32–37.
66 Sibai BM, Mercer BM, Schiff E, Friedman SA. Aggressive versus expectant management of severe preeclampsia at 28 to 32 weeks' gestation: a randomized controlled trial. *Am J Obstet Gynecol* 1994; 171: 818–822.
67 Odendaal HJ, Pattinson RC, Bam R, et al. Aggressive or expectant management for patients with severe preeclampsia between 28–34 weeks' gestation: a randomized controlled trial. *Obstet Gynecol* 1990; 76: 1070–1074.
68 Weinstein L. Syndrome of hemolysis, elevated liver enzymes, and low platelet count: a severe consequence of hypertension in pregnancy. *Am J Obstet Gynecol* 1982; 142: 159–167.
69 Pritchard JA, Cunningham FG, Pritchard SA. The Parkland Memorial Hospital protocol for the treatment of eclampsia: evaluation of 245 cases. *Am J Obstet Gynecol* 1984; 148: 951–963.
70 Wasserstrum N, Cotton DB. Hemodynamic monitoring in severe pregnancy-induced hypertension. *Clin Perinatol* 1986; 13: 781–799.
71 Joyce TH, Debnath KS, Baker EA. Preeclampsia: relationship of central venous pressure and epidural anesthesia. *Anesthesiology* 1979; 51: S297.
72 Graham C, Goldstein A. Epidural analgesia and cardiac output in severe preeclamptics. *Anaesthesia* 1980; 35: 709–712.
73 Jouppila P, Jouppila R, Hollman A, Koivula A. Lumbar epidural analgesia to improve intervillous blood flow during labor in severe preeclampsia. *Obstet Gynecol* 1982; 59: 158–161.
74 Gutsche B. The experts opine: is epidural block for labor and delivery and for cesarean section a safe form of analgesia in severe pre-eclampsia or eclampsia? *Surv Anesth* 1986; 30: 304–311.
75 Newsome LR, Bramwell RS, Curling PE. Severe preeclampsia: hemodynamic effects of lumbar epidural anesthesia. *Anesth Analg* 1986; 65: 31–36.
76 Cotton DB, Gonik B, Dorman KR. Cardiovascular alterations in severe pregnancy-induced hypertension: acute effects of intravenous magnesium sulfate. *Am J Obstet Gynecol* 1984; 148: 162–165.
77 Kirshon B, Moise KJ Jr, Cotton DB, et al. Role of volume expansion in severe preeclampsia. *Surg Gynecol Obstet* 1988; 167: 367–371.

78 Wasserstrum N, Kirshon B, Willis RS, et al. Quantitive hemodynamic effects of acute volume expansion in severe preeclampsia. *Obstet Gynecol* 1989; 73: 546–550.
79 Gonik B, Cotton DB. Peripartum colloid osmotic pressure changes: influence of intravenous hydration. *Am J Obstet Gynecol* 1984; 150: 90–100.
80 Cotton DB, Gonik B, Spillman T, Dorman KF. Intrapartum to postpartum changes in colloid osmotic pressure. *Am J Obstet Gynecol* 1984; 149: 174–177.
81 Jones MM, Longmire S, Cotton DB, et al. Influence of crystalloid versus colloid infusion on peripartum colloid osmotic pressure changes. *Obstet Gynecol* 1986; 68: 659–661.
82 Dorsett L. The intramuscular injection of magnesium sulphate for the control of convulsions in eclampsia. *Am J Obstet Gynecol* 1926; 11: 227–231.
83 Lazard EM. An analysis of 575 cases of eclamptic and pre-eclamptic toxemias treated by intravenous injections of magnesium sulphate. *Am J Obstet Gynecol* 1933; 26: 647–656.
84 Eastman NJ, Steptoe PP. The management of pre-eclampsia. *Can Med Assoc J* 1945; 52: 562–568.
85 Pritchard JA. The use of magnesium iron in the management of eclamptogenic toxemias. *Surg Gynecol Obstet* 1955; 100: 131–140.
86 Pritchard JA, Pritchard SA. Standardized treatment of 154 consecutive cases of eclampsia. *Am J Obstet Gynecol* 1975; 123: 543–552.
87 Shelley WC, Gutsche BB. Magnesium and seizure control. *Am J Obstet Gynecol* 1980; 136: 146–147.
88 Borges LF, Gucer G. Effect of magnesium on epileptic foci. *Epilepsia* 1978; 19: 81–91.
89 Pritchard JA. The use of magnesium sulfate in preeclampsia–eclampsia. *J Reprod Med* 1979; 23: 107–114.
90 Koontz WLL, Reid KH. Effect of parenteral magnesium sulfate on penicillin-induced seizure in foci in anesthetized cats. *Am J Obstet Gynecol* 1985; 153: 96–99.
91 Sibai BM, Spinnato JA, Watson DL, et al. Effect of magnesium sulfate on electroencephalographic findings in preeclampsia–eclampsia. *Obstet Gynecol* 1984; 64: 261–266.
92 Hallak M, Berman RF, Irtenkauf SM, Janusz CA, Cotton DB. Magnesium sulfate treatment decreases *N*-methyl-D-aspartate receptor binding in the rat brain: an autoradiographic study. *J Soc Gynecol Invest* 1994; 1: 25–30.
93 Hallak M. Effect of parenteral magnesium sulfate administration on excitatory amino acid receptors in the rat brain. *Magnes Res* 1998; 11: 117–131.
94 Belfort MA, Saade GR, Moise KJ. The effect of magnesium sulfate on maternal retinal blood flow in preeclampsia: a randomized placebo-controlled study. *Am J Obstet Gynecol* 1992; 167: 1548–1553.
95 Belfort M, Allred J, Dildy G. Magnesium sulphate decreases cerebral perfusion pressure in preeclampsia. *Hypertens Pregnancy* 2008; 27(4): 315–327.
96 Belfort MA, Varner MW, Dizon-Townson DS, Grunewald C, Nisell H. Cerebral perfusion pressure, and not cerebral blood flow, may be the critical determinant of intracranial injury in preeclampsia: a new hypothesis. *Am J Obstet Gynecol* 2002; 187: 626–634.
97 Sibai BM, Graham JM, McCubbin JH. A comparison of intravenous and intramuscular magnesium sulfate regimens in preeclampsia. *Am J Obstet Gynecol* 1984; 150: 728–733.
98 Pruett KM, Krishon B, Cotton DB, et al. The effects of magnesium sulfate therapy on Apgar scores. *Am J Obstet Gynecol* 1988; 159: 1047–1048.
99 Atkinson MW, Belfort MA, Saade GR, Moise K. The relation between magnesium sulfate therapy and fetal heart rate variability. *Obstet Gynecol* 1991; 83: 967–970.
100 Donaldson JO. The case against magnesium sulfate for eclamptic convulsions. *Int J Obstet Anesth* 1992; 1: 159–166.
101 Hutton JD, James DK, Stirrat GM, et al. Management of severe preeclampsia and eclampsia by UK consultants. *Br J Obstet Gynaecol* 1992; 99: 554–556.
102 Repke JT, Friedman SA, Kaplan PW. Prophylaxis of eclamptic seizures: current controversies. *Clin Obstet Gynecol* 1992; 35: 365–374.
103 Duley L, Johanson R. Magnesium sulphate for pre-eclampsia and eclampsia: the evidence so far. *Br J Obstet Gynaecol* 1994; 101: 565–567.
104 Lucas MJ, Leveno KJ, Cunningham FG. A comparison of magnesium sulfate with phenytoin for the prevention of eclampsia. *N Engl J Med* 1995; 333: 201–205.
105 Eclampsia Trial Collaborative Group. Which anticonvulsant for women with eclampsia? Evidence from the Collaborative Eclampsia Trial. *Lancet* 1995; 345: 1455–1463.
106 Coetzee EJ, Dommisse J, Anthony J. A randomised controlled trial of intravenous magnesium sulphate versus placebo in the management of women with severe pre-eclampsia. *Br J Obstet Gynaecol* 1998; 105: 300–303.
107 Chien PF, Khan KS, Arnott N. Magnesium sulphate in the treatment of eclampsia and pre-eclampsia: an overview of the evidence from randomised trials. *Br J Obstet Gynaecol* 1996; 103: 1085–1091.
108 Rey E, LeLorier J, Burgess E, Lange IR, Leduc L. Report of the Canadian Hypertension Society Consensus Conference: 3. Pharmacologic treatment of hypertensive disorders in pregnancy. *Can Med Assoc J* 1997; 157: 1245–1254.
109 Hypertensive disorders in pregnancy. In: Cunningham FG, Gant NF, Leveno KJ, Gilstrap LC, Hauth JC, Wenstrom KD, eds. *Williams' Obstetrics*. New York: McGraw-Hill, 2001.
110 American College of Obstetricians and Gynecologists. Diagnosis and management of preeclampsia and eclampsia. *Obstet Gynecol* 2002; 99(suppl): 159–167.
111 Duley L, Gulmezoglu AM, Henderson-Smart DJ. Anticonvulsants for women with pre-eclampsia (Cochrane Review). Cochrane Library. Oxford: Update Software, 2002, Issue 2.
112 Duley L, Gulmezoglu AM. Magnesium sulfate compared with lytic cocktail for women with eclampsia (Cochrane Review). Cochrane Library. Oxford: Update Software, 2002, Issue 2.
113 Duley L, Henderson-Smart D. Magnesium sulphate versus diazepam for eclampsia (Cochrane Review). Cochrane Library. Oxford: Update Software, 2002, Issue 2.
114 Duley L, Henderson-Smart D. Magnesium sulphate versus phenytoin for eclampsia (Cochrane Review). Cochrane Library. Oxford: Update Software, 2002, Issue 2.
115 Chesley LC. Parenteral magnesium sulfate and the distribution, plasma levels, and excretion of magnesium. *Am J Obstet Gynecol* 1979; 133: 1–7.
116 American College of Obstetricians and Gynecologists. *Hypertension in Pregnancy*. ACOG Technical Bulletin 219. Washington, DC: American College of Obstetricians and Gynecologists, 1996.
117 Bohman VR, Cotton DB. Supralethal magnesemia with patient survival. *Obstet Gynecol* 1990; 76: 984–985.
118 Mroczek WJ, Lee WR, Davidov ME. Effect of magnesium sulfate on cardiovascular hemodynamics. *Angiology* 1977; 28: 720–724.

119 Young BK, Weinstein HM. Effects of magnesium sulfate on toxemic patients in labor. *Obstet Gynecol* 1977; 49: 681–685.

120 Fontenot MT, Lewis DF, Frederick JB, et al. A prospective randomized trial of magnesium sulfate in severe preeclampsia: use of diuresis as a clinical parameter to determine the duration of postpartum therapy. *Am J Obstet Gynecol* 2005; 192: 1788–1793.

121 Naden RP, Redman CWG. Antihypertensive drugs in pregnancy. *Clin Perinatol* 1985; 12: 521–538.

122 Lubbe WF. Hypertension in pregnancy: whom and how to treat. *Br J Clin Pharmacol* 1987; 24: 15S–20S.

123 Zimmerman JL. Hypertensive crisis: emergencies and urgencies. In: Ayers SM, ed. *Textbook of Critical Care*. Philadelphia: WB Saunders, 1995.

124 Koch-Weser J. Hydralazine. *N Engl J Med* 1976; 295; 320–323.

125 Assali NS, Kaplan S, Oighenstein S, Suyemoto R. Hemodynamic effects of 1-hydrazinophthalazine (Apresoline) in human pregnancy: results of intravenous administration. *J Clin Invest* 1953; 32: 922–930.

126 Kuzniar J, Skret A, Piela A, et al. Hemodynamic effects of intravenous hydralazine in pregnant women with severe hypertension. *Obstet Gynecol* 1985; 66: 453–458.

127 Cotton DB, Gonik B, Dorman K, Harrist R. Cardiovascular alterations in severe pregnancy-induced hypertension: relationship of central venous pressure to pulmonary capillary wedge pressure. *Am J Obstet Gynecol* 1985; 151: 762–764.

128 Jouppila P, Kirkinen P, Koivula A, Ylikorkala O. Effects of dihydralazine infusion on the fetoplacental blood flow and maternal prostanoids. *Obstet Gynecol* 1985; 65: 115–118.

129 Liedholm H, Wahlin-Boll E, Hanson A, et al. Transplacental passage and breast milk concentrations of hydralazine. *Eur J Clin Pharmacol* 1982; 21: 417–419.

130 Spinnato JA, Sibai BM, Anderson GD. Fetal distress after hydralazine therapy for severe pregnancy-induced hypertension. *South Med J* 1986; 79: 559–562.

131 Cotton DB, Jones MM, Longmire S, et al. Role of intravenous nitroglycerin in the treatment of severe pregnancy-induced hypertension complicated by pulmonary edema. *Am J Obstet Gynecol* 1986; 154: 91–93.

132 Clark SL, Cotton DB. Clinical indications for pulmonary artery catheterization in the patient with severe preeclampsia. *Am J Obstet Gynecol* 1988; 158: 453–458.

133 Rubin AA, Roth FE, Taylor RM, Rosenkilde H. Pharmacology of diazoxide, an antihypertensive, non-diuretic benzothiadiazine. *J Pharmacol Exp Ther* 1962; 136: 344–352.

134 Thien T, Koene RAP, Schijf C, et al. Infusion of diazoxide in severe hypertension during pregnancy. *Eur J Obstet Gynecol Reprod Biol* 1980; 10: 367–374.

135 Waisman GD, Mayorga LM, Camera MI, et al. Magnesium plus nifedipine: potentiation of hypotensive effect in preeclampsia? *Am J Obstet Gynecol* 1988; 159: 308–309.

136 Fenakel K, Fenakel G, Appleman ZVI, et al. Nifedipine in the treatment of severe preeclampsia. *Obstet Gynecol* 1991; 77: 331–336.

137 Vermillion ST, Scardo JA, Newman RB, Chauhan SP. A randomized, double-blind trial of oral nifedipine and intravenous labetalol in hypertensive emergencies of pregnancy. *Am J Obstet Gynecol* 1999; 181: 858–861.

138 Aali BS, Nejad SS. Nifedipine or hydralazine as a first-line agent to control hypertension in severe preeclampsia. *Acta Obstet Gynecol Scand* 2002; 81: 25–30.

139 Belfort MA, Carpenter RJ Jr, Kirshon B, Saade GR, Moise KJ Jr. The use of nimodipine in a patient with eclampsia: color flow Doppler demonstration of retinal artery relaxation. *Am J Obstet Gynecol* 1993; 169: 204–206.

140 Belfort MA, Saade GR, Moise KJ Jr, et al. Nimodipine in the management of preeclampsia: maternal and fetal effects. *Am J Obstet Gynecol* 1994; 171: 417–424.

141 Belfort MA, Anthony J, Saade GR. Prevention of eclampsia. *Semin Perinatol* 1999; 23: 65–78.

142 Belfort MA, Saade GR, Yared M, et al. Change in estimated cerebral perfusion pressure after treatment with nimodipine or magnesium sulfate in patients with preeclampsia. *Am J Obstet Gynecol* 1999; 181: 402–407.

143 Lund-Johnson P. Short- and long-term (six year) hemodynamic effects of labetalol in essential hypertension. *Am J Med* 1983; 75: 24–31.

144 Lamming GD, Symonds EM. Use of labetalol and methyldopa in pregnancy-induced hypertension. *Br J Clin Pharmacol* 1979; 8: 217S–222S.

145 Michael CA. Use of labetalol in the treatment of severe hypertension during pregnancy. *Br J Clin Pharmacol* 1979; 8: 211S–215S.

146 Coevoet B, Leuliet J, Comoy E, et al. Labetalol in the treatment of hypertension of pregnancy: clinical effects and interactions with plasma renin and dopamine betahydroxylase activities, and with plasma concentrations of catecholamine. *Kidney Int* 1980; 17: 701.

147 Lunell NO, Hjemdahl P, Fredholm BB, et al. Circulatory and metabolic effects of a combined α- and β-adrenoceptor blocker (labetalol) in hypertension of pregnancy. *Br J Clin Pharmacol* 1981; 12: 345–348.

148 Riley AJ. Clinical pharmacology of labetalol in pregnancy. *J Cardiovasc Pharmacol* 1981; 3: S53–S59.

149 Mabie WC, Gonzalez AR, Sibai BM, Amon E. A comparative trial of labetalol and hydralazine in the acute management of severe hypertension complicating pregnancy. *Obstet Gynecol* 1987; 70: 328–333.

150 Pickles CJ, Symonds EM, Pipkin FB. The fetal outcome in a randomized double-blind controlled trial of labetalol versus placebo in pregnancy-induced hypertension. *Br J Obstet Gynaecol* 1989; 96: 38–43.

151 Michael CA. The evaluation of labetalol in the treatment of hypertension complicating pregnancy. *Br J Clin Pharmacol* 1982; 13: 127S–131S.

152 Lunell NO, Lewander R, Mamoun I, et al. Utero-placental blood flow in pregnancy-induced hypertension. *Scand J Clin Lab Invest* 1984; 169(suppl): 28–35.

153 Morgan MA, Silavin SL, Dormer KJ, et al. Effects of labetalol on uterine blood flow and cardiovascular hemodynamics in the hypertensive gravid baboon. *Am J Obstet Gynecol* 1993; 168: 1574–1579.

154 Belfort MA, Tooke-Miller C, Allen JC, Dizon-Townson D, Varner MA. Labetalol decreases cerebral perfusion pressure without negatively affecting cerebral blood flow in hypertensive gravidas. *Hypertens Pregn* 2002: 21(3): 185–197.

155 Herling IM. Intravenous nitroglycerin: clinical pharmacology and therapeutic considerations. *Am Heart J* 1984; 108: 141–149.

156 Cotton DB, Longmire S, Jones MM, et al. Cardiovascular alterations in severe pregnancy-induced hypertension: effects of intravenous nitroglycerin coupled with blood volume expansion. *Am J Obstet Gynecol* 1986; 154: 1053–1059.

157 Pasch T, Schulz V, Hoppelshauser G. Nitroprusside-induced formation of cyanide and its detoxification with thiosulfate during deliberate hypotension. *J Cardiovasc Pharmacol* 1983; 5: 77–85.
158 Strauss RG, Keefer JR, Burke T, Civetta JM. Hemodynamic monitoring of cardiogenic pulmonary edema complicating toxemia of pregnancy. *Obstet Gynecol* 1980; 55: 170–174.
159 Oates JA, Wood AJJ. Converting-enzyme inhibitors in the treatment of hypertension. *N Engl J Med* 1988; 319: 1517–1525.
160 Hurault de Ligny B, Ryckelynck JP, Mintz P, et al. Captopril therapy in preeclampsia. *Nephron* 1987; 46: 329–330.
161 Schubiger G, Flury G, Nussberger J. Enalapril for pregnancy-induced hypertension: acute renal failure in a neonate. *Ann Intern Med* 1988; 108: 215–216.
162 Barr M, Cohen M. ACE inhibitor fetopathy and hypocalvaria: the kidney–skull connection. *Teratology* 1991; 44: 485–495.
163 Hanssens M, Keirse MJ, Vankelecom F, van Assche FA. Fetal and neonatal effects of treatment with angiotensin-converting enzyme inhibitors in pregnancy. *Obstet Gynecol* 1991; 78: 128–135.
164 Ferris TF, Weir EK. Effect of captopril on uterine blood flow and prostaglandin E synthesis in the pregnant rabbit. *J Clin Invest* 1983; 71: 809–815.
165 Lindheimer MD, Katz AI. Current concepts. Hypertension in pregnancy. *N Engl J Med* 1985; 313: 675–680.
166 Connell H, Dalgleish JG, Downing JW. General anaesthesia in mothers with severe preeclampsia/eclampsia. *Br J Anaesth* 1987; 59: 1375–1380.
167 Hodgkinson R, Husain FJ, Hayashi RH. Systemic and pulmonary blood pressure during cesarean section in parturients with gestational hypertension. *Can Anaesth Soc J* 1980; 27: 389–394.
168 Ramos-Santos E, Devoe LD, Wakefield ML, Sherline DM, Metheny WP. The effects of epidural anesthesia on the Doppler velocimetry of umbilical and uterine arteries in normal and hypertensive patients during active term labor. *Obstet Gynecol* 1991; 77: 20–26.
169 Hogg B, Hauth JC, Caritis SN, et al. Safety of labor epidural anesthesia for women with severe hypertensive disease. National Institute of Child Health and Human Development Maternal–Fetal Medicine Units Network. *Am J Obstet Gynecol* 1999; 181: 1096–1101.
170 Head BB, Owen J, Vincent RD Jr, Shih G, Chestnut DH, Hauth JC. A randomized trial of intrapartum analgesia in women with severe preeclampsia. *Obstet Gynecol* 2002; 99: 452–457.
171 Swan HJC, Ganz W, Forrester JS, et al. Catheterization of the heart in man with the use of flow-directed balloon-tipped catheter. *N Engl J Med* 1970; 283: 447–451.
172 Dildy GA, Cotton DB. Hemodynamic changes in pregnancy and pregnancy complicated by hypertension. *Acute Care* 1988–89; 14–15: 26–46.
173 Dildy GA, Cotton DB. Management of severe preeclampsia and eclampsia. *Crit Care Clin* 1991; 7: 829–850.
174 Clark SL, Horenstein JM, Phelan JP, et al. Experience with the pulmonary artery catheter in obstetrics and gynecology. *Am J Obstet Gynecol* 1985; 152: 374–378.
175 Clark SL, Divon MY, Phelan JP. Preeclampsia/eclampsia: hemodynamic and neurologic correlations. *Obstet Gynecol* 1985; 66: 337–340.
176 Cotton DB, Lee W, Huhta JC, Dorman KF. Hemodynamic profile of severe pregnancy-induced hypertension. *Am J Obstet Gynecol* 1988; 158: 523–529.
177 Mitchell SE, Clark RA. Complications of central venous catheterization. *Am J Roentgenol* 1979; 133: 467–476.
178 Cotton DB, Benedetti TJ. Use of the Swan–Ganz catheter in obstetrics and gynecology. *Obstet Gynecol* 1980; 56: 641–645.
179 Kirshon B, Cotton DB. Invasive hemodynamic monitoring in the obstetric patient. *Clin Obstet Gynecol* 1987; 30: 579–590.
180 Gilbert WM, Towner DR, Field NT, Anthony J. The safety and utility of pulmonary artery catheterization in severe preeclampsia and eclampsia. *Am J Obstet Gynecol* 2000; 182: 1397–1403.
181 Belfort MA, Rokey R, Saade GR, Moise KJ. Rapid echocardiographic assessment of left and right heart hemodynamics in critically ill obstetric patients. *Am J Obstet Gynecol* 1994; 171(4): 884–892.
182 Belfort MA, Mares A, Saade G, Wen TS, Rokey R. Two-dimensional echocardiography and Doppler ultrasound in managing obstetric patients. *Obstet Gynecol* 1997; 90(3): 326–330.
183 Rokey R, Belfort MA, Saade GR. Quantitative echocardiographic assessment of left ventricular function in critically ill obstetric patients: a comparative study. *Am J Obstet Gynecol* 1995; 173(4): 1148–1152.
184 Chesley LC. Plasma and red cell volumes during pregnancy. *Am J Obstet Gynecol* 1972; 112: 440–450.
185 Hays PM, Cruikshank DP, Dunn LJ. Plasma volume determination in normal and preeclamptic pregnancies. *Am J Obstet Gynecol* 1985; 151: 958–966.
186 Bletka M, Hlavaty V, Trnkova M, et al. Volume of whole blood and absolute amount of serum proteins in the early stage of late toxemia of pregnancy. *Am J Obstet Gynecol* 1970; 106: 10–13.
187 Gallery EDM, Hunyor SN, Gyory AZ. Plasma volume contraction: a significant factor in both pregnancy-associated hypertension (preeclampsia) and chronic hypertension in pregnancy. *Q J Med* 1979; 48: 593–602.
188 Lees MM. Central circulatory response to normotensive and hypertensive pregnancy. *Postgrad Med J* 1979; 55: 311–314.
189 Rafferty TD, Berkowitz RL. Hemodynamics in patients with severe toxemia during labor and delivery. *Am J Obstet Gynecol* 1980; 138: 263–270.
190 Benedetti TJ, Cotton DB, Read JC, Miller FC. Hemodynamic observations in severe preeclampsia with a flow-directed pulmonary artery. *Am J Obstet Gynecol* 1980; 136: 465–470.
191 Phelan JP, Yurth DA. Severe preeclampsia. I. Peripartum hemodynamic observations. *Am J Obstet Gynecol* 1982; 144: 17–22.
192 Henderson DW, Vilos GA, Milne KJ, Nichol PM. The role of Swan–Ganz catheterization in severe pregnancy-induced hypertension. *Am J Obstet Gynecol* 1984; 148: 570–574.
193 Groenendijk R, Trimbos JBMJ, Wallenburg HCS. Hemodynamic measurements in preeclampsia: preliminary observations. *Am J Obstet Gynecol* 1984; 150: 232–236.
194 Hankins GDV, Wendell GD, Cunningham FG, Leveno KJ. Longitudinal evaluation of hemodynamic changes in eclampsia. *Am J Obstet Gynecol* 1984; 150: 506–512.
195 Clark SL, Cotton DB, Lee W, et al. Central hemodynamic observations in normal third trimester pregnancy. *Am J Obstet Gynecol* 1989; 161: 1439–1442.
196 Lund-Johansen P. The haemodynamic pattern in mild and borderline hypertension. *Acta Med Scand* 1983; 686(suppl): 15.
197 Sibai BM, Mabie BC, Harvey CJ, Gonzalez AR. Pulmonary edema in severe preeclampsia–eclampsia: analysis of thirty-seven consecutive cases. *Am J Obstet Gynecol* 1987; 156: 1174–1179.
198 Benedetti TJ, Kates R, Williams V. Hemodynamic observations in severe preeclampsia complicated by pulmonary edema. *Am J Obstet Gynecol* 1985; 152: 330–334.

199 Fein A, Grossman RF, Jones JG, et al. The value of edema fluid protein measurement in patients with pulmonary edema. *Am J Med* 1979; 67: 32–38.

200 Weil MN, Henning RJ, Puri VK. Colloid osmotic pressure: clinical significance. *Crit Care Med* 1979; 7: 113–116.

201 Benedetti TJ, Carlson RW. Studies of colloid osmotic pressure in pregnancy-induced hypertension. *Am J Obstet Gynecol* 1979; 135: 308–317.

202 Schannwell CM, Schmitz L, Schoebel FC, et al. Left ventricular diastolic function in pregnancy in patients with arterial hypertension. A prospective study with M-mode echocardiography and Doppler echocardiography. *Z Kardiol* 2001; 90: 427–436.

203 Desai DK, Moodley J, Naidoo DP, Bhorat I. Cardiac abnormalities in pulmonary oedema associated with hypertensive crises in pregnancy. *Br J Obstet Gynaecol* 1996; 103: 523–528.

204 Phillips RA, Diamond JA. Diastolic function in hypertension. *Curr Cardiol Rep* 2001; 3: 485–497.

205 Witlin AG, Mabie WC, Sibai BM. Peripartum cardiomyopathy: a longitudinal echocardiographic study. *Am J Obstet Gynecol* 1997; 177: 1129–1132.

206 Witlin AG, Mabie WC, Sibai BM. Peripartum cardiomyopathy: an ominous diagnosis. *Am J Obstet Gynecol* 1997; 176: 182–188.

207 Mabie WC, Ratts TE, Ramanathan KB, Sibai BM. Circulatory congestion in obese hypertensive women: a subset of pulmonary edema in pregnancy. *Obstet Gynecol* 1988; 72: 553–558.

208 Naidoo DP, Bhorat I, Moodley J, Naidoo JK, Mitha AS. Continuous electrocardiographic monitoring in hypertensive crises in pregnancy. *Am J Obstet Gynecol* 1991; 164: 530–533.

209 Bhorat IE, Naidoo DP, Rout CC, Moodley J. Malignant ventricular arrhythmias in eclampsia: a comparison of labetalol with dihydralazine. *Am J Obstet Gynecol* 1993; 168: 1292–1296.

210 Chesley LC, Duffus GM. Preeclampsia, posture, and renal function. *Obstet Gynecol* 1971; 38: 1–5.

211 Morris RH, Vassalli P, Beller PK, McCluskey RT. Immunofluorescent studies of renal biopsies in the diagnosis of toxemia of pregnancy. *Obstet Gynecol* 1964; 24: 32–46.

212 Sheehan HL. Renal morphology in preeclampsia. *Kidney Int* 1980; 18: 241–252.

213 Leduc L, Lederer E, Lee W, Cotton DB. Urinary sediment changes in severe preeclampsia. *Obstet Gynecol* 1991; 77: 186–189.

214 Gallery ED, Ross M, Gyory AZ. Urinary red blood cell and cast excretion in normal and hypertensive human pregnancy. *Am J Obstet Gynecol* 1993; 168: 67–70.

215 Krane NK. Acute renal failure in pregnancy. *Arch Intern Med* 1988; 148: 2347–2357.

216 Grunfeld JP, Pertuiset N. Acute renal failure in pregnancy. *Am J Kidney Dis* 1987; 9: 359–362.

217 Redman CWG, Beilin LJ, Bonner J. Renal function in preeclampsia. *J Clin Pathol* 1976; 10: 94–96.

218 Baker PN, Hacket GA. The use of urinary albumin–creatinine ratios and calcium–creatinine ratios as screening tests for pregnancy-induced hypertension. *Obstet Gynecol* 1994; 83: 745–749.

219 Clark SL, Greenspoon JS, Aldahl D, Phelan JP. Severe preeclampsia with persistent oliguria: management of hemodynamic subsets. *Am J Obstet Gynecol* 1986; 154: 490–494.

220 Kirshon B, Lee W, Mauer MB, Cotton DB. Effects of low-dose dopamine therapy in the oliguric patient with preeclampsia. *Am J Obstet Gynecol* 1988; 159: 604–607.

221 Lee W, Gonik B, Cotton DB. Urinary diagnostic indices in preeclampsia-associated oligura: correlation with invasive hemodynamic monitoring. *Am J Obstet Gynecol* 1987; 156: 100–103.

222 Pritchard JA, Weisman R, Ratnoff OD, Vosburgh GJ. Intravascular hemolysis, thrombocytopenia, and other hematologic abnormalities associated with severe toxemia of pregnancy. *N Engl J Med* 1954; 150: 89–98.

223 Stahnke E. Über das verhalten der blutplättchen bie eklampsie. *Zentralbl Gynäk* 1922; 46: 391.

224 Sheehan HL. Pathological lesions in the hypertensive toxemias of pregnancy. In: Hammond J, Browne FJ, Walstenholme GEW, eds. *Toxemias of Pregnancy, Human and Veterinary.* Philadelphia: Blakiston, 1950: 16–22.

225 Killam AP, Dillard SH, Patton RC, Pederson PR. Pregnancy-induced hypertension complicated by acute liver disease and disseminated intravascular coagulation. *Am J Obstet Gynecol* 1975; 123: 823–828.

226 Goodlin RC. Preeclampsia as the great imposter. *Am J Obstet Gynecol* 1991; 164: 1577–1581.

227 Sibai BM, El-Nazer A, Gonzalez-Ruiz A. Severe preeclampsia–eclampsia in young primigravid women: subsequent pregnancy outcome and remote prognosis. *Am J Obstet Gynecol* 1986; 155: 1011–1016.

228 Sibai BM, Mercer B, Sarinoglu C. Severe preeclampsia in the second trimester: recurrence risk and long-term prognosis. *Am J Obstet Gynecol* 1991; 165: 1408–1412.

229 Sibai BM, Taslimi MM, El-Nazer A, et al. Maternal–perinatal outcome associated with the syndrome of hemolysis, elevated liver enzymes, and low platelets in severe preeclampsia–eclampsia. *Am J Obstet Gynecol* 1986; 155: 501–509.

230 Oosterhof H, Voorhoeve PG, Aarnoudse JG. Enhancement of hepatic artery resistance to blood flow in preeclampsia in presence or absence of HELLP syndrome (hemolysis, elevated liver enzymes, and low platelets). *Am J Obstet Gynecol* 1994; 171: 526–530.

231 Arias F, Mancilla-Jimenez R. Hepatic fibrinogen deposits in preeclampsia. *N Engl J Med* 1976; 295: 578–582.

232 Shukla PK, Sharma D, Mandal RK. Serum lactate dehydrogenase in detecting liver damage associated with preeclampsia. *Br J Obstet Gynaecol* 1978; 85: 40–42.

233 Vardi J, Fields GA. Microangiopathic hemolytic anemia in severe preeclampsia. *Am J Obstet Gynecol* 1974; 119: 617–622.

234 Cunningham FG, Pritchard JA. Hematologic considerations of pregnancy-induced hypertension. *Semin Perinatol* 1978; 2: 29–38.

235 Gibson B, Hunter D, Neame PB, Kelton JG. Thrombocytopenia in preeclampsia and eclampsia. *Semin Thromb Hemost* 1982; 8: 234–247.

236 Cunningham FG, Lowe T, Guss S, Mason R. Erythrocyte morphology in women with severe preeclampsia and eclampsia. Preliminary observations with scanning electron microscopy. *Am J Obstet Gynecol* 1985; 153: 358–363.

237 Burrows RF, Hunter DJS, Andrew M, Kelton JG. A prospective study investigating the mechanism of thrombocytopenia in preeclampsia. *Obstet Gynecol* 1987; 70: 334–338.

238 Entman SS, Kambam JR, Bradley CA, Cousar JB. Increased levels of carboxyhemoglobin and serum iron as an indicator of increased red cell turnover in preeclampsia. *Am J Obstet Gynecol* 1987; 156: 1169–1173.

239 Hutt R, Ogunniyi SO, Sullivan MHF, Elder MG. Increased platelet volume and aggregation precede the onset of preeclampsia. *Obstet Gynecol* 1994; 83: 146–149.

240 Klechner HB, Giles HR, Corrigan JJ. The association of maternal and neonatal thrombocytopenia in high risk pregnancies. *Am J Obstet Gynecol* 1977; 128: 235–238.

241 Pritchard JA, Cunningham FG, Pritchard SA, Mason RA. How often does maternal preeclampsia–eclampsia incite thrombocytopenia in the fetus? *Obstet Gynecol* 1987; 69: 292–295.

242 Neiger R, Contag SA, Coustan DR. The resolution of preeclampsia-related thrombocytopenia. *Obstet Gynecol* 1991; 77: 692–695.

243 Martin JN, Blake PG, Perry KG, et al. The natural history of HELLP syndrome: patterns of disease progression and regression. *Am J Obstet Gynecol* 1991; 164: 1500–1513.

244 Bornstein E, Barnhard Y, Atkin R, Divon MY. HELLP syndrome: a rare, early presentation at 17 weeks of gestation. *Obstet Gynecol* 2007; 110(2 Pt 2): 525–527.

245 Messer RH. Symposium on bleeding disorders in pregnancy: observations on bleeding in pregnancy. *Am J Obstet Gynecol* 1987; 156: 1419–1420.

246 Goodlin RC, Mostello D. Maternal hyponatremia and the syndrome of hemolysis, elevated liver enzymes, and low platelet count. *Am J Obstet Gynecol* 1987; 156: 910–911.

247 Heyborne KD, Burke MS, Porreco RP. Prolongation of premature gestation in women with hemolysis, elevated liver enzymes and low platelets: a report of five cases. *J Reprod Med* 1990; 35: 53–57.

248 Clark SL, Phelan JP, Allen SH, Golde SH. Antepartum reversal of hematologic abnormalities with the HELLP syndrome. *J Reprod Med* 1986; 31: 70–72.

249 Sullivan CA, Magann EF, Perry KG, et al. The recurrence risk of the syndrome of hemolysis, elevated liver enzymes, and low platelets (HELLP) in subsequent gestations. *Am J Obstet Gynecol* 1994; 171: 940–943.

250 Sibai BM, Ramadan MK, Chari RS, Friedman SA. Pregnancies complicated by HELLP syndrome (hemolysis, elevated liver enzymes, and low platelets): subsequent pregnancy outcome and long-term prognosis. *Am J Obstet Gynecol* 1995; 172: 125–129.

251 Schwartz ML, Brenner W. Severe preeclampsia with persistent postpartum hemolysis and thrombocytopenia treated by plasmapheresis. *Obstet Gynecol* 1985; 65: 53S–55S.

252 Martin JN Jr, Rose CH, Briery CM. Understanding and managing HELLP syndrome: the integral role of aggressive glucocorticoids for mother and child. *Am J Obstet Gynecol* 2006; 195(4): 914–934.

253 Matchaba P, Moodley J. Corticosteroids for HELLP syndrome in pregnancy. *Cochrane Database Syst Rev* 2004; 1: CD002076.

254 Fonseca JE, Méndez F, Cataño C, Arias F. Dexamethasone treatment does not improve the outcome of women with HELLP syndrome: a double-blind, placebo-controlled, randomized clinical trial. *Am J Obstet Gynecol* 2005; 193(5): 1591–1598.

255 Rademaker L. Spontaneous rupture of liver complicating pregnancy. *Ann Surg* 1943; 118: 396–401.

256 Herbert WNP, Brenner WE. Improving survival with liver rupture complicating pregnancy. *Am J Obstet Gynecol* 1982; 142: 530–534.

257 Henny CP, Lim AE, Brummelkamp WH, et al. A review of the importance of acute multidisciplinary treatment following spontaneous rupture of the liver capsule during pregnancy. *Surg Gynecol Obstet* 1983; 156: 593–598.

258 Bis KA, Waxman B. Rupture of the liver associated with pregnancy: a review of the literature and report of two cases. *Obstet Gynecol Surv* 1976; 31: 763–773.

259 Goodlin RC, Anderson JC, Hodgson PE. Conservative treatment of liver hematoma in the postpartum period. A report of two cases. *J Reprod Med* 1985; 30: 368–370.

260 Smith LG, Moise KJ, Dildy GA, Carpenter RJ. Spontaneous rupture of liver during pregnancy: current therapy. *Obstet Gynecol* 1991; 77: 171–175.

261 Feliciano DV, Mattox KL, Jordan GL, et al. Management of 1,000 consecutive cases of hepatic trauma (1979–1984). *Ann Surg* 1986; 204: 438–445.

262 Lucas CE, Ledgerwood AM. Prospective evaluation of hemostatic techniques for liver injuries. *J Trauma* 1976; 16: 442.

263 Gardner WJ, Storer J. The use of the G suit in control of intra-abdominal bleeding. *Surg Gynecol Obstet* 1966; 123: 792–798.

264 Hunter SK, Martin M, Benda JA, Zlatnik FJ. Liver transplant after massive spontaneous hepatic rupture in pregnancy complicated by preeclampsia. *Obstet Gynecol* 1995; 85: 819–822.

265 Reck T, Bussenius-Kammerer M, Ott R, Muller V, Beinder E, Hohenberger W. Surgical treatment of HELLP syndrome-associated liver rupture: an update. *Eur J Obstet Gynecol Reprod Biol* 2001; 99: 57–65.

266 Sakala EP, Moore WD. Successful term delivery after previous pregnancy with ruptured liver. *Obstet Gynecol* 1986; 68: 124–126.

267 Greenstein D, Henderson JM, Boyer TD. Liver hemorrhage: recurrent episodes during pregnancy complicated by preeclampsia. *Gastroenterology* 1994; 106: 1668–1671.

268 Barrilleaux PS, Adair D, Johnson G, Lewis DF. Splenic rupture associated with severe preeclampsia. A case report. *J Reprod Med* 1999; 44: 899–901.

269 Marcovici I, Marzano D. Pregnancy-induced hypertension complicated by postpartum renal failure and pancreatitis: a case report. *Am J Perinatol* 2002; 19: 177–179.

270 Paternoster DM, Rodi J, Santarossa C, Vanin M, Simioni P, Girolami A. Acute pancreatitis and deep vein thrombosis associated with HELLP syndrome. *Minerva Ginecol* 1999; 51(1–2): 31–33.

271 Badja N, Troché G, Zazzo JF, Benhamou D. Acute pancreatitis and preeclampsia-eclampsia: a case report. *Am J Obstet Gynecol* 1997; 176: 707–709.

272 Goodlin RC. The effect of severe pre-eclampsia on the pancreas: changes in the serum cationic trypsinogen and pancreatic amylase. *Br J Obstet Gynaecol* 1987; 94: 1228.

273 Hibbard LT. Maternal mortality due to acute toxemia. *Obstet Gynecol* 1973; 42: 263–270.

274 Bell BA. A history of the study of cerebral edema. *Neurosurgery* 1983; 13: 724–728.

275 Kirby JC, Jaindl JJ. Cerebral CT findings in toxemia of pregnancy. *Radiology* 1984; 154: 114.

276 Miller JD. The management of cerebral edema. *Br J Hosp Med* 1979; 21: 152–165.

277 Weiss MH. Cerebral edema. *Acute Care* 1985; 11: 187–204.

278 Benedetti TJ, Quilligan EJ. Cerebral edema in severe pregnancy-induced hypertension. *Am J Obstet Gynecol* 1980; 137: 860–862.

279 Beeson JH, Duda EE. Computed axial tomography scan demonstration of cerebral edema in eclampsia preceded by blindness. *Obstet Gynecol* 1982; 60: 529–532.

280 Beal MF, Chapman PH. Cortical blindness and homonymous hemianopia in the postpartum period. *JAMA* 1980; 244: 2085–2087.

281 Beck RW, Gamel JW, Willcourt RJ, Berman G. Acute ischemic optic neuropathy in severe preeclampsia. *Am J Ophthalmol* 1980; 90: 342–346.

282 Hill JA, Devoe LD, Elgammal TA. Central hemodynamic findings associated with cortical blindness in severe preeclampsia. A case report. *J Reprod Med* 1985; 30: 435–438.

283 Seidman DS, Serr DM, Ben-Rafael Z. Renal and ocular manifestations of hypertensive disease of pregnancy. *Obstet Gynecol Surv* 1991; 46: 71–76.

284 Cunningham FG, Fernandez CO, Hernandez C. Blindness associated with preeclampsia and eclampsia. *Am J Obstet Gynecol* 1995; 172: 1291–1298.

285 Hinchey J, Chaves C, Appignani B, et al. A reversible posterior leukoencephalopathy syndrome. *N Engl J Med* 1996; 334: 494–500.

286 Kinsella CB, Milner M, McCarthy N, Walshe J. Sixth nerve palsy: an unusual manifestation of preeclampsia. *Obstet Gynecol* 1994; 83: 849–851.

287 Belfort MA, Anthony J, Saade GR, Allen JC Jr, Nimodipine Study Group. A comparison of magnesium sulfate and nimodipine for the prevention of eclampsia. *N Engl J Med* 2003; 348: 304–311.

288 Govan ADT. The pathogenesis of eclamptic lesions. *Pathol Microbiol (Basel)* 1961; 24: 561–575.

289 Douglas KA, Redman CWG. Eclampsia in the United Kingdom. *BMJ* 1994; 309: 1395–1399.

290 Saftlas AF, Olson DR, Franks AL, Atrash HK, Pokras R. Epidemiology of preeclampsia and eclampsia in the United States, 1979–1986. *Am J Obstet Gynecol* 1990; 163: 460–465.

291 Sibai BM, Abdella TN, Spinnato JA, et al. Eclampsia. V. The incidence of non-preventable eclampsia. *Am J Obstet Gynecol* 1986; 154; 561–566.

292 Sibai BM, Schneider JM, Morrison JC, et al. The late postpartum eclampsia controversy. *Obstet Gynecol* 1980; 55: 74–78.

293 Brown CEL, Cunningham FG, Pritchard JA. Convulsions in hypertensive proteinuric primiparas more than 24 hours after delivery: eclampsia or some other course. *J Reprod Med* 1987; 32: 449–503.

294 Lubarsky SL, Barton JR, Friedman SA, et al. Late postpartum eclampsia revisited. *Obstet Gynecol* 1994; 83: 502–505.

295 Lucas MJ, DePalma RT, Peters MT, et al. A simplified phenytoin regimen for preeclampsia. *Am J Perinatol* 1994; 11: 153–156.

296 Dunn R, Lee W, Cotton DB. Evaluation by computerized axial tomography of eclamptic women with seizures refractory to magnesium sulfate therapy. *Am J Obstet Gynecol* 1986; 155: 267–268.

297 Sibai BM, Spinnato JA, Watson DL, et al. Eclampsia. IV. Neurological findings and future outcome. *Am J Obstet Gynecol* 1985; 152: 184–192.

298 Cunningham FG, Gant NF. Management of eclampsia. *Semin Perinatol* 1994; 18: 103–113.

299 Sibai BM, Sarinoglu C, Mercer BM. Pregnancy outcome after eclampsia and long term prognosis. *Am J Obstet Gynecol* 1992; 166: 1757.

300 Lopez-Llera M. Complicated eclampsia: fifteen years experience in a referral medical center. *Am J Obstet Gynecol* 1982; 142: 28–35.

301 Chesley LC, Annitto JE, Cosgrove RA. The remote prognosis of eclamptic women. *Am J Obstet Gynecol* 1976; 124: 446–459.

302 Chesley LC. Remote prognosis. In: Chesley LC, ed. *Hypertensive Disorders in Pregnancy*. New York: Appleton-Century-Crofts, 1978: 421.

303 Browne JCM, Veall N. The maternal placental blood flow in normotensive and hypertensive women. *J Obstet Gynaecol Br Emp* 1953; 60: 141–147.

304 Dixon HG, Brown JCM, Davey DA. Choriodecidual and myometrial blood flow. *Lancet* 1963; ii: 369–373.

305 Lunell NO, Nylung LE, Lewander R, Sabey B. Uteroplacental blood flow in preeclampsia: measurements with indium-113m and a computer-linked gamma camera. *Clin Exp Hypertens* 1982; B1: 105–107.

306 Abdella TN, Sibai BM, Hays JM Jr, Anderson GD. Relationship of hypertensive disease to abruptio placentae. *Obstet Gynecol* 1984; 63: 365–370.

307 Hurd WW, Miodovnik M, Herzberg V, Lavin JP. Selective management of abruptio placentae: a prospective study. *Obstet Gynecol* 1983; 61: 467–473.

308 Eskenazi B, Fenster L, Sidney S, Elkin EP. Fetal growth retardation in infants of multiparous and nulliparous women with preeclampsia. *Am J Obstet Gynecol* 1993; 169: 1112–1118.

309 Wheeler TC, Graves CR, Troiano NH, Reed GW. Base deficit and oxygen transport in severe preeclampsia. *Obstet Gynecol* 1996; 87: 375–379.

310 Belfort MA, Saade GR, Wasserstrum N, et al. Acute volume expansion with colloid increases oxygen delivery and consumption but does not improve the oxygen extraction in severe preeclampsia. *J Matern-Fetal Med* 1995; 4: 57–64.

311 Habli M, Levine RJ, Qian C, Sibai B. Neonatal outcomes in pregnancies with preeclampsia or gestational hypertension and in normotensive pregnancies that delivered at 35, 36, or 37 weeks of gestation. *Am J Obstet Gynecol* 2007; 197(4): 406.

312 Bryant RD, Fleming JG. Veratrum viride in the treatment of eclampsia: II. *JAMA* 1940; 115: 1333–1339.

313 Chen CY, Kwek K, Tan KH, Yeo GS. Our experience with eclampsia in Singapore. *Singapore Med J* 2003; 44(2): 88–93.

314 Efetie ER, Okafor UV. Maternal outcome in eclamptic patients in Abuja, Nigeria – a 5 year review. *Niger J Clin Pract* 2007; 10(4): 309–313.

315 Harbert GM, Claiborne HA, McGaughey HS, et al. Convulsive toxemia. *Am J Obstet Gynecol* 1968; 100: 336–342.

316 Knight M; UKOSS. Eclampsia in the United Kingdom 2005. *Br J Obstet Gynaecol* 2007; 114(9): 1072–1078.

317 Lee W, O'Connell CM, Baskett TF. Maternal and perinatal outcomes of eclampsia: Nova Scotia, 1981–2000. *J Obstet Gynaecol Can* 2004; 26(2): 119–123.

318 Mabie WC, Ratts TE, Sibai BM. The central hemodynamics of severe preeclampsia. *Am J Obstet Gynecol* 1989; 161: 1443–1448.

319 Magpie Trial Collaboration Group. Do women with pre-eclampsia, and their babies, benefit from magnesium sulphate? The Magpie Trial: a randomised placebo-controlled trial. *Lancet* 2002; 359: 1877–1890.

320 Majoko F, Mujaji C. Maternal outcome in eclampsia at Harare Maternity Hospital. *Cent Afr J Med* 2001; 47: 123–128.

321 Onwuhafua PI, Onwuhafua A, Adze J, Mairami Z. Eclampsia in Kaduna State of Nigeria – a proposal for a better outcome. *Niger J Med* 2001; 10: 81–84.

322 Sibai BM. Eclampsia. VI. Maternal–perinatal outcome in 254 consecutive cases. *Am J Obstet Gynecol* 1990; 163: 1049–1054.

323 Zuspan FP. Treatment of severe preeclampsia and eclampsia. *Clin Obstet Gynecol* 1966; 9: 945–972.

324 Adetero OO. A sixteen year survey of maternal mortality associated with eclampsia in Ilorin, Nigeria. *Int J Gynecol Obstet* 1989; 30: 117–121.

325 Atkinson MW, Maher JE, Owen J, et al. The predictive value of umbilical artery Doppler studies for preeclampsia or fetal growth retardation in a preeclampsia prevention trial. *Obstet Gynecol* 1994; 83: 609–612.

326 Balla AK, Dhall GI, Dhall K. A safer and more effective treatment regime for eclampsia. *Aust NZ J Obstet Gynaecol* 1994; 34(2): 144–148.

35 Anaphylactoid Syndrome of Pregnancy (Amniotic Fluid Embolism)

Gary A. Dildy III[1], Michael A. Belfort[2] & Steven L. Clark[3]

[1]Maternal-Fetal Medicine, Mountain Star Division, Hospital Corporation of America, Salt Lake City, UT *and* Department of Obstetrics and Gynecology, LSU Health Sciences Center, School of Medicine in New Orleans, New Orleans, LA, USA
[2]Department of Obstetrics and Gynecology, Division of Maternal-Fetal Medicine, University of Utah School of Medicine, Salt Lake City, UT *and* HCA Healthcare, Nashville, TN, USA
[3]Women's and Children's Clinical Services, Hospital Corporation of America, Nashville, TN, USA

Introduction

Amniotic fluid embolism (AFE), an uncommon obstetric disorder, has a high case fatality rate and remains a leading cause of maternal mortality in industrialized countries [1–5]. Because of its rarity and absence of a gold standard for diagnosis, there is a 10-fold variation in estimates of incidence and a fivefold variation in estimates of mortality. AFE is classically characterized by hypoxia, hypotension or hemodynamic collapse, and coagulopathy. Despite numerous attempts to develop an animal model, AFE remains incompletely understood. Nevertheless, during the past decade, there have been several significant advances in our understanding of this enigmatic condition.

Historic considerations

The earliest written description of AFE is attributed to Meyer in 1926 [6]. The condition was not widely recognized, however, until the report of Steiner and Luschbaugh in 1941 [7]. These investigators described autopsy findings in eight pregnant women with sudden shock and pulmonary edema during labor. In all cases, squamous cells or mucin, presumably of fetal origin, were found in the pulmonary vasculature. In a follow-up report in 1969 by Liban and Raz [8], cellular debris was also observed in the kidneys, liver, spleen, pancreas, and brain of several such patients. Squamous cells also were identified in uterine veins of several control patients in this series, a finding confirmed in a report of Thompson and Budd [9] in a patient without AFE. It should be noted, however, that in the initial description of Steiner and Luschbaugh [7], seven of the eight patients carried clinical diagnoses other than AFE (including sepsis and unrecognized uterine rupture) and were not materially different from the diagnoses of their control patients without these specific histologic findings. Only one of the eight patients in the classic AFE group died of "obstetric shock" without an additional clinical diagnosis. Thus, the relevance of this original report to patients presently dying of AFE after the exclusion of other diagnoses is questionable.

Since the initial descriptions of AFE, several hundred case reports have appeared in the literature. Although most cases were reported during labor, sudden death in pregnancy has been attributed to AFE under many widely varying circumstances, including cases of first- and second-trimester abortion [10–13]. In 1948, Eastman, in an editorial review, stated, "Let us be careful not to make [the diagnosis of AFE] a waste basket for cases of unexplained death in labor" [14].

Experimental models

The first animal model of AFE was that of Steiner and Luschbaugh (1941) [7], who showed that rabbits and dogs could be killed by the intravenous injection of heterologous amniotic fluid and meconium. Several subsequent reports of AFE in experimental animals have yielded conflicting results (Table 35.1) [7,15–31]. In most series, experimental injection of amniotic fluid had adverse effects, ranging from transient alterations in systemic and pulmonary artery pressures in dogs, sheep, cats, and calves to sudden death in rabbits. Only two of these studies, however, involved pregnant animals, and in most, heterologous amniotic fluid was used. In several studies, the effects of whole or meconium-enriched amniotic fluid were contrasted with those of filtered amniotic fluid. A pathologic response was obtained only in particulate-rich amniotic fluid in four such studies, whereas three reports demonstrated physiologic changes with filtered amniotic fluid as well. Data produced with the models involving particulate-enriched amniotic fluid may have little relevance to the human model, because the concentration of particulate matter injected has been many times greater than that present in human amniotic fluid, even in the presence of meconium. In the four

Critical Care Obstetrics, 5th edition. Edited by M. Belfort, G. Saade, M. Foley, J. Phelan and G. Dildy.

Table 35.1 Animal models of amniotic fluid embolism.

Effects										
Reference	**Year**	**Animal**	**Anesthetized**	**Pregnant**	**Filtered AF**	**Whole AF**	**AF species**	**Hemodynamic changes**	**Coagulopathy**	**Autopsy**
Steiner & Luschbaugh [7]	1941	Rabbit/dog	No	No	No	Yes	Human	NE (death)	No	Debris in PA
Cron et al. [15]	1952	Rabbit	No	No	NE	Yes	Human	NNE (death)	No	Debris in PA
Schneider [16]	1955	Dog	No	No	NE	Yes	Human	NE (death)	5 of 8	Debris in PA
Jacques et al. [17]	1960	Dog	Yes	No	NE	Yes	Human/dog	Yes	Fibrinogen 12 of 13	Debris in PA
Halmagyi et al. [18]	1962	Sheep	Yes	No	No	Yes	Human	Yes	No	NE
Attwood & Downing [19]	1965	Dog	Yes	No	Yes	Yes	Human	Yes	4 of 12	NE
Stolte et al. [21]	1967	Monkey	Yes	Yes	No	No	Human/ monkey	No	1 of 12	NE
MacMillan [22]	1968	Rabbit	No	No	No	Yes	Human	NE (death)	2 of 12	Minimal debris, hemorrhage
Reis et al. [20]	1969	Sheep	Yes	Yes	Yes	Yes	Sheep	Yes	No	Normal
Dutta et al. [23]	1970	Rabbit	Yes	No	NE	Yes	Human	NE (death)	No	Minimal debris, massive infarction
Adamsons et al. [24]	1971	Monkey	Yes	Yes	NE	No	Monkey	No	No	NE
Kitzmiller & Lucas [25]	1972	Cat	Yes	No	No	Yes	Human	Yes	No	NE
Spence & Mason [27]	1974	Rabbit	No	Yes	No	No	Rabbit	No	No	NE
Reeves et al. [26]	1974	Calf	No	No	NE	Yes	Calf	Yes		
Azegami & Mori [28]	1986	Rabbit	No	No	No	Yes	Human	NE (death)	No	Pulmonary edema, debris in PA
Richards et al. [29]	1988	Rat*	Yes	No	Yes	NE	Human	Coronary flow		
Hankins et al. [30]	1993	Goat	Yes	Yes	Yes	Yes	Goat	Yes	No	NE
Petroianu et al. [31]	1999	Mini-pig	Yes	Yes	Yes	Yes	Mini-pig		Yes	Debris in PA

* Isolated heart preparation.

AF, amniotic fluid; BP, blood pressure; CO, cardiac output; CVP, central venous pressure; LAP, left atrial pressure; NE, not examined; P, pulse; PA, pulmonary artery; PAP, pulmonary artery pressure; PCWP, pulmonary capillary wedge pressure; PVR, pulmonary vascular resistance; RR, respiratory rate; SVR, systemic vascular resistance.

studies in which injections of amniotic fluid into the arterial and venous systems were compared, three showed toxic effects with both arterial and venous injection, implying a pathologic humoral substance or response. In studies in which autopsy was performed, pulmonary findings ranged from massive vascular plugging with fetal debris (after embolization with particulate-enriched amniotic fluid) to normal.

In contrast, the only two studies carried out in primates showed the intravenous injection of amniotic fluid to be entirely innocuous without effects on blood pressure, pulse, or respiratory rate [21,24]. In one study, the volume of amniotic fluid infused would, in the human, represent 80% of the total amniotic fluid volume. A carefully controlled study in the goat model using homologous amniotic fluid demonstrated hemodynamic and clinical findings similar to that seen in humans, including an initial transient rise in pulmonary and systemic vascular resistance and myocardial depression [30]. These findings were especially prominent when the injectate included meconium. Importantly, the initial phase of pulmonary hypertension in all animal models studied has been transient and in survivors has resolved within 30 minutes [32]. Because most attempts at the development of an animal model of AFE have involved the injection of tissue from a foreign species, the resultant physiologic effects may have limited clinical relevance to the human condition and must be interpreted with caution.

Clinical presentation

Hemodynamic alterations

In humans, an initial transient phase of hemodynamic change involving both systemic and pulmonary vasospasm leads to a more often recognized secondary phase involving principally hypotension and depressed ventricular function [5,33–35].

Figure 35.1 demonstrates in a graphic manner the depression of left ventricular function seen in five patients monitored with pulmonary artery catheterization. The mechanism of left ventricular failure is uncertain. Work in the rat model by Richards

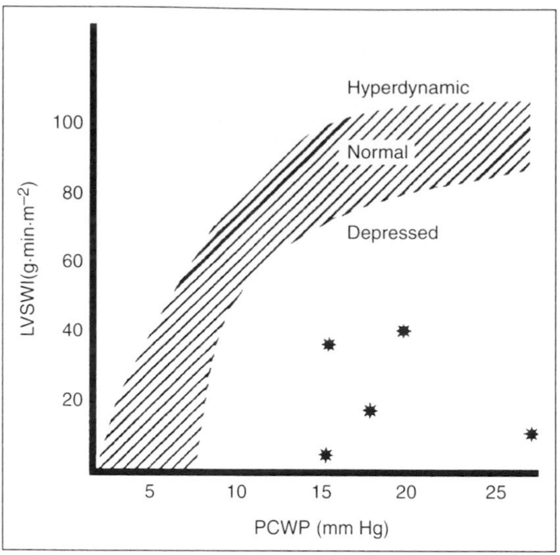

Figure 35.1 Modified Starling curve, demonstrating depressed left ventricular function in five patients with amniotic fluid embolism. LVSWI, left ventricular stroke work index; PCWP, pulmonary capillary wedge pressure. From Clark 1988 [34].

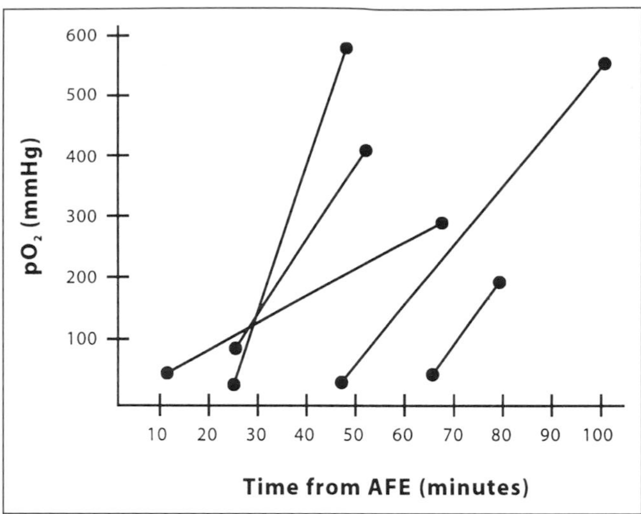

Figure 35.2 Resolution of hypoxia after amniotic fluid embolism (AFE). Unpublished data from Clark 1995 [5].

et al. [29] suggests the presence of possible coronary artery spasm and myocardial ischemia in animal AFE. On the other hand, the global hypoxia commonly seen in patients with AFE could account for left ventricular dysfunction. The *in vitro* observation of decreased myometrial contractility in the presence of amniotic fluid also suggests the possibility of a similar effect of amniotic fluid on myocardium [36].

Pulmonary manifestations

Patients suffering AFE typically develop rapid and often profound hypoxia, which may result in permanent neurologic impairment in survivors of this condition. This hypoxia is likely due to a combination of initial pulmonary vasospasm and ventricular dysfunction. A case report of transesophageal echocardiography findings during the hyperacute stage of AFE revealed acute right ventricular failure and suprasystemic right-sided pressures [37]. In both animal models and human experience, however, this initial hypoxia is often transient. Figure 35.2 details arterial blood gas findings in a group of patients with AFE for whom paired data are available. Initial profound shunting and rapid recovery are seen. In survivors, primary lung injury often leads to acute respiratory distress syndrome and secondary oxygenation defects.

Coagulopathy

Patients surviving the initial hemodynamic insult may succumb to a secondary coagulopathy [5,38]. The exact incidence of the coagulopathy is unknown. Coagulopathy was an entry criterion for inclusion in the initial analysis of the National AFE Registry; however, several patients submitted to the registry who clearly had AFE did not have clinical evidence of coagulopathy [5]. In a similar manner, a number of patients have been observed who developed an acute obstetric coagulopathy alone in the absence of placental abruption and suffered fatal exsanguination without any evidence of primary hemodynamic or pulmonary insult [38].

As with experimental investigations into hemodynamic alterations associated with AFE, investigations of this coagulopathy have yielded contradictory results. Amniotic fluid has been shown *in vitro* to shorten whole blood clotting time, to have a thromboplastin-like effect, to induce platelet aggregation and release of platelet factor III, and to activate the compliment cascade [39,40]. In addition, Courtney and Allington [41] showed that amniotic fluid contains a direct factor X-activating factor. Although confirming the factor X-activating properties of amniotic fluid, Phillips and Davison [42] concluded that the amount of procoagulant in clear amniotic fluid is insufficient to cause significant intravascular coagulation, a finding disputed by the studies of Lockwood et al. [43] and Phillips and Davidson [42].

In the experimental animal models discussed previously, coagulopathy has likewise been an inconsistent finding. Thus, the exact nature of the consumptive coagulopathy demonstrated in humans with AFE is yet to be satisfactorily explained. The powerful thromboplastin effects of trophoblast are well established. The coagulopathies associated with severe placental abruption and that seen with AFE are probably similar in origin and represent activation of the coagulation cascade following exposure of the maternal circulation to a variety of fetal antigens with varying thromboplastin-like effects [5].

Pathophysiology

In an analysis of the National AFE Registry, a marked similarity was noted between the clinical, hemodynamic, and hematologic manifestations of AFE and both septic and anaphylactic shock [5]. Clearly, the clinical manifestations of this condition are not identical; fever is unique to septic shock, and cutaneous manifestations are more common in anaphylaxis. Nevertheless, the marked similarities of these conditions suggest similar pathophysiologic mechanisms.

Detailed discussions of the pathophysiologic features of septic shock and anaphylactic shock are presented elsewhere in this text. Both of these conditions involve the entrance of a foreign substance (bacterial endotoxin or specific antigens) into the circulation, which then results in the release of various primary and secondary endogenous mediators (Figure 35.3). Similar pathophysiology has also been proposed in non-pregnant patients with pulmonary fat embolism. It is the release of these mediators that results in the principal physiologic derangements characterizing these syndromes. These abnormalities include profound myocardial depression and decreased cardiac output, described in both animals and humans; pulmonary hypertension, demonstrated in lower primate models of anaphylaxis; and disseminated intervascular coagulation, described in both human anaphylactic reactions and septic shock [44–53]. Further, the temporal sequence of hemodynamic decompensation and recovery seen in experimental AFE is virtually identical to that described in canine anaphylaxis [49]. An anaphylactoid response is also well described in humans and involves the non-immunologic release of similar mediators [44]. It is also intriguing that, on admission to hospital, 41% of patients in the AFE registry gave a history of either drug allergy or atopy [5].

The ability of arachidonic acid metabolites to cause the same physiologic and hemodynamic changes observed in human AFE has been noted [54]. Further, in the rabbit model of AFE, pretreatment with an inhibitor of leukotriene synthesis has been shown to prevent death [28]. These experimental observations further support the clinical conclusions of the National AFE Registry analysis that this condition involves the anaphylactoid release of endogenous mediators, including arachidonic acid metabolites, which result in the devastating pathophysiologic sequence seen in clinical AFE [5].

Earlier anecdotal reports suggested a possible relationship between hypertonic uterine contractions or oxytocin use and AFE. Although disputed on statistical grounds by Morgan [1], this misconception persisted in some writings until recently. The historic anecdotal association between hypertonic uterine contractions and the onset of symptoms in AFE was further clarified by the analysis of the National Registry [5]. These data demonstrated that the hypertonic contractions commonly seen in association with AFE appear to be a result of the release of catecholamines into the circulation as part of the initial human hemodynamic response to any massive physiologic insult. Under these circumstances, norepinephrine, in particular, acts as a potent uterotonic agent [5,55]. Thus, while the association of hypertonic contractions and AFE appears to be valid, it is the physiologic response to AFE that causes the hypertonic uterine activity rather than the converse. Indeed, there is a complete cessation of uterine blood flow in the presence of even moderate uterine contractions; thus, a tetanic contraction is the least likely time during an entire labor process for any exchange between maternal and fetal compartments [56]. Oxytocin is not used with increased frequency in patients suffering AFE compared with the general population, nor does oxytocin-induced hyperstimulation commonly precede this condition [5]. Thus, several authorities, including the American College of Obstetricians and Gynecologists, have concluded that oxytocin use has no relationship to the occurrence of AFE [1,5,57]. A recent population-based cohort study of approximately 3 million deliveries in Canada reported a statistically significant association of labor induction with AFE [58], however the same investigators did not observe this association in another population-based cohort of approximately 3 million deliveries in the US [59], casting doubt regarding any clinically significant relationship between labor stimulation and AFE.

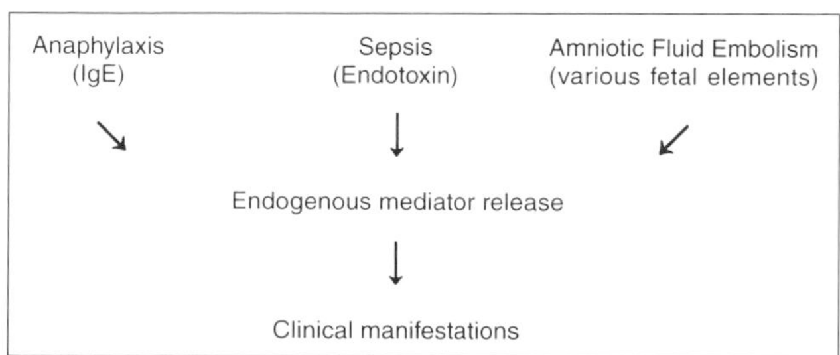

Figure 35.3 Proposed pathophysiologic relation between AFE, septic shock, and anaphylactic shock. Each syndrome also may have specific direct physiologic effects. (Reproduced by permission from Clark SL, Hankins GVD, Dudley DA et al. Amniotic fluid embolism: analysis of the national registry. *Am J Obstet Gynecol* 1995; 172: 1158–1169.)

The syndrome of AFE appears to be initiated after maternal intravascular exposure to various types of fetal tissue. Such exposure may occur during the course of normal labor and delivery; after potentially minor traumatic events, such as appropriate intrauterine pressure catheter placement; or during cesarean section. Because fetal-to-maternal tissue transfer is virtually universal during the labor and delivery process, actions by healthcare providers, such as intrauterine manipulation or cesarean delivery, may affect the timing of the exposure. No evidence exists, however, to suggest that exposure itself can be avoided by altering clinical management. Simple exposure of the maternal circulatory system to even small amounts of amniotic fluid or other fetal tissue may, under the right circumstances, initiate the syndrome of AFE. This understanding explains the well-documented occurrence of fatal AFE during first-trimester pregnancy termination at a time when neither the volume of fluid nor positive intrauterine pressure could be contributing factors [11]. Whereas much has been written about the importance to the fetus of an immunologic barrier between the mother and the antigenically different products of conception, little attention has been paid to the potential importance of this barrier to maternal well-being. The observations of the National Registry as well as cumulative data for the past several decades suggest that breaches of this barrier may, under certain circumstances and in susceptible maternal–fetal pairs, be of immense significance to the mother as well [5].

Previous experimental evidence in animals and humans unequivocally demonstrates that the intravenous administration of even large amounts of amniotic fluid *per se* is innocuous [21,24,60]. Further, the clinical findings described in the National Registry are not consistent with an embolic event as commonly understood (Table 35.2). Thus, the term "amniotic fluid embolism" itself appears to be a misnomer. In the National Registry analysis, the authors suggested that the term "amniotic fluid embolism" be discarded and the syndrome of acute peripartum hypoxia, hemodynamic collapse, and coagulopathy should be designated in a more descriptive manner, as "anaphylactoid syndrome of pregnancy."

Clinical presentation

Clinical signs and symptoms noted in patients with AFE are described in Table 35.2. In a typical case, a patient in labor, having just undergone cesarean delivery or immediately following vaginal delivery or pregnancy termination, suffers the acute onset of profound hypoxia and hypotension followed by cardiopulmonary arrest. The initial episode often is complicated by the development of a consumptive coagulopathy, which may lead to exsanguination, even if attempts to restore hemodynamic and respiratory function are successful. It must be emphasized, however, that in any individual patient any of the three principal phases (hypoxia, hypotension, or coagulopathy) may either dominate or be entirely absent [5,38,61]. Clinical variations in this syndrome may be related to variations in either the nature of the antigenic exposure or maternal response. The differential diagnosis is summarized in Table 35.3.

Table 35.2 Signs and symptoms noted in patients with amniotic fluid embolism.

Sign or symptom	No. of patients (%)
Hypotension	43 (100)
Fetal distress*	30 (100)
Pulmonary edema or ARDS†	28 (93)
Cardiopulmonary arrest	40 (87)
Cyanosis	38 (83)
Coagulopathy‡	38 (83)
Dyspnea§	22 (49)
Seizure	22 (48)
Atony	11 (23)
Bronchospasm¶	7 (15)
Transient hypertension	5 (11)
Cough	3 (7)
Headache	3 (7)
Chest pain	1 (2)

* Includes all live fetuses *in utero* at time of event.

† Eighteen patients did not survive long enough for these diagnoses to be confirmed.

‡ Eight patients did not survive long enough for this diagnosis to be confirmed.

§ One patient was intubated at the time of the event and could not be assessed.

¶ Difficult ventilation was noted during cardiac arrest in six patients, and wheezes were auscultated in one patient.

Reproduced by permission from Clark SL, Hankins GVD, Dudley DA. Amniotic fluid embolism: analysis of a national registry. *Am J Obstet Gynecol* 1995; 172: 1158–1169.

Maternal outcome is dismal in patients with AFE syndrome. In documented "classic" cases, the overall maternal mortality rate appears to be 60–80% [5,32]. Only 15% of patients survive neurologically intact. In a number of cases, following successful hemodynamic resuscitation and reversal of disseminated intravascular coagulation, life-support systems were withdrawn because of brain death resulting from the initial profound hypoxia. In patients progressing to cardiac arrest, only 8% survive neurologically intact [5]. In the National Registry database, no form of therapy appeared to be consistently associated with improved outcome. A large series of patients in whom the diagnosis of AFE was obtained from the discharge summary reported a 26% mortality rate. Notably, however, many patients in this series lacked one or more potentially lethal clinical manifestation of the disease classically considered mandatory for diagnosis, thus casting the diagnosis into doubt. However, if one assumes that the discharge diagnosis of these patients was accurate, these data suggest improved outcome for those women with milder forms of the disease [61]. Samuelsson and colleagues [62], using the Swedish Cause of Death Register, found that the case fatality rate for AFE was high and remained unaltered (42–48%) during the decades spanning the 1970s through 1990s. Reported maternal mortality rates are summarized in Table 35.4.

Neonatal outcome is similarly poor. If the event occurs prior to delivery, the neonatal survival rate is approximately 80%; only half of these fetuses survive neurologically intact [5]. Fetuses surviving to delivery generally demonstrate profound respiratory acidemia. Although at the present time no form of therapy appears to be associated with improved maternal outcome, there is a clear relationship between neonatal outcome and event-to-delivery interval in those women suffering cardiac

Table 35.3 Differential diagnosis of amniotic fluid embolism.

Air embolus
Anaphylaxis
Anesthetic toxicity
Myocardial infarction
Peripartum cardiomyopathy
Placental abruption
Pulmonary aspiration
Septic shock
Transfusion reaction
Venous thromboembolism

Table 35.4 Summary of published amniotic fluid embolism case series.

Series	Methodology	Period	AFE Incidence (1 per x births)	Maternal Mortality
Morgan 1979 [1]	Literature review	1926–1979	8,000–80,000	233/272 (86%)
Hogberg 1985 [4]	Swedish Birth Registry	1951–1980	83,000*	8/12 (66%)**
Burrows [90]	Royal Women's Hospital, Brisbane, Australia	1984–1993	6,579	2/9 (22%)
Clark 1995 [5]	U.S. Registry	1988–1994	N/A	28/46 (61%)
Gilbert 1999 [61]	California population database of 1,094,248 singleton births	1994–1995	20,646	14/53 (26%)
Tuffnell 2005 [89]	U.K. Registry	1997–2004	N/A	13/44 (30%)
Kramer 2006 [58]	Canadian population based cohort of 3,018,781 deliveries	1991–2002	16,667	24/180 (13%)
Samuelsson 2007 [62]	Swedish Cause of Death Register from 2,961,000 deliveries	1973–1999	51,947	25/57 (44%)
Abenhaim 2008 [59]	U.S. population based cohort study of 2,940,362 births	1998–2003	12,987	49/227 (22%)

* Incidence of fatal cases
** years 1972–1980

Table 35.5 Cardiac arrest-to-delivery interval and neonatal outcome.

Interval (min)	Survival	Intact survival
<5	3/3	2/3 (67%)
5–15	3/3	2/3 (67%)
16–25	2/5	2/5 (40%)
26–35	3/4	1/4 (25%)
36–54	0/1	0/1 (0%)

Reproduced by permission from Clark SL, Hankins GVD, Dudley DA. Amniotic fluid embolism: analysis of the national registry. *Am J Obstet Gynecol* 1995; 172: 1158–1169.

arrest (Table 35.5) [5]. Similar findings were reported by Katz et al. [63] in patients suffering cardiac arrest in a number of different clinical situations.

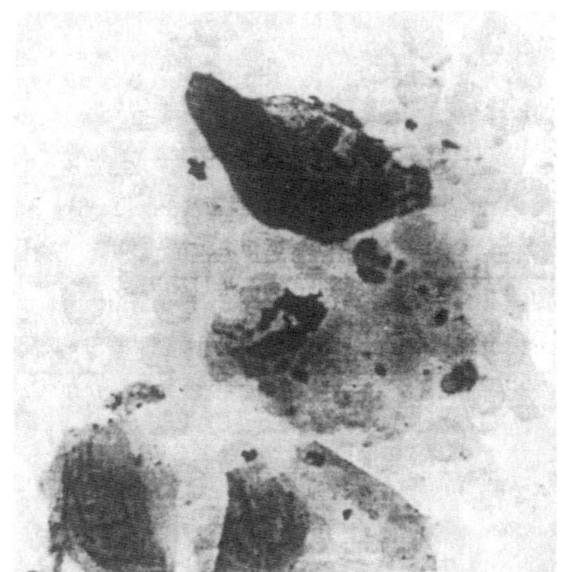

Figure 35.4 Squamous cells recovered from the pulmonary arterial circulation of a pregnant patient with class IV rheumatic mitral stenosis (magnification, ×1000). From Clark 1986 [66].

Diagnosis

In the past, histologic confirmation of the clinical syndrome of AFE was often sought by the detection of cellular debris of presumed fetal origin either in the distal port of a pulmonary artery catheter or at autopsy [32]. Several studies conducted during the past decade, however, suggest that such findings are commonly encountered, even in normal pregnant women (Figure 35.4) [64–67]. In the analysis of the National AFE Registry, fetal elements were found in roughly 50% of cases in which pulmonary artery catheter aspirate was analyzed and in roughly 75% of patients who went to autopsy [5]. The frequency with which such findings are encountered varies with the number of histologic sections obtained. In addition, multiple special stains often are required to document such debris [32]. Thus, the diagnosis of AFE remains a clinical one; histologic findings are neither sensitive nor specific. It is interesting to note that similar conclusions have been drawn regarding the diagnostic significance of histologic findings in patients with pulmonary fat embolism [68].

Other putative markers for AFE, such as serum tryptase [69], pulmonary mast cell antitryptase [70], serum TKH-2 antibody to fetal antigen sialyl Tn [71], pulmonary TKH-2 antibody to fetal antigen sialyl Tn [72], serum complement [69], and plasma zinc coproporphyrin I [73], have been studied but as of yet provide no definitive means of diagnosing or excluding AFE.

Treatment

For the mother, the end-result of therapy remains disappointing, with a high mortality rate. In the National Registry, we noted no difference in survival among patients suffering initial cardiac arrest in small rural hospitals attended by family practitioners compared with those suffering identical clinical signs and symptoms in tertiary-level centers attended by board-certified anesthesiologists, cardiologists, and maternal–fetal medicine specialists. Nevertheless, several generalizations can be drawn.

1 The initial treatment for AFE is supportive. Cardiopulmonary resuscitation is performed if the patient is suffering from a lethal dysrhythmia. Oxygen should be provided at high concentrations.

2 In the patient who survives the initial cardiopulmonary insult, it should be remembered that left ventricular failure is commonly seen. Thus, volume expansion to optimize ventricular preload is performed, and if the patient remains significantly hypotensive, the addition of an inotropic agent such as dopamine seems most appropriate. In patients who remain unstable following the initial resuscitative efforts, pulmonary artery catheterization may be of benefit to guide hemodynamic manipulation.

3 Although no evidence exists to document the benefit of corticosteroids in patients with AFE, the similarities between AFE and anaphylaxis proposed in the National Registry suggest that the administration of high doses of corticosteroids could be a consideration. In the absence of any data to suggest the benefit of this, however, steroid treatment is not mandated by standard of care; in fact since the original suggestion of corticosteroid therapy by the authors of the National Registry report, we have reviewed several cases where death resulted despite early high-dose steroid treatment.

4 In antepartum cases of AFE, careful attention must be paid to the fetal condition. In a mother who is hemodynamically unstable but has not yet undergone cardiorespiratory arrest, maternal considerations must be weighed carefully against those of the fetus. The decision to subject such an unstable mother to a major abdominal operation (cesarean section) is a difficult one, and each case must be individualized. However, it is axiomatic in these situations that where a choice must be made, maternal well-being must take precedence over that of the fetus.

5 In mothers who have progressed to frank cardiac arrest, the situation is different. Under these circumstances, maternal survival is extremely unlikely, regardless of the therapy rendered. In such women, it is highly unlikely that the imposition of cesarean section would significantly alter the maternal outcome. Even properly performed cardiopulmonary resuscitation (difficult at best in a pregnant woman) provides only a maximum of 30% of normal cardiac output. Under these circumstances, it is fair to assume that the proportion of blood shunted to the uterus and other splanchnic distributions approaches nil. Thus, the fetus will be, for practical purposes, anoxic at all times following maternal cardiac arrest, even during ideal performance of cardiopulmonary resuscitation. Because the interval from maternal arrest to delivery is directly correlated with newborn outcome, perimortum cesarean delivery should be initiated immediately on the diagnosis of maternal cardiac arrest in patients with AFE, assuming sufficient personnel are available to continue to provide care to the mother and deliver the baby [5,63]. For the pregnant patient, the standard ABC of cardiopulmonary resuscitation should be modified to include a fourth category, D: delivery.

New modalities for the treatment of AFE, such as high-dose steroids [5], extracorporeal membrane oxygenation with intra-aortic balloon counterpulsation [74], continuous hemodiafiltration [75,76], cardiopulmonary bypass [77,78], recombinant factor VIIa [79,80], and nitric oxide [81] have been reported in survivors but are thus far of limited cumulative experience or demonstrated benefit.

There are limited data on risk of recurrence in a subsequent pregnancy for women who experience AFE; fewer than a dozen cases are reported in the published literature [82–87]. At present, it appears that the risk of recurrence is low.

Despite many advances in the understanding of this condition, AFE or anaphylactoid syndrome of pregnancy remains enigmatic and in most cases is associated with dismal maternal and fetal outcomes, regardless of the quality of care rendered. Thus, AFE remains unpredictable, unpreventable, and, for the most part, untreatable. Further insight into this rare, but lethal, disorder may be forthcoming from the UK Obstetric Surveillance System (UKOSS), a joint initiative of the Royal College of Obstetricians and Gynaecologists and the National Perinatal Epidemiology Unit, which goal is to describe the epidemiology of a variety of uncommon disorders of pregnancy [88].

References

1 Morgan M. Amniotic fluid embolism. *Anaesthesia* 1979; 34: 29.
2 Kaunitz AM, Hughes JM, Grimes DA. Causes of maternal mortality in the United States. *Obstet Gynecol* 1985; 65: 605.
3 Grimes DA. The morbidity and mortality of pregnancy: still a risky business. *Am J Obstet Gynecol* 1994; 170: 1489.
4 Hogberg U, Joelsson I. Amniotic fluid embolism in Sweden, 1951–1980. *Gynecol Obstet Invest* 1985; 20(3): 130–137.
5 Clark SL, Hankins GDV, Dudley DA, et al. Amniotic fluid embolism: analysis of a national registry. *Am J Obstet Gynecol* 1995; 172: 1158.
6 Meyer JR. Embolia pulmonar amniocaseosa. *Bras/Med* 1926; 2: 301–303.
7 Steiner PE, Luschbaugh CC. Maternal pulmonary embolism by amniotic fluid. *JAMA* 1941; 117: 1245.
8 Liban E, Raz S. A clinicopathologic study of fourteen cases of amniotic fluid embolism. *Am J Clin Pathol* 1969; 51: 477.
9 Thomson WB, Budd JW. Erroneous diagnosis of amniotic fluid embolism. *Am J Obstet Gynecol* 1963; 91: 606.
10 Resnik R, Swartz WH, Plumer MH, Benirschke K, Stratthaus ME. Amniotic fluid embolism with survival. *Obstet Gynecol* 1976; 47: 295–298.
11 Guidotti RJ, Grimes DA, Cates W. Fatal amniotic fluid embolism during legally induced abortion in the United States, 1972–1978. *Am J Obstet Gynecol* 1981; 141: 257.
12 Cromley MG, Taylor PJ, Cummings DC. Probable amniotic fluid embolism after first trimester pregnancy termination. *J Reprod Med* 1983; 28: 209.

13 Meier PR, Bowes WA. Amniotic fluid embolus-like syndrome presenting in the second trimester of pregnancy. *Obstet Gynecol* 1983; 61(suppl): 31.
14 Eastman NJ. Editorial comment. *Obstet Gynecol Surv* 1948; 3: 35.
15 Cron RS, Kilkenny GS, Wirthwein C, et al. Amniotic fluid embolism. *Am J Obstet Gynecol* 1952; 64: 1360.
16 Schneider CL. Coagulation defects in obstetric shock: meconium embolism and defibrination. *Am J Obstet Gynecol* 1955; 69: 748.
17 Jacques WE, Hampton JW, Bird RM, et al. Pulmonary hypertension and plasma thromboplastin antecedent deficiency in dogs. *Arch Pathol* 1960; 69: 248.
18 Halmagyi DFJ, Starzecki B, Shearman RP. Experimental amniotic fluid embolism: mechanism and treatment. *Am J Obstet Gynecol* 1962; 84: 251.
19 Attwood HD, Downing SE. Experimental amniotic fluid embolism. *Surg Gynecol Obstet* 1965; 120: 255.
20 Reis RL, Pierce WS, Behrendt DM. Hemodynamic effects of amniotic fluid embolism. *Surg Gynecol Obstet* 1969; 129: 45.
21 Stolte L, van Kessel H, Seelen J, et al. Failure to produce the syndrome of amniotic fluid embolism by infusion of amniotic fluid and meconium into monkeys. *Am J Obstet Gynecol* 1967; 98: 694.
22 MacMillan D. Experimental amniotic fluid embolism. *J Obstet Gynaecol Br Comwlth* 1968; 75: 8.
23 Dutta D, Bhargava KC, Chakravarti RN, et al. Therapeutic studies in experimental amniotic fluid embolism in rabbits. *Am J Obstet Gynecol* 1970; 106: 1201.
24 Adamsons K, Mueller-Heubach E, Myer RE. The innocuousness of amniotic fluid infusion in the pregnant rhesus monkey. *Am J Obstet Gynecol* 1971; 109: 977.
25 Kitzmiller JL, Lucas WE. Studies on a model of amniotic fluid embolism. *Obstet Gynecol* 1972; 39: 626.
26 Reeves JT, Daoud FS, Estridge M, et al. Pulmonary pressor effects of small amounts of bovine amniotic fluid. *Respir Physiol* 1974; 20: 231.
27 Spence MR, Mason KG. Experimental amniotic fluid embolism in rabbits. *Am J Obstet Gynecol* 1974; 119: 1073.
28 Azegami M, Mori N. Amniotic fluid embolism and leukotrienes. *Am J Obstet Gynecol* 1986; 155: 1119.
29 Richards DS, Carter LS, Corke B, et al. The effect of human amniotic fluid on the isolated perfused rat heart. *Am J Obstet Gynecol* 1988; 158: 210.
30 Hankins GDV, Snyder RR, Clark SL, et al. Acute hemodynamic and respiratory effects of amniotic fluid embolism in the pregnant goat model. *Am J Obstet Gynecol* 1993; 168: 1113.
31 Petroianu GA, Altmannsberger SH, Maleck WH, et al. Meconium and amniotic fluid embolism: effects on coagulation in pregnant minipigs. *Crit Care Med* 1999; 27: 348.
32 Clark SL. New concepts of amniotic fluid embolism: a review. *Obstet Gynecol Surv* 1990; 45: 360.
33 Clark SL, Montz FJ, Phelan JP. Hemodynamic alterations in amniotic fluid embolism: a reappraisal. *Am J Obstet Gynecol* 1985; 151: 617.
34 Clark SL, Cotton DB, Gonik B, et al. Central hemodynamic alterations in amniotic fluid embolism. *Am J Obstet Gynecol* 1988; 158: 1124.
35 Girard P, Mal H, Laine JR, et al. Left heart failure in amniotic fluid embolism. *Anesthesiology* 1986; 64: 262.
36 Courtney LD. Coagulation failure in pregnancy. *BMJ* 1970; 1: 691.
37 Shechtman M, Ziser A, Markovits R, Rozenberg B. Amniotic fluid embolism: early findings of transesophageal echocardiography. *Anesth Analg* 1999; 89: 1456.
38 Porter TF, Clark SL, Dildy GA, Hankins GDV. Isolated disseminated intravascular coagulation and amniotic fluid embolism. Society of Perinatal Obstetricians 16th Annual Meeting, Poster Presentation, Kona, Hawaii, January 1996.
39 Ratnoff OD, Vosburgh GJ. Observations of the clotting defect in amniotic fluid embolism. *N Engl J Med* 1952; 247: 970.
40 Beller FK, Douglas GW, Debrovner CH, et al. The fibrinolytic system in amniotic fluid embolism. *Am J Obstet Gynecol* 1963; 87: 48.
41 Courtney LD, Allington LM. Effect of amniotic fluid on blood coagulation. *Br J Haematol* 1972; 113: 911.
42 Phillips LL, Davidson EC. Procoagulant properties of amniotic fluid. *Am J Obstet Gynecol* 1972; 113: 911.
43 Lockwood CJ, Bach R, Guha A, et al. Amniotic fluid contains tissue factor, a potent initiator of coagulation. *Am J Obstet Gynecol* 1991; 165: 1335.
44 Parker CW. In: *Clinical Immunology*. Philadelphia: WB Saunders, 1980: 1208.
45 Smith PL, Kagey-Sobotka A, Bleecker ER, et al. Physiologic manifestations of human anaphylaxis. *J Clin Invest* 1980; 66: 1072.
46 Smedegard G, Revenas B, Lundberg C, Arfors KE. Anaphylactic shock in monkeys passively sensitized with human reaginic serum. I. Hemodynamics and cardiac performances. *Acta Physiol Scand* 1981; 111: 239.
47 Enjeti S, Bleecker ER, Smith PL, et al. Hemodynamic mechanisms in anaphylaxis. *Circ Shock* 1983; 11: 297.
48 Silverman HJ, van Hook C, Haponik EF. Hemodynamic changes in human anaphylaxis. *Am J Med* 1984; 77: 341.
49 Kapin MA, Ferguson JL. Hemodynamic and regional circulatory alterations in dog during anaphylactic challenge. *Am J Physiol* 1985; 249: H430.
50 Lee WP, Clark SL, Cotton DB, et al. Septic shock during pregnancy. *Am J Obstet Gynecol* 1988; 159: 410.
51 Raper RF, Fisher MM. Profound reversible myocardial depression after anaphylaxis. *Lancet* 1988; i: 386.
52 Wong S, Dykewicz MS, Patterson R. Idiopathic anaphylaxis: a clinical summary of 175 patients. *Arch Intern Med* 1990; 150: 1323.
53 Parrillo JE. Pathogenic mechanisms of septic shock. *N Engl J Med* 1993; 328: 1471.
54 Clark SL. Arachidonic acid metabolites and the pathophysiology of amniotic fluid embolism. *Semin Reprod Endocrinol* 1985; 3: 253.
55 Paul RH, Koh BS, Bernstein SG. Changes in fetal heart rate: uterine contraction patterns associated with eclampsia. *Am J Obstet Gynecol* 1978; 130: 165.
56 Towell ME. Fetal acid–base physiology and intrauterine asphyxia. In: Goodwin JW, Godden JO, Chance GW, eds. *Perinatal Medicine*. Baltimore: Williams and Wilkins, 1976: 200.
57 American College of Obstetricians and Gynecologists. Prologue. Amniotic fluid embolism syndrome. In: *Obstetrics*, 3rd edn. Washington, DC: American College of Obstetricians and Gynecologists, 1993: 94.
58 Kramer MS, Rouleau J, Baskett TF, Joseph KS, Maternal Health Study Group of the Canadian Perinatal Surveillance System. Amniotic-fluid embolism and medical induction of labour: a retrospective population-based cohort study. *Lancet* 2006; 368: 1444–1448.
59 Abenhaim HA, Azoulay L, Kramer MS, et al. Incidence and risk factors of amniotic fluid embolisms: a population-based study on 3 million births in the United States. *Am J Obstet Gynecol* 2008; 199(1): 49.

60 Sparr RA, Pritchard JA. Studies to detect the escape of amniotic fluid into the maternal circulation during parturition. *Surg Gynecol Obstet* 1958; 107: 550.

61 Gilbert WM, Danielsen B. Amniotic fluid embolism: decreased mortality in a population-based study. *Obstet Gynecol* 1999; 93: 973.

62 Samuelsson E, Hellgren M, Högberg U. Pregnancy-related deaths due to pulmonary embolism in Sweden. *Acta Obstet Gynecol Scand* 2007; 86: 435–443.

63 Katz VJ, Dotters DJ, Droegemueller W. Perimortem cesarean delivery. *Obstet Gynecol* 1986; 68: 571.

64 Plauche WC. Amniotic fluid embolism. *Am J Obstet Gynecol* 1983; 147: 982.

65 Covone AE, Johnson PM, Mutton D, et al. Trophoblast cells in peripheral blood from pregnant women. *Lancet* 1984; i: 841.

66 Clark SL, Pavlova Z, Horenstein J, et al. Squamous cells in the maternal pulmonary circulation. *Am J Obstet Gynecol* 1986; 154: 104.

67 Lee W, Ginsburg KA, Cotton DB, Kaufman RH. Squamous and trophoblastic cells in the maternal pulmonary circulation identified by invasive hemodynamic monitoring during the peripartum period. *Am J Obstet Gynecol* 1986; 155: 999.

68 Gitin TA, Seidel T, Cera PJ, et al. Pulmonary microvascular fat: the significance? *Crit Care Med* 1993; 21: 664.

69 Benson MD, Kobayashi H, Silver RK, Oi H, Greenberger PA, Terao T. Immunologic studies in presumed amniotic fluid embolism. *Obstet Gynecol* 2001; 97: 510–514.

70 Fineschi V, Gambassi R, Gherardi M, Turillazzi E. The diagnosis of amniotic fluid embolism: an immunohistochemical study for the quantification of pulmonary mast cell tryptase. *Int J Legal Med* 1998; 111: 238–243.

71 Ohi H, Kobayashi H, Sugimura M, Terao T. [A new method for diagnosis of amniotic fluid embolism by means of monoclonal antibody TKH-2 that recognizes mucin-type glycoprotein, a component in meconium.] *Nippon Sanka Fujinka Gakkai Zasshi* 1992; 44: 813–819.

72 Oi H, Kobayashi H, Hirashima Y, Yamazaki T, Kobayashi T, Terao T. Serological and immunohistochemical diagnosis of amniotic fluid embolism. *Semin Thromb Hemost* 1998; 24: 479–484.

73 Kanayama N, Yamazaki T, Naruse H, Sumimoto K, Horiuchi K, Terao T. Determining zinc coproporphyrin in maternal plasma – a new method for diagnosing amniotic fluid embolism. *Clin Chem* 1992; 38: 526–529.

74 Hsieh YY, Chang CC, Li PC, Tsai HD, Tsai CH. Successful application of extracorporeal membrane oxygenation and intra-aortic balloon counterpulsation as lifesaving therapy for a patient with amniotic fluid embolism. *Am J Obstet Gynecol* 2000; 183: 496–497.

75 Weksler N, Ovadia L, Stav A, Ribac L, Iuchtman M. Continuous arteriovenous hemofiltration in the treatment of amniotic fluid embolism. *Int J Obstet Anesth* 1994; 3: 92–96.

76 Kaneko Y, Ogihara T, Tajima H, Mochimaru F. Continuous hemodiafiltration for disseminated intravascular coagulation and shock due to amniotic fluid embolism: report of a dramatic response. *Intern Med* 2001; 40: 945–947.

77 Esposito RA, Grossi EA, Coppa G, et al. Successful treatment of postpartum shock caused by amniotic fluid embolism with cardiopulmonary bypass and pulmonary artery thromboembolectomy. *Am J Obstet Gynecol* 1990; 163: 572–574.

78 Stanten RD, Iverson LI, Daugharty TM, Lovett SM, Terry C, Blumenstock E. Amniotic fluid embolism causing catastrophic pulmonary vasoconstriction: diagnosis by transesophageal echocardiogram and treatment by cardiopulmonary bypass. *Obstet Gynecol* 2003; 102: 496–498.

79 Lim Y, Loo CC, Chia V, Fun W. Recombinant factor VIIa after amniotic fluid embolism and disseminated intravascular coagulopathy. *Int J Gynaecol Obstet* 2004; 87: 178–179.

80 Prosper SC, Goudge CS, Lupo VR. Recombinant factor VIIa to successfully manage disseminated intravascular coagulation from amniotic fluid embolism. *Obstet Gynecol* 2007; 109: 524–525.

81 McDonnell NJ, Chan BO, Frengley RW. Rapid reversal of critical haemodynamic compromise with nitric oxide in a parturient with amniotic fluid embolism. *Int J Obstet Anesth* 2007; 16: 269–273.

82 Clark SL. Successful pregnancy outcomes after amniotic fluid embolism. *Am J Obstet Gynecol* 1992; 167: 511.

83 Duffy BL. Does amniotic fluid embolism recur? *Anaesth Intens Care* 1998; 26: 333.

84 Collier C. Recurring amniotic fluid embolism. *Anaesth Intens Care* 1998; 26: 599–600.

85 Stiller RJ, Siddiqui D, Laifer SA, Tiakowski RL, Whetham JC. Successful pregnancy after suspected anaphylactoid syndrome of pregnancy (amniotic fluid embolus). A case report. *J Reprod Med* 2000; 45: 1007.

86 Demianczuk CE, Corbett TF. Successful pregnancy after amniotic fluid embolism: a case report. *J Obstet Gynaecol Can* 2005; 27: 699–701.

87 Abecassis P, Benhamou D. Is amniotic fluid embolism likely to recur in a subsequent pregnancy? *Int J Obstet Anesth* 2006; 15: 90.

88 Knight M, Kurinczuk JJ, Tuffnell D, Brocklehurst P. The UK Obstetric Surveillance System for rare disorders of pregnancy. *Br J Obstet Gynaecol* 2005; 112: 263–265.

89 Tuffnell DJ, Johnson H. Amniotic fluid embolism: the UK register. *Hosp Med* 2000; 61: 532–534.

90 Burrows A, Khoo SK. The amniotic fluid embolism syndrome: 10 years' experience at a major teaching hospital. *Aust N Z J Obstet Gynaecol* 1995; 35(3): 245–50.

36 Systemic Lupus Erythematosus and Antiphospholipid Syndrome

T. Flint Porter[1] & D. Ware Branch[2]

[1]Department of Obstetrics and Gynecology, University of Utah Health Science UT *and* Maternal-Fetal Medicine, Urban Central Region, Intermountain Healthcare, Salt Lake City, UT, USA
[2]Department of Obstetrics and Gynecology, University of Utah Health Sciences Center *and* Women and Newborns Services, Intermountain Healthcare, Salt Lake City, UT, USA

Introduction

Systemic lupus erythematosus (SLE) is a chronic inflammatory condition that affects virtually every organ system. With an increased prevalence among women of reproductive age, it is the autoimmune disease most commonly encountered during pregnancy. The majority of women with stable, uncomplicated SLE tolerate pregnancy well with relatively few serious obstetric complications. However, women with poorly controlled disease and/or serious SLE-related end-organ disease are at substantial risk for maternal morbidity and even mortality, as well as several adverse obstetric outcomes. Antiphospholipid syndrome (APS) is another autoimmune condition associated with several adverse pregnancy outcomes. Anticoagulation prophylaxis reduces the risk of thromboembolism and fetal death but the incidence of pre-eclampsia, uteroplacental insufficiency, and preterm birth remain high.

Management of both SLE and APS during pregnancy requires vigilance for signs and symptoms of disease exacerbation, aggressive immunosuppressive treatment when needed, and careful assessment of fetal well-being. A multidisciplinary approach is essential and should include the rheumatologist, obstetrician, and if renal disease is present, the patient's nephrologist.

Systemic lupus erythematosus in pregnancy

Background

The prevalence of SLE varies depending on the population under study but generally ranges between 5 and 125 per 100 000 and affects women 5–10 times more often than men [1,2]. The peak age of onset in young women occurs between their late teens and early 40s [3]. The prevalence among ethnic groups, such as those with African or Asian ancestry, is highest and the disease appears to be more severe when compared to white patients. Familial studies indicate that genetic susceptibility to lupus involves several complex gene polymorphisms. Russell and colleagues [4] reported a linkage between susceptibility to lupus in family members and disequilibrium in polymorphisms located on the long arm of chromosome 1, 1q23–24. Genes coding for C-reactive protein (CRP), actively involved in apoptosis, have been mapped to this area and CRP levels are commonly low in patients with lupus. Another familial study suggested that a single nucleotide polymorphism within the programmed cell death 1 gene (*PDCD1*) is associated with the development of the disease in both European and Mexican populations [5].

SLE exacerbation (flare) during pregnancy

Based on published reports, flare occurs in about 30–60% of pregnant patients with lupus. Renal disease and disease activity appear to increase the rate of flare during pregnancy. There is a split of opinion about whether pregnancy itself predisposes to lupus flare [2]. All studies are hampered by the fact that many of the most common signs and symptoms of lupus flare also occur in normal pregnancy. Some studies show higher rates of flare in pregnant women compared to non-pregnant controls, even when disease is inactive at the time of conception [6–11]. Others report no difference in rates of flare in women with well-controlled disease, whether treated or untreated, and non-pregnant women. [12–18]. Importantly, in nearly all studies, flares during pregnancy are reported to be mild to moderate in nature and easily treated with glucocorticoids.

Women with pre-existing renal disease, even when inactive, are undoubtedly at greatest risk for SLE flare during pregnancy [3,9]. Pregnancy may predispose to deterioration of renal function, especially for women with active lupus nephritis (LN) and/or renal insufficiency before conception [19–21]. Tandon and colleagues [22] reported that LN patients with inactive renal disease showed changes in disease activity and deterioration in renal function during pregnancy that were similar to those in non-pregnant patients with active LN. Overall, about one-third of

Critical Care Obstetrics, 5th edition. Edited by M. Belfort, G. Saade, M. Foley, J. Phelan and G. Dildy.

women with renal disease experience flare during pregnancy, fewer than 25% have worsening renal function, and only 10% of have permanent deterioration. Renal deterioration appears to be less severe in women with inactive LN in the 6 months before conception [9,14,19,21,23,24].

Pulmonary hypertension arises in up to 14% of patients with lupus, and even mildly raised pulmonary artery pressures can be seen in 37% of patients [25]. Though fortunately rare during pregnancy, pulmonary hypertension confers an unacceptably high risk of maternal death and patients should be counseled accordingly.

Obstetric complications in women with SLE

Women with SLE are at risk for several obstetric complications, sometimes resulting in serious maternal and perinatal morbidity. Between 20 and 30% of women with SLE have pregnancies complicated by pre-eclampsia [10,21,26]. Uteroplacental insufficiency resulting in intrauterine growth restriction (IUGR) or small for gestational age neonates occurs in 12–40% of lupus pregnancies [6,9,12,26,27]. The risk of IUGR is highest for women with renal insufficiency and/or hypertension [28,29]. Preterm birth is also more common in pregnancies complicated by SLE [7–10,12,26]. Most of preterm deliveries in women with SLE probably occur iatrogenically because of disease exacerbation and/or obstetric complications, though a higher risk of preterm premature rupture of membranes has been reported. The likelihood of serious obstetric complications is highest for women with poorly controlled disease, renal disease and/or chronic hypertension, and APS [10,21,27,28,31,32]. Chronic steroid use may also contribute to higher rates of pre-eclampsia and IUGR.

Pregnancy loss is thought to be more prevalent among women with SLE, with rates ranging from 10 to 50% [11,16,17,29,33]. First-trimester loss occurs in about 20% of lupus pregnancies, not markedly higher than the general population [34]. However, stillbirth (after 20 weeks of gestation) rates are elevated in several studies [9,14,21,35,36]. In one series, 20% of losses occurred during the second or third trimester [35]. Disease activity increases the likelihood of pregnancy loss [9,14] with one study reporting live births in 64% of women with active disease within 6 months of conception, compared to 88% in women with quiescent disease [21]. In the Hopkins Lupus Pregnancy Cohort, increased lupus activity did not increase the risk for miscarriage, but the stillbirth rate was threefold higher [36]. The timing of lupus activity affects the pregnancy loss rate, with activity early in pregnancy being the most dangerous. Proteinuria, thrombocytopenia, and hypertension in the first trimester are each independent risk factors for pregnancy loss. Women with these risk factors have a 30–40% chance of suffering a pregnancy loss [37]. Accordingly, pregnancy loss is more likely if SLE is diagnosed during the index pregnancy [38,39].

Renal insufficiency is also important; one group reported fetal loss in 50% of pregnancies complicated by moderate to severe renal insufficiency as defined by serum creatinine >1.5 mg/dL [21] and in 40% with pre-existing proteinuria as defined by >300 mg/24 h or a creatinine clearance <100 mL/min [30].

Not surprisingly, the most important risk factor for pregnancy loss in women with SLE is coexisting APS. In one series of pregnant women with SLE, the presence of antiphospholipid antibodies had a positive predictive value for pregnancy loss of 50% [40]. In another, positive predictive value increased to over 85% if women with SLE also had a fetal death in a prior pregnancy [32].

Neonatal lupus erythematosus

Neonatal lupus erythematosus (NLE) is a rare condition of the fetus and neonate, occurring in 1 of 20 000 of all live births and in fewer than 5% of all women with SLE [41]. Dermatological NLE is most common and is described as erythematous, scaling annular or elliptical plaques occurring on the face or scalp, analogous to the subacute cutaneous lesions in adults. Lesions appear in the first weeks of life, probably induced by exposure of the skin to ultraviolet light, and may last for up to 6 months [42]. Hypopigmentation may persist for up to 2 years. A small percentage of affected infants will go on to have other autoimmune diseases later in life [42]. Hematological NLE is rare and may be manifest as autoimmune hemolytic anemia, leukopenia, thrombocytopenia and hepatosplenomegaly.

Cardiac NLE lesions include congenital complete heart block (CCHB) and the less frequently reported endocardial fibroelastosis. Endomyocardial fibrosis caused by NLE leads to interruption of the conduction system, especially in the area of the atrioventricular node. The diagnosis is typically made around 23 weeks of gestation [43] when a fixed bradycardia, in the range of 60–80 beats/min, is detected during a routine prenatal visit. Fetal echocardiography reveals complete atrioventricular dissociation with a structurally normal heart. The prognosis varies but in the most severe cases, hydrops fetalis develops *in utero*. Because the endomyocardial damage is permanent, a pacemaker may be necessary for neonatal survival. In the largest series of 113 cases diagnosed before birth, 19% died, of which 73% died within 3 months of delivery [43]. In that same series, the 3-year survival was 79%. Cutaneous manifestations of NLE have also been reported in infants with CCHB [42].

Not all women who give birth to babies with NLE have been previously diagnosed with an autoimmune disorder [42,44]. However, in one study, 7 of 13 previously asymptomatic mothers who delivered infants with dermatologic NLE were later diagnosed with one of several autoimmune disorders [42]. Surprisingly, asymptomatic women who deliver infants with CCHB are less likely to later develop an autoimmune disorder than those with dermatologic manifestations alone [44].

Fetal immunologic damage is probably caused by maternal autoantibodies that cross the placenta and bind to fetal tissue [45–49]. Anti-Ro/SSA antibodies are found in 75–95% mothers who deliver babies with NLE [43,45,50]. A smaller percentage have anti-La/SSB, and some have both [50]. Dermatological NLE has also been associated with anti-U1RNP without anti-Ro/SSA or anti-La/SSB [50,51]. Of mothers with SLE who are serologically positive for anti-Ro/SSA antibodies, 15% will have infants affected with dermatological SLE; the proportion who deliver infants with CCHB is much smaller. However, once a woman with SLE and anti-Ro/SSA antibodies delivers one infant with CCHB, her risk for recurrence is at least two- to threefold higher than other women with anti-SSA/Ro-SSB/La antibodies who have never had an affected child [45].

There is no known *in utero* therapy that completely reverses fetal CCHB secondary to SLE. However, there is some evidence that treatment with glucocorticoids, plasmapheresis, intravenous immune globulin or some combination thereof, may slow the progression of prenatally diagnosed CCHB or at least prevent recurrence in a future pregnancy [52]. *In utero* treatment with dexamethasone was felt to slow disease progression in one case report of hydrops secondary to CCHB [53]. In one retrospective study, maternally administered dexamethasone appeared to prevent progression from second-degree block to third-degree block [54]. In a large series of 87 pregnancies at risk for NLE, mothers who received corticosteroids before 16 weeks of gestation were less likely to deliver infants with CCHB compared to mothers who received no therapy [55]. However, there was no benefit to treatment when CCHB was diagnosed *in utero*. *In utero* treatment with digoxin is not beneficial for prenatally diagnosed CCHB [56].

Diagnosis of SLE and detection of SLE exacerbation (flare)

Thorough and frequent clinical assessment remains essential for the timely and accurate detection of SLE flare [2]. In pregnancy, detection is more difficult because many of the typical signs and symptoms associated with flare are considered normal (Table 36.1). The SLE disease activity index (SLEDAI) has been modified for pregnancy with several caveats to rule out normal pregnancy complications and thereby more accurately identify true SLE activity [2,43]). The most common presenting symptom in both flare and new onset disease is extreme fatigue. Fever, weight loss, myalgia and arthralgia are also very common [57]. In pregnancy, skin rashes are more frequent than musculoskeletal manifestations [8]. Patients with LN exhibit worsening proteinuria along with pyuria, hematuria and urinary casts. Not surprisingly, SLE flare in pregnant women with LN is easily confused with the development of pre-eclampsia/eclampsia syndromes (Table 36.2).

Serological evaluation of SLE disease activity may be beneficial in confirming flare in confusing cases. However, no study has found serial laboratory testing superior to thorough clinical assessment and if flare is suspected, treatment should not be reserved only for women with positive serologic evaluation. Even so, the most specific serologic sign of SLE flare is an elevation in anti-double-stranded DNA (anti-ds DNA) which precedes lupus flare in more than 80% of patients [58–60]. In pregnancy, elevated anti-ds DNA titers have also been shown to correlate with the need for preterm delivery [61] and in combination with aCL antibodies, with an increased risk of fetal loss.

Serial evaluation of complement levels has been suggested as method of predicting SLE flare during pregnancy. Devoe [62] reported that SLE flare was signaled by a decline of C3 and C4 into the subnormal range and Buyon [63] reported that the physiologic rise in C3 and C4 levels normally seen during pregnancy did not occur in women with active disease. The same group reported that activation of the alternative complement pathway

Table 36.1 Common symptoms in pregnancy that may mimic lupus flare.

Constitutional	• Debilitating fatigue; may worsen throughout pregnancy
Skin	• Palmar erythema • Facial blush due to increased estrogen levels.
Face	• Melasma; photosensitive rash over cheeks and forehead
Hair	• Increased hair thickness and growth • Hair loss postpartum
Pulmonary	• Increased respiratory rate secondary to increased progesterone levels. • Dyspnea
Musculoskeletal	• Back pain ○ Relaxin loosens sacroiliac joint and pubis ○ Gravid uterus increases lumbar lordosis • Joint effusions
Central Nervous System	• Headache, normal in pregnancy as well as in preeclampsia

Table 36.2 Preeclampsia versus Lupus Flare.

	Preeclampsia	SLE Flare
Risk Factors		
• 1st Pregnancy	Yes	No
• History of preeclampsia	Yes	No
• Multiple gestation	Yes	No
• Lupus nephritis	Yes	Yes
• Gestational age	After 20 weeks'	Anytime
Laboratory Findings		
• Urine sediment	Negative	Positive
• Coombs	Negative	Sometimes positive
• Complement (C3 & C4)	Normal	Usually low
• Anti-DS DNA antibodies	Negative	Usually positive
• Serum uric acid	Elevated	Normal
Physical Findings		
• Rash	Absent	Sometimes present
• Alopecia	Absent	Sometimes present
• Mouth ulcers	Absent	Sometimes present
• Arthritis	Absent	Sometimes present
• Serositis	Absent	Sometimes present

accompanies flare during pregnancy [63] and that a combination of low C3, C4, or CH50 levels accompanied by an elevation in complement split products is useful in detecting flare during pregnancy [63]. The results of other studies of complement activation in pregnant women with SLE have either been inconsistent or not predictive of SLE flare [11,64,65]. Lockshin [66] reported normal concentrations of the Cls–C1 inhibitor complex in pregnant patients with hypocomplementemia which suggests poor synthesis of complement components rather than excessive consumption.

Laboratory confirmation of SLE flare is probably most helpful in women with active LN in whom proteinuria, hypertension and evidence of multiorgan dysfunction may easily be confused with pre-eclampsia. Both elevated anti-ds DNA titers and urinary sediment with cellular casts and hematuria weigh in weigh in favor of active LN. An increase in proteinuria in women with pre-existing LN should not necessarily raise an alarm until it doubles [57]. Pre-eclampsia is more likely in women with decreased levels of antithrombin-III [67,68]. Complement concentrations are not helpful because activation may also occur in women with pre-eclampsia [69]. In the most severe and confusing cases, the diagnosis can be confirmed only with renal biopsy. However, in reality, concerns about maternal and fetal well-being often prompt delivery, rendering the distinction between the SLE flare and pre-eclampsia clinically moot.

Medications used for SLE during pregnancy

Glucocorticoids

The group of drugs most commonly given to pregnant women with SLE is the glucocorticoid preparations, both as maintenance therapy and in "bursts" to treat suspected SLE flares. The doses used in pregnancy are the same as those in non-pregnant patients. Pregnancy *per se* is not an indication to reduce the dose of glucocorticoids, though a carefully monitored reduction in dosage may be reasonable in appropriately selected women whose disease appears to be in remission. Some groups have recommended prophylactic glucocorticoid therapy during pregnancy [17,24,70] but no controlled studies have shown this practice to be prudent or necessary in women with inactive SLE. Moreover, good maternal and fetal outcomes are achieved without prophylactic treatment of women with stable disease [13]. In contrast, glucocorticoid treatment of women with active disease and/or elevated anti-ds DNA titers has been shown to result in fewer relapses and better pregnancy outcomes [14,58].

While glucocorticoids have a low potential for teratogenesis [71], they are not without risk during pregnancy. Patients requiring chronic maintenance therapy are best treated with prednisolone or methylprednisolone because of their conversion to relatively inactive forms by the abundance of 11-,B-ol dehydrogenase found in the human placenta. Glucocorticoids with fluorine at the 9a position (dexamethasone, betamethasone) are considerably less well metabolized by the placenta and chronic use during pregnancy should be avoided. Both have been associated with untoward fetal effects [72]. Maternal side effects of chronic glucocorticoid therapy are the same as in non-pregnant patients and include weight gain, striae, acne, hirsutism, immunosuppression, osteonecrosis and gastrointestinal ulceration. During pregnancy, chronic glucocorticoid therapy has also been associated with an increased risk of pre-eclampsia [35,73–75], uteroplacental insufficiency [75], and glucose intolerance [73,74]. Women chronically treated with glucocorticoids should be screened for gestational diabetes at 22–24, 28–30 and 32–34 weeks of gestation.

Hydroxychloroquine

Hydroxychloroquine (HCQ) has been proven to decrease the risk of SLE flare, improve the prognosis of SLE nephritis, and prevent death [76–79]. It also has the lowest side-effect profile of any medication available to treat SLE and is well tolerated by most patients. In the past, many patients and their physicians discontinued hydroxychloroquine in pregnancy because of concerns about teratogenicity including ototoxicity [80] and eye damage [81]. However, an accumulating body of evidence suggests that hydroxychloroquine can be used safely for the treatment of SLE during pregnancy [82–86] and is in fact superior to glucocorticoids for women who require maintenance therapy during pregnancy [87]. An expert panel of international physicians have recommended the continuation of HCQ during pregnancy [79].

Immunosuppressants

Azathioprine (Imuran) is probably the safest immunosuppressant medication taken during pregnancy. The fetal liver does not have the enzyme required to metabolize azathioprine into its active form [79]. Series of pregnancies exposed to azathioprine for inflammatory bowel disease or renal transplants show no significant increase in fetal abnormalities among renal transplant patients. Nearly 40% of the offspring were small for gestational age. But this may also have been due to the underlying illness and/or contemporaneous treatment with glucocorticoids [78,79]. Most authorities recommend continuation of azathioprine treatment during pregnancy [57]. Cyclophosphamide is reportedly teratogenic in both animal [88] and human studies [89,90] and should be avoided during the first trimester. Thereafter, cyclophosphamide should be used only in unusual circumstances such as in women with severe, progressive proliferative glomerulonephritis [1]. Methotrexate is well known to kill chorionic villi and cause fetal death and its use should be scrupulously avoided.

NSAID preparations

The most common types of analgesics used in the treatment of SLE are non-steroidal anti-inflammatory drugs (NSAIDs). Unfortunately, their use in pregnancy should be avoided after the first trimester because they readily cross the placenta and block prostaglandin synthesis in a wide variety of fetal tissues. Though short-term tocolytic therapy with indomethacin appears to be safe [91,92], chronic use has been associated with a number of untoward fetal effects and, when used after 32 weeks, may result in constriction or closure of the fetal ductus arteriosus [93].

Long-term use of all NSAIDs has been associated with decreased fetal urinary output and oligohydramnios as well as neonatal renal insufficiency [79]. Given these risks, chronic use of adult dosages of aspirin and other NSAIDs should be avoided during pregnancy. Acetaminophen- and narcotic-containing preparations are acceptable alternatives if analgesia is needed during pregnancy.

Other treatments

Several new treatment regimens including cyclosporin, high-dose intravenous immune globulin (IVIG), mycophenolate mofetil, and thalidomide have been studied in the treatment of non-pregnant patients with SLE [1]. Only IVIG has been used during pregnancy without reports of adverse fetal effects. Obviously, thalidomide is strictly contraindicated during pregnancy because of its known potent teratogenicity. Complete immunoablative therapy followed by bone marrow stem cell transplantation has also been studied in patients with the most severe, unresponsive SLE [1].

Treatment of SLE flare during pregnancy

Mild to moderate symptomatic exacerbations of SLE without CNS or renal involvement may be treated with initiation of glucocorticoids or an increase in the dose of glucocorticoids. Relatively small doses of prednisone (e.g. 15–30 mg/day) will result in improvement in most cases. For severe exacerbations without CNS or renal involvement, doses of 1.0–1.5 mg/kg/day of prednisone in divided doses should be used, and a good clinical response can be expected in 5–10 days. Thereafter, glucocorticoids may be tapered by several different approaches (Table 36.3).

Severe exacerbations, especially those involving the CNS or kidneys, are treated more aggressively, usually with intravenous pulse glucocorticoid therapy The initial regimen involves a daily intravenous dose of methylprednisolone at 10–30 mg/kg (about 500–1000 mg) for 3 to 6 days. Thereafter, the patient is treated with 1.0–1.5 mg/kg/day of prednisone in divided doses, rapidly tapered over the course of 1 month. One can expect that 75% of patients will respond favorably to this approach. This regimen may be repeated every 1–3 months in severe cases as an alternative to cytotoxic drugs.

Table 36.3 Suggested Methods for Tapering Prednisone.

1. Consolidate to a single morning dose of prednisone. Reduce the daily dose by 10% per week, as tolerated. When a dose of 20 to 30 mg/day is reached, reduce by 2.5-mg increments per week. If the patient remains asymptomatic at a dose of 15 mg/day, reduce the dose by 1-mg increments per week to a dose of 5 to 10 mg/day.
2. Consolidate to a single morning dose of prednisone. Taper to 50 to 60 mg/day by reducing the dose 10% per week. Thereafter eliminate the alternate-day dose by tapering it 10% per week, as tolerated. Thereafter, taper the remaining every other day dose by 10% per week, as tolerated.

Intravenous immunoglobin (IVIg) is another option for moderate to sever flare and is particularly helpful in controlling hematologic and renal disease [94,95]. There are few reports of IVIG use for SLE flare during pregnancy. However, the safety of IVIG in pregnancy has been well documented in its frequent use for other conditions in pregnancy including including alloimmune thrombocytopenia, immunologic thrombocytopenia purpurpa, and red blood cell antigen alloimmunization.

In non-pregnant patients, both cyclophosphamide and mycophenolate mofetil (MMF) may be used in severe SLE exacerbations to control disease, reduce irreversible tissue damage, and reduce glucocorticoid doses [96–98]. In particular, severe proliferative lupus nephritis may be treated more effectively with cyclophosphamide, usually in combination with glucocorticoids [96]. Their use during pregnancy should be avoided, particularly during the first trimester [57].

Antiphospholipid syndrome in pregnancy

The diagnosis of APS is based on the presence of one or more characteristic thrombotic or obstetric features of the condition; laboratory testing for antiphospholipid antibodies (aPLs) is used to confirm or refute the diagnosis. The International Consensus Statement was recently updated in 2006 and provides simplified criteria for the diagnosis of APS [99]. Patients with bona fide APS must manifest at least one of two clinical criteria (vascular thrombosis or pregnancy morbidity) and at least one of two laboratory criteria (positive lupus anticoagulant (LAC) or medium to high titers of IgG or IgM isotype anticardiolipin (aCL) antibodies, and/or IgG or IgM isotype anti β_2-glycoprotein I-antibodies, confirmed on two separate occasions, at least 6 weeks apart. Thrombosis may be either arterial or venous and must be confirmed by an imaging or Doppler study or by histopathology. Pregnancy morbidity is divided into three categories: (i) otherwise unexplained fetal death (10 weeks' gestation or greater); (ii) preterm birth (34 weeks gestation) for severe pre-eclampsia or placental insufficiency; or (iii) three or more otherwise unexplained, consecutive pre-embryonic or embryonic pregnancy losses. Autoimmune thrombocytopenia and amaurosis fugax are often associated with APS but are not considered sufficient diagnostic criteria. APS may exist as an isolated immunologic derangement (primary APS) or in combination with other autoimmune diseases (secondary APS), most commonly SLE.

The pathogenesis of antiphospholipid syndrome

The mechanism(s) by which aPLs cause thrombosis is complex and involves alterations in the coagulation cascade, platelets, and endothelial function. Interference with normal hemostasis occurs via interaction with phospholipids or phospholipid-binding protein components such as β_2-glycoprotein I (which has anticoagulant properties), prostacyclin, prothrombin, protein C, annexin V, and tissue factor [100]. Antiphospholipid antibodies also appear to activate endothelial cells, indicated by increased expression of adhesion molecules, secretion of cytokines, and production of arachidonic acid metabolites [101]. The findings that some aCLs cross-react with oxidized low-density lipoprotein [102] and that human aCLs bind to oxidized, but not reduced, cardiolipin [103] imply that aPLs may participate in oxidant-mediated injury of the vascular endothelium. They also bind perturbed cells, such as activated platelets [104] or apoptotic cells [105], which typically lose normal membrane symmetry and express anionic phospholipids on their surface.

Some APS-related pregnancy complications, particularly fetal loss, are probably related to abnormal placental function due to narrowing and thrombosis in decidual spiral arteries [106–108]. These abnormalities might result from thrombosis during the development of normal maternoplacental circulation via interference with trophoblastic annexin V [108] or by impairing trophoblastic hormone production or invasion [109]. Thrombosis as a mechanism for earlier pregnancy loss seems less likely.

Whether aPLs *per se* are the cause of adverse obstetric outcomes is also a matter of debate. Investigators working with murine models have found that passive transfer of aPLs results in clinical manifestations of APS, including fetal loss and thrombocytopenia [110–112]. aPLs have also been demonstrated to have a procoagulant effect [113]. It is not until recently that investigations into aPL-related pregnancy loss have focused on a role for the complement system, a component of the innate immune system, which has been shown to cause and perpetuate obstetric complications [114–117]. Studies in a mouse model have shown that passive transfer of aPL antibodies results in activation of the complement cascade, in turn leading to an increase in complement activation fragments which are extremely deleterious to the fetus [115,116]. Follow-up studies have found that inactivation and inhibition of the complement cascade prevent fetal loss and growth restriction even after addition of aPL antibodies [116]. TNF-α, an inflammatory factor released via complement activation, may also play a role as TNF-α deficient mice fail to have pregnancy loss when treated with aPLs [118].

Clinical features of APS during pregnancy

Venous thrombotic events (VTEs) associated with aPLs include deep venous thrombosis (DVT) and acute pulmonary emboli (APE); cerebral vascular accidents and transient ischemic attacks are the most common arterial events. A meta-analysis of 18 studies examining the thrombotic risk among SLE patients with LAC, found odds ratios (ORs) of 6.32 (95% CI 3.71–10.78) for VTE and 11.6 (95% CI 3.65–36.91) for recurrent VTE [119]. By contrast aPLs were associated with a lower OR of 2.50 (1.51–4.14) for an acute VTE, and 3.91 (95% CI 1.14–13.38) for recurrent VTE. A meta-analysis of studies in the general population identified a range of ORs for arterial and venous thromboses in patients with LAC of 8.6–10.8 and 4.1–16.2, respectively [120]. The comparable numbers for aCL were 1–18 and 1–2.5. Up to 30% of patients may have recurrence, supporting the use of long-term prophylaxis [121]. The risk of VTE in pregnancy and the puerperium may be as high as 5% despite treatment [122].

In the original description of APS, the sole obstetric criterion for diagnosis was fetal loss (>10 menstrual weeks gestation) [123,124]. At least 40% of pregnancy losses reported by women with LA or medium to high positive IgG aCL occur in the fetal period [122,125–127]. LACs are associated with fetal loss after the first trimester, with ORs ranging from 3.0 to 4.8 while ACA display a wider range of ORs, 0.86–20.0 [120]. APS-related pregnancy loss has also been extended to include women with early recurrent pregnancy loss (RPL) including those occurring in the pre-embryonic (<6 menstrual weeks of gestation) and embryonic periods (6–9 menstrual weeks of gestation) [99]. In serologic evaluation of women with RPL, 10–20% have detectable aPLs [128–133]. Women with APS followed prospectively also have demonstrated high rates of premature delivery for gestational hypertension or pre-eclampsia and uteroplacental insufficiency as manifested by fetal growth restriction, oligohydramnios, and non-reassuring fetal surveillance [122,134].

Women with APS identified because of a prior fetal death and/or thromboembolism seem to have more serious complications in subsequent pregnancies than those with early RPL [135]. Prospective treatment trials of APS during pregnancy have been comprised mainly of women with early RPL and no other APS-related medical problems [130–132,136–138]. Accordingly, the rates of obstetric complications were relatively low with fetal death, pre-eclampsia, and preterm birth occurring in 4.5% (0–15%), 10.5% (0–15%), and 10.5% (5–40%), respectively. Only 1 of 300 women suffered a thrombotic event and no neonatal deaths due to complications of prematurity were reported. Based on these data, it seems unlikely that early RPL, fetal death, and preterm birth resulting from severe pre-eclampsia or placental insufficiency are a result of the same pathophysiologic mechanism.

Treatment of antiphospholipid syndrome during pregnancy

Treatment goals for APS during pregnancy should include: (i) improvement in maternal and fetal/neonatal outcome by preventing pregnancy loss, pre-eclampsia, placental insufficiency, and preterm birth; and (ii) reduction or elimination of thromboembolism. Early enthusiasm for treatment with glucocorticoids to reduce the risk of pregnancy loss waned after publication of a small, randomized trial found maternally administered heparin to be as effective as prednisone [136]. Contemporary management (Table 36.4) should include treatment with either unfractionated heparin or low molecular weight heparin (LMWH) plus low dose aspirin (LDA) at 50–80 mg per day. [130–132,136–139]. A meta-analysis of trials using unfractionated heparin and LDA [140] reported a 54% improvement in the live birth rate. Another using enoxaparin treatment resulted in an increased live birth rate, as compared to LDA (RR 10.0, 95% CI 1.56–64.20) [140]. Despite treatment, other aPL-related adverse pregnancy outcomes still occur. In a prospective observational study of 150 women treated with LDA and either unfractionated heparin or enoxaparin after embryonic cardiac activity was identified to

Table 36.4 Subcutaneous Heparin Regimens Used for Antiphospholipid Syndrome During Pregnancy (132–134, 138–141).

Prophylactic Regimens

Recommended in women with no history of thrombotic events – diagnosis of recurrent preembryonic and embryonic loss or prior fetal death or early delivery because of severe preeclampsia or severe placental insufficiency

Standard Heparin

7,500–10,000 U every 12 hours in the first trimester, 10,000 U every 12 hours in the second and third trimesters

Low Molecular Weight Heparin

1) Enoxaparin 40 mg once daily or dalteparin 5000 U once daily
2) Enoxaparin 30 mg every 12 hours or dalteparin 5000 U every 12 hours

Anticoagulation Regimens

Recommended in women with a history of thrombotic events

Standard Heparin

Every 8–12 hours adjusted to maintain the midinterval heparin levels* in the therapeutic range

Low Molecular Weight Heparin

1) Weight adjusted (enoxaparin 1 mg/kg every 12 hours or dalteparin 200 U/kg every 12 hours)
2) Intermediate dose (enoxaparin 40 mg once daily or dalteparin 5000 U once daily until 16 weeks of gestation and every 12 hours from 16 weeks onwards

* Heparin levels = anti factor Xa levels. Women without a lupus anticoagulant in whom the activated partial thromboplastin time (aPTT) is normal can be observed using the aPTT.

either pregnancy loss or 34 weeks, the live birth rate was 71%, gestational hypertension occurred in 17%, abruption in 7% and IUGR in 15% [141].

The safe and effective dose of heparin anticoagulation during pregnancy for women with APS is debated but should depend on individual patient history. Because of their substantial risk of recurrence [84,142,143], most authorities recommend full, adjusted dose anticoagulation during pregnancy for women with APS and a history of thromboembolism [144,145]. In contrast, women diagnosed with APS *without* a history of thromboembolism are probably less likely to have a first episode during pregnancy. Women with early RPL alone, without a history of thromboembolism, have been treated with both low-dose prophylaxis and adjusted-dose anticoagulation regimens [140]. Live rates have exceeded 70% using either strategy [130,136]. Women with a history of fetal death alone may be at higher risk for thromboembolism during pregnancy [146] and should probably receive higher doses of heparin prophylaxis. It has been recommended to treat such women with generous thromboprophylaxis (e.g, 15 000–20 000 units of standard heparin or 60 mg of enoxaparin in divided doses daily) [122,136,147].

Women with APS should be counseled about the potential risks of heparin therapy during pregnancy including heparin-induced osteoporosis and heparin-induced thrombocytopenia (HIT). Osteoporosis resulting in fracture occurs in 1–2% of women treated during pregnancy [148]. Women treated with heparin should be encouraged to take daily supplemental calcium and vitamin D (e.g. prenatal vitamins). It also seems prudent to encourage daily axial skeleton weight-bearing exercise (e.g. walking). Immune-mediated HIT is much less common but potentially more serious. Most cases have their onset 3–21 days after heparin initiation and are relatively mild in nature [149]. A more severe form of HIT paradoxically involves venous and arterial thromboses resulting in limb ischemia, cerebrovascular accidents, and myocardial infarctions, as well as venous thromboses [150]. It may occur in up to 0.5% of patients treated with unfractionated sodium heparin [149]. Low molecular weight heparin (LMWH) is much less likely to be associated with HIT, compared with unfractionated sodium heparin [151].

Other pregnancy complications associated with APS occur in spite of appropriate treatment [122,141]. In a recent observational study of 107 pregnancies complicated by APS, pre-eclampsia occurred in 20%, preterm birth in 24%, and growth restriction in 15% of treated women [141].

Pregnancy losses continue to occur in 20–30% of cases in spite of heparin prophylaxis being given [122,136,139]. Several alternative therapies have been suggested in these so-called refractory cases. Glucocorticoids, often in high doses, have sometimes been added to regimens of heparin and low-dose aspirin. While there are anecdotal reports of success, this practice has never been studied in appropriately designed trials and the combination of glucocorticoids and heparin may increase the risk of osteoporotic fracture [136]. Hydroxychloroquine has been shown to diminish the thrombogenic properties of aPL in a murine thrombosis model [152]. There are few case reports and no trials of APS patients being treated during pregnancy with hydroxychloroquine.

Intravenous gammaglobulin (IVIG) has been reported to improve outcome in women with APS who have previously failed treatment with heparin and LDA [153]. However, in randomized controlled trials, the live birth rates in women receiving IVIG treatment during pregnancy were lower when compared to live birth rates in women receiving LDA and LMWH [154]. In another small trial, IVIG added to heparin and LDA was not superior to heparin and LDA alone [155]. Thus, IVIG is not recommended as first-line therapy for APS.

Healthy women with recurrent embryonic and pre-embyronic loss and low titers of aPL do not require treatment [156]. The controlled trial of Pattison and colleagues [131] included a majority of such women and found no difference in live birth rates using either low-dose aspirin or placebo.

Postpartum and catastrophic antiphospholipid syndrome

Catastrophic antiphospholipid syndrome is a rare but devastating syndrome characterized by multiple simultaneous vascular occlusions throughout the body, often resulting in death. The diagnosis should be suspected if at least three organ systems are affected

Table 36.5 Proposed Protocol For Acute Treatment of Catastrophic Antiphospholipid Syndrome (159, 161, 162).

1. Intravenous heparin should be initiated and adjusted to achieve an activated partial thromboplastin time (aPTT) 2–3 times greater than the mean. Heparin levels may be necessary for women with the LAC because they demonstrate a prolonged aPTT without anticoagulation.
2. Intravenous methylprednisolone should be initiated at a dosage of 10–30 mg/kg/day.
3. Plasmapheresis should be initiated with the replacement of 40 mL of plasma per kilogram of body weight or up to 3 liters per exchange. This should be repeated three times weekly for 2 to 6 weeks. The simultaneous administration of immunosuppressive agents may block potential rebound in production of autoantibodies.

and confirmed if there is histolopathologic evidence of acute thrombotic microangiopathy affecting small vessels. Renal involvement occurs in 78% of patients. Most have hypertension and 25% eventually require dialysis. Other common manifestations described by Asherson [157] include adult respiratory distress syndrome (66%), cerebral microthrombi and microinfarctions (56%), myocardial microthrombi (50%), dermatologic abnormalities (50%), and disseminated intravascular coagulation (25%). Death from multiorgan failure occurs in 50% of patients [157]. The pathophysiology of catastrophic antiphospholipid syndrome is poorly understood. However, the onset may be presaged by several factors including infection, surgical procedures, discontinuation of anticoagulant therapy, and the use of drugs such as oral contraceptives [157–159].

Early and aggressive treatment of catastrophic APS is necessary to avoid death. Patients should be transferred to an intensive care unit where supportive care can be provided. Hypertension should be aggressively treated with appropriate antihypertensive medication. While no treatment has been shown to be superior to another, a combination of anticoagulants (usually heparin) and steroids plus either plasmapheresis or intravenous immune globulin has been successful in some patients [157,159,160] (Table 36.5). Streptokinase and urokinase have also been used to treat acute vascular thrombosis [157]. Women suspected of catastrophic APS during pregnancy should probably be delivered.

References

1 Ruiz-Irastorza G, Khamashta MA, Castellino G, Hughes GR. Systemic lupus erythematosus. *Lancet* 2001; 357: 1027–1032.

2 Ruiz-Irastorza G, Khamashta MA. Evaluation of systemic lupus erythematosus activity during pregnancy. *Lupus* 2004; 13: 679–682.

3 D'Cruz DP, Khamashta M, Hughes GRV. Systemic lupus erythematosus. *Lancet* 2007; 369: 587–596.

4 Russell AI, Cunninghame Graham DS, Shepherd C, et al. Polymorphism at the C-reactive protein locus influences gene expression and predisposes to systemic lupus erythematosus. *Hum Mol Genet* 2004; 13: 137–147.

5 Prokunina L, Castillejo-Lopez C, Oberg F, et al. A regulatory polymorphism in PDCD1 is associated with susceptibility to systemic lupus erythematosus in humans. *Nat Genet* 2002; 32: 666–669.

6 Ruiz-Irastorza G, Lima F, Alves J, et al. Increased rate of lupus flare during pregnancy and the puerperium: a prospective study of 78 pregnancies. *Br J Rheumatol* 1996; 35(2): 133–138.

7 Petri M, Howard D, Repke J. Frequency of lupus flare in pregnancy. The Hopkins Lupus Pregnancy Center experience. *Arthritis Rheum* 1991; 34: 1538–1545.

8 Petri M. Hopkins Lupus Pregnancy Center: 1987 to 1996. *Rheum Dis Clin North Am* 1997; 23(1): 1–13.

9 Johns KR, Morand EF, Littlejohn GO. Pregnancy outcome in systemic lupus erythematosus (SLE): a review of 54 cases. *Aust NZ J Med* 1998; 28(1): 18–22.

10 Kleinman D, Katz VL, Kuller JA. Perinatal outcomes in women with systemic lupus erythematosus. *J Perinatol* 1998; 18(3): 178–182.

11 Wong KL, Chan FY, Lee CP. Outcome of pregnancy in patients with systemic lupus erythematosus. A prospective study. *Arch Intern Med* 1991; 151(2): 269–273.

12 Aggarwal N, Sawhney H, Vasishta K, Chopra S, Bambery P. Pregnancy in patients with systemic lupus erythematosus. *Aust NZ J Obstet Gynaecol* 1999; 39(1): 28–30.

13 Derksen RH, Bruinse HW, de Groot PG, Kater L. Pregnancy in systemic lupus erythematosus: a prospective study. *Lupus* 1994; 3(3): 149–155.

14 Georgiou PE, Politi EN, Katsimbri P, Sakka V, Drosos AA. Outcome of lupus pregnancy: a controlled study. *Rheumatology (Oxf)* 2000; 39: 1014–1019.

15 Huong DL, Wechsler B, Vauthier-Brouzes D, Beaufils H, Lefebvre G, Piette JC. Pregnancy in past or present lupus nephritis: a study of 32 pregnancies from a single centre. *Ann Rheum Dis* 2001; 60(6): 599–604.

16 Lockshin MD, Reinitz E, Druzin ML, Murrman M, Estes D. Lupus pregnancy. Case-control prospective study demonstrating absence of lupus exacerbation during or after pregnancy. *Am J Med* 1984; 77: 893–898.

17 Mintz R, Niz J, Gutierrez G, Garcia-Alonso A, Karchmer S. Prospective study of pregnancy in systemic lupus erythematosus: results of a multidisciplinary approach. *J Rheumatol* 1986; 13: 732–739.

18 Urowitz MB, Gladman DD, Farewell VT, Stewart J, McDonald J. Lupus and pregnancy studies. *Arthritis Rheum* 1993; 36(10): 1392–1397.

19 Bobrie G, Liote F, Houillier P, Grunfeld JP, Jungers P. Pregnancy in lupus nephritis and related disorders. *Am J Kidney Dis* 1987; 9: 339–343.

20 Carmona F, Font J, Moga I, et al. Class III-IV proliferative lupus nephritis and pregnancy: a study of 42 cases. *Am J Reprod Immunol* 2005; 53: 182–188.

21 Hayslett JP, Lynn RI. Effect of pregnancy in patients with lupus nephropathy. *Kidney Int* 1980; 18: 207–220.

22 Tandon A, Ibanez D, Gladman DD, Urowitz MB. The effect of pregnancy on lupus nephritis. *Arthritis Rheum* 2004; 50: 3941–3946.

23 Germaine S, Nelson-Piercy C. Lupus nephritis and renal disease in pregnancy. *Lupus* 2006; 15: 148–155.

24 Le Huong D, Wechsler B, Vauthier-Brouzes D, et al. Outcome of planned pregnancies in systemic lupus erythematosus: a prospective study on 62 pregnancies. *Br J Rheumatol* 1997; 36(7): 772–777.

25 Johnson SR, Gladman DD, Urowitz MB, Ibanez D, Granton JT. Pulmonary hypertension in systemic lupus. *Lupus* 2004; 13: 506–509.

26 Yasmeen S, Walkins EE, Field NT, et al. Pregnancy outcomes in women with systemic lupus erythematosus. *J Matern Fetal Med* 2001; 10: 91–96.

27 Packham DK, Lam SS, Nichols K, et al. Lupus nephritis and pregnancy. *Quart J Med* 1992; 83: 315–324.

28 Julkunen H, Jouhikainen T, Kaaja R, et al. Fetal outcome in lupus pregnancy: a retrospective case-control study of 242 pregnancies in 112 patients. *Lupus* 1993; 2: 125.

29 Rahman P, Gladman DD, Urowitz MB. Clinical predictors of fetal outcome in systemic lupus erythematosus. *J Rheumatol* 1998; 25(8): 1526–1530.

30 Fine LG, Barnett EV, Danovitch GM, et al. Systemic lupus erythematosus in pregnancy. *Arch Intern Med* 1981; 94: 667–677.

31 Oviasu E, Hicks J, Cameron JS. The outcome of pregnancy in women with lupus nephritis. *Lupus* 1991; 1: 19–25.

32 Ramsey-Goldman R, Kutzer JE, Kuller LH, Guzick D, Carpenter AB, Medsger TA. Pregnancy outcome and anti-cardiolipin antibody in women with systemic lupus erythematosus. *Am J Epidemiol* 1993; 138: 1057–1069.

33 Le Huong D, Wechsler B, Vauthier-Brouzes D, et al. Outcome of planned pregnancies in systemic lupus erythematosus: a prospective study on 62 pregnancies. *Br J Rheumatol* 1997; 36(7): 772–777.

34 Clark CA, Spitzer KA, Nadler JN, et al. Preterm deliveries in women with systemic lupus erythematosus. *J Rheumatol* 2003; 30(10): 2127–2132.

35 Lockshin MD, Qamar T, Druzin ML. Hazards of lupus pregnancy. *J Rheumatol* 1987; 14: 214.

36 Clowse ME, Magder LS, Witter F, et al. The impact of increased lupus activity on obstetric outcomes. *Arthritis Rheum* 2005; 52(2): 514–521.

37 Clowse ME, Magder LS, Witter F, et al. Early risk factors for pregnancy loss in lupus. *Obstet Gynecol* 2006; 107(2 Pt 1): 293–299.

38 Imbasciati E, Surian M, Bottino W, et al. Lupus nephropathy and pregnancy. *Nephron* 1984; 36: 46–51.

39 Jungers P, Dougados M, Pelissier C, et al. Lupus nephropathy and pregnancy. *Arch Intern Med* 1982; 142: 771–776.

40 Englert HJ, Derue GM, Loizou S, et al. Pregnancy and lupus: prognostic indicators and response to treatment. *Quart J Med* 1988; 66(250): 125–136.

41 Lockshin MD, Bonfa E, Elkon D, Druzin ML. Neonatal lupus risk to newborns of mothers with systemic lupus erythematosus. *Arthritis Rheum* 1988; 31: 697–701.

42 Neiman AR, Lee LA, Weston WL, Buyon JP. Cutaneous manifestations of neonatal lupus without heart block: characteristics of mothers and children enrolled in a national registry. *J Pediatr* 2000; 137: 674–680.

43 Buyon JP, Hiebert R, Copel J, et al. Autoimmune-associated congenital heart block: demographics, mortality, morbidity and recurrence rates obtained from a national neonatal lupus registry. *J Am Coll Cardiol* 1998; 31(7): 1658–1666.

44 Lawrence S, Luy L, Laxer R, Krafchik B, Silverman E. The health of mothers of children with cutaneous neonatal lupus erythematosus differs from that of mothers of children with congenital heart block. *Am J Med* 2000; 108: 705–709.

45 Buyon JP, Winchester RJ, Slade SG, et al. Identification of mothers at risk for congenital heart block and other neonatal lupus syndromes in their children: comparison of enzyme-linked immunosorbent asay and immunoblot for measurement of anti-SS-A/Ro and anti-SS-B/La antibodies. *Arthritis Rheum* 1993; 36: 1263–1273.

46 Lee LA, Gaither KK, Coulter SN, et al. Pattern of cutaneous immunoglobulin G deposition in subacute cutaneous lupus erythematosus is reproduced by infusing purified anti-Ro (SSA) autoantibodies into human skin-grafted mice. *J Clin Invest* 1989; 83: 1556–1562.

47 McCauliffe DP. Neonatal lupus erythematosus: a transplacentally acquired autoimmune disorder. *Semin Dermatol* 1995; 14: 47–53.

48 Scott JS, Maddison PJ, Taylor MV, et al. Connective tissue disease, antibodies to ribonucleoprotein and congenital heart disease. *N Engl J Med* 1983; 309: 209–212.

49 Taylor PV, Scott JS, Gerlis LM, Path FRC, Esscher E, Scott O. Maternal antibodies against fetal cardiac antigens in congenital complete heart block. *N Engl J Med* 1986; 315: 667–672.

50 Lee LA, Frank MB, McCubbin VR, Reichlin M. Autoantibodies of neonatal lupus erythematosus. *J Invest Dermatol* 1994; 102: 963–966.

51 Provost TT, Watson R, Gammon WR. Neonatal lupus syndrome associated with U_1RNP (nRNP) antibodies. *N Engl J Med* 1987; 316: 1135–1138.

52 Kaaja R, Julkunen H, Ammala P, et al. Congenital heart block: successful prophylactic treatment with intravenous gamma globulin and corticosteroid therapy. *Am J Obstet Gynecol* 1991; 165: 1333–1334.

53 Carreira PE, Gutierrez-Larraya F, Gomez-Reino JJ. Successful intrauterine therapy with dexamethasone for fetal myocarditis and heart block in a woman with systemic lupus erythematosus. *J Rheumatol* 1993; 20(7): 1204–1207.

54 Saleeb S, Copel J, Friedman D, Buyon JP. Comparison of treatment with fluorinated glucocorticoids to the natural history of autoantibody-associated congenital heart block: retrospective review of the research registry for neonatal lupus. *Arthritis Rheum* 1999; 42(11): 2335–2345.

55 Shinohara K, Miyagawa S, Fujita T, Aono T, Kidoguchi K. Neonatal lupus erythematosus: results of maternal corticosteroid therapy. *Obstet Gynecol* 1999; 93(6): 952–957.

56 Eronen M, Heikkila P, Teramo K. Congenital complete heart block in the fetus: hemodynamic features, antenatal treatment, and outcome in six cases. *Pediatr Cardiol* 2001; 22(5): 385–392.

57 Clowse ME. Lupus activity in pregnancy. *Rheum Dis Clin North Am* 2007; 33: 237–252.

58 Bootsma H, Spronk PE, Derksen R, et al. Prevention of relapses in systemic lupus erythematosus. *Lancet* 1995; 345: 1595–1599.

59 Clowse MEB, Magder LS, Petri M. Complement and double-stranded DNA antibodies predict pregnancy outcomes in lupus patients. *Arthritis Rheum* 2004; 50(9 Suppl): S408.

60 Ter Borg EJ, Horst G, Hummel EJ, Limburg PC, Kallenberg CG. Measurement of increases in anti-double-stranded DNA antibody levels as a predictor of disease exacerbation in systemic lupus erythematosus. A long-term, prospective study. *Arthritis Rheum* 1990; 33(5): 634–643.

61 Tomer Y, Viegas, OAC, Swissa M, Koh SCL, Shoenfeld Y. Levels of lupus autoantibodies in pregnant SLE patients: correlations with disease activity and pregnancy outcome. *Clin Exper Rheumatol* 1996; 14: 275–280.

62 Devoe LD, Loy GL. Serum complement levels and perinatal outcome in pregnancies complicated by systemic lupus erythematosus. *Obstet Gynecol* 1984; 63: 796–800.

63 Buyon JP, Tamerius J, Ordorica S, Young B, Abramson SB. Activation of the alternative complement pathway accompanies disease flares in systemic lupus erythematosus during pregnancy. *Arthritis Rheum* 1992; 35(1): 55–61.

64 Abramson SB, Buyon JP. Activation of the complement pathway: comparison of normal pregnancy, pre-eclampsia, and systemic lupus erythematosus during pregnancy. *Am J Reprod Immunol* 1992; 28(3–4): 183–187.

65 Adelsberg BR. The complement system in pregnancy. *Am J Reprod Immunol* 1983; 4: 38–44.

66 Lockshin MD, Bonfa E, Elkon D, Druzin ML. Neonatal lupus risk to newborns of mothers with systemic lupus erythematosus. *Arthritis Rheum* 1988; 31: 697–701.

67 Weiner CP, Brandt J. Plasma antithrombin III activity: an aid in the diagnosis of pre-eclampsia-eclampsia. *Am J Obstet Gynecol* 1982; 142(3): 275–281.

68 Weiner CP, Kwaan HC, Xu C, Paul M, Burmeister L, Hauck W. Antithrombin III activity in women with hypertension during pregnancy. *Obstet Gynecol* 1985; 65(3): 301–306

69 Mellembakken JR, Hogasen K, Mollnes TE, Hack CE, Abyholm T, Videm V. Increased systemic activation of neutrophils but not complement in pre-eclampsia. *Obstet Gynecol* 2001; 97(3): 371–374.

70 Tincani A, Faden D, Tarantini M, et al. Systemic lupus erythematosus and pregnancy: a prospective study. *Clin Exp Rheumatol* 1992; 10(5): 439–446.

71 Brooks PM, Needs CJ. Antirheumatic drugs in pregnancy and lactation. *Baillière's Clin Rheumatol* 1990; 4: 157.

72 National Institutes of Health. *Antenatal Corticosteroids Revisited: Repeated Doses*. NIH Consensus Statement. Bethesda, MD: National Institutes of Health, 2000; 17: 1–10.

73 Laskin CA, Bombardier C, Hannah ME, et al. Prednisone and aspirin in women with autoantibodies and unexplained recurrent fetal loss. *N Engl J Med* 1997; 337(3): 148–153.

74 Vaquero E, Lazzarin N, Valensise H, et al. Pregnancy outcome in recurrent spontaneous abortion associated with antiphospholipid antibodies: a comparative study of intravenous immunoglobulin versus prednisone plus low-dose aspirin. *Am J Reprod Immunol* 2001; 45(3): 174–179.

75 Rayburn WF. Connective tissue disorders and pregnancy. Recommendations for prescribing. *J Reprod Med* 1998; 43(4): 341–349.

76 Alarcon GS, McGwin G Jr, Bastian HM, et al. Systemic lupus erythematosus in three ethnic groups. VII [correction of VIII]. Predictors of early mortality in the LUMINA cohort. LUMINA Study Group. *Arthritis Rheum* 2001; 45(2): 191–202.

77 Canadian Hydroxychloroquine Study Group. A randomized study of the effect of withdrawing hydroxychloroquine sulfate in systemic lupus erythematosus. *N Engl J Med* 1991; 324(3): 150–154.

78 Kasitanon N, Fine DM, Haas M, et al. Hydroxychloroquine use predicts complete renal remission within 12 months among patients treated with mycophenolate mofetil therapy for membranous lupus nephritis. *Lupus* 2006; 15(6): 366–370.

79 Ostensen Khamashta M, Lockshin M, et al. Anti-inflammatory and immunosuppressive drugs and reproduction. *Arthritis Res Ther* 2006; 8: 209–228.

80 Hart C, Naughton RF. The ototoxicity of chloroquine phosphate. *Arch Otolaryngol* 1964; 80: 407.

81 Nylander U. Ocular damage in chloroquine therapy. *Acta Ophthalmol (Copenh)* 1967; 45(Suppl 92): 5.

82 Buchanan NM, Toubi E, Khamashta MA, Lima F, Kerslake S, Hughes GR. Hydroxychloroquine and lupus pregnancy: review of a series of 36 cases. *Ann Rheum Dis* 1996; 55: 486–488.

83 Costedoat-Chalumeau N, Amoura Z, Duhaut P, et al. Safety of hydroxychloroquine in pregnant patients with connective tissue diseases: a study of one hundred thirty-three cases compared with a control group. *Arthritis Rheum* 2003; 48(11): 3207–3211.

84 Khamashta MA, Buchanan NM, Hughes GR. The use of hydroxychloroquine in lupus pregnancy: the British experience. *Lupus* 1996; 5(Suppl 1): S65–66.

85 Klinger G, Morad Y, Westall CA, et al. Ocular toxicity and antenatal exposure to chloroquine or hydroxychloroquine for rheumatic diseases. *Lancet* 2001; 358(9284): 813–814.

86 Motta M, Tincani A, Faden D, Zinzini E, Chirico G. Antimalarial agents in pregnancy. *Lancet* 2002; 359(9305): 524–525.

87 Levy RA, Vilela VS, Cataldo MJ, et al. Hydroxychloroquine (HCQ) in lupus pregnancy: double-blind and placebo-controlled study. *Lupus* 2001; 10(6): 401–404.

88 Ujhazy E, Balonova T, Durisova M, et al. Teratogenicity of cyclophosphamide in New Zealand white rabbits. *Neoplasma* 1993; 40: 45.

89 Enns GM, Roeder E, Chan RT, Ali-Khan Catts Z, Cox VA, Golabi M. Apparent cyclophosphamide (cytoxan) embryopathy: a distinct phenotype? *Am J Med Genet* 1999; 86(3): 237–241.

90 Kirshon B, Wasserstrum N, Willis R, Herman GE, McCabe ER. Teratogenic effects of first-trimester cyclophosphamide therapy. *Obstet Gynecol* 1988; 72(3 Pt 2): 462–464.

91 Macones GA, Robinson CA. Is there justification for using indomethacin in preterm labor? An analysis of neonatal risks and benefits. *Am J Obstet Gynecol* 1997; 177(4): 819–824.

92 Vermillion ST, Newman RB. Recent indomethacin tocolysis is not associated with neonatal complications in preterm infants. *Am J Obstet Gynecol* 1999; 181(5 Pt 1): 1083–1086.

93 Pryde PG, Besinger RE, Gianopoulos JG, Mittendorf R. Adverse and beneficial effects of tocolytic therapy. *Semin Perinatol* 2001; 25(5): 316–340.

94 Rauova L, Lukac J, Levy Y, Rovensky J, Shoenfeld Y. High-dose intravenous immunoglobulins for lupus nephritis – a salvage immunomodulation. *Lupus* 2001; 10(3): 209–213.

95 Zandman-Goddard G, Levy Y, Shoenfeld Y. Intravenous immunoglobulin therapy and systemic lupus erythematosus. *Clin Rev Allergy Immunol* 2005; 29(3): 219–228.

96 Austin HA, Balow JE. Treatment of lupus nephritis. *Semin Nephrol* 2000; 20(3): 265–276.

97 Nossent HC, Koldingsnes W. Long-term efficacy of azathioprine treatment for proliferative lupus nephritis. *Rheumatology* 2000; 39(9): 969–974.

98 Sesso R, Monteiro M, Sato E, Kirsztajn G, Silva L, Ajzen H. A controlled trial of pulse cyclophosphamide versus pulse methylprednisolone in severe lupus nephritis. *Lupus* 1994; 3(2): 107–112.

99 Miyakis S, Lockshin MD, Atsumi T, et al. International consensus statement on an update of the classification criteria for definite antiphospholipid syndrome (APS). *J Thromb Haemost* 2006; 4: 295–306.

100 Levine J, Branch DW, Rauch J. The antiphospholipid syndrome. *N Engl J Med* 2002; 346: 752–763.

101 Merani PL, Raschi E, Camera M, et al. Endothelial activation by aPL: a potential pathogenetic mechanism for the clinical manifestations of the syndrome. *J Autoimmun* 2000; 15: 237–240.

102 Vaarala O, Alfthan G, Jauhiainen M, Leirisalo-Repo M, Aho K, Palosuo T. Crossreaction between antibodies to oxidised low-density lipoprotein and to cardiolipin in systemic lupus erythematosus. *Lancet* 1993; 341: 923–925.
103 Hörkkö S, Miller E, Dudl E, et al. Antiphospholipid antibodies are directed against epitopes of oxidized phospholipids: recognition of cardiolipin by monoclonal antibodies to epitopes of oxidized low density lipoprotein. *J Clin Invest* 1996; 98: 815–825.
104 Shi W, Chong BH, Chesterman CN. b2-Glycoprotein I is a requirement for anticardiolipin antibodies binding to activated platelets: differences with lupus anticoagulants. *Blood* 1993; 81: 1255–1262.
105 Price BE, Rauch J, Shia MA, et al. Anti-phospholipid autoantibodies bind to apoptotic, but not viable, thymocytes in a beta 2-glycoprotein I-dependent manner. *J Immunol* 1996; 157: 2201–2208.
106 De Wolf F, Carreras LO, Moerman P, Vermylen J, van Assche A, Renaer M. Decidual vasculopathy and extensive placental infarction in a patient with repeated thromboembolic accidents, recurrent fetal loss, and a lupus anticoagulant. *Am J Obstet Gynecol* 1982; 142: 829–834.
107 Erlendsson K, Steinsson K, Johannsson JH, et al. Relation of antiphospholipid antibody and placental bed inflammatory vascular changes to the outcome of pregnancy in successive pregnancies of 2 women with systemic lupus erythematosus. *J Rheumatol* 1993; 20: 1779–1785.
108 Rand JH, Wu X-X, Andree HAM, et al. Pregnancy loss in the antiphospholipid-antibody syndrome – a possible thrombogenic mechanism. *N Engl J Med* 1997; 337: 154–160.
109 Di Simone N, Meroni PL, del Papa N, et al. Antiphospholipid antibodies affect trophoblast gonadotropin secretion and invasiveness by binding directly and through adhered beta2-glycoprotein I. *Arthritis Rheum* 2000; 43: 140–150.
110 Blank M, Cohen J, Toder V, et al. Induction of anti-phospholipid syndrome in naive mice with mouse lupus monoclonal and human polyclonal anti-cardiolipin antibodies. *Proc Natl Acad Sci USA* 1991; 88: 3069–3073.
111 Branch DW, Dudley DJ, Mitchell MD, et al. Immunoglobulin G fraction from patients with antiphospholipid antibodies cause fetal death in Balb/C mice: a model for autoimmune fetal loss. *Am J Obstet Gynecol* 1990; 163: 210–216.
112 Chamley LW, Pattison NS, McKay EJ. The effect of human anticardiolipin antibodies on murine pregnancy. *J Reprod Immunol* 1994; 27: 123–134.
113 Pierangeli SS, Liu XW, Barker JH, Anderson G, Harris EN. Induction of thrombosis in a mouse model by IgG, IgM and IgA immunoglobulins from patients with the antiphospholipid syndrome. *Thromb Haemost* 1995; 74: 1361–1367.
114 Girardi G, Berman J, Redecha P, et al. Complement C5a receptors and neutrophils mediate fetal injury in the antiphospholipid syndrome. *J Clin Invest* 2003; 112: 1644–1654.
115 Holers VM, Girardi G, Mo L, et al. Complement C3 activation is required for antiphospholipid antibody-induced fetal loss. *J Exp Med* 2002; 195(2): 211–220.
116 Salmon J, Girardi G. Antiphospholipid antibodies and pregnancy loss: a disorder of inflammation. *J Reprod Immunol* 2008; 77: 51–56.
117 Xu C, Mao D, Holers VM, et al. A critical role for murine complement regulator crry in fetomaternal tolerance. *Science* 2000; 287: 498–501.
118 Berman J, Girardi G, Salmon JE. TNF-alpha is a critical effector and a target for therapy in antiphospholipid antibody induced pregnancy loss. *J Immunol* 2005; 174: 485–490.
119 Wahl D, Guillemin F, de Maistre E, et al. Risk for venous thrombosis related to antiphospholipid antibodies in systemic lupus erythematosus – a meta-analysis. *Lupus* 1997; 6(5): 467–473.
120 Galli M, Luciani D, Bertolini G, Barbui T. Anti-beta 2-glycoprotein I, antiprothrombin antibodies, and the risk of thrombosis in the antiphospholipid syndrome. *Blood* 2003; 102(8): 2717–2723.
121 Crowther MA, Ginsberg JS, Julian J, et al. A comparison of two intensities of warfarin for the prevention of recurrent thrombosis in patients with the antiphospholipid antibody syndrome. *N Engl J Med* 2003; 349(12): 1133–1138.
122 Branch DW, Silver RM, Blackwell JL, et al. Outcome of treated pregnancies in women with antiphospholipid syndrome: an update of the Utah experience. *Obstet Gynecol* 1992; 80: 614–620.
123 Asherson RA, Cervera R, de Groot PG, et al. Catastrophic Antiphospholipid Syndrome Registry Project Group. Catastrophic antiphospholipid syndrome: international consensus statement on classification criteria and treatment guidelines. *Lupus* 2003; 12: 530–534.
124 Harris EN. Syndrome of the black swan. *Br J Rheumatol* 1987; 26: 324–326.
125 Branch DW. Immunologic disease and fetal death. *Clin Obstet Gynecol* 1987; 30: 295–311.
126 Oshiro BT, Silver RM, Scott JR, et al. Antiphospholipid antibodies and fetal death. *Obstet Gynecol* 1996; 87: 489–493.
127 Pattison NS, Chamley LW, McKay EJ, et al. Antiphospholipid antibodies in pregnancy: prevalence and clinical associations [see comments]. *Br J Obstet Gynecol* 1993; 100: 909–913.
128 Branch DW, Silver R, Pierangeli S, van Leeuwen I, Harris EN. Antiphospholipid antibodies other than lupus anticoagulant and anticardiolipin antibodies in women with recurrent pregnancy loss, fertile controls, and antiphospholipid syndrome. *Obstet Gynecol* 1997; 89: 549–555.
129 Clifford K, Rai R, Watson H, Regan L. An informative protocol for the investigation of recurrent miscarriage: preliminary experience of 500 consecutive cases. *Hum Reprod* 1994; 9: 1328–1332.
130 Kutteh WH. Antiphospholipid antibody-associated recurrent pregnancy loss: treatment with heparin and low-dose aspirin is superior to low-dose aspirin alone. *Am J Obstet Gynecol* 1996; 174: 1584–1589.
131 Pattison NS, Chamley LW, Birdsall M, Zanderigo AM, Liddell HS, McDougall J. Does aspirin have a role in improving pregnancy outcome for women with the antiphospholipid syndrome? A randomized controlled trial. *Am J Obstet Gynecol* 2000; 183: 1008–1012.
132 Rai R, Cohen H, Dave M, Regan L. Randomised controlled trial of aspirin and aspirin plus heparin in pregnant women with recurrent miscarriage associated with phospholipid antibodies (or antiphospholipid antibodies). *BMJ* 1997; 314: 253–257.
133 Yetman DL, Kutteh WH. Antiphospholipid antibody panels and recurrent pregnancy loss: prevalence of anticardiolipin antibodies compared with other antiphospholipid antibodies. *Fertil Steril* 1996; 66: 540–546.
134 Lima F, Khamashta MA, Buchanan NM, Kerslake S, Hunt BJ, Hughes GR. A study of sixty pregnancies in patients with the antiphospholipid syndrome. *Clin Exp Rheumatol* 1996; 14: 131–136.

135 Branch DW. Antiphospholipid antibodies and reproductive outcome: the current state of affairs. *J Reprod Immunol* 1998; 38(1): 75–87.
136 Cowchock FS, Reece EA, Balaban D, Branch DW, Plouffe L. Repeated fetal losses associated with antiphospholipid antibodies: a collaborative randomized trial comparing prednisone with low-dose heparin treatment. *Am J Obstet Gynecol* 1992; 166(5): 1318–1323.
137 Granger KA, Farquharson RG. Obstetric outcome in antiphospholipid syndrome. *Lupus* 1997; 6(6): 509–513.
138 Silver RK, MacGregor SN, Sholl JS, Hobart JM, Neerhof MG, Ragin A. Comparative trial of prednisone plus aspirin versus aspirin alone in the treatment of anticardiolipin antibody-positive obstetric patients. *Am J Obstet Gynecol* 1993; 169(6): 1411–1417.
139 Empson M, Lassere M, Craig JC, Scott JR. Recurrent pregnancy loss with antiphospholipid antibody: a systematic review of therapeutic trials. *Obstet Gynecol* 2002; 99(1): 135–144.
140 Empson M, Lassere M, Craig J, Scott J. Prevention of recurrent miscarriage for women with antiphospholipid antibody or lupus anticoagulant. *Cochrane Database Syst Rev* 2005; 2: CD002859.
141 Backos M, Rai R, Baxter N, Chilcott IT, Cohen H, Regan L. Pregnancy complications in women with recurrent miscarriage associated with antiphospholipid antibodies treated with low dose aspirin and heparin. *Br J Obstet Gynaecol* 1999; 106(2): 102–107.
142 Rivier G, Herranz MT, Khamashta MA, Hughes GR. Thrombosis and antiphospholipid syndrome: a preliminary assessment of three antithrombotic treatments. *Lupus* 1994; 3(2): 85–90.
143 Rosove MH, Brewer PM. Antiphospholipid thrombosis: clinical course after the first thrombotic event in 70 patients. *Ann Intern Med* 1992; 117(4): 303–308.
144 American College of Obstetricians and Gynecologists. *Thromboembolism in Pregnancy*. ACOG Practice Bulletin No. 19. Washington, DC: American College of Obstetricians and Gynecologists, 2000.
145 Ginsberg JS, Greer I, Hirsh J. Use of antithrombotic agents during pregnancy. *Chest* 2001; 119(1 Suppl): 122S–131S.
146 Erkan D, Merrill JT, Yazici Y, Sammaritano L, Buyon JP, Lockshin MD. High thrombosis rate after fetal loss in antiphospholipid syndrome: effective prophylaxis with aspirin. *Arthritis Rheum* 2001; 44(6): 1466–1467.
147 Welsch S, Branch DW. Antiphospholipid syndrome in pregnancy. Obstetric concerns and treatment. *Rheum Dis Clin North Am* 1997; 23(1): 71–84.
148 Dahlman TC. Osteoporotic fractures and the recurrence of thromboembolism during pregnancy and the puerperium in 184 women undergoing thromboprophylaxis with heparin. *Am J Obstet Gynecol* 1993; 168(4): 1265–1270.
149 Kelton JG. Heparin-induced thrombocytopenia: an overview. *Blood Rev* 2002; 16(1): 77–80.
150 Warkentin TE, Kelton JG. Delayed-onset heparin-induced thrombocytopenia and thrombosis. *Ann Intern Med* 2001; 135(7): 502–506.
151 Warkentin TE, Levine MN, Hirsh J, et al. Heparin-induced thrombocytopenia in patients treated with low-molecular-weight heparin or unfractionated heparin. *N Engl J Med* 1995; 332(20): 1330–1335.
152 Edwards MH, Pierangeli S, Liu X, Barker JH, Anderson G, Harris EN. Hydroxychloroquine reverses thrombogenic properties of antiphospholipid antibodies in mice. *Circulation* 1997; 96(12): 4380–434.
153 Clark AL, Branch DW, Silver RM, Harris EN, Pierangeli S, Spinnato JA. Pregnancy complicated by the antiphospholipid syndrome: outcomes with intravenous immunoglobulin therapy. *Obstet Gynecol* 1999; 93(3): 437–441.
154 Triolo G, Ferrante A, Ciccia F, et al. Randomized study of subcutaneous low molecular weight heparin plus aspirin versus intravenous immunoglobulin in the treatment of recurrent fetal loss associated with antiphospholipid antibodies. *Arthritis Rheum* 2003; 48: 728–731.
155 Branch DW, Peaceman AM, Druzin M, et al. A multicenter, placebo-controlled pilot study of intravenous immune globulin treatment of antiphospholipid syndrome during pregnancy. The Pregnancy Loss Study Group. *Am J Obstet Gynecol* 2000; 182(1 Pt 1): 122–127.
156 Cowchock S, Reece EA. Do low-risk pregnant women with antiphospholipid antibodies need to be treated? Organizing Group of the Antiphospholipid Antibody Treatment Trial. *Am J Obstet Gynecol* 1997; 176(5): 1099–1100.
157 Asherson RA, Khamashta MA, Ordi-Ros J, et al. The "primary" antiphospholipid syndrome: major clinical and serological features. *Medicine (Baltimore)* 1989; 68: 366–374.
158 Camera A, Rocco S, de Lucia D, et al. Reversible adult respiratory distress in primary antiphospholipid syndrome. *Haematologica* 2000; 85(2): 208–210.
159 Schaar CG, Ronday KH, Boets EP, van der Lubbe PA, Breedveld FC. Catastrophic manifestation of the antiphospholipid syndrome. *J Rheumatol* 1999; 26(10): 2261–2264.
160 Gomez-Puerta JA, Cervera R, Espinosa G, et al. Catastrophic antiphospholipid syndrome during pregnancy and puerperium: maternal and fetal characteristics of 15 cases. *Ann Rheum Dis* 2007; 66: 740–746.

37 Trauma in Pregnancy

James W. Van Hook

Department of Obstetrics and Gynecology, Division of Maternal-Fetal Medicine, University of Cincinnati College of Medicine, Cincinnati, OH, USA

Introduction

Acts of violence, accidental injury, and war make trauma in pregnancy a global problem. In the United States alone, major trauma affects up to 8% of pregnant patients, with life-threatening maternal injuries complicating 3–4 per 1000 deliveries [1] and is the leading cause of non-obstetric maternal death in the United States [2,3]. The US maternal death rate, secondary to trauma, was recently reported at 1.9/1000 live births [4], and abuse of a pregnant woman occurs in as many as 10% of pregnancies [5]. Thus, a multidisciplinary approach for the management of pregnant trauma victims is of great importance. In this chapter, we will discuss trauma itself and outline issues that relate to diagnosis, care and treatment of the pregnant trauma victim and her fetus.

Maternal physiologic adaptations applicable to trauma during pregnancy

Physiologic adjustments of pregnancy can have a significant impact on the pathophysiologic responses to trauma exhibited by the mother and her fetus. At the same time the physiologic changes of pregnancy may alter the clinician's ability to accurately diagnose the extent of the trauma and can influence maternal outcome. Although thoroughly reviewed throughout this text, the reiteration of physiologic changes of pregnancy as they may relate to the pregnant trauma patient are an important component of any discussion of trauma during gestation. The primary physiologic changes, applicable to the pregnant trauma victim, are summarized in Table 37.1. Key considerations peculiar to pregnancy include recognition of the expanded intravascular volume and its affect on cardiovascular changes and the recognition of hypovolemia. Additionally the gravid uterus may alter the mechanism of injury such as penetrating abdominal trauma and may affect certain diagnostic or therapeutic interventions such as thoracostomy tube placement and direct peritoneal lavage. Next we will review several aspects of pregnancy physiologic changes as they relate to traumatic injury.. Aortocaval compression, for example, by mid-pregnancy or later necessitates consideration of supine positioning of the gravid trauma victim. These and other related issues make the use of the expertise of the obstetrician, the trauma specialist and other subspecialists to optimize care of the pregnant accident victim.

Critical Care Obstetrics, 5th edition. Edited by M. Belfort, G. Saade, M. Foley, J. Phelan and G. Dildy.

Management of trauma

The American College of Surgeons has long advocated a standardized approach to the initial management of the trauma victim [42]. Resuscitation is based upon a systematic survey and intervention method. A modified basic algorithm for initial resuscitation of the pregnant trauma patient is provided in Figure 37.1.

Primary survey

The primary survey encompasses the immediate evaluation of the pregnant or non-pregnant trauma patient. The initials "A-B-C-D-E" are used to describe the steps of the primary survey (Figure 37.1) [1,6,7,8]. Little is different in performing the primary survey during pregnancy as compared to the non-pregnant individual. Foremost in the primary survey is stabilization of a proper airway ("A"). If an adequate functioning airway is not present, chin lift (with a stabilized neck and cervical spine) and oral or nasal airway insertion may be necessary. Early endotracheal intubation by qualified personnel must be performed if the just-described measures fail. Because of the potential for aspiration, intubation should be more aggressively pursued in the pregnant trauma victim than in her non-pregnant counterpart [9]. After airway stabilization, adequate respiration ("B") must be established. Supplemental oxygen is given as necessary and its adequacy assessed via pulse oximetry. Arterial blood gas determination, if

Table 37.1 Trauma-related maternal adaptation to pregnancy.

Parameter	Change	Implications
Plasma volume	Increases by 45–50%	Relative maternal resistance to limited blood loss
Red cell mass	Increases by 30%	Dilutional anemia
Cardiac output	Increases by 30–50%	Relative maternal resistance to limited blood loss
Uteroplacental blood flow	20–30% shunt	Uterine injury may predispose to increased blood loss Increased uterine vascularity
Uterine size	Dramatic increase	Increased incidence of uterine injury with abdominal trauma Change in position of abdominal contents Supine hypotension
Minute ventilation	Increases by 25–30%	Diminished P_aCO_2 Diminished buffering capacity
Functional residual volume	Decreased	Predisposition to atelectasis and hypoxemia
Gastric emptying	Delayed	Predisposition to aspiration

See text for sources of data.

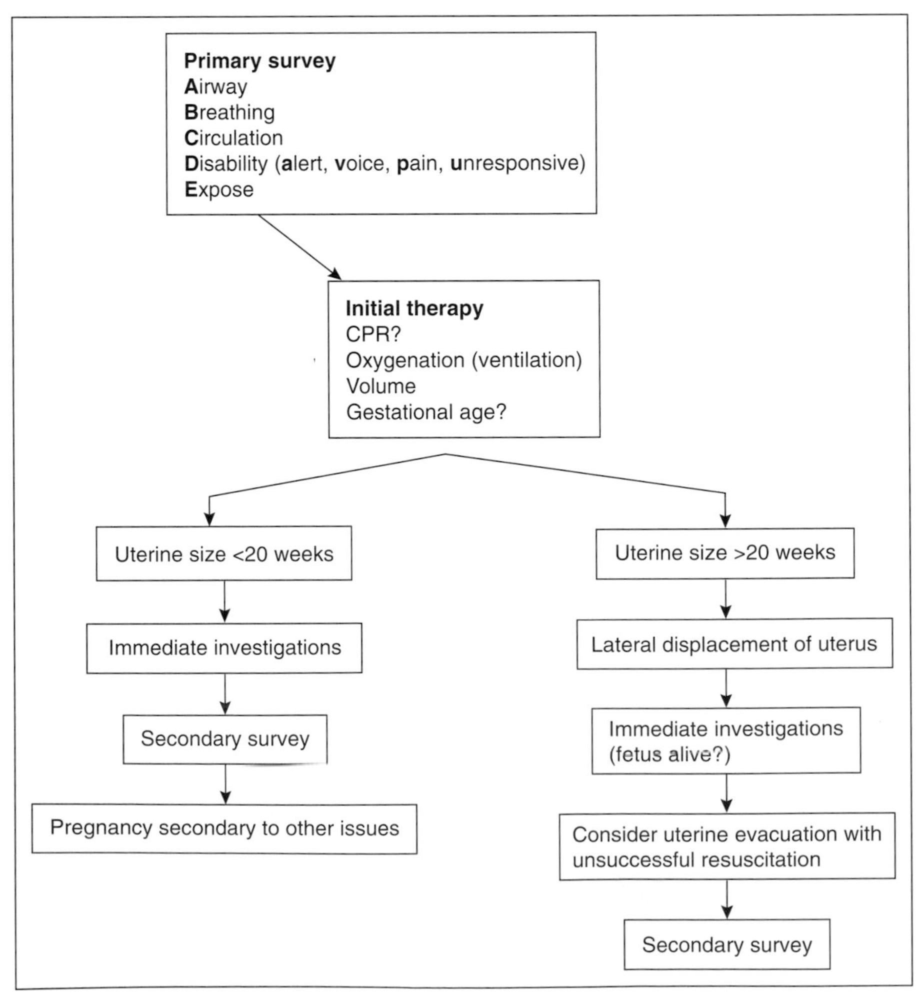

Figure 37.1 Initial resuscitation of the pregnant trauma patient. CRP, cardiopulmonary resuscitation. (See text for sources of data.)

obtained, must be interpreted in reference to what is normally found during pregnancy. A decreased serum bicarbonate level may be indicative of significant risk for fetal loss. One series reported that initial serum bicarbonate levels were significantly lower (16.4 ± 3.0 mEq/L versus 20.3 ± 2.2 mEq/L) in pregnant major trauma victims in which fetal loss was noted [10].

"C" refers to circulation. Pulse quality, blood pressure, and capillary refill are basic clinical determinants of the adequacy of perfusion. As mentioned earlier, clinical evaluation of maternal intravascular homeostasis is altered by the underlying physiologic changes of pregnancy. Also, fetal effects from maternal hypovolemia are not addressed by basic hemodynamic physical diagnosis [10–13]. In any case, because of the ongoing hemorrhage often present in any severely-injured trauma patient, immediate assessment and treatment of hypovolemia must be provided. In nearly all trauma cases, a large-bore (14 or 16G) intravenous (IV) access should be established Customarily, patients with multiple trauma should have a large-bore IV inserted in both an upper and lower extremity. Central venous access is not immediately indicated, provided adequate peripheral access can be established. An appropriately sized peripheral IV (14 or 16G) will provide the ability to rapidly instill large amounts of volume. Hypotension in the trauma patient is assumed to be hypovolemia until proven otherwise. Because of the blood volume changes described previously, it is not uncommon for pregnant patients to seemingly "tolerate" 1500–2000 mL of blood loss with only subtle hemodynamic changes. [1] Splanchnic and uterine blood flow may be, but are not always, compromised [12,13], and deterioration of the patient can develop rapidly with additional blood loss. Initial therapy for hypotension found during the primary survey is the rapid infusion of up to 2000 mL of crystalloid solution and preparation for blood transfusion as necessary. Cardiopulmonary resuscitation in the pregnant trauma victim, discussed in other chapters, is begun if no pulses are palpated.

Up to this point in the primary survey, obstetric, and non-obstetric management is very similar. However, at this stage of the resuscitation process, attention to great vessel compression by the gravid uterus must be addressed in pregnancies beyond 20 weeks gestation. In multiple trauma, because of potential vertebral injury, patients are generally placed on a rigid spinal "board" and usual methods for avoiding aortocaval compression (e.g. lateral roll, lateral tilt, etc.) are not possible. Manual lateral displacement of the uterus is performed to alleviate aortocaval compression. Alternatively, if the gravid trauma patient is on a trauma backboard, the entire board should be tilted 15° for stabilization of the vertebral column [6,14].

The letter "D" in the sequence stands for "disability". With any trauma, early neurological evaluation is undertaken. A rapid assessment is by the "A-V-P-U" method (*a*lert; *v*oice; *p*ain; *u*nresponsive) [6]. The Glasgow Coma Scale (GCS) can also be used (Table 37.2) [15,16]. A GCS of 8 or less may be indicative of significant ongoing neurologic pathology [17,18]. Use of the GCS allows general prognostication regarding the rate of craniotomy. In one non-obstetric study of level one trauma patients, subjects with a GCS of less than 8 had a 19% rate of craniotomy, those with GCS between 8 and 13 had a 9% rate of craniotomy, and victims who presented with a GCS of greater than 13 had a 3% need for craniotomy [19].

Table 37.2 Glascow Coma Scale.

	Points
Eye-opening response (E-score)	
Spontaneous (already open and blinking)	4
Opens in response to speech	3
Opens in response to pain (not to face)	2
No response	1
Verbal response (V-score)	
Oriented and appropriate response	5
Confused response	4
Inappropriate wording	3
Incomprehensible words	2
No response	1
Motor response (M-score)	
Obeys command	6
Localizes pain	5
Withdraws from pain	4
Flexion response to pain	3
Extension response to pain	2
No response	1

The Glasgow Coma Scale is the sum of scores in the three areas listed. A GCS score >8 is consistent with coma. Caregivers need to consider intubated patients' inability to speak.
Referenced in text.

Assessment of the patient with trauma in the fashion just described will immediately identify significant cardiovascular or central nervous system dysfunction. The next step in the evaluation is to expose ("E") the patient. "Expose" means completely undressing the patient and examining her from head to toe. The back is examined for entrance or exit wounds, the extremities are briefly palpated, and any obvious visible injuries are noted.

At this stage, the pregnant patient must undergo some preliminary determination of gestational age, the presence or absence of labor, and attempted measurement of fetal heart rate. Because of the potential for both fetal viability and the supine hypotension effects previously described, pregnancies greater than 20–24 weeks gestation evoke different management concerns than do gestations at less than the midpoint of pregnancy. Therefore, the crucial primary obstetric assessment of the pregnant trauma victim relates to a basic determination of gestational age of the pregnancy. For the patient undergoing CPR, perimortem cesarean section may be necessary. As stated previously, issues regarding mechanism of injury, abruption, preterm labor, and aortocaval compression all become important at or after the midpoint of pregnancy. Fetal heart activity may be addressed via direct auscultation or through the use of limited brief ultrasound (see FAST evaluation section). However, it should be emphasized that initial management of the pregnant patient should be the same as in the non-pregnant individual. This means that maternal health trumps fetal health. Once the pregnant trauma victim is stabilized, attention can then turn to assessing and managing fetal health. A key point to remember is that the leading cause of fetal mortality in trauma is maternal mortality, and rapid recognition and resuscitation reduce maternal mortality.

Investigations

At the conclusion of the primary survey, critical resuscitation is under way, major injuries are identified, and a general idea about the status of the pregnancy itself is known. At this juncture in management, diagnostic testing is ordered. *Immediate investigations* include necessary imaging studies, laboratory evaluation, and ancillary examination. "Fingers and/or tubes" should be placed in every orifice. Particular attention should be paid to the maternal bladder. Catheterization is undertaken and if gross hematuria is noted on the perineum, consideration of bladder, urethral, ureteral, renal or uterine trauma is essential. Evaluation for ruptured fetal membranes, cervical dilatation, vaginal bleeding, and fetal malpresentation is accomplished at this time. Cervical spine and other necessary radiographs are not contraindicated in the pregnant trauma victim. If otherwise indicated, pregnant trauma patients with multiple injuries should be considered candidates for chest and cervical vertebral radiographs. Other immediate investigations may include blood gas analysis, complete blood count, coagulation studies, serum electrolytes, and serum glucose determinations.

Measurement of fetomaternal hemorrhage (FMH) is also important and especially in Rhesus-negative (Rh-negative) [20] gravidas. The Kleihauer–Betke citric acid elution stain (KB) test can identify as little as 0.1 mL of fetal cells in the maternal circulation. The incidence of fetal–maternal hemorrhage is four- to fivefold higher in pregnant women who have experienced trauma than in uninjured controls. Therefore, 10–30% of pregnant trauma cases have some evidence of fetal/maternal admixture of blood [21,22]. Rh-negative gravidas who may be carrying an Rh-positive fetuses need Rh-immune globulin (RIG). In order to calculate the appropriate dose of RIG in the Rh-negative patient with evidence of FMH, Rose et al describe the following formula [23]:

$$(\text{number of fetal cells}/\text{number of adult cells}) \times \text{maternal red cell volume} = \text{fetal cells in maternal circulation}$$

One mL of RIG (300 µg) is used for each 15 mL of fetal cells or 30 mL of fetal blood detected. The mean volume of FMH is usually less than 15 mL of blood and over 90% exhibit less than 30 mL of FMH. Therefore, in the majority of such patients, 300 µg of RIG will suffice. Measurement of RIG in the maternal circulation on the day following administration via indirect Coombs assay should be weakly positive, thereby reflecting some residual "unused" RIG. If the follow-up indirect Coombs is negative, additional RIG may be needed [24–27]. Finally, even in the absence of detectable fetal cells in the Rh-negative and previously non-immunized trauma victim, administration of a 300-µg dose of RIG should be considered anyway, given the significant risk of FMH in the presence of trauma coupled with the relatively small amount of fetal blood required to sensitize the Rh-negative mother [14]. In addition to the use for maternal alloimmunization evaluation of the Rh-negative patient, FMH may also be a marker for occult or active placental abruption or uterine rupture, albeit less reliably than fetal heart rate monitoring or clinical signs [21,22,57]. Use of the KB test for issues other than RHIG administration testing should generally be for secondary or confirmatory evaluation of suspected conditions associated with FMH.

Secondary survey and treatment

At the conclusion of the primary survey, a second "top to bottom" physical assessment is made. This point in the resuscitation is ideal for a more extensive fetal evaluation. Earlier efforts were aimed at: (i) general evaluation of fetal age and presence of life; (ii) ascertainment of the appropriateness of perimortem cesarean section during unsuccessful CPR; (iii) minimizing the effects of uterine compression on maternal resuscitation; and (iv) indirect fetal resuscitation through successful maternal hemodynamic resuscitation. During the secondary survey, however, specific fetal investigations are indicated. Identification of vaginal bleeding, ruptured fetal membranes, preterm labor, placental abruption, direct uterine or fetal injury, and/or fetal distress are accomplished.

Fetal evaluation

Fetal injury or death from maternal trauma occurs by several mechanisms. Pearlman and Tintinalla (1990) noted a 41% fetal loss rate with life-threatening maternal injuries and a 1.6% fetal loss rate with non-life-threatening maternal injuries. More recently (2001), Weiss and colleagues, in a review of US birth certificate data, demonstrated a rate of fetal death from maternal trauma of 3.7 fetal deaths per 100 000 live births. Motor vehicle accidents were the leading cause of fetal traumatic death (2.3 fetal deaths per 100 000 live births) [28]. Generally, fetal loss is correlated with the severity of maternal injury; but unfortunately, lethal fetal injury has been encountered in the absence of significant maternal injury [29].

Placental abruption complicates up to 5% of otherwise minor injuries and up to 50% of major injuries during pregnancy [7,14,29,30]. Placental abruption is also a frequent cause of fetal death from trauma. The relatively inelastic placenta is thought to shear secondary to deformation of the much more elastic myometrium. Another possible mechanism is that placental abruption from traumatic injury may be a manifestation of placental fracture or laceration – again from decelerative force and/or direct injury. Uterine tenderness, uterine contractions, vaginal bleeding, and fetal heart rate abnormalities are clinical hallmarks of placental abruption. The association of contractions with traumatic placental abruption has been investigated by Williams (1990) and Pearlman. In the Williams' study of pregnant trauma patients placental abruption did not occur in women who did not have uterine contractions, or who had contractions at a frequency of less than 1 every 10 minutes after 4 hours of fetal monitoring. Whereas Pealman found no abruptions in the absence of uterine activity. In patients with more frequent contractions, nearly 20% had placental abruption. Other fetal heart rate abnormalities, such as bradycardia, late decelerations, and tachycardia were also frequently seen in patients who had experienced abruption [31]. Current evidence suggests that a period of continuous fetal monitoring is usually advisable in most cases of trauma during pregnancy of greater than 22–24 weeks' gestation. In those patients that are clinically unstable, prolonged monitoring is usually indicated [32]. Finally, placental abruption may be associated with a consumptive coagulopathy and, if so, it will be additive to other trauma-associated coagulopathies [33].

Thus, placental abruption is manifested by the presence of uterine activity within 4 hours of the traumatic event. In effect, the delayed manifestation of placental abruption is highly improbable and is often a delay in diagnosis rather than one of manifestation. The majority of catastrophic events occur much sooner. Patients with regular uterine contractions, or fetal heart rate abnormalities should be monitored until resolution of such findings. In patients without uterine contractions, fetal heart rate abnormalities, or other objective signs or symptoms of abruption it is suggested that a period of 2–6 hours of monitoring will suffice [32,34]. Electronic fetal monitoring is the preferred method to detect an abruption in the pregnant trauma victim of sufficient gestational age to warrant fetal monitoring. Ultrasonography is not a sensitive enough modality to diagnose many cases of placental abruption [32,35].

In the woman actively undergoing resuscitation, continuous electronic fetal monitoring of the potentially viable fetus is also a useful indicator of fetal response to and adequacy of resuscitation. Fetal heart rate monitoring has been useful for the identification of maternal hypovolemia [36]. Given the relatively large uteroplacental perfusion requirements during pregnancy, coupled with the poor placental autoregulation in the face of hypotension, the fetoplacental unit often may manifest pathophysiologic alterations in the absence of any obvious maternal manifestations of hypovolemia. The risk of fetal loss is directly related to the degree of maternal hemorrhagic shock [10]. Hence, aggressive volume replacement and shock treatment, coupled with continuous electronic fetal monitoring, is indicated in the gravid trauma victim who is otherwise a candidate for fetal monitoring.

The fetal patient

Direct fetal injuries and fractures complicate less than 1% of blunt traumatic injury during pregnancy [37,38]. The uterus of the early pregnant and non-pregnant patient is well protected by the bony pelvis. Direct fetal injury from blunt abdominal trauma often involves the fetal skull and head and is seen in the third trimester in patients with pelvic fractures [29]. This mechanism of injury may be due to the frequent occurrence of engagement of the fetal head within the confines of the bony pelvis late in pregnancy [39]. Decelerative injury to the unengaged fetal head may also occur [40].

Very few diagnostic or therapeutic interventions are *absolutely* contraindicated in the pregnant trauma victim with life-threatening injuries. While the effects of high doses of ionizing radiation on the fetus may be pronounced, the degree and amount of fetal exposure from routinely obtained conventional or computerized tomography (CT) radiography is considerably less. While an absolute lower threshold of safe exposure to ionizing radiation is not known, animal and human data show little or no risk to the fetus from up to 0.1 Gy or more of ionizing radiation [41–43]. A single pelvic film delivers less than 0.01 Gy to the fetus. Although fetal exposure is higher with CT scans or pyelography, they should not be avoided if needed to evaluate and treat the mother [29]. Despite the requirement to use fluoroscopy in conjunction with the technique, angiography may also be relatively beneficial to the pregnant trauma victim because of its ability to produce hemostasis [44]. As a general guideline for the practitioner, the maximum recommended dose by the National Council on Radiation Protection During Pregnancy is 0.5 cGy. Exposure levels of less than 5–15 cGy appear to have a relatively low risk of teratogenicity [43].

Few medications produce harmful fetal effects, and most teratogens impact only early pregnancy. With the supposition that fetal survival and well-being is directly related to maternal survival and well-being, most medically necessary interventions applied to the pregnant trauma victim are indicated for both maternal and fetal well-being. As a general guide, we would recommend an assessment of the risk versus benefit of medical therapy, and would consult available sources on whatever medications are to be used [45]. Tetanus toxoid administration and tetanus immune globulin are not contraindicated in the gravid trauma victim. Administration should be identical to that for the non-pregnant trauma patient.

As stated previously in this chapter, diagnostic ultrasound is not as sensitive as electronic fetal monitoring in the diagnosis of abruption [29,30,35]. Obstetric ultrasound is useful during the secondary evaluation of the pregnant trauma victim for measurement of fetal biometric indices, screening for direct trauma, and to aid in the biophysical assessment of the fetus.

Volume resuscitation in pregnancy

Volume replacement in pregnancy merits special consideration. By virtue of her young age, and the volume changes inherent in normal pregnancy, the pregnant woman may not exhibit clinically significant symptomatology of blood loss until 1500–2000 mL is lost. Blood loss greater than 2000 mL often produces rapid maternal deterioration. Because fetal status is a sensitive indicator of maternal hemodynamic homeostasis, fetal compromise may occur at maternal blood losses significantly less than

2000 mL. Fetal heart rate changes may be an early indicator of maternal hypovolemia. Initial treatment of suspected hypovolemia should consist of rapid infusion of isotonic crystalloid solution (normal saline or lactated Ringer's solution). Blood products should be considered in trauma with ongoing hemorrhage greater than 1000 mL. Type- and Rh-specific blood should be available as soon as possible. Until blood is available, isotonic crystalloid solutions is replaced at a rate of 3 cc for each cc of estimated blood loss [6]. While some feel that whole blood may be preferable to packed red blood cells, it is generally not available. Component therapy should not be given empirically, except perhaps in the case of massive exsanguination. Recent experience with the use of recombinant activated factor VII in trauma and massive exsanguination may make factor VIIa a choice to consider in the resuscitation of difficult to control bleeding in pregnant trauma victims [46,47]. Limited pregnancy data suggest efficacy in HELLP syndrome and uterine rupture [48,49]. Although stabilization of the patient is usually recommended prior to surgical treatment, catastrophic traumatic hemorrhage may necessitate concomitant volume and component resuscitation together with immediate surgical control of hemorrhage.

Initial resuscitation goals include restoration of maternal vital signs, normalization of fetal heart rate, and resumption of normal urine output. It should be reemphasized that up to a 20% reduction in uteroplacental blood flow can occur without changes in maternal blood pressure. Maternal resuscitation should be taken in the context of fetal resuscitation during pregnancy [29,50].

Perimortem cesarean section

Under normal circumstances, cesarean section in the trauma victim is reserved for the usual obstetric indications and is performed at gestational ages consistent with fetal viability. Unique clinical circumstances may alter these guidelines somewhat when perimortem cesarean section is considered during unsuccessful maternal cardiopulmonary resuscitation (CPR). Uterine evacuation may be indicated for either maternal or fetal reasons, or both. The issue of perimortem cesarean section is addressed in other chapters of this text. Katz et al. have reviewed (1986) and recently updated (2005) known reported experience with perimortem cesarean section [51,52]. A modified algorithm for perimortem cesarean section in the face of major trauma is listed in Figure 37.2.

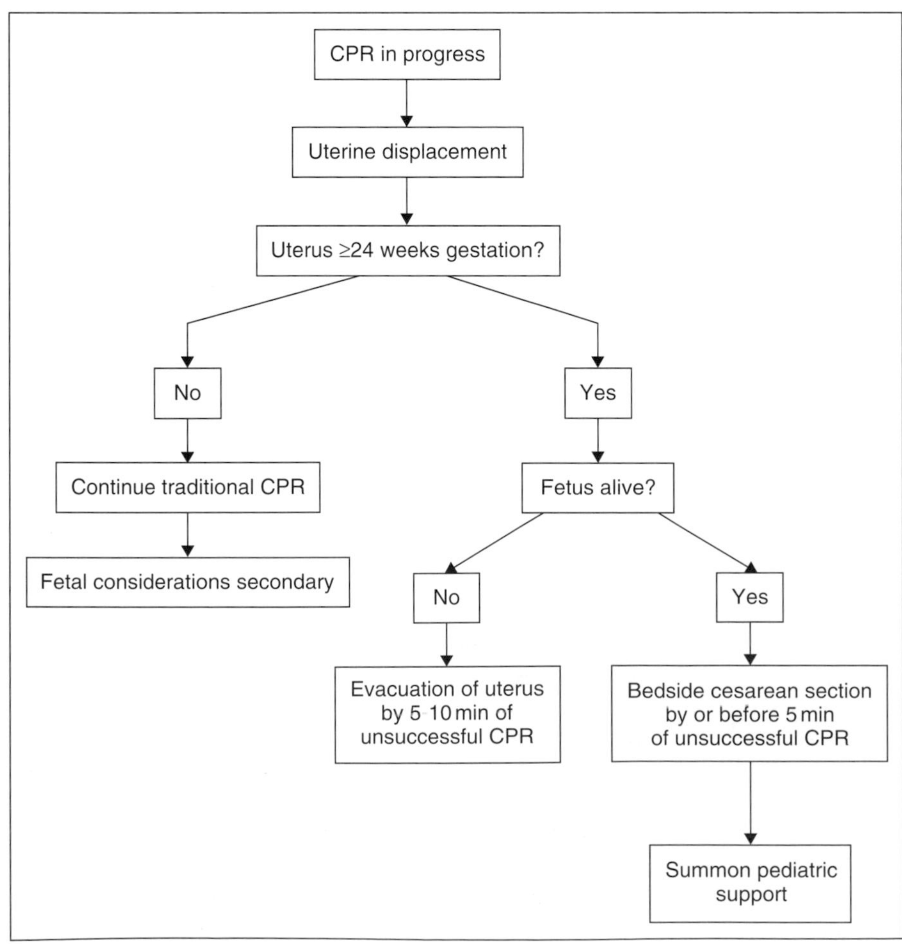

Figure 37.2 Perimortem cesarean section. (From Katz VL, Dotters DJ, Droegemueller W. Perimortem cesarean delivery. *Obstet Gynecol* 1986; 68: 571.)

Manifestations of trauma during pregnancy

Blunt abdominal trauma

Motor vehicle accidents account for a large portion of severe blunt obstetric trauma. Other lesser causes of blunt abdominal trauma include accidental falls and intentional trauma (violence) [20,22,32,53,54]. During the third trimester of pregnancy, the fetus is more vulnerable to injury due to the thinning of the uterine wall and a reduction in the amniotic fluid volume. Engagement of the fetal head into the maternal pelvis predisposes the fetus to head trauma associated with pelvic injury [55].

Motor vehicle accidents

Passenger restraint systems reduce maternal and fetal injury in motor vehicle accidents (MVAs). In accidents where occupant restraints were not used, the most common cause of fetal death was maternal death [56]. Expulsion from the vehicle and the presence of coexisting head trauma portend poor maternal and fetal outcome. To illustrate, Crosby and Costiloe (1971) noted a 33% mortality in unrestrained gravid automobile accident victims compared to a 5% mortality in those pregnant victims using two-point restraints (traditional lap belt) [56]. The fetal death rate was also lower in the restraint group. The three-point restraint system (lap and shoulder belt) limits "jack-knifing" of the gravid abdomen during sudden deceleration. Furthermore, Pearlman and associates noted that the proper use of seat belts was the best predictor of maternal and fetal outcome in crashes controlled for severity of collision [57]. In the properly restrained pregnant occupant, placental abruption rather than maternal death was the greatest cause of fetal death. The use of airbags, in conjunction with proper positioning of the mother and correctly placed and used three point restraints afford the best protection to the pregnant mother and her unborn child. At present, the National Highway Traffic Safety Administration does not consider pregnancy as a reason to deactivate the airbags [58]. This is supported by the work of Moorcroft et al. who concluded that, for all frontal impacts, it is safer for the pregnant occupant of an automobile to be properly belted via three-point restraint in a seat in proper apposition to a impact specific deployable airbag [59]. In MVAs, the majority of fetal deaths occur in conjunction with relatively minor maternal injury and most are due to placental abruption [32,60–62]. Less frequently, fetal death can be associated with fetal skull fracture and intracranial hemorrhage [55]. To protect against fetal injury, the lap belts should be positioned low across the bony pelvis instead of over the mid or upper uterine fundus. Incorrect placement of the lap belt over the uterine fundus could result in an increase in direct force transmission to the uterus during decelerative trauma. Close proximity to airbags markedly increases the transmural forces applied to the maternal abdomen and uterus [59]. The transmission of direct force may result in placental abruption [63]. Shoulder belts should be adjusted for comfort to lie above the gravid uterus and be located between below the breasts [66]. Although fetal injury and death have been attributed to lap belts, restraint systems are still recommended and in most states are mandatory [32]. Available data from crash test dummy simulations of restrained collision during pregnancy suggest that there does not appear to be extraordinary force transmission to the pregnant uterus when seat belts are properly placed [32,64,65,66].

Fetal manifestations of blunt trauma

The severity of blunt abdominal trauma is associated with the likelihood of placental abruption. Trauma-induced placental abruption is manifested by the appearance of contractions within 4 hours of the traumatic event. The severity of the trauma and mechanism of injury does not directly correlate with the incidence or severity of fetomaternal hemorrhage. Relatively minor direct blunt abdominal trauma may infrequently produce placental abruption and/or fetomaternal hemorrhage.

Evaluation of the blunt abdominal trauma victim

Evaluation of the pregnant patient with blunt abdominal trauma is similar to that for the non-pregnant patient. However, and depending on the gestational age, the gravid uterus may alter the typical patterns of injury seen in blunt trauma. For example, bowel injury is less frequent in the pregnant blunt trauma victims when compared to their non-pregnant counterparts [21]; whereas hepatic and splenic injury are more frequent during pregnancy. In cases of severe blunt abdominal trauma, hemodynamically significant hepatic and/or splenic injuries [9,14] can be seen in up to 25% of victims. Upper abdominal pain, referred shoulder pain, sudden onset of pain, and elevated transaminases suggest hepatic or splenic injury.

Abdominal ultrasound is particularly useful in the identification of intraperitoneal fluid collections secondary to hemorrhage in these cases. Over the last several years, the evaluation of traumatic blunt abdominal injury has changed to often include the FAST exam ("Focused Assessment with Sonography for Trauma") [67,68]. The FAST exam consists of a four-part brief evaluation of the pericardium, perihepatic (RUQ), perisplenic (LUQ), and pelvic regions via ultrasound. Use of the FAST exam, therefore, allows rapid initial bedside assessment for the presence of free fluid in the abdomen and the presence of a pericardial effusion. In the blunt abdominal and/or chest trauma, FAST examination is a useful screen for the presumptive presence of intra-abdominal hemorrhage, traumatic or non-traumatic pleural effusions, or for corroboration of a suspected hemopericardium. Sensitivity and specificity in experienced hands demonstrate up to 100% sensitivity and specificity for the evaluation of abdominal hemorrhage in the hypertensive blunt trauma victim [69,70].

The use of FAST in the female patient frequently will demonstrate intra-abdominal hemorrhage via a fluid collection in the pouch of Douglas. FAST examination has been shown to be an effective tool for use during pregnancy. Brown and colleagues (2005) reported on the accuracy of FAST in 102 pregnant trauma victims. Sensitivity and specificity for the determination of intra-abdominal hemorrhage were 80% and 100%, respectively [71].

Other methods used to assess the presence and severity of intra-abdominal bleeding include CT radiography and diagnostic peritoneal lavage. Hemodynamically stable patients with ultrasound-identified abdominal fluid may have characterization of the fluid source and nature through the use of CT scanning [72,73]. The sensitivity and specificity of abdominal ultrasonography to detect intraperitoneal fluid associated with intra-abdominal lesions have been demonstrated to be similar to those seen in non-pregnant individuals. Patients with no intraperitoneal fluid visible by ultrasound are usually at low risk of having intra-abdominal lesions requiring immediate operative management.

CT radiography scanning may aid diagnosis in less obvious cases. Hemodynamically stable patients with the ultrasound-identified abdominal fluid may have characterization of the fluid source and nature through use of CT scanning. Embolization or hepatic lobe resection, coupled with packing and local control may ameliorate hepatic hemorrhage. Splenectomy is generally the preferred treatment for splenic rupture. Other indications for exploratory laparotomy in the pregnant patient with blunt abdominal trauma include hemodynamic instability with suspected active bleeding, viscus perforation, infection, and fetal distress in the viable gestation.

Direct peritoneal lavage (DPL) may also be used in pregnancy. However, the open technique should nearly always be the method of choice in pregnancy beyond the first trimester of pregnancy. The FAST examination reduces the necessity for DPL (Figure 37.3) and its usefulness is limited to cases with conflicting FAST and CT results [71] is markedly reduced [71]. Theoretically the procedure-associated risks of DPL may often be avoided. Its mention here in this chapter is merely for completeness. Criteria for a positive DPL include aspiration of at least 10 mL of gross blood, a bloody lavage effluent, a serum amylase of >175 IU/dL, a red blood cell count of >100 000/mm^3, a white blood cell count of >500/mm^3 or the detection of bile, gastrointestinal contents or bacteria [74]. Fetal outcome is not adversely affected by the performance of a DPL during pregnancy. However, FAST examination often makes DPL a less-used diagnostic modality in pregnant trauma evaluation.

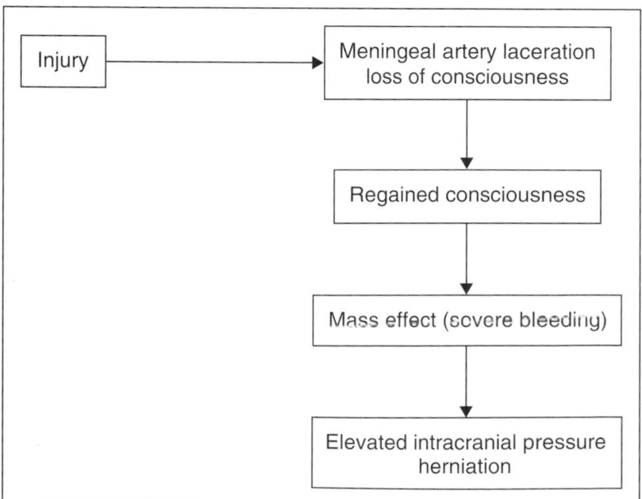

Figure 37.3 Sequence of events associated with acute epidural hemorrhage.

Unstable patients with FAST, DPL and/or CT findings may have surgical treatment directed toward the abdomen. Unstable patients with an expanding abdomen should generally not have definitive therapy delayed by these evaluative tests. Figure 37.4 outlines a suggested use of FAST, DPL, and CT examinations in blunt abdominal trauma.

Maternal volume changes and pregnancy-associated intra-abdominal anatomical alterations may mask significant intra-abdominal injuries. For example, Baerga et al. [75] found that 44% of pregnant abdominal trauma victims who eventually required laparotomy for intra-abdominal pathology were initially asymptomatic. The presence of maternal hypotension (systolic blood pressure <90 mmHg) and tachycardia may represent late findings. Consequently, the risk of pregnancy loss is much higher in such cases [75]. Rib or pelvic fractures in the pregnant trauma victim should heighten one's suspicion for hepatic, splenic, genitourinary, uterine, or other abdominal injury [1,76]. Uterine rupture may also occur and is more likely in patients with a history of prior cesarean section. In patients without a surgically scarred uterus, uterine rupture often involves the posterior aspect of the uterus [55].

Another leading cause of blunt abdominal trauma is physical abuse during pregnancy. It is estimated that between 1 in 6 and 1 in 10 pregnant women will experience physical or sexual abuse at some time during pregnancy. In addition to blunt abdominal trauma, other injuries commonly occur on the face, neck, and proximal extremities. Serious fetal injury or death may not always be related to the degree of maternal injury from physical abuse. In one analysis of fetal death from maternal injury secondary to interpersonal violence, 5 of 8 fetal deaths occurred in those that otherwise appeared to be minimally injured [76]. Providers must maintain an index of suspicion for physical or sexual abuse during pregnancy [77–79].

Traumatic uterine rupture

Uterine rupture is a relatively infrequent complication of blunt traumatic injury during pregnancy. The incidence does tend to increase with advancing gestational age and the severity of direct traumatic abdominal force of injury. Most traumatic uterine rupture involves the uterine fundus. Other locations and degrees of uterine injury may be found. At least one case of complete transection of the gravid uterus has been reported as a result of blunt vehicular trauma combined with incorrect seat belt positioning [80]. Principles of management and repair of uterine rupture secondary to trauma are similar to those used in treatment of non-traumatic uterine rupture. As reviewed later in this chapter, pelvic fractures as a result of blunt trauma during pregnancy may result in significant retroperitoneal bleeding. Regarding delivery route in a future pregnancy, the past presence

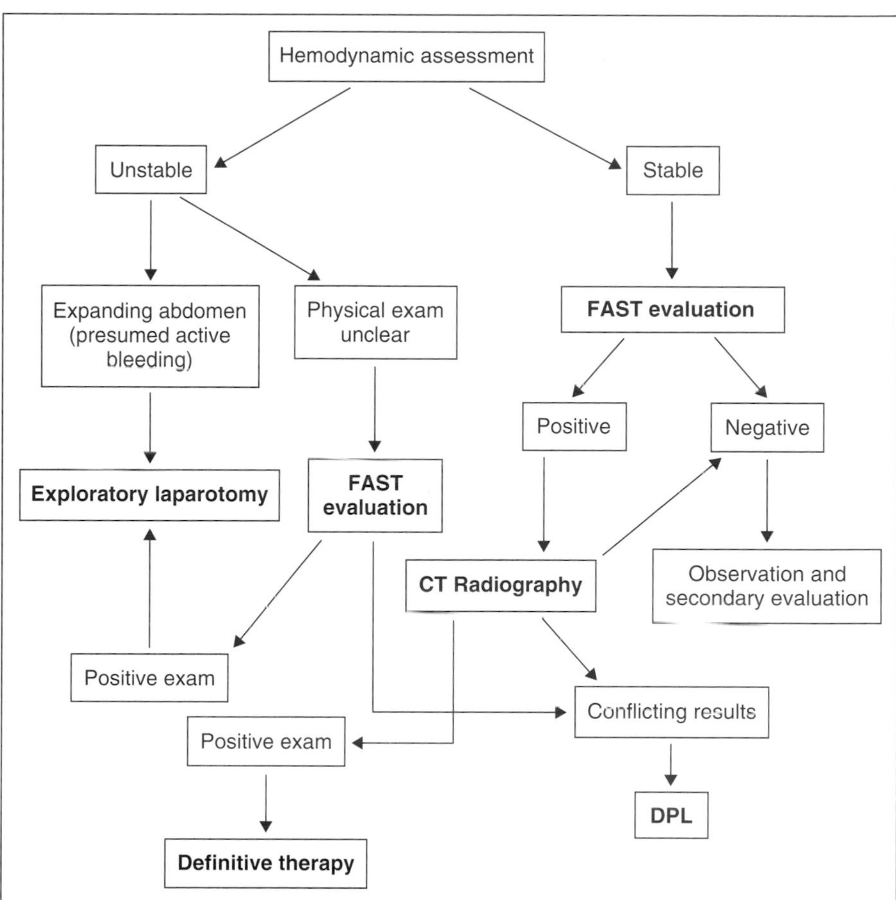

Figure 37.4 Diagnostic abdominal evaluation – blunt trauma, CT. CT, radiograph; FAST, focused assessment with sonography for trauma; DPL, direct peritoneal lavage.

of a pelvic fracture is not an absolute contraindication for vaginal delivery. Provided pelvic architecture is not substantially disrupted and the old fracture is not unstable, safe vaginal delivery is often possible.

Penetrating abdominal trauma

The two most common types of penetrating abdominal injury are stab and gunshot wounds. As with blunt trauma, pregnancy often changes the usual manifestations of penetrating abdominal injury. The gravid uterus displaces lower abdominal organs cephalad. Therefore, after the first trimester, the gravid uterus is somewhat protective of other intra-abdominal organs. Accordingly, reported maternal mortality is lower from abdominal gunshot wounds than it is in non-pregnant adults (3.9% versus 12.5%). Fetal mortality (71%), however, is high [81]. Reported data from abdominal stab wounds were similar in that fetal mortality was high (42%) and maternal mortality was not seen [82]. The reduced maternal mortality, yet high fetal loss, from penetrating abdominal injury are probably due to the gravid uterus shielding other abdominal contents from the force of the penetrating projectile when the impact of the shell or penetrating object is below the uterine fundus [1,29,81,82]. In contrast, upper abdominal penetrating injuries are more likely to produce small bowel injury in the advanced gravida than would occur in non-pregnant victims.

Gunshot wounds

Management of gunshot wounds to the pregnant abdomen includes general resuscitation measures outlined previously. Particular attention should be paid to the pathway of the projectile. Entry and exit wounds must both be identified. If the missile has not exited the abdomen, radiographic localization aids bullet location and injury prognostication. Gunshot projectiles that enter into the uterus often will remain *in utero*. Penetrating trauma occurring anteriorly and above the uterine fundus or from the maternal back carries a high risk of extrauterine visceral injuries. Patients in whom the missile entered anteriorly and below the uterine fundus often do not have maternal visceral involvement [83]. Fetal death may be direct or indirect. Most authors recommend abdominal exploration for all extrauterine intra-abdominal gunshot wounds and most intrauterine wounds. Experience from the Middle East conflict and other reports suggest an individualized approach to intrauterine injuries [9,84]. Awwad and colleagues advocate conservative management in anterior abdominal entry wounds which enter below the uterine fundus [85]. Posterior abdominal wounds, upper abdominal wounds, fetal or maternal compromise, or uterine location of projectile in cases of gunshot wound are not, according to Awwad, optimal for expectant management. We generally advocate surgical exploration of the pregnant intra-abdominal gunshot wound victim, although individualized circumstances may permit a modified approach [86,112].

Stab wounds

Abdominal stab wounds generally are less serious than gunshot wounds. Because of less likelihood for "collateral damage", many pregnant stab wound victims will not have abdominal organ damage that requires surgical repair. Because of the compartmentalization that occurs with advanced pregnancy, the mechanism of injury changes with abdominal stab wounds during pregnancy. Small bowel involvement is more frequent with upper abdominal stab wounds during pregnancy [10,14]. Also, the upper abdomen is the most frequent site of abdominal stab wounds during pregnancy, comprising some two out of three anterior abdominal penetrating wounds [9]. Because of the propensity for small intestinal injury and the potentially catastrophic effects of diaphragmatic involvement with up to a 66% mortality with thoracic herniation and strangulation of small intestine, most recommend exploration of upper abdominal stab wounds during pregnancy.

Depending on the gestational age of the pregnancy, lower abdominal stab wounds during pregnancy may involve the uterus, fetus, uteropelvic vessels, or urinary bladder. An individualized approach to management is suggested. FAST evaluation, CT radiography, and possibly DPL are useful to evaluate intra-abdominal bleeding [29]. Amniocentesis and ultrasound may help in the evaluation of intrauterine bleeding. Urinary bladder involvement may be determined by radiographic evaluation [9]. Actual abdominal cavity entry can be determined through direct exploration of the wound or the performance of a wound fistulogram [87]. While not all lower abdominal stab wounds need to be explored, a very high index of suspicion for the need to explore the abdomen should be maintained.

Direct uterine injury

During exploratory laparotomy for penetrating abdominal trauma, the uterus must be carefully inspected for injury. If direct uterine perforation is noted in the presence of a living term fetus, abdominal delivery is probably warranted. Less extensive uterine or adnexal injury or the presence of intrauterine fetal death does not necessarily dictate emptying of the uterus [88]. Likewise, the uterus should not necessarily be emptied via cesarean section or hysterectomy during surgery for non-uterine injuries. In cases in which direct uterine injury is found and the fetus is alive, premature, but potentially viable, cesarean section may be obvious for fetal or maternal hemorrhage or intrauterine infection [1,9,89]. These are incredibly difficult cases and will require an assessment of the risk : benefit ratio of expectant management versus delivery by cesarean section specific to the best estimate of gestational age, of fetal injury, and of both the maternal and fetal prognosis if left undelivered.

Other obstetric considerations for delivery also apply in that direct uterine injury to the active uterine segment probably necessitates eventual cesarean section as the preferred route of delivery. Injury to the lower uterine segment with delayed delivery probably needs to be approached on an individual case-by-case basis.

In cases of direct uterine injury, preterm labor may be treated with tocolytics, although betasympathomimetics and non-steroidal anti inflammatory agents generally should be avoided because of their effects upon maternal hemodynamics and platelet function, respectively [90,91]. From a hemodynamic perspective, magnesium sulfate would probably be the drug of choice for treatment of preterm labor in the circumstance of maternal trauma. General consensus is probably not present regarding preference and/or indicated use of tocolytics for idiopathic preterm labor. Therefore, little non-anecdotal data are available to make an evidence-based recommendation on the use of tocolytics for the treatment of preterm labor in the pregnant trauma patient. It is obvious to state that maternal instability, non-reassuring fetal status, or active uterine bleeding are generally contraindications to tocolytic therapy.

Victims of penetrating trauma should receive tetanus prophylaxis as needed. In the previously immunized patient with no booster within the last 5 years, 0.5 mL of tetanus toxoid is administered. If the patient has not been previously immunized, the toxoid is administered in conjunction with tetanus immunoglobulin at a dose of 500 U intramuscularly [92].

Chest trauma

Thoracic trauma represents a particular challenge to the clinician caring for the pregnant trauma victim. There is a paucity of information regarding thoracic trauma (or its management) during pregnancy. In the United States, chest trauma accounts for 1 in 4 trauma deaths annually. Recognition and stabilization of chest trauma is vital, because less than 10% of blunt chest trauma and less than 30% of penetrating chest injuries require immediate thoracotomy [6,74]. Most cases of thoracic trauma initially respond to non-surgical stabilization. Effective stabilization ultimately results in improved operative outcome if surgery is required. A basic understanding of the types of chest trauma will help the obstetric member of the trauma team function more effectively in the overall resuscitation of the injured gravida.

Classification of chest trauma

Chest trauma can be classified functionally or mechanistically. Mechanistically, thoracic trauma is subdivided into blunt and penetrating injuries (much like abdominal trauma). More immediately important is the recognition of immediately life-threatening chest trauma, with differentiation of life-threatening trauma from potentially serious, but less immediately life-threatening subtypes of chest trauma. In this discussion we will generally divide chest trauma into immediately life-threatening and non-life-threatening subtypes [6,84].

Table 37.3 Life-threatening chest injuries.

Immediately life threatening	Initial treatment*
Airway obstruction	Airway control
Open pneumothorax	Injury site control and thoracotomy tube
Tension pneumothorax	Needle thoracostomy
Flail chest	Supportive (± intubation)
Cardiac tamponade	Volume therapy and pericardiocentesis
Severe myocardiac damage	Inotropic support and treatment of dysrhythmias

* Qualified consultants should be involved in the care of any chest trauma patient. These treatment recommendations are guidelines. Each case should be individualized.

The primary survey of a trauma patient will identify several types of life-threatening thoracic trauma. When identified, life-threatening injuries require expedient management. Fortunately, many immediately life-threatening injuries can be initially managed by oxygen administration, mechanical ventilation, needle pneumothoracocentesis, or tube thoracostomy (chest tube) placement. Life-threatening chest injuries (Table 37.3) include airway obstruction, open pneumothorax, massive hemothorax, tension pneumothorax, flail chest, cardiac tamponade, and blunt trauma-mediated severe myocardial dysfunction (blunt cardiac injury).

Airway management

Airway obstruction should be managed initially as described elsewhere in this text with CPR, and then systematically with early intubation or cricothyroidotomy, if required. Cervical spine protection by neck stabilization and jaw thrust is vital during intubation of any patient with an unevaluated cervical spine. In pregnancy, the additional increased risk of aspiration of gastric contents may necessitate the more aggressive use of endotracheal intubation or surgical airway control. The requirement for oxygenation and effective pulmonary gas exchange precedes all other aspects of resuscitation [18,93].

Tension pneumothorax

Tension pneumothorax develops when a one-way flow of gas collects in the pleural space. Intrapleural pressure increases progressively with each inspiration. When intrapleural pressure increases to a level higher than great vessel pressures, hemodynamic instability can result. The clinical diagnosis of a tension pneumothorax is made by a combination of respiratory distress, hypotension, tachycardia, diminished or absent breath sounds, possible jugular venous distention, and tracheal deviation. The differential diagnosis of tension pneumothorax includes massive hemothorax (similar thoracic pathophysiology and treatment) and pericardial tamponade (much less common) [94]. Radiographic confirmation of a suspected tension pneumothorax is usually only useful for postmortem correlation [95].

In addition to trauma, other causes of tension pneumothorax include central line placement, bullous emphysema, and mechanical ventilation. Regardless of its etiology, immediate recognition and treatment of a tension pneumothorax or massive hemothorax is vital. Needle thoracostomy, performed in the second intercostal space–mid-clavicular line, will convert a tension pneumothorax to a simple pneumothorax. Definitive treatment is by insertion of a thoracostomy tube in the affected hemithorax. For this indication, a thoracostomy tube is usually placed in the fifth intercostal space (nipple level), anterior to the mid-axillary line [96]. Additional care during pregnancy must be taken, because of the normally elevated diaphragm [1]. Inadvertent abdominal insertion of a chest tube with the resultant diaphragmatic, hepatic, or splenic injury is potentially more likely during pregnancy. Particular attention to this potentially catastrophic complication must be heeded if additional thoracostomy tubes are placed in locations other than the anterior mid-axillary fifth intercostal space and especially if such tubes are placed in lower intercostal spaces. To reduce the chance of abdominal placement, consideration should be taken to place the thoracostomy tube at least one interspace higher than usual.

Hemothorax

Massive hemothorax is initially treated by thoracostomy tube placement as previously described. To facilitate drainage of thoracic blood, the chest tube should be directed inferiorly (after its insertion in the mid-axillary fifth intercostal space). Once again, care should be taken to avoid abdominal entry. A large chest tube (i.e. 38 French) is usually recommended. If the initial volume of blood drained from the tube is ≥1500 mL, early thoracotomy is probably necessary. Continued loss of 300 mL or more per hour from the chest tube may also indicate the need of a thoracotomy. Other temporizing measures such as volume replacement, transfusion, and potential use of cell-saving autotransfusion should be initiated until the patient is evaluated by a qualified thoracic trauma surgeon [94,97,98].

Open pneumothorax

Open pneumothorax is often referred to as a "sucking chest wound". If the size of the opening to the hemothorax is near to or greater than the size of the tracheal diameter, physics dictates that air will preferentially enter the chest through the chest wall rather than through the trachea during inspiratory attempts. Consequently, to temporarily restore effective ventilation, a large occlusive dressing is placed upon the open injury. Ultimately, thoracostomy tube placement at a site distal to the thoracic entry wound and surgical repair is required [74].

Cardiac tamponade

Cardiac tamponade has been mentioned previously in our discussion of tension pneumothorax. Tamponade usually occurs with penetrating injuries, and is less common than tension pneumothorax. Catastrophic hypotension and, ultimately, pulseless electrical activity (electromechanical disassociation) result from cardiac tamponade. Because of non-compliance of the pericardial sac, a relatively small amount of rapidly collected blood will cause hemodynamic compromise. Diagnosis is possible by clinical features (Becks' triad: venous pressure elevation, decreased arterial pressure, and muffled heart tones), radiographic examination (enlarged cardiac silhouette), or echocardiography. Unfortunately, as with tension pneumothorax, time is often not available to definitively diagnose cardiac tamponade. Pericardiocentesis by a qualified operator is a life-saving temporizing measure. Rapid volume infusion will also often temporarily alleviate the problem. As with thoracostomy tube placement, pericardiocentesis should be undertaken with recognition of the fact that the pregnant patient's diaphragm is normally elevated. Definitive treatment of pericardiocentesis is usually by the opening of the pericardium by a qualified thoracic trauma surgeon [99,100].

Flail chest

Flail chest occurs secondary to trauma-mediated separation of a part of the bony chest wall from the remaining thorax. Respiratory failure from pain-induced atelectasis and underlying pulmonary contusion is produced by flail chest [101,102]. Paradoxical movement of part of the chest during respiration, direct physical examination of the chest and radiographic evaluation lead to the diagnosis of this condition. Intubation and mechanical ventilation may be required in the flail chest victim with intractable hypoxemia or other injuries [93,94].

Blunt cardiac injury

Massive chest trauma can produce intrinsic myocardial damage. Myocardial contusion, myocardial ischemia from hypoperfusion, or underlying substance abuse all may cause or contribute to myocardial injury. Because trauma-mediated myocardial injury may not occur *per se* in association with a contusion itself, the term "myocardial contusion" has been supplanted by the more accurate term "blunt cardiac injury" (BCI). Although usually diagnosed during the secondary survey, potentially lethal dysrhythmias can also be noted during the primary survey. These dysrhythmias may be produced by the initial injury or from reperfusion of the injured myocardium. Standard treatment of such dysrhythmias is recommended to reduce the likelihood of malignant degeneration of the rhythm or cardiac arrest [103–106]. Patients at a lower risk of life-threatening dysrythmia development can be determined through the use of ECG screening. A troponin I level of less than 1.5 ng/mL 8 hours after injury is also consistent with stable prognosis [107].

Other thoracic traumatic injuries

The secondary survey may also uncover evolving life-threatening thoracic injuries, although *usually* the progression of such injuries is less fulminant than when they are diagnosed during the primary survey. Potentially lethal secondary survey injuries include pulmonary or myocardial contusion, aortic esophageal disruption, tracheal or bronchial rupture, and traumatic diaphragmatic rupture [6].

Pulmonary contusion is a very frequent complication of blunt chest trauma [74]. Progressive hypoxemia results from the secondary effects of the contusion. Typically, respiratory failure from pulmonary contusion progresses insidiously and is often not immediately present. A diffuse radiographic injury pattern is characteristic of pulmonary contusion. Careful clinical monitoring, frequent blood gas analysis, and a low threshold for intubation and mechanical ventilation in the patient with a severe pulmonary contusion help reduce mortality [8,106,107].

The increased frequency of traumatic diaphragmatic rupture in association with upper abdominal injury during pregnancy needs to be considered in any pregnant chest or upper abdominal trauma victim [14].

Traumatic aortic rupture frequently occurs in conjunction with motor vehicle accidents or falls from great heights [106]. Aortic rupture mechanistically occurs from the relative fixation of the aorta, thereby reducing its ability to move or flex with sudden deceleration. This produces tearing of one or more of the layers of the vessel. The clinical manifestation of aortic rupture is variable and depends on the extent of the rupture. For example, patients with unconfined lesions or transections usually exsanguinate before or shortly after arrival to the hospital, while patients with contained hematomas are more frequently alive at hospital presentation. Diagnosis of the contained aortic rupture may be more difficult because it may often be associated with modest hypotension, especially with lesions near the ligamentum arteriosum. Mediastinal widening, obliteration of the aortic knob, or first or second rib fractures may suggest an aortic rupture [97,106,122]. Ultrasound, magnetic resonance imaging, or CT radiography may assist in the diagnosis of aortic rupture, but angiography is the definitive diagnostic procedure for traumatic aortic rupture [6,108]. In the context of trauma management of the pregnant patient, medically necessary radiographic studies should not be deferred if required for the diagnosis and/or treatment of maternal life-threatening injuries.

Tracheobronchial tree injuries (TBI) may produce sudden airway obstruction. A high clinical index of suspicion, especially in cases of refractory pneumothorax, subcutaneous emphysema, or blast injuries is necessary for timely diagnosis. Operative intervention is frequently necessary in patients with TBI [94,108,109].

Esophageal trauma is often an insidious feature of chest trauma. It is usually, but not always, associated with penetrating chest trauma. Esophageal rupture is suspected in any patient with severe epigastric injury, substernal trauma, pneumothorax without chest wall injury, and/or in patients with continued particulate material in their thoracostomy tube drainage. Esophagoscopy or contrast studies confirm the diagnosis. Death may result directly from hemorrhage or from unrelenting mediastinitis [6,110,111].

While thoracic trauma should be evaluated by a thoracic specialist familiar with chest trauma management, an understanding of the ramifications of potentially lethal chest trauma often will allow the obstetrician to recognize and stabilize the chest trauma victim.

Head trauma

Approximately 50% of all trauma deaths are associated with head injury. Over 60% of motor vehicle-associated trauma deaths occur as a result of head trauma [6]. In a recent review of pregnant trauma deaths in Cook County (Illinois), approximately 10% of maternal trauma deaths were directly due to head injury [112].

Several aspects of cranial and cerebral physiology and pathophysiology are very important in head trauma victims. The brain is one of the most carefully protected organs of the body; the calvarium and cerebrospinal fluid cushion the brain from minor trauma. However, in severe trauma, these two otherwise protective features may contribute to or precipitate brain injury. The brain has poor tolerance of diminished perfusion with little or no metabolic reserve in brain tissues. Global cerebral oxygen consumption of at least 1.5 mL/100 g/min must be maintained to prevent injury. Oxygen delivery to the brain is determined by blood pressure, blood oxygen content, blood flow distribution, and relative perfusion pressure. Because the closed space of the calvarium is occupied by blood, cerebrospinal fluid, and brain volume, intracranial pressure is a function of all three components, referred to as the Monro–Kellie doctrine. Cerebral edema results in increased brain volume, thereby producing elevated intracranial pressure. Traumatic collections of blood in the cranial vault will similarly increase intracranial pressure. Often, both of these mechanisms are present in the head trauma victim [113,114].

Cerebral autoregulation in traumatic injury

Cerebral autoregulation is normally maintained over a wide range of blood pressures. Extremes of blood pressure, such as hypotension found in the multiple trauma victim, taxes the brain's ability to autoregulate. When coupled with cerebral edema and/or intracranial bleeding, hypotension further aggravates the inability of the brain to autoregulate. When the injured brain loses its ability to autoregulate, self-perpetuation of the brain injury occurs. Finally, because the cranium is a closed system, propagation of elevated extravascular cerebral pressure transmurally causes the driving pressure in the cerebral circulation to be significantly decreased. In that flow is directly determined by a change in pressure, diminished cerebral perfusion pressure (mean arterial blood pressure – intracranial pressure) causes decreased effective cerebral blood flow. Cerebral mass lesions will therefore diminish cerebral perfusion pressure in proportion to their size even in the face of normal blood pressure. It should thus be obvious that acute brain injury is often self-perpetuating and when in evolution and is poorly tolerated by the fastidious neuronal cells. Cell death and permanent injury may result. The therapeutic goal of acute cerebral resuscitation is to limit cell death by regulated reperfusion to non-functioning, but still viable brain tissue (*ischemic penumbra*). The clinician's ability to accomplish this goal is often limited [115,116].

Another feature of brain injury is the concept of secondary, or reperfusion, injury. An initial insult produces the loss of autoregulation described above. Unfortunately, reperfusion of the injured area may occur in the presence of absent or diminished autoregulation. Injury is either mechanically (through edema) or metabolically (through inappropriate substrate production) produced through reperfusion [117].

In order to avoid or limit permanent cerebral injury, specific cerebral resuscitation must be carried out in the head trauma victim. The sooner resuscitation is begun, the greater the chance injured, but living, neuronal tissue will survive [117–119].

Brain injury mechanism in trauma

Penetrating head injuries produce injury by obvious mechanisms. With blunt head trauma, especially in deceleration events, movement of the brain occurs first in one direction with a secondary rebound movement in the opposite direction producing a *coup–countercoup* effect. Closed head injuries can occur without significant injury of the cutaneous tissues and calvarium through bruising or contusion of the brain at *coup* or *countercoup* sites. Intracerebral hemorrhage from traumatic brain injury often results from severe contusion. Subdural or epidural hematomas are produced by direct laceration or tearing of subdural or epidural vessels, respectively [6,116].

Primary management of traumatic brain injury

Initial management of suspected brain injury starts with the basic "ABCs" discussed previously. Profound hypotension, defined as systolic blood pressure less than 60 mmHg in non-pregnant individuals, may cause or contribute to altered consciousness. Correction of hypotension is important. While possible, hypotension as a result of the neurologic insult is uncommon. Until proven otherwise, hypotension in the presence of head injury is usually from other causes. Severe hypertension in the comatose trauma victim may be centrally mediated. This "Cushing response" is also characterized by bradycardia and a diminished respiratory rate [113]. Altered levels of consciousness may also be produced by alcohol or drug ingestion. Toxicological assessment is recommended in most trauma patients with altered levels of consciousness. Conversely, an altered level of consciousness should never be totally attributed to alcohol or other drug ingestion alone unless completely proven otherwise. Finally, other medical conditions such as hypoglycemia may occasionally be seen coincidental with trauma.

A baseline and ongoing mental assessment is necessary as a frame of reference in all trauma patients. The "A-V-P-U" mini exam (Figure 37.1) is a brief primary survey tool. In the secondary survey, more extensive evaluation, such as by the Glasgow Coma scale (GCS) is recommended (Table 37.2) [15,16]. A score of 8 or less is indicative of the diagnosis of coma and is classified as severe head injury [6,114,118]. If the GCS is from 9 to 12, the injury is classified as moderate. GCS scores greater than 12 are classified as minor head injuries [108,116]. Once again, the GCS and other neurologic examinations need to be performed frequently so trends in neurologic response can be identified. A decrease in the GCS score of 2 or more points is indicative of

Table 37.4 Classification of acute head trauma.

Diffuse brain injury
A. Concussion
B. Diffuse axonal injury

Focal brain injury
A. Contusion
B. Hemorrhage/hematoma
 1. Parenchymal hemorrhage
 2. Meningeal hemorrhage/hematoma
  a. Acute epidural hemorrhage/hematoma
  b. Subarachnoid hemorrhage/hematoma

Skull fractures
A. Simple fracture
B. Basilar skull fracture
C. Depressed skull fracture

deterioration [108]. Irrespective of the GCS score, unequal pupils, unequal motor findings, open head injury with leaking cerebrospinal fluid or exposed brain tissue, and/or the presence of a depressed skull fracture also indicate severe head injury. Finally, if headache severity dramatically increases, pupillary size increases unilaterally, or lateralizing weakness is noted to develop, particular concern is warranted.

Appropriate immediate investigations of the head trauma victim may include roentgenograms (X-ray), CT radiography, and neurologic or neurosurgical consultation. Sedation and/or paralysis is delayed until the consultant examines the patient, if possible. Generally, all patients with moderate or severe head injury should be radiographically evaluated for cervical spine fracture. Conversely, skull roentgenograms are often not helpful [108] as physical examination or CT imaging provide more reliable information and higher-quality data. CT imaging is a vital tool in the evaluation of head injuries and except for women with minor injuries, all head-injured patients require CT imaging. Severe injury dictates imaging as soon as possible. However, it is important to adequately monitor the victim while she undergoes imaging. Once C-spine fractures are ruled out, the 20+ week gestation pregnant patient is placed in left lateral tilt during the scanning [9]. Head injuries can be simply classified into the categories of diffuse brain injury, focal brain injury, and skull fractures (Table 37.4) [6,8,116].

Diffuse brain injury

Diffuse brain injury can be classified as a concussion or diffuse axonal injury. Concussion is produced from widespread brief interruption of global brain function. Although confusion, headache, dizziness, etc., are often present in the recovering concussion victim, any persistent neurologic abnormalities in the patient with a presumed concussion must be investigated for other etiologies. Many authors feel that the patient with 5 minutes or more of lost consciousness should be observed in the hospital for at least 24 hours [120]. Other criteria that differentiate mild concussion (less likelihood of sequelae) from the more severe classic concussion include the presence or absence of loss of consciousness itself, the duration of amnesia, and the presence of persistent memory deficit. Diffuse axonal injury (DAI), more commonly known as "closed head injury", is produced by widespread global brain injury or the cerebral edema resulting from diffuse brain injury [118]. Prolonged coma is the hallmark of DAI. CT imaging will show cerebral edema without focal lesions. Nearly 50% of coma-producing brain injuries are caused by DAI. DAI is classified clinically into mild, moderate, and severe categories [121]. Severe DAI carries a 50% mortality. Long-term supportive care and control of intracranial hypertension are the only treatment for the condition. Partial or complete recovery is possible, but permanent coma ("chronic vegetative state") is often an inexorable consequence of severe DAI.

Focal brain injury

Focal brain injuries are those in which damage occurs in a relatively local area. Types of focal brain injury include contusions, hemorrhages, and hematomas. Because focal injuries may produce a mass effect and damage underlying normal brain tissue, rapid diagnosis and treatment of focal brain injuries may improve outcome and recovery.

Contusions are usually caused by deceleration *coup–countercoup* trauma as previously described. Although contusions can occur anywhere, they are most commonly found in the tips of the frontal and temporal lobes. In addition to producing deficits from focal injury, delayed bleeding and edema can produce injury from mass effects [116]. Prolonged observation is recommended. If neurologic deterioration is detected and is thought to be from a mass effect, surgery may be indicated.

Hemorrhages and hematomas can be functionally classified into those occurring in the meningeal or parenchymal regions of the brain. Parenchymal hemorrhage includes intracerebral hematomas, impalement injuries and missile (bullet) wounds. Meningeal hemorrhage is further classified as acute epidural hemorrhage, acute subdural hematoma, or subarachnoid hemorrhage.

Acute epidural hemorrhage (AEH) usually occurs from tears in the middle meningeal artery. Although found in 1% or less of coma-producing acute brain injuries, AEH can be rapidly progressive and fatal. Figure 37.3 describes the usual sequence of events associated with AEH. It is important to note that the patient with AEH may display an intervening period of lucidity prior to a rapid deterioration from massive rebleeding of the lesion [143]. If surgically treated early, the prognosis is good (91% survival) [118]. If not evacuated until hemiparesis and pupil fixation, the prognosis is poor. AEH is, in effect, "the vasa previa" of acute brain injury. Rapid recognition and treatment yields markedly improved results.

Subarachnoid hemorrhage (SAH) produces bleeding in the subarachnoid space. Meningeal irritation occurs with the resulting symptoms of headache and/or photophobia. Because the subarachnoid space is much larger than the epidural space, bleeding does not usually rapidly progress to death. Although bloody spinal fluid is a hallmark of SAH, CT scanning has basically replaced lumbar puncture in the diagnosis of SAH. Evacuation is sometimes not required. If evacuation is not performed, treatment is supportive. Meningeal irritation can produce unwanted cerebral artery vasospasm. Cerebral artery vasospasm may be diagnosed by clinical ascertainment of neurological deficit, with either empiric treatment and/or confirmation via transcranial Doppler velocitometry and/or cerebral arteriography. Treatment of cerebral artery vasospasm involves volume loading, vasopressor-induced hypertension and calcium channel blocker therapy with nimodipine. Refractory treatment of vasospasm has been advocated by the use of angiographically instilled papaverine and/or calcium channel blocking agents or direct balloon angioplasty [114,119,122]. Clear-cut consensus on optimal treatment is still pending [123].

Acute subdural hematoma (SDH) is one of the more common causes of serious brain hemorrhage. SDHs commonly occur from rupture of bridging veins between the cerebral cortex and dura; but, may also occur from direct laceration of the brain or cortical arteries. The clinical presentation of SDH often depends upon the rapidity of expansion of the hematoma. Rapidly expanding hematomas carry a poorer prognosis than do stable, chronic SDHs. Early evacuation of rapidly growing SDHs may favorably impact the 60% mortality that SDH carries [20,118,120]. Others advocate early (within 4 hours of injury) evacuation of subdural hematomas greater than 1 cm in diameter that are associated with a shift in midline brain structures. Patients with subdural hematomas of less than 5 mm with only mild or absent neurologic symptoms may be candidates for expectant management.

Intracerebral hematomas can occur anywhere in the brain. Symptoms and outcome depend upon the size and location. Intraventricular and intracerebellar hemorrhages portend poor outcome. With impalement injuries the missile or projectile should be left in place until neurosurgical evaluation is obtained. Bullet wounds should be mapped as to entrance and potential exit. CT radiography may help the localization process of any remaining missile fragments. Non-penetrating bullet wounds may result in significant blunt trauma [118,125].

Skull fractures are relatively common and may or may not be associated with severe brain injury. Because skull fractures may be an indicator that significant energy dispersal occurred on the cranial vault, most patients with seemingly uncomplicated skull fractures should still be observed in the hospital with serial neurosurgical evaluations.

Skull fractures

Different types of skull fractures have different clinical considerations. Linear non-depressed skull fractures that traverse suture lines or vascular arterial grooves may be associated with epidural hemorrhage, whereas depressed skull fractures may require operative elevation of the bony fragment. On the other hand, open skull fractures nearly always require early operative intervention. Basilar skull fractures may not immediately be apparent clinically. Anterior basilar skull fractures may predispose to inadvertent placement of a nasogastric tube into the intracranial space [116].

Skull fractures typical require cranial CT scanning and physical exam. Skull X-rays are usually not helpful for the initial evaluation of head injury. Attempt at precise delineation of skull fractures should not delay recognition and treatment of other head injuries.

Head trauma: general principles

Mainstays in the treatment of head trauma include maintenance of brain perfusion, reduction of cerebral edema, elimination or reduction of hemorrhage, and prevention of infection. Patients with evolving symptomatology or unremitting coma need to be evaluated immediately for potential neurosurgical intervention. Maintenance of normal arterial blood pressure will aid the often impaired cerebral autoregulation seen with head trauma. Normalization of blood glucose will help supply cerebral metabolic needs. Hyperglycemia is to be avoided, as it is as undesirable as hypoglycemia [114,120].

Figure 37.5 outlines a general scheme for severe head injury triage and features of high-, moderate-, and low-risk lesions. It should be noted that a lateralizing defect and GCS ≤8 requires immediate evaluation for surgical treatment. Intracranial pressure (ICP) monitoring has been long advocated as a measure to improve outcome in traumatic brain injury. There is clearly a split of opinion with regard to the indications and effectiveness of ICP monitoring. The current consensus recommendations propose ICP monitoring be used in comatose patients with GCS scores of 8 or less after resuscitation who also demonstrate pathologic CT radiographic abnormalities. In those patients with a GCS of 8 or less without CT abnormalities, ICP monitoring is indicated if two or more of the following are present: age >40 years, unilateral or bilateral posturing, and systolic blood pressure less than 90 mmHg at any time since injury [117,126,127]. Abnormal intracranial pressure (ICP) is medically treated with controlled hyperventilation, mannitol administration, barbiturate coma, loop diuretics, volume restriction, and head-up positioning [117]. When ICP monitoring is employed, measurements above 20–25 mmHg generally necessitate treatment strategies to lower ICP.

Hyperventilation works to transiently decrease ICP by reducing cerebral blood flow. If used, hyperventilation should be undertaken to a P_aCO_2 endpoint of 26–28 mmHg [128], although the appropriate level for pregnancy is not established. Hyperventilation is *not* effective in "prophylaxis" against elevated ICP [6,112,129]. If hyperventilation is abruptly discontinued, ICP may rise rapidly. Current data refute the long-held clinical practice of using aggressive hyperventilation for the treatment or prevention of intracranial hypertension. In non-pregnant patients, sustained hyperventilation is associated with the least favorable outcome. Hyperventilation's impact is probably mediated through reduction in cerebral blood flow in normal brain parenchyma surrounding damaged neural tissue. Hyperventilation

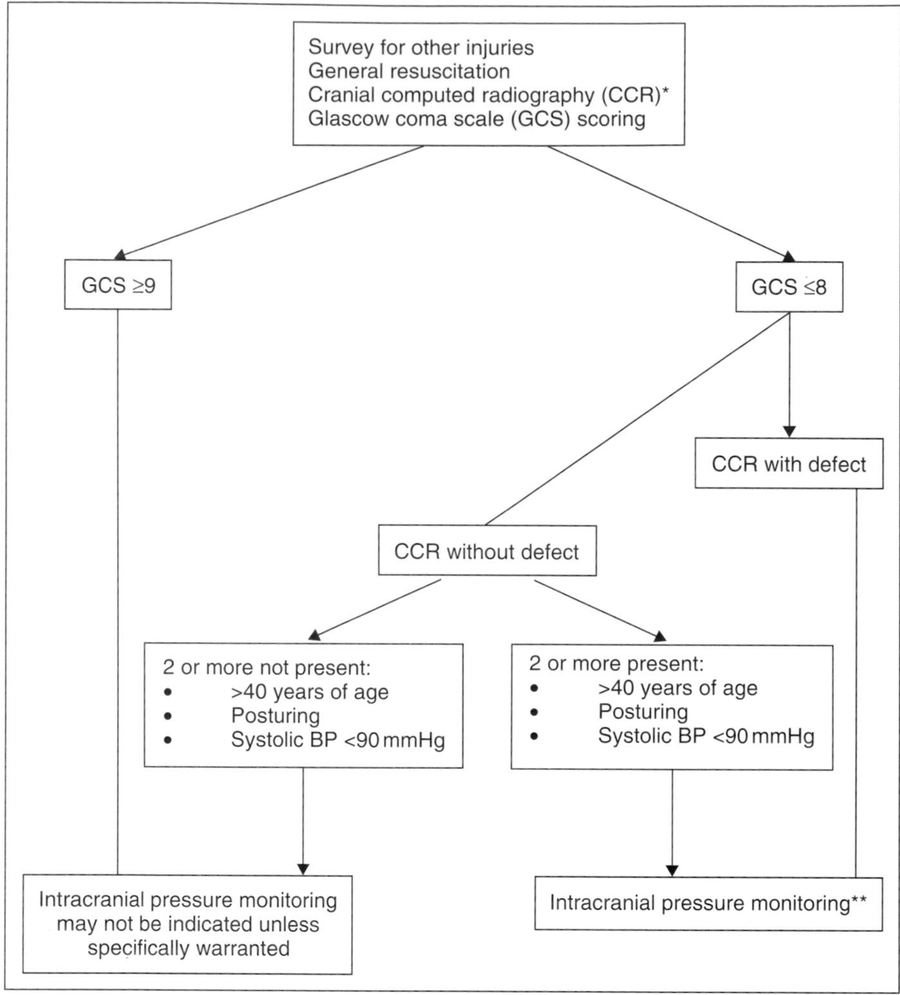

Figure 37.5 Initial evaluation of the comatose trauma victim. *Neurosurgical consultation liberally indicated during the evaluation of the comatose trauma victim. **A lateralizing defect with GCS <8 may necessitate expedited surgical exploration (sources as referenced in text).

is no longer recommended and should be avoided, if possible, within the first 24 hours following acute brain injury. If used at all, the technique is reserved for temporary treatment of severe intractable intracranial hypertension. The effects of normal pregnancy (compensated respiratory alkalosis) on CO_2-mediated regulation of cerebral blood flow are not known.

Mannitol functions as a hyperosmotic diuretic. Doses of 0.5–1 g/kg body weight are typically used as primary treatment of intracranial hypertension [130]. Frequent monitoring of serum osmolality is needed, and mannitol should be withheld if osmolality is greater than 315–320 mOsm/L. Treatment may be directed at maintaining ICP at less than 20–25 mmHg. Alternatively, cerebral perfusion pressure-directed treatment (CPP = mean arterial pressure − ICP) may be instituted using mannitol and peripheral vasoconstrictors to increase mean peripheral arterial pressure. At present, there is no standard recommendation for CPP nor is there a recommendation as to the most effective way for achieving a particular CPP treatment endpoint. Mannitol can theoretically affect uteroplacental perfusion and/or fetal volume homeostasis. However, given the grave circumstances for which mannitol is used in severe head trauma, the benefits of its administration far outweigh these risks [9,116]. Diuresis with furosemide or other loop diuretics may also be used. Overhydration, especially with hypotonic solutions, should be avoided. Head-up positioning at 20° may marginally reduce hydrostatic pressure.

Barbiturate coma has been utilized as a treatment of refractory intracranial hypertension. The technique probably works by reducing cerebral oxygen consumption [118,119]. Corticosteroids are not indicated for therapy of cerebral edema from trauma [120,131]. Other less successful treatments of refractory intracranial hypertension include hypothermia, decompressive craniotomy, hypertonic saline, and a variety of investigational neuroprotective agents. Research is ongoing in this area of neurotrauma.

Delivery considerations in brain trauma

The best route of delivery in the patient with acute brain injury is unknown [132]. The original large series addressing the issue in patients with non-traumatic brain injury was in 1974 by Hunt et al. [132]. Regardless, limited data are available as to the recommended route of delivery in patients with traumatic or atraumatic brain injury. Individualized therapy and consultation with a neurologist and/or a neurosurgeon are recommended.

Rapid diagnosis, early neurosurgical intervention and meticulous attention to support measures offer the best hope for a favorable outcome in patients with severe brain injuries. Comanagement with consultants, appropriate and timely use of cranial CT scans, and serial neurologic examination may reduce mortality and morbidity in brain trauma. Improvement in maternal outcome offers the best hope for improved fetal outcome.

Traumatic orthopedic injury

Very limited information has been published specifically on fracture management complicating pregnant traumatic injury. Just as the care of a complicated pregnancy requires the expertise of a qualified obstetrician and gynecologist or maternal-fetal medicine subspecialist, specific management of skeletal fractures is beyond the scope of this text and warrants specific management by the appropriately trained and credentialed orthopedic specialist. However, several important points and issues may help the obstetric provider care for the pregnant trauma patient with multiple fractures.

In the initial assessment of the victim with orthopedic injury, only acute extremity injury and unstable pelvic fracture with fracture-related hemorrhage are typically immediate life-threatening injuries which would require emergency department or immediate operating room treatment [133]. Acute extremity hemorrhage is managed according to the site of hemorrhage and degree of bleeding and the injury itself. An unstable pelvic fracture or dislocation may result in marked pelvic hemorrhage. If faced with a patient with an unstable bleeding pelvic fracture, most orthopedic specialists recommend placement of an external pelvic fixator to reduce pelvic volume and to stabilize the pelvic ring. Hemorrhage is generally controlled so as to allow successful resuscitation and focus on other injuries [134]. Other chapters of this book outline the importance of deep venous thrombosis (DVT) prophylaxis: DVT prophylaxis is very important in the patient with orthopedic injury.

Orthopedic urgencies (after and/or not at the exclusion of primary resuscitation and life-saving measures) generally include management of amputation or devascularization, and debridement of open fractures. Necessity for amputation of the severely mangled extremity is directly related to the age of the victim, the degree of skeletal or soft tissue injury, the degree of systemic hypotension/shock, and the degree of and duration of limb ischemia. Re-attachment of a severed limb is possible and should be considered as appropriate after primary stabilization has occurred [135].

Open fracture debridement and fixation will help relieve pain and may improve long-term outcome. Early, but non-immediate fracture fixation allows earlier mobilization. Fixation and repair of a femur fracture is usually not an immediate concern during resuscitation of the trauma victim with a concomitant head injury. However, it is recommended that repair of the femur fracture should be accomplished relatively early. The underlying rationale is that outcome is improved in the stable head injury patient when the femur fracture is addressed within 3–5 days after the injury [136]. Placement of pins to stabilize fractures does not appear to increase the incidence of acute respiratory distress syndrome (previously held opinion was that embolic marrow showering occurred as a consequence of bone manipulation from hardware placement).

One serious manifestation of severe injury of extremities is acute, compartment syndrome (ACS). ACS is causes by tissue edema and/or bleeding increasing the intramural pressure within a fascial compartment. ACS is not an infrequent complication of traumatic skeletal injury. Up to 17% of patients with a tibial fracture secondary to a motor vehicle accident may develop ACS [137]. Clinical features of the diagnosis include severe pain, tenderness, and swelling of the involved extremity. Loss of distal pulses is a late finding. Tonometry of an affected fascial compartment may be used to supplant clinical diagnosis. Treatment is by fasciotomy, and, outcome is improved if the diagnosis is made early [138].

As stated previously, published experience with the specific management of traumatic orthopedic injury in pregnancy is lacking. However, the general principles discussed in this section may serve to provide a basis of management during pregnancy. Multidisciplinary care is helpful in the management of complex cases.

Spinal trauma in pregnancy

Spinal cord injury has both immediate and long-term implications for trauma victim. As related earlier in this chapter, neck and back stabilization is paramount during the extraction, transport, and initial resuscitative phases of any patient with suspected neck or back injury. Use of back boards and neck stabilization during intubation are crucial to the preservation of whatever potential function remains and for the prevention of further spinal cord trauma. As with other traumatic injury, avoidance of systemic hypotension is associated with better neurological outcome after traumatic spinal injury.

Suspected neck or back traumatic injury necessitates both cervical spine radiography and careful evaluation of the spine via CT radiography. When specific radiographic screening techniques are utilized, the combination of three-view cervical spine X-ray and CT radiography have an over 99% negative predictive value in ruling out significant spinal injury [139,140]. Identified injuries need to be stabilized under the care of a skilled neurosurgeon. Surgical strategy in these cases is beyond the scope of this text. Opinion is divided regarding early (postresuscitation and immediate treatment of acutely life-threatening injuries) surgical repair of spinal cord injury patients. Another unanswered question is that concerning the use of corticosteroids. Several randomized and non-randomized trials have been conducted in order to answer the question as to whether systemic corticosteroid administration results in improved neurological outcome in traumatic spinal injury. Opinion is divided over corticosteroid use in blunt spinal injury [140,141]. It does appear that corticosteroids are not beneficial in penetrating spinal injury (such as gunshot wounds) [142]. If used at all, therapy should be begun within 8 hours following injury.

Several manifestations of autonomic instability may be seen in the spinal injury victim. The patient with recent cervical or thoracic spinal cord complete transection has a loss of sympathetic outflow. Vagal afferent and efferent innervation is preserved through the intact vagus nerve, with the result being systemic hypotension and bradycardia from unbalanced parasympathetic stimulation. Heat dissipation increases and oliguria may result. Initial treatment with isotonic fluid resuscitation may not be totally effective. Vasopressors and/or pressor inotropes (dopamine) may be required. In the non-pregnant patient, a target mean arterial blood pressure (MAP) of at least 85–90 mmHg is optimal for best neurologic outcome [140,143]. Since published data are limited in pregnant populations, individualized guidance using fetal heart rate monitoring in the potentially viable fetus may be required.

In the non-acute setting, incomplete transections above T5 through T6 may place the patient at risk from autonomic dysreflexia. Afferent stimulation from a hollow viscus often produces marked catecholamine release with marked hypertension and other sympathetic sequelae. Uterine stimulation from labor, bladder distention, constipation, or superficial stimulation of the skin below the level of the lesion may produce this condition [144,145]. For the laboring patient, epidural or spinal anesthesia may ameliorate the unopposed afferent stimulation. Treatment of hypertension via direct-acting agents or ganglionic blockade may be necessary in patients who do not have epidural or spinal anesthesia [140].

Long-term care of the patient with a catastrophic spinal injury is beyond the aim of this chapter. Severe impairment may result in lifelong challenges for the spinal injury victim.

Conclusion

Trauma during pregnancy poses a special and immediate challenge to the obstetrician and to the emergency room provider. Generally speaking, most diagnostic and therapeutic modalities relating to trauma care should not be avoided or modified during pregnancy. Co-management, with input from obstetric and non-obstetric services, functions to insure appropriate care of the pregnant trauma victim and her fetus.

References

1 Laverly JP, Staten-McCormick M. Management of moderate to severe trauma in pregnancy. *Obstet Gynecol Clin North Am* 1995; 22: 69.

2 Vainer MW. Maternal mortality in Iowa from 1952 to 1986. *Surg Obstet Gynecol* 1989; 168: 555.

3 Fildes J, Reed L, Jones N, Martin M, Barrett J. Trauma: the leading cause of maternal death. *J Trauma* 1992; 32: 643.

4 Sachs BP, Brown DAT, Driscoll SG, et al. Maternal mortality Massachusetts: trends and prevention. *N Engl J Med* 1987; 316: 667.

5 Satin A, Hemsell DL, Stone IC, et al. Sexual assault in pregnancy. *Obstet Gynecol* 1991; 77: 710.

6 American College of Surgeons, Committee on Trauma. *Advanced Trauma Life Support*, 7th edn. Chicago: First Impressions, 2004.

7 Vaizey CJ, Jacobson MJ, Cross FW. Trauma in pregnancy. *Br J Surg* 1994; 81: 1406.

8 American College of Surgeons. *Advanced Trauma Life Support for Doctors – Faculty Manual*, 7th edn. Chicago: First Impressions, 2004.

9 Kuhlman RS, Cruikshank DP. Maternal trauma during pregnancy. *Clin Obstet Gynecol* 1994; 37: 274.

10 Scorpio RJ, Esposito TJ, Smith LG, Gens DR. Blunt trauma during pregnancy: factors affecting fetal outcome. *J Trauma* 1992; 32: 213.

11 Hoff WS, d'Amelio LF, Tinkhoff GH, et al. Maternal predictors of fetal demise during pregnancy. *Surg Gynecol Obstet* 1991; 172: 175.

12 Dilts PV, Brintzman CR, Kirschbaum TH, et al. Uterine and systemic hemodynamic inter-relationships and their response to hypoxia. *Am J Obstet Gynecol* 1967; 103: 38.

13 Greiss F. Uterine vascular response to hemorrhage during pregnancy. *Obstet Gynecol* 1966; 27: 408.

14 Hankins GDV, Barth WH, Satin AJ. Critical care medicine and the obstetric patient. In: Ayres SM, Grenuik A, Holbrook PR, Shoemaker WC, eds. *Textbook of Critical Care*, 3rd edn. Philadelphia: WB Saunders, 1995: 50–64.

15 Jennett B, Teasdale G, Braakman R, et al. Prognosis of patients with severe head injury. *Neurosurgery* 1979; 4: 283.

16 Teasdale G, Jennett B. Assessment of coma and impaired consciousness: a practical scale. *Lancet* 1974; 1: 81.

17 Baxt WG, Moody P. The differential survival of trauma patients. *J Trauma* 1987; 27: 602.

18 Rutherford EJ, Nelson LD. Initial assessment of the multiple trauma patient. In: Ayres SM, Grenuik A, Holbrook PR, Shoemaker WC, eds. *Textbook of Critical Care*, 3rd edn. Philadelphia: WB Saunders, 1995: 1382–1389.

19 Winchell RJ, Hoyt DB, Simons RK. Use of computed tomography of the head in the hypotensive blunt-trauma patient. *Ann Emerg Med* 1995; 25: 737.

20 National Blood Transfusion Service Immunoglobulin Working Party. *Recommendations for the use of anti-D immunoglobulin*. 1991: 137–145.

21 Pearlman MD, Tintinalli JE, Lorenz RP. Blunt trauma during pregnancy. *N Engl J Med* 1990; 323: 1609.

22 Goodwin TM, Breen MT. Pregnancy and fetomaternal hemorrhage after noncatastrophic trauma. *Am J Obstet Gynecol* 1990; 162: 665.

23 Rose PG, Strohm PL, Zuspan FP. Fetomaternal hemorrhage following trauma. *Am J Obstet Gynecol* 1985; 153: 844.

24 Bowman JM. Management of Rh-isoimmunization. *Obstet Gynecol* 1978; 52: 1.

25 Laml T, Egermann R, Lapin A, Zekert M, Wagenbichler P. Fetomaternal hemorrhage after a car accident: a case report. *Acta Obstet Gynecol Scand* 2001; 80: 480.

26 American College of Obstetricians and Gynecologists. *Practice Bulletin No. 282. Prevention of RhD Alloimmunization*. Washington, DC: American College of Obstetricians and Gynecologists, 1999.

27 Boyle J, Kim J, Walerius H, Samuels P. The clinical use of the Kleihauer–Betke test in Rh positive patients. *Am J Obstet Gynecol* 1996; 174: 343.
28 Weiss HB, Songer TJ, Fabio A. Fetal deaths related to maternal injury. *JAMA* 2001; 286: 1863–1868.
29 Fries MH, Hankins GDV. Motor vehicle accident associated with minimal maternal trauma, but subsequent fetal demise. *Ann Emerg Med* 1989; 18: 301.
30 Pearlman MD, Tintinalli JE, Lorenz RP. A prospective controlled study of outcome after trauma during pregnancy. *Am J Obstet Gynecol* 1990; 162: 1502.
31 Williams JK, McClain L, Rosemursy AS, Colorado NM. Evaluation of blunt abdominal trauma in the third trimester of pregnancy: *Obstet Gynecol* 1990; 75: 33.
32 American College of Obstetricians and Gynecologists. *Obstetric Aspects of Trauma Management. Technical Bulletin No. 251.* Washington, DC: American College of Obstetricians and Gynecologists, 1998.
33 Pritchard JA, Brekken AL. Clinical and laboratory studies on severe abruptio placentae. *Am J Obstet Gynecol* 1967; 97: 681.
34 Higgins SD, Garite TJ. Late abruptio placentae in trauma patients: implications for monitoring. *Obstet Gynecol* 1987; 63(Suppl): 510.
35 Dahmus MA, Sibai BM. Blunt abdominal trauma: are there predictive factors for abruptio placentae or maternal-fetal distress? *Am J Obstet Gynecol* 1993; 169: 1054.
36 Katz JD, Hook R, Baragh PG. Fetal heart rate monitoring in pregnant patients undergoing surgery. *Am J Obstet Gynecol* 1976; 125: 267.
37 Evrard JR, Sturmer WQ, Murray EJ. Fetal skull fracture from an automobile accident. *Am J Forensic Med Pathol* 1998; 10: 232.
38 Hartl R, Ko K. In utero skull fracture: case report. *J Trauma* 1996; 41: 549.
39 Palmer JD, Sparrow OC. Extradural hematoma following intrauterine trauma. *Injury* 1994; 25: 671.
40 Weyerts LK, Jones MC, James HE. Paraplegia and congenital fractures as a consequence of intrauterine trauma. *Am J Med Genet* 1992; 43: 751.
41 Hall EJ. Scientific view of low-level radiation risks. *Radiographics* 1991; 11: 509.
42 Shepard TH. *Catalog of Teratogenic Agents*, 7th edn. Baltimore, MD: Johns Hopkins, 1992.
43 American College of Obstetricians and Gynecologists. *Guidelines for Diagnostic Imaging During Pregnancy. Committee Opinion No. 299.* Washington, DC: American College of Obstetricians and Gynecologists, 2004.
44 Ben-Menachem Y, Handel SF, Ray RD, et al. Embolization procedures in trauma, a matter of urgency. *Semin Intervent Radiol* 1985; 2: 107.
45 Briggs GG, Freeman RK, Jaffe SJ. *A Reference Guide to Fetal and Neonatal Risk – Drugs in Pregnancy and Lactation*, 6th edn. Baltimore, MD: Williams and Wilkins, 2001.
46 Martinowitz U, Kenet G, Segal E, et al. Recombinant activated factor VII for adjunctive hemorrhage control in trauma. *J Trauma* 2001; 51: 431.
47 O'Neill PA, Bluth M, Gloster ES, et al. Successful use of recombinant activated factor VII for trauma-associated hemorrhage in a patient without preexisting coagulopathy. *J Trauma* 2002; 52: 400.
48 Dart BW, Cockerham T, Torres C, Kipikasa JH, Maxwell RA. A novel use of recombinant factor VIIa in HELLP syndrome associated with spontaneous hepatic rupture and abdominal compartment syndrome. *J Trauma* 2004; 57: 171.
49 Boehlen F, Morales MA, Fontana P, Ricou B, Irion O, Moerloos P. Prolonged treatment of massive postpartum haemorrhage with recombinant factor VIIa: case report and review of the literature. *Br J Obstet Gynaecol* 2004; 111: 284.
50 Boba A, Linkie DM, Plotz EJ. Effects of vasopressor administration and fluid replacement on fetal bradycardia and hypoxia induced by maternal hemorrhage. *Obstet Gynecol* 1966; 27: 408.
51 Katz VL, Dotters DJ, Droegemueller W. Perimortem cesarean delivery. *Obstet Gynecol* 1986; 68: 571.
52 Katz V, Balderston K, DeFreest M. Perimortem cesarean delivery: were our assumptions correct? *Am J Obstet Gynecol* 2005; 192: 1916.
53 Morris JA, Rosenbower TJ, Jurkovich GJ, et al. Infant survival after cesarean section for trauma. *Ann Surg* 1996; 223: 481.
54 Rothenberger D, Quattlebaum FW, Perry JF Jr, et al. Blunt maternal trauma: a review of 103 cases. *J Trauma* 1978; 18: 173.
55 Kimball IM. Maternal fetal trauma. *Semin Pediatr Surg* 2001; 10(1): 32–34.
56 Crosby WM, Costiloe JP. Safety of lap belt restraints for pregnant victims of automobile collisions. *N Engl J Med* 1971; 284: 632.
57 Pearlman MD, Klinich KD, Schneider LW, et al. A comprehensive program to improve safety for pregnant women and fetuses in motor vehicle crashes: a preliminary report. *Am J Obstet Gynecol* 2000; 182: 1554.
58 National Conference on Medical Indications for Air Bag Disconnection, George Washington University Medical Center. *Final Report*. 1997. Available at: http://dmses.dot.gov/docimages/pdf24/29064_web.pdf.
59 Moorcroft DM, Dunn SM, Stizel JD, Duma GG. *The Effect of Pregnant Occupant Position and Belt Placement on the Risk of Fetal Injury*. Warrendale, PA: SAE International, 2004.
60 Agran PF, Dunkle DE, Winn DG, Kent D. Fetal death in motor vehicle accidents. *Ann Emerg Med* 1987; 16: 1355.
61 Lane PL. Traumatic fetal death. *J Emerg Med* 1989; 7: 433
62 Stafford PA, Biddinger PW, Zumwalt RE. Lethal intrauterine fetal trauma. *Am J Obstet Gynecol* 1988; 159: 485
63 Bunai Y, Nagai A, Nakamura I, Ohya I. Fetal death from abruptio placentae associated with incorrect use of a seatbelt. *Am J Forensic Med Pathol* 2000; 21(3): 207.
64 Griffiths M, Hillman G, Usherwood M. Seat belt injury in pregnancy resulting in fetal death. A need for education? Case reports. *Br J Obstet Gynaecol* 1991; 98: 320.
65 Pearce M. Seat belts in pregnancy. *BMJ* 1992; 304: 586.
66 Pearlman MD, Viano D. Automobile crash simulation with first pregnant crash test dummy. *Am J Obstet Gynecol* 1996; 175: 977.
67 Rozycki GS, Shackford SR. Ultrasound: what every trauma surgeon should know. *J Trauma* 1996; 40: 1.
68 Scalea TM, Rodriguez A, Chiu WC, et al. Focused assessment with sonography for trauma (FAST): results from an international consensus conference. *J Trauma* 1999; 46: 466.
69 Rozycki GS,Gallard RB, Feliciano DV, Schmidt JA, Pennington SD. Surgeon performed ultrasound for the assessment of truncal injuries: lessons learned from 1540 patients. *Ann Surg* 1998; 228: 557.
70 Rozycki GS, Feliciano DV, Schmidt JA, et al. The role of the surgeon performed ultrasound in patients with possible cardiac wounds. *Ann Surg* 1996; 223: 737.

71 Brown MA, Sirlin CB, Farahmand N, Hoyt DB, Casola, G. Screening sonography in pregnant patients with blunt abdominal trauma. *J Ultrasound Med* 2005; 24:175.

72 Sirlin C, Casola G, Brown M, et al. US of blunt abdominal trauma: importance of free pelvic fluid in women of reproductive age. *Radiology* 2001; 219: 229.

73 Goodwin H, Holmes J, Wisner D. Abdominal ultrasound examination in pregnant blunt trauma patients. *J Trauma* 2001; 50(4): 689.

74 Hoyt DB, Coimbra R, Winchell RJ. Management of acute trauma. In: Townsend CM, Beauchamp RD, Evers BM, Mattox KL, eds. *Sabiston Textbook of Surgery*, 16th edn. Philadelphia: WB Saunders, 2001; 311–344.

75 Baerga VY, Zietlow S, Scott P, Bannom M, Harsem W, Illstrup D. Trauma in pregnancy. *Mayo Clin Proc* 2000; 75(12): 1243.

76 Poole GV, Martin JN, Perry KG, Griswold JA, Lambert J, Rhodes RS. Trauma in pregnancy: the role of interpersonal violence. *Am J Obstet Gynecol* 1996; 174: 1873.

77 Guth AA, Pachter I. Domestic violence and the trauma surgeon. *Am J Surg* 2000; 179:134.

78 Newberger EH, Barkan SE, Lieberman ES, et al. Abuse of pregnant women and adverse birth outcomes. Current knowledge and implications for practice. *JAMA* 1992; 267: 2370.

79 Parker B, McFarlane J, Soeken K. Abuse during pregnancy: effects on maternal complications and birth weight in adult and teenage women. *Obstet Gynecol* 1994; 84: 323.

80 McCormick RD. Seat belt injury: case of complete transection of pregnant uterus. *J Am Osteopathic Assoc* 1968; 67: 1139.

81 Sandy EA, Koerner M. Self-inflicted gunshot wound to the pregnant abdomen: report of a case and review of the literature. *Am J Perinatol* 1989; 6: 30.

82 Sakala EP, Kost DD. Management of stab wounds to the pregnant uterus. A case report and review of the literature. *Obstet Gynecol Surv* 1988; 43: 319.

83 Stone IK. Trauma in the obstetric patient. *Obstet Gynecol Clin North Am* 1999; 26: 459.

84 Del Rossi AJ, ed. Blunt thoracic trauma. *Trauma Quart* 1990; 6(3): 1.

85 Awwad JT, Azar GB, Seoud MA, Mroueh AM, Karam KS. High-velocity penetrating wounds of the gravid uterus: review of 16 years of civil war. *Obstet Gynecol* 1994; 83: 59.

86 Grubb DK. Non-surgical management of penetrating uterine trauma in pregnancy – a case report. *Am J Obstet Gynecol* 1992; 166: 583.

87 Cornell WP, Ebert PA, Zvidma GD. X-ray diagnosis of penetrating wounds of the abdomen. *J Surg Res* 1976; 5: 142.

88 Franger AL, Buschbaum HJ, Peaceman AM. Abdominal gunshot wounds in pregnancy. *Am J Obstet Gynecol* 1989; 29: 1628.

89 Edwards R, Bennet B, Ripley D, et al. Surgery in the pregnant patient. *Curr Probl Surg* 2001; 38(4): 274.

90 Hankins GDV. Complications of beta-sympathomimetic tocolytic agents. In: Clark SL, Cotton DB, Hankins GDV, Phelan JP, eds. *Critical Care Obstetrics*, 2nd edn. Boston: Blackwell Scientific, 1991: 223–250.

91 Caritis SN, Kuller JA, Watt-Morse ML. Pharmacologic options for treating preterm labor. In: Rayburn WF, Zuspan FP, eds. *Drug Therapy in Obstetrics and Gynecology*, 3rd edn. St Louis: Mosby Year Book, 1992; 74–89.

92 American College of Obstetricians and Gynecologists. *Committee Opinion No. 282. Immunization during pregnancy*. Washington, DC: American College of Obstetricians and Gynecologists, 2003.

93 Barone JE, Pizzi WS, Nealon TF Jr, et al. Indications for intubation in blunt chest trauma. *J Trauma* 1986; 26: 334.

94 Wilson RF. Thoracic injuries. In: Ayres SM, Grenvik A, Holbrook PR, Shoemaker WC, eds. *Textbook of Critical Care*. Philadelphia: WB Saunders, 1995: 1429–1438.

95 Weaver WD, Cobb LA, Hallstrom AP, et al. Factors influencing survival after out of hospital cardiac arrest. *J Am Coll Cardiol* 1986; 7: 752.

96 Feliciano DV. Tube thoracostomy. In: Benumof JL, ed. *Clinical Procedures in Anesthesia and Intensive Care*. Philadelphia: JB Lippincott, 1992; 305–314

97 Mattox KL. Approaches to trauma involving the major vessels of the thorax. *Surg Clin North Am* 1989; 69: 77.

98 Mansour MA, Moore EE, Moore FA, et al. Exingent post-injury thoracotomy. Analysis of blunt versus penetrating trauma. *Surg Gynecol Obstet* 1992; 175: 97.

99 Shoemaker WC, Carey JS, Yao ST, et al. Hemodynamic alterations in acute cardiac tamponade after penetrating injuries of the heart. *Surgery* 1970; 67: 754.

100 Shoemaker WC. Algorithm for early recognition and management of cardiac tamponade. *Crit Care Med* 1975; 3: 59.

101 Rene G, Mattox K, Beall A. Recent advances in operative management of massive chest trauma. *Ann Thorac Surg* 1973; 16: 52.

102 Sankaran S, Wilson RF. Factors affecting prognosis in patients with flail chest. *J Thorac Cardiovasc Surg* 1976; 60: 402.

103 Paone RF, Peacock JB, Smith DLT. Diagnosis of myocardiac contusion. *South Med J* 1993; 86.

104 Mattox KL, Flint LM, Carrico CJ. Blunt cardiac injury (formerly termed "myocardiac contusion") (editorial). *J Trauma* 1992; 33: 649.

105 Frazee RC, Mucha P, Fainell MB, et al. Objective evidence of blunt cardiac trauma. *J Trauma* 1986; 26: 510.

106 Biffl WL, Herzig D. Thoracic trauma. In: Fink MP, Abraham E, Vincent JL, Kochanek PM, eds. *Textbook of Critical Care*, 5th edn. Philadelphia: Elsevier Saunders, 2005: 2077–2087.

107 Velmahos GC, Karaiskakis M, Salim A, et al. Normal electrocardiography and serum troponin I levels preclude the presence of clinically significant blunt cardiac injury. *J Trauma* 2003; 54: 45–51.

108 Barton RG. *Initial approach to the injured patient*. In: Abrams JH, Druck P, Cerra FB, eds. *Surgical Critical Care*, 2nd edn. Boca Raton, FL: Taylor and Francis, 2005: 63–80.

109 Taskinen SO, Salo JA, Halttunen PEA, et al. Tracheobronchial rupture due to blunt chest trauma: a follow-up study. *Ann Thorac Surg* 1989; 48: 846.

110 Jones WG, Ginsberg RJ. Esophageal perforation: a continuing challenge. *Ann Thorac Surg* 1992; 53: 534.

111 Tilanus HW, Bossuyt P, Schattenkeck ME, et al. Treatment of oesophageal perforation: a multivariate analysis. *Br J Surg* 1991; 78: 582.

112 Fildes J, Reed L, Jones N, Martin M, Barrett J. Trauma: the leading cause of maternal death. *J Trauma* 1992; 32: 643.

113 Hayek DA, Veremakis C. Intracranial pathophysiology of brain injury. *Problems Crit Care* 1991; 5: 135.

114 Deitch EA, Sarawati DD. Intensive care unit management of the trauma patient. *Crit Care Med* 2006; 34: 2294.

115 Robertson CS, Contant CF, Gokaslan ZL, et al. Cerebral blood flow, arteriovenous oxygen difference and outcome in head injured patients. *J Neurol Neurosurg Psychiatry* 1992; 55: 594.

116 Rabadi MH, Jordan BD. Maternal head trauma during pregnancy. In: Hainline B, Devinsky O, eds. *Neurologic Complications of Pregnancy*, 2nd edn. Philadelphia: Lippincott Williams and Wilkins, 2002: 75–85.

117 Brain Trauma Foundation, American Association of Neurological Surgeons, Congress of Neurological Surgeons, Joint Section on Neurotrauma and Critical Care. *Guidelines for the Management of Severe Traumatic Brain Injury: Cerebral Perfusion Pressure*. New York: Brain Trauma Foundation, 2003.

118 Bullock R, Ward JD. Management of head trauma. In: Ayres SM, Granuik A, Holbrook PR, Shoemaker WC, eds. *Textbook of Critical Care*. Philadelphia: WB Saunders, 1995: 1449–1457.

119 Brain Trauma Foundation, American Association of Neurological Surgeons, Joint Section on Neurotrauma and Critical Care. Intracranial pressure treatment threshold. *J Neurotrauma* 2000; 17: 493.

120 Durbin CG. Management of traumatic brain injury: have we learned what works? *Crit Care Alert* 2001; 9(6): 63.

121 Judy KD. Craniotomy. In: Lanken PN, Hanson CW, Manaker S, eds. *The Intensive Care Unit Manual*. Philadelphia: WB Saunders, 2001: 979–986.

122 American Nimodipine Study Group. Clinical trial of nimodipine in acute ischemic stroke. *Stroke* 1992; 23: 3.

123 Schmid-Elaesser R, Kunz M, Zausinger S, Prueckner S, Briegel J, Steiger H. Intravenous magnesium versus nimodipine in the treatment of patients with aneurismal subarachnoid hemorrhage: a randomized study. *Neurosurgery* 2006; 58: 1054.

124 Gennarelli TA, Thibault LE. Biomechanics of acute subdural hematoma. *J Trauma* 1982; 22: 680.

125 Bullock R, Teasdale GM. Surgical management of traumatic intracranial hematomas. In: Breakman R, ed. *Handbook of Clinical Neurology – Head Injury*. Amsterdam: Elsevier, 1990: 259–297.

126 Brain Trauma Foundation, American Association of Neurological Surgeons, Joint Section on Neurotrauma and Critical Care. Hyperventilation. *J Neurotrauma* 2000; 17: 513.

127 Muizelear JP, Wei EP, Kontos HA, et al. Mannitol causes compensatory cerebral vasoconstriction and vasodilation on response to blood viscosity changes. *J Neurosurg* 1983; 59: 822.

128 Enevoldsen EM, Jensen FT. Autoresolution and CO2 responses of cerebral blood flow in patients with acute head injury. *J Neurosurg* 1978; 48: 689.

129 Muizelear JP, Maramou A, Ward JD, et al. Adverse effects of prolonged hyperventilation in patients with severe head injury: a randomized clinical trial. *J Neurosurg* 1991; 75: 731.

130 Wakai A, Roberts I, Schierhout G. Mannitol for acute traumatic brain injury. *Cochrane Database Syst Rev* 2005;4: CD001049.

131 Dearden NM, Gibson JS, McDowell DG, et al. Effect of high dose dexamethasone on outcome from severe head injury. *J Neurosurg* 1986; 64: 81.

132 Hunt HB, Schifrin BS, Suzuki K. Ruptured berry aneurysms and pregnancy. *Obstet Gynecol* 1974; 43: 827.

133 Flynn WJ, Bone L. *Fractures in blunt multiple trauma*. In: Abrams JH, Druck P, Cerra FB, eds. *Surgical Critical Care*, 2nd edn. Boca Raton, FL: Taylor and Francis, 2005: 81–86.

134 Bone L. Management of polytrauma. In: Chapman M, ed. *Operative Orthopedics*. Philadelphia: Lippincott, 2002: 417–430.

135 Court-Brown C, McQueen M, Tornetta P. *Orthopedic Surgery Essentials*. Philadelphia: Lippincott, 2006: 482–491.

136 Giannoudic P, Veysi V, Pape HC, Smith M. When should we operate on major fractures in patients with severe head injuries? *Am J Surg* 2002; 183: 261.

137 Gulli B, Templeton D. Compartment syndrome of the lower extremity. *Orthop Clin North Am* 1994; 25: 677.

138 Besman A, Kirton O. Pelvic and major long bone fractures. In: Fink MP, Abraham E, Vincent JL, Kochanek PM, eds. *Textbook of Critical Care*, 5th edn. Philadelphia: Elsevier Saunders, 2005: 299–300.

139 Brohi K, Wilson-MacDonald J. Evaluation of unstable cervical spine injury: a six year experience. *J Trauma* 2000; 49: 76.

140 Bottini A. *Spinal cord injury*. In: Abrams JH, Druck P, Cerra FB, eds. *Surgical Critical Care*, 2nd edn. Boca Raton, FL: Taylor and Francis, 2005: 245–267.

141 Bracken MD, Shepard MJ, Collins WF, et al. A randomized controlled trial of methylprednisolone or naloxone in the treatment of acute spinal cord injury. *N Engl J Med* 1990; 322: 1405.

142 Heary RF, Vaccaro AR, Mesa JJ, et al. Steroids and gunshot wounds to the spine. *Neurosurgery* 1997; 41: 576.

143 Jallo G. Neurosurgical management of penetrating spinal injury. *Surg Neurol* 1997; 47: 328.

144 Baker EB, Cardenas DD. Pregnancy in spinal cord injured women. *Arch Phys Med Rehabil* 1996; 77: 501.

145 Baker EB, Cardenas DD, Benedetti TJ. Risks associated with pregnancy in spinal cord injured women. *Obstet Gynecol* 1992; 80: 425.

38 Thermal and Electrical Injury

Cornelia R. Graves
Tennessee Maternal-Fetal Medicine PLC, Nashville, *and* Vanderbilt University, Nashville, TN, USA

Introduction

Most burns are caused by exposure to a thermal, chemical, or electrical source. Recent studies have estimated that approximately 7% of women of reproductive age are seen for treatment of major burns. In the United States, most burns during pregnancy are due to industrial accidents [1]. Unfortunately, a recent proliferation of clandestine methamphetamine labs, especially in rural areas, has emerged as a new cause of burns in this age group [2].

Maternal and perinatal morbidity and mortality increase as the total body surface area burned increases [3–5] (Figure 38.1). In the non-pregnant population, recent advances in treatment have reduced mortality rates and improved the quality of life in burn survivors. This has been translated into improved survival for both mother and fetus. Due to the complicated clinical nature of the process, a multidisciplinary approach is required to achieve the best results.

Classification

Burns are classified by degree based on the depth of the burn into the skin and also by the amount of surface area involved. Partial-thickness injury includes first- and second-degree burns; third-degree burns are full thickness.

First-degree or superficial burns involve the epidermis only. The skin is erythematous and painful to touch. The best example of this type of burn is a sunburn. These types of burns require topical treatment only.

Second-degree burns involve death and destruction of portions of the epidermis and part of the corium or dermis. A superficial burn is typically characterized by fluid-filled blisters. A deep partial-thickness burn may form eschar. On initial evaluation, it may be difficult to assess the depth of the injury. These burns are painful, but enough viable tissue is left for healing to take place without grafting.

Third-degree or full-thickness burns involve the dermis and the corium (dermis) and extend into the fat layer or further. The skin has a thick layer of eschar and may or may not be painful depending on the amount of damage done to the surrounding nerves [3].

In addition to the thickness of the burn, the part of the body burned, concurrent injuries, and past medical history may also affect outcome.

Estimation of total body surface area (TBSA) involved in a burn may be determined in two ways: "the rule of nines" or the Lund–Browder chart [6]. The rule of nines divides the body into sections that allows for quick estimation of the burn area and is especially useful in emergency situations (Table 38.1). The Lund–Browder chart also divides the body into sections but is more accurate as it takes into account changes in body surface area related to patient age. In both methods only second- and third-degree burns are estimated. A chart specific to pregnancy has not been developed [6].

Minor burns involve less than 10% of TBSA, are no more than partial thickness in depth, and are otherwise uncomplicated. Burns are considered major if the patient has a history of chronic illness, if the burn involves the face, hands, or perineum, if there is concurrent injury, or if the burn is caused by electrical injury [7]. Critical burns encompass greater than 40% of TBSA and are associated with major morbidity and mortality. Severe burns involve 20–39% of TBSA; moderate burns involve 10–19% of TBSA [8].

Thermal burns

Thermal injuries during pregnancy usually occur at home and are most often caused by flame burns or hot scalding liquids. This type of burn commonly involves smoke inhalation injury. The burn only involves the area of the body that was in direct contact with the cause of the injury. Thermal burns are classified based on the degree of injury as described above [3,9].

Critical Care Obstetrics, 5th edition. Edited by M. Belfort, G. Saade, M. Foley, J. Phelan and G. Dildy.

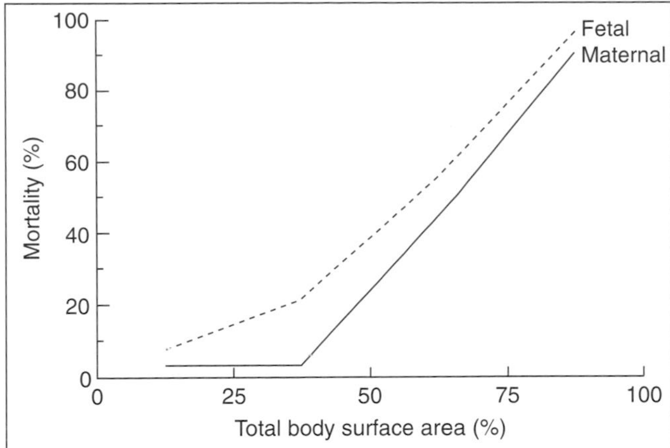

Figure 38.1 Maternal and perinatal morbidity and mortality increase as the total body surface area burned increases [7].

Table 38.1 The rule of nines.

Anatomic area	Percentage of body surface area
Head	9
Upper extremities	9 (each)
Lower extremities	9 (each)
Anterior trunk	18
Posterior trunk	18
Neck	1

Small burns are classified as less than 20% of total body surface area.

Chemical burns

The amount of injury to the skin from a chemical burn is dependent on several factors: (i) the concentration of the chemical; (ii) the duration of exposure to the chemical; (iii) the amount of chemical involved; (iv) the type of chemical; and (v) the effect of the chemical on the skin or exposed area. Unlike thermal burns, the degree of injury is directly related to the duration of exposure. Flushing of the skin or exposed area should be accomplished as soon as possible after exposure. While water is usually the flushing medium of choice, a careful history should be taken as water may actually potentiate the injury when used with certain chemicals such as phosphorus.

Electrical burns

The passage of high-voltage electrical energy through tissues results in thermal injury [10] and a burn that involves not only the skin and subcutaneous tissues but also all other tissue in the path of the current. The amount of damage to the tissues depends on the characteristics of the electrical current.

The burn area usually involves an entry and an exit site. The amount of underlying tissue, muscle, and nerve damage can be extremely difficult to assess. Electrical current may be delivered as a wave or alternating pattern called alternating current (AC), or as direct current (DC). Current is created when the flow of electricity, measured by voltage, meets resistance. When this flow encounters resistance it generates current, measured by amperage. The higher the current, the more severe is the injury.

Alternating current is more dangerous than direct current as it can cause tonic muscle contractions and the victim may be unable to release the source of electrical energy. Since different parts of the body provide varying degrees of resistance, the damage caused by electricity can vary. As the same current can generate varying amounts of heat, damage is based on the resistance it encounters [3].

Electrical injury can occur through four mechanisms. Direct contact with the electrical source results in injury to the skin in contact with the source and the surrounding subcutaneous tissues. Arcing of electricity usually occurs across joint areas as electrical charge is transferred. This results in cutaneous burns in areas not involved with entry or the exit site. Conduction burns occur when the current is conducted through another medium such as water to another body area. Secondary ignition burns occur when the electrical source ignites a flammable material.

The most common causes of electrical burns include occupational hazards, household appliances, and lightning.

There is scarce information regarding fetal outcome after accidental electric shock in pregnancy. A prospective cohort study noted that in most cases accidental electric shock occurring during day-to-day life during pregnancy does not pose a major fetal risk [11].

Maternal concerns

There are a number of physiologic changes that occur during pregnancy. These changes can make the management of the burn patient especially challenging. This section will address these changes and their relationship to maternal complications.

Cardiovascular system

During pregnancy, cardiac output and plasma volume are increased. Systemic vascular resistance is decreased to compensate for the increased circulatory volume. Colloid osmotic pressure is decreased in the vascular spaces. This high-flow, low-resistance state is essential for maintaining perfusion to the uterus and for increasing oxygen delivery to the fetus. A loss of integrity of the skin results in a loss of body water. This loss is more exaggerated in pregnancy due to the decreased colloid osmotic pressure. Therefore, the pregnant burn patient is at increased risk of losing cardiac output and circulatory volume, which are essential for maintaining a stable hemodynamic profile.

Pulmonary system

Increased oxygen delivery and consumption are the hallmark changes in the pulmonary system during pregnancy. Respiratory rate, tidal volume, and minute volume are increased. These changes lead to a state of relative hyperventilation. Arterial blood gases reflect higher resting oxygen tension and lower resting carbon dioxide tension (~30 mmHg) than that seen in the non-pregnant state.

Oxygen delivery is facilitated by the increased cardiac output and circulating red cell volume. Oxygen needs of the placenta and fetus increase oxygen consumption, making the patient susceptible to hypoxemia if oxygen delivery decreases.

As many thermal and chemical inhalation injuries involve the pulmonary system, early evaluation is warranted. Burns involving the face, neck, or chest may also involve damage to the respiratory passages, leading to compromise of the airway. As the trachea tends to be more edematous, especially during the third trimester of pregnancy, consideration should be given to early intubation in any case where there is potential damage to the airway.

Integumentary system

The skin is the organ system most often involved in burns. The skin serves as a barrier to infection and a regulator of fluid, electrolyte, and thermal balance. During pregnancy, the skin is also expected to adapt to changes in body habitus. Severe burns involving the trunk of the patient before or during early pregnancy may lead to problems with skin expansion, especially during the second and third trimester when the abdomen must expand to accommodate the growing fetus [12]. A longitudinal study of seven patients with circumferential truncal burns sustained during childhood reveal one case of scar tissue breakdown in the third trimester. Burn treatment of all seven patients included excision and split-thickness skin grafts [13]. Cultured epidermal autograft has also been used successfully in pregnancy in the case of severe burns over a large surface area when the patient has a shortage of skin suitable for grafting [14]. A recent case report described using the naturally expanded skin of pregnancy to reconstruct the abdominal wall to allow for future pregnancies to proceed without discomfort [15].

Management strategies

Management of burns in the general patient can be divided into four periods: the resuscitation period (0–36 hours post injury), the postresuscitation period (2–5 days post injury), the inflammation–infection period (from 6 days to post wound closure), and rehabilitation [16].

Resuscitation period

The primary treatment goal of the patient suffering a large burn is the avoidance of complications related to fluid and electrolyte deficits in the period immediately after the burn. Cardiovascular and pulmonary support is crucial.

Estimation of TBSA and the severity of the burns are the first steps toward management. While there are many formulas for calculating fluid replacement based on TBSA, the modified Brooke formula [17] and the Parkland formula [18] are two of the most frequently used. Initial management includes placement of a Foley catheter to monitor renal perfusion. In patients with a history of cardiac or pulmonary disease, those with combined cutaneous and pulmonary injury, or in patients unresponsive to initial resuscitative efforts, a pulmonary artery catheter should be considered to help with management of fluid balance.

Early intubation is recommended in those patients with suspected inhalation injury as inflammation and development of tissue edema in the airway may make intubation difficult. Chemical damage of the respiratory passages may require intubation to provide the adequate pulmonary toilet necessary for healing. Pulmonary injury in a pregnant woman adds to the complexity of managing a burn patient since hypoxia may lead to uterine contractions and fetal compromise and these concerns must be anticipated [19].

Serial chemical and electrolyte studies should be performed. Care should be taken to monitor glucose carefully, since hypoglycemia can occur as the patient tries to regulate her body temperature. Arterial blood gases should be obtained immediately, as should a complete blood cell count, blood cultures when indicated, and a coagulation panel. When X-ray examinations are indicated abdominal shielding should be used when possible. Tetanus toxoid is not contraindicated in pregnancy and should be given if indicated.

Crystalloid is given in the form of lactated Ringer's at a rate of 4 mL/kg per % of body burn during the first 24 hours. For example, in a 65-kg patient with TBSA burn of 50%, 13 000 mL of fluid would be required. Half of this volume should be given over the first 8 hours, the remaining half over the next 16 hours in divided increments [20]. Red cell replacement may be required and can be used for volume expansion as well as for increasing oxygen-carrying capacity. The hematocrit may be falsely elevated in the face of volume depletion and is not a reliable indicator of volume status. The use of more sophisticated methods of fluid volume monitoring is usually indicated. Urinary output should be maintained at approximately 100 mL/h by judicious volume expansion. Hypoproteinemia secondary to losses from the burn area and the decreased colloid osmotic pressure of pregnancy may be associated with massive tissue edema during the resuscitation period.

The wound should be treated daily with debridement, cleansing, and topical antibacterial creams. As the hypercoaguable state of pregnancy is aggravated by the endothelial damage and immobility of the burn victim, prophylactic heparin or sequential compression devices are recommended to decrease the risk of deep venous thrombosis.

Postresuscitation period

This period typically begins 2–5 days after the injury has taken place. If the patient is hemodynamically stable and oxygen delivery is adequate, operative management of the wound can begin. It is important to accomplish excision of the burned tissue and closure of the skin at this time before inflammation and infection occur. This usually takes the form of a series of short surgical procedures since hypothermia is always a concern. To combat infection, topical antibiotic administration and frequent wound cultures (to determine specific bacterial colonization) are carried out. Intravenous antibiotics are specifically targeted to those organisms identified in culture. A consumptive coagulopathy may occur during this period, requiring blood component therapy replacement. When interpreting the coagulation profile during pregnancy, it should be remembered that fibrinogen levels are increased and that fibrinogen in the normal range may be a sign of an early coagulopathy.

Inflammation–infection period

The hypermetabolic response to injury begins at about 4–5 days after injury and peaks at about 7–10 days [21]. Cardiac output is often more than doubled in order to keep pace with the necessary increase in oxygen demand. Carbon dioxide production is also increased, and this can lead to rapid deterioration in respiratory status as the injured lung may be unable to exchange gases satisfactorily. The difficulty in differentiating a hypermetabolic state from sepsis or pregnancy-related processes can make diagnosis during this period extremely difficult. The injured lung is also at increased risk for pneumonia secondary to hypoxia, atelectasis, mucous plugging, and increased tissue edema. In addition to all of the pathologic processes, the decreased colloid osmotic pressure of pregnancy further contributes to the development of acute respiratory distress syndrome (ARDS).

Adequate nutritional support is crucial during this period. Supplementation via the gastrointestinal route is optimal. Parenteral nutrition may also be needed to meet caloric demands. When calculating nutritional needs it is important to remember that the metabolic demands of pregnancy are increased and early nutritional assessment is recommended. A true measurement of caloric needs can be obtained from indirect calorimetry and this technique may be required to adequately address the nutritional situation.

The burn wound is best managed by the use of topical antibiotics. Silver sulfadiazine is most commonly used and is not contraindicated in pregnancy. *Staphylococcus aureus* is the most common bacterium responsible for wound infection; however, Gram-negative organisms, especially *Pseudomonas aeruginosa*, may also be cultured [22]. Once infection has been ruled out or treated, skin grafting can take place if needed. This is usually accomplished 2–3 weeks after the injury.

Rehabilitation

Active range of motion exercises in the burn patient should be instituted as soon as possible to prevent loss of muscle and loss of joint function. In the parturient, movement of the lower extremities and early ambulation is important for another reason as well, since it can prevent the formation of deep venous thrombosis. Current recommendations for the prevention of thromboembolism in the high-risk pregnancy including the use of low-dose heparin or sequential compression stockings [23,24] should be implemented. Left lateral recumbent positioning helps to increase blood flow to the fetus and avoid maternal hypotension. The route of delivery should be based on obstetric considerations. Some authors advocate proceeding with urgent delivery in term patients who have sustained critical burns [1,25].

Maternal complications

Acute renal failure

Acute renal failure presenting as oliguria or anuria is not uncommon in the burn patient. Prerenal azotemia occurs frequently because underestimation of the extent of the injury may lead to an underestimation of volume status. In the pregnant patient, assessment of vital signs alone may be insufficient as the increased maternal cardiac output and increased volume status associated with pregnancy may mask signs of hemodynamic compromise. Treatment should be aimed at maintaining adequate intravascular volume. In the patient who is unresponsive to reasonable fluid replacement, hemodynamic monitoring should be instituted to assist in aggressive fluid replacement. Low-dose dopamine is not contraindicated in pregnancy.

In the electrical burn patient, deep tissue injury may not be readily apparent. Massive muscle injury, common in the electrical burn patient, may lead to the production of myoglobin. Myoglobin, a breakdown product of necrotic muscle, is directly toxic to the renal tubule. Hypovolemia may assist in potentiating renal injury in patients with myoglobinuria. Hyperkalemia can accompany myoglobinuria and may be life-threatening. The diagnosis of myoglobinuria can be easily performed at the bedside. The presence of reddish-brown urine and a negative urine dipstick for hemoglobin confirms the presence of myoglobin. Treatment should be undertaken to maintain urine output through volume replacement. Mannitol may also be used to aid in increasing urinary output. This is one condition in which the use of bicarbonate should be considered in all intravenous fluids in order to alkalize the urine and assist in the excretion of myoglobin.

Sepsis/ARDS

Sepsis is a major cause of death in burn patients. It has been estimated that approximately half of all deaths from burns are due to complications from infection and pneumonia. The most common causes of infection include *S. aureus*, *Enterococcus*, *Candida albicans*, and *Pseudomonas* species. The regular use of wound biopsies as well as tissue and blood cultures has allowed for the more specific and controlled use of systemic antimicrobial and antifungal agents. Aggressive efforts are needed to prevent sepsis since this may lead to multisystem end-organ failure.

Multisystem end-organ failure in the burn patient has a mortality rate of nearly 100%. The immunosuppressive effects of pregnancy, as well as host compromise secondary to injury, may make the parturient especially susceptible to the development of septic complications. Recognition of appropriate treatment is crucial. In interpreting pulmonary artery catheter values, the hyperdynamic state of pregnancy must be considered and taken into account, and this is certainly an area where obstetricians can assist their critical care colleagues.

During pregnancy, the development of sepsis frequently leads to the development of ARDS. As mentioned above, changes in the respiratory system during pregnancy may make the lung susceptible to injury. Smoke inhalation injury associated with massive fluid shifts during the postresuscitation period may predispose the patient to bacterial colonization and the development of pneumonia. As respiratory failure is the leading cause of death in the burn patient, early recognition of respiratory distress is imperative. Early intubation and the use of positive end-expiratory pressure may prevent further injury. While parameters have not been established for pregnancy, it is my opinion that intubation be strongly considered in patients with a respiratory rate of greater than 40/min, a P_aO_2 of less than 80 mmHg, or a P_aCO_2 of greater than 40 mmHg. Given the physiologic changes of pregnancy, P_aO_2 and P_aCO_2 levels that would be otherwise tolerated in a non-pregnant individual are unacceptable in pregnancy. A sustained P_aO_2 of less than 60 mmHg will lead to fetal distress, and a sustained P_aCO_2 of greater than 40 mmHg will affect placental gas exchange and lead to fetal acidosis. The frequently employed strategies of permissive hypoventilation and hypoxia/hypercapnia may not be possible in a pregnant woman if there is concern about fetal health. Obviously the maternal condition takes precedence and fetal outcome may in some cases be disregarded, especially in non-viable fetuses. In other cases, however, early delivery may be required in order to allow institution of permissive ventilation strategies for the mother. This is another area where the obstetrician is often of great value to the critical care team.

Fractures

Evaluation for skeletal trauma should occur early in the assessment in patients experiencing electrical injury. Increased tetany of the muscles during electrocution may result in long bone fractures as well as fractures of the vertebral column. Appropriate radiologic investigation should not be delayed or avoided because of the pregnant state.

Mortality

Maternal mortality in industrial countries following burn injury is related to the severity of the injury and the potential for complications. Maternal mortality is lower than 5% when less than 50% of TBSA is affected, and greater than 100% when more than 80% of TBSA is involved. In developing areas, the risk of maternal and fetal death may approach 100% when greater than 40% of the TBSA is involved [5].

Fetal complications

Preterm labor

Preterm labor and delivery usually ensue within the first few days after significant thermal injury. Prostaglandin levels are uniformly increased in the burn patient. Inadequate volume resuscitation may also lead to a decrease in uteroplacental perfusion and tissue hypoxia. These factors combine to increase the incidence of preterm labor and delivery. As burn patients are at great risk for complications from tocolytic therapy, care should be taken to individualize care for each patient. Because β-mimetics are associated with increased capillary permeability and electrolyte imbalances, it has been suggested that the safest tocolytic agent in these patients may be parenteral magnesium sulfate [26]. Corticosteroids should be administered to those patients between 24 and 34 weeks if appropriate and infection is not a major concern. In a retrospective review, 100% of patients with critical burns delivered their fetus within the first 7 days after their injury [27].

Monitoring

External fetal monitoring should be instituted when the fetus is potentially viable. This is generally around 24 weeks [28]. If the abdominal burns are present, a sterile transducer cover should be used to reduce the risks of infection. Not only can fetal assessment provide important information about fetal well-being, but it may also assist in maternal resuscitation [29]. If fetal stress is noted, optimizing maternal fluid resuscitation and oxygen delivery capacity may result in improvement of the fetal heart rate tracing, thereby avoiding unnecessary delivery. In the event of maternal cardiac arrest, one should consider intervention on behalf of the fetus at 4 minutes into the resuscitative efforts and attempt to deliver the fetus within 5 minutes of the maternal code [30].

Pregnancy loss

Several authors have noted an increase in the spontaneous abortion rate in patients who experience burns during the first trimester. In one study, four of six patients who were injured during this period miscarried [31]. Some authors have advocated therapeutic terminations in patients with severe burns in the first trimester; however, there are no data to associate this with improved maternal outcome [32].

Fetal distress and stillbirths

Fetal distress secondary to hypoxia and uteroplacental insufficiency may necessitate the need for emergent delivery. For this reason, all parturients with a viable fetus should have fetal monitoring instituted if at all possible. Perinatal morbidity is directly related to the severity of the burn. When less than 40% of TBSA is involved, the perinatal mortality rate is approximately 25%; when 50% of TBSA is involved, the perinatal mortality rate increases to 50%; and when greater than 80% of TBSA is involved, 100% of fetuses are usually lost (see Figure 38.1).

Conclusions

While massive burn injury is relatively uncommon during pregnancy, it is associated with significant maternal and neonatal morbidity and mortality. Aggressive resuscitation and therapeutic measures aimed at stabilizing the mother and the fetus as well as collaborative care between the surgical and obstetric team are necessary to optimize outcome.

References

1 Guo S, Greenspoon JS, Kahn AM. Management of burn injuries during pregnancy. *Burns* 2001; 27: 394–397.
2 Danks RR, Wibbenmeyer LA, Faucher LD, et al. Metamphetamine-associate burn injuries: a retrospective analysis. *J Burn Care Rehabil* 2005; 25(5): 425–429.
3 Caine R, Lefcourt N. Patients with burns. In: Clochesy J, Breu C, Cardin S, et al, eds. *Critical Care Nursing*. Philadelphia: WB Saunders, 1993: 183.
4 Akhtar MA, Mulawkar PM, Kulkarni HR. Burns in pregnancy: effect on maternal and fetal outcomes. *Burns* 1994; 20: 351–355.
5 Maghsoudi H, Samnia R, Garadaghi A et al. Burns in pregnancy. *Burns* 2006; 32: 246–250.
6 Demling RH. Burn management. In: Wilmore D, ed. *Pre- and Postoperative Care*. New York: Scientific American, 1991.
7 Polko LE, McMahon MJ. Burns in pregnancy. *Obstet Gynecol Surv* 1999; 54: 131.
8 Reiss G. Thermal injuries. In: Lopez-Veigo MA, ed. *The Parkland Trauma Handbook*. St Louis: Mosby, 1994: 389.
9 Gang RK, Bajec J, Tahboub M. Management of thermal injury in pregnancy: an analysis of 16 patients. *Burns* 1992; 18: 317–320.
10 Holliman CJ, Saffle JR, Kravitz M, et al. Early surgical decompression in the management of electrical injuries. *Am J Surg* 1982; 144: 733–739.
11 Einarson A, Bailey B, Inocencion G, et al. Accidental electric shock in pregnancy: a prospective cohort study. *Am J Obstet Gynecol* 1997; 176: 678–681.
12 Widgerow AD, Ford TD, Botha M. Burn contracture preventing uterine expansion. *Ann Plast Surg* 1991; 27: 269–271.
13 McCauley RL, Stenberg BA, Phillips LG, et al. Long-term assessment of the effects of circumferential truncal burns in pediatric patients on subsequent pregnancies. *J Burn Care Rehabil* 1991; 12: 51–53.
14 Barillo DJ, Nangle NE, Farrell K. Preliminary experience with cultured epidermal autograft in a community hospital burn unit. *J Burn Care Rehabil* 1992; 13: 158–165.
15 Webb JC, Baack BR, Osler TM, et al. A pregnancy complicated by mature abdominal burns scarring and its surgical solution: a case report. *J Burn Care Rehabil* 1995; 16: 276–279.
16 Demling RH. Management of the burn patient. In: Grenvik A, Holbrook PR, Shoemaker WC, eds. *Textbook of Critical Care*, 3rd edn. Philadelphia: WB Saunders, 1995: 1499.
17 Pruitt BA Jr, Mason AD Jr, Moncrief JA. Hemodynamic changes in the early postburn patient: the influence of fluid administration and of a vasodilator. *J Trauma* 1971; 11: 36–46.
18 Baxter CR. Guidelines for fluid resuscitation. *J Trauma* 1981; 21: 687–689.
19 Pimental L. Mother and child trauma in pregnancy. *Emerg Med Clin North Am* 1991; 9: 549.
20 Georgiade G, Pederson C. Burns. In: Sabiston DC, ed. *Essentials of Surgery*. Philadelphia: WB Saunders, 1987: 122.
21 Alexander J. The role of infection in the burn patient. In: Boswick J, ed. *The Art and Science of Burn Care*. Rockville, MD: Aspen Publishers, 1987: 103.
22 Boss WK, Brand DA, Acampora D, et al. Effectiveness of prophylactic antibiotics in the outpatient treatment of burns. *J Trauma* 1985; 25: 244–247.
23 Mabrouk AR, El-Feky AE. Burns during pregnancy: a gloomy outcome. *Burns* 1997; 23: 596–600.
24 American College of Obstetricians and Gynecologists. *Practice Bulletin No. 84. Prevention of Deep Vein Thrombosis and Pulmonary Embolism*. Washington, DC: American College of Obstetricians and Gynecologists, 2007.
25 Ullmann Y, Blumenfield Z, Hakim M, et al. Urgent delivery, the treatment of choice in term pregnant women with extended burn injury. *Burns* 1997; 23: 157–159.
26 Unsur V, Oztopcu C, Atalay C, et al. A retrospective study of 11 pregnant women with thermal injuries. *Eur J Obstet Gynecol Reprod Biol* 1996; 64: 55–58.
27 Rayburn W, Smith B, Feller I, Varner, M, Cruikshank D. Major burns during pregnancy: effects on fetal well-being. *Obstet Gynecol* 1984; 63: 392–395.
28 Kuhlmann RS, Cruikshank DP. Maternal trauma during pregnancy. *Clin Obstet Gynecol* 1994; 37: 274–293.
29 Pacheco L, Gei AF, VanHook JW, et al. Burns in pregnancy. *Obstet Gynecol* 2005; 106: 1210–1212.
30 Katz V, Balderston K, DeFreest M. Perimortem cesarean delivery: were our assumptions correct? *Am J Obstet Gynecol* 2005; 192: 1916.
31 Jain ML, Garg AK. Burns with pregnancy: a review of 25 cases. *Burns* 1993; 19: 166–167.
32 Lippin Y, Shvoron A, Tsur H. Therapeutic abortion in a severely burned woman. *J Burn Care Rehabil* 1993; 14: 398.

39 Overdose, Poisoning and Envenomation During Pregnancy

Alfredo F. Gei[1] & Victor R. Suarez[2]

[1]Department of Obstetrics and Gynecology, Methodist Hospital in Houston, Houston, TX, USA
[2]Maternal-Fetal Medicine Attending, Advocate Christ Medical Center, Chicago, IL, USA

All substances are poisons.
Paracelsus (1493–1541)

Definitions

Although the terms poisoning and overdose are frequently used interchangeably, poisoning denotes the morbid state produced by the exposure of a toxic agent (poison) that, because of its chemical action, causes a functional disturbance (renal failure or hepatitis, for example) and/or structural damage (chemical burn, for example) [1]. Overdose or overdosage, refers to a state produced by the excess or abuse of a drug or substance [1]. Consequently overdoses can be considered as a particular type of poisoning. Whereas the former suggests an intentional exposure, and the second connotes unintentional or unknown toxic exposure, in the following text we will use the terms poisoning or overdose with respect to the ingestion of chemical agents or drugs and medications, respectively. Envenomations are a particular type of toxic exposure resulting from the human contact with biologic substances (venoms or toxins) produced in specialized glands or tissues from animals, usually by cutaneous or transdermal (parenteral) injection (bee and scorpion stings, snake bites, etc.).

Scope of the problem

Toxic exposures

It is estimated that every year up to 7.2 million poisonings could occur in the USA, for a rate of approximately 8.2 exposures per thousand population [2]. A little over 50% of those toxic exposures occur in women, and more than 300 000 of the poisonings take place in women of reproductive age. Although toxic exposures are overall more frequent in children, the age distribution of the fatal exposures peaks in the late reproductive years [2]. Studies performed in Emergency Departments have shown that up to 6.3% of the consulting female patients may have an unrecognized pregnancy, even when the patient's history is not suggestive of such [3]. For this reason, it has been recommended that a pregnancy test should be part of the evaluation of any woman of child-bearing age presenting with an overdose or poisoning [4].

Pregnancy and medications

Independent of comorbid conditions, pregnancy increases the average intake of medications among women [5,6]. This period in a woman's life should be therefore considered a predisposing condition for adverse effects of medications, including overdosing. Fortunately though, as shown in Table 39.1, the incidence of poisoning during pregnancy is low, likely due to an increased awareness of potentially adverse side effects of medications upon the fetus, though significant cultural and geographical variations exist worldwide [7,8,9].

Toxic exposures during pregnancy

Poisoning is a significant global public health problem. According to World Health Organization data, in 2002 an estimated 350 000 people died worldwide from unintentional poisoning [10]. In 2000, unintentional poisoning was the ninth most common cause of death globally in young adults (15–29 years) [11]. In 2005 in the USA, 8438 cases of toxic exposures during pregnancy were reported to the country's 61 Poison Control Centers [2]. The temporal distribution during pregnancy is approximately equal along the different trimesters, with a slight predominance of the second trimester (Table 39.1). Since 1993, the number of toxic exposures accounted for by pregnant patients has increased in a parallel fashion to the total number of exposures reported (Table 39.1) [12]. The majority of the toxic exposures occurring during pregnancy are acute (86.6% for 1999) and due to a single substance (90.6%). The most frequent route of exposure is oral (50.3%), followed by inhalation (30%) and dermal (10.3%). Although the majority of patients were treated on-site, 4.9% of

Critical Care Obstetrics, 5th edition. Edited by M. Belfort, G. Saade, M. Foley, J. Phelan and G. Dildy.

Table 39.1 Toxic exposures during pregnancy reported to the Poison Control Centers in the USA: 1993–2000. Between 1993 and 2001, the number of toxic exposures during pregnancy represent only a fraction of the exposures reported nationwide (0.3–0.4%). Overall, during this time period, both the total number of exposures and the ones reported by pregnant women have increased steadily by a factor of 1.6–10% per year. The distribution of toxic exposures per trimester of pregnancy has been stable over the past 9 years, with a slightly higher predominance of the second over the other two trimesters.

Year	Total	Pregnant *N* (%)	Trimester* First (%)	Second (%)	Third (%)
1993	1751476	6443 (0.36)	32	38	30
1994	1926438	6147 (0.32)	31	38	31
1995	2023089	6484 (0.32)	30	39	31
1996	2155952	7103 (0.33)	30	39	31
1997	2192088	7250 (0.33)	31	38	31
1998	2241082	8120 (0.36)	32	38	30
1999	2201156	8980 (0.40)	32	38	30
2000	2168248	8438 (0.38)	32	38	31
2001	2267979	7588 (0.33)	32	38	30

* Of those with known gestational age.
(Source: 1993, 1994, 1995, 1996, 1997, 1998, 1999, 2000 and 2001 (in press) From Litovitz TL, Klein-Schwartz W, Martin E et al. American Annual Reports of the American Association of Poison Control Centers Toxic Exposure Surveillance System. *Am J Emerg Med* 1999;17:435–487) [173,197–199]

the exposures resulted in moderate to major effects and 3.4% required admission to a critical care facility. No deaths were reported in this series [13].

During pregnancy, drug overdose frequently is part of a suicide gesture [14,15]. Less often, it is the result of an attempt to induce abortion. Even though most of the exposures during pregnancy are accidental (77.9% for 1999), almost one-fifth (18.0%) are intentional; either related to a suicide attempt (or gesture) or as the result of drug abuse or misuse [13]. More than 95% of suicide gestures involve ingestion of a combination of drugs. When the exposure reported occurred with more than one substance, the risk of a suicide attempt (as the mechanism for the exposure) was three times higher than when a single substance was the toxic agent (odds ratio 3.1, 95% CI 2.75–3.49).The risk of suicidal exposure was also three times higher in pregnant teenagers than for other age groups (odds ratio 3.1, 95% CI 2.79–3.49) [16]. Approximately 1% of suicide gestures in a gravid woman will result in a maternal death [17]. The consideration of a suicide attempt as the mechanism of the poisoning or overdose is extremely important when evaluating and treating these patients (see Figure 39.1, acetaminophen poisoning in a teenager).

Toxicologic considerations in pregnancy

The poisoned pregnant woman poses particular challenges to the obstetrician as well to the emergency physicians and toxicology experts. Most of these challenges are the result of the variable effect with which the physiologic changes of pregnancy may influence the absorption, distribution and metabolic disposition of different potentially toxic agents (Table 39.2) [12].

Overall, there is little information on the appropriate treatment of poisoning in pregnancy, and the use of antidotes raises ethical and medicolegal questions [18]. Several instances have been reported where treatment has been withheld from women because of their gravid condition, with catastrophic results for both mother and fetus [19,20,21].

A developing fetus brings forth the considerations and concerns for latent and delayed effects, including teratogenesis and developmental issues on the conceptus. Up to a certain extent, although the pregnant patient goes through an episode of overdose or poisoning during pregnancy, the fetus would continue to be exposed to the toxic agent and environment, sometimes for several weeks. Once the acute compromise of the pregnant patient resolves, a specific discussion on those regards is in most cases warranted and proper follow-up need to be considered [12].

Evaluation of the poisoned pregnant patient

Although both the poisoning and the pregnancy can be concealed or unknown at the time of the patient presentation or initial consultation, the most common scenario is that of a pregnant woman in her second trimester with a history of an acute exposure to a known toxic agent. The ideal setting for the evaluation of these patients is the Emergency Department, as the situation can range from a very straightforward and of no consequence to a life-threatening and very complex one, requiring a multidisciplinary team and elaborate forms of treatment. The algorithms presented in Figure 39.2 summarize suggested guidelines of evaluation and management of pregnant patients with a known or suspected toxic exposure, regardless of the agent(s) in question. Specific comments are made on the most relevant aspects [12].

Initial evaluation

The initial assessment should determine in a matter of seconds if the patient is conscious or unconscious and, if so, whether she is in cardiac or respiratory arrest (Figure 39.2a). The management of the latter conditions in pregnancy differs very little from the ones on non-pregnant patients with the exception of two additional considerations, as follows.

- Special positioning with a pelvic tilt or wedge to the left and/or the manual displacement of the uterus off the midline to the left is recommended, to relieve the aorto-caval compression by the gravid uterus and improve venous blood return.
- If evaluated by Emergency Room physicians, a prompt consult to the Obstetric Service is recommended, as these patients need an expert assessment of the gestational age and eventually the capability to proceed with a bedside cesarean if the resuscitative efforts are not successful within 5 minutes of the cardiac arrest (see Figure 39.2b, unconscious algorithm) [22,23].

The rapid removal of all clothes (including footwear) is critical. The personnel involved in the patient care should handle the

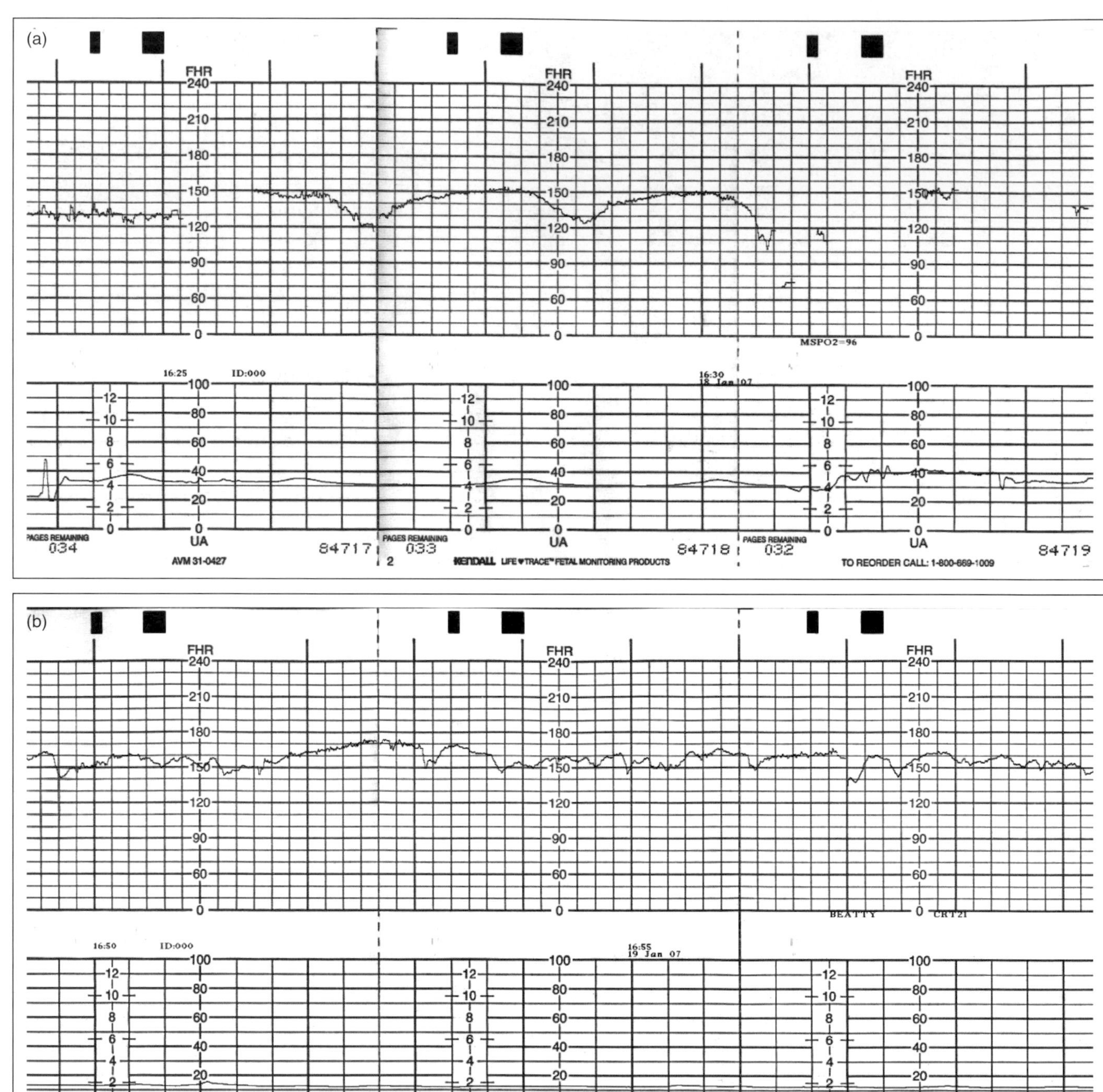

Figure 39.1 Electronic fetal monitoring tracings of a patient with acetaminophen overdose: 17-year-old primigravida with history of bipolar disorder (without treatment) who presented to Labor and Delivery with severe nausea and vomiting, icterus and anion gap metabolic acidosis. An empty bottle of Tylenol was found at home. (a) On arrival; 25 weeks; maternal pH 7.14/bicarbonate of 4 mmol/L. (b) Hours later after aggressive hydration (maternal pH 7.44). (c) At 39 5/7 weeks, after spontaneous onset of labor.

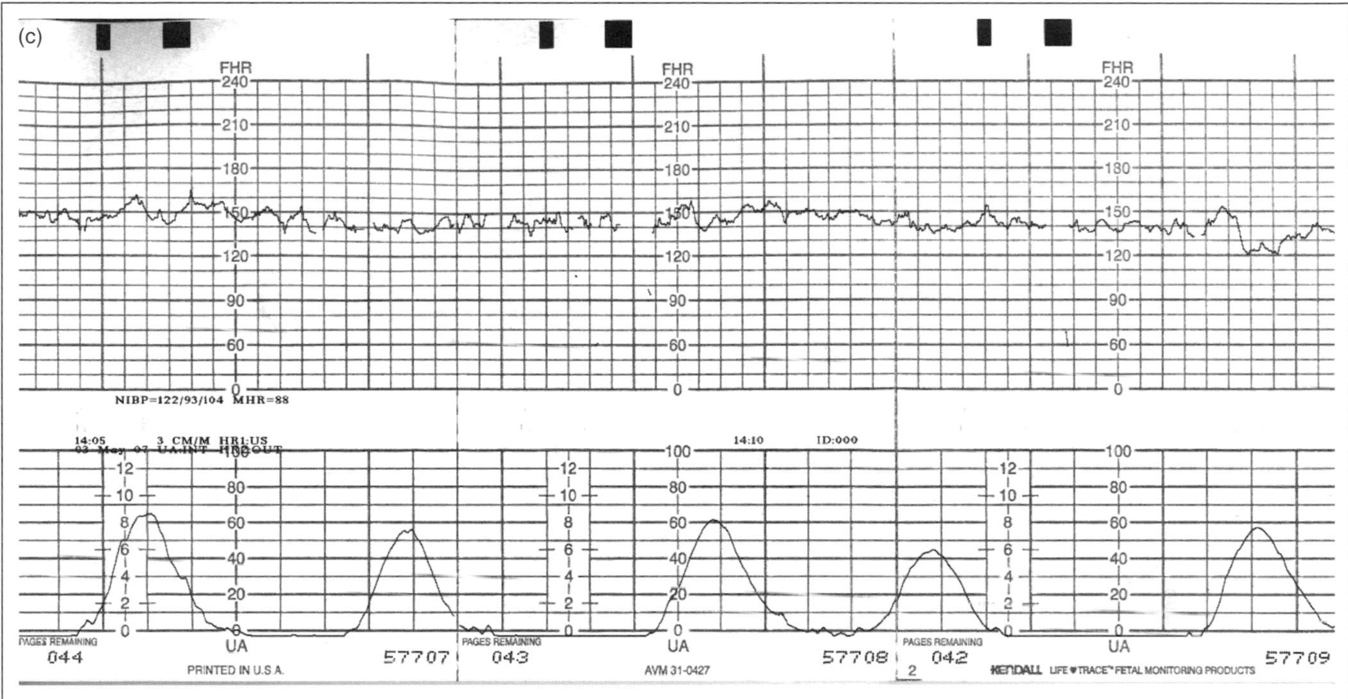

Figure 39.1 *Continued.*

clothes with gloves and set them aside in a labeled plastic bag. Absorption of toxins, organic chemicals, and industrial compounds through the skin is generally the rule rather than the exception. The garments can potentially be used for sampling later and should not be disposed of.

In the unconscious patient with a history of or suspected toxic exposure, trauma should be strongly considered and cervical spine injury should be stabilized until it can be evaluated and cleared by the Emergency Room or trauma physicians.

Altered mental status

- If the patient is unconscious but hemodynamically stable or conscious but disoriented, the diagnosis of "altered mental status" is made.
- Hypoxemia and hypoglycemia should immediately be considered as possible etiologies and oxygen (via a face mask) and a parenteral glucose infusion (1 g/kg or 50 g of 50% glucose) need to be started without delay, even before the diagnosis is confirmed through an arterial blood gas and a glucose determination [24]. Forcing oral intake in a patient with altered mental status is actively discouraged.
- The use of padded restraints, the insertion of an indwelling bladder catheter, and intravenous sedation may be required for the management of uncooperative and belligerent patients. The use of sedatives should ideally be delayed until the toxic agent(s) of exposure is identified to avoid unforeseeable interactions and possibly further central nervous system (CNS) depression. Most institutions have special policies regarding the documentation of the indications, the extent and the duration for physical restraints.
- Other components of the so-called "coma-cocktail" (thiamine, naloxone, and flumazenil) should not be given routinely but selectively and as considered appropriate by the treating physicians. Specific recommendations for the use of these medications can be seen in Table 39.3.

Secondary evaluation

- History-taking is of fundamental importance and every effort should be made to obtain as much information from as many sources as possible (patient, her relatives or friends, and the paramedic personnel if she was brought by ambulance to the Emergency Department). In addition to the obstetric and general history, specific questions to be asked regarding the toxic exposure are: the time of exposure, substances exposed to, the amount of exposure (including strength of prescription, if pills or medications), route of exposure, treatment prior to arrival (including emetics, dilutants and adsorbants), vomit (number and content) or diarrhea (number and content), and symptoms since the exposure.
- A high degree of caution needs to be exercised with the interpretation of the histories, as the information obtained can be contradictory and, in the case of suicide attempts/gestures, even deceitful (Figure 39.1). As a rule of thumb, the most severe history of (worse) exposure obtained should be used as a clinical parameter to guide the initial treatment.

Table 39.2 Physiological changes of pregnancy and their toxicological impact.

System/gestational change	Toxicological implication
Digestive	*Pros:*
Pica	• Window of opportunity for gastric lavage potentially longer
Decreased intra-esophageal pressure	*Cons:*
Delayed gastric emptying	• Increased risk of exposure
Delayed transit time	• Increased gastric absorption
Hepatic flow unchanged	• Increased risk of aspiration
Reduced hepatic enzymatic activity	• Increased enteral absorption
	• Increased risk of hepatotoxicity
Respiratory	*Pros:*
Hyperemia of upper respiratory tract	• Higher sensitivity to hypoxemia and hypercarbia (protective against respiratory depression)
Increased minute ventilation	*Cons:*
Decreased residual lung volume	• Increased absorption of inhaled agents
Increased diffusing capacity	
Circulatory	*Pros:*
30–50% increase in cardiac output	• Dilutional effect
50% increase in plasma volume	*Cons:*
25% decrease in serum albumin	• Higher concentrations in organs with rich perfusion (uterus, placental bed, kidneys, skin)
Increased oxygen consumption	• Higher free fraction of toxins and higher placental passage
Renal	*Pros:*
Increase in glomerular filtration rate	• Increased renal clearance of protein bound and unbound substances
Increased tubular reabsorption	*Cons:*
	• Increased nephrotoxicity potential
Skin	*Cons:*
Increased surface	• Increased absorption of contact agents
Increased blood flow	
Uterus/placenta	*Pros:*
Volume increased by 2000% at term	• Maternal protection for certain exposures
Increased blood perfusion	*Cons:*
Pronounced liposolubility	• Fetal exposure to toxic agents
Others	*Pros:*
Body mass:	• Larger distribution volumes
• Increased by 25% at term	*Cons:*
Oxygen consumption:	• Potential for re-exposure during third trimester
• Increased by 20%	
Fat:	
• Increased storage	
• Third-trimester mobilization	

(Reproduced by permission from Gei AF, Saade GR. Poisoning during pregnancy and lactation. In: Yankowitz J, Niebyl J., eds. Drug Therapy in Pregnancy, 3rd edn. Philadelphia: Lippincott, Williams and Wilkins, 2001.)

• Some groups of agents produce a complex of signs and symptoms that can be recognized as a typical syndrome (toxidrome) [25,26]. Knowledge of such toxidromes is particularly useful when information about the substance is not available. A list of the most common toxidromes is shown in Table 39.4. Other physical findings that are useful in the recognition of a toxic exposure are outlined in Table 39.5.

• Pregnant victims of poisoning or envenomations have particular issues to be considered in the interpretation of test results and treatment of the poisoning (see Table 39.6).

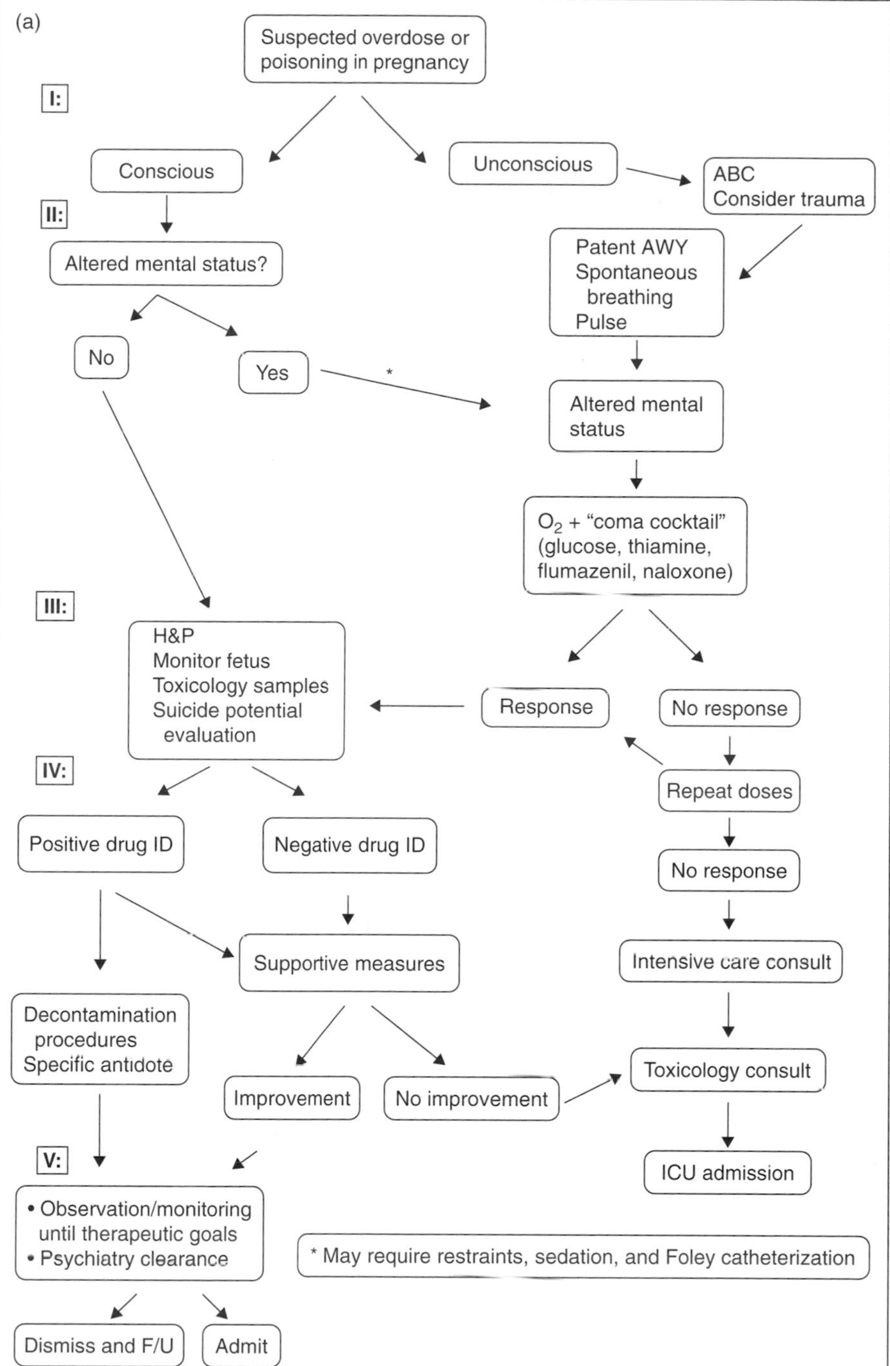

Figure 39.2 (a) Guidelines for evaluation and management of pregnant patients with a known or suspected toxic exposure. (b) Guidelines for the evaluation of the unconscious pregnant patient with a known or suspected toxic exposure. During 1999 1085 suicidal toxic exposures among pregnant women were reported to American Poison Control Centers. This represents 12% of the toxic exposures reported during pregnancy for that year and less than 1% of the suicide attempts by poisoning reported to the American Association of Poison Control Centers. The substances most frequently involved were acetaminophen (alone or in combination with decongestants and antihistamines; 35.5%), nonsteroidal anti-inflammatory drugs (15.2%), selective serotonin-reuptake inhibitors (SSRIs; 8.8%), and benzodiazepines (7.1%). *May require restraints, sedation, and Foley catheterization. ACLS, advanced cardiac life support; AWY, airway; CPR, cardiopulmonary resuscitation; C/S, cesarean section; EKG, electrocardiogram; F/U, follow-up; GA, gestational age; H&P, history and physical; OD, overdose. Reproduced with permission from Gei AF, Saade GR. Poisoning during pregnancy and lactation. In: Yankowitz J, Niebyl J. *Drug Therapy in Pregnancy*, 3rd edn. Philadelphia: Lippincott, Williams and Wilkins, 2001.

• Some patients would require observation and management in an intensive care setting (see Table 39.7).

Toxic identification

• The collection of samples for toxicology is of paramount importance in the identification of the toxic agent(s) causing the exposure, to predict the severity and to implement and monitor specific treatment/antidotes. As a general rule, at least one sample of all biologic fluids should be obtained, and saved for toxicology analysis (see Tables 39.8 and 39.9). Depending on the clinical circumstances, these will include blood, urine, saliva, vomit, gastric lavage fluid, feces, cerebrospinal fluid,

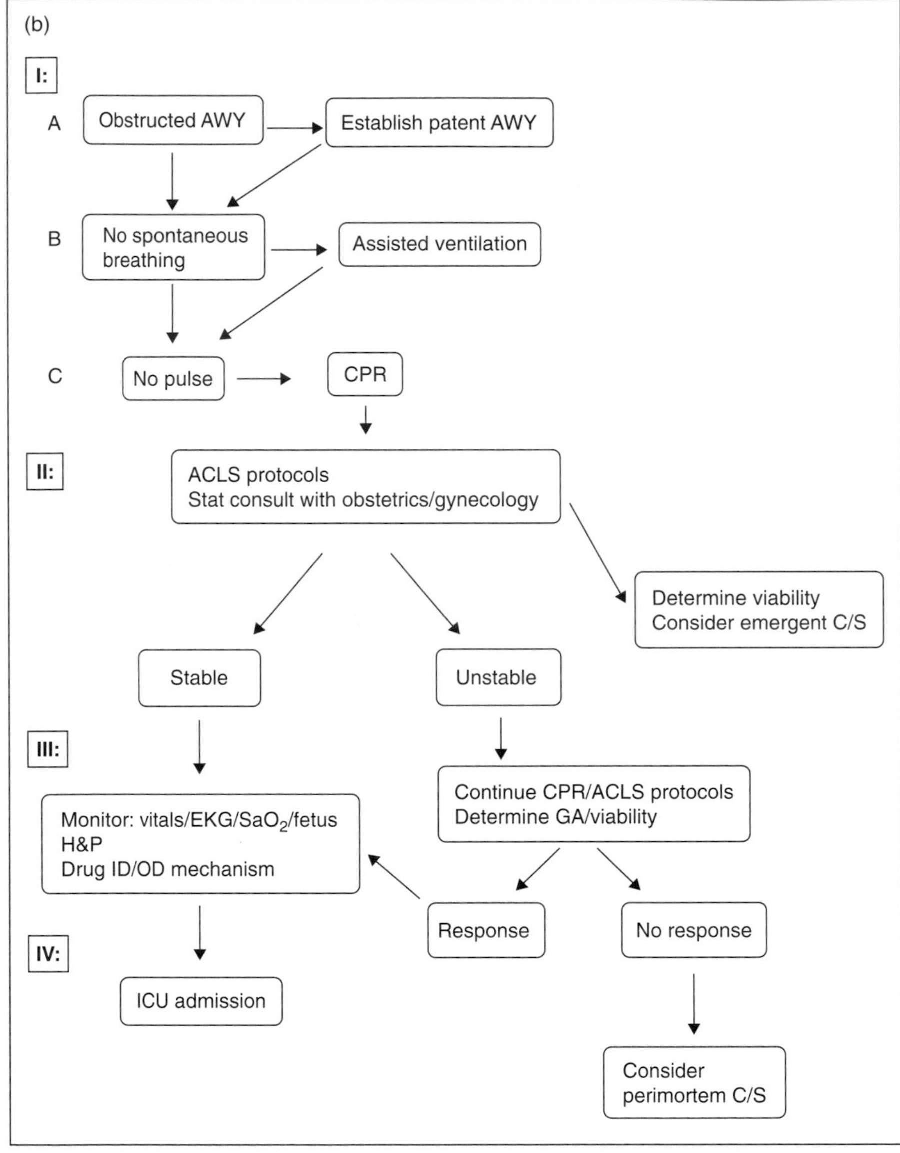

Figure 39.2 *Continued.*

amniotic fluid if collected, and meconium if the patient delivers soon after admission. Occasionally the analysis of an arterial blood gas and basic chemistry will detect an anion gap [AG=(Na^++K^+)−(Cl^-+HCO_3^-); normal outside pregnancy 12 ± 4 mEq/l; for pregnancy 8.5 ± 2.9 mEq/l; postpartum 10.7 ± 2.5 mEq/l] or osmolar gap (normal −5 to +15 mOsm/l) which will assist in the differential diagnosis of acidosis and suggest the possibility of a poisoning or overdose (see Tables 39.10 and 39.11) [27,28,29].

• The mainstay of treatment for all poisonings is supportive therapy. For some toxic agents, three additional strategies can be implemented to: (a) decrease the exposure (*decontamination procedures*), (b) enhance elimination (diuresis, hemofiltration, hemoperfusion, hemodyalisis, and plasmapheresis), or (c) counteract the toxicity of the agent (antidotes). The specific measures to enhance elimination and the use of antidotes are particular for every toxic substance and will be discussed as appropriate in the corresponding section (see Tables 39.12, 39.13, 39.14, 39.15 and 39.16).

Decontamination procedures

Skin

Substances that can cause significant systemic toxicity through transdermal absorption include: organophosphate insecticides, organochlorines, nitrates, and industrial aromatic hydrocarbons. Organophosphates in particular can pass through intact skin at a remarkable speed, without causing any specific skin sensation of burning or itching. In theory, pregnancy, as shown in Table 39.2, predisposes to such toxicity, given the physiologic increase in skin perfusion throughout gestation.

Table 39.3 Altered mental status: indications for antidote treatment in pregnancy.

Naloxone (Narcan)	Altered mental status (AMS) associated with: • miosis • respiratory rate less than 12 or • circumstantial evidence of opioid use/abuse	2 mg (IV, IM, ET, IL); onset of action: 1–3 min. May repeat if no response is noted after 3–5 min (maximal effect is observed within 5–10 min) • An IV drip or repeated doses are given as needed • Higher doses may be necessary to reverse methadone, diphenoxylate, propoxyphene, butorphanol, pentazocine, nalbuphine, designer drugs, or veterinary tranquilizers • Caution in cardiovascular disease; may precipitate withdrawal symptoms in patients with opiate addiction
Thiamine (vitamin B_1, thiamilate)	AMS in patient with risk factors for B_1 deficiency: • ethanol abuse • malnutrition • hyperemesis gravidarum • eating disorder • total parenteral nutrition • AIDS • cancer • dialysis requirement	100 mg daily IV/IM for up to 2 weeks • Administer before or with dextrose-containing fluids (100 mg/L of fluid)
Flumazenil (Romazicon)	AMS with: • suspected or known benzodiazepine exposure and no contraindication for antidote use (hypersensitivity, use of benzodiazepine for control of life-threatening condition, intracranial pressure or seizure disorder), coexposure to tricyclic antidepressant or chronic benzodiazepine use • check EKG to rule out conduction disturbances, which would suggest the presence of tricyclics	0.2 mg (2 mL) given IV over 30 s; a second dose of 0.3 mg (3 mL) can be given over another 30 s • Further doses of 0.5 mg (5 mL) can be given over 30 s at 1-min intervals up to a total dose of 3 mg (although some patients may require up to 5 mg) • If the patient has not responded 5 min after receiving a cumulative dose of 5 mg, the major cause of sedation is probably not due to benzodiazepines and additional doses of flumazenil are likely to have no effect • For resedation, repeated doses may be given at 20-min intervals; no more than 1 mg (given as 0.5 mg/min) at any one time and no more than 3 mg in any 1 h should be administered

The skin should be flushed thoroughly with warm soapy water. It may be worthwhile to use an industrial shower (as is used for corrosive exposure) to thoroughly rinse the entire body. A rare exception to immediate decontamination with water would be the exposure to agents that may react violently with it (e.g. the chemical may ignite, explode, or produce toxic fumes with water). Examples include: chlorosulfonic acid, titanium tetrachloride, and calcium oxide.

Gastrointestinal [30,31,32,33]

Several strategies can be useful, as described below.

Dilution

Lacking from alternatives (see below), 200–300 ml of milk may be given orally (not through gastric tubes) in caustic ingestions (acids or alkalis).

Emesis

Considered the second choice after lavage as the preferred method for gastric emptying. The dose in adults is 30 ml of ipecac with water and repeated in 15–30 minutes if vomiting is not induced. Indicated in ingestions of drugs that can form gastric concretions: salicylates, meprobamate, barbiturates, glutethimide, or drugs that can delay the gastric emptying: tricyclics, narcotics, salicylates, or conditions producing adynamic ileus (see Table 39.12).

Its use is controversial for the following reasons:

1 not immediately effective;

2 the effect may persist for 2 hours, delaying the administration of adsorbants;

3 unlikely to be effective within several hours after the ingestion (more than 1–2 hours with exceptions);

4 not proven to be better than lavage;

5 several contraindications: caustic ingestion; altered mental status; inability to protect airway, seizures or seizure potential, hemorrhagic diathesis, hematemesis, ingestion of drugs that can lead to rapid change in the patient's condition (tricyclics, β-blockers, PCP, isoniazid);

6 has no value in ethanol intoxication and certain hydrocarbon ingestions;

7 in case of failure to induce emesis (about 5% of cases), the stomach should be evacuated by other means, since ipecac can be cardiotoxic (theoretical risk).

Recently published guidelines recommend the use of ipecac syrup when in the absence of contraindications (above) it can be

Table 39.4 The most common toxic syndromes.

Class of drug	Common signs	Common causes
Anticholinergics	Dementia with mumbling speech Tachycardia Dry flushed skin Dilated pupils (mydriasis) Myoclonus Temperature slightly elevated Urinary retention Decreased bowel sounds Seizures/dysrhythmias (severe cases)	Antihistamines Antiparkinsonian medications Atropine Scopolamine Amantadine Antipsychotics Antidepressants Antispasmodics Mydriatics Skeletal muscle relaxants Some plants (i.e. jimson weed)
Sympathomimetics	Delusions Paranoia Tachycardia Hypertension Hyperpyrexia Diaphoresis Piloerection Mydriasis Hyperreflexia Seizures/dysrhythmias (severe cases)	Cocaine Amphetamines Methamphetamines and derivatives Over-the-counter decongestants (phenylpropanolamine, ephedrine, pseudoephedrine) NB: Caffeine and theophylline overdoses have similar findings, except for organic psychiatric signs
Opiate/sedatives	Coma Respiratory depression Constricted pupils (miosis) Hypotension Bradycardia Hypothermia Pulmonary edema Decreased bowel sounds Hyporeflexia Needle marks	Narcotics Barbiturates Benzodiazepines Ethchlorvynol Glutethimide Methyprylon Methaqualone Meprobamate
Cholinergics	Confusion/CNS depression Weakness Salivation Lacrimation Urinary and fecal incontinence Gastrointestinal cramping Emesis Diarrhea Diaphoresis Muscle fasciculations Bronchospasm	Organophosphate and carbamate insecticides Physostigmine Edrophonium Some mushrooms (*Amanita muscaria*; *Amanita pantherina*, *Inocybe* spp., *Clitocybe* spp.)

(From Briggs GG, Freeman RK, eds. Drugs in pregnancy and lactation, 4th edn. Baltimore: Williams and Wilkins, 1994; and Doyon S, Roberts JR. Reappraisal of the "coma cocktail". Dextrose, flumazenil, naloxone and thiamine. *Emerg Clin of N Am*, 1994;12:301–316.)

Table 39.5 Physical findings in poisoning.

Pupils	*Breath odor*	
Dilation	Acetone:	Acetone, chloroform, ethanol, isopropyl alcohol, salicylates
Alkaloids	Acrid or pear-like:	Chloral hydrate, paraldehyde
Aminophylline	Bitter almonds:	Cyanide
Anticholinergics	Carrots:	Cicutoxin (water hemlock)
Antihistaminics	Garlic:	Arsenic, organophosphates, phosphorus, selenium, thallium
Barbiturates	Mothballs:	Camphor, naphthalene, paradichlorobenzene
Carbon monoxide	Pungent aromatic:	Ethchlorvynol (Placidyl)
Cocaine	Violets:	Turpentine
Cyanide	Wintergreen:	Methyl salicylate
Ergot		
Ethanol	*Reflexes*	
Ethylene glycol	Depressed	
Glutethimide	Antidepressants	
LSD	Barbiturates	
Methaqualone	Benzodiazepines	
Mushrooms	Chloral hydrate	
Phenothiazines	Clonidine	
Phenytoin	Ethanol	
Quinine	Ethchlorvynol	
Reserpine	Glutethimide	
Sympathomimetics	Meprobamate	
Toluene	Narcotics	
Tricyclics	Phenothiazines	
Withdrawal states	Tricyclic antidepressants	
Constriction	Valproic acid	
Acetone	Hyperreflexia	
Barbiturates	Amphetamines	
Benzodiazepines	Carbamazepine	
Caffeine	Carbon monoxide	
Chloral hydrate	Cocaine	
Cholinergics	Cyanide	
Cholinesterase inhibitors	Haloperidol	
Clonidine	Methaqualone	
Codeine	Phencyclidine	
Ethanol	Phenothiazines	
Meprobamate	Phenytoin	
Opiates (except meperidine)	Propoxyphene	
Organophosphates	Propranolol	
Phencyclidine	Strychnine	
Phenothiazines	Tricyclic antidepressants	
Propoxyphene		
Sympatholytics		

(Data for "Breath odor" from Olson K. Poisoning and drug overdose, 2nd edn. Norwalk, CT: Appleton and Lange, 1994.)

administered within 30–90 minutes of an ingestion with a substantial risk of serious toxicity to the victim and no alternative to decrease gastrointestinal (GI) absorption is available (or effective) and a delay of greater than 1 hour to an emergency medical facility is anticipated [34].

Gastric lavage

Indicated when emesis is inappropriate or contraindicated, the patient is comatose or mentally altered, the substance ingested has the potential for seizures or when the substance ingested is lethal and/or rapidly absorbed (i.e. delay for emesis can result in

Table 39.6 Factors to consider in the clinical management of the pregnant poison patient.

Supine hypotensive syndrome
Lower potential to resist acidosis in pregnancy
Need for preservation of a maternal P_aO_2 of at least 60–70 mmHg for fetal oxygenation
Increased maternal cardiac output and oxygen consumption
Increased renal clearance of antidotes and therapeutic drugs
Different "normal" values of blood tests such as BUN and creatinine
Effects of various resuscitative drugs on the uteroplacental circulation and myometrium
Increased potential for gastric aspiration in pregnant women and heightened need for airway protection

Table 39.7 Quantitative toxicology testing.

Test	Time to sample postingestion	Repeat sample	Implication positive test
Acetaminophen	4 h	None	Blood level Nomogram and N-acetylcysteine
Carbamazepine	2–4 h	2–4 h	Repetitive doses of activated charcoal/hemoperfusion
Carboxyhemoglobin	Immediate	2–4 h	100% oxygen
Cholinesterase blood RBC	Immediate	12–24 h	Confirm exposure to insecticide
Digoxin	2–4 h	2–4 h	Digoxin antibody fragments (Fab)
Ethanol	0.5–1 h	Not necessary	If negative, not ethanol intoxication; if positive, inconclusive (tolerance)
Ethylene glycol	0.5–1 h	2 h	Ethanol therapy, hemodialysis, sodium bicarbonate
Heavy metals	First 24 h	2–4 h	Chelation therapy, dialysis
Iron	2–4 h (chewable/liquid preparation absorbed faster)	2–4 h	Serum iron 350 μg use deferoxamine
Isopropanol	0.5–1 h	2 h	Supportive-care hemodialysis
Lithium	2–4 h	4 h	Hemodialysis
Methanol	0.5–1 h	2 h	Ethanol therapy folinic acid, $NaHCO_3$, hemodialysis
Methemoglobin	Immediate	1–2 h	Methylene blue
Phenobarbital	1–2 h	4–6 h	Alkaline diuresis Repeated activated charcoal; hemoperfusion
Phenytoin	1–2 h	4–6 h	Supportive care Repeated activated charcoal
Salicylates	2–4 h	2–4 h	Serum and urine alkalinization Repeated activated charcoal, hemodialysis
Theophylline	1-h peak at 12–36 h	1–2 h	Repeat activated charcoal, hemoperfusion

2-PAM, pralidoxime; ABGs, arterial blood gases; Fab, fragment antigen-binding; PT, prothrombin time; PTT, partial thromboplastin time.
(Reproduced by permission from Mowry JB, Furbee RB, Chyka PA. Poisoning. In: Chernow B, Borater DC, Holaday JW, et al., eds. The Pharmacological Approach to the Critically Ill Patient, 3rd edn. Baltimore: Williams and Wilkins, 1995.)

Table 39.8 Time intervals for detecting drugs in urine after use.

Drug	Detectable after use
Alcohol	24 h
Amphetamines	48 h
Barbiturates	
Short-acting	48 h
Long-acting	7 days
Benzodiazepines	72 h
Cocaine	72 h
Marijuana	
Single use	72 h
Chronic use	30 days

(Reproduced by permission from Thorp J. Management of drug dependency, overdose, and withdrawal in the obstetric patient. *Obstet Gynecol Clin N Am* 1995;22:131–142).

Table 39.9 Compounds for which hemoperfusion is appropriate.

Acetaminophen	Chloroquine	Heptabarbital	Procainamide
Amanita toxins	Creatinine	Meprobamate	Quinalbital
Ammonia	Cyclobarbital	Methaqualone	Quinidine
Amobarbital	Demeton	Methotrexate	Salicylates
Barbital	Digoxin	Methyprylon	Secobarbital
Bromide	Dimethoate	Nitrostigmine	Theophylline
Butabarbital	Diquat	Paraquat	Thyroxine
Camphor	Disopyramide	Parathion	Tricyclic antidepressant
Carbon tetrachloride	Ethanol	Pentobarbital	Triiodothyronine
Carbamazepine	Ethchlorvynol	Phenobarbital	Uric acid
Chloral hydrate	Glutethimide	Phenytoin	

Table 39.10 Compounds for which dialysis is an appropriate consideration.

Acetaminophen	Chloride	Gallamine	Nitrofurantoin
Aluminum	Chromate	Gentamicin	Ouabain
Amanita toxin	Cimetidine	Glutethimide	Paraquat
Amikacin	Cisplatin	Hydrogen ions	Penicillin
Ammonia	Citrate	Iodide	Phenobarbital
Amobarbital	Colistin	Iron desferrioxamine	Phosphate
Amoxicillin	Creatinine	Isoniazid	Potassium
Amphetamines	Cyclobarbital	Isopropyl alcohol	Primidone
Ampicillin	Cyclophosphamide	Kanamycin	Procainamide
Aniline	Cycloserine	Lactate	Quinidine
Arsenic	Demeton	Lead edetate	Quinine
Azathioprine	Diazoxide	Lithium	Salicylates
Barbital	Dimethoate	Magnesium	Sodium
Borate	Diquat	Mannitol	Streptomycin
Bromide	Diisopyramide	Meprobamate	Strontium
Butabarbital	Ethambutol	Methanol	Sulfonamides
Calcium	Ethanol	Methaqualone	Theophylline
Camphor	Ethchlorvynol	Methotrexate	Thiocyanate
Carbenicillin	Ethionamide	Methyldopa	Ticarcillin
Carbon tetrachloride	Ethylene glycol	Methylprednisolone	Tobramycin
Cephalosporins	Flucytosine	Methyprylon	Trichloroethylene
Chloral hydrate	Fluoride	Metronidazole	Urea
Chloramphenicol	5-Fluorouracil	MAO inhibitors	Uric acid
Chlorate	Fosfomycin	Neomycin	Water

death). It is contraindicated in ingestion of caustics and in hemorrhagic diathesis. It has the advantages that can be performed immediately on arrival of the patient; takes only 15–20 minutes to complete and facilitates the administration of charcoal.

A large gastric tube (Ewald, Lavaculator®, and others) size 36–40 F should be passed orally with lubricant. Consideration for intubation needs to be made in patients with depressed mental status, altered gag reflex, and seizures or seizure potential. The patient needs to be placed in Trendelenburg or sitting position and aspiration prior to lavage needs to be made to confirm placement of the tube (collect sample for analysis). Lavage is made with normal saline or water in runs of 1.5 ml/kg (up to 200 ml) until clear and then with at least one more liter. Some recommend slight movement changes of the patient or position changes to dislodge potential residues of medications or undisolved pills.

Adsorption (activated charcoal)

Activated charcoal is a finely divided powder made by pyrolysis of carbonaceous material. It consists of small particles with an internal network of pores that adsorb substances. It is indicated after gastric emptying procedures (successful or not) and in repeated doses (2–4 hours) for drugs with enterohepatic circulation (theophylline, digoxin, nor and amitryptiline, salicylates, benzodiazepines, phenytoin, and phenobarbital for example). This effect has been called GI dialysis. Activated charcoal may be used immediately after ipecac (does not interfere with its action; some authors actually think this is the best way to give it) and

Table 39.11 Antidotes.

Poison	Antidote	Dosage
Acetaminophen	N-Acetylcysteine	140 mg/kg PO, followed by 70 mg/kg/4 h × 17 doses
Anticholinergics (atropine)	Physostigmine salicylate	0.5–2.0 mg IV (IM) over 2 min every 30–60 min prn
Anticholinesterases (organophosphates)	Atropine sulfate Pralidoxime (2-PAM) chloride	1–5 mg IV (IM, SQ) every 15 min prn 1 g IV (PO) over 15–30 min every 8–12 h × 3 doses prn
Benzodiazepines	Flumazenil (British data)	1–2 mg IV (for respiratory arrest)
Carbon monoxide	Oxygen	100%, hyperbaric
Cyanide	Amyl nitrite Sodium nitrite Sodium thiosulfate	Inhalation pearls for 15–30 s every minute 300 mg (10 mL of 3% solution) IV over 3 min, repeated in half dosage in 2 h if persistent toxicity 12.5 g (50 mL of 25% solution) IV over 10 min, repeated in half dosage in 2 h if persistent toxicity
Digoxin	Antidigoxin Fab fragments	—
Ethylene glycol	Ethanol	0.6 g/kg ethanol in D5W IV (PO) over 30–45 min, followed initially by 110 mg/kg/hr to maintain blood level of 100–150 mg/dL
Extrapyramidal signs	Diphenhydramine HCl	25–50 mg IV (IM, PO) prn
	Benztropine mesylate	1–2 mg IV (IM, PO) prn
Heavy metals (arsenic, copper, gold, lead, mercury)	Chelator Calcium disodium edetate (EDTA) Dimercaprol (BAL) Penicillamine	 1 g IV (IM) over 1 h every 12 h 2.5–5.0 mg/kg IM every 4–6 h 250–500 mg PO every 6 h
Heparin	Protamine	1 mg/100 units heparin and for every 60 min after heparin, halved dose
Iron	Desferrioxamine mesylate	1 gIM (IV at a rate of ≤15 mg/kg/hr if hypotension) every 8 h prn (maximum 80 mg/kg in 24 h)
Isoniazid	Pyridoxine	Gram per gram ingested; 5 g, if INH dose unknown
Magnesium sulfate	Calcium glutamate	2–3 g IV over 5 min (in 30-mL D10)
Methanol	Ethanol	See ethylene glycol
Methemoglobinemia (nitrites)	Methylene blue	1–2 mg/kg (0.1–0.2 mL/kg 1% solution) IV over 5 min, repeated in 1 h prn
Opiates/narcotics	Naloxone HCl	0.4–2.0 mg IV (IM, SQ, ET) prn
Warfarin	Phytonadione/vitamin K	0.5 mg/min IV (in NS or D5W)

2-PAM, pralidoxime; ET, endotracheal; IM, intramuscularly; INH, isoniazid; NS, normal saline; PO, by mouth; prn, as circumstances may require; SQ, subcutaneously. (From Thorp J. Management of drug dependency, overdose, and withdrawal in the obstetric patient. *Obstet Gynecol Clin N Am* 1995;22:222–228; and Roberts JM. Pregnancy related hypertension. In: Creasy RK, Resnick R, eds. Maternal-fetal Medicine: Principles and Practice, 3rd edn. Philadelphia: WB Saunders, 1994:804–843.)

N-acetylcysteine. It is contraindicated in caustic ingestions and ineffective in ingestion of elemental metals (iron for example), some pesticides (malathion, DDT), cyanide, ethanol, and methanol.

The typical dose is 30–100 g in adults (or 1 g/kg) and is usually given with a cathartic (50 ml of 70% sorbitol or 30 g of magnesium sulfate) in order to accelerate the transit time of the complex toxin–charcoal. A superactivated charcoal formulation, capable of adsorbing two to three times the conventional capacity of the charcoal, is available.

Neutralizing agents

In some poisonings a neutralizing agent instead of charcoal is preferable for instillation (see Table 39.13).

Cathartics

Used as adjunctive treatment with charcoal. These agents should be used only when indicated. They are contraindicated in diarrhea, dehydration, electrolyte imbalances, abdominal trauma, intestinal obstruction and ileus. The agent most frequently used in poisoning treatment is sorbitol because of the onset of action

Table 39.12 Indications for ipecac syrup.

Gastric concretion formation
Salicylates
Meprobamate
Barbiturates
Glutethimide
Gastric emptying delay (pregnancy)
Tricyclics
Narcotics
Salicylates
Conditions producing adynamic ileus

Table 39.13 Poisoning in which a specific neutralizing agent is preferable to activated charcoal.

Mercury	Sodium formaldehyde (20 g) converts HgCl to less soluble metallic mercury
Iron	Iodium bicarbonate (200–300 mL) converts ferrous iron to ferrous carbonate
Iodine	Starch solution (75 g of starch in 1 L of water; continue until aspirate is no longer blue)
Strychnine, nicotine, quinine, physostigmine	Potassium permanganate (1:10 000)

Table 39.14 Substances most frequently involved in adult exposures (>19 years).

Substance	No.	% of all adult exposures	As cause of mortality
Analgesics	92 245	13.3	1
Sedatives/hypnotics/antipsychotics	67 946	9.8	3
Cleaning substances	66 384	9.5	12
Antidepressants	55 429	8.0	2
Bites/envenomations	55 145	7.9	19
Alcohols	37 451	5.4	6
Food products, food poisoning	35 860	5.2	20
Cosmetics and personal care products	33 511	4.8	18
Chemicals	31 738	4.6	10
Pesticides	31 285	4.5	15
Cardiovascular drugs	28 941	4.2	5
Fumes/gases/vapors	27 486	3.9	9
Hydrocarbons	27 419	3.9	16
Antihistamines	19 570	2.8	11
Anticonvulsants	17 851	2.6	7
Antimicrobials	17 683	2.5	14
Stimulants and street drugs	17 423	2.5	4
Plants	17 261	2.5	17
Cough and cold preparations	16 866	2.4	18

(From Litovitz TL, Klein-Schwartz W, White S, et al. 2000. Annual report of the American Association of Poison Control Centers Toxic Exposure Surveillance System. *Am J Emerg Med* 2001;19(5):337–95.)

Table 39.15 Stages of acetaminophen toxicity.

Phase	Time	Symptoms
I	0–24 h	Gastrointestinal symptoms (anorexia, nausea, vomiting), malaise, diaphoresis
II	24–48 h	Clinical improvement, but abnormal liver function tests
III	72–96 h	Peak hepatotoxicity with encephalopathy, coagulopathy, and hypoglycemia
IV	7–8 days	Death, or recovery from hepatic failure (begins within 5 days and usually progresses to complete resolution within 3 months)

Table 39.16 Criteria for consideration of admission to the intensive care unit.

Mechanical ventilation required
Vasopressor support necessary
Arrhythmia management or need for hemodialysis
Signs of severe poisoning
Worsening signs of toxicity
Predisposing underlying medical conditions
Potential for prolonged absorption of toxin
Potential for delayed onset of toxicity
Invasive procedures or monitoring needed
Antidotes with potential for serious side effects
Suicidal patients requiring observation

(less than an hour), duration of effect (8–12 hours) and no interaction with charcoal. Oil cathartics are contraindicated because they can be aspirated and can increase the absorption of hydrocarbons. Complications can result from overaggressive use (fluid and electrolyte imbalances) [35].

Whole-bowel irrigation

Consists of the administration of polyethylene-glycol at a rate of 500–2000 ml/hour orally or through a nasogastric tube with the purpose of cleaning the bowel of whole or undisolved pills. May be helpful in clearing the GI tract of iron, lead, zinc lithium, delayed-release formulations not adsorbed by charcoal, very delayed onset of treatment or drug packets of illicit drugs [36]. The procedure takes 3–5 hours and may be complicated by bowel perforation or obstruction, ileus or GI hemorrhage.

SPECIFIC AGENTS

More than 250 000 drugs and commercial products are available for ingestion [37,38]. Table 39.14 lists the most frequent causes of morbidity and mortality from poisoning in adults in the USA [2]. Figure 39.3 details the classes of drugs most frequently used in suicide attempts among 1085 pregnant women in 1999 [16].

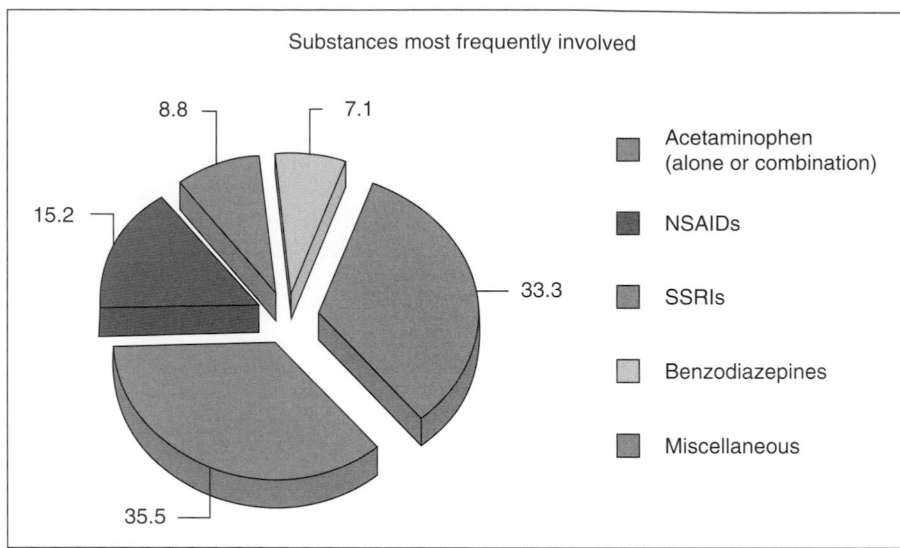

Figure 39.3 Suicide attempts during pregnancy by poisoning or overdose: report from a National Database, 1999 NSAIDs, nonsteroidal anti-inflammatory drugs; SSRIs, selective serotonin-reuptake inhibitors.

The general characteristics and management of selected toxic exposures during pregnancy are discussed in further detail in the sections below, arranged in alphabetical order by drug name.

In the USA all consults and reports of exposure can be made to the number: +1-800-222-1222.

Acetaminophen

Toxicology

- Common proprietary names: Alka-Seltzer® (some presentations); Anacin®; Benadryl® (some presentations); Comtrex®; Contac®; Coricidin®; Darvocet; Dimetapp®; Drixoral®; Esgic®; Excedrin (aspirin-free)®; Fioricet®; Goody's Body Pain Relief®; Lortab®; Midol®; Midrin®; Nyquil®; Pamprin®; Panadol®; Parafon®; Percocet®; Phenaphen®; Robitussin®; Sudafed®; Tavist®; Thera-Flu®; Triaminic®; Tylenol®, Tempra®; Unisom®; Vicodin®; Wygesic®
- FDA classification: B [39]
- As a cause of morbidity: 1 (other analgesics included) [2]
- As a cause of mortality: 1 (other analgesics included) [2]
- Most frequent route of exposure: ingestion
- Most frequent reason for exposure: unintentional overdose

Metabolism

Acetaminophen is metabolized in the liver to nontoxic sulfate (52%) and glucuronide (42%) forms and then excreted by the kidneys. Approximately 4% is metabolized by the hepatic cytochrome oxidase P450 system, resulting in a toxic reactive intermediate. This toxic metabolite is conjugated with glutathione and excreted in the urine as nontoxic mercaptourate. Two percent of acetaminophen is excreted unchanged. In an overdose, the hepatic glutathione stores are depleted and the toxic intermediates become covalently bound to hepatic cellular proteins, resulting in hepatocellular necrosis [40].

Serum half-life

The serum half-life of acetaminophen in pregnancy is 3.7 hours, and the pharmacokinetics (absorption, metabolism, and renal clearance) are similar in the pregnant and nonpregnant states [41,42].

Lethal dosage

The lethal dosage is in excess of 150 mg/kg or 15 g in the healthy adult and primarily involves hepatotoxicity [40,43]. The lethality of acetaminophen is not only directly related to the dose, but to other factors such as age, nutritional status, and other compounds ingested. Renal failure, myocardial depression, and pancreatitis also have been observed in acute overdoses.

Maternal considerations

In general, the primary short-term problem of acetaminophen overdose is hepatocellular necrosis, which peaks at 72–96 hours. Cardiac, renal, and pancreatic complications rarely occur, but appropriate monitoring should be instituted. Perhaps the most serious long-term consequence is residual liver damage.

Symptoms

Nausea; vomiting; anorexia; right upper quadrant pain. The symptoms of acetaminophen toxicity have been divided into four stages (Table 39.15).

Signs

Icterus; right upper quadrant abdominal tenderness; lethargy; evidence of bleeding.

Diagnostic tests

Blood: acetaminophen level (at 4 or more hours after ingestion); transaminases (elevated); lactic dehydrogenase (LDH) (elevated); prothrombin time (prolonged); amylase (elevated); lipase (elevated); creatinine (elevated); urinalysis. Plasma acetaminophen level (obtained 4 or more hours after ingestion) can be plotted on a Rumack–Matthew nomogram (Figure 39.4). A level drawn less than 4 hours after ingestion may be falsely low resulting from a partial absorption.

Electrocardiogram (EKG): nonspecific ST/T changes.

Short-term problems

Oliguria; pancreatitis; hypotension; myocardial ischemia and necrosis. Premature contractions; potential for premature delivery.

Long-term problems

Diffuse hepatic necrosis (potential for 1–2% late mortality)

Fetal and neonatal considerations

General

Acetaminophen crosses the placenta; the fetus is at risk of poisoning, particularly late in pregnancy [44]. Unless severe maternal toxicity develops, acetaminophen overdose does not appear to increase the risk for adverse pregnancy outcome [45]. Placental transfer of therapeutic levels of N-acetylcysteine has been documented in humans and provides evidence of a direct antidotal effect of N-acetylcysteine in the fetus [46].

Signs

Decreased fetal movements; decreased beat to beat variability; absence of fetal heart rate accelerations; falling baseline heart rate (see Figure 39.1).

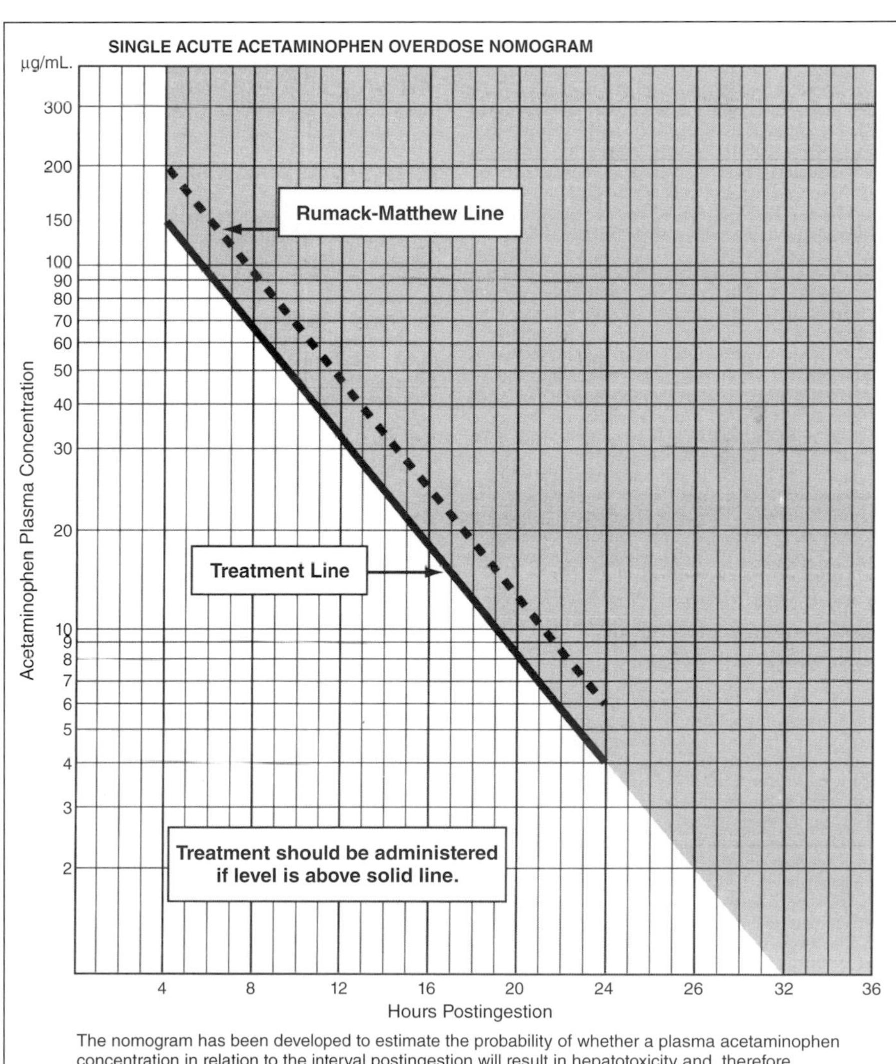
SINGLE ACUTE ACETAMINOPHEN OVERDOSE NOMOGRAM
μg/mL.
300
200
150
100
90
80
70
60
50
40
30
20
10
9
8
7
6
5
4
3
2
Acetaminophen Plasma Concentration
Rumack-Matthew Line
Treatment Line
Treatment should be administered if level is above solid line.
4
8
12
16
20
24
26
32
36
Hours Postingestion
The nomogram has been developed to estimate the probability of whether a plasma acetaminophen concentration in relation to the interval postingestion will result in hepatotoxicity and, therefore, whether acetylcysteine therapy should be administered.
CAUTIONS FOR USE OF THIS CHART:
1. Time coordinates refer to time postingestion.
2. Graph relates only to plasma concentrations following a signle, acute overdose ingestion.
3. The Treatment Line is plotted 25% below the Rumack-Matthew Line to allow for potential errors in plasma acetaminophen assays and estimated time from ingestion of an overdose.

Figure 39.4 Nomogram for acetaminophen toxicity. (Modified from Rumack RH, Matthew H. Acetaminophen poisoning and toxicity. *Pediatrics* 1975; 55: 871). Reproduced by permission of McNeil Pharmaceuticals.

Teratogenic potential
No support for association; potential for fetal liver damage (hepatocellular necrosis); increased risks of spontaneous abortion and stillbirth. Case control studies have not found an evidence of increased malformations after prenatal acetaminophen [47]. A report on 300 overdoses during pregnancy did not suggest an increase in adverse pregnancy outcome attributable to the drug ingestion [48].

Fetal distress potential
Yes; reported [49]. There is a relationship between pregnancy outcome and the interval between drug exposure and administration of N-acetylcysteine, with an increase in the incidence of spontaneous abortion and stillbirth as the interval increases [50,51].

Indications for delivery
Nonreassuring fetal condition unresponsive to medical therapy or in the presence of deteriorating maternal condition.

Neonatal period
Hyperbilirubinemia.

Management guidelines

In regards to acetaminophen poisoning, pregnant patients should be managed no differently than nonpregnant patients.

Supportive
Induced emesis may be indicated for home treatment of a large dose (>100 mg/kg or ≈6 g). Gastric lavage+activated charcoal (1 g/kg in water or sorbitol).

Specific measures/antidotes
• N-acetylcysteine (Mucomyst®), a glutathione substitute or precursor, is used as an effective antidote to acetaminophen toxicity. Indications for antidotal use are as follows.

a If the ingestion is known to be greater than 4 g (or 100 mg/kg; whichever is less) [52].

b If acetaminophen levels (at 4 or more hours after exposure) are 150 µg/ml or greater (993 umol/l),

c When exposure to other hepatotoxics or history of liver disease is associated to the acetaminophen exposure (including ethanol, carbamazepine and isoniazide).

d While the results of the acetaminophen levels are back if not be available by 7–8 hours after the exposure.

• Oral: methionine (2.5 g every 4 hours × 4 doses) or N-acetylcysteine (category B) (140 mg/kg loading followed by 70 mg/kg every 4 hours for 17 doses);

• Parenteral (preferred in pregnancy): N-acetylcysteine: 150 mg/kg in 200 ml of 5% dextrose over 15 minutes or 100 mg/kg in 1000 ml 5% dextrose over 16 hours. The best results are obtained when therapy is started within 16 hours of the overdose, but N-acetylcysteine is still indicated up to 24 hours after ingestion of the overdose [53]. In those presentations after 8 hour of exposure consider using a 48 or 72 hour protocol [43].

• In selected circumstances, hemoperfusion and hemodialysis have been found to be effective, but these techniques are not usually indicated.

• Intensive care unit (ICU) admission if hepatic failure or encephalopathy (see Table 39.16).

Monitoring
Vital signs/mental status/intake and output; Blood: transaminases, prothrombin time and acetaminophen level every 4 hours (first 24 hours), then daily or as indicated. Other tests if originally abnormal or drawn less than 4 hours since exposure; EFM: indicated.

Therapeutic goals
Asymptomatic patient; normal liver function tests (transaminases and prothrombin time).

Disposition considerations
Consider Psychiatry evaluation for all exposures. Contemplate induction of labor in third trimester cases with severe exposures. May discharge after 72–96 hours from exposure if therapeutic goals met.

Follow-up
Caution the patient about possibility of spontaneous abortion, premature delivery, and risk of stillbirth. Counsel against the use potential hepatotoxics. Consider serial biophysical profiles in viable pregnancies and severe exposure (value not established). Clinical follow-up may include a social worker, obstetrician, hepatologist, and psychiatrist [43,52,53,54].

Amphetamines

Toxicology

Amphetamines are a group of sympathomimetic drugs (derivates of phenylethylamine) used to stimulate the CNS via norepinephrine- (noradrenalin-) and dopamine-mediated pathways. Although the precise mechanism of action is unknown, proposed mechanisms have included presynaptic release of catecholamines, direct postsynaptic stimulation, and inhibition of monoamine oxidase. These drugs are used frequently for appetite suppression, to treat narcolepsy, or for illicit recreational reasons. Approximately 200 designer phenylethylamine derivatives have been described [55].

Metabolism
Amphetamines are weak bases with a pK_a of 9.9 and are metabolized in the liver. Both active metabolites and free amphetamines are excreted in the urine. Chronic abusers develop tolerance to amphetamines and may ingest lethal doses without effect. Thus,

most cases of fatal intoxication seen are of people who are not chronic abusers.

Lethal dose

The lethal dose in adults is 20–25 mg/kg. Smaller doses, however, have been known to be fatal [56].

• Examples/other names: amphetamine sulfate (Benzedrine®) also known as "blues", "sulfate", "purple hearts", "black beauties", "truck drivers," or "uppers"; dextroamphetamine (Dexedrine®); methamphetamine (Methedrine®] also known as "ice"; methylamphetamine (desoxyephedrine known as "speed", "crank", "crystal meth"); mescaline; phenylpropanolamine; Ritalin®; Adderall®; 3,4-methylenedioxyamphetamine (MDA) also known as "Adam"; 3,4-methylenedioxethamphetamine (MDEA) also known as "Eve"; methylbenzodiolbutanamine (MDMB); 3,4-methylenedioxymethamphetamine (MDMA) also known as "ecstasy" or the "love drug", "X", "E", "XTC", "hug", "beans"; others: 2C-T2, 2C-T7 also known as "Triptasy" or "Beautiful"; Ma Huang (contains ephedrine); Khat (contains cathine: norpseudoephedrine) also known as "Abyssinian tea", "miraa", "graba," or "African salad"; methcathinone also known as "Jeff" or "mulka".
• FDA classification: C
• As a cause of morbidity: 17* [2]
• As a cause of mortality: 4* [2]
• Most frequent route of exposure: oral; occasionally mucous membranes (snorting, smoking and suppositories); rarely injected.
• Most frequent reason for exposure: unintentional overdose

Maternal considerations

Pregnant women who use MDMA tend to be young, single, and report psychological morbidity, and have a clustering of risk factors that may compromise the pregnancy and fetus. Smoking, heavy alcohol intake, and polysubstance drug use, combined with a higher than expected rate of unplanned pregnancies, increases the risk of fetal exposure to potentially harmful substances [57].

Consider in the differential diagnosis of congestive heart failure, myocardial infarction, and ventricular arrhythmias among young patients [58].

Symptoms

See Table 39.17.

Signs

Restlessness; anxiety; agitation. Also remarkable for life-threatening vital signs: tachycardia; hypertension; hyperthermia; muscle tension; bruxism and involuntary jaw clenching (latter two are clues to MDMA use). The differential diagnoses include sedative/hypnotic withdrawal syndrome (especially ethanol) and neuroleptic malignant syndrome.

*Other stimulants included.

Table 39.17 Signs and symptoms of amphetamine overdose.

Mild toxicity
Respiratory (tachypnea)
Cardiovascular (tachycardia, mild hypertension, chest pain, palpitations)
Gastrointestinal (abdominal cramping, nausea, vomiting, diarrhea)
Sympathetic stimulation (mild hyperpyrexia, dry mouth, mydriasis, diaphoresis, hyperreflexia)
Central nervous system symptoms (dizziness, hyperactivity, irritability, confusion, and panic)
Severe toxicity
Cardiovascular (severe hypertension with intracranial hemorrhage, tachyarrhythmias, ventricular tachycardia or fibrillation, hypotension, and cardiovascular collapse)
Severe hyperthermia (associated with coagulopathies, rhabdomyolysis, and renal failure)
Metabolic (systemic acidosis)
Central nervous system (convulsions, delirium, psychosis, usually in chronic abusers with paranoia, delusions, and hallucinations, coma)

Diagnostic tests

Blood levels correlate partly with both clinical status and mortality risk, secondary to the development of tolerance.

Short-term problems

Short-term problems are manifested by cardiovascular changes such as severe hypertension, tachyarrhythmias, and cardiovascular collapse. Possibility for a hemorrhagic or ischemic stroke.

Long-term problems

The potential long-term consequence of chronic abuse are psychosis, parkinsonism, and an increased risk of cardiovascular diseases [58,59,60,61].

Fetal considerations

Signs

Intrauterine growth restriction. Possibility for threatened preterm labor and antepartum hemorrhage [62,63].

Teratogenic potential

Presently, there is no evidence that these drugs are associated with an increase in the frequency of major and/or minor congenital malformations in humans [39,64,65,66]. Correcting for confounding factors (tobacco, alcohol), however, babies of amphetamine abusers have significantly decreased birth weight, length, and head circumference [64]. Infants exposed to methamphetamine and/or cocaine have significantly greater frequency of prematurity, intrauterine growth retardation, placental hemorrhage, and anemia [39,67,68].

Fetal distress potential
Possible. Neonatal cerebral injuries have been reported among infants exposed *in utero* [69].

Indications for delivery
Obstetric indications.

Neonatal period
Neonatal amphetamine- and methamphetamine-withdrawal syndromes have been described [66,68,70].

Management considerations

Supportive
With amphetamine overdose, the therapeutic goal is to provide primarily supportive care until the patient is stabilized. A cool, quiet environment will decrease external stimulation and potential for further physical agitation. Obtain a basal temperature.

Specific measures/antidotes
- Gastric emptying, followed by charcoal instillation and cathartic administration for oral overdoses. Consider a vaginal exam for the possibility of "body stuffing". Forced acid diuresis is indicated in severe toxicity to enhance renal excretion.
- The most appropriate choice for sedation are benzodiazepines [diazepam: 10 mg intravenously (IV); cumulative doses may exceed 100 mg]. Use restraints as needed to prevent injury to the patient or others. Symptomatic therapy for psychosis and agitation can best be treated with haloperidol (chlorpromazine may increase the half-life of amphetamines and cause greater respiratory depression) or diazepam. Along with these complications, seizures may be terminated with diazepam, and recurrent seizures may be treated with phenytoin.
- Cardiovascular complications such as arrhythmias and hypertension can be managed with propranolol and haloperidol or chlorpromazine, respectively.
- Severe or refractory hypertension may require phentolamine or nitroprusside. β-Blockers should be avoided for the potential of unopposing the α-adrenergic effects and worsening the hypertension. Volume depletion, hypotension, and hyperthermia need to be treated aggressively with IV fluids (≈20 ml/kg). Refractory hypotension may be due to catecholamine depletion and may require a direct-acting agent such as norepinephrine.
- Hyperthermia is an ominous sign. Haloperidol or chlorpromazine and active cooling should be used to manage temperatures in excess of 38.9°C.
- Hemodialysis may be useful for life-threatening cases that are unresponsive to supportive care, with acidemia, or in patients with renal compromise (renal failure or hyperkalemia). Lethargic, obtunded, or patients with altered mental status need a head computed tomography (CT) scan to rule out hemorrhage or infarction.

Monitoring
Includes EKG, blood pressure (BP), temperature, respiratory rate and blood gases, electrolytes, creatine kinase, urine myoglobin levels, and fetal heart rate and uterine activity, when applicable.

Therapeutic goals
Asymptomatic patient. Normal vital signs. Urine output of at least 1 ml/kg/h. Consider prolonged observation for "body stuffers".

Discharge considerations
Drug counselor, psychiatry, and social worker consults recommended. Evaluate for sexually transmitted diseases.

Follow-up
Clinical follow-up may include a social worker, obstetrician, and psychiatrist. Subsequently, she should be monitored for evidence of preterm labor, placental hemorrhage, and intrauterine growth restriction [59,61,71,72,73,74].

Antidepressants

Toxicology

Antidepressant drugs (imipramine, amitriptyline, Doxepin, trimipramine, trazadone, fluoxetine) may produce three major toxidromes: anticholinergic crisis, cardiovascular failure, or seizure activity. A patient may experience one or all three of these toxic effects, depending on the dose and the drug taken. Patients who initially are awake may abruptly lose consciousness and/or develop seizures without warning. The signs and symptoms associated with antidepressant overdose are illustrated in Table 39.18.

Table 39.18 Signs and symptoms of antidepressant overdose.

Signs	Symptoms
Tachycardia	Blurred vision
Dry skin and mucous membranes	Dysarthria
Blisters	Visual hallucinations
Mydriasis	Sedation
Divergent strabismus	Delirium
Decreased bowel sounds	Sedation
Urinary retention	Coma
Increased muscular tone	
Hyperreflexia	
Myoclonic activity	
Rapid loss of consciousness	
Seizures	
Cardiac dysrhythmias	
Hypotension	
Pulmonary edema	

The safety profile of the selective serotonin-reuptake inhibitors (SSRIs) in overdose is favorable. SSRI efficacy for mood and anxiety disorders, relatively weak effect on the cytochrome P450 system, and tolerability profile and safety in overdose are factors that contribute to make it a first-line agent during pregnancy [75,76].

Bupropion hydrochloride is a new antidepressant that differs clinically and pharmacologically from the tricyclic antidepressants and the monoamine oxidase inhibitors. Bupropion is devoid of cardiovascular effects (e.g. impaired intracardiac conduction, reduced myocardial contractility, decreased peripheral resistance, orthostatic hypotension) in both human and animal studies. The drug is nonsedating and antagonizes the effects of commonly used sedatives, such as alcohol and diazepam.

- Examples/other names: Imipramine; amitriptyline, doxepin, trimipramine; trazadone; fluoxetine; Anafranil®; Asendin®; Celexa®; Effexor®; Elavil®; Etafron®; Lexapro®; Limbitrol®; Norpramin®; Pamelor®; Paxil®; Prozac®; Sinequan®; Surmontil®; Tofranil®; Triavil®; Vivactil®; Wellbutrin®; Zoloft®
- FDA classification: C/D depending on the specific medication.
- As a cause of morbidity: 4 [2]
- As a cause of mortality: 3 [2]
- Most frequent route of exposure: ingestion
- Most frequent reason for exposure: intentional overdose

Maternal considerations

Symptoms

Dry mouth; urinary retention; delirium (see Table 39.19).

Signs

Agitation; mydriasis; hyperthermia; tachycardia; dry axilla; myoclonus; rapid loss of consciousness; seizures; cardiac dysrrhytmias. Some patients do not show evidence of toxicity (see Table 39.19).

Diagnostic tests

EKG: sinus tachycardia with prolonged PR, QRS, and QT intervals. Prolongation of the QRS segment greater than 0.12 is a reliable indicator of serious cardiovascular and neurologic toxicity (with the exception of amoxapine). In addition, bradyarrhythmias carry a bad prognosis. Additional EKG changes include atrioventricular block and ventricular tachycardia. Although drug levels can be obtained, these are not generally useful in the acute management of an overdose. Arterial blood gases, electrolytes, glucose, and complete blood count also are helpful.

Table 39.19 Barbiturates commonly associated with overdose.*

Type	Duration of action	Drug
Ultra-short-acting (methohexital)	20 min	Thiopental, thiamylal
Short-acting	3 h	Pentobarbital, secobarbital, hexobarbital
Intermediate-acting	3–6 h	Amobarbital, butabarbital, aprobarbital,
Long-acting	6–12 h	Barbital, phenobarbital, mephobarbital Primidone

* Lethal dosage: short-acting, ingestion of 3 g (lethal level, 3.5 mg/dL); long-acting, ingestion of 5 g (lethal level, 8 mg/dL) [89].

Short-term problems

Short-term problems include cardiac dysrrhythmias, seizures, urinary retention, GI hypomotility, aspiration pneumonitis, and acute respiratory distress syndrome (ARDS).

Long-term problems

Long-term problems include rhabdomyolysis, brain damage, and multisystem failure.

Fetal considerations

The effects of antidepressants on the fetus are variable.

Signs

Abnormal electronic fetal heart rate monitoring [77].

Teratogenic potential

A recent association of paroxetine with congenital malformations including anencephaly, craniosynostosis, and omphalocele has been reported [78,79].

Fetal distress potential

Yes.

Indications for delivery

While the potential for fetal distress exists due to maternal seizures, hypotension, or dysrhythmias, cesarean delivery is reserved for the usual obstetric indications.

Neonatal period

Tachypnea, cyanosis, irritability, urinary retention, paralytic ileus, seizures as a manifestation of SSRI withdrawal syndrome [80,81]. An association between paroxetine and the development of persistent pulmonary hypertension of the newborn has also been reported [82].

Management considerations

Supportive

With antidepressant overdose, the therapeutic goal is to prevent complications in the first 24 hours after a significant ingestion.

Once decontamination has been initiated, supportive therapy is warranted to maintain the airway, and, if necessary, mechanical ventilation should be instituted. Agitation, seizures, hyperthermia, hypotension, and arrhythmias should be treated. Because painful interventions and patient movement can precipitate seizures, such stimuli should be avoided.

Specific measures/antidotes

• The first step is decontamination with activated charcoal and a cathartic. A gastric lavage (30% excreted into stomach) should also be performed. Because of the risk of sudden onset of seizures, induced emesis is contraindicated.

• If the patient manifests coma, seizures, QRS greater than 0.1 second, ventricular arrhythmias, or hypotension, alkalinization therapy with IV sodium bicarbonate is indicated. To alkalinize the patient, one ampule (44–50 mEq) of sodium bicarbonate should be given IV slowly over 1–5 minutes (1–3 mEq/kg). This is followed by an infusion at 0.5 mEq/kg/h to maintain an arterial pH of 7.45–7.55.

• If perfusion is compromised or there is hypotension despite bicarbonate therapy, phenytoin, 100 mg over 3 minutes, should be considered.

• A split of opinion exists regarding the use of physostigmine salicylate (usually given as a 2-mg bolus over 2 min) because it may precipitate convulsions or ventricular tachycardia. In situations in which there is doubt as to the cause of the coma, or in patients with altered mental status and serious respiratory compromise, physostigmine may be considered.

• Antiarrhythmics are used to control dysrhythmia.

• Hypotension refractory to volume expansion is best treated with an α-agonist such as norepinephrine or phenylephrine, rather than with dopamine.

• If seizures are not immediately controlled with anticonvulsants, muscle relaxation with a nondepolarizing long-acting agent (pancuronium, norcuronium) should be instituted to avoid hyperthermia and lactic acidosis. An electroencephalogram (EEG) may be required to evaluate the effectiveness of the anticonvulsant therapy.

• Forced diuresis, dialysis, and hemoperfusion are generally ineffective.

Monitoring

At least 6 hours of cardiac monitoring.

Therapeutic goals

During therapy, 12 hours of maternal and fetal cardiac monitoring is recommended in asymptomatic pregnant patients. If there are signs of significant maternal toxicity, 24 hours in an intensive care setting appears warranted.

Discharge considerations

Prior to the discharge of the patient, a final dose of charcoal should be considered. In addition, the patients will need to be evaluated for suicide potential.

Follow-up

Observe (or make arrangements for outpatient monitoring) for 72 hours, because deaths from the original overdose have been reported up to 3 days after ingestion. Clinical follow-up may include a social worker, obstetrician, and a psychiatrist [61,83,84].

Aspirin

Toxicology

• Common names: Alka-Seltzer®; Ascriptin®; BC Powder®; Bufferin®; Darvon®; Ecotrin®; Excedrin®; Fiorinal®; Goody's Body Pain Relief®; Norgesic®; Pepto-Bismol®; Percodan®; Soma®; Talwin®

• FDA classification: C (D if full dose used in third trimester)

• As a cause of morbidity: 1* [2]

• As a cause of mortality: 1* [2]

• Main route of exposure: oral

• Main mechanism of exposure: intentional

Metabolism

Absorption of salicylates occurs in the stomach and small intestine. Both salicylic acid and acetylsalicylic acid are pharmacologically active but salicylic acid is the predominant form in plasma. There is a decrease of protein binding from ≈90 to 75% at toxic concentrations. It is metabolized to inactive forms of salicyluric acid and glycine or glucuronic acid conjugates. As the concentration increases two of the five metabolic pathways of elimination become saturated. At therapeutic doses only a small amount is excreted in the urine, but this increases at toxic doses (particularly at higher urinary pH values). The distribution of salicylates into the tissues increases as the pH decreases. The principal pathophysiologic mechanism in salicylate poisoning is interference with aerobic metabolism by means of uncoupling of mitochondrial oxidative phosphorylation.

Serum half life

At therapeutic doses: 4 hours; with toxic plasma levels: 15–29 hours.

Lethal dosage

Greater than 150 mg/kg (serious toxicity >300 mg/kg) [85,86].

Maternal considerations

Symptoms

None; nausea, vomiting; abdominal pain; tinnitus; decreased audition; dyspnea.

Signs

Hyperventilation; altered mental status; flushing; diaphoresis; hyperpirexia; GI bleeding; petechiae; bruising; hypovolemia; pulmonary edema; seizures; ARDS; coma.

Diagnostic tests

Blood: ABGs: respiratory alkalosis; compensated metabolic acidosis or metabolic acidosis; increased anion gap (greater than 14 mEq/l; Table 39.20); salycilate levels; creatinine; blood urea

*Other analgesics included.

Table 39.20 Causes for an increased or decreased anion gap.

Increased anion gap
Lactic acidosis:
Beta-adrenergic drugs
Caffeine
Carbon monoxide
Cyanide
Hydrogen sulfide
Ibuprofen
Iron
Isoniazid
Phenformin
Salicylates
Seizures
Theophylline
Other:
Benzyl alcohol
Ethanol (ketoacidosis)
Ethylene glycol
Exogenous organic and mineral acids
Formaldehyde
Methaldehyde
Methanol
Toluene
Decreased anion gap
Bromates
Lithium
Nitrites

nitrogen; electrolytes, glucose; complete blood count; prothrombin and partial thromboplastin times; urinalysis: specific gravity, volume and ferric chloride test (bedside colorimetric test: add 10% $FeCl_3$ in equal amounts to a 1 ml of urine at least 2 hours after ingestion: purple to purple brown indicates salicylate presence). Chest X ray: pulmonary edema.

Short-term problems
Volume depletion; shock; hemorrhage; seizures.

Long-term problems
Prolonged pregnancy; prolonged labor; higher risk of peripartum hemorrhage.

Fetal considerations
Salicylates cross the placenta freely and can concentrate on the fetus at higher concentrations, particularly CNS [87].

Signs
Constriction of ductus arteriosus; growth restriction.

Teratogenic potential
No, with the exception of a possible association of human intake during the first trimester and the development of gastroschisis [88].

Fetal distress potential
Yes.

Indications for delivery
Nonreassuring fetal condition. Avoidance of instruments during delivery is recommended (risk for cephalohematomata and intracranial bleeding).

Neonatal period
Hyperbilirubinemia; clinical evidence of thrombocytopenia.

Management considerations
Supportive
Generous IV fluid replacement (glucose-containing solutions); if hypotension is refractory, may use plasma or blood. May need a pulmonary artery catheter to manage fluid administration. If assisted ventilation required, hyperventilation (16–20/min) as needed to keep pCO_2 around 35 mmHg. Keep glycemia above 90 mg/dl.

Specific measures/antidotes
- Induced emesis not recommended.
- Gastric lavage (even if more than 4 hours have elapsed since ingestion).
- Forced alkaline diuresis (3 ampules of 40% sodium bicarbonate (50 ml/43 mEq of sodium) in 1 liter of 5% dextrose plus 40 mEq of KCl) at 2–3 ml/kg/h; goal: 5–10 ml/min of urine with pH of 7.5.
- Administer vitamin K 10 mg IV or intramuscularly (IM) (aspirin inhibits vitamin K).
- Hemodyalisis may be indicated (severe acidosis of hypotension refractory to optimal supportive care, Severe CNS symptoms (seizures); pulmonary edema; renal failure; salicylate level greater than 90 mg/dl (6.6 mmol/l); inability to alkalinize urine and/or no improvement with decontamination and urine alkalinization.

Monitoring
Vital signs/mental status/intake and output/EKG/oxymetry. Blood: ABGs+potassium every 2–4 hours (monitor alkalinization). Serial determination of salicylate levels (every 2 hours) until declining trend noted and levels fall below 30 mg/dl (2.2 mmol/l). Serial blood glucose. Urine: pH every hour. If fetus is viable consider informing the neonatology or pediatrics service of the potential delivery of a salicylate-exposed infant.

Therapeutic goals
Asymptomatic patient; level under 30 mg/dl (2.2 mmol/l) more than 2 hours after exposure.

Disposition considerations
May discharge if asymptomatic, appropriate treatment administered, decreasing serum levels and absence of electrolyte or acid-base imbalance. Contemplate induction of labor in third trimester exposures in severe exposures.

Follow-up

Establish. Consider evaluation of fetal growth. Consider psychiatry evaluation of all ingestions [85,86,87].

Barbiturates

Toxicology

Barbiturates are weak acids with pK_a values ranging between 7.2 and 8.0 (see Table 39.19) [89]. The more lipid-soluble drugs have a faster onset but shorter duration of action. Barbiturates cause CNS depression and in toxic doses depress other excitable tissues (skeletal, cardiac, and smooth muscle) [60]. The short-acting agents cause more potent CNS depression, are more toxic, and are more commonly abused. The quantity of drug ingested and the blood level may not correlate with the clinical status, because chronic abusers develop tolerance [60]. The patient's clinical condition is the best predictor of morbidity and mortality in cases of barbiturate toxicity. Death occurs from cardiopulmonary depression and is seen only in deeply comatose patients.

• Includes medications used as anticonvulsants, hypnotics, and sedatives.
• Common names and examples: amobarbital; barbital; butabarbital; pentobarbital; phenobarbital; secobarbital; thiamylal; thiopental; Amytal®; Arco-Lase®; Butisol®; Donnatal®; Esgic®; Fioricet®; Fiorinal®; Luminal®; Membaral®; Nembutal®; Phrenilin®; Sedapap®; Tuinal®; Veronal®
• FDA classification: D (most of them)
• As a cause of morbidity: 2*, 14† [2]
• As a cause of mortality: 2*, 7† [2]
• Most frequent route of exposure: ingestion
• Most frequent reason for exposure: unintentional overdose; acute or chronic

Maternal considerations

Barbiturate use by adolescents has increased gradually in the past several years, often used to treat unpleasant effects of illicit stimulants, to reduce anxiety, and to get "high". Maternal complications arise from either acute intoxication, chronic addiction of mother and fetus or barbiturate withdrawal. Signs and symptoms of the acute toxicity are illustrated in Table 39.21. Barbiturate withdrawal is characterized by insomnia, excitement, delirium, hallucinations, toxic psychosis, tremors, nausea and vomiting, orthostatic hypotension, and seizures. This condition may not present until 48–72 hours after the last dose but must be considered whenever managing a chronic abuser, because deaths have been reported with severe withdrawal reactions (see Table 39.22) [90].

Symptoms

Weakness; fatigue; sleepiness (see Table 39.22).

*Sedatives, hypnotics, and antipsychotics.
†Anticonvulsants.

Table 39.21 Signs and symptoms of barbiturate overdose.

Central nervous system
Mild intoxication: drowsiness
Moderate intoxication: CNS depression, slurred speech, ataxia, nystagmus, and miosis
Severe intoxication: extraocular motor palsies, absent corneal reflexes, sluggish pupillary reaction, mydriasis, absent deep tendon reflexes, absent Babinski sign, and coma. A flatline EEG has been reported

Respiratory system
Respiratory depression (typically three times the hypnotic dose) [60,196]
Aspiration pneumonia, atelectasis, pulmonary edema, and bronchopneumonia also have been reported

Cardiovascular system
Hypotension, low cardiac output, and direct myocardial depression [60,196]
Other
Hypothermia due to depressed thermal regulation in the brainstem
Cutaneous bullae (barb-burns) over pressure points [196]
Decreased GI motility
Renal failure due to cardiovascular shock or rhabdomyolysis

Table 39.22 Therapy for maternal drug withdrawal.

Drugs	Therapy
Alcohol	Barbiturates Pentobarbital sodium (short-acting) followed by phenobarbital (longer-acting) Benzodiazepines (cleared slowly by fetus)
Amphetamines	Tricyclic antidepressants (severe depression)
Barbiturates	Barbiturates: 200 mg pentobarbital sodium IV or by mouth to test for physical dependence (short-acting), followed by phenobarbital (withdrawal equivalent, 30 mg phenobarbital/100 mg of short-acting). Estimated dose of phenobarbital is administered by mouth every 8 h (maximum daily dose, 500 mg; if toxicity, daily dose is halved; if withdrawal symptoms, 200 mg phenobarbital intramuscularly). Once stable, decrease daily dose by 30 mg
Benzodiazepine	Benzodiazepine: slow tapering over a 1–2-week period Barbiturates (see Barbiturates in text) Withdrawal equivalents: 30 mg phenobarbital/100 mg chlordiazepoxide or 50 mg diazepam
Opiates	Librium 10–25 mg by mouth every 8 h ± compazine, as warranted, for nausea/vomiting Methadone 10–20 mg intramuscularly Refractory withdrawal may require short-acting narcotics (morphine, meperidine, hydromorphine)

(From Stine RJ, Marcus RH. Toxicologic emergencies. In: Haddad LM, Winchester JF, eds. Clinical management of poisoning and drug overdose. Philadelphia: WB Saunders, 1983:297–342; and Thorp J. Management of drug dependency, overdose, and withdrawal in the obstetric patient. *Obstet Gynecol Clin N Am* 1995;22:131.)

Signs

Sedation; altered mental status; myosis; bradypnea; respiratory depression; ataxia; nystagmus; extraocular muscle palsies; dysarthria; hyporreflexia; incoordination; decreased bowel sounds; hypothermia; hypotension; cardiovascular collapse.

Diagnostic tests

Blood: complete blood cell count; electrolytes; glucose; creatinine and blood urea nitrogen; prothrombin time and partial thromboplastin time; phenobarbital level (in cases of suspected barbiturate overdose, blood levels may be useful for confirming the identity of the drug, although the quantitative level may not reflect the clinical status of the patient). Urinalysis: drug screen; pH.

Short-term problems

Respiratory failure; coma; anoxic encephalopathy (interpretation of EEGs is unreliable with abnormal levels of barbiturates). Maternal EKG, respiratory rate, and peripheral oxygen saturation, as well as fetal heart rate monitoring, are recommended.

Long-term problems

Withdrawal syndrome is chronic user/abuser (insomnia; excitement; delirium; psychosis; seizures; hypotension).

Fetal considerations

Because barbiturates cross the placenta, the teratogenic potential depends on the agent and the category (most of the class D/Dm) [39]. Epileptic pregnant women taking phenobarbital in combination with other anticonvulsants have a two- to threefold greater risk of minor congenital defects in the fetus (estimated range of 10–20%) [39,91].

Signs

Potential for decreased beat-to-beat variability; bradycardia; abnormal biophysical profile in severe maternal poisoning.

Teratogenic potential

Split of opinion; usually risk is multifactorial and associated to the combination of the seizure disorder and the medication. Risk appears to be greater with the combination of phenytoin [39,91,92,93].

Fetal distress potential

The potential for fetal distress depends on maternal clinical status. In severe intoxication, cardiopulmonary depression (if respiratory depression, hypoxemia or cardiovascular collapse) may lead to fetal compromise.

Indications for delivery

Obstetric indications. Caution is suggested when interpreting fetal assessment techniques (electronic fetal monitoring and biophysical profile).

Postnatal

Fetal and neonatal addiction have been reported [94]. Neonatal withdrawal complications may occur 3–14 days after delivery in chronic users (average 6 days; up to 2 weeks later); and may require treatment [95,96]. Increased risk of hemorrhagic disease of the newborn [97]. May cause neonatal sedation of some breastfed infants (caution patients about it) [91].

Management considerations

With barbiturate overdose, the initial therapeutic goal is stabilization of maternal cardiopulmonary status. Because there are no specific antidotes the management focus is on gradual withdrawal to prevent abrupt withdrawal complications. Hypoxia and hypotension are the main determinants of a poor outcome [94,98,99].

Supportive

Respiratory support is the priority; measures needed may range from supplemental O_2 to endotracheal intubation and mechanical ventilation. Maintaining an adequate volume expansion and diuresis is critical.

Hypotension may be supported by oxygen and IV fluids. With severe hypotension, dopamine or norepinephrine may be required.

Hypothermia can be prevented with blankets, use of warm IV fluids and heated humidified oxygen if intubated. Core rewarming techniques or cardiopulmonary bypass may be required if the core temperature is under 32°C.

Specific measures/antidotes

- Gastric emptying (even after 8 hours of ingestion since there may be delayed gastric emptying associated to barbiturates) should be followed by the administration of charcoal and cathartic agents. Multiple doses of activated charcoal (every 4 hours) are recommended [97]. Because phenobarbital may form gastric concretions, endoscopic removal may be surgically necessary [98]. Induced emesis may be indicated if no significant depression.
- Forced alkaline diuresis recommended for symptomatic patients to enhance elimination (add potassium to the bicarbonate infusion as recommended under the aspirin-management section, above) particularly after ingestion of long-acting barbiturates (goal: 5–10 ml/min of urine with a pH ≈ 8.0) [60].
- Hemoperfusion (resin over charcoal) or hemodyalisis may be indicated in cases of toxic/lethal exposures (phenobarbital level of 100 µg/ml or 430 µmol/l), if uremia develops or for life-threatening overdoses refractory to supportive care [100]. Hemodialysis is useful in long-acting barbiturate overdose.
- No specific antidote. In chronic overdose, a decremental dosage regimen, beginning with 200 mg of phenobarbital every 6 hours should be used to prevent withdrawal complications in both mother and fetus.

Monitoring

Vital signs/mental status/airway/BP/oxygen saturation; electrolytes and serum calcium levels need to be followed. Severe toxicity requires management in an ICU [60].

Therapeutic goals

Asymptomatic patient; no need for supplemental oxygen or volume expansion; therapeutic or subtherapeutic level.

Discharge considerations

Dose adjustment if patient is epileptic. Psychiatry consult recommended if mechanism of exposure is deemed intentional. As part of the patient's ongoing care, drug rehabilitation should be considered.

Follow-up

Follow phenobarbital levels. Notify primary physician (obstetrician and neurologist) before discharge. Consider folate supplementation in chronic users and vitamin K administration to mothers during the last month of the pregnancy. Clinical follow-up with a social worker, obstetrician, and psychiatrist is warranted [60,99,100].

Benzodiazepines

Toxicology

Benzodiazepines are CNS depressants and are widely prescribed for their anxiolytic, muscle relaxant, anticonvulsant, and hypnotic effects.

Benzodiazepines are metabolized in the liver by demethylation (active metabolites) and/or conjugation (inactive metabolites) and are excreted in the urine (predominantly) and in the bile [101].

Gastrointestinal absorption is rapid and complete, while intramuscular absorption is erratic [98]. Benzodiazepines have a wide therapeutic index [98] and are relatively safe when taken orally and as a single agent [60]. Intravenous administration, however, has been associated with a 2% mortality rate from respiratory or cardiac arrest [98].

- Common names and examples: lorazepam; oxazepam; clonazepam; diazepam; temazepam; chlordiazepoxide; Ativan®; Centrax®; Dalmane®; Diastat®; Halcion®; Klonopin®; Librium®; Limbitrol®; ProSom®; Restoril®; Serax®; Tranxene®; Valium®; Versed®; Xanax®
- FDA classification: D
- As a cause of morbidity: 2* [2]
- As a cause of mortality: 2* [2]
- Most frequent route of exposure: ingestion
- Most frequent reason for exposure: intentional overdose

*Sedatives, hypnotics, and antipsychotics.

Maternal considerations

Symptoms

Drowsiness, ataxia, nystagmus, dysarthria, dizziness, weakness, and confusion. Occasionally, paradoxical irritability, excitation, or delirium may occur [102].

Signs

Lethargy, altered mental status; slurred speech; ataxia; brady or tachycardia; decreased bowel sounds; respiratory depression; hypotension; dyskinesia; acute dystonic reactions. Uncommonly, respiratory and/or circulatory depression may be present. Coma is the manifestation of severe overdose and/or a coingestion.

Diagnostic tests

Blood: complete blood count; electrolytes and glucose; toxicology screen (detects most of them except clonazepam). Serum levels are of no value in the emergent treatment as drug levels do not correlate with clinical status. Calculation of osmolal and anion gaps (Table 39.23) recommended if suspicion of coingestants and severe clinical manifestations. Urinalysis: drug screen; specific gravity.

Short-term problems

Respiratory depression; hypotension; anoxic encephalopathy (interpretation of EEGs is unreliable with abnormal levels of benzodiazepines).

Long-term problems

Tolerance to the sedative effects. Withdrawal syndrome (anxiety; insomnia; dysphoria; nausea; palpitations; fatigue; confusion; delirium; muscle twitching; seizures; psychosis) may appear after 1–7 days after abrupt cessation of benzodiazepines or after switching to a different benzodiazepine with different receptor activity. Seizures have been reported up to 12 days after withdrawal in chronic users [102].

Fetal considerations

Signs

Potential for decreased beat-to-beat variability; bradycardia; abnormal biophysical profile in severe maternal poisoning.

Table 39.23 Causes of increased osmolal gap.

Methanol (mol. wt = 32)
Ethanol (mol. wt = 46)
Acetone (mol. wt = 58)
Isopropyl alcohol (mol. wt = 60)
Ethylene glycol (mol. wt = 62)
Propylene glycol (mol. wt = 76)
Mannitol (mol. wt = 182)
Ethyl ether
Magnesium
Renal failure without dialysis
Severe alcoholic or lactic ketoacidosis

Teratogenic potential
Majority of the evidence does not support it. The teratogenic potential of these agents generally falls in category C/D/Xm [39]. In one study, chlordiazepoxide (category D) was associated with a fourfold increase in congenital anomalies [103]. However, others have not found such associations [104,105]. Diazepam (category D) has been reported to be associated with oral clefts [106,107]. More recently retrospective and prospective studies have been unable to find an association between diazepam use during pregnancy and facial clefts or other defects in the offspring, even among those patients exposed to high doses [108,109,110].

Fetal distress potential
Only in the presence of severe maternal toxicity and secondary to maternal hypovolemia or hypoxemia.

Indications for delivery
Obstetric indications. Caution is suggested when interpreting fetal assessment techniques (electronic fetal monitoring and biophysical profile).

Postnatal
Potential for neonatal hypotonia, impaired temperature regulation, lethargy, and apnea needing resuscitation measures [111]. Risk of neonatal withdrawal may produce seizures 2–6 days after delivery. High-dose or recent use prior to delivery has been associated with birth depression and withdrawal stigmata in neonates, the latter occurring up to 6 days after delivery [110,112].

Management considerations

Wide therapeutic index; low lethal potential if isolated poison. Investigate the possibility of coingestion (particularly alcohol and tricyclics). The therapeutic goal with benzodiazepine overdose is supportive care and gradual withdrawal of the benzodiazepines in long-term abusers.

Supportive
Respiratory assistance may be required; crystalloid infusion to maintain adequate volume; dopamine and norepinephrine infusions may be required in refractory hypotension. If severe toxicity is present, respiratory and cardiovascular support may be needed.

Specific measures/antidotes
• The first step is gastric emptying followed by activated charcoal and cathartics (50–60 g of activated charcoal in sorbitol: 1 g/kg) and repeated (25–30 g) every 4 hours (the sorbitol added only every 12 hours). Induced emesis not recommended.
• Flumazenil (Romazicon®; category C); give if vital signs are no stable, tricyclic coingestion excluded and if no history of chronic use or abuse of benzodiazepines (possibility of inducing seizures) (see Table 39.3).
• If the patient develops seizures, IV injection of benzodiazepine may be required to terminate withdrawal seizures, followed by a gradual withdrawal of the agent [102]. An alternative treatment for seizure control is phenobarbital.

Monitoring
Vital signs/mental status/oxymetry/intermittent fetal heart rate monitoring. Repeat drug levels not indicated.

Therapeutic goals
Asymptomatic patient; normal mental status without benzodiazepine antagonism (at least more than 4 hours since last dose of flumazenil); normal bowel sounds; completed decontamination procedures; no evidence of coingestion; reassurant fetal condition; consults completed.

Discharge considerations
Investigate chronic use/abuse of benzodiazepines. Consider drug counselor, psychiatry, and social worker evaluations. As part of the patient's ongoing care, drug rehabilitation should be considered.

Follow-up
Notify primary care physician (obstetrician, psychiatry). Clinical follow-up with a social worker, obstetrician, and psychiatrist is warranted [102,109,113].

Carbon monoxide

Toxicology

Carbon monoxide (CO) is a tasteless, colorless, odorless gas. It is a by-product of cigarette smoking (the most common source of CO exposure), automobile exhaust, opens fires, kerosene stoves, and heating systems (heaters or furnaces) in improperly ventilated areas. An unusual source of CO poisoning is paint removers that contain methylene chloride, which can be absorbed by the respiratory tract and be metabolized to CO over a delayed period of time. CO is absorbed rapidly through the respiratory tract. Hemoglobin's affinity for CO is 250–300 times greater than for oxygen. In addition it binds to myoglobin with a 40-fold greater affinity than that of oxygen, which may be related to some of the cardiac effects seen in this type of poisoning [114,115,116].
• Examples: fires, motor vehicle fumes, heat stoves
• As a cause of morbidity: 13* [2]
• As a cause of mortality: 9* [2]
• Main route of exposure: inhalation
• Reasons for exposure: unintentional; intentional (suicide attempt)

Maternal considerations

Maternal signs and symptoms relate to the reduction of the oxygen carrying capacity of hemoglobin as it is bound by CO

*Includes vapors, fumes, and other gases.

Table 39.24 Signs and symptoms of carbon monoxide overdose.*

Signs	Symptoms
Vasodilation	Headache
Disturbed judgment	Shortness of breath
Collapse	Nausea
Coma	Dizziness
Convulsions	Visual disturbances
Cheyne–Stokes respiration	Weakness

* Signs and symptoms will vary depending on the concentration of carboxyhemoglobin.

(Table 35.24). Given their higher oxygen extraction ratios the heart and CNS are responsible for most of the presenting features [115].

Symptoms
Depends on concentration (%COHb): headache; shortness of breath; nausea; dizziness; dim vision; weakness; chest pain (see Table 39.24).

Signs
Vasodilation; confusion; disturbed judgement; tachypnea; tachycardia; collapse; dysrhythmias; hypotension; non-cardiogenic pulmonary edema; myocardial ischemia; coma; seizures; Cheyne–Stokes respirations; "cherry-red" discoloration is clinically rare.

Diagnostic tests
EKG: sinus tachycardia, ST depression, atrial fibrillation, prolonged PR and QT intervals; AV or bundle branch block.; ABGs: %COHb (correlates with symptoms and signs). A metabolic acidosis implies significant exposure with resultant tissue hypoxia Others: complete blood count, transaminases, electrolytes, creatinine, urinalysis. Chest X-ray (if respiratory symptoms). Head CT (if coma, seizures, or focal neurologic deficits). If the patient was rescued from a fire, consider obtaining a cyanide level (hydrogen cyanide is a common fire intoxicant).

Short-term problems
Short-term concerns with CO poisoning include myocardial ischemia or infarction, rhabdomyolysis, renal failure, pulmonary edema, blindness, and hearing loss.

Long-term problems
Delayed CNS toxicity (perivascular infarction; demyelination of basal ganglia) on comatose or acidotic patients on arrival. Delayed problems include CNS toxicity due to perivascular infarction and demyelination of basal ganglia. This is usually seen in patients who are comatose or acidotic on arrival to the hospital [115,117,118].

Fetal considerations
CO crosses the placenta and has a higher affinity for fetal than adult hemoglobin. As a result, fetal concentrations of CO are 10% to 15% higher than those in the mother. Maximal concentrations of CO in fetal blood are found after about 4 hours of the exposure. Maternal COHb levels are a poor predictor of fetal toxicity and maternal wellbeing might be misleadingly reassuring of the fetal condition [118,119].

Signs
Nonreassuring fetal condition: decreased variability; decelerations [120].

Teratogenic potential
Although the teratogenic potential is unclear, fetal brain damage and subsequent developmental delays may be seen [116,121]. Some cases of CO poisoning severe enough to cause maternal symptoms have been associated with premature birth, neurologic deficits and anomalies (CNS, skeletal, clefts) in surviving infants [116,119,120,122].

Fetal distress potential
Yes; high. Increased risk of fetal demise with chronic exposure [123]. Fetal death or permanent neurological damage can occur in the absence of severe maternal symptoms [119,120]. The fetal prognosis is difficult to estimate.

Indications for delivery
Obstetric indications; nonreassuring fetal condition despite adequate maternal therapy.

Management considerations
The half-life of CO in a healthy adult breathing 21% oxygen is 4–5 hours. This time is reduced to 80–90 minutes when breathing 100% oxygen. Hyperbaric oxygen (100%) reduces the half-life to less than 30 minutes [115]. Pulse oxymetry inaccurately reflects oxygen saturation (cannot differentiate carboxyhemoglobin from oxyhemoglobin) [61]. Given the fetal considerations above, a more aggressive management approach is indicated during pregnancy [117].

Specific measures/antidotes
- Oxygen (100%) should be administered via a tight-fitting nonrebreathing mask and continued for a period equal to five times the duration that it took for the maternal CO levels to normalize [117,124].
- Hyperbaric oxygen is indicated if COHb is greater than 15% (versus more than 40% in the nonpregnant state), signs of nonreassuring fetal condition any neurologic signs in the mother (altered mental status; coma; focal neurologic deficits; seizures) or history of loss of consciousness [56,61,118].

Monitoring
Admit if COHb greater than 10% in pregnant patients; impaired mentation or metabolic acidosis with any presenting COHb level.

Any pregnant woman who is exposed to CO and has a potentially viable fetus should be monitored for a minimum of 12 hours. If cardiovascular complications are present, she should be admitted to the ICU. Such complications are expected in nonpregnant patients with a COHb greater than 15%. This level is lower in pregnant women (COHb 10%). Additionally, each patient's mental state and acid-base status should be monitored.

Therapeutic goals

COHb <5% and no symptoms. Reassuring antenatal fetal condition as appropriate according to the gestational age.

Discharge considerations

Identification (and avoidance) of source of exposure if not obvious (social work consult may be helpful). Suicidal potential evaluation (psychiatry consult) if circumstances suggest such possibility. Counsel on potential long-term effects on fetus.

Follow-up

Establish. Consider follow-up of intrauterine growth and fetal anatomy [61,115,117,118].

Cocaine

Toxicology

Cocaine is a naturally occurring agent that is legally available for use as a topical anesthetic. It is more commonly used illegally as a CNS stimulant with a street-sample purity of 15–60% [125]. It is principally used in one of two forms: either as the hydrochloride salt ("snorted" intranasal or IV) or as an alkaloid ("crack," "free base"). Illegally produced cocaine is frequently adulterated with foreign substances such as lactose, mannitol, lidocaine, and/or procaine [125].

Cocaine is absorbed through mucous membranes and can be inhaled, smoked, swallowed, injected IV, IM, or subcutaneously, or placed in the vagina or rectum [126]. Lethal overdoses can be taken via any route but are more likely with parenteral use or "freebasing" (smoking purified cocaine) or by the accidental rupture of a container of cocaine in "body packers" [127].

Cocaine is a sympathomimetic with direct cardiovascular stimulant activity that causes hypertension and vasoconstriction (see Table 39.4). It has both direct and indirect cardiotoxic effects (sensitizing the myocardium to epinephrine (adrenalin) and norepinephrine) [128]. It is detoxified by liver and plasma cholinesterase. Though the biologic half-life is 0.5–1.5 hours vascular catastrophes can occur several weeks after its use [129].

- Examples/other names: "crack"; "rock"; "blow"; "snow"; "liquid lady": alcohol+cocaine; "speedball": heroine+cocaine
- FDA classification: X (C if used as a local anesthetic) [39]
- As a cause of morbidity: 17* [2]
- As a cause of mortality: 4* [2]
- Most frequent route of exposure: inhalation
- Most frequent reason for exposure: unintentional overdose

*Includes other stimulants and street drugs.

Maternal considerations

The fetus, infant, and pregnant woman experience slower metabolism and elimination [127,130]. The peak effects of cocaine in nonpregnant women occur within 3–5 minutes IV or at 60–90 minutes orally.

Symptoms

Mild-to-moderate toxicity is manifested by nausea, vomiting, abdominal pain, headache, apprehension, dysphoria, confusion, and hallucinations [60]. Other symptoms include: anxiety, dizziness, chest pain, respiratory difficulty, and palpitations. Specific during pregnancy: threatened preterm labor; vaginal bleeding; preterm premature rupture of membranes [131].

Signs

Agitation; altered mental status (up to frank psychosis); tachycardia; hypertension; hyperthermia; mydriasis; tachypnea; diaphoresis; hyperactive bowel sounds; pulmonary edema; uterine contractions (up to tetany); vaginal bleeding. Severe toxicity is manifested by psychotic behavior, seizures, coma, ventricular arrhythmias (myocardial ischemia/infarction), hypertension (severe), circulatory collapse, pulmonary edema and respiratory depression, ARDS ("crack lung"), pneumomediastinum, rhabdomyolysis, hyperthermia, and hepatic infarction [129]. Death may occur rapidly from respiratory depression and/or circulatory collapse [114].

Diagnostic tests

Rectal and vaginal exams indicated to rule out occult drug packing. Blood: complete blood count; electrolytes and glucose; creatinine and blood urea nitrogen; creatine phosphokinase (CPK) and isofractions; myoglobin; troponin I (most specific in cocaine users); amylase; lipase and liver-function tests. Urine: microhematuria; myoglobinuria; EKG: tachycardia; ischemia; ST elevation (up to 43% of patients with chest pain); acute myocardial infarction. Chest X ray: pulmonary edema, pulmonary infarction. Consider other X rays surveys if history of recent traveling (possibility of body packing). CT and lumbar puncture if seizures. Cocaine is detectable in blood within 24 hours of ingestion and in urine for several days (see Table 39.8).

Short-term problems

Arrhythmias; myocardial infarction; seizures; pulmonary infarction; intracranial hemorrhage or infarcts; visceral infarcts; preterm delivery; abruptio placentae. Cerebral infarction is more common among alkaloidal cocaine users, and hemorrhagic stroke is seen more frequently in IV cocaine hydrochloride use. Cerebral catastrophes can occur within minutes of the use of cocaine [132].

Long-term problems

Malnutrition; sexually transmitted diseases; growth restriction; stillbirth; pre-eclampsia; risk for fetal neurodevelopmental delay (when cocaine is a component of a polydrug abuse). Long-term problems include the aftermath of intracranial hemorrhage or infarction and rhabdomyolysis [58,129,132].

Fetal considerations

Cocaine has high water and lipid solubility, a low molecular weight, and a low degree of ionization, all of which facilitate its passage across the placenta and into the fetus [130]. Cocaine infusion is associated with a decrease in uterine blood flow, leading to fetal hypoxic damage in the short term and to intrauterine growth retardation over time [128,133].

In pregnancy, there is a significant increase in the incidence of preterm labor (25–30% vs 12–17%) and anemia (57 vs 39%) [134]. There is also a higher incidence of pregnancy-induced hypertension (25 vs 4%) [134] and abruptio placentae [135]. Meconium aspiration, preeclampsia, premature rupture of membranes, and fetal distress are all increased [134,136].

Signs

Fetal tachycardia; decreased beat-to-beat variability; bradycardia; late decelerations [127].

Teratogenic potential

Controversial data; there is no agreement on whether cocaine increases the risk of structural malformations. The teratogenic potential for cocaine falls into category C. For nonmedicinal use, cocaine is classified as category X [39]. Urinary tract malformations (hydronephrosis, hypospadias, prune-belly syndrome), congenital heart defects (transposition of the great vessels, hypoplastic right-heart, ventricular septal defect, patent ductus arteriosus), and skull defects (exencephaly, encephalocele) have been associated with cocaine use in pregnancy [137,138]. Potential for growth restriction and restriction of fetal brain growth [138].

Fetal distress potential

Yes; secondary to uterine hyperstimulation, uterine vasoconstriction, abruption placentae, uterine rupture, and/or maternal seizures. Up to 13% of women who used cocaine during pregnancy develop an abruption, which may be sudden, unpredictable, and catastrophic. The incidence of abruptio placentae-related stillbirths in cocaine users can be 10 times higher than that of drug-free control women [130,135,139,140].

Indications for delivery

Nonreassuring fetal condition despite adequate supportive maternal care; severe abruptio placentae and severe growth restriction.

Postnatal

Risk of withdrawal syndrome (seizures; cardiovascular collapse); antenatal notification of the neonatology service recommended. Cocaine has been shown to be associated with significantly increased perinatal distress hypotonia and significantly lower 5-minute Apgar scores [135]. Postnatally, perinatal, or newborn cerebrovascular accidents may be found in neonates with a positive cocaine screening test [135,141]. The pathology of these injuries may include, intraventricular hemorrhage, echodensities known to be associated with necrosis, and cavitary lesions particularly in the basal ganglion, frontal lobes, and posterior fossa [69]. The risk of necrotizing enterocolitis is also higher among neonates exposed to cocaine [142,143].

Management considerations

The initial therapeutic goal is to stabilize and support the patient for 24 hours. In addition, most patients require symptomatic management of specific problems [60]. In selected circumstances, overdose victims or users will suffer from seizures, arrhythmias, hyperthermia, hypertension, hypotension, behavioral problems, and rhabdomyolysis.

Supportive

Hydration (forced alkaline diuresis if myoglobinuria detected or if creatinine elevated on arrival) to maintain the urine output at ≈3 ml/kg/h.

Physical restraints may be required for patients with significant psychomotor agitation as a temporizing measure to facilitate chemical sedation [129].

Admit to an ICU if seizures, ventricular arrhythmias, or hyperthermia.

Specific measures/antidotes

- Activated charcoal and whole bowel irrigation may decrease absorption if history of ingestion ("stuffing").
- Benzodiazepines (diazepam 5–10 mg IV or lorazepam 2–4 mg IV) are the first line of treatment for supraventricular arrhythmias, hypertension, ischemic chest pain, behavioral problems, and seizures.
- Lidocaine (1.5 mg/kg IV bolus followed by infusion of 2 mg/min) and alkalinization are the treatments of choice for ventricular arrhythmias. Defibrillation is indicated if hemodynamically unstable. Avoid use of β-blockers for the treatment of arrhythmias or hypertension (may worsen hypertension and coronary vasoconstriction, and induce seizures).
- Phenobarbital (25–50 mg/min up to 10–20 mg/kg) is the second choice for seizures and propofol the third. Status epilepticus may require paralysis and ventilation.
- In severe cases of hypertension (after diazepam or lorazepam), the use of nitroprusside or phentolamine may be needed for control.
- Hyperthermia is managed with external cooling. This is especially important in pregnancy to protect the fetus.
- In cases of hypotension, treatment with IV fluids should be initiated. For refractory hypotension, dopamine or norepinephrine may be required.

• In ischemic chest pain, may also use nitroglycerine (0.4 mg sublingually every 5 minutes and IV continuous drip thereafter) and in refractory cases: phentolamine 1 mg IV (repeat in 5 min).
• Heparinize if ischemic chest pain (5000 IU IV bolus+1000 I/h infusion).
• External cooling is needed to control hyperthermia (neuromuscular blockade may be needed in severe cases).
• Rhabdomyolysis is treated with maintenance and alkalinization of urine flow with IV fluids and sodium bicarbonate infusion (see doses under aspirin poisoning, above). Hemodyalisis may be indicated for renal failure secondary to myoglobinuria.
• No specific antidote available.

Monitoring

Vitals/mental status/oxymetry/cardiac for at least 24 hours after the exposure. Consider repeat EKGs and cardiac enzymes every 6 hours if significant exposure, risk factors for coronary artery disease or chest pain on arrival. Evaluation may include EKG, BP, temperature, blood gases, chest X-ray, renal and liver function tests, prothrombin and partial thromboplastin times and platelets, hemoglobin/hematocrit, and urinalysis for myoglobin.

Therapeutic goals

Asymptomatic patient; normal laboratory values; no contractions or bleeding; reassuring fetal condition; more than 24 hours of observation. Consults obtained (see below).

Disposition considerations

Drug counselor, psychiatry, and social worker consults recommended. Evaluate for sexually transmitted diseases.

Follow-up

Establish since a high proportion of these patients do not have (or have an erratic) prenatal care. Consider follow-up of fetal growth. On discharge, the patient will need clinical follow-up with a social worker, obstetrician, or psychiatric service. Fetal follow-up will require ultrasound evaluations to monitor fetal growth and anatomy. Once the fetus is potentially viable, assessment of fetal well-being is warranted. In addition, evaluation of the newborn for cerebral, urologic, and GI sequelae is indicated [61,127,129].

Ethanol

Toxicology

Ethanol is the most frequently ingested toxin in the world [144]. Ethanol is a colorless, odorless, volatile, liquid hydrocarbon. It is fully miscible in water and is lipid-soluble. It diffuses readily across lipid membranes, accounting for its multiorgan effects [145]. It is rapidly absorbed from the GI tract with approximately 20% absorbed in the stomach and the remainder in the small intestine. No specific receptor for ethanol has been identified and the mechanism of action leading to intoxication remains the subject of debate [145]. Ethanol is primarily (>90%) eliminated by the liver via enzymatic oxidation, with 5–10% excreted unchanged by the kidneys, lungs, and sweat. Ethanol is metabolized via at least three different pathways: alcohol dehydrogenase (ADH) located in the cytosol of the hepatocytes; the microsomal ethanol-oxidizing system (MEOS or CYP2E1), located in the endoplasmatic reticulum; and the peroxidase-catalase system, associated with the hepatic peroxisomes [145]. In adults, the average rate of ethanol metabolism is 100–125 mg/kg/h (up to 175 in habitual drinkers). As a result of an hourly metabolism of 7–10 g, the concentrations of ethanol fall 15–20 mg/dl/h with considerable individual variation [145].

Clinical presentation may vary with acute and/or chronic ethanol abuse or withdrawal. In addition consumption of illegally produced ethanol ("moonshine") can result in a methanol, lead, or arsenic poisoning [145]. Only acute overdosage is considered here.

• Examples/other names: alcohol; ethylic alcohol; "booze"
• FDA classification: D (X if used in large amounts or for prolonged periods)
• As a cause of morbidity: 7 [2]
• As a cause of mortality: 6 [2]
• Most frequent route of exposure: ingestion
• Most frequent reason for exposure: unintentional overdose

Maternal considerations

Clinical presentation may vary with acute and/or chronic ethanol abuse or withdrawal. Will consider here the acute overdose (see Table 39.22 for treatment of alcohol withdrawal). A systematic approach to the inebriated patient will help the clinician avoid potential pitfalls as they may present to a medical facility with a broad range of diagnostic possibilities and many serious conditions [144].

Symptoms

With acute alcohol overdosage, the signs and symptoms vary depending on the severity of intoxication and may include euphoria, incoordination, impaired judgment, and altered mental status. Social inhibitions are loosened. As such, aggressive or boisterous behavior is commonly seen.

Signs

As above plus flushed facies, diaphoresis, tachycardia, hypotension, hypothermia, ataxia, abnormal reflexes, nystagmus, altered mental status, mydriasis, impaired judgment and reflexes, and a characteristic breath smell. The presence of an ethylic breath is an unreliable means of ascertaining whether a person is intoxicated or whether ethanol was recently consumed [145]. In severe overdose, bradycardia, hypotension, respiratory depression, hypoglycemia, hypothermia, and coma are seen.

Diagnostic tests

Blood work: complete blood count, glucose, electrolytes, blood urea nitrogen, creatinine, transaminases, lipase, prothrombin time, magnesium, calcium, ketones, acetone, ammonia, and alcohol level. Patients with anion gap metabolic acidosis should have urine ketones and serum lactate concentration analysis as metabolic acidosis resulting from ethanol intoxication is uncommon (see Table 39.20). A high acetone level may suggest isopropanol intoxication. Clinically significant lactic acidosis due to ethanol can be related to a seizure, infection, hypoxia, or hypoperfusion states [144].

Consider arterial blood gases if altered mental status or respiratory distress, depression, or hypoxemia suspected on pulse oxymetry. Consider a drug screen if altered mental status or history of trauma. If aspiration is suspected, a chest x-ray should be obtained. History of head trauma and comatose patients with concentrations of alcohol under 300 mg/dl and those with levels above 300 mg/dl who fail to improve after a period of observation should have a head CT, followed by a lumbar puncture if needed [145].

Short-term problems

The most important short-term problems of a severe overdose are respiratory depression, pulmonary aspiration, hypoglycemia, and coma. Less frequently, GI bleeding, atrial arrhythmias, or rhabdomyolysis are encountered.

Long-term problems

Long-term problems are both organic and social. Organic problems include pancreatitis, hepatitis, cirrhosis, hepatic encephalopathy, portal hypertension, GI bleeding, anemia, thiamine deficiency, alcoholic ketoacidosis, systemic hypertension, decreased resistance to infection, hypomagnesemia, hypokalemia, and hypophosphatemia. Alcohol abuse is an important risk factor for intracerebral hemorrhage, particularly hemorrhagic stroke [58]. Alcohol is the leading cause of non-ischemic cardiomyopathy [58]. Social problems are manifested by malnutrition, isolation, depression, or suicide attempts.

Fetal considerations

Signs

Decrease in fetal heart rate accelerations and variability (nonreactivity of electronic fetal heart rate tracing); suppression of fetal breathing movements, electrocorticographic activity, and electro-oculographic activity [39,146,147].

Teratogenic potential

Fetal alcohol syndrome (FAS): (a) craniofacial dysmorphology (short palpebral fissures, hypoplastic philtrum, flattened maxilla); (b) prenatal and postnatal growth deficiencies (body length more than weight); (c) CNS dysfunction (including mental retardation and behavioral abnormalities); and (d) major organ system abnormalities (mainly cardiac, urogenital and hemangiomas) in 30–40% and probably more of the infants exposed. Other features are: ptosis, strabismus, epicanthal folds, myopia, microphtalmia, short upturned nose, posterior rotation of ears, poorly formed concha, hypotonia, poor coordination, and microcephaly. Diagnosis may be delayed until 9–12 months of age [148].

Fetal distress potential

Not likely unless the acute intoxication is complicated by trauma or maternal respiratory compromise (aspiration or depression). Transient nonreactivity to fetal movements or to external stimuli has been described in acute intoxications [146]. Yet a threefold increase in the risk of stillbirth has been described for women who drink more than four drinks per week during pregnancy [149].

Indications for delivery

Obstetric indications. Allow metabolism of alcoholic load before acting upon nonreassuring tracings of electric fetal monitoring.

Postnatally

Postnatally, the potential for withdrawal syndrome in neonates should be considered and the infant carefully monitored [148]. Because ethanol passes freely into breast milk, there is the potential for sedation and dose-related psychomotor and developmental delay in breast-fed infants. For ethanol, which cannot be measured in hair or meconium, accumulation of its fatty acid ethyl esters in meconium is emerging as a promising test for heavy maternal drinking in the second part of pregnancy [150]. Maternal ethanol use during pregnancy has been associated with an increase in childhood leukemia, particularly for the development of acute nonlymphocytic leukemia [148,151] and possibly other neoplasias.

Management considerations

With ethanol overdose, the therapeutic goal is to prevent acute complications in the first 6–8 hours following admission. Elimination occurs at a fixed rate.

Supportive

Protection of the airway because of the possibility of gastric aspiration or respiratory depression. Treatment of coma and seizures if they occur. If arriving with altered mental status immediate investigation for reversible causes (hypoxemia, hypoglycemia, and opioid intoxication) is warranted. Supplemental oxygen, intravenous dextrose (0.5–1 mg/kg), thiamine (100 mg), and naloxone should be administered if clinically indicated (see Table 39.3) [145].

Specific measures/antidotes

- Although the first step in ethanol overdose is decontamination, its use will depend on the proximity to the ingestion. Emesis is not indicated unless a substantial ingestion has occurred within minutes of presentation or other drug ingestion is suspected. Gastric lavage is indicated if intake of large amounts occurred within 30–45 minutes of presentation. Charcoal does not efficiently adsorb ethanol; it may be useful if other drugs were (or suspected to be) ingested.

• If trauma is suspected cervical spine immobilization should be instituted and the injury specifically ruled out.
• There is no specific antidote for ethanol; flumazenil and naloxone may alleviate respiratory depression in an inconsistent manner (anecdotal arousal after use of naloxone). Glucose and thiamine should be given routinely to ethanol overdose patients.
• Hemodyalisis may be considered in severe ethanol intoxication associated with respiratory failure or coma.

Monitoring
Continuous pulse oxymetry if the patient is asleep or initial reading is abnormal.

Therapeutic goals
Sobriety; no acute complications in 6–8 hours of observation. Ponder admission for social reasons. Other indications for hospital admission are: persistently abnormal vital signs, persistently abnormal mental status, mixed overdose, concomitant trauma, ethanol withdrawal or associated disease process (pancreatitis, GI hemorrhage, etc.).

Discharge considerations
Clinical re-evaluation should be performed to avoid missing injuries initially masked by the intoxication. Social worker, drug counseling, and psychiatry evaluations may be helpful prior to discharge. Consider folate supplementation. On discharge, clinical follow-up may involve a social worker, drug counselor, obstetrician, and/or psychiatrist.

Follow-up
Fetal follow-up will require ultrasound evaluations to monitor fetal growth [144,145].

Iron

Toxicology
Iron supplements are available as the iron salts: ferrous gluconate, ferrous sulfate, and ferrous fumarate, and as the nonionic preparations carbonyl iron and polysacchararide iron. Their concentrations of elemental iron may vary from 12 to 98%. Under normal conditions the oral bio-availability of inorganic iron is less than 10%. It is not known whether in overdoses this percentage is actually higher. In overdose peak concentrations are thought to occur 2–6 hours after ingestion. Toxic effects of iron poisoning occur at doses of 10–20 mg/kg of elemental iron. The lethal dose of elemental iron is 200–300 mg/kg [152,153].

Iron can generate oxidative stress and inhibit several metabolic enzymes (including mitochondrial oxidative phosphorilation) causing local caustic injury and metabolic acidosis. The damage to the GI tract allows iron ions to enter the systemic circulation, bind to circulating proteins, and eventually allowing "free iron" to be deposited in most major organs affecting metabolism and local dysfunction of the GI, hepatic, cardiovascular and CNS [152,153].

• Examples/common names: ferrous gluconate; ferrous fumarate; ferrous sulfate/Chromagen®; Feosol®, Fergon®; Ferro-Folic®; Ferro-Grad®; Ferlecit®; Iberet®; Irospan®; Megadose®; Nephrofer®; Nephrovite®; Prenate®; Slow Fe®; Trinsicon®
• FDA classification: A
• As a cause of morbidity: 2* [67]
• As a cause of mortality: rare
• Most frequent route of exposure: ingestion
• Most frequent reason for exposure: intentional overdose; suicidal gesture

Maternal considerations
Four physiopathologic stages of iron overdose have been recognized: (a) direct corrosive insult to the intestinal mucosa; (b) a quiescent phase (which may not occur in severe overdoses); (c) systemic organ failure, characterized by a worsening of the GI hemorrhage, cardiovascular collapse, and severe metabolic acidosis; (d) GI sequelae as a result of intestinal scarring weeks after the ingestion [152,154].

Symptoms
Indigestion; abdominal pain; nausea; vomiting; hematemesis; diarrhea, hematochezia.

Signs
As above+bloody stools; tachycardia; fever; lethargy; shock and acidosis in severe cases. Rarely icterus, hypoglycemic symptoms, coagulopathy.

Diagnostic tests
Complete blood count: leukocytosis; anemia, or hemoconcentration. Serum iron levels: normal: 50–175 μg/dl; mild-to-moderate toxicity generally manifests at levels of 350–500 μg/dl. Hepatotoxicity usually is observed at levels higher than 500 μg/dl. Levels higher than 1000 μg/dl are associated with severe toxicity and potential mortality. Caveats: A single iron concentration may not represent a peak concentration; repeat every 2 hours for the first 6–8 hours. Samples drawn too early or too late post-overdose may be unreliable. Other tests: serum electrolytes (anion gap metabolic acidosis; see Table 39.20); blood urea nitrogen and creatinine; glucose (mild hyperglycemia); liver function tests, including coagulation profile; ABGs if patient's mental status is altered or in shock.

Abdominal X-ray: radiopaque pills may guide further GI decontamination (their absence does not exclude potential toxicity).

Short-term problems
Shock; hemorrhage; hepatic failure; pulmonary edema/hemorrhage; disseminated intravascular coagulation.

*Intentional overdoses during pregnancy.

Long-term problems
GI scarring; small intestine infarction; hepatic necrosis; achlorhydria.

Fetal considerations

Signs
Uterine contractions may be associated to maternal hypovolemia and shock.

Teratogenic potential
None specific. In a review of 61 cases of obstetric iron overdose it was found that a peak iron level greater than or equal to 400 µg/dl was not associated with increased risk of spontaneous abortion, preterm delivery or congenital anomalies. However, patients with evidence of organ failure due to iron toxicity were more likely to spontaneously abort or deliver preterm [154,155].

Fetal distress potential
None unless associated with maternal acidosis, hypovolemia, dehydration or bleeding.

Indications for delivery
Obstetric indications.

Management considerations

Pregnancy should not alter therapy for acute iron overdose. If the patient condition is stable the need for treatment begins from the estimation the amount of ingested elemental iron [156].

When calculating the dose ingested use prepregnancy (not current) weight [157]. Deferoxamine administered in the third trimester is not associated with perinatal complications and is potentially life saving [18,158].

Supportive
Initial stabilization must include supplemental oxygen, airway assessment and establishment of intravenous access. Assess hemodynamic status and start vigorous intravenous hydration through 2 large bore IVs if indicated. Consider early orogastric intubation in lethargic patients for airway protection.

Specific measures/antidotes

- Ipecac emesis recommended within the first 30–60 minutes in the conscious patient if lavage is not available (and the patient has not started vomiting on her own). The uses of bicarbonate in the gastric lavage or enteral deferoxamine are currently not recommended. Activated charcoal is ineffective in adsorbing iron [157].
- The presence and location of radiopaque pills on an abdominal radiograph can help guide lavage (see caveats above). If pills are past the pylorus a lavage will be unlikely. If lavage is performed, a post-lavage radiograph is recommended.
- Whole-bowel irrigation (polyethylene glycol: at 1.5–2 l/h; decrease rate by 50% if not tolerated) may be required if gastric lavage is ineffective in removing pill fragments or pills are seen past the stomach [152,153].
- Endoscopy or surgery may be occasionally required to remove iron tablets adherent to the gastric mucosa [153].
- Deferoxamine (category C medication) is a specific chelator of ferric iron (≈9 µg of free iron per 100 mg) with resulting formation of ferrioxamine, which is renally excreted (redish-brown color). It should be given at a dose of 15 mg/kg/h as an intravenous infusion for up to 24 hours. It is recommended for ingestions of >60 mg/kg of elemental iron; peak serum irons >350 µg/dl; toxic appearance, lethargy, hypotension, signs of shock and metabolic acidosis. If prolonged infusion is deemed necessary, consider a hiatus of 12 hours to allow the elimination of ferrioxamine.
- The use of deferoxamine may be associated to hypotension. Hypovolemia should be corrected with crystalloids before initiation of chelation [152].
- Hemodialysis may be required in the presence of associated or toxic renal failure.

Monitoring
Serum iron levels every 4–6 hours until within normal range.

Therapeutic goals
Normal serum iron levels. Admit patients who ingested in excess of 60 mg of elemental iron; those with symptomatic ingestions of lower amounts; patients with levels in excess of 350 µg/dl regardless of symptoms or those with positive radiographs (if obtained) [152]. Admission to an ICU is indicated if serum iron level that exceed 1000 µg/dl; coma, shock or metabolic acidosis.

May discontinue deferoxamine when the patient is asymptomatic, the anion gap acidosis has resolved, the urine color undergoes no further change and/or with serum iron levels <100 µg/dl.

Discharge considerations
Asymptomatic patients are unlikely to develop symptoms after more than 6 hours of the ingestion. Be mindful of patients that appeared to have recovered from the GI toxicity as they might be in the quiescent stage of the intoxication. Evaluate suicidal potential in all patients (psychiatry consult).

Follow-up
Establish multidisciplinary prenatal care if not already done (obstetrician, social worker and/or psychiatrist). A follow-up with gastroenterology may be indicated 2 weeks after the ingestion to assess integrity of the GI tract [152,153,154,156,157].

Organophosphates (and carbamates)

Toxicology

Organophosphates and carbamates are cholinesterase-inhibiting chemicals used predominantly as pesticides. Some forms are used as nerve gases in chemical warfare (Sarin, VX) [159,160]. Collectively they are responsible for about 4 million poisonings and 300 000 deaths worldwide per year [161].

These insecticides are in general extremely well absorbed from the lungs, GI tract, skin, mucous membranes, and conjunctiva following inhalation, ingestion, or topical contact [162]. Carbamates in general (Carboryl® and Bendiocarb® for example) do not enter the CNS, and enzyme inhibition is reversible in minutes to hours resulting in limited toxicity. Organophosphates permanently inactivate acetylcholinesterase and penetrate the CNS leading to greater toxicity and need for antidote administration [61].

Cholinergic poisoning, which can be acute or chronic, is caused by the accumulation of acetylcholine at synapses exerting deleterious effects on three systems: muscarinic, nicotinic and CNS [61].

Although pesticide exposure is ubiquitous, special consideration should be taken with immigrants and seasonal farm workers, particularly in medically underserved areas.

- Examples/other names: Dichlorvos®, Diazinon®, Dimethoate®, Malathion®; Parathion®; Quinalphos®, Sarban®; nerve gases: tabun (GA); sarin (GB); soman (GD); VX
- As a cause of morbidity: 8 [2]
- As a cause of mortality: 15 [2]
- Most frequent route of exposure: ingestion
- Most frequent reason for exposure: accidental exposure/intentional overdose

Maternal considerations

The majority of agents show some signs and symptoms of toxicity within 6–12 hours after the exposure (exception of highly liposoluble: fenthion, difenthion, and chlorfenthion) [159]. The latter compounds may require several exposures before the person becomes symptomatic because the agent is stored in the adipose tissue depressing cholinesterase activity in an additive manner [159].

Symptoms

Nausea; vomiting; blurred vision; headache; dizziness; respiratory difficulty; abdominal pain (cramping usually); diarrhea; urinary incontinence; coma (see Table 39.4).

Signs

Agitation; altered mental status; fever; myosis; fasciculations or tremors; sialorrhea; bronchorrhea; bronchospasm; pulmonary edema; tachy- or bradycardia; hypo- or hypertension; respiratory arrest; coma (see Table 39.4). Some compounds may give a "garlic-like" breath smell; other may have a solvent-type smell.

Diagnostic tests

Blood: complete blood count (leukocytosis possible); electrolytes and glucose (hypokalemia and hyperglycemia); amylase (might be elevated); decrease of 80–90% of erythrocyte cholinesterase (correlates better with synaptic inhibition). Urine: drug screen (intentional use can coexist with cocaine). EKG: tachycardia; bradycardia; AV block or various degrees; QT prolongation; asystole.

Short-term problems

Bronchorrhea, bronchospasm and respiratory failure; aspiration pneumonia; ventricular arrhythmias; pancreatitis; ARDS.

Long-term problems

Hepatic failure: three kinds of neurologic sequelae described: (a) prolonged memory impairment, peripheral neuropathy, personality change have been reported; (b) relapse after apparent recovery is known as "intermediate syndrome" has been described 24–96 hours after resolution of the acute cholinergic crisis and manifesting as muscular paralysis (including respiratory failure) developing after recovery from the cholinergic phase (explained by the hepatic metabolism to more toxic compounds within 72 hours of the exposure); (c) organophosphate-induced delayed neurotoxicity (OPIDN) is a sensorimotor polyneuropathy occurring 1–3 weeks after exposure and may mimic Guillain–Barre syndrome; recovery may take 12–15 months and might not be complete.

Fetal considerations

These compounds cross the placenta.

Signs

Potential for preterm delivery [161]. Mild decreases in duration of pregnancy have been reported [163].

Teratogenic potential

Not enough evidence (one case reported of multiple anomalies after exposure to oxydemeton-methyl at 4 weeks). Association between pesticides and male genital anomalies has not been confirmed [164]. Possible effects on neurobehavioral development has not been studied [165].

Fetal distress potential

Yes; from maternal hypoxia or low placental perfusion associated to maternal bradycardia. Fetotoxicity and fetal death has been reported [166]. Organic brain dysfunction has also been described [165].

Indications for delivery

Obstetric indications. Nonreassuring fetal condition.

Management considerations

Patients will remain clinically ill as long as there is active toxin available to bind to any free cholinesterase and depress its activity to less than 20% [159].

Organophosphates can penetrate latex gloves and health care personnel should wear nitrile or neoprene (chemical-resistant) gloves, water-resistant gowns, and eye shields to prevent a secondary exposure [159].

Supportive

Respiratory: administer 100% oxygen. The airway is best protected by early endotracheal intubation. Only nondepolarizing neuromuscular blockers should be used due to prolonged paralysis with succinylcholine.

Specific measures/antidotes

• Decontamination: all forms of carbamates and organophosphates may persist on the human body and clothing and footwear (particularly leather). They need to be removed and discarded as toxic waste [159]. Aspiration of gastric contents is indicated if ingestion occurred within the past hour and the patient is not vomiting. Activated charcoal is administered if no contraindications.

• If the exposure has been cutaneous the patient needs to be washed down with copious amounts of water. Shaving the head might be necessary for oily insecticides. The water and other body fluids should be considered potentially toxic and deactivated with chlorine bleach (4–5%).

• Atropine (category C) 2 mg (0.05 mg/kg) IV (or IM if no IV access established yet) in repeated doses controls muscarinic effects (nausea, vomiting, bradycardia, salivation, bronchorrhea, bronchospasm) but does not reverse nicotinic effects. The dose can be repeated every 5 minutes until muscarinic findings subside. Large doses of atropine may be needed in patients expose to more liposoluble compounds. A continuous infusion of atropine (0.05 mg/kg/h) can be started and titrated to effect and then slowly withdrawn. The end-point of atropinization is drying of the tracheobronchial tree and the ability to oxygenate (mydriasis is not a contraindication).

• Pralidoxime chloride (2-PAM chloride) (category C) is required for muscle weakness (nicotinic effect). 2-PAM chloride allows for reactivation of the cholinesterases if given before irreversible binding of the toxin (time not fully known; usually within 24–48 hours depending on the agent, but may be attempted even later). The usual dose is 1–2 g IV (may be given IM if IV access not established) over 10–20 minutes (may cause neuromuscular blockade if administered too fast) followed by an infusion of 200–500 mg/h (World Health Organization-recommended doses are: 30 mg/kg or more as a bolus and more than 8 mg/kg/h as an infusion for 7 days or until recovery).

• Diazepam IV can be used for seizures (phenobarbital being the second-line therapy).

Monitoring

Any symptomatic patient should be admitted for at least 24 hours. Any evidence of nicotinic symptoms or airway compromise requires an ICU setting until all signs have resolved [159]. Pulse oximetry; respiratory frequency; cholinesterase levels every 12–24 hours until cholinergic effects resolve.

Therapeutic goals

Asymptomatic patient with normal levels of erythrocyte cholinesterase.

Discharge considerations

More than 72 hours after significant exposure and 24 hours after the last atropine; stable cholinesterase level; easy accessibility to the hospital. Caution patients about recurring symptoms: an intermediate syndrome of respiratory paralysis, weakness, and depressed reflexes has been described 24–96 hours after the resolution of the severe cholinergic crisis [61].

Follow-up

Establish multidisciplinary prenatal care if not already done (obstetrician, social worker, and/or psychiatrist; monitor acetylcholinesterase activity level until normal after discharge (5 weeks to 4 months in untreated patients) [159,167]. Ensure that workplace has been inspected and meet approved standards [159]. Workers should not be re-exposed to organophosphates until acetylcholinesterase levels are more than 75% [61,159,162,168].

Envenomations during pregnancy

Venomous animals are a significant health problem for rural populations in many parts of the world. The medically important venomous animals consist of six major groups: cnidarians (e.g. jelly fish, anemones, and corals), venomous fish, sea snakes, scorpions, spiders, hymenoterans (e.g. bee, wasps, ants), and venomous terrestrial snakes. An animal classified as venomous possesses a special apparatus for injecting venom (snakes, scorpions, etc.). Unlike venomous animals, poisonous animals possess toxins that are dispersed in their body tissues and are activated when the animal is ingested [169]. Terrestrial venomous snakes are the most important group of venomous animals.

During 1999, 524 cases of bites or stings during pregnancy were reported to occur to the American Poison Control Centers. This represents 5.9% of all the toxic exposures occurring during pregnancy reported nationally in 1999. Moderate effects (more pronounced or prolonged than minor effects, usually requiring some form of treatment) were seen in only 5.1%; however, the rate increased to 13.1% when the envenomation was by a spider bite. No major effects (life-threatening or resulting in residual disability or disfigurement) were reported in this series [170].

Snakebites

Snakebite is a largely unrecognized public health problem that presents significant challenges for medical management. It has been estimated that worldwide about 2.5 million people are envenomed per year, and over 125 000 die from this cause [171].

More than 6000 people are reported to sustain snakebites annually in the USA with nearly half from poisonous species [172]. In the USA snakebites during pregnancy are fortunately an uncommon event. In 1999, ophidic accidents represented 3.5% of all the stings and bites reported to American Poison Control Centers [173]. That year the majority of snakebites during pregnancy arose from envenomations by snakes in the Crotalidae family (pit vipers) (see Table 39.25). Common pit vipers in the

Table 39.25 Snake envenomation during pregnancy by type of snake and maternal effects, US: 1999.

Type of snake	No.	Minor effect	Moderate effects	Major effects	No. follow-up
Copperhead	2	2 (100%)	0	0	0
Rattlesnake	3	2 (67%)	0	1 (33%)	0
Nonpoisonous	8	3 (37%)	0	0	5 (63%)
Unknown snake	5	3 (60%)	1 (20%)	0	1 (20%)
Total	18	10 (56%)	1 (5%)	1 (5%)	6 (34%)

Minor effects are signs or symptoms developing from the exposure but minimally bothersome and generally resolving without residual disability. A *moderate effect* is one that is more pronounced or prolonged than minor effects, usually requiring some form of treatment. *Major effects* are life-threatening signs or symptoms of the exposure that result in significant disability or disfigurement.

(Reproduced by permission from Toxic Exposure Surveillance System (TESS). Exposures in Pregnant Women, 1999. AAPCC 2000.)

USA include the rattlesnakes (*Sistrurus* and *Crotalus* spp.) and the moccasins snakes: cotton-mouths (*Agkistrodon piscivorus*) and copperheads (*Agkistrodon contortrix*). Overall, rattlesnakes cause two-thirds of all bites by identified venomous snakes in the USA.

Venom usually is injected into subcutaneous tissue via fangs; occasionally, intramuscular or intravenous injection can occur. Dry bites (no envenomation) occur in as many as 50% of strikes. Venom generally is composed of several digestive enzymes and spreading factors, which result in local and systemic injury.

The venom may be cytotoxic, hematotoxic, neurotoxic, rhabdomyolytic, cardiotoxic, nephrotoxic, or may cause an autoimmune reaction (complement activation). In general, viper (Crotalidae spp.) venom is mainly cytotoxic, whereas elapid venom is mainly neurotoxic, colubrid venom predominantly hemotoxic, and sea snake venom chiefly myotoxic [174].

Subdivision of symptoms into local, autopharmacological, antihemostatic, neurological, muscular, cardiac, and renal effects help to stage the patient. In conjunction with information on geographical distribution, habitat, and behavior of the snake, the clinical pattern of symptoms and signs is useful to identify the culprit of the envenomation [169]. Clinically, local effects most commonly predominate, progressing from pain and edema to ecchymosis and bullae. Hematologic abnormalities, including benign defibrination with or without thrombocytopenia, may result, but severe generalized bleeding is uncommon. Local or diffuse myotoxicity may result in complications such as compartment syndrome or rhabdomyolysis. Neurotoxins produce neuromuscular blockade and nerve conduction. Prodromal symptoms of neurotoxicity (drowsiness, hypersalivation, diaphoresis, fasciculations and circumoral paresthesias) are often followed by specific effects on cranial nerves. Progressive respiratory paralysis is the most serious neurotoxic effect [174]. Other rare general effects include cardiotoxicity, fasciculations, and shock.

In the event of snakebite during pregnancy, all patients should be transported (left lateral decubitus since a maternal death after snakebite has been reported for presumptive supine hypotensive syndrome) to a medical care facility with appropriate fetal and maternal monitoring capabilities. Priorities for evaluation and resuscitation should not differ from those established for the patient who is not pregnant. As with multiple other critical situations, the best chance for fetal survival is maternal survival [174].

Local measures include positive identification of the type of snake and rapid transport to definitive medical care. There is no universally applicable method to reliably delay the transport of venom from the bite site to the systemic circulation [169]. Calming the patient, immobilization, and splinting of the extremity bitten are crucial. A loose constriction bandage may be used to delay spread of the venom by compressing lymphatic vessels. If care is available within 60 minutes, wound incision and suctioning are not recommended. Unfortunately negative pressure venom extraction devices have shown no benefit [175]. Tourniquets are not recommended as they can contribute to severe tissue destruction [169]. Local and supportive measures for poisonous snakebite include careful cleaning of the wound, maintaining the extremity in neutral position, supportive care, potential use of antibiotics, and tetanus prophylaxis [174]. Circumferential measurement at several points along the affected limb should be started shortly after the patient's arrival and repeated hourly until progression has ceased [172].

In general indications for antivenom use are: (a) hypotension or other signs and symptoms of autopharmacological reactions, (b) hemostatic abnormalities or spontaneous systemic bleeding, (c) paralysis, (d) rhabdomyolysis, (e) cardiovascular signs and symptoms, and (f) renal compromise [169]. In local envenomation, antivenom is indicated if: (a) the species involved is known to cause local tissue necrosis, (b) there is swelling involving more than half of the bitten limb, (c) there is rapidly progressive swelling, and (d) there are bites on fingers and/or toes [169]. Although there is no universal grading system for snakebites, a I–IV grading scale is clinically useful as a guide to antivenom administration (Table 39.26).

When considering the use of antivenom, the risk of adverse reaction to its administration must be weighed against the benefits of reducing venom toxicity. In general, antivenom should

Table 39.26 Grading of snakebite poisoning.

Grade	Envenomation	Skin effects	Symptoms	Lab abnormalities
I	None	1 inch of edema or erythema, puncture wounds	None	None
II	Minimal	1–5 inch of edema or erythema within first 12 h	None	None
III	Moderate	6–12 inch of edema or erythema within first 12 h	Minimal (nausea, vomiting, paresthesias, metallic taste, and fasciculations)	Platelets < 90 000/μL Fibrinogen < 100 mg/dL) PT > 14 s CK > 500–1000 U/L
IV	Severe	Rapidly involves the entire part; potential compartment syndrome	Systemic effects may include shock, diffuse or life-threatening bleeding, renal failure, respiratory difficulty, and altered mental status	Platelets < 20 000/μL Any abnormal coagulation parameter associated with potentially life-threatening bleeding Rhabdomyolysis Myoglobinuric renal failure

PT, prothrombin time; CK, creatine kinase.
(From Wood JT, Hoback WW, Green TW. Poisonous snakebites resulting in lack of venom poisoning. *Va Med Monthly* 1955;82:130; and Dunnihoo DR, Rush BM, Wise RB, Brooks GG, Otterson WN. Snake bite poisoning in pregnancy: a review of the literature. *J Reprod Med* 1992;37:653–658.)

not be given in the field because of the risk of severe allergic complications. Hypersensitivity reactions are common with antivenin use (23–56%) [172]. Skin testing (which may be unreliable) and careful monitoring must be available and used when antivenin is given.

The quality of the antivenoms and its frequency of severe side effects (nearly 50% of patients treated) makes monitoring and treatment of side effects an important part of the management of these patients.

Crotalidae polyvalent immune Fab antivenom (CroFab or FabAV, a sheep-derived antigen-binding fragment) is more specifically tailored for crotalids of North America and is less allergenic than equine-derived whole immunoglobulin antivenoms.

With pit viper poisoning, antivenin is usually recommended for grade III or IV bites. Crotalidae polyvalent immune Fab antivenom effectively controls the effects of envenomation; however, initial control of coagulopathy is difficult to achieve in some cases, and recurrence or delayed-onset hematotoxicity is not uncommon [176]. Because copperheads carry a lesser potent venom, their bites usually do not require antivenin.

Fasciotomies may be required occasionally but only after confirmation of the presumptive diagnosis of compartment syndrome (pressures above 30 mmHg) and adequate treatment with antivenom [172].

In their review of snakebites during pregnancy, Dunnihoo et al [177]. reported an overall fetal wastage of 43% and a maternal mortality of 10%. Bleeding diathesis resulted from pit viper envenomation. Possible mechanisms for the fetal losses may be anoxia associated with shock, bleeding into the placenta and uterine wall and uterine contractions initiated by the venom [174]. Although the specific effects of venom on the human fetus are unknown, there is evidence that snake venom may cross the placenta affecting the fetus even without evidence of envenomation in the mother [178]. The effects of venom on the human fetus are unknown. Venom exposure during pregnancy may result in teratogenesis, fetal growth retardation, or even mutagenesis. It is also undetermined what effect the different types of venom, the amount and the route of exposure have on the fetus. Snake venom has uterotonic properties and fetal wastage during early gestation may be due to intrauterine bleeding, hypoxia and pyrexia [174,179]. The absence of short-term and long-term variability in the fetal heart rate is an ominous sign and along the lack of fetal movements, suggest depression of the CNS of the fetus [174].

We were unable to find any English-language reports of coral snakes (characterized by a black snout and an alternating pattern of black, yellow, and red) envenomation during pregnancy. Coral snakes and sea snakes of the Elapidae family are much less efficient in injecting venom into large prey; thus, their poor efficiency at envenomation, coupled with their relatively small size and shy nature, may play a role in the paucity of information concerning these snake bites during pregnancy. Coral snake bites often show little local reaction. Systemic effects may be delayed for several hours. Because of the neurotoxicity of coral snake venom, coral snake antivenin is usually recommended for its victims. Of note, the net effect of these neurotoxins is a curare like syndrome, thus contraindicating the use of magnesium sulfate as a tocolytic if patient develops preterm labor.

Occasionally, a victim will present with the bite of a rare, exotic snake. Most zoos or poison control centers have specific information on unusual breeds of snakes. Timely consultation is highly recommended [180].

Spider bites

In the USA, spider bites during pregnancy are reported four times more frequently than snake bites (see Tables 39.25 and 39.27). In the USA only two types of poisonous spider bites are of concern: the black widow and the brown recluse. These spiders bite only when trapped or crushed against the skin [181].

The adult female black widow spider (*Latrodectus mactans*) has a highly neurotoxic venom (α-latrotoxin), which destabilizes the cell membranes and degranulates nerve terminals resulting in massive norepinephrine and acetylcholine release into synapses, causing excessive stimulation and fatigue of the motor endplate and muscle [172,182].

Membrane receptors that bind α-latroxin have been identified: neurexin and latrophilin/CIRL (calcium-independent receptor for α-latrotoxin). Although the nervous system is the primary target of low doses of α-latrotoxin, cells of other tissues (placenta, kidney, spleen, ovary, heart, and lung) are also susceptible to the toxic effects of α-latrotoxin because of the presence of CIRL-2, a low-affinity receptor of the toxin [183]. Although it is known that this venom does not affect the CNS due to its inability to cross the blood–brain barrier, it is not known whether it crosses the placenta or has direct fetal effects [182].

The diagnosis of a black widow spider bite is mainly clinical. The venom does not contain inflammagens so the site of the envenomation is usually unremarkable except for a small circle of erythema and induration [172,182]. Within about one hour of the incident (minutes to hours), patients develop an autonomic and neuromuscular syndrome characterized by hypertension, tachycardia, and diaphoresis, abdominal pain and tenderness, and back, chest, or lower extremity pain (painful muscle spasms and cramping), and weakness [181,184,185,186]. Muscle cramping is a characteristic finding associated with black widow envenomation [172]. Other symptoms include: perspiration, nausea, vomiting, diarrhea, sialorrhea, and headache [182]. The neuromuscular manifestation of the envenomation progress over several hours and then subside over 2–3 days [185]. The evaluation of these patients may include a complete blood count, abdominal ultrasound or CT, EKG, and creatine kinase (CPK) to evaluate acute abdominal and chest pain syndromes.

General supportive management (airway protection, breathing and circulation per advanced cardiac life support protocols) must be instituted promptly. Most black widow spider envenomations may be managed with opioid analgesics and sedative-hypnotics. A specific antivenin for black widow bites is available. Although it results in resolution of most symptoms 30 minutes after administration and has been shown to decrease the need for hospitalization significantly, it should be cautiously restricted for severe envenomations, due to hypersensitivity, anaphylaxis, serum sickness reactions, and even risk of death [1,185,187]. Antivenom should be considered when envenomation seriously threatens pregnancy or precipitates potentially limb- or life-threatening effects (e.g. severe hypertension, unstable angina). As is the case with snake antivenoms, it should be given only in the hospital setting for the possibility of anaphylactic reactions [172]. The antivenin is derived from horse serum must be diluted (in 2.5 ml of normal saline) and administered slowly (200 ml over an hour) after skin testing and antihistamines to reduce acute adverse reactions to the antivenom [182]. One to two vials are generally sufficient to counteract the nanomolar concentrations of circulating black widow spider venom; however additional dosing may be necessary in patients who do not demonstrate adequate recovery [188]. Symptoms have been shown to improve within 1 hour of

Table 39.27 Insect and arthropod envenomation by category of exposure and maternal effects, US: 1999.

Category of exposure	Total	No effect	Minor effects	Moderate effects	No follow-up
Ants/fire ants	14	1 (7.1%)	3 (21.4%)	3 (21.4%)	7 (50%)
Bee/wasp/hornet	66	1 (1.5%)	23 (34.8%)	1 (1.5%)	41 (62.1%)
Miscellaneous insects	97	6 (6.1%)	31 (31.9%)	3 (3.1%)	56 (57.7%)
Caterpillar/centipede	9	1 (11.1%)	4 (44.4%)	0	4 (44.4%)
Scorpion	165	1 (0.6%)	67 (40.6%)	3 (1.8%)	94 (56.9%)
Ticks	11	0	5 (45.4%)	0	6 (54.5%)
Black widow spider	22	2 (9.1%)	11 (50%)	5 (22.7%)	4 (18.1%)
Brown recluse spider	23	0	7 (30.4%)	3 (13.0%)	13 (56.5%)
Other spiders	77	0	20 (25.9%)	8 (10.3%)	49 (63.6%)
Miscellaneous arthropods	41	0	13 (31.7%)	1 (2.4%)	27 (65.8%)
Total:	524	12 (2.3%)	184 (35.1%)	27 (5.1%)	301 (57.4%)

Minor effects are signs or symptoms developing from the exposure but minimally bothersome and generally resolving without residual disability. A *moderate effect* is one that is more pronounced or prolonged than minor effects, usually requiring some form of treatment. *Major effects* (exposure resulting in life-threatening signs or symptoms or results in significant disability or disfigurement) were not reported in this series.

(From Gei AF, Van Hook JW, Olson GL, Saade GR, Hankins GDV. Arthropod envenomations during pregnancy. Report from a national database—1999. (Abstract no. 0662). Annual Meeting of the Society for Maternal–Fetal Medicine, Reno, Nevada, 2001.)

antivenom administration and for as long as 48 hours after envenomation [182,188].

Analgesics (morphine) and benzodiazepines (midazolam) are effective adjuvant treatment for the neuromuscular symptoms [172,184]. Calcium gluconate is no longer recommended for black widow spider envenomation [1]. Antibiotics are not indicated unless specific signs of cellulitis are noted. A booster of the tetanus toxoid should be given following a black widow spider bite.

In the particular case of pregnancy, black widow envenomations can mimic acute intra-abdominal processes [186,189] and preeclampsia (abdominal pain, headache, hypertension, and proteinuria) [182]. Hospitalization and treatment with specific antivenom is recommended given that maternal mortality has been postulated to be as high as 5% [174,186].

In 1999, 22 bites by black widow spiders were reported to Poison Control Centers in the USA (Table 39.27). Half of the women reported only minor effects and another five women (18.7%) reported effects requiring some form of treatment. The outcome was not known in four cases [170].

Loxosceles spiders have a worldwide distribution in temperate and tropical regions. There are approximately 50 recognized Loxosceles species in North America [190]. *Loxosceles recluse* is perhaps the best known member of the family and along with *Loxosceles deserta* are endemic and responsible for the majority of documented bites. Characteristic violin-shaped markings on their backs have led brown recluses to also be known as "fiddle-back spiders" though these markings may not be visible without magnification and may vary according to spider variable color. In South America, the more potent venom of the species *Loxosceles laeta* is responsible for systemic loxoscelism and several deaths each year. The usual habitat of the brown recluse is in dark closet corners and the sides of cardboard boxes and can infest in large numbers. Although not aggressive, the spider will bite when trapped [190].

The venom of these spiders has variable toxicity depending on the species. It contains at least nine enzymes, consisting of various lysins (facilitating venom spread), hyaluridonidase, and sphingomyelinase D, which causes cell membrane injury and lysis, thrombosis, local ischaemia, and chemotaxis [172,190]. *Loxosceles* venom is also capable of inducing systemic intravascular clotting, which can result in hemolysis and renal failure [190].

Although most bites are asymptomatic, envenomation can begin with severe burning pain (characteristic of these envenomations) and itching that progresses to vesiculation (single clear or hemorrhagic vesicle) with violaceous necrosis and surrounding erythema, and ultimately ulcer formation and necrosis (dermonecrotic arachnidism) (see Figure 39.5). The differential diagnosis includes arterial injection injury, herpes simplex, Stevens–Johnson syndrome, vasculitis, purpura fulminans, necrotizing fasciitis, and toxic epidermal necrolysis among others [190].

Loxoscelism is the term used to describe the systemic clinical syndrome caused by envenomation from the brown spiders.

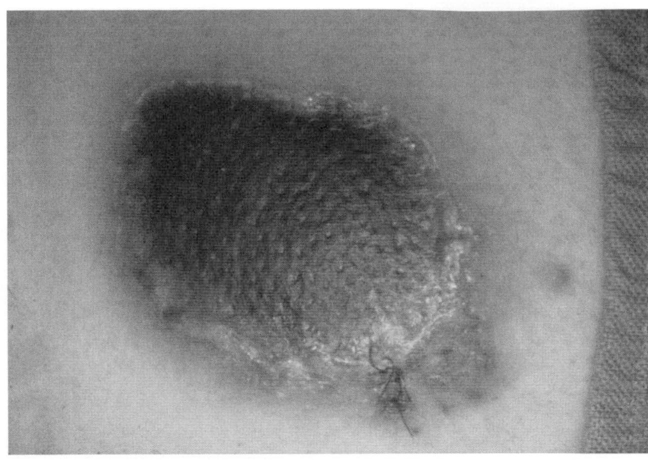

Figure 39.5 Effects of *Loxosceles* reclusa bite. (Photograph courtesy of Dr. Ramon L. Sanchez; Galveston, Texas.)

Systemic involvement, although uncommon, occurs within 24–72 hours of the bite more frequently in children than in adults. These systemic envenomations may be life threatening, and present with fever, constitutional symptoms (low-grade fevers, diarrhea, vomiting), petechial eruptions, thrombocytopenia, and hemolysis with hemoglobinuric renal failure, seizures or coma, and usually associated with minimal skin changes [191]. This presentation is more common seen after a bite by *L. laeta*, prevalent in Peru, Chile, and part of Brazil [190].

Treatment of envenomations is hindered by the delayed presentation of the victims to a medical facility and overdiagnosis. Unfortunately by the time a necrotic ulcer develops it may be too late for interventions. The treatment of local envenomations is mainly conservative (immobilization and elevation, application of ice, local wound care, tetanus prophylaxis, analgesics, and close follow-up). The application of ice in theory decreases the damage and inflammation and local spread of the venom through vasoconstriction (application of heat results in more severe damage). Severe brown recluse spider bites produce dermonecrosis within 72–96 hours. Early surgical management in general has been found to be ineffective and sometimes harmful as an initial management technique [172,190]. Skin grafting may be necessary after 4–6 weeks of standard therapy or until the lesion borders are well defined.

Given its leukocyte inhibiting properties, dapsone has frequently been recommended for the treatment of local lesions. However, because of the potential for adverse effects associated with dapsone use, especially in the setting of glucose-6-phosphate dehydrogenase deficiency, hypersensitivity, cross-reactivity with sulfa allergies and methemoglobinemia, appropriate caution should be exercised if using this medication. To date, no well-controlled studies have shown dapsone to affect clinical outcome in human brown recluse envenomations; therefore, it is not routinely recommended [172,190].

Other treatments, such as colchicine, steroids, antivenom, nitroglycerin patches, hyperbaric oxygen, and surgical excision, have been reported but insufficient data exist to support their clinical use [190]. Intradermal anti-loxosceles Fab fragments have been shown to attenuate dermonecrotic arachnidism in a rabbit model when given up to 4 hours after venom inoculation [192]. This treatment has not yet been applied clinically [190]. Antivenom is not commercially available for *Loxosceles reclusa*. There are four sources of commercial *Loxosceles* antivenoms, none of which is available in the USA [190]. In countries where antivenom is available the usual indication is systemic loxoscelism and it is likely that its use is capable of decrease the size of the lesion.

Systemic envenomation requires supportive care and treatment of arising complications, corticosteroids to stabilize red blood cell membranes, and support of renal function.

Patients with an isolated dermal lesion who will be discharged home should be instructed to watch carefully for a change in the color of the urine because the can develop a delayed systemic reaction [190].

Anderson [193] reported five cases of envenomation by *Loxosceles reclusa* in pregnant patients. He concluded that no special risks or complications resulted from being bitten by the brown recluse during pregnancy when managed only with low-dose prednisone. No instances of hemolysis, disorders of coagulation, or renal damage were reported in this case series. In 1999, 23 bites by brown recluse spiders were reported to Poison Control Centers nationwide. Of those bites, the outcome is unknown in the majority (13) and moderate effects (more pronounced or prolonged than minimal; usually requiring some form of treatment) were reported in three cases [170].

Scorpions

Over 650 species of scorpions are known to cause envenomation (mostly to children under 10 years); they are endemic mostly in arid and tropical areas. In developing countries scorpion stings are associated with mortality ratios of up to 0.2% [194]. Different venoms and clinical presentations are seen across the different species. Systemic envenoming is caused by members of the genera *Centruroides* (found in Southwest USA and Mexico), *Tityus* (Brazil and Trinidad), *Androctonus*, *Buthus*, *Leiurus*, and *Nebo* (North Africa, Near and Middle East); *Hemiscorpius* (Iran and Iraq); *Parabuthus* (South Africa), and *Mesobuthus* (Indian subcontinent) [169]. The scorpion of primary concern in the USA is *Centruroides exilicauda* (formerly *sculpturatus*) which has a sting that is potentially fatal [195].

In general scorpion stings produce an immediate sharp, burning pain that may be followed by numbness extending beyond the sting site. Regional lymph node swelling may also occur. Less frequently ecchymosis and lymphangitis develop [195]. Scorpion envenomations and snake bites can be graded similarly. A grade I envenomation is characterized by local pain whereas remote pain and/or paresthesias remote from the sting site characterize a grade II envenomation. The most important clinical effects of envenomations are neuromuscular and neuroautonomic [175]. A grade III envenomation is characterized by either cranial/autonomic or somatic skeletal neuromuscular dysfunction, including blurred vision, nystagmus, hypersalivation, tongue fasciculations, dysphagia, slurred speech, respiratory distress; restlessness and severe involuntary shaking or jerking of extremities that may be mistaken for a seizure. A grade IV combines cranial/autonomic and somatic nerve dysfunction [175].

Most commonly, an inflammatory local reaction occurs with the envenomation, which is treated with wound debridement and cleaning, tetanus prophylaxis, and antihistamines [185]. Antivenom is recommended for grade III and IV envenomations [195]. In Israel and India control of the overstimulated autonomous system has been successfully achieved with the use of β-blockers (prazosin), calcium-channel blockers (nifedipine), and angiotensin-converting enzyme (ACE) inhibitors (captopril) [169].

In 1999, 165 scorpion envenomations were reported by pregnant women in the USA. In those patients with known outcome, minor symptoms were predominant. No life-threatening symptoms or signs were reported (see Table 39.27) [170].

Summary

1. Poisoning during pregnancy represent a third of a percent of all toxic exposures reported in the USA.
2. The number of reported toxic exposures has increased by about 25% over the past 6 years both in the pregnant and non-pregnant population.
3. Although slightly more frequent during the second trimester, toxic exposures during pregnancy are reported with similar frequency in all trimesters.
4. The emergency treatment and stabilization of the mother should take priority over the monitoring and treatment of the fetus.
5. A prompt consultation with the obstetric service is recommended in the emergent management of the compromised poisoned pregnant patient. The goals of this consult are: (a) the assessment of fetal viability and (b) the decision/skill to proceed with an emergent or perimortem cesarean section, if the resuscitative efforts are not successful and/or the patient's condition worsens.
6. The mechanism of exposure needs to be sought and established, since intentional toxic exposure usually indicates severe social, emotional and/or psychiatric pathology. When identified, the need for additional and aggressive intervention (hospital admission, social and psychiatry consults, etc.) may prevent a potentially fatal recurrence.
7. Insect and arthropod exposures are not uncommon during pregnancy. The majority of these envenomations resulted in minor or no effects. Moderate effects are more likely when the cause of the exposure is a spider bite than with other arthropod exposures, including scorpion and bee stings.

8. Regardless of their severity, all toxic exposures need to be reported to the respective Poison Control Center (+1-800-222-1222).

References

1 Clark RF, Wethern-Kestner S, Vance MV et al. Clinical presentation and treatment of black widow spider envenomation: a review of 163 cases. *Ann Emerg Med* 1992; 21: 782–787.

2 Lai MW, Klein-Schwartz W, Rodgers GC et al. 2005 Annual Report of the American Association of Poison Control Centers National Poisoning and Exposure Database. *Clin Toxicol* 2005; 44(6): 803–932.

3 Stengel CL, Seaburg DC, MacLeod BA. Pregnancy in the emergency department: Risk factors and prevalence among all women. *Ann Emerg Med* 1994; 24: 697–700.

4 Jones JS, Dickson K, Carlson S. Unrecognized pregnancy in the overdosed or poisoned patient. *Am J Emerg Med* 1997; 15: 538–541.

5 CGDUP. Medication during pregnancy: an intercontinental cooperative study. *Int J Gynaecol Obstet* 1992; 39: 185–196.

6 Bakker MK, Jentink J, Vroom F et al. Drug prescription patterns before, during and after pregnancy for chronic, occasional and pregnancy-related drugs in the Netherlands. *Br J Obstet Gynaecol* 2006; 113: 559–568.

7 Lacroix I, Damase-Michel C, Lapeyre-Mestre M et al. Prescription of drugs during pregnancy in France. *Lancet* 2000; 356: 1735–1736.

8 Andrade SE, Gurwitz JH, Davis RL et al. Prescription drug use in pregnancy. *Am J Obstet Gynecol* 2004; 191: 398–407

9 Malm H, Martikainen J, Klaukka T et al. Prescription of hazardous drugs during pregnancy. *Drug Saf* 2004; 27: 899–908.

10 World Health Organization. *The World Health Report 2002 – Reducing Risks, Promoting Healthy Life*. Geneva: World Health Organization, 2002. http://www.who.int/whr/2002/en/whr2002_annex2.pdf.

11 Peden M, Mc Gee K, Krug E, eds. *Injury. A Leading Cause of the Global Burden of Disease*. 2000. Geneva: World Health Organization, 2002. http://www.whqlibdoc.who.int/publications/2002/9241562323.pdf.

12 Gei AF, Saade G. Poisoning during pregnancy and lactation. In: Yankowitz J, Niebyl JR, eds. *Drug Therapy in Pregnancy*. Philadelphia: Lippincott, Williams & Wilkins, 2001: 271.

13 Gei AF, Locksmith GJ, Saade GR, Hankins GDV. *Toxic exposures during pregnancy: Report from a national database – 1999* (Abstract # 0146). 2001 Annual Meeting of the Society for Maternal-Fetal Medicine, Reno, Nevada.

14 Rogers BD, Lee RV. Drugs abuse. In: Burrow GN, Ferris TF, eds. *Medical Complications During Pregnancy*, 3rd edn. Philadelphia: WB Saunders, 1988: 570–581.

15 Gilstrap L III, Little BB. *Drugs and Pregnancy*. New York: Elsevier, 1992.

16 Gei AF, Suarez VR, Goodrum L, Saade GR, Hankins GDV. Suicide attempts during pregnancy by poisoning or overdose. Report from a national database – 1999 (Abstract # 0623). 2001 Annual Meeting of the Society for Maternal-Fetal Medicine, Reno, Nevada.

17 Bayer MJ, Rumack BH. Poisoning and Overdose. Aspen Systems, 1983.

18 McElhatton PR, Roberts JC, Sullivan FM. The consequences of iron overdose and its treatment with desferrioxamine in pregnancy. *Hum Exp Toxicol* 1991; 10: 251–259.

19 Richards S, Brooks SHE. Ferrous sulphate poisoning in pregnancy (with apofibrinogenaemia as a complication). *West Indian Med J* 1966; 15: 134–140.

20 Strom RL, Schiller P, Seeds AE et al. Fatal iron poisoning in a pregnant female: case report. *Minnesota Med* 1976; 59: 483–489.

21 Olenmark M, Biber B, Dottori O et al. Fatal iron intoxication in late pregnancy. *Clin Toxicol* 1987; 25: 347–359.

22 Kloeck A, Cummins RO, Chamberlain D et al. Special Resuscitation Situations. An Advisory Statement from the International Liaison Committee on Resuscitation. *Circulation*, 1997; 95: 2196–2210.

23 American Heart Association. Cardiac arrest associated with pregnancy. *Circulation* 2005; 112: IV-150–IV-153.

24 Hoffman JR, Schriger DL, Votey SR et al. The empiric use of hypertonic dextrose in patients with altered mental status: a reappraisal. *Ann Emerg Med* 1992; 21: 20–4.

25 Noji E, Kelen G. *Manual of Toxicologic Emergencies*. St. Louis: Year Book Medical, 1989.

26 Davis CO, Wax PM. Focused Physical examination/toxidromes. In: Ford MD, Delaney KA, Ling LJ et al., eds. *Clinical Toxicology*, 1st edn. Philadelphia: W.B. Saunders Company, 2001.

27 Borak J. Anion and osmolar gaps. In: Viccellio P, ed. *Emergency Toxicology*, 2nd edn. Philadelphia: Lippincott-Raven Publishers, 1998: Chapter 12.

28 Eldridge DL, Dobson T, Brady W, Holstege CP. Utilizing diagnostic investigations in the poisoned patient. *Med Clin N Am* 2005: 89: 1079–1105.

29 Akbari A, Wilkes P, Lindheimer M et al. Reference intervals for anion gap and strong ion difference in pregnancy: a pilot study. *Hypertens Pregnancy* 2007; 26: 111–119.

30 Kulig K. Gastrointestinal decontamination. In: Ford MD, Delaney KA, Ling LJ, eds. *Clinical Toxicology*. Philadephia: WB Saunders, 2001: 34.

31 Heard K. Gastrointestinal decontamination. *Med Clin N Am* 2005; 89: 1067–1078.

32 Christophersen AJ, Hoegberg LC. Techniques used to prevent gastrointestinal absorption. In: *Goldfrank's Toxicologic Emergencies*, 8th edn. New York: McGraw Hill, 2006: 109.

33 Olson KR. *Poisoning and Drug Overdose*, 5th edn. New York: Appleton and Lange, 2007.

34 Manoguerra AS, Cobaugh DJ. Guideline on the use of ipecac syrup in the Out-of-Hospital management of ingested poisons. *Clin Toxicol* 2005; 1: 1–10.

35 Adams BK, Mann MD, Aboo A et al. The effects of sorbitol on gastric empyting half-times and small intestinal transit after drug overdose. *Am J Emerg Med* 2006; 24: 130–132.

36 Tenenbein M. Position statement: whole bowel irrigation. American Academy of Clinical Toxicology; European Association of Poison Centres and Clinical Toxicologists. *J Toxicol Clin Toxicol* 1997; 35: 753–762.

37 Olson K. *Poisoning and Drug Overdose*, 2nd edn. Norwalk, CT: Appleton and Lange, 1994.

38 Weisman RS, Howland MA, Flomenbaum NE. The toxicology laboratory. In: Goldfrank LR, Flomenbaum NE, Lewin NA et al.

Goldfrank's Toxicologic Emergencies, 4th edn. Norwalk, CT: Appleton and Lange, 1990: 45–46.

39 Briggs GG, Freeman RK, Yaffe SJ, eds. *Drugs in Pregnancy and Lactation*, 6th edn. Philadelphia: Lippincott Williams and Wilkins, 2002.

40 Peterson RG, Rumack BH. Toxicity of acetaminophen overdose. *JACEP* 1978; 7: 202.

41 Reynolds JR, Howland MA, Weisman RS. Pharmacokinetic and toxicokinetic principles. In: Goldfrank LR, Flomenbaum NE, Lewin NA et al., eds. *Goldfrank's Toxicologic Emergencies*, 4th edn. Norwalk, CT: Appleton and Lange, 1990: 29–38.

42 Rayburn W, Shukla U, Stetson P et al. Acetaminophen pharmacokinetics: comparison between pregnant and nonpregnant women. *Am J Obstet Gynecol* 1986; 155: 1353–1356.

43 Rowden AK, Norvell J, Eldridge DL et al. Updates on acetaminophen toxicity. *Med Clin N Am* 2005; 89: 1145–1159.

44 Levy G, Garretson LK, Socha DM. Evidence of placental transfer of acetaminophen. *Pediatrics* 1975; 55: 895.

45 Kozer E, Koren G. Management of paracetamol overdose: current controversies. *Drug Safety* 2001; 24: 503–512.

46 Horowitz RS, Dart RC, Jarvie DR et al. Placental transfer of N-Acetylcysteine following human maternal acetaminophen toxicity. *Clin Toxicol* 1997: 35: 447–451.

47 Reprotox. Acetaminophen. Last updated: December 2006. www.reprotox.org (accessed May 2007).

48 McElhatton PR, Sullivan FM, Volans GN. Paracetamol overdose in pregnancy analysis of the outcomes of 300 cases referred to the Teratology Information Service. *Reprod Toxicol* 1997; 11: 85–94.

49 Haibach H, Akhter JE, Muscato MS. Acetaminophen overdose with fetal demise. *Am J Clin Pathol* 1984; 82: 240–242.

50 Lumir J, Main DM, Landon MB et al. Maternal acetaminophen overdose at 15 weeks of gestation. *Obstet Gynecol* 1986; 67: 750–751.

51 Riggs BS, Bronstein AC, Kuling K et al. Acute acetaminophen overdose during pregnancy. *Obstet Gynecol* 1989; 74: 247–253.

52 Dart RC, Erdman AR, Olson KR et al. Acetaminophen poisoning: an evidence-based consensus guideline for out-of-hospital management. *Clin Toxicol* 2006; 44: 1–18.

53 Rumack BH, Peterson RC, Koch GG, Amara IA. Acetaminophen overdose: 662 cases with evaluation of oral acetylcysteine treatment. *Arch Intern Med* 1981; 141: 380.

54 Zed PJ, Krenzelok EP. Treatment of acetaminophen overdose. *Am J Health-Syst Pharm* 1999; 56: 1081–1091.

55 Haroz R, Greenberg MI. Emerging drugs of abuse. *Med Clin N Am* 2005; 89: 1259–1276.

56 Haddad LM, Winchester JF, eds. *Clinical Management of Poisoning and Drug Overdose*, 2nd edn. Philadelphia: W.B. Saunders, 1990.

57 Ho E, Karimi-Tabesh L, Koren G. Characteristics of pregnant women who use ecstasy (3, 4-methylenedioxymethamphetamine). *Neurotoxicol Teratol* 2001; 23(6): 561–567.

58 O'Connor AD, Rusyniak DE, Bruno A. Cerebrovascular and cardiovascular complications of alcohol and sympathomimetic drug abuse. *Med Clin N Am* 2005: 89: 1343–1358.

59 Perrone J. Amphetamines. In: Viccellio P, ed. *Emergency Toxicology*, 2nd edn. Philadelphia: Lippincott-Raven Publishers, 1998: 899.

60 Stine RJ, Marcus RH. Toxicologic emergencies. In: Haddad LM, Winchester JF, eds. *Clinical Management of Poisoning and Drug Overdose*. Philadelphia: WB Saunders, 1983: 297–342.

61 Zimmerman JL. Poisonings and overdoses in the intensive care unit: General and specific management issues. *Crit Care Med* 2003; 31: 2794–2801.

62 Thaithumyanon P, Limpongsanurak S, Praisuwanna P et al. Perinatal effects of amphetamine and heroin use during pregnancy on the mother and infant. *J Med Assoc Thai* 2005; 88: 1506–1513.

63 Smith LM, LaGasse LL, Derauf C et al. The infant development, environment, and lifestyle study: effects of prenatal methamphetamine exposure, polydrug exposure, and poverty on intrauterine growth. *Pediatrics* 2006; 118: 1149–1156.

64 Little BB, Snell LM, Klein VR et al. Cocaine abuse during pregnancy: maternal and fetal implication. *Obstet Gynecol* 1989; 72: 157–160.

65 Biggs GG, Samaon JH, Crawford DJ. Lack of abnormalities in a newborn exposed to amphetamine during gestation. *Am J Dis Child* 1975; 129: 249–250.

66 Reprotox. *Amphetamines*. Last updated: April 2006. www.reprotox.org (accessed May 2007).

67 Rayburn W, Anonow R, Delay B et al. Drug overdose during pregnancy: an overview from a metropolitan poison control center. *Obstet Gynecol* 1984; 64: 611.

68 Oro AS, Dixon SD. Perinatal cocaine and methamphetamine exposure: maternal and neonatal correlates. *J Pediatr* 1987; 111: 571–578.

69 Dixon SD, Bejar R. Echoencephalographic findings in neonates associated with maternal cocaine and methamphetamine use: incidence and clinical correlates. *J Pediatr* 1989; 115: 770–778.

70 Sussman S. Narcotic and methamphetamine use during pregnancy: effect on newborn and infants. *Am J Dis Child* 1965; 106: 325–330.

71 Henry JA. Amphetamines. In: Ford MD, Delaney KA, Ling LJ, Erickson T, eds. *Clinical Toxicology*, 1st edn. Philadelphia: W.B. Saunders Company, 2001: 620.

72 Kashani J, Ruha AM. Methamphetamine toxicity secondary to intravaginal body stuffing. *J Toxicol Clin Toxicol* 2004; 42: 987–989.

73 Semple SJ, Grant I, Patterson TL. Female methamphetamine users: social characteristics and sexual risk behavior. *Women Health* 2004; 40: 35–50.

74 Chiang WK. Amphetamines. In: *Goldfrank's Toxicologic Emergencies*, 8th edn. New York: McGraw Hill, 2006: 1118.

75 MacQueen G. Born L. Steiner M. The selective serotonin reuptake inhibitor sertraline: its profile and use in psychiatric disorders. *CNS Drug Rev* 2001; 7: 1–24.

76 Mourilhe P, Stokes PE. Risks and benefits of selective serotonin reuptake inhibitors in the treatment of depression. *Drug Safety* 1998; 18: 57–82.

77 Gimovsky ML. Fetal heart rate monitoring casebook. *J Perinatol* 1995; 15: 246–249.

78 Berard A, Ramos E, Rey E et al. First trimester exposure to paroxetine and risk of cardiac malformations in infants: the importance of dosage. *Birth Defects Res B Dev Reprod Toxicol* 2007; 80: 18–27.

79 Reprotox. Paroxetine. Last updated: June 2007. www.reprotox.org (accessed June 2007).

80 Sanz EJ, De las Cuevas C, Kiuru A et al. Selective serotonin reuptake inhibitors in pregnant women and neonatal withdrawal syndrome: a database analysis. *Lancet* 2005; 365: 482–487.

81 Alwan S, Reefhuis J, Rasmussen SA et al. Use of selective serotonin-reuptake inhibitors in pregnancy and the risk of birth defects. *N Engl J Med* 2007; 356: 2684–2692.

82 Chambers CD, Hernandez-Diaz S, Van Marter LJ et al. Selective serotonin-reuptake inhibitors and risk of persistent pulmonary hypertension of the newborn. *N Engl J Med* 2006; 354: 579–587.
83 Pentel PR, Keyler DE. Cyclic antidepressants. In: Ford MD, Delaney KA, Ling LJ, Erickson T. eds. *Clinical Toxicology*, 1st edn. Philadelphia: W.B. Saunders Company, 2001: 515.
84 Nelson LS, Erdman AR, Booze LL et al. Selective serotonin reuptake inhibitor poisoning: an evidence-based consensus guideline for out-of-hospital management. Practice Guideline. *Clin Toxicol* 2007; 45: 315–332.
85 Donovan JW, Akhtar J. Salicylates. In: Ford MD, Delaney KA, Ling LJ et al., eds. *Clinical Toxicology*, 1st edn. Philadelphia: W.B. Saunders Company, 2001: 275.
86 O'Malley GF. Emergency department management of the salicylate-poisoned patient. *Emerg Med Clin North Am* 2007; 25: 333–346
87 Chyka PA, Erdman AR, Christianson G et al. Salicylate Poisoning: *an Evidence-Based Consensus Guideline for Out-of-Hospital Management. Practice Guideline*. American Association of Poison Control Centers 2006. www.aapcc.org (accessed May 2007).
88 Reprotox. *Aspirin*. Last updated: May 2007. www.reprotox.org (accessed May 2007).
89 Winchester JF, Gelfand MC, Knepshield JH, Schreiner GE. Dialysis and hemoperfusion of poisons and drugs update. *Trans Am Soc Artif Intern Organs* 1977; 23: 762.
90 Victor M, Adams RD. Barbiturates. In: Isselbacher KS, Adams RD, Braunswald E, et al., eds. *Principles of Internal Medicine*, 9th edn. New York: McGraw-Hill, 1980: 982–985.
91 Reprotox. *Phenobarbital*. Last updated: May 2007. www.reprotox.org (accessed May 2007).
92 Holmes LB, Wyszynski DF, Lieberman E. The AED (antiepileptic drug) pregnancy registry: a 6 year experience. *Arch Neurol* 2004; 61: 673–678.
93 Kjaer D, Horvath-Puho E, Christensen J et al. Use of phenytoin, phenobarbital, or diazepam during pregnancy and risk of congenital abnormalities: a case-time-control study. *Pharmacoepidemiol Drug Saf* 2007; 16: 181–188.
94 Shubert PJ, Savage B. Smoking, alcohol and drug abuse. In: James DK, Stein RJ, Weiner CP et al., eds. *High Risk Pregnancy Management Options*. Philadelphia: WB Saunders, 1994: 51–66.
95 Desmond MM, Schwanecke PP, Wilson GS et al. Maternal barbiturate utilization and neonatal withdrawal symptomatology. *J Pediatr* 1972; 80: 190–197.
96 Coupey SM. Barbiturates. *Pediatrics in Review* 1997; 18: 260–264.
97 Bleyer WA, Skinner AL. Fatal neonatal hemorrhage after maternal anticonvulsant therapy. *JAMA* 1976; 235: 826–827.
98 Shannon BE, Jenkins JL, Loscalzo J. Poisoning and ingestion. In: Jenkins JL, Loscalzo J, eds. *Manual of Emergency Medicine–Diagnosis and Treatment*, 2nd edn. 1995: 417–469.
99 Schiebel N, Vicas I. Barbiturates. In: Ford MD, Delaney KA, Ling LJ et al., eds. *Clinical Toxicology*, 1st edn. Philadelphia: W.B. Saunders Company, 2001: 569.
100 Berg MJ, Berlinger WG, Goldberg MJ et al. Acceleration of the body clearance of phenobarbital by oral activated charcoal. *N Engl J Med* 1982; 507: 642.
101 Hardman JG, Limbird LE, eds. *Goodman & Gilman's The Pharmacological Basis of Therapeutic*, 9th edn. New York: McGraw-Hill, 1996.
102 MacGregor SN, Keith LG. Drug abuse during pregnancy. In: Rayburn RF, Zuspan FP, eds. *Drug Therapy in Obstetrics and Gynecology*, 3rd edn. St. Louis: Mosby Year Book, 1992: 164–189.
103 Milkovich L, van den Berg BJ. Effects of prenatal meprobamate and chlordiazepoxide, hydrochloride in human embryonic and fetal development. *N Engl J Med* 1974; 291: 1268–1271.
104 Hartz SC, Heinonen OP, Shapiro S et al. Antenatal exposure to meprobamate and chlordiazepoxide in relation to malformations, mental development and childhood mortality. *N Engl J Med* 1975; 292: 726–728.
105 Czeizel AE, Rockenbauer M, Sorensen HT et al. A population-based case-control study of oral chlordiazepoxide use during pregnancy and risk of congenital abnormalities. *Neurotoxicol Teratol* 2004; 26: 593–598.
106 Saxen I, Saxen L. Association between maternal intake of diazepam and oral clefts. *Lancet* 1975; 2: 498.
107 Safra MJ, Oakley JP. Association between cleft lip with and without cleft palate and prenatal exposure to diazepam. *Lancet* 1975; 2: 478.
108 Czeizel A. Lack of evidence of teratogenicity of benzodiazepine drugs in Hungary. *Reprod Toxicol* 1987–1988; 1: 183–188.
109 Cerqueira MJ, Olle C, Bellart J et al. Intoxication by benzodiazepines during pregnancy. *Lancet* 1988; 1(8598): 1341.
110 Reprotox. *Diazepam*. Last updated: May 2007. www.reprotox.org (accessed May 2007).
111 Malgorn G, Leboucher B, Harry P et al. Benzodiazepine poisoning in a neonate: clinical and toxicokinetic evaluation following enterodyalisis with activated charcoal. *Arch Pediatr* 2004; 11: 819–821.
112 Athinarayanan P, Pieroy SH, Nigan SK et al. Chlordiazepoxide withdrawal in the neonate. *Am J Obstet Gynecol* 1976; 124: 212–213.
113 Farrell SE. Benzodiazepines. In: Ford MD, Delaney KA, Ling LJ, Erickson T. eds. *Clinical Toxicology*, 1st edn. Philadelphia: W.B. Saunders Company, 2001: 575.
114 Balaskas TN. Common poisons. In: Gleicher N, Elkayam U, Galgraith RM et al., eds. *Principles and Practice of Medical Therapy in Pregnancy*, 2nd edn. Norwalk, CT: Appleton and Lange, 1992.
115 Chale SN. Carbon monoxide poisoning. In: Viccellio P, ed. *Emergency Toxicology*, 2nd edn. Philadelphia: Lippincott-Raven Publishers, 1998: 979.
116 Reprotox. Carbon monoxide. Last updated: April 2007. www.reprotox.org (accessed May 2007).
117 Tomaszewski C. Carbon monoxide poisoning. Ford MD, Delaney KA, Ling LJ et al. eds. *Clinical Toxicology*, 1st edn. Philadelphia: W.B. Saunders Company, 2001: 657.
118 Kao LW, Nanagas KA. Carbon monoxide poisoning. *Med Clin N Am* 2005: 89: 1161–1194.
119 Greingor JL, Tosi JM, Ruhlmann S et al. Acute carbon monoxide intoxication during pregnancy. One case report and review of the literature. *Emerg Med J* 2001; 18: 399–401.
120 Aubard Y, Magne I. Carbon monoxide poisoning in pregnancy. *Br J Obstet Gynaecol* 2000; 107(7): 833–838.
121 Alehan F, Erol I, Onay OS. Cerebral palsy due to nonlethal maternal carbon monoxide intoxication. *Birth Defects Res A Clin Mol Teratol* 2007; Jun 21.
122 Koren G, Sharav T, Pastuzak A. A multicenter, prospective study of fetal outcome following accidental carbon monoxide poisoning in pregnancy. *Reprod Toxicol* 1991; 5: 397–403.
123 Mishra V, Retherford RD, Smith KR. Cooking smoke and tobacco smoke as risk factors for stillbirth. *Int J Environ Health Res* 2005; 15: 397–410.

124 Longo LD. The biological effects of carbon monoxide on the pregnant woman, fetus, and newborn infant. *Am J Obstet Gynecol* 1977; 129: 69–103.

125 Gay GR. Clinical management of acute and chronic cocaine poisoning. *Ann Emerg Med* 1982; 11: 562.

126 Grinspoon L, Bakalan JB. Adverse effects of cocaine: selected issues. *Ann NY Acad Sci* 1981; 326: 125.

127 Cordero, DR, Medina C, Helfgott A. Cocaine body packing in pregnancy. *Ann Emerg Med* 2006; 48: 323–325.

128 Zuckerman B, Frank DA, Hingson R et al. Effects of maternal marijuana and cocaine use on fetal growth. *N Engl J Med* 1989; 320: 762–768.

129 Hollander JE, Hoffman RS. Cocaine. In: Ford MD, Delaney KA, Ling LJ, Erickson T. eds. *Clinical Toxicology*, 1st edn. Philadelphia: W.B. Saunders Company, 2001: 613.

130 Bingol N, Fuchs M, Diaz V. Teratogenicity of cocaine in humans. *J Pediatr* 1987; 110: 93–96.

131 Ney JA, Dooley SL, Keith LG et al. The prevalence of substance abuse in patients with suspected preterm labor. *Am J Obstet Gynecol* 1990; 162: 1562–1565.

132 Levine B, ed. *Principles of Forensic Toxicology*. Washington DC: American Association of Clinical Chemistry, 1999.

133 Neerhof MG, MacGregor SN, Retzky SS et al. Cocaine abuse during pregnancy: peripartum prevalence and perinatal outcome. *Am J Obstet Gynecol* 1989; 161: 633–638.

134 Gillogley KM, Evans AT, Hansen RL et al. The perinatal impact of cocaine, amphetamine and opiate use detected by universal intrapartum screening. *Am J Obstet Gynecol* 1990; 163: 1535–1542.

135 Chasnoff IJ, Burns KA, Burns WJ. Cocaine use in pregnancy: perinatal morbidity and mortality. *Neurotoxicol Teratol* 1987a; 9: 291–293.

136 Matera C, Warren WB, Moomjy M, Fink DJ, Fox HE. Prevalence of use of cocaine and other substances in an obstetric population. *Am J Obstet Gynecol* 1990; 163(3):797–801.

137 Briggs GG, Freeman RK, eds. *Drugs in Pregnancy and Lactation*, 4th edn. Baltimore: Williams and Wilkins, 1994.

138 Reprotox. Cocaine. Last updated: January 2005. www.reprotox.org (accessed May 2007).

139 Chasnoff IJ, Griffith DR, MacGregor S et al. Temporal patterns of cocaine use in pregnancy: perinatal outcome. *JAMA* 1989; 261: 1741–1744.

140 Hsu, CD, Chen S, Feng TI et al. Rupture of uterine scar with extensive maternal bladder laceration after cocaine abuse. *Am J Obstet Gynecol* 1992; 167: 129–130.

141 Chasnoff IJ, MacGregor S. Maternal cocaine use and neonatal morbidity. *Pediatr Res* 1987b; 21: 356.

142 Telsey AM, Merrit TA, Dixon SD. Cocaine exposure in a term neonate: necrotizing enterocolitis as a complication. *Clin Pediatr* 1988; 27: 547–550.

143 Lopez SL, Taeusch HW, Findlay RD et al. Time of onset of necrotizing enterocolitis in newborn infants with known prenatal cocaine exposure. *Clin Pediatr* 1995; 34: 424–429.

144 Otten EJ, Prybys KM, Gesell LB. Ethanol. In: Ford MD, Delaney KA, Ling LJ et al. eds. *Clinical Toxicology*, 1st edn. Philadelphia: W.B. Saunders Company, 2001: 605.

145 Yip L. Ethanol. In: *Goldfrank's Toxicologic Emergencies*, 8th edn. New York: McGraw Hill, 2006: 1147.

146 Halmesmaki E, Ylikorkala O. The effect of maternal ethanol intoxication on fetal cardiotocography: a report of four cases. *Br J Obstet Gynaecol* 1986; 93: 203–205.

147 Brien JF, Smith GN. Effects of alcohol (ethanol) on the fetus. *J Dev Physiol* 1991; 15: 21.

148 Reprotox. Ethanol. Last updated: November 2005. www.reprotox.org (accessed May 2007).

149 Kesmodel U, Wisborg K, Olsen SF et al. Moderate alcohol intake during pregnancy and the risk of stillbirth and death in the first year of life. *Am J Epidemiol* 2002; 155: 305–312.

150 Koren G. Chan D. Klein J. Karaskov T. Estimation of fetal exposure to drugs of abuse, environmental tobacco smoke, and ethanol. *Therapeutic Drug Monitoring* 2002; 24(1): 23–55.

151 Van Duija CM, van Steensel-Moll HA, Coebergh JW et al. Risk factors for childhood acute non-lymphocytic leukemia association with maternal alcohol consumption during pregnancy. *Cancer Epidemiol Biomarkers Prev* 1994; 3: 457.

152 Schiavone FM. Metals: Iron intoxication. In: Viccellio P, ed. *Emergency Toxicology*, 2nd edn. Philadelphia: Lippincott-Raven Publishers, 1998: 391.

153 Perrone J, Hoffman RS. Toxic ingestions in pregnancy: abortifacient use in a case series of pregnant overdose patients. *Academic Emergency Medicine*, 1997; 4: 206–209.

154 Tran T, Wax JR, Philput C et al. Intentional iron overdose in pregnancy-management and outcome. *J Emerg Med* 2000; 18: 225–228.

155 Reprotox. Iron. Last updated: November 2006. www.reprotox.org (accessed May 2007).

156 Tenenbein M. Iron. In: Ford MD, Delaney KA, Ling LJ, Erickson T. eds. *Clinical Toxicology*, 1st edn. Philadelphia: W.B. Saunders Company, 2001: 305.

157 Manoguerra AS, Erdman AR, Booze LL et al. Iron ingestion: an evidence-based consensus guideline for out-of-hospital management. *Clin Toxicol* 2005: 43; 553–570.

158 Tran T, Wax JR, Steinfeld JD et al. Acute intentional iron overdose in pregnancy. *Obstet Gynecol* 1998; 92(4 Pt 2): 678–680.

159 Aaron CK. Organophosphates and carbamates. In: Ford MD, Delaney KA, Ling LJ, Erickson T, eds. *Clinical Toxicology*, 1st edn. Philadelphia: W.B. Saunders Company, 2001: 819.

160 Zimmerman JL. Poisonings and overdoses in the intensive care unit: general and specific management issues. *Crit Care Med* 2003; 31(12): 2794–2801.

161 Solomon GM, Moodley J. Acute chlorpyrifos poisoning in pregnancy: a case report. *Clin Toxicol* 2007; 45: 416–419.

162 Clark RF. Insecticides: Organic phosphorus compounds and carbamates. In: *Goldfrank's Toxicologic Emergencies*, 8th edn. New York: McGraw Hill, 2006: 1497.

163 Eskenazi B, Harley K, Bradman A et al. Association of in utero organophosphate pesticide exposure and fetal growth and length of gestation in an agricultural population. *Environ Health Perspect* 2004; 112: 1116–1124.

164 Bhatia R et al. Organochlorine pesticides and male genital anomalies in the child health and development studies. *Environ Health Perspect* 2005; 113(2): 220–224.

165 Reprotox. Malathion. Last updated: February 2007. www.reprotox.org (accessed May 2007).

166 Sebe A, Satar S, Alpay R et al. Organophosphate poisoning associated to fetal death: A case study. *Mt Sinai J Med* 2005; 72: 354–456.

167 Osmundson M. Insecticides and pesticides. In: Viccellio P, ed. *Emergency Toxicology*, 2nd edn. Philadelphia: Lippincott-Raven Publishers, 1998: 401.

168 Okumura T. Organophosphate poisoning in pregnancy. *Ann Emerg Med* 1997; 29: 299.

169 Junghanss T, Bodio M. Medically important venomous animals: biology, prevention, first aid, and clinical management. *Clin Infect Dis* 2006; 43: 1309–1317.

170 Gei AF, Van Hook JW, Olson GL, Saade GR, Hankins GDV. Arthropod envenomations during pregnancy. Report from a national database – 1999 (Abstract # 0662). 2001 Annual Meeting of the Society for Maternal-Fetal Medicine, Reno, Nevada.

171 Chippaux JP. Snake-bites: appraisal of the global situation. *Bull WHO* 1998, 76: 515–524.

172 Singletary EM, Rochman AS, Arias JC et al. Envenomations. *Med Clin N Am* 2005; 89: 1195–1224.

173 Litovitz TL, Klein-Schwartz W, White S et al. 1999 Annual Report of the American Association of Poison Control Centers Toxic Exposure Surveillance System. *Am J Emerg Med* 2000; 18(5): 517–574.

174 Pantanowitz L, Guidozzi F. Management of snake and spider bite in pregnancy. *Obstet Gynecol Surv* 1996; 51: 615–620.

175 Bush SP, Hegewald KG, Green SM et al. Effects of a negative pressure venom extraction device (Extractor) on local tissue injury after artificial rattlesnake envenomation in a porcine model. *Wilderness Env Med* 2000; 11: 180–188.

176 Ruha AM, Curry SC, Beuhler M et al. Initial postmarketing experience with crotalidae polyvalent immune Fab for treatment of rattlesnake envenomation. *Ann Emerg Med* 2002; 39(6): 609–615.

177 Dunnihoo DR, Rush BM, Wise RB, Brooks GG, Otterson WN. Snake bite poisoning in pregnancy: a review of the literature. *J Reprod Med* 1992; 37: 653–658.

178 James RF. Snakebite in pregnancy. *Lancet* 1985; 2: 731.

179 Parrish HM, Khan MS. Snakebite during pregnancy. Report of 4 cases. *Obstet Gynecol* 1996; 27: 468–471.

180 Gold BS, Pyle P. Successful treatment of neurotoxic king cobra envenomation in Myrtle Beach, South Carolina. *Ann Emerg Med* 1998; 32: 736–738.

181 Wilson DC, King LE Jr. Spiders and spider bites. *Dermatol Clin* 1990; 8: 277–286.

182 Sherman RP, Groll JM, Gonzalez DI, Aerts MA. Black widow spider (Latrodectus mactans) envenomation in a term pregnancy. *Curr Surg* 2000; 57: 346–348.

183 Ichtchenko K, Bittner MA, Krasnoperov V et al. A novel ubiquitously expressed alpha-latrotoxin receptor is a member of the CIRL family of G-protein-coupled receptors. *J Biol Chem* 1999; 274: 5491–5498.

184 Rauber A. Black widow spider bites. *J Toxicol Clin Toxicol* 1983–1984; 21: 473–485.

185 Binder LS. Acute arthropod envenomation. Incidence, clinical features and management. *Med Toxicol* 1989; 4: 163–173.

186 Scalzone JM, Wells SL. Latrodectus mactans (black widow spider) envenomation: an unusual cause for abdominal pain in pregnancy. *Obstet Gynecol* 1994; 83: 830–831.

187 Heard K, O'Malley GF, Dart RC. Antivenom therapy in the Americas. *Drugs* 1999; 58: 5–15.

188 Rangan C. Emergency Department evaluation and treatment for children with arthropod envenomations: immunologic and toxicologic considerations. *Clin Ped Emerg Med* 2007; 8: 104–109.

189 Torregiani F, La Cavera C. Differential diagnosis of acute abdomen and latrodectism. *Minerva Chirurgica* 1990, 45: 303–305.

190 Hogan CJ, Barbaro KC, Winkel K. Loxoscelism: Old obstacles, new directions. *Ann Emerg Med* 2004; 46: 462–464.

191 Forks TP. Brown recluse spider bites. *J Am Board Fam Pract* 2000; 13: 415–423.

192 Gomez HF, Miller MJ, Trachy JW et al. Intradermal anti-Loxosceles Fab fragments attenuate dermonecrotic arachnidism. *Acad Emerg Med* 1999; 6: 1195–202.

193 Anderson PC. Loxoscelism threatening pregnancy: five cases. *Am J Obstet Gynecol* 1991; 165: 1454–1456.

194 Nouira S, Boukef R, Nciri N et al. A clinical score predicting the need for hospitalization in scorpion envenomation. *Am J Emerg Med* 2007; 25: 414–419.

195 Steen CJ, Carbonaro PA, Schwartz RA. Arthropods in dermatology. *J Am Acad Dermatol* 2004; 50: 819–842.

196 Roberts JM. Pregnancy related hypertension. In: Creasy RK, Resnik R, eds. *Maternal-Fetal Medicine: Principles and Practice*, 3rd edn. Philadelphia: WB Saunders, 1994: 804–843.

197 Litovitz TL, Felberg L, Soloway RA et al. 1994 Annual Report of the American Association of Poison Control Centers Toxic Exposure Surveillance System. *Am J Emerg Med* 1995; 13: 551–597.

198. Litovitz TL, Klein-Schwartz W, Martin E et al. 1998 American Annual Report of the American Association of Poison Control Centers Toxic Exposure Surveillance System. *Am J Emerg Med* 1999; 17: 435–487.

199 Litovitz TL, Klein-Schwartz W, White S et al. 2000 Annual report of the American Association of Poison Control Centers Toxic Exposure Surveillance System. *Am J Emerg Med* 2001; 19(5): 337–395.

40 Hypovolemic and Cardiac Shock

Scott Roberts

Department of Obstetrics and Gynecology, The University of Texas Southwestern Medical Center (UTSMC) at Dallas, TX, USA

Introduction

Hemorrhage is one of the leading causes of pregnancy-related mortality in the United States (2.0/100 000 live births) second only to embolism (2.3/100 000 live births) (Table 40.1) [1]. Almost 99% of maternal deaths occur in developing countries. Immediate postpartum hemorrhage (PPH), defined as excessive blood loss within 24 hours after childbirth, is the single most important cause of maternal death worldwide, accounting for almost half of all postpartum maternal deaths in developing countries [2,3].

In the United States, hemorrhage was the leading cause of death after stillbirth (from abruptions and uterine rupture), and accounted for 93% of deaths associated with ectopic pregnancies. Hemorrhage was also prominent as a cause of death in pregnancies ending in induced or spontaneous abortion (21.8%) [1]. These deaths are mediated through hypovolemic shock which is also responsible for a number of other serious non-fatal complications, including acute renal failure, acute respiratory distress syndrome (ARDS), and more rarely, postpartum pituitary necrosis. The parturient undergoes several important physiologic adaptations during pregnancy to protect her from the bleeding expected at the time of delivery. Peripartum complications can occur quickly and since the uterus receives a blood flow of 450–650 mL/min quick, decisive, and coordinated action on the part of the practitioner and supporting staff can be life-saving [4]. Shock is perhaps best defined as reduced tissue oxygenation resulting from poor perfusion [5]. Low flow or unevenly distributed flow from hypovolemia and disproportionate vasoconstriction are major causes of inadequate tissue perfusion in the acutely ill patient with circulatory dysfunction or shock. In hemorrhagic shock, the disparity is a result of blood loss that leads to both compensatory neurohormonal activation as well as the release of various endogenous mediators, which may aggravate the primary physiologic effects of hypovolemia [6–8]. Because the purpose of the circulation is to provide oxygen and oxidative substrates for metabolic requirements, insufficient tissue perfusion and oxygenation to support body metabolism is the common circulatory problem of acute critical illness. This inadequate perfusion leads to local tissue hypoxia, organ dysfunction, multiple organ failure, and death.

Blood flow to the capillary beds of various organs is controlled by arterioles, which are resistance vessels that in turn are controlled by the CNS. On the other hand, 70% of the total blood volume is contained in venules, capacitance vessels controlled by humoral factors. Hypovolemic shock evolves through several pathophysiologic stages as body mechanisms combat acute blood volume loss (Table 40.2). The diagnosis of shock is most often made by the presence of hypotension, oliguria, acidosis, and collapse in the late stage, when therapy is frequently ineffective. Early in the course of massive hemorrhage, there are decreases in mean arterial pressure (MAP), cardiac output (CO), central venous pressure (CVP), pulmonary capillary wedge pressure (PCWP), stroke volume and work, mixed venous oxygen saturation, and oxygen consumption. Increases are seen in systemic vascular resistance (SVR) and arteriovenous oxygen content differences. These latter changes serve to improve tissue oxygenation when blood flow is reduced [9]. Catecholamine release also causes a generalized increase in venular tone, resulting in an autotransfusion effect from the capacitance reservoir. These changes are accompanied by compensatory increases in heart rate, SVR and pulmonary vascular resistance, and myocardial contractility. Redistribution of CO and blood volume occurs via selective arteriolar constriction mediated by the CNS. This results in diminished perfusion to the kidneys, gut, skin, and uterus, with relative maintenance of blood flow to the heart, brain, and adrenal glands. In the pregnant patient, such redistribution may result in fetal hypoxia and distress, even before the mother becomes overtly hypotensive. In such situations, the uterus is, from a teleologic viewpoint, relatively less important than the essential life-saving organs systems. Regardless of the absolute maternal BP,

Critical Care Obstetrics, 5th edition. Edited by M. Belfort, G. Saade, M. Foley, J. Phelan and G. Dildy.

Table 40.1 Causes of pregnancy-related death, by outcome of pregnancy and pregnancy-related mortality ratios (PRMR*) – United States, 1991–1999.

Cause of death	Outcome of pregnancy (% distribution)							All outcomes (n = 4200)	
	Livebirth (n = 2519)	Stillbirth (n = 275)	Ectopic (n = 237)	Abortion† (n = 165)	Molar (n = 14)	Undelivered (n = 438)	Unknown (n = 552)	Percent	PRMR
Embolism	21.0	18.6	2.1	13.9	28.6	25.1	18.3	**19.6**	**2.2**
Hemorrhage	2.7	21.1	93.3	21.8	7.1	8.7	8.7	**17.2**	**2.0**
PIH§	19.3	20.0	0	0.6	0	12.3	11.8	**15.7**	**1.8**
Infection	11.7	18.9	2.5	33.9	14.3	11.0	12.9	**12.6**	**1.5**
Cardiomyopathy	10.1	5.1	0.4	1.8	0	3.4	11.2	**8.3**	**1.0**
CVA¶	5.7	0.7	0	1.2	0	3.9	8.5	**5.0**	**0.6**
Anesthesia	1.8	0.7	1.3	9.7	0	0	0.4	**1.6**	**0.2**
Other**	17.1	14.9	0.4	16.4	50.0	33.6	27.9	**19.2**	**2.3**
Unknown	0.6	0	0	0.6	0	2.1	0.4	**0.7**	**0.1**
Total††	**100.0**	**100.0**	**100.0**	**100.0**	**100.0**	**100.0**	**100.0**	**100.0**	**100.0**

* Pregnancy-related deaths per 100 000 livebirths.
† Includes spontaneous and induced abortions.
§ Pregnancy-induced hypertension.
¶ Cerebrovascular accident.
** The majority of the other medical conditions were cardiovascular, pulmonary, and neurologic problems.
†† Percentages might not add to 100.00 because of rounding.
From Centers for Disease Control and Prevention. Pregnancy-related mortality surveillance – United States, 1991–1999. *MMWR* 2003; 52: 55–62.

Table 40.2 Clinical classification of maternal hemorrhage.

Class	Blood loss (mL)	Volume deficit (%)	Signs and symptoms
I	≤1000	15	Orthostatic tachycardia (↑ 20 bpm)
II	1001–1500	15–25	↑ HR 100–120 bpm Orthostatic changes (↓ 15 mmHg) Cap refill >2 sec Mental changes
III	1501–2500	25–40	↑ HR (120–160 bpm) Supine ↓ BP ↑ RR (30–50 rpm) Oliguria
IV	>2500	>40	Obtundation Oliguria-anuria CV collapse

BP, blood pressure; bpm, beats per minute; CV, cardiovascular; rpm, respirations per minute; RR, respiratory.
From Eisenberg M, Copass MK, eds. *Emergency Medical Therapy*. Philadelphia: WB Saunders, 1982: 40.

significant maternal shock is highly unlikely in the absence of fetal distress [10]. Peripheral vasoconstriction caused by the adrenomedullary stress response is an initial reaction to blood loss that maintains pressure in the presence of decreasing flow. This vasoconstriction, however, is disparate and leads to unevenly distributed microcirculatory flow. These early changes precede the development of organ failure. In the presence of continued hypovolemia, the stress response may result in poor tissue perfusion, tissue hypoxia, covert clinical shock, organ dysfunction, ARDS, and other organ failure [11,12].

As the blood volume deficit approaches 25%, such compensatory mechanisms become inadequate to maintain CO and arterial pressure. At this point, small additional losses of blood result in rapid clinical deterioration, producing a vicious cycle of cellular death and vasoconstriction, organ ischemia, loss of capillary membrane integrity, and additional loss of intravascular fluid volume into the extravascular space [13,14].

Increased platelet aggregation is also found in hypovolemic shock. Aggregated platelets release vasoactive substances, which cause small vessel occlusion and impaired microcirculatory perfusion. These platelet aggregates can embolize to the lungs and be a factor contributing to respiratory failure, which is often seen following prolonged shock.

Physiologic changes in preparation for pregnancy blood loss

The pregnant woman undergoes profound physiologic changes to prepare for the blood loss that will occur at the time of parturition. By the end of the second trimester of pregnancy, the maternal blood volume has increased by 1000–2000 mL [15]. The maternal CO increases by 40–45% while total peripheral resistance decreases [16]. This decreased peripheral resistance results from hormonal factors (progesterone, and prostaglandin metabolites such as prostacyclin) that reduce overall vasomotor tone and from the development of a low-resistance arteriovenous shunt through the placenta. The decreased peripheral resistance is maximal in the second trimester. About 20–25% of the maternal CO goes to the placental shunt to yield a blood flow of approximately 500 mL/min. Placental blood flow is directly proportional to the uterine perfusion pressure, which in turn is proportional to systemic BP. Any decrease in maternal CO results in a proportionate decrease in placental perfusion. The uterine arterioles are very sensitive to exogenous vasopressor substances but because of an incompletely understood pregnancy-related stimulus of the renin–angiotensin system, the vasopressor effect of angiotensin appears to be blunted during pregnancy [17]. Thus, during her pregnancy, the mother has been prepared for a blood volume loss of up to 1000 mL. Following a normal spontaneous vaginal delivery, a first-day postpartum hematocrit usually is not altered significantly from the admission hematocrit. In practice, blood loss at delivery is often underestimated. Actual measurements show that the average blood loss after normal spontaneous vaginal delivery is over 600 mL [18]. With a postpartum blood loss of less than 1000 mL, the parturient's vital signs may reflect acute blood loss (i.e., hypotension and tachycardia).

During the antepartum period, the obstetrician must be concerned with both patients. Fetal oxygenation decreases in proportion to the decrease in maternal CO. The catecholamine output from the mother's adrenal medulla may preferentially increase arteriolar resistance of the spiral arterioles in the placental bed, thus further decreasing oxygenation. Under such circumstances, the fetus may be in jeopardy, even though compensatory mechanisms maintain stable maternal vital signs. Thus, even in the absence of overt hypotension, the healthcare team must act quickly to preserve fetal well-being by expanding the intravascular volume of an antepartum patient who has lost a significant amount of blood.

Although all vital organs receive increased blood flow during pregnancy, three organs (other than the placenta) are particularly susceptible to damage when perfusion pressure decreases as a result of hemorrhagic shock. These organs are the anterior pituitary gland, the kidneys, and the lungs. During pregnancy, the anterior pituitary enlarges and receives increased blood flow. Under the condition of shock, blood flow is shunted away from the anterior pituitary gland. As a result, the anterior pituitary gland may undergo ischemic necrosis. Sheehan and Murdoch first described the syndrome of hypopituitarism secondary to postpartum hypotension as result of hemorrhage [19]. This condition is now a rare complication in modern obstetrics. The clinical presentation can vary, but secondary amenorrhea resulting from loss of pituitary gonadotrophs is usually present. In severe cases, thyrotropic and adrenotropic pituitary hormones also may be deficient. A typical or partial deficiency syndrome of both anterior and posterior pituitary hormones has been reported. Hypovolemia from any cause leads to reduced renal perfusion, which can result in acute tubular necrosis. In one series, hemorrhage and hypovolemia were precipitating factors in 75% of obstetric patients with acute renal failure [20]. Prompt blood and fluid replacement is essential in order to avoid such sequelae. Lung injury may result from hypovolemic shock [21]. In the non-pregnant state, a critical cardiac output exists below which oxygen extraction becomes impaired, and this critical oxygen delivery has been implicated in the pathogenesis of ARDS in humans. The question of a critical oxygen delivery point in human pregnancy is unclear although it has been suggested as a component of the pathology of severe pre-eclampsia [22]. Evans and colleagues presented evidence that in the pregnant sheep model, such a critical cardiac output does not exist [23].

Causes of obstetric hemorrhage

Any disruption in the integrity of the maternal vascular system during pregnancy has the potential for devastating blood loss. As an overview, ectopic pregnancy is the leading cause of life-threatening obstetric hemorrhage in the first half of gestation (see Table 40.1). Beyond the first trimester, antepartum obstetric hemorrhage usually results from a disruption of the placental attachment site (involving either a normally implanted placenta or placenta previa) or uterine rupture (spontaneous or trauma related). During the intrapartum period, the likelihood of clinical shock is enhanced in patients with pre-eclampsia. Because of the intravascular volume depletion associated with this condition, even the usual blood loss associated with delivery may result in clinical instability. Another pathophysiologic change often associated with pre-eclampsia is thrombocytopenia, which when severe, may contribute to postpartum blood loss [24].

Most serious obstetric hemorrhage occurs in the postpartum period. The most common cause is uterine atony following placental separation. Under normal conditions, shortening myometrial fibers act as physiologic ligatures around the arterioles of the placental bed. Thus, uterine atony with failure of myometrial contraction results in arterial hemorrhage. Factors that predispose a patient to uterine atony include precipitous or prolonged labor, oxytocin augmentation, magnesium sulfate infusion, chorioamnionitis, enlarged uterus resulting from increased intrauterine contents, and operative deliveries [10,25].

Table 40.3 Common causes of obstetric hemorrhage.

Antepartum and intrapartum
Placental abruption
Uterine rupture
Placenta previa
Postpartum
Retained placenta
Uterine atony
Uterine rupture
Genital tract trauma
Coagulopathy

Table 40.4 Central hemodynamic changes.

	Non-pregnant	Pregnant
Cardiac output (L/min)	4.3 ± 0.9	6.2 ± 1.0
Heart rate (beats/min)	71 ± 10.0	83 ± 10.0
Systemic vascular resistance (dyne/cm/sec^{-5})	1530 ± 520	1210 ± 266
Pulmonary vascular resistance (dyne/cm/sec^{-5})	119 ± 47.0	78 ± 22
Colloid oncotic pressure (mmHg)	20.8 ± 1.0	18.0 ± 1.5
Colloid oncotic pressure – pulmonary capillary wedge pressure (mmHg)	14.5 ± 2.5	10.5 ± 2.7
Mean arterial pressure (mmHg)	86.4 ± 7.5	90.3 ± 5.8
Pulmonary capillary wedge pressure (mmHg)	6.3 ± 2.1	7.5 ± 1.8
Central venous pressure (mmHg)	3.7 ± 2.6	3.6 ± 2.5
Left ventricular stroke work index (g/m/m^{-2})	41 ± 8	48 ± 6

Reproduced with permission from Clark S, Cotton D, Lee W, et al. Central hemodynamic assessment of normal term pregnancy. *Am J Obstet Gynecol* 1989; 161: 1439–1442.

Obstetric trauma is another common cause of postpartum hemorrhage. Cervical and vaginal lacerations are more common with midpelvic operative deliveries, and as a consequence of an extension of a uterine incision for cesarean birth. Other causes of postpartum hemorrhage (Table 40.3) include uterine inversion, morbidly adherent placenta (accreta/percreta), amniotic fluid embolism, retroperitoneal bleeding from either birth trauma or episiotomy, and coagulopathies of various causes [10,25,26].

Management of hypovolemic shock in pregnancy

Fundamentally the most important and prerequisite management tool in approaching hypovolemic shock is a complete understanding of maternal blood volume and how that volume is affected by pregnancy. In 1989, Clark et al. presented central hemodynamic parameters of normal-term pregnancy and contrasted them with non-pregnant values (Table 40.4). The calculation and demonstration of a 50% increased blood volume in term pregnancy was delineated by Pritchard et al. in 1965 [15].

So we are to understand that the average pregnant woman has 4.5–5 L of total blood volume, not 3–3.5 L as in the non-pregnant state. Further, there is a rise in CO of 50% in the term patient, a result of an increased heart rate and stroke volume. There is also a dramatic decrease in SVR and pulmonary vascular resistance. Clark et al. were not able to document increases in left ventricular contractility and we are left with the knowledge that pregnancy is not a hyperdynamic state, but rather a finely written (evolved) and adapted symphony of perfect resilience and capacity to perpetuate the gestation. Excesses have also been built into the system to withstand the blood loss of labor and delivery. After delivery, the low resistance placental shunt is turned off and a process of autotransfusion helps to replenish lost volume from the delivery phase. We are fortunate to have reproduction occur at the zenith of human health in the early adult years.

Oxygenation

The most frequent cause of maternal death from shock is inadequate respiratory exchange leading to multiple organ failure [11]. The duration of relative tissue hypoxia is important in the accumulation of byproducts of anaerobic metabolism. Thus, increasing the partial pressure of oxygen across the pulmonary capillary membrane by giving 8–10 L of oxygen per minute by tight-fitting mask may forestall the onset of tissue hypoxia and is a logical first priority. Also, increasing the partial pressure of oxygen in maternal blood will increase the amount of oxygen carried to fetal tissue [27]. If the airway is not patent, or the tidal volume is inadequate, the clinician should not hesitate to perform endotracheal intubation and institute positive-pressure ventilation to achieve adequate oxygenation.

Studies in adult critical care indicate that tissue oxygen debt resulting from reduced tissue perfusion is the primary underlying physiologic mechanism that subsequently leads to organ failure and death [28,29]. It seems that early identification and treatment of hypovolemic shock and its inciting cause is imperative to improving outcome. One approach commonly used to assist the clinician is to classify the degree of hemorrhage from I to IV based on the patient's signs and symptoms (Table 40.2).

Volume replacement

Protracted shock appears to cause secondary changes in the microcirculation; and these changes affect circulating blood volume. In early shock, there is a tendency to draw fluid from the interstitial space into the capillary bed. As the shock state progresses, damage to the capillary endothelium occurs and is manifested by an increase in capillary permeability. Capillary permeability further accentuates the loss of intravascular volume. This deficit is reflected clinically by the disproportionately large volume of fluid necessary to resuscitate patients in severe shock. Sometimes, the amount of fluid required for resuscitation is twice the amount indicated by calculation of blood loss volume. Prolonged hemorrhagic shock also alters active transport of ions at the cellular level, and intracellular water decreases.

As can be appreciated from Table 40.3 most instances of hypovolemic shock in obstetrics are hemorrhagic and immediate. Although optimal measurements of this process may certainly document its severity, quick action and volume replacement is essential to optimizing outcome of the patient. The two most common crystalloid fluids used for resuscitation are 0.9% sodium chloride and lactated Ringer's solution. Both have equal plasma volume-expanding effects. The large volumes of required crystalloids can markedly diminish the colloid osmotic pressure (COP). Fluid resuscitation in young, previously healthy patients can be accomplished safely with modest volumes of crystalloid fluid and with little risk of pulmonary edema. The enormous volumes of crystalloids necessary to adequately resuscitate profound hypovolemic shock, however, will reduce the gradient between the COP and PCWP and may contribute to the pathogenesis of pulmonary edema [30].

Unfortunately, only 20% of infused crystalloid solution remains intravascular after 1 hour in the critically ill patient. Their use should be limited to immediate resuscitation and perfusion as the clinician orders and awaits the arrival of blood products. Crystalloid solutions such as lactated ringers and normal saline also help to replenish intracellular water and electrolytes, and help to correct metabolic derangement created by the hemorrhagic and resuscitative event [31]. Recently, data supporting the use of colloid solutions (e.g. 5% albumin) in the active resuscitation of patients have come under re-evaluation. No trial or analysis has purported to show any benefit for the use of colloids over crystalloids and some have suggested increased mortality with the use of colloids [32].

The most effective replacement therapy for lost blood volume is its replacement with whole blood. The immediacy of obstetric hemorrhage may, at times, demand this.

Modern blood transfusion practice emphasizes the use of cell components or component hemotherapy rather than whole blood. Red blood cells are administered to improve oxygen delivery in patients with decreased red cell mass resulting from hemorrhage. A National Institutes of Health (NIH) consensus conference concluded that transfusion of fresh frozen plasma (FFP) was inappropriate for volume replacement or as a nutritional supplement [33]. In the past, up to 90% of FFP use was for volume replacement. The other 10% was for the following conditions approved by the NIH consensus conference: replacement of isolated coagulation factor deficiencies, reversal of coumarin effect, antithrombin III deficiency, immunodeficiency syndromes, and treatment of thrombotic thrombocytopenic purpura. The current concern for excessive use of FFP is at least threefold. Firstly, the high profile of cost containment has caused blood banks to reevaluate use of blood products and the time involved in their preparation. Second, the routine use of FFP compromises the availability of raw material for preparation of factor VIII concentrates for hemophiliacs. Third, with regard to recipient safety, the risk of FFP includes disease transmission, anaphylactoid reactions, alloimmunization, and excessive intravascular volume [34].

Massive blood replacement is defined as transfusion of one total blood volume within 24 hours. The NIH consensus conference report noted that pathologic hemorrhage in the patient receiving a massive transfusion is caused more frequently by thrombocytopenia than by depletion of coagulation factors. This finding was demonstrated in a prospective study of 27 massively transfused patients in whom levels of factors V, VII, and IX and fibrinogen could not be correlated with the number of units of whole blood transfused [35]. A study of combat casualties suggested the thrombocytopenia was more important than depletion of coagulation factors as a cause of bleeding in massively transfused patients [36]. In this report, restoration of the prothrombin times (PT) and partial thromboplastin times (PTT) to normal with FFP had little effect on abnormal bleeding; however, platelet transfusions were effective. There is no evidence that routine administration of FFP per a given number of units of RBCs decreases transfusion requirements in patients who are receiving multiple transfusion and who do not have documented coagulation defects [37]. Thus, during massive blood replacement, correction of specific coagulation defects (fibrinogen levels <150 mg/dL) and thrombocytopenia (platelet count <30 000/mL) will minimize further transfusion requirements. With massive obstetric hemorrhage (the usual reason for hypovolemic shock) coagulation factors as well as red blood cells are lost. Specific replacement with PRBC's and crystalloid solution may lead to dilutional coagulopathy and subsequently more blood loss.

In acute hemorrhagic shock, central venous pressure (CVP) or pulmonary capillary wedge pressure (PCWP) reflect intravascular volume status and may be useful in guiding fluid therapy. In the critically ill patient, however, CVP may be a less reliable indicator of volume status due to compliance changes in the vein walls [38]. The clinician must use resources on hand to correct the volume deficiency. Central hemodynamic monitoring equipment, and personnel to introduce and maintain it, are not commonly present in the obstetric delivery suite or labor area. Again, we digress to the obstetrician's fundamental knowledge of maternal volume in pregnancy, and how that may be authenticated by her current condition (e.g. pre-eclampsia or abruption).

In the absence of diuretic use (an unusual if not proscribed therapy during the conduct of labor and delivery, or preparations for elective cesarean delivery); urine output measured with indwelling Foley catheter and drainage will provide approximate and important information about maternal volume and intravascular status in real time. The operative or treating physician's time is best confined to eliminating the focus of hemorrhage and relying on simple and adequate techniques for assessing patient response to resuscitation measures. Serial hematocrit, platelets, fibrinogen, PT, and PTT can monitor the hemoglobin and coagulation integrity in the maternal vascular tree. Urine flow should be maintained between 30 and 60 cc/h.

Initial type and screening of labor and delivery patients can provide valuable information if the need for blood replacement arises in hemorrhagic morbidity. Type-specific blood to the patient with Coombs negative blood screens is associated with an acceptably low level of incompatibility of 0.01% [39].

Pharmacologic agents

During the antepartum and intrapartum periods, only correction of maternal hypovolemia will maintain placental perfusion and prevent fetal compromise. Although vasopressors may temporarily correct hypotension, they do so at the expense of uteroplacental perfusion. Thus, vasopressors are not used in the treatment of obstetric hemorrhagic shock.

Further evaluation

After the patient's oxygenation and expansion of intravascular volume have been accomplished and her condition is beginning to stabilize, it is essential for the healthcare team to evaluate the patient's response to therapy, to diagnose the basic condition that resulted in circulatory shock, and to consider the fetal condition. Serial evaluation of vital signs, urine output, acid–base status, blood chemistry, and coagulation status aid in this assessment. In select cases, placement of a pulmonary artery catheter should be considered to assist in the assessment of cardiac function and oxygen transport variables. In general, however, central hemodynamic monitoring is not necessary in simple hypovolemic shock.

Evaluation of the fetal cardiotocograph may indicate fetal distress during an acute hemorrhagic episode. As a rule, maternal health trumps fetal health. This means that delivery, under these circumstances, should not be considered until maternal condition has been stabilized. Once the pregnant woman is stabilized and the fetus continues to demonstrate persistent signs of fetal distress, the clinician should then consider delivery. It is important to realize that as the maternal hypoxia, acidosis, and underperfusion of the uteroplacental unit are being corrected, the fetus may recover. Serial evaluation of the fetal status and *in utero* resuscitation are preferable to emergency delivery of a depressed infant from a hemodynamically unstable mother.

Hemostasis

In certain situations, such as uterine rupture with intraperitoneal bleeding, definitive surgical therapy may need to be instituted before stabilization can be achieved. With postpartum hemorrhage resulting from uterine atony that has not responded to the conventional methods of uterine compression and dilute intravenous oxytocin, the physician should consider intramuscular methergine or 15 methyl prostaglandin $F_{2\alpha}$. The latter is administered as a 250-μg dose, which may be repeated as necessary for up to a maximum of eight doses at 15–90-min intervals.

In a small series of patients, rectal administration of misoprostol, a PGE_1 analogue, has been found effective in the treatment of uterine atony [40]. Other data indicate that rectal misoprostol is no more effective than intravenous oxytocin in preventing postpartum hemorrhage [41]. In a systematic review oxytocin and aroyl preparations delivered in the third stage of labor were more effective than rectal misoprostol in the prevention of postpartum hemorrhage [42].

In cases of persistent vaginal bleeding, careful exploration of the vagina, cervix, and uterus is performed. The clinician looks for retained products of conception or lacerations. For hemorrhage resulting from uterine atony that has failed to respond to the previously described conservative measures, as well as in cases of extensive placenta accreta or uterine rupture not amenable to simple closure, laparotomy and hysterectomy may be indicated. If the patient does desire future fertility and is clinically stable, uterine artery ligation or stepwise uterine devascularization has been favorably described [43,44].

The fundus compression suture as described by B-Lynch has also been reported to abate uterine hemorrhage in many cases [45]. Rarely, hypogastric artery ligation is surgically necessary. Balloon occlusion and embolization of the internal iliac arteries have also been described in cases of placenta percreta [46,47]. A good discussion of many of these techniques, as well as a more comprehensive discussion of techniques for achieving medical and surgical hemostasis in patients with postpartum bleeding, have been described elsewhere [48,49].

It should be emphasized that preventable surgical death in obstetrics may, on occasion, represent an error in judgment and a reluctance to proceed with laparotomy or hysterectomy, rather than deficiencies in knowledge or surgical technique. Proper management of serious hemorrhage requires timely medical and surgical decision-making as well as meticulous attention to the aforementioned principles of blood and volume replacement.

Cardiogenic shock

This type of shock is caused by failure of the heart as an effective pump. In the obstetric patient this most often occurs in the patient with pre-existing myocardial disease, peripartum cardiomyopathy, congenital or acquired valvular heart disease, and certain cardiac arrhythmias. It is important to remember that ischemic changes in the heart may be induced in the settling of hypovolemic and septic shock [50].

Common causes of cardiogenic pulmonary edema in pregnancy are diastolic heart failure due to chronic hypertension and obesity, leading to left ventricular hypertrophy [51,52]. Cyanotic congenital heart disease leads to ischemic changes with increasing right to left shunting due to normal decreases in systemic vascular resistance in pregnancy [53]. Patients with Eisenmenger syndrome can develop right heart failure and cardiogenic shock as pulmonary hypertension worsens temporarily [54].

Pathogenesis

Cardiogenic shock is characterized by systemic hypoperfusion in the setting of an adequate intravascular volume. Hemodynamic criteria include sustained hypertension (i.e. systolic blood pressure <90 mmHg), reduced cardiac index (<2.2 L/min/m^2), and an elevated filling pressure (pulmonary capillary wedge pressure >18 mmHg).

Cardiogenic shock is characterized by a vicious cycle in which decreased myocardial contractility, usually due to ischemia, results in reduced cardiac output and arterial pressure. The cycle continues with hypoperfusion of the myocardium and further depression of maternal cardiac output. Systolic myocardial dysfunction reduces stroke volume and, together with diastolic dysfunction, leads to elevated LV end-diastolic pressure and PCWP as well as to pulmonary congestion. Reduced coronary perfusion leads to worsening ischemic and progressive myocardial dysfunction and a rapid downward spiral, which, if uninterrupted, is often fatal [55].

Due to the unstable condition of these patients, supportive therapy must be initiated simultaneously with diagnostic evaluation. In this circumstance, clinical evaluation of the patient is important in helping to establish a diagnosis and to guide patient management. Blood work including baseline ABG, cardiac troponin, metabolic profile, hematocrit, and live enzymes should be sent to the lab. ECG, chest X-ray, and echocardiogram should be obtained. There is a split of opinion with respect to the use of pulmonary artery catheterization in patients with suspected cardiogenic shock. However, many clinicians believe that the use of the pulmonary artery catheter provides diagnostic clarity and guidance for clinical management [56–59].

Acute myocardial infarction

Acute myocardial infarction in pregnancy is a rare event. Recent studies place the incidence at 2.8–6.2 per 100 000 deliveries [60,61]. The three strongest independent predictors of myocardial infarction in one population were chronic hypertension, diabetes, and advanced maternal age [60]. Case fatality rates have been estimated from 5.1% to 37%; and the most dangerous time for the gravida is in the last trimester of gestation or puerperium [60–62]. Women who sustain an infarction less than 2 weeks prior to labor are at especially high risk of death [64]. Myocardial infarction is more common during the third trimester or puerperium of the first or second pregnancies [65].

Patients typically present with ischemic chest pain in the presence of an abnormal ECG and elevated specific cardiac troponin I. Initially the maternal condition should be stabilized by medical management. Nitroglycerin and morphine sulfate should be administered. Oxygen is also a potent vasodilator and should be administered initially by nasal cannula. Ventricular arrhythmia may occur and if left unchecked, can lead to cardiogenic shock or sudden cardiac death. Ventricular defibrillation should be effective in this case. Lidocaine should be started to prevent arrhythmias. In the case where left ventricular dysfunction occurs as a result of ischemic changes, intra-aortic balloon pump has been used to improve left ventricular output and coronary artery perfusion [66,67]. Calcium channel blockers and β-blockers may be used to help decrease afterload.

Pregnancy-associated spontaneous coronary artery dissection (P-SCAD) is the most common cause of myocardial infarction in the immediate postpartum period. In one report 78% of women with peripartum P-SCAD had no risk factors for coronary artery disease and 84% of lesions involved the left anterior descending artery [68]. Successful treatment includes coronary stenting and emergency bypass grafting [69,70]. One review of P-SCAD management concluded that approximately one-third of women could be managed medically with antiplatelet therapy and β-blocker administration and achieve excellent clinical and angiographic results [71].

Women who have evidence of atherosclerotic or intracoronary thrombosis are candidates for coronary stenting or the administration of tissue plasminogen activator (TPA). This large molecular weight molecule should not cross the placenta and has been used successfully in thrombolysis of intracoronary thrombosis during pregnancy [72]. However, TPA is contraindicated in the early postpartum period because the risk of postpartum hemorrhage is greater than the risk of angioplasty and coronary artery stenting. The foregoing discussion should emphasize the usefulness of early coronary angiography after acute myocardial infarction in pregnancy.

Peripartum cardiomyopathy

Peripartum cardiomyopathy (PPCM) is cardiomyopathy that develops in the last gestational month of pregnancy or in the first 5 months postpartum. By definition, it requires that there be no identifiable cause for heart failure and no identifiable heart disease. It is rare in the United States (1 in 3000 to 1 in 15 000) but more prevalent in Africa (1 in 3000), and Haiti (1 in 350).

Risk factors include, but are not limited to, the following: older women, obesity, multiparous mothers with multifetal gestation [73], and may also include pre-eclampsia and severe hypertension during pregnancy [74]. Prior to delivery PPCM presents as a patient with NYHA class III or IV functional status [75]. Patients who present after delivery often have dramatic signs of congestive heart failure. Symptoms may include, but are not limited to, dyspnea, orthopnea, persistent weight retention or weight gain, peripheral edema, nocturnal cough, and profound fatigue postpartum. Evaluation of left ventricular size and systolic function should be performed with echocardiography. Every attempt should be made to rule out other causes of cardiomyopathy. Cunningham et al. evaluated 28 cases of peripartum heart failure of obscure etiology and was able to ascribe underlying causes to all but 7 (25%). The majority of cases on this cohort were due to underlying chronic hypertension, obesity, and forme fruste mitral stenosis that were eliminated by thorough evaluation. In this study, peripartum heart failure was usually precipitated by, or may even have been caused by, a constellation of complications common to pregnancy, namely pre-eclampsia, cesarean delivery, anemia, and infection [76].

Treatment of peripartum cardiomyopathy is similar to the treatment of acute and chronic heart failure due to other causes of left ventricular systolic dysfunction. Patients who are congested but have adequate perfusion will require treatment with intravenous diuretics alone or in combination with vasodilators such as nitroglycerin or nitroprusside. Patients with diminished perfusion will require augmentation of their cardiac output with inotropic agents such as dobutamine [77]. Beta-blockers are used, since high heart rate, arrhythmias, and sudden death often occur with PPCM. Digitalis, an inotropic agent, is also safe during pregnancy and may help to maximize contractility and rate control. Because of the high incidence of thromboembolism in these patients, the use of heparin is considered medically necessary, followed by warfarin (when not pregnant) in those with left ventricular ejection fractions less than 35%. After pregnancy is over, ACE inhibitors are used to reduce afterload by vasodilatation. Angiotensinogen receptor blockers may be substituted for those patients intolerant of ACE inhibitors.

The acute treatment aims to reduce preload and afterload, and increase contractility. In the setting of cardiogenic shock, invasive hemodynamic monitoring may be helpful in making decisions regarding maternal responses to therapy and the need for additional therapeutics. Since an immune pathogenesis has been postulated, immune modulation with intravenous immunoglobulin has been proposed [77,78]. However, no consistent benefit has been demonstrated. If patients remain in cardiogenic shock despite aggressive medical therapy, additional therapies to maintain circulatory support and organ perfusion should be considered. Intra-aortic balloon counterpulsation can be used acutely. Where resources exist, left ventricular assist devices and heart transplantation may be used if clinically indicated [79,80].

Mitral stenosis

Rheumatic mitral stenosis (MS) is the most common clinically significant valvular abnormality in pregnant women and may be associated with pulmonary congestion, edema, and atrial arrhythmias during pregnancy or soon after delivery. The contracted valve impedes blood flow from the left atrium to the ventricle. The left atrium is dilated, left atrial pressure is chronically elevated, and significant passive pulmonary hypertension may develop. Twenty-five per cent of women have cardiac failure for the first time during pregnancy [81]. This has been confused with peripartum cardiomyopathy [76].

With significantly tight MS (surface area <2.5 cm^2) symptoms usually develop [82]. The most common complaint is dyspnea and others may include, but are not limited to, fatigue, palpitations, cough, and hemoptysis. Tachycardia shortens diastolic filling time and increases the mitral gradient, which raises left atrial and pulmonary venous and capillary pressures and may result in pulmonary edema. Sinus tachycardia is often treated with β-blockers. Atrial tachyarrhythmias, including fibrillation,

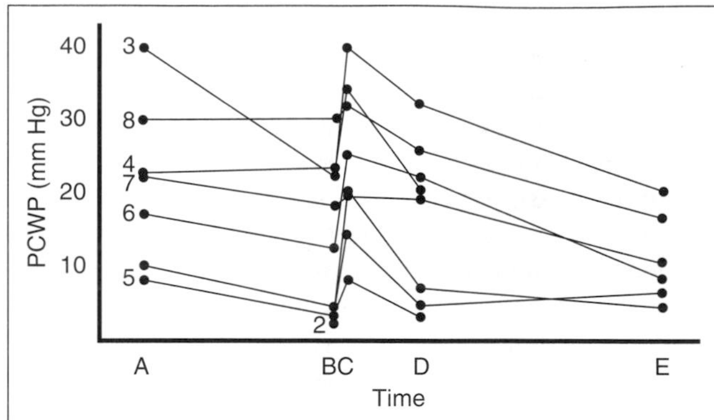

Figure 40.1 Intrapartum alterations in pulmonary capillary wedge pressure (PCWP) in eight patients with mitral stenosis. (a) First-stage labor; (b) second-stage labor, 15–30 min before delivery; (c) 5–15 min post partum; (d) 4–6 h post partum; (e) 18–24 h post partum. (Reproduced with permission from Clark SL, Phelan JP, Greenspoon J, et al. Labor and delivery in the presence of mitral stenosis: central hemodynamic observations. *Am J Obstet Gynecol* 1985; 152: 986.)

are common in mitral stenosis and should be treated aggressively with intravenous verapamil (5–10 mg) or cardioversion, if necessary. Because of the increased risk of systemic embolism in patients with mitral stenosis and atrial fibrillation, anticoagulant therapy is indicated.

Intrapartum, carefully controlled epidural anesthesia with attention to minimizing preload will decrease anxiety, which causes tachycardia and pulmonary congestion. Choice of route of delivery should be left to the patient as both vaginal delivery and elective cesarean are obstetrically acceptable options. Assuming the patient does not elect a cesarean using a regional anesthetic, instrumental vaginal delivery should be considered to shorten the second stage. Once delivered, the low resistance uterine shunt disappears and "autotransfusion" may bring about pulmonary edema (Figure 40.1).

During pregnancy diuretic therapy may be used to decrease preload along with prophylactic β-blockers to slow the heart rate response to activity and anxiety [83]. Acute pulmonary edema in pregnancy may also occur with the use of tocolytics, preeclampsia, and fluid overload [84].

Arrhythmias

Management of cardiac arrest attributable to life-threatening ventricular tachyarrhythmias is essential to prevent sudden cardiac death in the mother and fetus. This requires a correct diagnosis and is usually possible with a 12-lead surface ECG. Clinical errors can occur in circumstances where medical personnel believe that a young healthy woman is unlikely to develop a life-threatening ventricular arrhythmia. Ventricular tachycardia (VT) is rare in pregnant women but can originate from either the right or left ventricle in structurally normal hearts [85,86]. If the pregnant patient has structural heart disease VT carries a poor prognosis [87].

Acutely, it is important to determine whether VT is hemodynamically stable or unstable. If at any time the patient becomes unstable or there is evidence of fetal compromise direct-current (DC) countershock (50–100 J) should be delivered immediately [88]. Conservative therapy is appropriate for sustained VT and stable hemodynamics. Acute therapy should be initiated with procainamide (50–100 mg intravenously). Another potential antiarrhythmic drug is lidocaine. Neither is known to be teratogenic. Life-threatening ventricular fibrillation (VF) or ventricular flutter can occur in any stage of pregnancy and is associated with a high risk of sudden cardiac death [89]. In these patients DC defibrillation is the method of choice (100–360 J). Prompt cardiopulmonary resuscitation and early defibrillation by either DC countershock or an automated external defibrillator significantly improves the likelihood of successful resuscitation from VF [89,90]. The implantable cardioverter-defibrillator (ICD) is an excellent approach to terminal tachyarrhythmias and prevents sudden death [91].

Ventricular premature beats (VPBs) in pregnant women with structurally normal hearts are benign and do not usually require therapy [87]. Exacerbating chemical stimulants (e.g. caffeine, cocaine) should be eliminated, and cardiology and maternal–fetal medicine consultation should be considered. If patients remain highly symptomatic a selective β-blocker such as metoprotol may be used.

Aortic dissection

Acute aortic dissection may occur in pregnancy in association with severe hypertension due to pre-eclampsia, coarctation of the aorta, or connective tissue disease such as Marfan's syndrome [92,93]. Although rare, aortic dissection during pregnancy accounts for 50% of all dissections in women under 40 years of age [94]. Classic symptoms include severe retrosternal and/or abdominal pain. The patient may present with cardiogenic shock due to aortic incompetence or hemopericardium and tamponade. Diagnosis is made with computed tomography or transesophageal echocardiography. Maternal outcome is poor with mortality as high as 25% [93,95]. If the dissection is limited to the descending aorta some patients can be managed successfully to term and surgery performed postpartum.

Before 28 weeks gestation, aortic repair with the fetus kept *in situ* is warranted, given the high mortality (80%) of non-operative treatment in this setting [93,96]. After 32 weeks gestation (fetal viability) primary cesarean followed by repair is appropriate [93,95]. Controlled vaginal delivery with regional anesthesia has been described [95]. Management between 28 and 32 weeks is controversial. If there is hemodynamic instability or non-reassuring fetal status, then cesarean followed by operative repair should be affected. Epidural anesthesia reduces increases in vessel shear stress (cardiac output) and wall tension (mean arterial blood pressure) associated with labor. The combined α- and β-blocker labetolol can be titrated (1–10 mg/kg/min) to allow rapid control of mean arterial blood pressure during labor and delivery. A split of opinion exists as to the optimal anesthetic for cesarean delivery in these patients. General anesthesia may be indicated in anticoagulated patients, but the hypertensive response to intubation and surgical stimulation may increase cardiovascular stress, promoting rupture or progression of a pre-existing dissection [65].

Summary

Cardiogenic shock is quite different from hypovolemic shock, the latter requiring increased preload and the former inotropic support and decreased afterload. Cardiogenic shock occurs infrequently and calls for consultation, timely decision-making, and diagnostic integration. Pulmonary congestion is the usual presenting symptom and has multiple etiologies. Although there is a split of opinion as to the effectiveness of invasive hemodynamic monitoring, accurate diagnosis as to the etiology of heart failure is essential and many experts feel comfortable with this diagnostic modality. Others have demonstrated that non-invasive echocardiographic modalities to estimate cardiac parameters are reasonably accurate [97]. Obstetricians should have a working knowledge of maternal hemodynamics in pregnancy and should avail themselves of frequent cardiology and maternal–fetal medicine consultation. Responding to postpartum hemorrhage should be fairly straightforward in most but not all instances. Cardiogenic shock (and its imitators) should be suspected in the setting of pulmonary congestion and myocardial infarction. In many of these circumstances, timely consultation and a multidisciplinary approach can enhance maternal and fetal outcome.

References

1 Center for Disease Control and Prevention. Pregnancy-related mortality surveillance – United States. *MMWR* 2003; 52 (Suppl 2): 1991–1999.

2 McCormick M, Sanghvi H, Kinzie B. Preventing postpartum hemorrhage in low-resource settings. *Int J Gynecol Obstet* 2002; 77: 267–275.

3 Li X, Fortney J, Katelchuk M, et al. The postpartum period: the key to maternal mortality. *Int J Gynecol Obstet* 1996; 54: 1–10.

4 Edman C, Toofanian A, MacDonald P, et al. Placental clearance rate of maternal plasma and rostenedione through placental estradiol formation. *Am J Obstet Gynecol* 1981; 141: 1029–1037.

5 Shoemaker W. Diagnosis and treatment of shock and circulatory dysfunction. In: Grenvik A, Ayers S, Holbrook P, Shoemaker W, eds. *Textbook of Critical Care*, 4th edn. Philadelphia: WB Saunders: 2000.

6 Pullicino E, Carli F, Poole S, et al. The relationship between circulating concentrations of interleukin-6, tumor necrosis factor, and the acute phase response to elective surgery and accidental injury. *Lymphokine Res* 1990; 9: 231–238.

7 Abraham E. Physiologic stress and cellular ischemia: relationship to immunosuppression and susceptibility to sepsis. *Crit Care Med* 1991; 19: 613–618.
8 Hoch R, Rodriguez R, Manning T, et al. Effects of accidental trauma on cytokine and endotoxin production. *Crit Care Med* 1993; 21: 839–845.
9 Bassin R, Vladeck B, Kim S, et al. Comparison of hemodynamic responses of two experimental shock models with clinical hemorrhage. *Surgery* 1971; 69: 722–729.
10 Clark SL. Shock in the pregnant patient. *Semin Perinatol* 1990; 14: 52–58.
11 Shoemaker W, Appel P, Kram HB. Role of oxygen debt in the development of organ failure, sepsis, and death in high risk surgical patients. *Chest* 1992; 102: 208–215.
12 Shoemaker W, Appel P, Kram HB. Hemodynamic and oxygen transport responses in survivors and nonsurvivors of high risk surgery. *Crit Care Med* 1993; 21: 977–990.
13 Shoemaker WC. Pathophysiologic basis for therapy for shock and trauma syndromes: use of sequential cardiorespiratory measurements to describe natural histories and evaluate possible mechanisms. *Semin Drug Treat* 1973; 3: 211–229.
14 Slater G, Vladeck B, Bassin R, et al. Sequential changes in the distribution of cardiac output in various stages of experimental hemorrhagic shock. *Surgery* 1973; 73: 714–722.
15 Pritchard JA. Changes in the blood volume during pregnancy and delivery. *Anesthesiology* 1965; 26: 393.
16 Clark S, Cotton D, Lee W, et al. Central hemodynamic assessment of normal term pregnancy. *Am J Obstet Gynecol* 1989; 161: 1439–1442.
17 Greiss FC. Uterine vascular response to hemorrhage during pregnancy and delivery. *Anesthesiology* 1965; 26: 393.
18 Pritchard J, Baldwin R, Dickey JC, et al. Blood volume changes in pregnancy and the puerperium, 2. Red blood cell loss and changes in apparent blood volume during and following vaginal delivery, cesarean section, and cesarean section plus total hysterectomy. *Am J Obstet Gynecol* 1962; 84: 1271.
19 Sheehan H, Murdoch R. Postpartum necrosis of the anterior pituitary: pathologic and clinical aspects. *Br J Obstet Gynaecol* 1938; 45: 456.
20 Smith K, Browne J, Shackman R, et al. Renal failure of obstetric origin. *Br Med Bull* 1968; 24: 49.
21 Mabie WC, Barton JR, Sibai BM. Adult respiratory syndrome in pregnancy. *Am J Obstet Gynecol* 1992 Oct; 167(4 pt 1): 950–957.
22 Belfort M, Anthony J, Saade G, et al. The oxygen consumption: oxygen delivery curve in severe preeclampsia: evidence for a fixed oxygen extraction state. *Am J Obstet Gynecol* 1993; 169: 1448–1455.
23 Evans W, Capelle S, Edelstone DI. Lack of a critical cardiac output and critical systemic oxygen delivery during low cardiac output in the third trimester in the pregnant sheep. *Am J Obstet Gynecol* 1996; 175: 222–228.
24 Haddad B, Barton JR, Livingston JC, et al. Risk factors for adverse maternal outcomes among women with HELLP (hemolysis, elevated liver enzymes, and low platelet count) syndrome. *Am J Obstet Gynecol* 2000 Aug; 183(2): 444–448.
25 Naef R, Chauhan S, Chevalier S, et al. Prediction of hemorrhage at cesarean delivery. *Obstet Gynecol* 1994; 83: 923–926.
26 Zelop C, Harlow B, Frigoletto FD, et al. Emergency peripartum hysterectomy. *Am J Obstet Gynecol* 1993; 168: 1443–1448.
27 Dildy G, Clark S, Loucks CA. Intrapartum fetal pulse oximetry: the effects of maternal hyperoxia on fetal arterial oxygen saturation. *Am J Obstet Gynecol* 1994; 171: 1120–1124.
28 Thangathurai D, Charbonnet C, Wo C, Shoemaker WC, et al. Intraoperative maintenance of tissue perfusion prevents ARDS. *New Horiz* 1996; 4: 466–474.
29 Taylor RW. Pulmonary Artery Catheter Consensus Conference Participants: Pulmonary Artery Catheter Consensus Conference consensus statement. *Crit Care Med* 1997; 25: 910.
30 Harms B, Kramer GC, Bodai BI. The effect of hypoproteinemia and pulmonary and soft tissue edema formation. *Crit Care Med* 1981; 9: 503.
31 Chiao J, Minei J, Shires G, et al. In vivo myocyte sodium activity and concentration during hemorrhagic shock. *Am J Physiol* 1990; 258: R684–R689.
32 SAFE Study Investigators. A comparison of albumin and saline for fluid resuscitation in the intensive care unit. *N Engl J Med* 2004; 350: 2247–2256.
33 National Institutes of Health Consensus Development Conference. Fresh frozen plasma. Indications and risks. *JAMA* 1985; 253: 551–553.
34 Oberman HA. Uses and abuses of fresh frozen plasma. In: Garrity A, ed. *Current Concepts in Transfusion Therapy*. Arlington, VA: American Association of Blood Banks, 1985.
35 Counts R, Haisch C, Simon TL, et al. Hemostasis in massively transfused trauma patients. *Ann Surg* 1979; 190: 91–99.
36 Miller R, Robbins T, Tong MJ, et al. Coagulation defects associated with massive blood transfusions. *Ann Surg* 1971; 174: 794–801.
37 Mannucci P, Federici A, Sirchia G. Hemostasis testing during massive blood replacement: a study of 172 cases. *Vox Sang* 1982; 42: 113–123.
38 Shippy C, Appel P, Shoemaker WC. Reliability of clinical monitoring to assess blood volume in critically ill patients. *Crit Care Med* 1984; 12: 107–112.
39 Boral L, Hill S, Apollon CJ, et al. The type and antibody screen, revisited. *Am J Clin Pathol* 1979; 71: 578–581.
40 O'Brien P, El-Refaey H, Gordon A, et al. Rectally administered misoprostol for the treatment of postpartum hemorrhage unresponsive to oxytocin and ergotomine: a descriptive study. *Obstet Gynecol* 1998; 92: 212–214.
41 Gerstenfeld T, Wing DA. Rectal misoprostol versus intravenous oxytocin for the prevention of postpartum hemorrhage after vaginal delivery. *Am J Obstet Gynecol* 2001; 185: 878–882.
42 Villar J, Gülmezoglu A, Hofmeyr GJ, et al. Systematic review of randomized controlled trials of misoprostol to prevent postpartum hemorrhage. *Obstet Gynecol* 2002; 100: 1301–1312.
43 AbdRabbo SA. Stepwise uterine devascularization: a novel technique for management of uncontrolled postpartum hemorrhage with preservation of the uterus. *Am J Obstet Gynecol* 1994; 171: 694–700.
44 O'Leary JA. Uterine artery ligation in the control of postcesarean hemorrhage. *J Reprod Med* 1995; 40: 189–193.
45 B-Lynch C, Coker A, Lawal AH, et al. The B-Lynch surgical technique for the control of massive postpartum hemorrhage: an alternative to hysterectomy? *Br J Obstet Gynaecol* 1997; 104: 372–375.
46 Dubois J, Burel L, Brignon A, et al. Placenta percreta: balloon occlusion and embolization of the internal iliac arteries to reduce intraoperative blood loss. *Am J Obstet Gynecol* 1997; 176: 723–726.
47 Shih J, Liu K, Shyu MK. Temporary balloon occlusion of the common iliac artery: new approach to bleeding control during cesarean hyster-

ectomy for placenta percreta. *Am J Obstet Gynecol* 2005; 193: 1756–1758.

48 Dildy GA. Postpartum hemorrhage: new management options. *Clin Obstet Gynecol* 2002; 45: 330–344.

49 Gilstrap LC, Cunningham FG, Vandorsten JP, eds. *Operative Obstetrics*, 2nd edn. New York: McGraw-Hill.

50 Karpati P, Rossignal M, Pirot M, et al. High incidence of myocardial ischemica during postpartum hemorrhage. *Anesthesiology* 2004; 100: 30–36.

51 Jessup M, Brozena S. Heart failure. *N Engl J Med* 2003; 348: 2007–2018.

52 Kenchaiak S, Evans J, Levy D, Wilson P, et al. Obesity and the risk of heart failure. *N Engl J Med* 2002; 347: 305–313.

53 Shime J, Mocurski E, Hastings D, et al. Congenital heart disease in pregnancy: short and long-term implications. *Am J Obstet Gynecol* 1987; 156: 313.

54 Weiss B, von Segesser L, Alon E, et al. Outcome of cardiovascular surgery and pregnancy: a systematic review of the period 1984–1996. *Am J Obstet Gynecol* 1998; 179: 1643.

55 Hochman J, Ingbar D. Cardiogenic shock and pulmonary edema. In: Kasper D, Braunwald E, Hauser S, et al, eds. *Harrison's Principles of Internal Medicine*, 16th edn. New York: McGraw-Hill, 2005.

56 Harvey S, Harrison D, Singer M, Ashcroft J. Assessment of the clinical effectiveness of pulmonary artery catheters in management of patients in intensive care (PAC-Man): a randomized controlled trial. *Lancet* 2005; 366: 472–477.

57 Simini B. Pulmonary artery catheters in intensive care. *Lancet* 2005; 366: 435–436.

58 Stevenson L, ESCAPE Investigators and ESCAPE Study Coordinators. Evaluation study of congestive heart failure and pulmonary artery catheterization effectiveness. *JAMA* 2005; 294: 1625–1633.

59 Hall JB. Searching for evidence to support pulmonary artery catheter use in critically ill patients. *JAMA* 2005; 294: 1693–1694.

60 Ladner H, Danielson B, Gilbert W. Acute myocardial infarction in pregnancy and the puerperium: a population-based study. *Obstet Gynecol* 2005; 105: 480–484.

61 James A, Jamison M, Biswas M, et al. Acute myocardial infarction in pregnancy: a United States population-based study. *Circulation* 2006; 113: 1564–1571.

62 Badui E, Enisco R. Acute myocardial infarction during pregnancy and puerperium: a review. *Angiology* 1996; 47: 739–756.

63 Hawkins G, Wendel G Jr, Leveno KJ, Stoneheim J. Myocardial infarction during pregnancy: a review. *Obstet Gynecol* 1985; 65: 139–146.

64 Esplin S, Clark SL. Ischemic heart disease and myocardial infarction during pregnancy. *Contemp OB/GYN* 1999; 44: 27.

65 Ray P, Murphy GJ, Shutt LE. Recognition and management of maternal cardiac disease in pregnancy. *Br J Anaesth* 2004; 93: 428–439.

66 Allen J, Wewers MD. Acute myocardial infarction with cardiogenic shock during pregnancy: treatment with intra-aortic balloon counterpulsation. *Crit Care Med* 1990; 18: 888–889.

67 Ko W, Ho H, Chu SH. Postpartum myocardial infarction resured with an intra-aortic balloon pump and extracorporal membrane oxygenator. *Int J Cardiol* 1998; 63: 81–84.

68 McKechnie R, Patel D, Eitzman D, et al. Spontaneous coronary artery dissection in a pregnant woman. *Obstet Gynecol* 2001; 98: 899–902.

69 Hoppe U, Beukelmann D, Bohm M, Erdmann E. A young mother with severe chest pain. *Heart* 1998; 79: 205.

70 Lewis R, Makie W, Burlew B, Sibai BM. Biventricular assist device as a bridge to cardiac transplantation in the treatment of peripartum cardiomyopathy. *South Med J* 1997; 90: 955–958.

71 Maeder M, Ammann P, Drack G, Rickli H. Pregnancy-associated spontaneous coronary artery dissection. *Z Kardiol* 2005; 94: 829–835.

72 Schumacher B, Belfort M, Card RJ. Successful treatment of myocardial infarction during pregnancy with tissue plasminogen activator. *Am J Obstet Gynecol* 1997; 176: 716–719.

73 Lang R, Lampert M, Poppas A, et al. Peripartum cardiomyopathy. In: Elkayam U, Gleicher N, eds. *Cardiac Problems in Pregnancy*, 3rd edn. New York: Wiley-Liss, 1998.

74 Lampert M, Lang RM. Peripartum cardiomyopathy. *Am Heart J* 1995; 130: 860–870.

75 Phillips S, Wames CS. Peripartum cardiomyopathy: current therapeutic perspectives. *Curr Treat Options Cardiovasc Med* 2004; 6: 481–488.

76 Cunningham F, Pritchard J, Hawkins G, et al. Peripartum heart failure: cardiomyopathy or confounding cardiovascular events? *Obstet Gynecol* 1986; 67: 157.

77 Bozkurt B, Villanueva F, Holubkov R, et al. Intravenous immune globulin in the therapy of peripartum cardiomyopathy. *J Am Coll Cardiol* 1999; 34: 177–180.

78 McNamara D, Halubkov R, Starling RC, et al. Controlled trial of intravenous immunoglobulin in recent onset dilated cardiomyopathy. *Circulation* 2001; 103: 2254–2259.

79 Phillips S, Warnes CA. Peripartum cardiomyopathy: current therapeutic perspectives. *Curr Treat Options Cardiovasc Med* 2004; 6: 481–488.

80 Aziz T, Burgess M, Acladiom NN, et al. Heart transplantation for peripartum cardiomyopathy: a report of three cases and a literature review. *Cardiovasc Surg* 1999; 7: 565–567.

81 Caulin-Glaser T, Serato JF. Pregnancy and cardiovascular disease. In: Burrow C, Duffy TP, eds. *Medical Complications During Pregnancy*, 5th edn. Philadelphia: Saunders, 1999.

82 Desai D, Adanlauvo M, Naidou DP, et al. Mitral stenosis in pregnancy: a four year experience at King Edward II hospital, Durban, South Africa. *Br J Obstet Gynaecol* 2000; 107: 953.

83 Silva A, Shah AM. Moderate mitral stenosis in pregnancy: the haemodynamic impact of duress. *Heart* 2005; 91: e3.

84 Saisione A, Ivester T, Largoya M, et al. Acute pulmonary edema in pregnancy. *Obstet Gynecol* 2003; 101: 511–515.

85 Rabiely G, Prystawsky E, Zipes D, et al. Clinical and electrophysiological findings in patients with repetitive mono morphic ventricular tachycardia and otherwise normal electro-cardiogram. *Am J Cardiol* 1982; 50: 459–468.

86 Page R, Shenasa H, Evans J, et al. Radiofrequency catheter oblation of idiopathic recurrent ventricular tachycardia with a right bundle branch block, left axis pattern pace. *Clin Electrophysiol* 1993; 16: 327–336.

87 Chow T, Galvin J, McGovern B. Antiarrhythmic drug therapy in pregnancy and lactation. *Am J Cardiol* 1998; 82: 581–621.

88 Trappe HJ. Acute therapy of maternal and fetal arrhythmia during pregnancy. *J Intens Care Med* 2006; 21: 305–315.

89 Trappe HJ. Long-term outcomes of out-of-hospital cardiac arrest after successful early defibrillation. *Intensiv Medizin* 2005; 42: 311–316.

90 Trappe HJ. Early defibrillation: where are we? *Dtsch Med Wochenschr* 2005; 130: 685–688.

91 Natule A, Davidson T, Geiger M, Newby K. Implantable cardioventer-defibrillators and pregnancy. A safe combination? *Circulation* 1997; 96: 2808–2812.
92 Plunkett M, Bond L, Geiss DM. Staged repair of acute type aortic dissection and correlation in pregnancy. *Ann Thorac Surg* 2000; 69: 1945–1947.
93 Zeebregts C, Schepeus M, Hamceteman T, Morshires N, de la Riviere AB. Acute aortic dissection complicating pregnancy. *Ann Thorac Surg* 1997; 64: 1345–1348.
94 Katy N, Cullen J, Morout M, et al. Aortic dissection during pregnancy: treatment by emergency caesarean section immediately followed by operative repair of the dissection. *Am J Cardiol* 1984; 54: 699–701.
95 Lipscomb K, Clayton-Smith J, Clarke B, et al. Outcome of pregnancy in women with Marfan's syndrome. *Br J Obstet Gynaecol* 1997; 104: 201–206.
96 Weiss B, von Segesser L, Alou F, et al. Outcome of cardiovascular surgery and pregnancy: a systematic review of the period 1984–1996. *Am J Obstet Gynecol* 1998; 179: 1643–1653.
97 Belfort M, Rokey R, Saade G, Moise KJ. Rapid echocardiographic assessment of left and right heart hemodynamics in critically ill obstetric patients. *Am J Obstet Gynecol* 1994; 171: 884–892.

41 Septic Shock

Errol R. Norwitz[1] & Hee Joong Lee[2]

[1]Department of Obstetrics and Gynecology, Tufts University School of Medicine and Tufts Medical Center, Boston, MA, USA
[2]Department of Obstetrics and Gynecology, The Catholic University of Korea, Seoul, Korea

Introduction

Shock is a generalized physiologic state characterized by a significant reduction in tissue perfusion resulting in decreased tissue oxygen delivery. Although the effects of inadequate tissue perfusion are initially reversible, prolonged oxygen deprivation leads to generalized cellular hypoxia, end-organ damage, multiple organ system failure, and death [1]. For these reasons, prompt recognition and appropriate management of shock is crucial. Any classification scheme simplifies the complex pathophysiology underlying the many individual causes of shock. Three broad types of shock are recognized characterized by one of three primary physiologic derangements: (i) decreased preload (hypovolemic shock); (ii) pump failure (cardiogenic shock); and (iii) a severe drop in systemic vascular resistance with a compensatory increase in cardiac output (known as distributive or vascular shock) (Table 41.1).

Septic shock describes the constellation of clinical findings that results from the systemic inflammatory response to an infectious insult (defined in Table 41.2). It is characterized by an inability of the host to maintain vascular integrity and fluid homeostasis resulting in inadequate tissue oxygenation and circulatory failure. The spectrum of host response ranges from simple sepsis to septic shock with multiple-organ system dysfunction and death. Patients with septic shock require early and aggressive intervention, and often succumb despite timely and appropriate therapy. The annual incidence of sepsis is estimated at 50–95 cases per 100 000, and has increased over the past 20 years by 9% per annum [2]. Sepsis accounts for 2% of overall hospital admissions. Roughly 9% of patients with sepsis progress on to severe sepsis, and 3% of those with severe sepsis develop septic shock [3]. Septic shock accounts for approximately 10% of admissions to non-coronary intensive care units (ICUs) and is the 13th leading cause of death in the United States. Its incidence appears to be increasing [4]. After correcting for the increased age of the population, the rate of septic shock reported by the Centers for Disease Control and Prevention of the United States (CDC) more than doubled between 1979 and 1987. Moreover, this increased rate of septic shock was observed regardless of age group or geographic area [5].While improvements in care have led to a decrease in septic shock mortality rates over the past two decades [6,7], the overall number of patients dying from sepsis is growing as more patients are affected. Moreover, despite improvements in ICU care, the mortality rate from septic shock remains at 40–50% in most series [8], and an additional 20% of hospital survivors may succumb within the following year [9]. Short-term mortality appears to be related to the number of organ systems affected. The average risk of death increases by 15–20% with failure of each additional organ system [10]. If there is evidence of renal, pulmonary, and cerebral dysfunction, mortality may be as high as 70% [2]. Although septic shock remains an uncommon event in the obstetric population, factors that contribute to the increased rate of sepsis in the general population are also more common in women of reproductive age. Additionally, because maternal mortality is so uncommon, sepsis remains an important overall cause of maternal mortality [11].

Systemic inflammatory response syndrome

The systemic inflammatory response syndrome (SIRS) describes a generalized inflammatory response of the host to a variety of insults. Its etiology is not limited to infection, since burn injuries, trauma, and inflammatory conditions (such as pancreatitis) can elicit a similar clinical picture. It is characterized by two or more of the following cardinal signs: (i) a body temperature less than 36°C or more than 38°C; (ii) a pulse rate greater than 90 beats per minute (bpm); (iii) tachypnea manifesting as a respiratory rate exceeding 20 breaths per minute or a P_aCO_2 less than 32 mmHg; and/or (iv) a circulating leukocyte count less than 4000/μL, greater than 12 000/μL, or more than 10% immature

Critical Care Obstetrics, 5th edition. Edited by M. Belfort, G. Saade, M. Foley, J. Phelan and G. Dildy.

Table 41.1 Pathophysiology and hemodynamic profile of shock states.

Type of shock	Physiologic variable				Causes
	Preload	Pump function	Afterload	Tissue perfusion	
	Clinical measurement				
	Pulmonary capillary wedge pressure	Cardiac output	Systemic vascular resistance	Mixed venous oxygen saturation	
Hypovolemic shock	(↓)	↓	↑	↓	Hemorrhage Fluid loss
Cardiogenic shock	↑	(↓)	↑	↓	Cardiomyopathy Arrhythmias Valvular disease Obstruction
Distributive (vasodilatory) shock	↓ or ↔	↑	(↓)	↑	Septic shock Toxic shock syndrome Anaphylaxis Drug/toxin reaction Myxedema coma Neurogenic shock Burn shock

Adapted from Gaieski D, Manaker S. General evaluation and differential diagnosis of shock in adults. UpToDate, 2007. The primary pathophysiologic defect for each type of shock is highlighted.

forms on the differential count. A consensus committee in 1991 concluded that evidence of SIRS in the setting of suspected or proven infection should be regarded as diagnostic of *sepsis* [12].

Severe sepsis is diagnosed when SIRS is associated with organ dysfunction, tissue hypoperfusion, and/or hypotension. Useful indicators of tissue hypoperfusion include lactic acidosis, oliguria, or an acute alteration in mental status. Hypotension may not be present if the patient is on exogenous vasopressor support. Other features of severe sepsis may include acute lung injury (acute respiratory distress syndrome [ARDS]), coagulopathy, thrombocytopenia, and acute renal, liver, or cardiac failure [1,12,13]. Multiple-organ system dysfunction syndrome (MODS) is the terminal phase of this spectrum, represented by the progressive physiologic deterioration of interdependent organ systems such that homeostasis cannot be maintained without active intervention. If hypotension and reduced tissue perfusion persists despite adequate fluid resuscitation, then a diagnosis of *septic shock* (severe sepsis with cardiovascular failure) should be made. Refractory hypotension is defined as a systolic blood pressure less than 90 mmHg, mean arterial pressure less than 65 mmHg, or a decrease of 40 mmHg in systolic blood pressure compared to baseline which is unresponsive to a crystalloid fluid challenge of 20–40 mL/kg.

Pathophysiology of septic shock

Infection with a pathogenic organism results in cellular activation of monocytes, macrophages, and neutrophils and induction of a proinflammatory cascade triggered by interaction between the organism and a number of pathogen recognition receptors in the host [14]. The proinflammatory mediators, in turn, induce a systemic response (characterized by tachycardia, tachypnea, and hypotension) and – if excessive or uncontrolled – can lead to end-organ dysfunction, including ARDS and acute renal failure [15]. In such patients, the severity of the clinical presentation [16] and the mortality rate [8] is dependent largely on the vigor of the host's inflammatory response and *not* on the virulence of the inciting infection.

For the most part, Gram-negative sepsis has been the model used to study this phenomenon in experimental animals. In this model, endotoxin – a complex lipopolysaccharide (LPS) present in the cell wall of aerobic Gram-negative bacteria that is released at the time of the organism's death – appears to be a critical factor in inducing the pathophysiologic derangements associated with septic shock [11]. A similar mechanism may also be responsible for the development of shock in the setting of Gram-positive sepsis [17]. Indeed, Cleary et al. [18] demonstrated that patients

Table 41.2 Definitions.*

	Definition	Is a positive blood/tissue culture required for the diagnosis?
Infection	A microbial phenomenon characterized by an inflammatory response to the presence of micro-organisms or the invasion of normally sterile host tissue by those organisms	Yes
Bacteremia	The presence of viable bacteria in the blood	Yes
Systemic inflammatory response syndrome (SIRS)	SIRS is a widespread inflammatory response to a variety of severe clinical insults. This syndrome is clinically recognized by the presence of two or more of the following: – Temperature >38°C or <36°C – Heart rate >90 beats/min – Respiratory rate >20 breaths/min or $PaCO_2 < 32$ mmHg – WBC >12,000 cells/mm^3, <4000 cells/mm^3 or with >10% immature (band) forms	Yes
Sepsis	Sepsis is the systemic response to infection. Thus, in sepsis, the clinical signs describing SIRS are present together with definitive evidence of infection. In contrast to the lactic acidosis typically associated with septic shock, early sepsis may be associated with acute respiratory alkalosis due to stimulation of ventilation	No (a clinical diagnosis)
Severe sepsis	Sepsis is considered severe when it is associated with organ dysfunction, hypoperfusion or hypotension. The manifestations of hypoperfusion may include, but are not limited to, lactic acidosis, oliguria or an acute alteration in mental status	No (a clinical diagnosis)
Septic shock	Septic shock is sepsis with hypotension despite adequate fluid resuscitation combined with perfusion abnormalities that may include, but are not limited to, lactic acidosis, oliguria or an acute alteration in mental status. Patients who require inotropic or vasopressor support despite adequate fluid resuscitation are in septic shock. Septic shock is one of the forms of vasodilatory or distributive shock. It results from a marked reduction in systemic vascular resistance, often associated with an increase in cardiac output	No (a clinical diagnosis)

* Data from: American College of Chest Physicians and Society of Critical Care Medicine. Consensus Conference: Definitions for sepsis and organ failure and guidelines for the use of innovative therapies in sepsis. *Crit Care Med* 1992; 20: 864; Balk RA. Severe sepsis and septic shock. Definitions, epidemiology, and clinical manifestations. *Crit Care Clin* 2000; 16: 179; Levy MM, Fink MP, Marshall JC, et al. 2001 SCCM/ESICM/ACCP/ATS/SIS International Sepsis Definitions Conference. *Crit Care Med* 2003; 31: 1250.

infected with *Streptococcus pyogenes* are only at risk of developing septic shock if the isolates from the patients were able to produce exotoxin. Exotoxins released by *Clostridium perfringens*, *Staphylococcus aureus*, and Group A β-hemolytic streptococcus can cause rapid and extensive tissue necrosis and gangrene, especially of the postpartum uterus, leading to profound cardiovascular collapse and maternal death [19,20]. In addition to exotoxin, Gram-positive microorganisms also release peptidoglycans and lipoteichoic acid which can induce the production of proinflammatory mediators associated with sepsis [21]. The clinical presentation of septic shock is generally not helpful in identifying the underlying pathogenic mechanism.

Although the response of the host innate immune system is generally similar for all microorganisms, there are some pathogen-specific responses [17,22,23]. For example, highly antigenic toxins released by some *Staphylococcus* and *Streptococcus* species can directly activate T-lymphocytes without involving intermediate antigen-processing cells such as macrophages [24]. This abbreviated mechanism of T-lymphocyte activation may explain the rapid progression and fulminant clinical course seen with some Gram-positive bacterial infections.

The series of events initiated by endotoxin is presented schematically in Figure 41.1. The first event is a local activation of the immune system at the site of infection in an attempt to confine its spread. If the ability to contain the infection is lost, systemic activation of effector cells leads to the production of proinflammatory cytokines with widespread systemic effects and end-organ injury [25]. In this way, the initial infectious insult primes the immune system for an exaggerated and disproportionate response to any subsequent insult [26–30] with an outpouring of copious amounts of proinflammatory mediators [31]. Activation of the complement cascade also plays a central role in activation of the immune system [32] and can itself lead to the hemodynamic changes characteristic of sepsis in animal models [33].

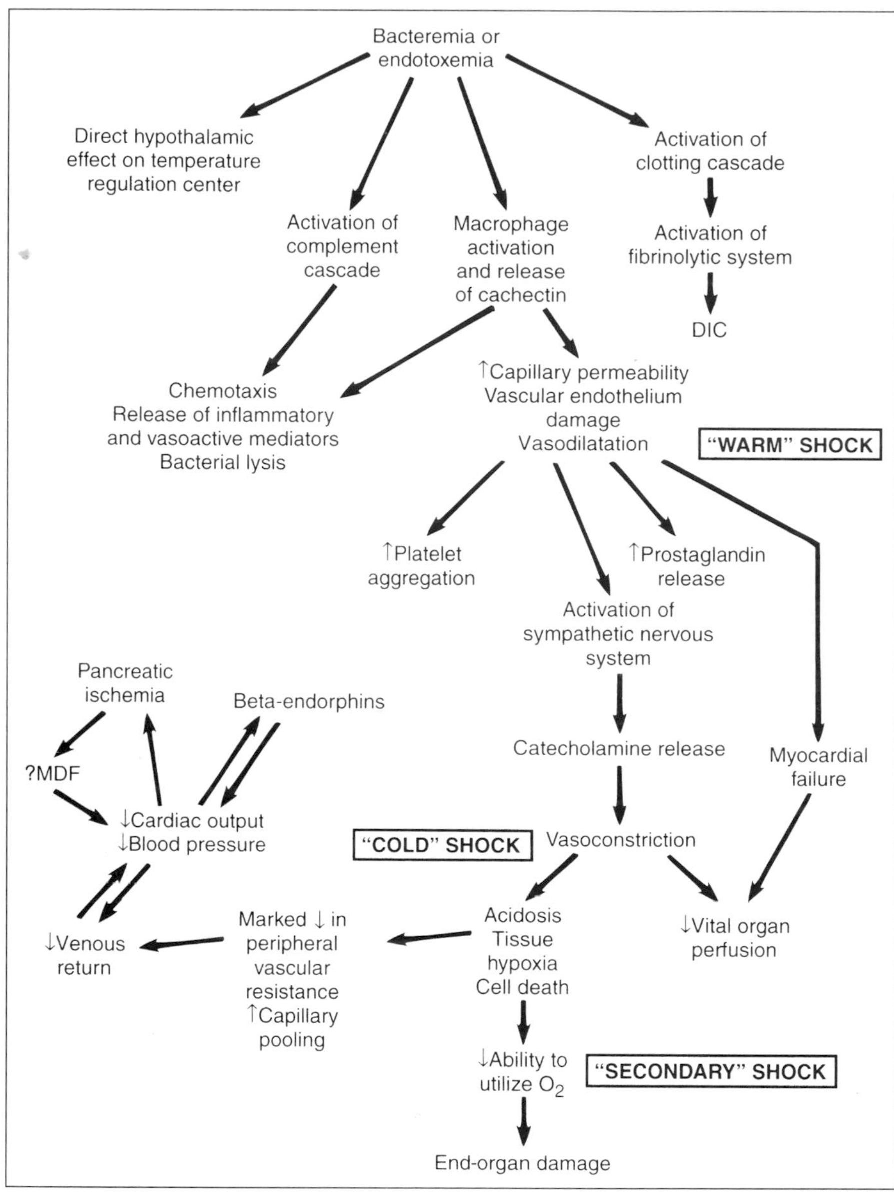

Figure 41.1 Pathophysiology of septic shock. DIC, disseminated intravascular coagulopathy; MDF, Myocardial depressant factor; O_2, oxygen.

Various proinflammatory mediators have been implicated in the pathogenesis of septic shock. Several lines of experimental evidence in both humans and animal models support a central role for tumor necrosis factor-α (TNF-α) in the pathophysiology of sepsis [34]. Large amounts of TNF-α are produced in response to LPS administered to healthy human subjects [35,36] and administration of either endotoxin or TNF-α provokes similar physiologic derangements to that seen in sepsis [37]. Elevated levels of TNF-α in animals are associated with irreversible shock and death [38,39], and infusion of TNF-α into experimental animals produces the pulmonary, renal, and gastrointestinal histopathology observed at autopsy in septic patients [40,41]. In similar experimental models, early and adequate administration of anti-TNF-α antiserum is able to protect against the development of sepsis leading to decreased mortality [42,43]. At a cellular level, LPS bound to a carrier protein interacts with pattern recognition molecules or receptors on the surface of target cells, such as CD14 and Toll-like receptors (TLRs). Activation of these receptors induces transcription of inflammatory and immune response genes typically by way of nuclear factor-κB (NFκB)-mediated mechanisms. Activation of this signal transduction cascade triggers the production and release of endogenous mediators, such as TNF-α and interleukin-1β (IL-1β), which amplify the LPS signal and transmit it to other cells and tissues. Currently, more than 10 TLR isoforms have been described in humans and the list of their specific microbial ligands is growing [44]. The presence of numerous TLR complexes on the surface of immune cells allows these cells to recognize many conserved microbial molecules. Lipopolysaccharide also binds to soluble CD14 to facilitate interaction with tissues lacking the CD14 receptor, such as vascular endothelium [45]. The production of TNF-α, in turn, stimulates the secretion of interleukins, prostaglandins, leukotrienes, and other inflammatory mediators. These inflammatory products cause the clinical symptoms associated with sepsis as well as capillary leak, hypotension, and activation of the coagulation system [46]. In a rabbit model of IL-1β-induced hypotension, the lung was the primary organ injured. Although both cytokines were able to produce massive pulmonary damage, TNF-α produced more injury than IL-1β. Moreover, these studies suggested that TNF-α and IL-1β may act synergistically to disrupt vascular endothelial integrity [47]. Additional evidence for the role of cytokines in mediating lung injury in ARDS includes the increased production of IL-1β and TNF-α by lung macrophages in response to LPS administration [48] and the *in vivo* observation that alveolar macrophages from ARDS patients produce increased amounts of IL-1β [49].

Vascular endothelium is a metabolically active tissue that exerts a pivotal role in the regulation of underlying vascular smooth muscle tone, the maintenance of vessel integrity and fluidity of blood, and the regulation of leukocyte adhesion. Maintenance of vascular homeostasis is regulated in large part by production of nitric oxide (originally identified as endothelium-derived relaxing factor) [50]. TNF-α stimulation of macrophages causes a sustained increase in nitric oxide production resulting in profound effects on vascular tone and permeability. This nitric oxide excess, in turn, leads to microvascular damage, vascular hyporeactivity, and multiorgan dysfunction likely through induction of apoptosis [51]. Cyclooxygenase is also activated, and the elaboration of prostaglandins contributes to the misdistribution of blood flow [52].

Stimulation of endothelial cells by several cytokines including IL-1α, IL-1β, and TNF-α results in endothelial activation, and alters the structural and metabolic functions of the endothelium. Rather than its usual anticoagulant properties, the endothelial lining of blood vessels becomes a procoagulant surface with upregulation of adhesion molecule expression, increased production of chemoattractant and vasoactive substances, and decreased expression of anticoagulants. Specifically, there is evidence of activation of the extrinsic pathway of the coagulation cascade with increased production of tissue factor (a critical promoter of the procoagulant pathway) and suppression of a number of key anticoagulant factors, including thrombomodulin, heparan sulfate, and protein C. In the normal state, few adhesion molecules are expressed on vascular endothelium. After activation by proinflammatory mediators, increased amounts of P-selectin, E-selectin, intercellular adhesion molecule-1, and other adhesion molecules are expressed on the surface of vascular endothelial cells. Leukocytes adhere and transmigrate into the inflamed tissues. This mechanism is designed to confine and localize the infection, but may also lead to endothelial dysfunction with capillary leakage. Systemic endothelial activation, with its associated outpouring of proinflammatory mediators and cytokines, facilitates the inflammatory cascade and worsens the clinical syndrome. As our understanding of this process grows, opportunities will be identified for targeted intervention to abort this systemic inflammatory cascade that leads to progressive multiorgan dysfunction [53].

Tumor necrosis factor-α and activated complement fragments attract neutrophils whose products exacerbate endothelial injury [54]. This results in altered ability of the host to maintain tissue perfusion through regulation of blood pressure, cardiac output (CO), and systemic vascular resistance (SVR) [15]. The production of IL-1β by macrophages also promotes procoagulant activity, which results in fibrin deposition in the microvasculature leading to further perturbations of organ perfusion [55–57]. Activation of the microvasculature endothelium by TNF-α and IL-1β produces capillary leak and increased leukocyte receptor expression. Leukocyte migration and activation result in release of vasoactive substances such as histamine, serotonin, and bradykinin. These substances, in turn, increase capillary permeability, induce endothelial damage, and promote vasodilation [26]. Neutrophil activation stimulates a respiratory burst with increased production and release of lysosomal enzymes and toxic oxygen species such as superoxide, hydroxyl, and peroxide radicals. This can have deleterious effects on the vasculature as well as other organs and is especially detrimental in the lung, where it is felt to play a key role in the pathogenesis of ARDS [50]. Stimulation of neutrophils by activated complement fragments also leads to leukotriene secretion, further affecting capillary permeability and blood flow distribution [57]. At the same time, the damage to the vascular endothelium stimulates platelet aggregation. Complement activation ensues, with microthrombus formation and fibrin deposition leading to further derangements of perfusion [58].

As discussed above, disruption of the endothelium and vascular smooth muscle is a well-recognized component of septic shock. This results also in a blunting of the response to vasoactive drugs. Because these effects can be blocked in experimental animal models by treatment with inhibitors of nitric oxide synthesis, alterations in nitric oxide metabolism are felt to play a role in the development of refractoriness to endogenous catecholamines and exogenous vasopressors [59]. The elaboration of inflammatory mediators may also affect sympathetic vasomotor tone resulting in impaired vasoconstriction to sympathetic stimulation. The combination of a leaky vasculature and loss of smooth muscle tone results in refractory hypotension [59,60].

An intact sympathetic reflex response to a local inflammatory event may produce profound vasoconstriction in some organ systems leading to a reduction in tissue perfusion [26]. Alternatively, a localized loss of control of vascular tone can result in a failure of arterioles to dilate in response to physiologic vasoactive substances such as histamine and bradykinin [61], leading to increased capillary leak and intravascular fluid depletion. The net result is a marked reduction in peripheral vascular resistance with extensive capillary pooling of blood. Cellular hypoxia and acidosis further disrupt the ability of individual cells to utilize available oxygen [62], leading to worsening tissue and organ damage.

Direct effects of bacterial immunologic complexes are also thought to play an important role in tissue injury [63]. Immune complex precipitants have been identified within the lung vasculature and are thought to contribute to the development of ARDS. Similarly, focal areas of acute tubular necrosis seen in the kidney have been associated with the deposition of inflammatory infiltrates.

Disseminated intravascular coagulopathy (DIC) frequently complicates septic shock. DIC involves activation of both the coagulation and fibrinolytic cascades leading to depletion of circulating coagulation factors (a consumptive coagulopathy). Tissue factor is released by TNF-α stimulation of monocytes and by exposure of subendothelial tissue factor following injury to the vascular endothelium with activation of the extrinsic pathway. Microvasculature fibrin deposition compromises end-organ perfusion. At the same time, TNF-α also inhibits the production and action of regulatory proteins such as protein C, thereby amplifying the procoagulant state. Although its role in DIC is not significant, activation of the intrinsic pathway provides a powerful stimulus to the production of kinins, such as bradykinin, thus contributing to hypotension and disruption of vascular homeostasis. Derangements in the coagulation system are magnified by the ability of endotoxin to rapidly activate and then suppress fibrinolysis, which again appears to be mediated by TNF-α [64].

Table 41.3 Clinical features of septic shock.

Early (warm) shock
Altered mental status
Peripheral vasodilation (warm skin, flushing)
Tachypnea or shortness of breath
Tachycardia
Temperature instability
Hypotension
Increased cardiac output and decreased peripheral resistance
Late (cold) shock
Peripheral vasoconstriction (cool, clammy skin)
Oliguria
Cyanosis
ARDS
Decreased cardiac output and decreased peripheral resistance
Secondary (irreversible) shock
Obtundation
Anuria
Hypoglycemia
Disseminated intravascular coagulation
Decreased cardiac output and decreased peripheral resistance
Myocardial failure

Clinical presentation of septic shock

The clinical presentation of shock varies with the type and cause, but several features are common including hypotension (defined as systolic blood pressure less than 90 mmHg), cool clammy skin and oliguria (due to redistribution of blood), changes in mental status (confusion, delirium, or coma), and metabolic acidosis. *Sepsis* refers to a clinical syndrome that encompasses a variety of host responses to systemic infection. As discussed above, the clinical spectrum of sepsis depends primarily on the host response to infection rather than the severity of the infection itself [16,65]. Because the clinical manifestations of sepsis can be recapitulated experimentally by infusing proinflammatory mediators (such as interleukins and TNF-α), an exaggerated host inflammatory response is felt to be central to its pathophysiology [43,47]. Although various risk factors have been identified and scoring systems developed, there is as yet no effective method to predict which patients will progress from bacteremia to septic shock and MODS [66]. In general, however, more severe inflammatory responses appear to be accompanied by progressively greater mortality rates [67]. The timing of onset of infection may also influence the clinical outcomes. A recent study showed that patients who developed septic shock within 24 hours of ICU admission were more severely ill but had better outcomes than patients who became hypotensive later during their ICU stay [68].

The clinical manifestations of septic shock fall into three broad categories, which correlate with progressive physiologic derangement (summarized in Table 41.3). *Early (warm) shock* is characterized by a hyperdynamic circulation and decreased SVR. The hallmark of *late (cold) shock* is abnormal tissue perfusion and oxygenation due to regional (peripheral) vasoconstriction and myocardial dysfunction. *Secondary (irreversible) shock* is frequently a terminal condition associated with multiple-organ system dysfunction. Each phase represents a continued downward progression in the course of this disease process.

In the early phase of septic shock, bacteremia is heralded typically by shaking chills, a sudden rise in temperature, tachycardia, and warm extremities. Although the patient may appear ill, the diagnosis of septic shock may be elusive until hypotension is evident. In addition, patients may present initially with nonspecific complaints such as malaise, nausea, vomiting, or even profuse diarrhea. Abrupt alterations in behavior and mental status changes, which have been attributed to a reduction in cerebral blood flow, may also herald the onset of septic shock. Tachypnea or dyspnea may be present with no objective findings on physical examination. These symptoms likely represent a direct effect of endotoxin on the respiratory center and may precede the development of clinical ARDS.

Laboratory findings are highly variable during the early stages of septic shock. The circulating WBC count may initially be depressed, although a marked leukocytosis is a more common finding. Although there may be a transient increase in circulating blood glucose levels due to catecholamine release, hypoglycemia is more likely to prevail later due to hepatic dysfunction and a reduction in gluconeogenesis. Evidence of a decreased platelet count, decreased fibrinogen, elevated fibrin split products, and elevated prothrombin time may suggest the presence of DIC. Initial arterial blood gas may show an initial transient respiratory alkalosis due to tachypnea, but this is likely to evolve with time into a metabolic acidosis with increased circulating levels of lactic acid resulting from tissue hypoxia.

In the setting of undiagnosed and untreated septic shock, profound and progressive myocardial depression will develop with a marked reduction in CO and SVR [69]. This will manifest clinically as cold extremities, oliguria, and peripheral cyanosis. Prolonged tissue hypoxia will lead to worsening metabolic acidosis, electrolyte imbalance, DIC, and mental status changes, which with time will become irreversible. The etiology of this myocardial depression is not clear. In contrast to patients with myocardial failure due structural heart disease or myocardial infarction [70], extensive studies in both humans and animal point to a circulating myocardial depressant factor or toxin as the cause of myocardial depression rather than an alteration in coronary flow or insufficient myocardial oxygenation [71]. In support of this hypothesis, infusion of endotoxin in healthy human subjects results in a decrease in myocardial performance and left ventricular dilation similar to that seen in patients with septic shock [72].

Echocardiography in women with septic shock may be helpful. Cardiac output and cardiac index (CI) are initially increased in women with septic shock due to a profound decrease in SVR and a compensatory increase in heart rate. However, this increase in CO is typically inadequate to meet the patient's metabolic needs. As a result, with time, both the left and right ventricles dilate, and the ejection fraction decreases [72]. Cardiac output is maintained despite the low ejection fraction because ventricular dilatation permits a normal stroke volume. The limitation in cardiac performance and ejection fraction is greater than that seen in equally ill non-septic patients [73]. Ventricular compliance is also affected in women with sepsis as evidenced by a decreased ability of the myocardium to response to an increase in preload [74].

To better understand the hemodynamic response to sepsis, Parker & Parillo [69] studied 20 subjects with septic shock. By conventional criteria, 95% of the patients would have been classified as hyperdynamic, but 10 of the 20 (50%) had abnormally depressed ejection fractions that could not be accounted for by differences in preload, afterload, or positive end-expiratory pressure (PEEP). In the acute phase of septic shock, dilatation of the left ventricle appears to represent an adaptive response that confers a survival advantage, since it allows for the CO to be maintained in the face of a declining ejection fraction [73]. Two discrete subsets of patients were identified based on their response to volume loading: those who respond with ventricular dilation and increased CO (better prognosis) and those who respond with increased pulmonary capillary wedge pressure (PCWP) and no increase in CO (poorer prognosis) [75]. Cardiac depression of similar magnitude and frequency has also been reported in obstetric patients with septic shock managed with pulmonary artery (PA) catheters [76].

Predisposing factors in obstetrics

The ability of both Gram-positive and Gram-negative organisms to systematically activate the inflammatory cascade has particular relevance in the obstetric patient, in whom mixed polymicrobial infections are commonly identified [77]. Although Gram-negative coliforms make up a significant portion of the organisms recovered in bacteremic obstetric patients, other organisms, including aerobic and anaerobic streptococci, *Bacteroides fragilis*, and *Gardnerella vaginalis*, are found frequently. Septic shock in pregnancy associated with legionella pneumonia has also been described [78]. As in other areas of medicine, the number of cases of obstetric sepsis associated with Group A streptococcus appears to be increasing [79].

Pregnancy has been described as an immunocompromised state, although little objective evidence exists comparing the ability of pregnant and non-pregnant individuals to process bacterial antigens and elicit an appropriate immune response. Pregnant women remain at risk for common medical and surgical illnesses (such as pneumonia and appendicitis) as well as conditions unique to pregnancy (for example, intra-amniotic infection and septic abortion), all of which may result in sepsis. If the pregnancy is not the cause of the infection, delivery is not generally indicated. Supportive care should include control of fever with antipyretics, cooling blankets, or both. The fetus should be resuscitated *in utero* with correction of maternal acidosis, hypoxemia, and systemic hypotension, which will usually improve any abnormalities in the fetal heart tracing. Although genital tract infections are common on an obstetric service [80–82], septic shock in this same population tends to be an uncommon event. When an obstetric patient has clinical evidence of local infection, the incidence of bacteremia is approximately 8–10% [77,83–86]. Overall, rates of bacteremia of 7.5 per 1000 admissions to the obstetrics and gynecology services at two large teaching hospitals have been reported [83,84]. More striking is that patients with bacteremia rarely progress to develop more significant complications, including septic shock. Ledger and colleagues [83] identified only a 4% rate of septic shock in pregnant patients with bacteremia. This value is in agreement with that of other investigators, who have reported a 0–12% incidence of septic shock in bacteremic obstetric and gynecologic patients [77,83–87]. Obstetric conditions that have been identified as predisposing to the development of septic shock are listed in Table 41.4 [84,87,88–92].

The physiologic changes that accompany pregnancy may place the gravida at greater risk for morbidity than her non-pregnant counterpart. Elevation of the diaphragm by the gravid uterus, delayed gastric emptying, and the emergent nature of many intubations in obstetrics dramatically increases the risk of aspiration pneumonitis (Mendelson's syndrome). Although the pregnant patient has been previously identified as being at increased risk of pulmonary sequelae from systemic infection such as pyelonephritis, the pathophysiologic mechanisms have been known only for the past decade [93]. Hemodynamic investigation in normal women using flow-directed PA catheters has quantified the physiologic alterations that place the patient at increased risk for pulmonary injury. Pregnancy decreases the gradient between colloid osmotic pressure (COP) and PCWP [94]. This increases the propensity for pulmonary edema if pulmonary capillary permeability changes or the PCWP increases. In the critically ill, non-pregnant patient, decreases in the COP–PCWP gradient predict an increased propensity for pulmonary edema [95,96,97]. The intrapulmonary shunt fraction (Q_S/Q_T) is also increased in normal pregnancy [98], which may further increase the risk of pulmonary morbidity.

Fortunately, mortality from septic shock, which is extremely high in the setting of bacteremia in other medical and surgical specialties, tends to be an infrequent event in obstetrics and gynecology. The incidence of death from sepsis is estimated at 0–3% in obstetric patients as compared with 10–81% in non-obstetric patients [83,84,90,99]. Suggested reasons for this observation of a more favorable outcome in pregnant woman include: (i) younger age group; (ii) transient nature of the bacteremia; (iii) type of organisms involved; (iv) a primary site of infection (pelvis) that is more amenable to both surgical and medical intervention; and (v) lack of associated medical diseases that could adversely impact the prognosis for recovery. Evidence in support of the latter explanation comes from earlier studies demonstrating increased mortality in septic non-pregnant patients with underlying comorbid disease [100].

Table 41.4 Bacterial infections associated with septic shock in the obstetric population.

	Incidence (%)
Chorioamnionitis	0.5–1.0
Postpartum endometritis	
– After cesarean delivery	0.5–85
– After vaginal delivery	<10
Urinary tract infection	1–4
Pyelonephritis	1–4
Septic abortion	1–2
Necrotizing fasciitis (postoperative)	<1
Toxic shock syndrome	<1

Pregnancy and septic shock

The pregnant host may be different from the traditional septic shock host in ways other than the difference in microbiologic pathogens involved. Physiologic adaptations to pregnancy designed to promote favorable maternal and fetal outcome occur in almost every organ system (summarized in Table 41.5) [94,98,101–103]. Some of these changes, such as a dramatic increase in pelvic vascularity, promote maternal survival after infection. They may also influence the presentation and course of septic shock in the gravida, although this idea has received little attention in the published literature. On the other hand, other physiologic adaptations to pregnancy (e.g. ureteral dilatation) may predispose the gravid female to more significant infectious morbidity than her non-pregnant counterpart.

In an animal model of endotoxin-induced septic shock, Beller and coworkers [104] compared pregnant and non-pregnant responses to fixed doses of LPS. The pregnant animals had a much more pronounced respiratory and metabolic acidosis than did the controls, and they died significantly faster than did non-pregnant controls due primarily to cardiovascular collapse.

Table 41.5 Hemodynamic and ventilatory parameters in pregnancy.

	Non-pregnant	Pregnant	Relative change
Cardiac output (L/min)	4.3	6.2	+43%
Heart rate (bpm)	71	83	+17%
Systemic vascular resistance (dyne/sec/cm^5)	1530	1210	+21%
Pulmonary vascular resistance (dyne/sec/cm^5)	119	78	+34%
COP (mmHg)	20.8	18.0	+14%
COP–PCWP gradient (mmHg)	14.5	10.5	+18%
Mean arterial pressure (mmHg)	86.4	90.3	No change
Central venous pressure (mmHg)	3.7	3.6	No change
PCWP (mmHg)	6.3	7.5	No change
Left ventricular stroke work index (g/m/m^2)	41	48	No change

From Clark SL, Cotton DB, Lee W, et al. Central hemodynamic assessment of normal term pregnancy. *Am J Obstet Gynecol* 1989; 161: 1439–1442.

COP, colloid osmotic pressure; PCWP, pulmonary capillary wedge pressure.

Although the increased susceptibility to endotoxin-mediated injury in pregnant animals is a consistent observation in the literature [104–106], different animal species appear to succumb to different physiologic aberrations. As such, caution is warranted in applying the results of animal studies to critically ill pregnant women.

It is interesting to note that, in experimental animal models, the fetus is more resistant to the deleterious effects of endotoxin than is the mother. Bech-Jansen et al. [105] demonstrated that, although blood flow to the uterus declined out of proportion to maternal hypotension, the fetal sheep was able to tolerate endotoxin doses tenfold higher than those proven to be lethal in adult pregnant sheep. Indeed, the fetal circulation was not affected until the adult's condition was terminal. The investigators suggest that this protective effect is due to the immature status of the fetal vascular responsiveness. In contrast, Morishima et al. [106] administered endotoxin to pregnant baboons and observed rapid and profound fetal asphyxia, acidemia, and death in concert with maternal circulatory collapse. The investigators concluded that the rapid deterioration in fetal wellbeing was due primarily to maternal factors such as hypotension and increased myometrial activity, both of which contributed to a reduction in placental perfusion. Although the pathophysiologic basis for the increased susceptibility to endotoxin-mediated injury during gestation remains speculative, published data suggest that a pregnant woman should be considered a compromised host. The response of the parturient to an infectious stimulus probably represents the combined effects of alterations in her physiology as well as enhanced responsiveness to the effects of endotoxin. Although the fetus is likely more resistant to the effects of endotoxin than the mother, alterations in uteroplacental flow can lead to hypoxia, acidosis, placental abruption, fetal cerebral injury (including intracranial hemorrhage and global hypoxic injury), and fetal demise.

As expected in an uncommon condition, the available human data regarding septic shock in human pregnancy are limited. Data describing contemporary ICU management of the septic obstetric patient, including invasive hemodynamic monitoring, are even more scarce. Published studies tend to be small and heterogenous and suffer from significant ascertainment bias. The hemodynamic alterations seen in this patient population have been described in a review of women with sepsis in pregnancy whose management was guided by a PA catheter [76]. In this series, maternal morbidity was 20%. Similar to the non-pregnant patient, septic shock in pregnant women was accompanied by an overall decrease in SVR, although the absolute SVR measurement varied widely depending on the stage of shock at which the PA catheter was initially inserted. At presentation, a normal to increased CO and decreased SVR were observed. Those patients who ultimately survived demonstrated an increase in mean arterial pressure (MAP), SVR, and left ventricular stroke work index (LVSWI) in response to therapy. Indeed, LVSWI appeared to be the best measure of cardiac function and predictor of outcome. Longitudinal measurements of SVR also proved to be useful in monitoring the progress of therapy. Response to treatment was reflected in normalization of the SVR [76]. These findings are consistent with physiologic patterns observed in non-pregnant septic shock patients [107].

Diagnosis of septic shock in pregnancy

Early diagnosis of septic shock is critical to improve outcome. There is no definitive diagnostic test, and a high index of clinical suspicion in the appropriate clinical setting is needed to confirm the diagnosis. A rapid and focused history and examination should be performed (see Table 41.6). The patient is rarely able to provide any history. As such, historical data are often obtained from relatives and available medical records. The patient's recent complaints, activities prior to presentation, and general physical condition may hold valuable information about the primary cause of shock. A battery of laboratory tests should be sent in an effort to identify potential causes for shock and early signs of organ failure. These are summarized in Table 41.6. Blood type and cross-matching should also be done, especially if the hematocrit is low, in anticipation of blood transfusion. Initial blood count may demonstrate an increase in hematocrit due to increased vascular permeability and hemoconcentration, and initial fluid resuscitation may result in a decrease in hematocrit. Although leukocytosis with a left shift (increase in immature white blood cells) may suggest the diagnosis of bacterial infection, these tests have a poor sensitivity and specificity. Indeed, overwhelming septic shock may be associated with leucopenia. Thrombocytopenia may be an early sign of DIC and is an independent predictor of multiorgan failure and poor outcome. Although non-specific, an elevated D-dimer level is associated with the development of septic shock and death, and declining levels in response to therapy are a good prognostic feature [108,109]. Elevated and increasing circulating lactate levels in patients admitted with septic shock are associated with poor prognosis and can be used to guide response to therapy [110]. Blood culture yields increase with greater blood volume and the number of specimens collected. Multiple specimens from varying sites can also be useful in distinguishing true pathogens from contaminants. Therefore, patients being evaluated for septic shock should have at least two blood cultures obtained from separate sites [111–113]. If infection of an indwelling line is suspected, the catheter should be removed as soon as possible and the tip cultured. Gram stain and culture of secretions from any potential site of infection (such as urine, sputum, and cerebrospinal fluid) should be performed. Provisional results from these collections are often the only immediately available data to aid in the selection of antimicrobial therapy.

Identification of a pathogenic organism from blood or tissue culture in the appropriate clinical setting will usually confirm a diagnosis of septic shock. However, culture results often take 24–48 hours to come back and, even then, are negative in up to 30% of cases of suspected septic shock. While this may

Table 41.6 Diagnosis of septic shock.

History
Presenting complaints
Activities/travel prior to presentation
Food and medicine allergies
Recent changes in medications
Potential acute or chronic drug intoxication
Pre-existing medical diseases
Immunosuppression (such as HIV disease)
Hypercoagulable conditions
Physical examination
ENT examination: evidence of scleral jaundice; dry conjunctivae and mucous membranes; pinpoint pupils; dilated and fixed pupils; nystagmus
Neck examination: jugular venous distension; carotid bruits; meningeal signs
Pulmonary system: tachypnea; shallow breaths; crackles (rales); consolidation; egophony; absent breath sounds; rub
Cardiovascular system: irregular rhythm; tachycardia; bradycardia; S3 gallop; ventricular heave; murmurs; distant heart sounds; rub; pulsus paradoxus
Abdomen: distension; tenderness; rebound; guarding; absence of or high-pitched bowel sounds; pulsatile masses; hepatosplenomegaly; ascites
Rectal examination: decreased tone; bright red blood; melena; Hemoccult-positive stool
Extremities: swollen calf; palpable cord; unequal intensity of pulses or disparity of blood pressure between upper extremities
Neurologic examination: agitation; confusion; delirium; obtundation; coma
Skin: cold, clammy or warm, hyperemic skin; rashes; petechiae; urticaria; cellulitis
Laboratory evaluation
Complete blood count with differential count
Basic chemistry tests
Liver function tests
Amylase and lipase (to diagnose pancreatitis)
Coagulation profile, including fibrinogen and fibrin split products
Lactate
Cardiac enzymes
Arterial blood gases
Toxicology screen (blood and urine)
Chest radiograph
Abdominal radiograph (to exclude intestinal obstruction)
Electrocardiogram
Urinalysis
Search for infection, if indicated (including blood culture, urine culture, chest radiograph, lumbar puncture)

be due to early and aggressive use of antibiotics, it is more likely because the systemic manifestations of sepsis result from toxic agents released by pathogens or proinflammatory cascades triggered by pathogens rather than from the pathogens themselves. Some investigators have recommended routine serum analysis for endotoxin. However, such tests have been shown to have limited diagnostic values and, although present in 30–40% of patients with Gram-negative sepsis, elevated serum levels of endotoxin can also be detected in patients with Gram-positive bacteremia.

High concentration of inflammatory mediators in serum or tissue may be helpful in confirming the diagnosis of culture-negative septic shock. Serum concentrations of procalcitonin are usually increased in sepsis, but may also increase in non-septic conditions, including post-cardiopulmonary bypass surgery and pancreatitis. Nevertheless, the high negative predictive value of a normal serum procalcitonin level (<0.25 μg/L) can be used to exclude a diagnosis of septic shock and thereby avoid unnecessary use of antibiotics [114,115]. Another marker, TREM-1 (triggering receptor expressed on myeloid cells-1) has been shown to be strongly and specifically expressed on the surface of neutrophils and macrophages from human tissues infected with bacteria or fungi [116,117]. Elevated concentrations of soluble TREM-1 in bronchoalveolar lavage fluid (>5 ng/L) are associated with ventilator-associated pneumonia, and plasma concentrations of soluble TREM-1 of 60 mg/L or more have been associated with infection in patients with systemic inflammatory response syndrome [118]. Some patients with septic shock will have inadequate adrenal reserves as evidenced by an inadequate response when challenged with either adrenocorticotropic hormone (ACTH) or corticotrophin-releasing hormone (CRH). Relative adrenal insufficiency, defined as an increase in serum cortisol level of less than or equal to 9 μg/dL measured 1 hour after administration of 250 μg of ACTH, is present in 56–77% of mechanically ventilated patients who have refractory septic shock [111,119,120,121]. Although many investigators include a need for vasopressors to maintain arterial pressure as an important criterion for the diagnosis of shock, incorporation of other criteria – such as low central venous oxygen saturation (<70%), direct non-invasive visualization of altered microcirculation, and/or impaired cardiovascular variability – could provide for earlier diagnosis [122].

Treatment of septic shock

Over 750 000 cases of sepsis occur in the United States each year, resulting in approximately 200 000 fatalities [123]. Unfortunately, even with optimal treatment, the mortality rate from severe sepsis or septic shock is approximately 40% [124] and can exceed 50–70% in the sickest patients [125,126]. Early recognition and management of septic shock is critical to optimize outcome. A significant reduction in septic shock-related mortality is seen if normal physiologic parameters can be achieved through the use of aggressive hemodynamic resuscitation within 6 hours of presentation [122].

Once recognized, goal-directed intervention for the management of septic shock should be instituted immediately with placement of a subclavian or internal jugular central venous catheter for monitoring central venous pressure (CVP) and central venous oxygen saturation ($S_{cv}O_2$). Initial management should include the following.

1 Improvement in functional circulating intravascular volume through the aggressive use of volume replacement and inotropic

support to treat hypotension as evidenced by meeting the targeted hemodynamic goals: CVP 8–12 mmHg, MAP ≥65 mmHg, $S_{cv}O_2$ >70%, and urine output ≥0.5 mL/kg/h [122,127].
2 Establishment and maintenance of an adequate airway to facilitate management of respiratory failure.
3 Assurance of adequate tissue perfusion and oxygenation as evidenced by normalization of mixed venous oxygenation, arterial lactate levels, and acid–base status.
4 Initiation of diagnostic evaluations to determine the septic focus and remove it, if possible (abscesses should be drained and extensive soft tissue infections should be debrided or amputated).
5 Institution of empiric antimicrobial therapy to eradicate the most likely pathogens. Although not currently recommended, future management algorithms will likely include treatment with anti-inflammatory mediators [128].

In pregnancy, the initial management should focus on maternal resuscitation even in the face of potential injury to the fetus. Because fetal compromise in the setting of septic shock results primarily from maternal cardiovascular decompensation, improvements in the maternal status should have an immediate positive effect on the fetal condition. Furthermore, any attempt to deliver the fetus by emergency cesarean in the setting of maternal hemodynamic instability due to septic shock may further increase the risk of maternal mortality. In a mother who is not adequately resuscitated or is hemodynamically unstable, a further decrease in intravascular volume due, for example, to excessive blood loss at the time of cesarean may result in irreversible hemodynamic decompensation. The only exception to this course of management is if the fetal compartment is the source of sepsis (chorioamnionitis). Under such circumstances, immediate cesarean to deliver the fetus and drain the infection is indicated.

Resuscitation

The first step in the management of the patient with septic shock is to assess the airway, respiration, and perfusion. Subsequently, efforts should be taken to restore the blood pressure to levels that perfuse core organs. Supplemental oxygen should be supplied to all patients with sepsis, and oxygenation monitored using continuous pulse oximetry. Intubation may be required for airway protection because encephalopathy and a depressed level of consciousness frequently complicate sepsis [129].

Volume expansion

The mainstay of the acute management of septic shock involves volume expansion and correction of absolute or relative hypovolemia [63,130–134]. Such therapy correlates closely with improvement in CO, oxygen delivery, and survival [135]. At times, considerable quantities of fluid are needed because of profound vasodilation, increased capillary permeability, and extravasation of fluid into the extravascular space. Serial measurements of blood pressure, heart rate, urine output, and hematocrit are conventionally used to assess the adequacy of intravascular volume. While these criteria are adequate for the initiation of volume resuscitation, they are unreliable in guiding optimal fluid and inotrope management in the patient with septic shock or multiple-organ system dysfunction [136]. The best means of monitoring this critical therapy is with the use of a flow-directed PA catheter [137,138]. Although CVP monitoring has been suggested as an acceptable alternative, available evidence suggests that CVP monitoring alone will give erroneous information in many cases because of discordance between the left- and right-sided pressures and that a flow-directed PA catheter should be used in all cases [139]. In addition, PA catheterization allows determination of CO and the calculation of variables related to oxygen delivery and utilization. These determinants cannot be made with standard CVP systems. Use of a PA catheter to optimize oxygen delivery and allow earlier intervention in the event of decompensation has been shown to decrease morbidity and mortality in high-risk surgical ICU patients [128,137].

A common endpoint for volume replacement is a PCWP of 14–16 mmHg, a point at which, according to Starling's law, ventricular performance is optimal. However, sepsis significantly alters Starling forces and ventricular performance. As such, rather than selecting a specific numerical value as an endpoint, therapy should be titrated to optimize cardiopulmonary performance [72,132,140]. PCWP is used as an indicator of left ventricular end-diastolic pressure (LVEDP). Left ventricular end-diastolic volume (LVEDV) and circulating intravascular volume are inferred from the PCWP. For a given volume, LVEDP will vary with left ventricular compliance, which is influenced by a multitude of factors in the septic patient [132,141]. Fluid resuscitation is a dynamic process, not an endpoint, and the value for PCWP that optimizes preload will vary from patient to patient. Therapy should be optimized for the individual patient by sequentially expanding intravascular volume until a plateau is reached where further volume challenge produces no incremental increase in CO [72]. An elevated PCWP may reflect an overexpanded intravascular space, a reduced left ventricular function, or both. The LVSWI can be used to differentiate between these two possibilities and select appropriate intervention. Information obtained from the PA catheter should be interpreted based on norms established for pregnancy rather than those derived from a nonpregnant population.

Controversy surrounds the debate about the optimal type of fluid to be used for volume expansion. Although isotonic crystalloid solutions such as normal saline are advocated most often, some investigators have recommended the use of colloid solutions (e.g. 5% normal human albumin) to maintain a normal COP–PCWP gradient [142]. Rackow et al. [133] have suggested that maintenance of the balance between COP and PCWP reduces the risk of pulmonary edema. Various colloid and crystalloid solutions have been studied. In one series, both were able to restore cardiac function and hemodynamic stability, but the use of crystalloid required 2–4 times as much volume to achieve the same hemodynamic endpoint. One liter of normal saline solution adds 275 mL to the plasma volume, whereas 1 L of 5% albumin will increase plasma volume by 500 mL. Crystalloids significantly decrease the COP and the COP–PCWP gradient with a commensurate increase in the potential for pulmonary edema. These findings are supported by the results of others who, in addition, found that the risk of pulmonary edema was lower in younger patients [95,97]. These authors concluded that younger, healthier patients are more able to tolerate crystalloid resuscitation. Colloids also have been shown to increase oxygen delivery and extraction [143]. Coupled with the decrease in COP and increased risk of pulmonary edema with massive infusion of crystalloids, further study in a homogenous group of patients is warranted. In clinical trials comparing crystalloid and colloid resuscitation, different endpoints and methodologies have been used, and the study groups were heterogenous, making comparisons between studies difficult [144]. Finfer et al. [145] found no difference in mortality between crystalloids and albumin fluid replacement in 7000 critically ill patients. With appropriate caution, the use of either crystalloid or colloid solutions for volume resuscitation in septic shock is appropriate. Moreover, in patients with low CVP and concurrent pulmonary edema, a colloid may be combined with a crystalloid to avoid a large volume of crystalloid and to rapidly achieve the CVP goal.

Vasoactive drug therapy

At times, fluid resuscitation proves inadequate in restoring optimal cardiovascular performance. In such cases, the use of vasoactive agents is indicated after restoration of adequate intravascular volume guided by a PA catheter. The most commonly used agent in this regard is dopamine hydrochloride. *Dopamine* is a drug with dose-dependent effects on dopaminergic, α-, and β-adrenergic receptors [146]. Myocardial performance after dopamine therapy is best evaluated using ventricular function curves, with the goal of maintaining a systemic CI above 3 L/min/m^2. In obstetric patients with septic shock, the dopamine infusion is usually started at 2–5 μg/kg/min and titrated against its effect on CO and blood pressure [147]. At very low doses (0.5–5.0 μg/kg/min), dopamine acts primarily on the dopaminergic receptors leading to vasodilation and improved perfusion of the renal and mesenteric vascular beds. As the dose increases (5.0–15.0 μg/kg/min), dopamine appears to act more selectively on the receptors of the heart. The β-adrenergic effects are responsible for improved myocardial contractility, stroke volume, and CO. With doses exceeding 20 μg/kg/min, α-receptor stimulation predominates, similar to that seen with a norepinephrine infusion, and result in generalized vasoconstriction with a reduction in tissue perfusion.

Inotropic support with *dobutamine* (2–10 μg/kg/min) may treat the myocardial depression and unmask hypovolemia. Dobutamine is an inotropic agent with fewer chronotropic effects than dopamine. It increases CI and oxygen delivery and decreases SVR, thereby improving perfusion [148]. Because the vasodilatory effect of dobutamine may worsen hypotension, it should be used in combination with vasopressors for patients with persistent hypotension. In addition, dobutamine may also exacerbate tachycardia. When a trial of dobutamine therapy is able to achieve the goals of CVP, MAP, and hematocrit but fails to increase $S_{cv}O_2$ above 70% or if dobutamine causes an exaggerated response such as significant tachycardia and hypotension, one should consider reducing systemic oxygen demand and consumption. Dobutamine is commonly combined with low-dose dopamine to improve myocardial performance and maintain renal perfusion in the ICU setting. Other vasoconstrictive drugs, including norepinephrine [10,149,150] and epinephrine [128,148,151,152], have been suggested as alternatives in dopamine-resistant shock. Epinephrine increases myometrial contractility, CI, blood pressure, and oxygen delivery. Oxygen debt is increased, possibly reflecting decreased tissue oxygenation, but hypotension is reversed by a balanced effect on both SVR and CO [148]. These hemodynamic improvements come at the expense of increased myocardial work and oxygen requirement [128], which has limited the use of epinephrine. Significant vasoconstriction and end-organ hypoperfusion are also of concern. If indicated, epinephrine can be started at a dose of 1–10 μg/min. Epinephrine increases MAP by increasing CO and stroke volume, but may impair splanchnic circulation and increase lactate production [153].

Early experiences using *norepinephrine* as a primary agent for inotropic support in septic shock were disappointing. Initial studies demonstrated that norepinephrine was able to reverse hypotension and oliguria more reliably than dopamine in patients with septic shock, and could effectively reverse shock in patients who failed dopamine therapy while avoiding the rebound tachycardia induced by dopamine [154]. Subsequent studies showed that norepinephrine had less of a detrimental effect on splanchnic perfusion and oxygen delivery than dopamine [155]. However, the profound and often excessive vasoconstriction induced by norepinephrine leads to marked reduction in organ perfusion [156], and it is this complication that has severely limited its use in septic shock. This is a particular concern in pregnancy, where reduction of placental perfusion may compromise fetal wellbeing. Catecholamines with more favorable side-effect profiles, such as dopamine, are therefore preferred over norepinephrine as first-line agents for the management of septic shock [154]. Norepinephrine should only be used as a second-line agent in cases of dopamine-resistant or refractory shock [149,150].

Microvascular shunting and organ hypoperfusion associated with the use of vasoactive agents can be difficult to recognize, and may only become apparent with deterioration of the patient's overall condition or evidence of increasing serum lactic acid concentrations [72]. Despite well-described limitations to this biochemical test, serial measurements of circulating lactic acid may be useful as an indicator of end-organ perfusion. Changes in calculated oxygen delivery and extraction are also helpful in assessing the adequacy of tissue perfusion and response to therapy. Of particular interest to the pregnant patient were the results of the study by Rolbin et al. [157] that demonstrated a decrease in uterine blood flow in hypotensive pregnant sheep treated with dopamine. Dopamine (and other vasoactive agents) may therefore compromise fetal well-being while concomitantly improving the maternal condition. For this reason, continuous fetal heart rate monitoring is recommended as a "marker" for end-organ (placental) perfusion in all pregnant women with a viable fetus (commonly regarded as greater than 24 weeks' gestation) requiring vasopressor therapy.

The ability of an individual to generate a hyperdynamic state in response to sepsis is associated with lower mortality rate [29,69,107,136]. Whether this reflects early and aggressive therapy or identifies patients with better underlying cardiovascular function who are then more responsive to intervention is not known. It is clear, however, that survivors are more responsive to initial inotropic therapy than non-survivors [143].

The observation that better cardiovascular performance is associated with improved survival has led some investigators to suggest that titration of inotropic support to supranormal values may improve outcome [158–163]. The desired hemodynamic profile typically includes a CI greater than 4.5 L/min/m^2 and an oxygen delivery (DO_2) rate greater than 600 mL/min/m^2. These recommendations represent median values for survivors, and have not been tested prospectively. This approach is controversial, and has been challenged by two recent large prospective randomized studies. Hayes et al. [164] were unable to demonstrate a decrease in mortality in patients who achieved normalization of SVo_2 or stated supraphysiologic hemodynamic goals as long as volume replacement was adequate and perfusion pressure was maintained. Similarly, a large multicenter European trial found that the targeted parameters were difficult to achieve, and the propensity to achieve them was primarily a function of the patient's age. These investigators were unable to demonstrate a decrease in mortality in patients who achieved supraphysiologic levels of cardiovascular performance regardless of group or reason for ICU admission [165]. These studies should not be interpreted as advocating a conservative approach to hemodynamic therapy in patients with septic shock. The apparently contradictory findings may be viewed as complementary. In susceptible patients, oxygen delivery, intravascular volume, and perfusion should be optimized to prevent progression to organ failure. In patients who develop shock, inotropic therapy should be directed toward maintenance of adequate CO and blood pressure with a view to maintaining perfusion and oxygenation [166]. Evidence of responsiveness to inotropic support and the ability to generate a hyperdynamic state early in the clinical course of septic shock are good prognostic features.

Additional evidence in support of early and aggressive intervention came from a recent study of goal-directed therapy in the treatment of sepsis and septic shock, which demonstrated a reduction in mortality from 46.5% to 35.5% [122]. In this study, aggressive resuscitation was begun as early as possible and typically while the patient was still in the emergency room. A detailed management algorithm was used to direct therapy with specific clinical endpoints for gauging therapeutic response, and the time interval between initial evaluation and initiation of therapy was extremely short. This publication does not contradict earlier randomized studies, but emphasizes the importance of intervening at the earliest possible time point prior to systemic decompensation and cardiovascular collapse. This study also emphasized the importance of continuous availability of experienced on-site intensivists if the outcome of such critically ill patients is to be optimized.

Oxygenation

Although pulmonary oxygenation can be relatively easily assessed by arterial blood gas determinations, oxygen consumption and utilization is a more difficult parameter to evaluate. The use of a PA catheter allows direct measurement and calculation of parameters relevant to oxygen delivery and consumption. Early in the course of shock, blood pressure may actually be normal due to peripheral vasoconstriction, because perfusion is disproportionately diverted from the renal and splanchnic circulations to maintain systemic blood pressure. Impairment of splanchnic perfusion may permit translocation of bacteria and toxins across the gastrointestinal mucosa, thereby worsening septic shock [31,167]. Oxygen delivery and tissue extraction are decreased in all forms of shock. If untreated, this will lead to increasing anaerobic metabolism and the development of progressive oxygen debt resulting in worsening lactic acidemia, organ dysfunction, and ultimately death [159]. A low $S_{cv}O_2$ coupled with an elevated lactate level suggests a mismatch between systemic oxygen delivery and oxygen consumption at the level of the tissues. When a low $S_{cv}O_2$ is identified, attention should be focused on interventions that can increase $S_{cv}O_2$ by increasing either oxygen-carrying capacity, CO, or arterial oxygen saturation. These interventions include blood transfusion, use of inotropic agents, and supplemental oxygen or mechanical ventilation [111].

Septic patients have increased metabolic needs for oxygen and, at the same time, a decreased ability to extract the oxygen that is delivered [168]. Peripheral tissue utilization of oxygen is frequently reduced, leading to tissue hypoxia [62]. Two possible mechanisms play a pivotal role in this phenomenon. First, there is evidence to suggest that cellular dysfunction during the later stages of septic shock can lead to underextraction of delivered oxygen. Mitochondrial and cellular dysfunction further decreases the ability to utilize oxygen [169–171]. Second, microvascular shunting and loss of autoregulation of blood flow may decrease local availability of oxygen [59,62]. Additionally, hypophosphatemia, alkalosis, and multiple blood transfusions all shift the oxyhemoglobin dissociation curve to the left, which result in a decrease in the availability of oxygen at the cellular level.

Tissue oxygen extraction can be assessed indirectly. Decreased tissue oxygen extraction is suggested by an increase in mixed venous oxygen saturation (S_vO_2) or decrease in arteriovenous oxygen content difference [168]. Actual peripheral oxygen consumption can be calculated using the Fick equation; the normal indexed non-pregnant range is 120–140 mL O_2/min/m^2 [172]. Because delivery far exceeds consumption, oxygen consumption is normally independent of oxygen delivery. In the septic patient, every effort should be taken to increase oxygen delivery until lactic acid concentrations return to normal [128,143]. Even in the absence of lactic acidosis, it is prudent to maintain excess oxygen delivery to avoid local reduction in tissue perfusion and subsequent organ dysfunction [31,110]. More recent studies suggest that therapy should be tailored according to the patient's needs, with blood lactate and S_vO_2 forming part of the management algorithm [173,174]. In an animal model of sepsis, anaerobic metabolism (suggestive of inadequate perfusion) was demonstrated in the gastrointestinal tract despite supranormal CO and oxygen delivery that was seemingly adequate for the rest of the body [25].

Acute respiratory distress syndrome

ARDS develops in 50% of patients with severe sepsis or septic shock. ARDS requiring ventilatory support has an overall mortality rate of approximately 50%, but may exceed 90% if caused or complicated by sepsis. Although generally younger and healthier, pregnant women with ARDS still have mortality of 25–40% [175,176]. The diagnosis of ARDS is typically made on the basis of progressive hypoxemia, with no evidence of heart failure (a normal PCWP), diffuse infiltrates on chest radiograph, and/or decreased pulmonary compliance [26,177,178]. With acute lung injury, there is recruitment of neutrophils to the site of inflammation by chemokines. As neutrophils accumulate, they initiate further tissue injury including widespread injury to alveolar epithelial cells and to the microvascular endothelium of the pulmonary vasculature. This results in increased pulmonary capillary permeability, surfactant loss or inactivation, diminished lung volume, and vascular shunting with resultant arterial hypoxemia [179]. The increased capillary permeability leads to further extravasation of fluid into the interstitial space with the development of progressive oxygen debt that contributes to multiple-organ system dysfunction and death.

The development of pulmonary hypertension increases the rate at which extravascular interstitial fluid collects and contributes to the progressive hypoxemia observed clinically in patients with ARDS. Pulmonary hypertension develops initially in response to neurohormonal mechanism, but structural changes soon develop in the pulmonary microvasculature in response to inflammatory byproducts released by the lung parenchyma [180]. During this later inflammatory fibrotic phase, ARDS is commonly associated with fever, leukocytosis, and decreased SVR, making it exceedingly difficult to distinguish from pneumonia and worsening sepsis [181,182].

The cornerstone of the treatment of ARDS involves intubation and ventilatory support to maintain adequate gas exchange at non-toxic levels of inspired oxygen. PEEP is often needed to accomplish this goal, and serial monitoring of arterial blood gases is essential with a view to maintaining a P_aO_2 of >60 mmHg and an oxygen saturation of >90% at an inspired oxygen content of <50%. Whether delivery will improve maternal oxygenation remains controversial [183,184]. The clinician must remember that, even in the face of overt pulmonary capillary leakage, intravenous hydration should be continued and adequate intravascular volume maintained to promote systemic perfusion. PEEP generates increased intrathoracic pressure and, at high pressures, may decrease venous return and consequently CO and organ perfusion, especially in patients who are volume depleted. PEEP can be used safely at low pressures (5–15 mmHg), but care should be taken when higher pressures are needed. High pressures may also result in overdistention of alveoli leading to falling compliance and barotrauma. When interpreting hemodynamic readings and assessing intravascular volume status, the clinician must keep in mind that PEEP can artificially increase PCWP measurements.

Recent advances in ventilator management and in our understanding of the role that overventilation plays in pulmonary injury and inflammation have lead to an improvement in outcome. Traditionally, supraphysiologic tidal volumes of 10–15 mL/kg body weight were used to ventilate ICU patients. In patients with ARDS, this led to a high rate of stretch-induced lung injury, high airway pressures, and barotrauma. Recent studies have demonstrated a significant reduction in mortality with the use of lower tidal volumes (6–7 mL/kg ideal body weight), although higher levels of PEEP and F_iO_2 were required and, interestingly, there was no observed decrease in barotrauma [185]. As our understanding of the pathophysiology of sepsis and ARDS evolves, incorporation into clinical practice of measures to avoid iatrogenic lung injury and inflammation, such as limiting stretch-induced injury, will serve to improve patient outcome [186].

Antimicrobial therapy

In concert with efforts to restore normal cardiovascular function and tissue oxygenation in patients with septic shock, an aggressive investigation should be initiated to identify the underlying infectious etiology. Because the course of septic shock can be rapid and fulminant, such a workup must be carried out without delay and empiric antimicrobial therapy should be started. Although there are insufficient data to conclude that delays of the order of hours are deleterious, administration of antibiotics within 4 hours of diagnosis has been associated with a lower mortality rate and more favorable outcome in patients with septic shock [187]. At times, the source of sepsis in a pregnant patient is obvious (such as chorioamnionitis or pyelonephritis). At other times, the etiology can be elusive (e.g. postpartum toxic shock syndrome, necrotizing fasciitis, or septic pelvic thrombophlebitis). The diagnostic work-up may include the microbiologic evaluation of specimens from blood, urine, sputum, and wound. Because vaginal cultures typically demonstrate mixed flora, sampling of the endometrial cavity is seldom useful [188]. In patients thought to have chorioamnionitis, transabdominal amniocentesis or cultures taken from a free-flowing internal pressure transducer catheter (IUPC) have been described, but are also of limited clinical utility [189]. Gram-stain of infected abortion materials or a sample taken from a deep fascial infection may be helpful in making the diagnosis of infection with *Clostridium perfringens* or Group A β-hemolytic streptococcus.

Empiric antibiotic therapy in pregnant patients with sepsis and septic shock should include coverage for a wide variety of both aerobic and anaerobic Gram-negative and Gram-positive bacteria, with particular attention to the likely source of infection [190]. Combination parenteral antimicrobial therapy is commonly recommended, such as a combination of ampicillin (2 g every 6 hours), an aminoglycoside appropriately dosed for patient weight and renal function, and clindamycin (900 mg every 8 hours). Other broad-spectrum treatment regimens are also acceptable, and clinicians should be familiar with the dosage and route of administration of all medications they prescribe as well as the potential adverse affects of each these drugs.

Community- and institution-specific sensitivities of common nosocomial pathogens should be considered in the choice of empiric therapy until culture results are available. For example, more than 90% of *E. coli* isolates have recently been shown to be susceptible to aminoglycosides, fluoroquinolones, and new-generation cephalosporins; but 9–17% were resistant to ciprofloxacin [191,192]. Additionally, the prevalence of community-acquired strains of *Streptococcus pneumoniae* that are resistant to penicillin, macrolide antibiotics, and/or trimethoprim-sulfamethoxazole has increased significantly [193–195]. There are no reports of vancomycin-resistant *Streptococcus pneumoniae*. In patients who previously received cephalosporin therapy, additional coverage specifically directed against enterococci may be warranted. In addition, if *Staphylococcus aureus* is a suspected pathogen, a semisynthetic penicillin may be substituted for ampicillin. Because nephrotoxicity is a well-established complication of aminoglycoside usage and septic patients may already have or are prone to renal compromise, monitoring of peak and trough aminoglycoside levels is imperative. When available, culture results and organism sensitivities should be used to more selectively guide subsequent antimicrobial therapy. Methicillin-resistant *Staphylococcus aureus* (MRSA) is the most common pathogen isolated in community-acquired skin and soft tissue infections. Most of these patients have no identified risk factors for MRSA. Antimicrobials with consistent activity against MRSA include vancomycin, trimethoprim-sulfamethoxazole, rifampin, daptomycin, and linezolid [196,197].

Critically ill patients are at risk for developing unusual sources of infection not commonly encountered by obstetricians, and careful physical examination as well as selective imaging studies are important in excluding uncommon sources. For example, sinusitis may result from prolonged intubation or nasogastric suction. Nosocomial pneumonia commonly develops in ICU patients, and is a major cause of mortality [198]. When broad-spectrum antibiotics are utilized, careful surveillance for resistant organisms and fungal infection is imperative.

Surgical therapy

Surgical extirpation of infected tissues (if possible) is important to ensure survival. In patients with suspected septic abortion, evacuation of the uterus should begin promptly after initiating antibiotics and stabilizing the patient. Septic shock in association with chorioamnionitis in a viable fetus is treated by delivery; this can be accomplished vaginally if maternal hemodynamic parameters are stable and delivery is imminent. Under certain circumstances and only after initial maternal resuscitation, cesarean delivery may be appropriate. This decision should be based on the chance of survival of the fetus and the risks to the mother if the nidus for infection is not removed rapidly. In the postpartum patient, hysterectomy may be indicated if microabscess formation is identified within myometrial tissues or if there is clinical evidence of deterioration in the patient's condition despite appropriate antibiotic therapy. Necrotizing soft tissue infection (fasciitis) can proceed rapidly to septicemia, profound hemoconcentration due to capillary leakage, circulatory collapse, and death. Early diagnosis, early and aggressive surgical debridement, antimicrobials, and supportive care in an ICU setting are all required for the successful treatment of necrotizing fasciitis [199,200]. When a diagnosis of septic pelvic thrombophlebitis is entertained, empiric treatment with heparin in combination with broad-spectrum antibiotics is appropriate. If this proves unsuccessful, surgical evaluation may be necessary [201].

Coagulation cascade

Disseminated intravascular coagulation frequently complicates septic shock, and most commonly results from activation of the coagulation cascade and depletion of coagulation factors (consumptive coagulopathy). Unless there is clinical evidence of bleeding or surgery is anticipated, aggressive attempt at correcting these laboratory defects is not usually recommended. With early and appropriate treatment of the underlying condition, the consumptive coagulopathy will resolve spontaneously. However, if the platelet count falls below 5000–10 000/mL, a platelet transfusion is recommended to prevent spontaneous hemorrhage.

Whenever thrombocytopenia occurs in the septic patient, the effect of heparin must be considered in the differential diagnosis. Heparin is commonly used in the ICU setting, and can cause thrombocytopenia via two mechanisms. The first, generally seen within 2–5 days after initiation of heparin therapy, is usually mild and of little clinical significance. The second, known as immune-mediated heparin-induced thrombocytopenia, is less common but of considerably more importance and may cause profound thrombocytopenia. This phenomenon occurs 7–15 days after initiation of heparin therapy and is independent of dose or route of administration [202]. If this diagnosis is suspected, all sources of heparin should be eliminated, including subcutaneous injections for deep venous thrombosis prophylaxis, flushing solutions of indwelling lines, and total parenteral nutrition (TPN) solutions. Platelet transfusions are not indicated for this condition.

Recent studies have demonstrated significant cross-talk between the coagulation and inflammatory cascades. In the setting of septic shock, the inflammatory response leads to systemic hypotension and tissue hypoperfusion. The resultant tissue hypoxia establishes a vicious cycle whereby localized cellular injury results in plugging of the microvasculature with cellular and fibrinous debris causing further cellular hypoxia and injury and release of endogenous mediators of inflammation and chemokines. The end result is a decrease in circulating concentrations of platelets, antithrombin III, protein C antigen and inhibitor, protein S, and factors VII and XII. Fibrinogen, thrombin–antithrombin (TAT) complexes, D-dimers, thrombomodulin, tissue-type plasminogen activator (tPA) activity and antigen, and other markers of the coagulation and thrombolytic cascades are increased. These perturbations in the coagulation and complement systems lead to further activation of the systemic inflammatory response [203]. Activation of the extrinsic pathway can further increase the coagulability of blood. Anticoagulation mediators are involved in the inflammatory process, and their depletion is frequently observed in patients with sepsis and ARDS. It is theorized that the lack of endogenous anticoagulants facilitates the production of microthrombi in the vasculature which, in turn, aggravates hypoperfusion and tissue hypoxia. Large-scale, randomized, clinical trials looking at the efficacy of inflammatory mediator inhibitor therapy to improve prognosis in the setting of sepsis with or without DIC are currently under way, but initial results have been disappointing [204].

Renal function

Renal function is best monitored with an indwelling catheter and serial creatinine and blood urea nitrate (BUN) determinations. Although acute tubular necrosis most often presents with oliguria, it may present as a high-output state. Regardless, tests of tubular function will demonstrate increased fractional excretion of sodium and impaired concentrating ability as evidenced by a urinary sodium concentration greater than 40 mEq/L and urine osmolality less than 400 mOsmol/kg, respectively. Serum creatinine concentrations also rise at a rate of 0.5–1.5 mg/dL per day [205]. Provided irreversible acute tubular necrosis has not occurred, correction of the hemodynamic and perfusion deficits should result in restoration of renal function. Table 41.7 lists various prognostic indicators of poor outcome in addition to renal parameters in patients with septic shock [26,107,134,135,172,206]. Daily hemodialysis or continuous hemofiltration with an ultrafiltration rate of 35–45 mL/kg per hour should be considered in septic patients with established acute renal failure who are not responding to expectant management [207,208].

Table 41.7 Prognostic indicators of poor outcome in septic shock.

Delay in initial diagnosis
Underlying debilitating disease process
Poor response to intravenous fluid resuscitation
Depressed cardiac output
Reduced oxygen extraction
Presence of ARDS or renal failure
High serum lactate (>4 mmol/L)
Reduced colloid osmotic pressure (<15 mmHg)

Gastrointestinal tract and nutrition

Although often overlooked, the gastrointestinal tract can be a reservoir of infection and a source of considerable morbidity to the ICU patient. Three interrelated areas requiring attention include provision for adequate nutrition, prevention or minimization of the effect of translocation of bacteria from the gut to the systemic circulation, and stress ulcer prophylaxis. All three relate directly to efforts aimed at maintaining adequate splanchnic circulation and the integrity of the gastrointestinal mucosa.

Sepsis provokes a catabolic state, the effects of which are especially pronounced in skeletal muscle, loose connective tissue, and intestinal viscera [25]. Metabolic alterations provoked by sepsis differ from starvation in that the compensatory mechanisms to preserve lean body mass in starvation are absent in sepsis [209]. Provision for adequate nutrition early in the patient's ICU course is essential. In addition to providing adequate calories, carbohydrates, lipids, protein, vitamins, and trace elements to prevent catabolism, restoration of adequate nutritional support has other beneficial effects. Inadequate nutrition is associated with significant immune impairment with suppression of both cellular and humoral immunity. The potential for alterations in immune function emphasizes the importance of providing adequate nutrition early in the course of sepsis. There are good animal evidence and preliminary human data to suggest that specific nutrients such as glutamine, arginine, and omega-3 fatty acids may have significant immunomodulatory functions [210].

Malnutrition has additional deleterious effects. It alters gastrointestinal mucosal integrity and promotes increases in endogenous gut flora. By itself, malnutrition does not promote translocation of bacteria and bacterial toxins into the circulation [211]. Sepsis increases the permeability of the gastrointestinal mucosa, and permeability increases with increasing severity of infection, an effect probably mediated by endotoxin [211,212]. When endotoxin is administered in the face of starvation or malnutrition, an increase in translocation of bacteria across the mucosa is observed, and this increase correlates with the duration of malnutrition [211].

The mucosa is highly susceptible to injury from hypotension because of its high metabolic rate. It is affected early when perfusion is directed away from the gastrointestinal tract to maintain central nervous system and cardiac perfusion. Ischemia interferes with mucosal function to prevent bacterial translocation into the systemic circulation [25,213]. Several investigators have suggested that gastric tonometry be used to follow intramucosal pH as an indicator of gastrointestinal and splanchnic perfusion. Mucosal pH has been correlated with perfusion, the propensity for mucosal injury, transmural migration of gut flora, and clinical outcome [167,214–216]. Clinical improvement in the patient's condition should be reflected in normalization of mucosal pH.

When selecting the optimal route to provide nutritional supplementation, the adage: "If the gut works, use it" should be borne in mind. Even in the face of nutritionally adequate replenishment, TPN is associated with impairment of host defenses and intrinsic gut immunity. Infectious complications are increased with TPN even when complications associated with central access and line sepsis are excluded [210]. The enteral route slows atrophy and maintains integrity of the mucosal barrier, especially if glutamine is provided. If adequate caloric replacement cannot be provided enterally, even small-volume enteral feeding with the remaining nutrition provided by TPN is better than TPN alone in promoting mucosal integrity and preventing atrophy [209]. Enteral nutrition can be provided to the intubated patient either through a needle catheter jejunostomy or through a small nasogastric tube advanced well into the duodenum.

Alterations in splanchnic perfusion, the patient's response to stress, and drugs administered to ICU patients can all promote ulceration and upper gastrointestinal bleeding. Prophylaxis against gastrointestinal ulceration is commonly provided in the form of either regular administration of antacids, H_2-receptor antagonists, or cytoprotective agents such as sucralfate. More than 50 trials have been performed to date with various endpoints and have all found a comparable protective effect regardless of which type of prophylaxis is used. A relative disadvantage of antacids and H_2-receptor antagonists is that they increase gastric pH, thereby promoting overgrowth of the normally sterile stomach with Gram-negative enteric pathogens. The risk of aspiration and nosocomial pneumonia is increased significantly by their use and has led some investigators to recommend sucralfate over antacids or H_2 blockers [216–222]. Although sucralfate is associated with a significant reduction in nosocomial pneumonias in intubated patients, adequate trials have not been conducted to demonstrate conclusively a reduction in overall mortality. Potential advantages of sucralfate in the pregnant patient include poor gastrointestinal absorption and lack of the potential systemic side effects associated with H_2 blockers. It has no effect on fertility, does not cross the placenta, and is not teratogenic [223]. Sucralfate should be considered a viable alternative for gastrointestinal ulcer prophylaxis in the pregnant ICU patient who can tolerate nasogastric medications.

Additional measures that require the attention of clinicians include the management of electrolyte imbalances, correction of metabolic acidosis, stabilization of coagulation defects, prophylaxis for deep venous thrombosis (with subcutaneous heparin, low molecular weight heparin, or pneumatic compression boots), and monitoring of renal function. Patients in septic shock may have either hypokalemia due to losses from the alimentary tract or hyperkalemia resulting from acute cation shifts in the face of acidosis or from renal failure. Lactic acidosis from anaerobic metabolism should be monitored serially and treated aggressively by increasing oxygen delivery and perfusion to peripheral tissues. Half-normal saline infusions with one to two ampules of sodium bicarbonate can be administered periodically to help correct severe acidosis, but is not generally recommended. Serum glucose levels may be elevated, normal, or depressed. If serum glucose levels are depressed, consideration should be given to administering intravenous glucose in combination with insulin to improve peripheral uptake of glucose. Van den Berghe et al. [224] published a prospective randomized trial assessing the benefit of aggressive glycemic control with insulin therapy in a group of 1548 critically ill patients. One group of patients was assigned to tight glycemic control (glucose 80–110 mg/dL) and the other group to concentrated control (insulin given only if blood glucose was >215 mg/dL). The mortality rate in the tight glycemic control group was reduced by 76% in patients with sepsis. Additional benefits from tight glycemic control included fewer ventilator days, less time in the ICU, and a reduced need for dialysis. The impact of tight glycemic control in the pregnant populations of critically ill patients, however, remains to be studied.

Controversial treatment modalities

Corticosteroids

The most controversial modality in the treatment of septic shock is the use of high-dose corticosteroids. Theoretic benefits of such treatment include stabilization of lysosomal membranes, inhibition of complement-induced inflammatory changes, and attenuation of the effects of cytokines and other inflammatory mediators. In an early trial, Sprung and coworkers [225] reported reversal of shock when steroids were given early in the course of sepsis. Although there was evidence of short-term improvement, overall mortality was not changed. Moreover, more than 25% of patients treated with steroids developed superinfections. Two large randomized, placebo-controlled, prospective studies subsequently demonstrated no benefit to the early administration of corticosteroids for either the treatment of severe sepsis and septic shock or for preventing progression to septic shock [226,227]. In light of these studies, there is currently no compelling reason to use corticosteroids in the treatment of septic shock, and many experts would recommend that their use should be reserved only for patients with documented adrenal insufficiency. Despite these data, the Surviving Sepsis Campaign Guidelines for the management of severe sepsis and septic shock still recommend the use of moderate doses of hydrocortisone pending the results of a large ongoing multicenter study [127].

Evidence of inadequate adrenal reserve in patients with septic shock is associated with increased morbidity (including prolonged requirement for vasopressor support) and morbidity. After a standard ACTH stimulation test, Annane et al. [119] randomized severely ill ICU patients with septic shock to corticosteroids (hydrocortisone 50 mg intravenously every 6 hours plus the mineralocorticoid, 9α-fludrocortisone, 50 μg orally once daily) or matching placebo for 7 days. Of all patients with adrenal insufficiency, those randomized to corticosteroids had a significantly lower 28-day adjusted mortality rate compared with those in the placebo group (53% vs 63%, respectively). No benefit was seen in patients with normal adrenal reserve. In light of these and other studies, some authorities suggest that patients with refractory shock or multiorgan dysfunction should be given low-dose corticosteroid replacement therapy if their ACTH stimulation test suggests adrenal insufficiency [111].

Another potential role for steroid therapy is to prevent ongoing lung injury in patients in the late fibroproliferative phase of ARDS. Several small case series have suggested that, although progression from lung injury to ARDS cannot be entirely prevented, steroids may be of some benefit in preventing pulmonary fibrosis and may accelerate recovery in patients with ARDS [181,182,228,229] Transient suppression of maternal immune function has been described following antepartum corticosteroid therapy to accelerate fetal pulmonary maturation prior to a preterm delivery [230]. This effect is clinically inconsequential and likely poses no maternal risk [231].

Prostaglandins

Prostaglandins have long been known to play a central role in septic shock, particularly in regulating regional blood flow. For example, Oettinger and colleagues [232] demonstrated increased production and decreased degradation of prostaglandin $F_{2\alpha}$ in severe sepsis. Other researchers have suggested that these alterations are associated with known endotoxin-induced pulmonary vascular changes [233]. Cefalo et al. [234] used prostaglandin synthetase inhibitors to successfully blunt these pathophysiologic responses in sheep. The same beneficial effects could be observed in other organ systems when experimental animals were pretreated with prostaglandin synthetase inhibitors prior to exposure to endotoxin [235–237]. Unfortunately, further clinical trials supporting the use of adjunctive anti-prostaglandin therapy have not been forthcoming and, as such, the routine use of these agents cannot be recommended at this time.

Immunotherapy

In 1984, Lachman et al. [238] demonstrated a reduction in both morbidity and mortality in obstetric and gynecologic patients with septic shock treated with anti-LPS immunoglobulin. Similar results were seen in preliminary studies in animal models and humans with septic shock using antibodies directed against endotoxin or specific inflammatory mediators such as TNF-α [42]. Despite this initial enthusiasm, however, subsequent large clinical studies using anti-endotoxin or anticytokine therapies to treat patients with septic shock have failed to demonstrate improvements in outcome [239–243]. Circulating endogenous inhibitors of proinflammatory cytokines have also been described, such as IL-1 receptor antagonist (IL-1ra) which antagonizes the systemic effects of IL-1β. In animal models, these circulating inhibitors decrease mortality in endotoxic shock. The interactions between these circulating antagonists and the proinflammatory cytokines on the molecular level and their impact on the clinical course of sepsis are only now beginning to be investigated. Their presence may explain the inconsistent results observed in clinical trials of exogenously administered inflammatory mediators [244].

Manipulation of the coagulation cascade

The results of a double-blind, placebo-controlled, multicenter, phase 3 clinical trial of *recombinant antithrombin III* treatment in critically ill ICU patients with sepsis were recently published [245]. Not only was there no improvement in overall survival, but there was a significant increase in the risk for hemorrhagic complications in patients who receiving the study drug along with heparin. As such, this intervention cannot be recommended at this time for patients with septic shock.

Early studies using *recombinant activated protein C* (drotrecogin alfa) to treat critically ill patients with severe sepsis and septic shock showed a significant reduction in overall mortality, but there was also a significant increase in the risk for bleeding complications, including two fatal intracranial hemorrhages [246]. The authors of this study calculated a rate of one serious bleeding event for every 66 patients treated compared with a 28-day survival benefit for one patient out of every 16 treated. In light of these and subsequent studies and consensus opinions [111,247,248], the Food and Drug Administration of the United States (FDA) recently approved the use of activated protein C in a well-defined subgroup of adult patients with severe sepsis or septic shock resistant to standard therapy who are at high risk of mortality (as evidenced by an APACHE II score of greater than or equal to 25) and who are at low risk of hemorrhagic side effects. Preliminary data suggest that early administration of recombinant activated protein C within 24 hours of presentation may be associated with better outcomes [249–252], but further studies are needed before this treatment can be recommended for patients presenting with septic shock.

As these examples illustrate, manipulation of the coagulation and inflammatory systems is not without risk. The patient groups studied are heterogenous and, as such, we are as yet unable to optimally individualize therapy. Currently, the recommended therapy for septic shock can be regarded as reactive rather than proactive. Early intervention has obvious advantages, but attempts to manipulate or modulate the inflammatory cascade or to abort systemic activation of the inflammatory response are in their infancy. There is likely no magic bullet or cocktail with which to treat severe sepsis and septic shock. As the intricacies of the activation and regulation of the inflammatory and coagulation cascades are elucidated, it becomes increasingly apparent that no single intervention or replacement of an individual coagulation factor can be expected to make a dramatic difference in outcome. However, a better understanding of these mechanisms in both health and disease will undoubtedly improve our ability to manage patients with severe sepsis and septic shock.

References

1 Bone RC, Balk RA, Cerra FB, et al. Definitions for sepsis and organ failure and guidelines for the use of innovative therapies in sepsis. *Chest* 1992; 101: 1644–1655.

2 Martin GS, Mannino DM, Eaton S, et al. The epidemiology of sepsis in the United States from 1979 through 2000. *N Engl J Med* 2003; 348: 1546.

3 Rangel-Frausto MS, Pittet D, Hwang T, Woolson RF, Wenzel RP. The dynamics of disease progression in sepsis: Markov modeling describing the natural history and the likely impact of effective anti-sepsis agents. *Clin Infect Dis* 1998; 27: 185–190.

4 Centers for Disease Control and Prevention. National Center for Health Statistics Mortality Patterns – United States, 1990. *Monthly Vital Stat Rep* 1993; 41: 5.

5 Centers for Disease Control and Prevention. Progress in chronic disease prevention. Chronic disease reports: deaths from nine types of chronic disease – United States, 1986. *MMWR* 1990; 39: 30.

6 Annane D, Aegerter P, Jars-Guincestre MC, Guidet B. Current epidemiology of septic shock: the CUB-Rea Network. *Am J Respir Crit Care Med* 2003; 1687: 165–172.

7 Friedman G, Silva E, Vincent JL. Has the mortality of septic shock changed with time? *Crit Care Med* 1998; 26: 2078–2086.

8 Brun-Buisson C, Doyon F, Carlet J, et al. Incidence, risk factors, and outcome of severe sepsis and septic shock in adults. A multicenter prospective study in intensive care units. *JAMA* 1995; 274: 968–974.

9 Annane D, Sebille V, Charpentier C, et al. Effect of treatment with low doses of hydrocortisone and fludrocortisone on mortality in patients with septic shock. *JAMA* 2002; 288: 862–871.

10 Wheeler AP, Bernard GR. Treating patients with severe sepsis. *N Engl J Med* 1999; 340: 207–214.

11 Gibbs CE, Locke WE. Maternal deaths in Texas, 1969 to 1973. A report of 501 consecutive maternal deaths from the Texas Medical Association's Committee on Maternal Health. *Am J Obstet Gynecol* 1976; 126: 687–692.

12 Levy MM, Fink MP, Marshall JC, et al. 2001 SCCM/ESICM/ACCP/ATS/SIS international sepsis definitions conference. *Intens Care Med* 2003; 29: 530–538.

13 Marshall JC, Cook DJ, Christou NV, et al. Multiple organ dysfunction score a reliable descriptor of a complex clinical outcome. *Crit Care Med* 1995; 23: 1638–1652.

14 Beutler B. Inferences, questions and possibilities in toll-like receptor signaling. *Nature* 2004; 430: 257–263.

15 Parrillo JE. Pathogenetic mechanisms of septic shock. *N Engl J Med* 1993; 328: 1471–1477.

16 Lynn WA, Cohen J. Science and clinical practice: management of septic shock. *J Infect* 1995; 30: 207–212.

17 Kwaan HM, Weil MH. Differences in the mechanism of shock caused by infections. *Surg Gynecol Obstet* 1969; 128: 37–45.

18 Cleary PP, Kaplan EL, Handley JP, et al. Clonal basis for resurgence of serious Streptococcus pyogenes disease in the 1980s. *Lancet* 1992; 339: 518–521.

19 Hoadley DJ, Marck EJ. Case records of the Massachusetts General Hospital. Weekly clinicopathological exercises. Case 28-2002. A 35-year-old long-term traveler with a rapidly progressive soft-tissue infection. *N Engl J Med* 2002; 347: 831.

20 Nathan L, Peters MT, Ahmed AM, et al. The return of life-threatening puerperal sepsis caused by group A streptococci. *Am J Obstet Gynecol* 1993; 169: 571.

21 Wang JE, Dahle MK, McDonald M, Foster SJ, Aasen AO, Thiemermann C. Peptidoglycan and lipoteichoic acid in gram-positive bacterial sepsis: receptors, signal transduction, biological effects, and synergism. *Shock* 2003; 20: 402–414.

22 Moine P, Abraham E. Immunomodulation and sepsis: impact of the pathogen. *Shock* 2004; 22: 297–308.

23 Yu SL, Chen HW, Yang PC, et al. Differential gene expression in gram-negative and gram-positive sepsis. *Am J Respir Crit Care Med* 2004; 169: 1135–1143.

24 Webb SR, Gascoigne NRJ. T-cell activation by superantigens. *Curr Opin Immunol* 1994; 6: 467–475.

25 Pinsky MR, Matuschak GM. Multiple systems organ failure: failure of host defense homeostasis. *Crit Care Clin* 1989; 5: 199–220.

26 Sugerman HJ, Peyton JWR, Greenfield LJ. Gram-negative sepsis. *Curr Probl Surg* 1981; 18: 405–475.

27 Van Bebber PT, Boekholz WKF, Goris RJ, et al. Neutrophil function and lipid peroxidation in a rat model of multiple organ failure. *J Surg Res* 1989; 47: 471–475.

28 Daryani R, Lalonde C, Zhu D, et al. Effect of endotoxin and a burn injury on lung and liver lipid peroxidation and catalase activity. *J Trauma* 1990; 30: 1330–1334.

29 Moore FA, Haenel JB, Moore EE, et al. Incommensurate oxygen consumption in response to maximal oxygen availability predicts postinjury multiple organ failure. *J Trauma* 1992; 33: 58–65.

30 Poggetti RS, Moore FA, Moore EE, et al. Liver injury is a reversible neutrophil-mediated event following gut ischemia. *Arch Surg* 1992; 127: 175–179.

31 Demling RH, Lalonde C, Ikegami K. Physiologic support of the septic patient. *Surg Clin North Am* 1994; 74: 637–658.

32 Fearon DT, Ruddy S, Schur PH, et al. Activation of the properdin pathway of complement in patients with gram-negative bacteremia. *N Engl J Med* 1975; 292: 937–940.

33 Schirmer WJ, Schirmer JM, Naff GB, et al. Systemic complement activation produces hemodynamic changes characteristic of sepsis. *Arch Surg* 1988; 123: 316–321.

34 Tracey KJ, Lowry SF, Cerami A. The pathophysiologic role of cachectin/TNF in septic shock and cachexia. *Ann Institut Pasteur Immunol* 1988; 139: 311–317.

35 Hesse DG, Tracey KJ, Fong Y, et al. Cytokine appearance in human endotoxemia and primate bacteremia. *Surg Gynecol Obstet* 1988; 166: 147–153.

36 Michie HR, Manogue KR, Spriggs DR, et al. Detection of circulating tumor necrosis factor after endotoxin administrations. *N Engl J Med* 1988; 318: 1481–1486.

37 Michie HR, Spriggs DR, Manogue KB, et al. Tumor necrosis factor and endotoxin induce similar metabolic responses in human beings. *Surgery* 1988; 104: 280–286.

38 Tracey KJ, Lowry SF, Fahey TJ III, et al. Cachectin/tumor necrosis factor induces lethal shock and stress hormone responses in the dog. *Surg Gynecol Obstet* 1987; 164: 415–422.

39 Mayoral JL, Schweich CJ, Dunn DL. Decreased tumor necrosis factor production during the initial stages of infection correlates with survival during murine gram-negative sepsis. *Arch Surg* 1990; 125: 24–27.

40 Tracey KJ, Beutler B, Lowry SF, et al. Shock and tissue injury induced by recombinant human cachectin. *Science* 1986; 234: 470–474.

41 Remick DG, Kunkel RG, Larrick JW, et al. Acute in vivo effects of human recombinant tumor necrosis factor. *Lab Invest* 1987; 56: 583–590.

42 Beutler B, Milsark IW, Cerami AC. Passive immunization against cachectin/tumor necrosis factor protects mice from lethal effect of endotoxin. *Science* 1985; 229: 869–871.

43 Tracey KJ, Fong Y, Hesse DG, et al. Anti-cachectin/TNF monoclonal antibodies prevent septic shock during lethal bacteriaemia. *Nature* 1987; 330: 662–664.
44 Yamamoto M, Takeda K, Akira S. TIR domain-containing adaptors define the specificity of TLR signaling. *Mol Immunol* 2004; 40: 861–868.
45 Lynn WA, Golenbock DT. Lipopolysaccharide antagonists. *Immunol Today* 1992; 13: 271–276.
46 Hageman JR, Caplan MS. An introduction to the structure and function of inflammatory mediators for clinicians. *Clin Perinatol* 1995; 22: 251–261.
47 Okusawa S, Gelfand JA, Ikejima T, et al. Interleukin 1 induces a shock-like state in rabbits: synergism with tumor necrosis factor and the effect of cyclooxygenase inhibition. *J Clin Invest* 1988; 81: 1162–1172.
48 Tabor DR, Burchett SK, Jacobs RF. Enhanced production of monokines by canine alveolar macrophages in response to endotoxin-induced shock (42681). *Proc Soc Exp Biol Med* 1988; 187: 408–415.
49 Jacobs RF, Tabor DR, Lary CH, et al. Interleukin-1 production by alveolar macrophages and monocytes from ARDS and pneumonia patients compared to controls. *Am Rev Respir Dis* 1988; 137: 228.
50 Hollenberg SM, Cunnion RE. Endothelial and vascular smooth muscle function in sepsis. *J Crit Care* 1994; 9: 262–280.
51 Sharshar T, Gray F, Lorin G, et al. Apoptosis of neurons in cardiovascular autonomic centres triggered by inducible nitric oxide synthase after death from septic shock. *Lancet* 2003; 362: 1799–1805.
52 Dinerman JL, Lowenstein CJ, Snyder SH. Molecular mechanisms of nitric oxide regulation: potential relevance to cardiovascular disease. *Circ Res* 1993; 73: 217–222.
53 Hack CE, Zeerleder S. The endothelium in sepsis: source of and a target for inflammation. *Crit Care Med* 2001; 29: S21–27.
54 Sriskandan S, Cohen J. Science and clinical practice: the pathogenesis of septic shock. *J Infect* 1995; 30: 201–206.
55 Bonney RJ, Humes JL. Physiological and pharmacological regulation of prostaglandin and leukotriene production by macrophages. *J Leukoc Biol* 1984; 35: 1–10.
56 Goetzl EJ, Payan DG, Goldman DW. Immunopathogenic roles of leukotrienes in human diseases. *J Clin Immunol* 1984; 4: 79–84.
57 Jacobs RF, Tabor DR. Immune cellular interactions during sepsis and septic injury. *Crit Care Clin* 1989; 5: 9.
58 Lee W, Cotton DB, Hankins GDV, et al. Management of septic shock complicating pregnancy. *Obstet Gynecol Surv* 1989; 16: 431.
59 Siegel JH, Greenspan M, del Guercio LRM. Abnormal vascular tone, defective oxygen transport and myocardial failure in human septic shock. *Ann Surg* 1967; 165: 504–517.
60 Sibbald WJ, Fox G, Martin C. Abnormalities of vascular reactivity in the sepsis syndrome. *Chest* 1991; 100: S155–S159.
61 Altura BM, Gebrewold A, Burton RW. Failure of microscopic meta-arterioles to elicit vasodilator responses to acetylcholine, bradykinin, histamine and substance P after ischemic shock, endothelial cells. *Microcirc Endothel Lymphat* 1985; 2: 121–127.
62 Duff JH, Groves AC, McLean AP, et al. Defective oxygen consumption in septic shock. *Surg Gynecol Obstet* 1969; 128: 1051–1060.
63 Knuppel RA, Rao PS, Cavanagh D. Septic shock in obstetrics. *Clin Obstet Gynecol* 1984; 27: 3–10.
64 Levi M, ten Cate H, van der Poll T, et al. Pathogenesis of disseminated intravascular coagulation in sepsis. *JAMA* 1993; 270: 975–979.
65 Bone RC. Sepsis syndrome: new insights into its pathogenesis and treatment. *Infect Dis Clin North Am* 1991;5: 793–805.
66 Bone RC, Sibbald WJ, Sprung CL. The ACCP-SCCM consensus conference on sepsis and organ failure. *Chest* 1992; 101: 1481–1483.
67 Rangel-Frausto MS, Pittet D, Costigan M, et al. The natural history of the systemic inflammatory response syndrome (SIRS). *JAMA* 1995; 273: 117–123.
68 Roman-Marchant O, Orellana-Jimenez CE, de Backer D, Melot C, Vincent JL. Septic shock of early or late onset: does it matter? *Chest* 2004; 126: 173–178.
69 Parker MM, Parillo JE. Septic shock: hemodynamics and pathogenesis. *JAMA* 1983; 250: 3324–3327.
70 Parrillo JE, Burch C, Shelhamer JH, et al. A circulating myocardial depressant substance in humans with septic shock: septic shock patients with a reduced ejection fraction have a circulating factor that depresses in vitro myocardial cell performance. *J Clin Invest* 1985; 76: 1539.
71 Marksad AK, Ona CJ, Stuart RC, et al. Myocardial depression in septic shock: physiologic and metabolic effect of a plasma factor on an isolated heart. *Circ Shock* 1979; 1(Suppl): 35.
72 Porembka DT. Cardiovascular abnormalities in sepsis. *New Horiz* 1993; 2: 324–341.
73 Parker MM, Shelhamer JH, Bacharach SL, et al. Profound but reversible myocardial depression in patients with septic shock. *Ann Intern Med* 1984; 100: 483–490.
74 Ognibene FP, Parker MM, Natanson C, et al. Depressed left ventricular performance: response to volume infusion in patients with sepsis and septic shock. *Chest* 1988; 93: 903–910.
75 Parrillo JE. Cardiovascular dysfunction in septic shock: new insights into a deadly disease. *Int J Cardiol* 1985; 7: 314.
76 Lee W, Clark SL, Cotton DB, et al. Septic shock during pregnancy. *Am J Obstet Gynecol* 1988; 159: 410–416.
77 Monif GRG, Baer H. Polymicrobial bacteremia in obstetric patients. *Obstet Gynecol* 1976; 48: 167–169.
78 Tewari K, Wold SM, Asrat T. Septic shock in pregnancy associated with legionella pneumonia: Case report. *Am J Obstet Gynecol* 1997; 176: 706–707.
79 Holm SE. Invasive group A streptococcal infections. *N Engl J Med* 1996; 335: 590–591.
80 Gibbs RS, Jones PM, Wilder CJ. Antibiotic therapy of endometritis following cesarean section: treatment successes and failures. *Obstet Gynecol* 1978; 52: 31–37.
81 Duff P. Pathophysiology and management of postcesarean endomyometritis. *Obstet Gynecol* 1986; 67: 269–276.
82 Balk RA, Bone RC. The septic syndrome: definition and clinical implications. *Crit Care Clin* 1989; 5: 1–8.
83 Ledger WJ, Norman M, Gee C, et al. Bacteremia on an obstetric-gynecologic service. *Am J Obstet Gynecol* 1975; 121: 205–212.
84 Blanco JD, Gibbs RS, Castaneda YS. Bacteremia in obstetrics: clinic course. *Obstet Gynecol* 1981; 58: 621–625.
85 Bryan CS, Reynolds KL, Moore EE. Bacteremia in obstetrics and gynecology. *Obstet Gynecol* 1984; 64: 155–158.
86 Reimer LG, Reller LB. Gardnerella vaginalis bacteremia: a review of thirty cases. *Obstet Gynecol* 1984; 64: 170–172.
87 Chow AW, Guze LB. Bacteroidaceae bacteremia: clinical experience with 112 patients. *Medicine* 1974; 53: 93–126.
88 Lowthian JT, Gillard LJ. Postpartum necrotizing fasciitis. *Obstet Gynecol* 1980; 56: 661–663.

89 Mariona FG, Ismail MA. Clostridium perfringens septicemia following cesarean section. *Obstet Gynecol* 1980; 56: 518–521.

90 Cavanagh D, Knuppel RA, Shepherd JH, et al. Septic shock and the obstetrician/gynecologist. *South Med J* 1982; 75: 809–813.

91 Lloyd T, Dougherty J, Karlen J. Infected intrauterine pregnancy presenting as septic shock. *Ann Emerg Med* 1983; 12: 704–707.

92 Duff P. Pyelonephritis in pregnancy. *Clin Obstet Gynecol* 1984; 27: 17–31.

93 Cunningham FG, Lucas MJ, Hankins GD. Pulmonary injury complicating antepartum pyelonephritis. *Am J Obstet Gynecol* 1987; 156: 797–807.

94 Clark SL, Cotton DB, Lee W, et al. Central hemodynamic assessment of normal term pregnancy. *Am J Obstet Gynecol* 1989; 161: 1439–1442.

95 Rackow EC, Fein IA, Leppo J. Colloid osmotic pressure as a prognostic indicator of pulmonary edema and mortality in the critically ill. *Chest* 1977; 72: 709–713.

96 Rackow EC, Fein IA, Siegel J. The relationship of the colloid osmotic-pulmonary artery wedge pressure gradient to pulmonary edema and mortality in critically ill patients. *Chest* 1982; 82: 433–437.

97 Weil MH, Henning RJ, Morissette M, et al. Relationship between colloid osmotic pressure and pulmonary artery wedge pressure in patients with acute cardiorespiratory failure. *Am J Med* 1978; 64: 643–650.

98 Hankins G, Clark S, Uckan E. Intrapulmonary shunt (QS/QT) and position in healthy third-trimester pregnancy. *Am J Obstet Gynecol* 1996; 174: 322A.

99 Weinstein MP, Murphy JR, Reller LB, et al. The clinical significance of positive blood cultures: a comparative analysis of 500 episodes of bacteremia and fungemia in adults. II. Clinical observations, with special reference to factors influencing prognosis. *Rev Infect Dis* 1983; 5: 54–70.

100 Freid MA, Vosti KL. The importance of underlying disease in patients with gram-negative bacteremia. *Arch Intern Med* 1968; 121: 418–423.

101 Metcalfe J, Ueland K. Maternal cardiovascular adjustments to pregnancy. *Prog Cardiovasc Dis* 1974; 16: 363–374.

102 Fletcher AP, Alkjaersig NK, Burstein R. The influence of pregnancy upon blood coagulation and plasma fibrinolytic enzyme function. *Am J Obstet Gynecol* 1979; 134: 743–751.

103 Pritchard JA, MacDonald PC, Gant NF, eds. Maternal adaption to pregnancy. In: *Williams Obstetrics*, 20th edn. Norwalk, CT: Appleton-Century-Crofts, 1997.

104 Beller JF, Schmidt EH, Holzgreve W, et al. Septicemia during pregnancy: a study in different species of experimental animals. *Am J Obstet Gynecol* 1985; 151: 967–975.

105 Bech-Jansen P, Brinkman CR 3rd, Johnson GH, et al. Circulatory shock in pregnant sheep. II: Effects of endotoxin on fetal and neonatal circulation. *Am J Obstet Gynecol* 1972; 113: 37–43.

106 Morishima HO, Niemann WH, James LS. Effects of endotoxin on the pregnant baboon and fetus. *Am J Obstet Gynecol* 1978; 131: 899–902.

107 Shoemaker WC, Montgomery ES, Kaplan E, et al. Physiologic patterns in surviving and nonsurviving shock patients. Use of sequential cardiorespiratory variables in defining criteria for therapeutic goals and early warning of death. *Arch Surg* 1973; 106: 630–636.

108 Kinasewitz GT, Yan SB, Basson B, et al. Universal changes in biomarkers of coagulation and inflammation occur in patients with severe sepsis, regardless of causative micro-organism. *Crit Care* 2004; 8: 82–90.

109 Shorr AF, Thomas SJ, Alkins SA, et al. D-dimer correlates with proinflammatory cytokine levels and outcomes in critically ill patients. *Chest* 2002; 121: 1262–1268.

110 Nguyen HB, Rivers EP, Knoblich BP, et al. Early lactate clearance is associated with improved outcome in severe sepsis and septic shock. *Crit Care Med* 2004; 32: 1637–1642.

111 Nguyen HB, River EP, Abrahamian FM, et al. Severe sepsis and septic shock; review of the literature and emergency department management guidelines. *Ann Emerg Med* 2006; 48: 28–54.

112 Cockerill 3rd FR, Wilson JW, Vetter EA, et al. Optimal testing parameters for blood cultures. *Clin Infect Dis* 2004; 38: 1724–1730.

113 Lamy B, Roy P, Carret G, et al. What is the relevance of obtaining multiple blood samples for culture? A comprehensive model to optimize the strategy for diagnosing bacteremia. *Clin Infect Dis* 2002; 35: 842–850.

114 Christ-Crain M, Jaccard-Stolz D, Bingisser R, et al. Effect of procalcitonin-guided treatment on antibiotic use and outcome in lower respiratory tract infections: cluster-randomised, single-blinded intervention trial. *Lancet* 2004; 363: 600–607.

115 Gattas DJ, Cook DJ. Procalcitonin as a diagnostic test for sepsis: health technology assessment in the ICU. *J Crit Care* 2003; 18: 52–58.

116 Colonna M, Facchetti F. TREM-1 (triggering receptor expressed on myeloid cells): a new player in acute inflammatory responses. *J Infect Dis* 2003; 187: S397–S401.

117 Gibot S, Cravoisy A, Levy B, Bene MC, Faure G, Bollaert PE. Soluble triggering receptor expressed on myeloid cells and the diagnosis of pneumonia. *N Engl J Med* 2004; 350: 451–458.

118 Gibot S, Kolopp-Sarda MN, Bene MC, et al. Plasma level of a triggering receptor expressed on myeloid cells-1: its diagnostic accuracy in patients with suspected sepsis. *Ann Intern Med* 2004; 141: 9–15.

119 Annane D, Sebille V, Troche G, Raphael JC, Gajdos P, Bellissant E. A 3-level prognostic classification in septic shock based on cortisol levels and cortisol response to corticotropin. *JAMA* 2000; 283: 1038–1045.

120 Cooper MS, Stewart PM. Corticosteroid insufficiency in acutely ill patients. *N Engl J Med* 2003; 348: 727–734.

121 Sam S, Corbridge TC, Mokhlesi B. Cortisol levels and mortality in sepsis. *Clin Endocrinol (Oxf)* 2004; 60: 29.

122 Rivers E, Nguyen B, Havstad S, et al. Early goal-directed therapy in the treatment of severe sepsis and septic shock. *N Engl J Med* 2001; 345: 1368–1377.

123 Angus DC, Linde-Zwirble WT, Lidicker J, et al. Epidemiology of severe sepsis in the United States: analysis of incidence, outcome, and associated costs of care. *Crit Care Med* 2001; 29: 1303.

124 Bernard GR, Wheeler AP, Russell JA, et al. The effects of ibuprofen on the physiology and survival of patients with sepsis. The Ibuprofen in Sepsis Study Group. *N Engl J Med* 1997; 336: 912.

125 Sasse KC, Nauenberg E, Long A, et al. Long-term survival after intensive care unit admission with sepsis. *Crit Care Med* 1995; 23: 1040.

126 Zeni F, Freeman B, Natanson C. Anti-inflammatory therapies to treat sepsis and septic shock: a reassessment. *Crit Care Med* 1997; 25: 1095.

127 Dellinger RP, Carlet JM, Masur H, et al. Surviving sepsis campaign guidelines for management of severe sepsis and septic shock. *Crit Care Med* 2004; 32: 858–873.

128 Lindeborg DM, Pearl RG. Recent advances in critical care medicine: inotropic therapy in the critically ill patient. *Int Anesthesiol Clin* 1993; 31: 49–71.
129 Ghosh S, Latimer RD, Gray BM, et al. Endotoxin-induced organ injury. *Crit Care Med* 1993; 21: S19.
130 Roberts JM, Laros RK. Hemorrhagic and endotoxic shock: a pathophysiologic approach to diagnosis and management. *Am J Obstet Gynecol* 1971; 110: 1041–1049.
131 Hawkins DF. Management and treatment of obstetric bacteremia shock. *J Clin Pathol* 1980; 33: 895–896.
132 Packman MI, Rackow EC. Optimum left heart filling pressure during fluid resuscitation of patients with hypovolemic and septic shock. *Crit Care Med* 1983; 11: 165–169.
133 Rackow EC, Falk JL, Fein IA, et al. Fluid resuscitation in circulatory shock: a comparison of the cardiorespiratory effects of albumin, hetastarch, and saline solutions in patients with hypovolemic and septic shock. *Crit Care Med* 1983; 11: 839–850.
134 Kaufman BS, Rackow EC, Falk JL. The relationship between oxygen delivery and consumption during fluid resuscitation of hypovolemic and septic shock. *Chest* 1984; 85: 336–340.
135 Weil MN, Nishijima H. Cardiac output in bacterial shock. *Am J Med* 1978; 64: 920–922.
136 Shippy CR, Appel PL, Shoemaker WC. Reliability of clinical monitoring to assess blood volume in critically ill patients. *Crit Care Med* 1984; 12: 107–112.
137 Shoemaker WC, Kram HB, Appel PL, et al. The efficacy of central venous and pulmonary artery catheters and therapy based upon them in reducing mortality and morbidity. *Arch Surg* 1990; 125: 1332–1337.
138 Swan HJ, Ganz W, Forrester J, et al. Catheterization of the heart in man with use of a flow-directed balloon-tipped catheter. *N Engl J Med* 1970; 283: 447–451.
139 Cotton DB, Gonik B, Dorman K, et al. Cardiovascular alterations in severe pregnancy-induced hypertension: relationship of central venous pressure to pulmonary capillary wedge pressure. *Am J Obstet Gynecol* 1985; 151: 762–764.
140 Rackow EC, Kaufman BS, Falk JL, et al. Hemodynamic response to fluid repletion in patients with septic shock: evidence for early depression of cardiac performance. *Circ Shock* 1987; 22: 11–22.
141 Lewis BS, Gotsman MS. Current concepts of left ventricular relaxation and compliance. *Am Heart J* 1980; 99: 101–112.
142 Haupt MT, Rackow EC. Colloid osmotic pressure and fluid resuscitation with hetastarch, albumin, and saline solutions. *Crit Care Med* 1982; 10: 159–162.
143 Shoemaker WC, Appel PL, Kram HB. Oxygen transport measurements to evaluate tissue perfusion and titrate therapy: dobutamine and dopamine effects. *Crit Care Med* 1991; 19: 672–688.
144 Wagner BKJ, d'Amelio LF. Pharmacologic and clinical considerations in selecting crystalloid, colloidal, and oxygen-carrying resuscitation fluids, part 2. *Clin Pharm* 1993; 12: 415–428.
145 Finfer S, Bellomo R, Boyce N, et al. A comparison of albumin and saline for fluid resuscitation in the intensive care unit. *N Engl J Med* 2004; 350: 2247–2256.
146 Rao PS, Cavanagh D. Endotoxic shock in the primate: some effects of dopamine administration. *Am J Obstet Gynecol* 1982; 144: 61–66.
147 Goldberg LI. Dopamine: clinical uses of an endogenous catecholamine. *N Engl J Med* 1974; 291: 707–710.
148 Bollaert PE, Bauer P, Audibert G, et al. Effects of epinephrine on hemodynamics and oxygen metabolism in dopamine-resistant septic shock. *Chest* 1990; 98: 949–953.
149 Desjars P, Pinaud M, Poptel G, et al. A reappraisal of norepinephrine therapy in human septic shock. *Crit Care Med* 1987; 15: 134–137.
150 Meadows D, Edwards JD, Wilkins RG, et al. Reversal of intractable septic shock with norepinephrine therapy. *Crit Care Med* 1988; 16: 663–666.
151 MacKenzie SJ, Kapadia F, Nimmo GR, et al. Adrenaline in treatment of septic shock: effects on hemodynamics and oxygen transport. *Intens Care Med* 1991; 17: 36–39.
152 Moran JL, O'Fathartaigh MS, Peisach AR, et al. Epinephrine as an inotropic agent in septic shock: a dose-profile analysis. *Crit Care Med* 1993; 21: 70.
153 De Backer D, Creteur J, Silva E, et al. Effects of dopamine, norepinephrine, and epinephrine on the splanchnic circulation in septic shock. Which is best? *Crit Care Med* 2003; 31: 1659–1667.
154 Martin C, Papazian L, Perrin G, et al. Norepinephrine or dopamine for the treatment of hyperdynamic septic shock? *Chest* 1993; 103: 1826–1831.
155 Marik PE, Mohedin M. The contrasting effects of dopamine and norepinephrine on systemic and splanchnic oxygen utilization in hyperdynamic sepsis. *JAMA* 1994; 272: 1354–1357.
156 Lucas CE. A new look at dopamine and norepinephrine for hyperdynamic septic shock. *Chest* 1994; 105: 7–8.
157 Rolbin SH, Levinson G, Shnider DM, et al. Dopamine treatment of spinal hypotension decreases uterine blood flow in the pregnant ewe. *Anesthesiology* 1979; 51: 37–40.
158 Shoemaker WC, Appel PL, Kram HB, et al. Prospective trial of supranormal values of survivors as therapeutic goals in high-risk surgical patients. *Chest* 1988; 94: 1176–1186.
159 Shoemaker WC, Appel PL, Kram HB. Role of oxygen debt in the development of organ failure sepsis, and death in high-risk surgical patients. *Chest* 1992; 102: 208–215.
160 Tuchschmidt J, Fried J, Astiz M, et al. Elevation of cardiac output and oxygen delivery improves outcome in septic shock. *Chest* 1992; 102: 216–220.
161 Boyd O, Grounds RM, Bennett ED. A randomized clinical trial of the effect of deliberate perioperative increase of oxygen delivery on mortality in high-risk surgical patients. *JAMA* 1993; 270: 2699–2707.
162 Yu M, Levy MM, Smith P, et al. Effect of maximizing oxygen delivery on morbidity and mortality rates in critically ill patients: a prospective, randomized, controlled study. *Crit Care Med* 1993; 21: 830–838.
163 Bishop MH, Shoemaker WC, Appel PL, et al. Prospective, randomized trial of survivor values of cardiac index, oxygen delivery, and oxygen consumption as resuscitation endpoints in severe trauma. *J Trauma* 1995; 38: 780–787.
164 Hayes MA, Timmins AC, Yau EH, et al. Elevation of systemic oxygen delivery in the treatment of critically ill patients. *N Engl J Med* 1994; 330: 1717–1722.
165 Gattinoni L, Brazzi L, Pelosi P, et al. A trial of goal-oriented hemodynamic therapy in critically ill patients. *N Engl J Med* 1995; 333: 1025–1032.
166 Hinds C, Watson D. Manipulating hemodynamic and oxygen transport in critically ill patients. *N Engl J Med* 1995; 333: 1074–1075.
167 Fiddian-Green RG, Haglund U, Gutierrez G, et al. Goals for the resuscitation of shock. *Crit Care Med* 1993; 21: S25–S31.

168 Tuchschmidt J, Oblitas D, Fried JC. Oxygen consumption in sepsis and septic shock. *Crit Care Med* 1991; 19: 664–671.

169 Rackow EC, Astiz ME, Weil MH. Cellular oxygen metabolism during sepsis and shock: the relationship of oxygen consumption to oxygen delivery. *JAMA* 1988; 259: 1989–1993.

170 Dantzker D. Oxygen delivery and utilization in sepsis. *Crit Care Clin* 1989; 5: 81–98.

171 Gutierrez G, Lund N, Bryan-Brown CW. Cellular oxygen utilization during multiple organ failure. *Crit Care Clin* 1989; 5: 271–287.

172 Shoemaker WC, Appel PL, Bland R, et al. Clinical trial of an algorithm for outcome prediction in acute circulatory failure. *Crit Care Med* 1983; 11: 165.

173 Pinsky MR, Vincent JL. Let us use the PAC correctly and only when we need it. *Crit Care Med* 2005; 33: 1119–1122.

174 Vincent JL. Hemodynamic support in septic shock. Guidelines for the management of severe sepsis and septic shock. International Sepsis Forum. *Intens Care Med* 2001; 27: S80–S92.

175 Catanzarite V, Willms D, Wong D, et al. Acute respiratory distress syndrome in pregnancy and the puerperium: causes, courses, and outcomes. *Obstet Gynecol* 2001; 97: 760.

176 Perry KG Jr, Martin RW, Blake PG, et al. Maternal outcome associated with adult respiratory distress syndrome. *Am J Obstet Gynecol* 1996; 174: 391.

177 Weg JG, Anzueto A, Balk RA, et al. The relation of pneumothorax and other air leaks to mortality in the acute respiratory distress syndrome. *N Engl J Med* 1998; 338: 341.

178 Ware LB, Matthay MA. The acute respiratory distress syndrome. *N Engl J Med* 2000; 342: 1334–1349.

179 Ware LB, Matthay MA. Alveolar fluid clearance is impaired in the majority of patients with acute lung injury and the acute respiratory distress syndrome. *Am J Respir Crit Care Med* 2001; 163: 1376–1383.

180 Bersten A, Sibbald WJ. Acute lung injury in septic shock. *Crit Care Clin* 1989; 5: 49–79.

181 Ashbaugh DG, Maier RV. Idiopathic pulmonary fibrosis in adult respiratory distress syndrome: diagnosis and treatment. *Arch Surg* 1985; 120: 530–535.

182 Meduri GU, Belenchia JM, Estes RJ, et al. Fibroproliferative phase of ARDS: clinical findings and effects of corticosteroids. *Chest* 1991; 100: 943–952.

183 Tomlinson MW, Caruthers TJ, Whitty JE, et al. Does delivery improve maternal condition in the respiratory-compromised gravida? *Obstet Gynecol* 1998; 91: 108.

184 Jenkins TM, Troiano NH, Graves CR, et al. Mechanical ventilation in an obstetric population: characteristics and delivery rates. *Am J Obstet Gynecol* 2003; 188: 439.

185 Petrucci N, Lacovelli W. Ventilation with lower tidal volumes versus traditional tidal volumes in adults for acute lung injury and acute respiratory distress syndrome. *Cochrane Database Syst Rev* 2004; 2: CD003844.

186 Acute Respiratory Distress Syndrome Network. Ventilation with lower tidal volumes as compared with traditional tidal volumes for acute lung injury and the acute respiratory distress syndrome. *N Engl J Med* 2000; 342: 1301–1308.

187 Houck PM, Bratzler DW, Nsa W, et al. Timing of antibiotic administration and outcomes for Medicare patients hospitalized with community-acquired pneumonia. *Arch Intern Med* 2004; 164: 637–644.

188 Duff P, Gibbs RS, Blanco JD, et al. Endometrial culture techniques in puerperal patients. *Obstet Gynecol* 1983; 61: 217–222.

189 Gibbs RS, Blanco JD, Hrilica VS. Quantitative bacteriology of amniotic fluid from women with clinical intraamniotic infection at term. *J Infect Dis* 1982; 145: 1–8.

190 MacArthur RD, Miller M, Albertson T, et al. Adequacy of early empiric antibiotic treatment and survival in severe sepsis: experience from the MONARCS trial. *Clin Infect Dis* 2004; 38: 284.

191 Garau J, Xercavins M, Rodriguez-Carballeira M, et al. Emergence and dissemination of quinolone-resistant *Escherichia coli* in the community. *Antimicrob Agents Chemother* 1999; 43: 2736–2741.

192 Gupta K, Sahm DF, Mayfield D, et al. Antimicrobial resistance among uropathogens that cause community-acquired urinary tract infections in women: a nationwide analysis. *Clin Infect Dis* 2001; 33: 89–94.

193 Thornsberry C, Sahm DF, Kelly LJ, et al. Regional trends in antimicrobial resistance among clinical isolates of *Streptococcus pneumoniae*, *Haemophilus influenzae*, and *Moraxella catarrhalis* in the United States: results from the TRUST Surveillance Program, 1999–2000. *Clin Infect Dis* 2002; 34: S4–S16.

194 Karlowsky JA, Thornsberry C, Jones ME, et al. Factors associated with relative rates of antimicrobial resistance among *Streptococcus pneumoniae* in the United States: results from the TRUST Surveillance Program (1998–2002). *Clin Infect Dis* 2003; 36: 963–970.

195 Doern GV, Brown SD. Antimicrobial susceptibility among community-acquired respiratory tract pathogens in the USA: data from PROTEKT US 2000–01. *J Infect* 2004; 48: 56–65.

196 Frazee BW, Lynn J, Charlebois ED, et al. High prevalence of methicillin-resistant *Staphylococcus aureus* in emergency department skin and soft tissue infections. *Ann Emerg Med* 2005; 45: 311–320.

197 Lewis JS 2nd, Jorgensen JH. Inducible clindamycin resistance in staphylococci. Should clinicians and microbiologists be concerned? *Clin Infect Dis* 2005; 40: 280–285.

198 Fagon JY, Chastre J, Vuagnat A, et al. Nosocomial pneumonia and mortality among patients in intensive care units. *JAMA* 1996; 275: 866–869.

199 Urschel JD. Necrotizing soft tissue infections. *Postgrad Med J* 1999; 75: 645.

200 Gallup DG, Meguiar RV. Coping with necrotizing fasciitis. *Contemp Ob/Gyn* 2004; 49: 38.

201 Collins CG. Suppurative pelvic thrombophlebitis. A study of 202 cases in which the disease was treated by ligation of the vena cava and ovarian vein. *Am J Obstet Gynecol* 1970; 108: 681–687.

202 Mei CT, Feeley TW. Coagulopathies and the intensive care setting. *Int Anesthesiol Clin* 1993; 31: 97–117.

203 Marshall JC. Inflammation, coagulopathy, and the pathogenesis of multiple organ dysfunction syndrome. *Crit Care Med* 2001; 29(Suppl): S99–S106.

204 Vincent JL. New therapeutic implications of anticoagulation mediator replacement in sepsis and acute respiratory distress syndrome. *Crit Care Med* 2000; 28: S83–S85.

205 Miller TR, Anderson RJ, Linas SL, et al. Urinary diagnostic indices in acute renal failure. *Ann Intern Med* 1978; 89: 47–50.

206 Hardaway RM. Prediction of survival or death of patients in a state of severe shock. *Surg Gynecol Obstet* 1981; 152: 200–206.

207 Ronco C, Bellomo R, Homel P, et al. Effects of different doses in continuous veno-venous haemofiltration on outcomes of acute renal failure: a prospective randomised trial. *Lancet* 2000; 356: 26–30.

208 Schrier RW, Wang W. Acute renal failure and sepsis. *N Engl J Med* 2004; 351: 159–169.

209 Wojnar MM, Hawkins WG, Lang CH. Nutritional support of the septic patient. *Crit Care Clin* 1995; 11: 717–733.

210 Mainous MR, Deitch EA. Nutrition and infection. *Surg Clin North Am* 1994; 74: 659–676.

211 Deitch EA, Winterton J, Li M, et al. The gut as a portal of entry for bacteremia: role of protein malnutrition. *Ann Surg* 1987; 195: 681–692.

212 Ziegler TR, Smith RJ, O'Dwyer ST, et al. Increased intestinal permeability associated with infection in burn patients. *Arch Surg* 1988; 123: 1313–1319.

213 Riddington DW, Venkatesh B, Boivin CM, et al. Intestinal permeability, gastric intramucosal pH, and systemic endotoxemia in patients undergoing cardiopulmonary bypass. *JAMA* 1996; 275: 1007–1012.

214 Gys T, Hubens A, Neels H, et al. Prognostic value of gastric intramural pH in surgical intensive care patients. *Crit Care Med* 1988; 16: 1222–1224.

215 Doglio GR, Pusajo JF, Egurrola MA, et al. Gastric mucosal pH as a prognostic index of mortality in critically ill patients. *Crit Care Med* 1991; 19: 1037–1040.

216 Sauve JS, Cook DJ. Gastrointestinal hemorrhage and ischemia: prevention and treatment. *Int Anesthesiol Clin* 1993; 31: 169–183.

217 Craven DE, Kunches LM, Kilinshy V, et al. Risk factors for pneumonia and fatality in patients receiving continuous mechanical ventilation. *Am Rev Respir Dis* 1986; 133: 792–796.

218 Bresalier RS, Grendell JH, Cello JP, et al. Sucralfate suspension versus titrated antacid for the prevention of acute stress-related gastrointestinal hemorrhage in critically ill patients. *Am J Med* 1987; 83: 110.

219 Cannon LA, Heiselman D, Gardner W, et al. Prophylaxis of upper gastrointestinal tract bleeding in mechanically ventilated patients. A randomized study comparing the efficacy of sucralfate, cimetidine, and antacids. *Arch Intern Med* 1987; 147: 2101–2106.

220 Driks MR, Craven DE, Celli BR, et al. Nosocomial pneumonia in intubated patients given sucralfate as compared with antacids or histamine type 2 blockers. *N Engl J Med* 1987; 317: 1376–1382.

221 Tryba M. Risk of acute stress bleeding and nosocomial pneumonia in ventilated intensive care unit patients: sucralfate versus antacids. *Am J Med* 1987; 83: 117–124.

222 Cook DJ, Reeve BK, Guyatt GH, et al. Stress ulcer prophylaxis in critically ill patients: resolving discordant meta-analyses. *JAMA* 1996; 275: 308–314.

223 Briggs GG, Freeman RK, Yaffe SJ, eds. Sucralfate: gastrointestinal agent. In: *A Reference Guide to Fetal and Neonatal Risk: Drugs in Pregnancy and Lactation*, 4th edn. Baltimore: Williams and Wilkins, 1995: 792.

224 Van den Berghe G, Wouters P, Weckers F, et al. Intensive insulin therapy in critically ill patients. *N Engl J Med* 2001; 345: 1359–1367.

225 Sprung CL, Caralis PV, Marcial EH, et al. The effects of high-dose corticosteroids in patients with septic shock. *N Engl J Med* 1984; 311: 1137–1143.

226 Bone RC, Fisher CJ Jr, Clemmer TP, et al. A controlled clinical trial of high-dose methylprednisolone in the treatment of severe sepsis and septic shock. *N Engl J Med* 1987; 317: 653–658.

227 Veterans Administration Systemic Sepsis Cooperative Study Group. Effect of high-dose glucocorticoid therapy on mortality in patients with clinical signs of systemic sepsis. *N Engl J Med* 1987; 317: 659.

228 Weigelt JA, Norcross JF, Borman KR, et al. Early steroid therapy for respiratory failure. *Arch Surg* 1985; 120(5): 536–540.

229 Hooper RG, Kearl RA. Established ARDS treated with a sustained course of adrenocortical steroids. *Chest* 1990; 97: 138–143.

230 Cunningham DS, Evan EE. The effects of betamethasone on maternal cellular resistance to infection. *Am J Obstet Gynecol* 1991; 165: 610.

231 Crowley PA. Antenatal corticosteroid therapy: a meta-analysis of the randomized trials, 1972 to 1994. *Am J Obstet Gynecol* 1995; 173: 322.

232 Oettinger WK, Walter GO, Jensen UM, et al. Endogenous prostaglandin F2 alpha in the hyperdynamic state of severe sepsis in man. *Br J Surg* 1983; 70: 237–239.

233 Vada P. Elevated plasma phospholipase A2 levels: correlation with the hemodynamic and pulmonary changes in gram-negative septic shock. *J Lab Clin Med* 1984; 104: 873.

234 Cefalo RC, Lewis PE, O'Brien WF, et al. The role of prostaglandins in endotoxemia: comparisons in response in the nonpregnant, maternal, and fetal model. *Am J Obstet Gynecol* 1980; 137: 53–57.

235 Rao PS, Cavanagh D, Gaston LW. Endotoxic shock in the primate: effects of aspirin and dipyridamole administration. *Am J Obstet Gynecol* 1981; 140: 914–922.

236 O'Brien WF, Cefalo RC, Lewis PE, et al. The role of prostaglandins in endotoxemia and comparisons in response in the nonpregnant, maternal, and fetal models. II. Alterations in prostaglandin physiology in the nonpregnant, pregnant, and fetal experimental animal. *Am J Obstet Gynecol* 1981; 139: 535–539.

237 Makabali GL, Mandal AK, Morris JA. An assessment of the participatory role of prostaglandins and serotonin in the pathophysiology of endotoxic shock. *Am J Obstet Gynecol* 1983; 145: 439–445.

238 Lachman E, Pitsoe SB, Gaffin SL. Antilipopolysaccharide immunotherapy in management of septic shock of obstetric and gynaecologic origin. *Lancet* 1984; 1: 981–983.

239 Greenman RL, Schein RMH, Martin MA, et al. A controlled clinical trial of E5 murine monoclonal IgM antibody to endotoxin in the treatment of gram-negative sepsis. *JAMA* 1991; 266: 1097–1102.

240 Wenzel RP. Monoclonal antibodies and the treatment of gram-negative bacteremia and shock. *N Engl J Med* 1991; 324: 486.

241 Ziegler EJ, Fisher CJ Jr, Sprung CL, et al. Treatment of gram-negative bacteremia and septic shock with HA-1A human monoclonal antibody against endotoxin. *N Engl J Med* 1991; 324: 429–436.

242 Warren HS, Danner RL, Munford RS. Anti-endotoxin monoclonal antibodies. *N Engl J Med* 1992; 326: 1153.

243 Natanson C, Hoffman WD, Suffredini AF, et al. Selected treatment strategies for shock based on proposed mechanisms of pathogenesis. *Ann Intern Med* 1994; 120: 771–783.

244 Goldie AS, Fearon KCH, Ross JA, et al. Natural cytokine antagonists and endogenous antiendotoxin core antibodies in sepsis syndrome. *JAMA* 1995; 274: 172–177.

245 Warren BL, Eid A, Singer P, et al. KyberSept Trial Study Group. Caring for the critically ill patients. High-dose antithrombin III in severe sepsis: a randomized controlled trial. *JAMA* 2001; 286: 1869–1878.

246 Bernard GR, Vincent JL, Laterre PF, et al. Efficacy and safety of recombinant human activated protein C for severe sepsis. *N Engl J Med* 2001; 344: 699–709.

247 Warren HS, Suffredini AF, Eichacker PQ, et al. Risks and benefits of activated protein C treatment for severe sepsis. *N Engl J Med* 2002; 347: 1027–1030.

248 Abraham E, Laterre PF, Garg R, et al. Drotrecogin alfa (activated) for adults with severe sepsis and a low risk of death. *N Engl J Med* 2005; 353: 1332–1341.

249 Johnston JA, Pulgar S, Ball DE, et al. The impact of timely drotrecogin alfa (activated) administration on hospital mortality and resource use. *Crit Care Med* 2003; 31: A73.

250 Verceles A, Schwarcz R, Birnbaum P, et al. Factors influencing survival in patients receiving activated protein C. *Crit Care Med* 2003; 31: A126.

251 Vincent JL, Levy MM, Macias WL, et al. Early intervention with drotrecogin alfa (activated) improves survival benefit. *Crit Care Med* 2003; 31: A123.

252 Wheeler A, Steingrub J, Linde-Zwirble W, et al. Prompt administration of drotrecogin alfa (activated) is associated with improved survival. *Crit Care Med* 2003; 31: A120.

42 Anaphylactic Shock in Pregnancy

Raymond O. Powrie
Department of Medicine, Obstetrics and Gynecology, Warren Alpert School of Medicine at Brown University, RI, USA

Introduction

Anaphylaxis is a serious potentially life-threatening allergic reaction that is rapid in onset and requires prompt treatment. The pathophysiology, precipitants, and management of anaphylaxis are similar in pregnant and non-pregnant patients so this chapter will largely focus on the general management of this condition but will highlight pregnancy specific concerns when appropriate.

Definitions

"Anaphylaxis" is a term that is often imprecisely used. It was coined in 1902 from the Greek words *ana* (meaning backwards) and *phylax* (meaning guard) to describe the phenomenon where an agent that was administered for its protective effect had instead the opposite effect and instead caused harm. Strictly speaking, anaphylaxis refers to IgE-mediated immediate ("type 1") hypersensitivity reactions to proteins (see Table 42.1) [1–3]. However, in clinical practice, such reactions are often difficult to distinguish from other types of severe allergic reactions that are not mediated by IgE. Such non-IgE-mediated reactions are correctly termed "anaphylactoid reactions". Although true anaphylaxis is more likely to cause hypotension and cardiac arrest than anaphylactoid reactions, the initial management of the two conditions is identical and the two terms will therefore be used interchangeably in this chapter.

Epidemiology

Anaphylactoid reactions are responsible for 1% of emergency room visits and perhaps 1000 deaths per year in the US. Between 0.05 and 2% of individuals will have an anaphylactoid reaction over the course of their lifetime. Anaphylactoid reactions are more likely to occur in hospitalized patients, with estimates of the frequency of anaphylaxis in hospital varying from 1 in 2700 to 1 in 5100 admissions [4,5]. The incidence of anaphylaxis in pregnant women is not known but there is no reason to believe that the incidence should be lower in this population, given both (i) the frequent need for both hospitalization and medications in this population and (ii) our present understanding of the immunologic changes in pregnancy.

Critical Care Obstetrics, 5th edition. Edited by M. Belfort, G. Saade, M. Foley, J. Phelan and G. Dildy.

Precipitants

Table 42.2 reviews the most commonly identified precipitants of anphylactoid reactions in adults. Despite this extensive list, in up to 60% of cases, the precipitating agent cannot be identified [6,7]. Some anaphylactic responses are only seen if the exposure is followed by physical exertion or exercise. Such a response is called "food-dependent, exercise-induced anaphylaxis" (FDEIAn).

There are over 50 case reports that detail anaphylaxis occurring in obstetric patients in relation to their antenatal/intrapartum care and some of these causes are also listed in Table 42.2.

Risk factors for anaphylaxis/anaphylactoid reactions

The following are some of the known risk factors for anaphylactoid reactions.

Gender

Women are more likely to have anaphylactoid responses in general and particularly to NSAIDs, latex and neuromuscular blockers. It is theorized that this relates to gender differences in antigen exposures, with women being more likely to have had prior exposures to antigens in cosmetics and skin-care products.

Table 42.1 Gell and Coombs classification of allergic reactions [30].

Type	Clinical manifestations	Mechanism
I. Anaphylactic, immediate-type hypersensitivity	True anaphylaxis as described in this chapter	Exposure to antigen causes release of histamine, leukotrienes and prostaglandins from mast cells or basophils. Usually an IgE-dependent reaction
II. Antibody-dependent cytotoxicity	Hemolytic anemia, Interstitial nephritis	Antigens or haptens that are closely associated with a cell bind to an antibody, which leads to cell death or tissue injury
III. Immune complex disease	Serum sickness	Formation or deposition of antigen-antibody complexes causes damage to vessels and tissue
IV. Cell-mediated or delayed hypersensitivity	Contact dermatitis	Tissue injury mediated by T cells which have been sensitized to antigens
V. Idiopathic	Maculopapular rash, Stevens–Johnson syndrome	Not known

Type of exposure

Parenteral exposure to antigens is much more likely to cause anaphylactoid reactions than is oral ingestion. Parenteral exposures may be less likely to present with hives and flushing and therefore anaphylaxis may be mistaken for other causes of hypotension [8]. Inhalational exposures can rarely lead to anaphylaxis and when this does occur, peanuts or latex are the most likely precipitants. Exposures to larger volumes of antigen are also more like to put a patient at risk than are smaller ones. Lastly, concomitant exposures to other antigens to which the patient may have an allergy also seem to put patients at increased risk.

History of prior exposures

Consistent exposure is less likely to cause anaphylactoid responses than intermittent ones.

History of previous anaphylactoid response

Anaphylactoid responses are more likely to occur in patients who have had anaphylaxis in the past. However, anaphylaxis does not predictably recur in every patient upon repeat exposure [9]. If it has been years since previous exposure to the precipitating antigen, IgE levels may have declined over time and the immune response may have become muted.

History of atopy

Patients with atopy are at increased likelihood of anaphylactoid reactions to most agents except for medications. Atopic and asthmatic individuals are also more likely to die when they do have anaphylaxis [10].

Pathophysiology

True anaphylaxis is caused by the release of inflammatory mediators from the degranulation of mast cells and basophiles. This degranulation occurs in response to the cross-linking of mast cells bound to IgE with a precipitating antigen. The mediators initially released include histamine, prostaglandins, leukotrienes, and platelet activating factor. Later, cytokines, interleukin 3 and 4 and tumor necrosis factor may be released. The anaphylactic response can also be associated with stimulation of complement C3a, C4a and C5a. Alternations in arachidonic acid metabolism may also contribute to the anaphylactic syndrome in some cases. These mediators induce pruritus, vasodilation and increased vascular permeability. They can also cause respiratory muscle contraction, autonomic nervous system stimulation, platelet aggregation, recruitment of inflammatory cells and increased gastrointestinal motility. All of these responses contribute to the variable clinical presentation of anaphylaxis.

Clinical presentation

Symptoms generally develop within 5–60 minutes of exposure to the inciting antigen. Parenteral administration leads to a more rapid response. Oral ingestion will take longer. In rare circumstances, onset may be delayed up to several hours [11]. The manifestations of anaphylaxis vary widely and are reviewed in Table 42.3. Fatalities from anaphylaxis generally occur due to cardiovascular collapse, and asphyxia from upper airway obstruction from edema or intractable bronchospasm.

Timing and length of reaction

Most cases of anaphylaxis have a single severe response that resolves with treatment over a few hours. Some patients have a protracted syndrome that lasts for 24–48 hours. Between 1 and 20% of cases of anaphylactoid responses will have an acute phase followed by a period of recovery and then a recurrence between 1 and 8 hours after the initial presentation. Reports of a second wave of symptoms occurring up to 72 hours after the initial exposure exist but are rare [12–14]. The pathophysiology underlying such biphasic responses remains unclear. Biphasic reactions appear to

Table 42.2 Some precipitants of anaphylactoid reactions in adults [27,31–39].

Class of agent	Specific agents	Comments
Medications True anaphylaxis to drugs requires previous exposure, but anaphylactoid responses can occur the first time a medication is administered	Antibiotics, especially β-lactams (penicillins and less commonly cephalosporins) Aspirin and other NSAIDs, particularly in patients with nasal polyps/chronic sinusitis and asthma Neuromuscular blockers Narcotics Antineoplastic compounds Insulin [40] ACE inhibitors [41]	4–10% of people who have received penicillins have penicillin-specific Ig E antibodies although very few of these patients will manifest anaphylaxis. Anaphylaxis from penicillins is said to occur in 0.04–0.2% of exposures, with death from anaphylaxis occurring in only 0.001% of all exposures. Most of these patients will have had prior exposure to penicillins but no documented allergy to it. Concerningly, one-third of patients who die of penicillin anaphylaxis do have a documented history of prior reactions to penicillin [42]. Although 20% of patients with PCN allergies will have laboratory or skin testing evidence of a cross-reaction to cephalosporins, only 1% will actually have a clinical reaction to cephalosporins. For this reason, it is now recommended that cephalosporins be withheld from patients with PCN allergies only if their response to PCN included hypotension or respiratory difficulty. Anaphylactoid responses to non-β-lactam antibiotics are uncommon. NSAIDs can produce anaphylactoid responses by a variety of mechanisms, some of which are specific to a single drug, while others can occur with several different NSAIDs [43,44]. Selective COX-2 inhibitors are less likely to cause anaphylactoid reactions than NSAIDs
Insect bites/stings	Tiatoma (kissing bugs or assassin bugs) and members of the order Hymenoptera [45] (yellowjackets, wasps, imported fire ants and harvester ants)	
Foods [23,46–48]	Seafood, fish, peanuts, tree nuts, vegetables such as carrots and celery, wheat and grain	Although most commonly seen in children, food allergies can begin at any age in life. Food allergies are more likely to have bad outcomes in patients with asthma. Anaphylactoid reactions to seafood are not related to iodine content but rather to tropomyosin proteins. Celery and carrot anaphylaxis is more common in patients with allergies to pollens. Wheat and grain are particularly likely to be associated with "food dependent, exercise-induced anaphylaxis" (FDEIAn)
Sulfiting agents	Sulfites (or sulfiting agents) are a group of simple chemicals that include sulfur dioxide and sulfite salts. Some of these agents are approved by the US FDA for use as food preservatives and to prevent food discoloration. Sulfites are most commonly found now in the following foods: dried soup mixes, vegetable juices, baked goods, canned or dried fish, dried fruit, relishes, shredded coconut, shrimp, lobster, scallops, olives, pickles, sauerkraut, dried noodle meals, molasses, gravies, potatoes, lemon and lime juice, jams and jellies, grape juice, wine, beer, maraschino cherries, dehydrated vegetables and fruit	In 1986 the US FDA prohibited the use of sulfites on fruits and vegetables meant to be eaten raw. They also required companies to list on product labels sulfiting agents that occur at concentrations of 10 ppm or higher, and any sulfiting agents that had a technical or functional effect in the food regardless of the amount present
Immunotherapy injections	Antigen exposures given by allergists to downregulate systemic response in patients with allergies	

Table 42.2 *Continued*

Class of agent	Specific agents	Comments
Radiocontrast media (RCM) [48–51]	Lower osmolarity RCM presently in use have a very low risk of inducing anaphylactoid reactions as compared to the high osmolality agents used in the past. Iso-osmolar agents make RCM reactions extremely unlikely and can be requested when a patient is felt to be at risk of such a reaction	RCM causes anaphylactoid reactions but not true anaphylaxis. The incidence of life-threatening reactions is <0.1%. Peak incidence is between the ages of 20 and 50 so it does occur in women of childbearing age. Anaphylactoid reactions to RCM are more likely if it has happened before but even with a prior history of reactions to RCM, the incidence runs between 16% and 44% with a subsequent exposure. Volume overload from administration of RCM can lead to cardiogenic pulmonary edema that is not a hypersensitivity response and is part of the differential diagnosis of respiratory failure in this setting [52]. There is no relationship between RCM reactions and shellfish allergies (which are generally due to reactions to tropomyosin proteins and not iodine). The only association between these two allergies is that persons who have anaphylaxis to any agent are more likely to have anaphylaxis to other agents. Pretreatment with steroids and an H1 atagonist such as diphenhydramine can ameliorate or prevent reactions in patients deemed to be at risk
Unusual causes described in obstetric patients	Seminal fluid Laminaria Oxytocic agents	Administration of syntocinon has been associated with anaphylactoid response but has generally been attributed to preservatives used in specific formulations such as chlorobutanol [55–59]
	Methotrexate Anesthetic agents including local anesthetic [53]	Anaphylaxis to MTX used intravenously to treat cancer has been reported [60]
	Colloids such as dextran, albumin	Dextran use has been associated with both maternal and fetal morbidity and mortality with an incidence of dextran-70 solution-induced anaphylactoid reactions of 1 in 383 [61–64]
	Exercise [54]	Exertion can precipitate anaphylaxis in some individuals and this includes the exertion of labor [65]
Blood products	Whole blood, serum, plasma, fractionated serum products or immunoglobulins can all provoke an anaphylactoid response	Blood products can cause an anaphylactoid response via type II or type III hypersensitivity reactions
Latex	Exposure to hard rubbers not usually significant Latex exposure can occur with gloves, intravenous tubing, Foley catheters, endotracheal tubes, dental dams, vial stoppers, condoms, adhesive dressings, and balloons. Exposure can occur through direct contact, aerosolization or inhalation	Latex allergies remain one of the leading causes of perioperative anaphylactoid reactions. Widespread use of powder-free and low latex protein gloves has decreased latex sensitization but it still does occur in healthcare workers and patients who have undergone multiple hospital procedures [26,66]. Infants with spina bifida are at increased risk of latex allergies and ideally should be delivered and cared for using non-latex materials

be more common with oral ingestions and in general the delayed second phase is less severe than the initial presentation.

Diagnosis

Anaphylaxis is a clinical diagnosis. Three proposed sets of criteria for the diagnosis of anaphylaxis are reviewed in Table 42.4.

Approach to anaphylaxis

Acute management [15–20]

The acute management of anaphylaxis is reviewed below and should proceed in a stepwise manner.

1 Provide oxygen and assess airway. Equipment for intubation and persons experienced with intubation should be brought to

Table 42.3 Manifestations of anaphylaxis [67].

Affected system	Symptoms/signs	Comments
Skin	Itching, flushing, sensation that skin is being pulled or burned, urticaria (hives) and angioedmea (88%)	
Psychologic	Sense of impending doom	
Respiratory	Shortness of breath, hoarseness, difficulty breathing/swallowing/ talking, choking, lump in throat, wheezing, stridor, laryngeal edema (50%). CXR may show hyperinflation, pulmonary edema or ARDS [67]. Intubated patients may have elevated airway pressures and increased airway resistance	
Cardiovascular	Faintness, palpitations, chest discomfort, syncope, tachycardia, bradycardia, ST/T changes on EKG, multiple PVCs, hypotension due to sudden hypovolemia. Shock will occur in up to 30%. Eventually fatal arrhythmias may occur	Hypotension occurs due to three factors: **1** sudden hypovolemia from third spacing of intravascular fluid from sudden changes in vascular permeability **2** vasodilation and **3** myocardial depression [1,15]. Although initially cardiac output may be increased, it will often decrease with progression of the syndrome. Systemic vascular resistance (SVR) is typically initially reduced in anaphylaxis. However, in severely hypovolemic patients vasoconstriction can occur and be so severe that there is no additional response to vasopresssors
Gastrointestinal	Metallic taste in mouth, nausea, vomiting, diarrhea, incontinence, abdominal bloating, abdominal and uterine cramping (30%)	
Fetal	Decreased fetal movement. Fetal heart rate monitor may also show late decelerations, tachycardia, diminished variability, bradycardia	

Table 42.4 Three distinct criteria for the diagnosis of anaphylaxis [15,16,26,68].

Criterion 1

Acute onset of an illness over minutes to hours with involvement of skin, mucosal tissue or both, e.g. hives, swollen lips/tongue/uvula, flushing with at least one of the following:
- respiratory compromise, e.g. dyspnea, wheezing, stridor, hypoxemia
- reduced blood pressure or symptoms of end-organ dysfunction suggestive of hypotension (e.g. syncope, incontinence, collapse, hypotonia)

Criterion 2

Two or more of the following after a potentially allergenic exposure:
- mucosa/skin involvement: urticaria, flushing, itching, tongue, lip or uvula swelling
- respiratory involvement: dyspnea, stridor, bronchospasm, hypoxia
- gastrointestinal involvement: abdominal pain, vomiting
- hemodynamic instability: hypotension, syncope, incontinence

Criterion 3

Drop in blood pressure (either <90 mmHg or >30 mmHg drop from baseline) minutes to hours after exposure to a known allergen for that patient

the bedside promptly if there is any evidence of airway compromise or facial or neck swelling. Pregnant women are difficult to intubate because of pregnancy-related changes in the airway and body habitus. Anaphylaxis-related airway edema may further contribute to the difficulty in establishing an airway in a pregnant patient. Therefore, if intubation is performed it should be done by the most experienced person available and with a plan in place for what will be done should the intubation fail (including being prepared for the possibility of emergency cricothyroidotomy).

2 Administer aqueous epinephrine 0.5 mg (0.5 mL of a 1 : 1000 (1 mg/mL) solution) intramuscularly into the lateral or anterior thigh. Epinephrine will both treat hypotension and help with bronchospasm and is the cornerstone of the initial medical management of anaphylaxis. There are no absolute contraindications to epinephrine in the setting of anaphylaxis. This dose of epinephrine may be repeated every 5 minutes as needed. Subcutaneous administration is acceptable but is associated with less rapid absorption and effect than an intramuscular or intravenous injection. If patient is on a β-blocker, the response to epinephrine may be dampened, and the patient may be given glucagon 1 mg intravenously as an alternate if epinephrine does not produce the desired effect. This dose of glucagon may be repeated as needed every 1 minute until a total of 5 mg has been given. Glucagon has chronotropic and inotropic effects on the heart that are not mediated through the β-receptors [21].

3 Ensure the patient has two large-bore (14–16 G) peripheral intravenous lines in place for fluid and medication administration and prepare to obtain central venous access. Typically 5–10 mL/kg of normal saline or Ringer's lactate should be administered in the first minutes of treatment although this will warrant monitoring in patients with renal or cardiac disease [22]. Pregnant women have a predisposition to pulmonary edema that also warrants extra attention to overall fluid balance. Use fluid boluses to maintain blood pressure above 90/60 mmHg, especially if the patient has not responded to epinephrine. Anaphylaxis is often associated with sudden and massive extravasation of fluid into the third space and patients may have profound intravascular volume depletion. In severe cases of anaphylaxis up to 7 L of fluid may need to be given to support blood pressure [23].

4 Remove the inciting antigen when possible. Consider use of a tourniquet to obstruct venous return from a limb that was exposed to the probable precipitating antigen when appropriate. The tourniquet should be released every 15 minutes to prevent ischemia.

5 Place the patient in the reverse Trendelenburg position lying on her left side to improve venous return.

6 Initiate cardiac and frequent blood pressure monitoring. Initially, these parameters should be measured no less frequently than every 5 minutes.

7 Administer an intravenous histamine H_1 blocker (typically diphenhydramine 25 mg IV over 3–5 min) and histamine H_2 blocker (typically ranitidine 1 mg/kg IV over 10–15 min).

8 Administer intravenous steroids (typically hydrocortisone 100 mg every 6 hours or methylprednisolone 1–2 mg/kg per day). These agents do not treat the acute symptoms of anaphylaxis but may have a role in preventing late-phase reactions. Because there are rare reports of biphasic reactions occurring as late as 72 hours after the initial exposure, many experts would continue steroids at a dose equivalent to this dose for a total of 4 days (typically prednisolone 50 mg daily).

9 If wheezing is present, administration of bronchodilators such as albuterol (2.5–5 mg in 3 mL saline via nebulizer) should be considered.

10 Place a fetal monitoring device on the patient. Several anecdotal reports of fetal injury or death in the setting of anaphylaxis despite prompt maternal blood pressure control have suggested that maternal blood pressure in anaphylaxis may be maintained at the expense of uterine (or splanchnic) flow. Evidence of fetal distress should be addressed by improving oxygen delivery through increasing oxygen administration, changing position of the mother, and increasing fluid administration. If there is ongoing evidence of maternal or fetal compromise, then vasopressor support (see below) should be introduced. Cesarean delivery should rarely be necessary but should be considered if the fetus is at a gestation where delivery may lead to a viable infant and the fetus demonstrates ongoing distress despite aggressive maternal resuscitation.

11 If blood pressure remains below 90/60 mmHg, begin administration of intravenous vasopressors. Patients who require this level of care or who have ongoing airway concerns after the initial treatment should be transferred promptly to an intensive care unit. Epinephrine can be given intravenously at a dose of 0.1 mg (1.0 mL of a 1 : 10 000 (1 mg/10 mL) solution) over several minutes and repeated every 5–10 minutes as needed. This medication should be given with the patient on a cardiac monitor and ideally through a central line to decrease the risk of tissue damage from extravasation. It can also be administered via an endotracheal tube (0.3–0.5 mg (3–5 mL of a 1 : 10 000 dilution)) if intravenous access is compromised. If continued boluses of epinephrine are needed, a continuous infusion can be given: 1 mL of 1 : 1000 dilution of epinephrine should be placed in 500 mL of normal saline and given at a rate of 1–4 micrograms per minute (0.05–0.1 μg/kg/min) and titrated to response. Some concern does exist about the effects of epinephrine use in pregnancy because of both a weak association with ventral hernias when used in the first trimester and its possible adverse effects on uterine blood flow. Because of these concerns, some authors have suggested a trial of terbutaline subcutaneously (typically 0.25 mg subcutaneously) as an alternative to epinephrine in pregnancy. However, the data supporting the efficacy of terbutaline in the treatment of anaphylaxis are minimal and therefore most experts would recommend the use of epinephrine as a first-line agent in treating anaphylaxis in pregnancy given the life-threatening nature of the condition. Studies in non-pregnant patients have shown that fatality rates are highest in patients in whom treatment with epinephrine is delayed [24–26]. Other vasopressors that may be helpful in patients with anaphylactic shock when epinephrine has failed include dopamine (5–20 μg/kg/min), norepinephrine (0.5–30 μg/min) or phenylephrine (30–180 μg/min). Vasopressin 10–40 IU IV has also been reported to be of assistance in refractory cases [15].

Management of the patient after the acute episode of anaphylaxis

Management after an anaphylactic reaction typically involves ongoing vasopressor support until the blood pressure no longer requires it. The acute symptoms and danger should usually have begun to resolve within 6 hours of the onset of the event. Steroids and antihistamines are typically continued for 72–96 hours and then can be discontinued.

Once the patient has been stabilized, a careful history should be taken to identify all exposures in the hours prior to the reaction. The patient should also be asked about any exertion prior to the onset of the event, including sexual activity.

Laboratory findings that may be drawn as soon as possible after the event to help confirm the diagnosis of an anaphylactoid response include serum levels of histamine and tryptase, both of which will be elevated in anaphylaxis [18,27]. Histamine will be elevated for up to 60 minutes and tryptase for up to 6 hours. Typically, several specimens should be obtained in the 6-hour period following the onset of anpahylaxis so that a pattern of elevation followed by decline may be observed. The assay for histamine can be falsely elevated from basophil activation of clotted blood in the test tube and has a very short half-life that limits its clinical use at many instructions. Therefore a 24-hour urine sample looking for the histamine metabolite N-methyl histamine may be a useful additional test to consider. Assays showing elevated levels of histamine or tryptase and its metabolites are indicative of anaphylaxis; however a normal assay does not preclude the diagnosis.

All patients who have had an anaphylactic event should be educated as to the seriousness of their condition and its propensity to recur. Patients should be provided a prescription for an epinephrine autoinjector and educated as to its use. The importance of this should be emphasized to the patient, as many patients will not fulfil their prescription or be willing to self-inject unless they clearly understand the nature of their condition [15,28,29]. Preloaded auto-injectors marketed in the US include EpiPen© and Twinject©. Twinject© has the advantage of offering two-dose devices that may be necessary to treat more severe reactions in adults.

Ideally, all patients who have had an episode of life-threatening anaphylaxis should be referred to an allergist for care and counseling regarding their condition. Allergists will often do skin and serum IgE tests to confirm or identify inciting antigens and consider the need for immunotherapy. Skin testing should only be done by allergists and should be delayed for at least 4 weeks so that mast cells in the skin have a chance to replenish their inflammatory mediators. Serum testing can, however, be done immediately [15].

Patients who have had anaphylaxis should be told to wear a MedicAlert bracelet or a similar device to avoid inadvertent exposure to a precipitating allergen. Patient with anaphylaxis who have been on a β-blocker should generally be switched to an alternate medication if at all possible because the β-blocker may decrease the efficacy of epinephrine given in a subsequent attack.

Table 42.5 The differential diagnosis of anaphylaxis.

Alternative diagnoses	Comments
Vasovagal response	Should generally be associated with bradycardia and pallor and no flushing, rash, itch, hives or wheezing
Anxiety	Hives and hypotension should not be present
Amniotic fluid embolism (AFE)	Initial presentation may be similar but AFE should not be associated with rash, itch or hives and is generally associated with DIC
Pulmonary edema in pregnancy	Pulmonary edema can occur in pregnancy in association with fluid overload, pre-eclampsia, infection or tocolytic administration. Onset will generally be gradual over several hours and not be associated with rash or hypotension
Medication effects other than allergies	Vancomycin, nicotinic acid, ACE inhibitors and alcohol can all cause flushing in susceptible individuals
Pulmonary embolism or any other cause of acute respiratory failure	Can cause sudden-onset tachycardia, respiratory failure (with or without wheeze) and hypotension but should not cause rash or itch
Scromboid poisoning [68]	Histamine-producing bacteria in fish such as spoiled tuna, mackerel and skipjack can cause gastrointestinal symptoms, flushing, headache, dizziness but not usually hives. This can be difficult to distinguish from anaphylaxis but is suggested by a clustering of cases related to a particular meal/restaurant
Vocal cord dysfunction	Young women can present with acute inspiratory stridor related to paradoxic vocal cord motion. This is more often seen in women with a preceding diagnosis of asthma. Stridor in this setting is typically only inspiratory which distinguishes it from the stridor seen with true airway edema which is typically both inspiratory and expiratory. Hypotension, uvular edema, rash should not be seen in these patients
Acute myocardial infarction, congestive heart failure	Less likely in this patient population but it is reasonable to obtain EKG, CXR and serial cardiac enzymes (troponin) in patients presenting with probable anaphylaxis. If concern exists for a cardiac cause, an echocardiogram should be ordered acutely
Miscellaneous	Flushing syndromes (carcinoid syndrome, medullary carcinoma of the thyroid, perimenopausal symptoms) pheochromocytoma Hemorrhagic/hypovolemic shock Septic shock Epiglottitis Status asthmaticus Foreign body aspiration Panic attacks Systemic mastocytosis

Differential diagnosis

The differential diagnosis of anaphylaxis is broad and is summarized in Table 42.5.

Conclusions

Anaphylaxis and anaphylactoid reactions are common in hospitalized patients. They are a medical emergency which warrant prompt administration of oxygen, intravenous fluids, epinephrine and removal of the inciting agent when possible. Management in pregnancy is unchanged from that for non-pregnant patients. The life-saving nature of epinephrine in this setting justifies its use even if there are concerns about its effects in general on placental flow. Patients who have had anaphylactic responses should be observed for at least 8 hours and placed on steroids because of a risk of a biphasic response in 48–72 hours. With prompt identification and management, both mother and fetus can expect to do well.

References

1 Sampson HA, Munoz-Furlong A, Bock SA, et al. Symposium on the definition and management of anaphylaxis: summary report. *J Allergy Clin Immunol* 2005; 115: 584.
2 Winbery SL, Lieberman PL. Anaphylaxis. *Immunol Allergy Clin North Am* 1995; 15: 447.
3 DeJarnatt AC, Grant JA. Basic mechanisms of anaphylaxis and anaphylactoid reactions. *Immunol Allergy Clin North Am* 1992; 12: 501.
4 Lieberman P, Camargo CA Jr, Bohlke K, et al. Epidemiology of anaphylaxis: findings of the American College of Allergy, Asthma and Immunology Epidemiology of Anaphylaxis Working Group. *Ann Allergy Asthma Immunol* 2006; 97: 596.
5 International Collaborative Study of Severe Anaphylaxis. An epidemiologic study of severe anaphylactic and anaphylactoid reactions among hospital patients: methods and overall risks. *Epidemiology* 1998; 9: 141.
6 Thong BY, Cheng YK, Leong, KP et al. Anaphylaxis in adults referred to a clinical immunology/allergy centre in Singapore. *Singapore Med J* 2005; 46: 529.
7 Webb LM, Lieberman P. Anaphylaxis: a review of 601 cases. *Ann Allergy Asthma Immunol* 2006; 97: 39.
8 Fisher MM, Doig GS. Prevention of anaphylactic reactions to anaesthetic drugs. *Drug Saf* 2004; 27: 393.
9 Reisman RE. Insect sting anaphylaxis. *Immunol Allergy Clin North Am* 1992; 12: 535.
10 Pumphrey R. Anaphylaxis: can we tell who is at risk of a fatal reaction? *Curr Opin Allergy Clin Immunol* 2004; 4: 285.
11 Stark BJ, Sullivan TJ. Biphasic and protracted anaphylaxis. *J Allergy Clin Immunol* 1986; 78: 76.
12 Lieberman P. Biphasic anaphylactic reactions. *Ann Allergy Asthma Immunol* 2005; 95: 217.
13 Brazil E, MacNamara AF. "Not so immediate" hypersensitivity – the danger of biphasic anaphylactic reactions. *J Accid Emerg Med* 1998; 15: 252.
14 Douglas DM, Sukenick E, Andrade P, Brown JS. Biphasic systemic anaphylaxis: an inpatient and outpatient study. *J Allergy Clin Immunol* 1994; 93: 977.
15 Yocum MW, Khan DA. Assessment of patients who have experienced anaphylaxis: a 3-year survey. *Mayo Clin Proc* 1994; 69: 16.
16 Sampson HA, Munoz-Furlong A, Campbell RL, et al. Second symposium on the definition and management of anaphylaxis: summary report – Second National Institute of Allergy and Infectious Disease/ Food Allergy and Anaphylaxis Network symposium. *J Allergy Clin Immunol* 2006; 117: 391.
17 Atkinson TP, Kaliner MA. Anaphylaxis. *Med Clin North Am* 1992; 76: 841.
18 Fisher M. Treatment of acute anaphylaxis. *BMJ* 1995; 311: 731.
19 Zaloga GP, Delacey W, Holmboe E, Chernow B. Glucagon reversal of hypotension in a case of anaphylactoid shock. *Ann Intern Med* 1986; 105: 65.
20 Lieberman P, Kemp SF, Oppenheimer J, et al. The diagnosis and management of anaphylaxis: an updated practice parameter. *J Allergy Clin Immunol* 2005; 115: S483.
21 Fisher MM. Clinical observations on the pathophysiology and treatment of anaphylactic cardiovascular collapse. *Anaesth Intens Care* 1986; 14: 17.
22 Clark S, Long AA, Gaeta TJ, Camargo CA Jr. Multicenter study of emergency department visits for insect sting allergies. *J Allergy Clin Immunol* 2005; 116: 643.
23 Sampson HA, Mendelson L, Rosen JP. Fatal and near-fatal anaphylactic reactions to food in children and adolescents. *N Engl J Med* 1992; 327: 380.
24 Clark S, Bock SA, Gaeta TJ, et al. Multicenter study of emergency department visits for food allergies. *J Allergy Clin Immunol* 2004; 113: 347.
25 Kill C, Wranze E, Wulf H. Successful treatment of severe anaphylactic shock with vasopressin. Two case reports. *Int Arch Allergy Immunol* 2004; 134: 260.
26 Bochner BS, Lichtenstein LM. Anaphylaxis. *N Engl J Med* 1991; 324: 1785.
27 Fisher M. Treatment of acute anaphylaxis. *BMJ* 1995; 311: 731.
28 Weiss ME, Adkinson NF. Immediate hypersensitivity reactions to penicillin and related antibiotics. *Clin Allergy* 1998; 18: 515.
29 Riedl MA, Casillas AM. Adverse drug reactions: types and treatment options. *Am Fam Physician* 2003; 68(9): 1781.
30 Pumphrey R. Anaphylaxis: can we tell who is at risk of a fatal reaction? *Curr Opin Allergy Clin Immunol* 2004; 4: 285.
31 Barnard JH. Studies of 400 Hymenoptera sting deaths in the United States. *J Allergy Clin Immunol* 1973; 52: 259.
32 Novembre E, Cianferoni A, Bernardini R, et al. Anaphylaxis in children: clinical and allergologic features. *Pediatrics* 1998; 101: E8.
33 Porsche R, Brenner ZR. Allergy to protamine sulfate. *Heart Lung* 1999; 28: 418.
34 Ditto AM, Harris KE, Krasnick J, et al. Idiopathic anaphylaxis: a series of 335 cases. *Ann Allergy Asthma Immunol* 1996; 77: 285.
35 Kemp SF, Lockey RF, Wolf BL, Lieberman P. Anaphylaxis: review of 266 cases. *Arch Intern Med* 1995; 155: 1749.
36 Horan RF, Sheffer AL. Exercise-induced anaphylaxis. *Immunol Allergy Clin North Am* 1992; 3: 559.
37 Ewan PW. Anaphylaxis. *BMJ* 1998; 316: 1442.

38 Tejedor A, Sastre DJ, Sanchez-Hernandez JJ, et al. Idiopathic anaphylaxis: a descriptive study of 81 patients in Spain. *Ann Allergy Asthma Immunol* 2002; 88: 313.
39 Dykewicz MS. Cough and angioedema from angiotensin-converting enzyme inhibitors: new insights into mechanisms and management. *Curr Opin Allergy Clin Immunol* 2004; 4: 267.
40 Idsoe O, Guthe T, Willcox RR, de Weck AL. Nature and extent of penicillin side-reactions, with particular reference to fatalities from anaphylactic shock. *Bull World Health Organ* 1968; 38(2): 159.
41 Brown AF, McKinnon D, Chu K. Emergency department anaphylaxis: a review of 142 patients in a single year. *J Allergy Clin Immunol* 2001; 108: 861.
42 Stevenson DD. Approach to the patient with a history of adverse reactions to aspirin or NSAIDs: diagnosis and treatment. *Allergy Asthma Proc* 2000; 21: 25.
43 Brown SG, Blackman KE, Stenlake V, Heddle RJ. Insect sting anaphylaxis; prospective evaluation of treatment with intravenous adrenaline and volume resuscitation. *Emerg Med J* 2004; 21: 149.
44 Clark S, Bock SA, Gaeta TJ, et al. Multicenter study of emergency department visits for food allergies. *J Allergy Clin Immunol* 2004; 113: 347.
45 Bock SA, Munoz-Furlong A, Sampson HA. Fatalities due to anaphylactic reactions to foods. *J Allergy Clin Immunol* 2001; 107: 191.
46 Novembre E, Cianferoni A, Bernardini R, et al. Anaphylaxis in children: clinical and allergologic features. *Pediatrics* 1998; 101: E8.
47 Bush WH. Treatment of systemic reactions to contrast media. *Urology* 1990; 35: 145.
48 Lieberman P. Anaphylactoid reactions to radiocontrast material. *Immunol Allergy Clin North Am* 1992; 12: 649.
49 Bush WH, Swanson DP. Acute reactions to intravascular contrast media: types, risk factors, recognition, and specific treatment. *AJR* 1991; 157: 1153.
50 Lieberman P, Kemp SF, Oppenheimer J, et al. The diagnosis and management of anaphylaxis: an updated practice parameter. *J Allergy Clin Immunol* 2005; 115: S483.
51 Browne IM, Birnbach DJ. A pregnant woman with previous anaphylactic reaction to local anesthetics: a case report. *Am J Obstet Gynecol* 2001; 185(5): 1253.
52 Tarlo SM. Natural rubber latex allergy and asthma. *Curr Opin Pulm Med* 2001; 7: 27.
53 Slater RM, Bowles BJM, Pumphrey RSH. Anaphylactoid reaction to oxytocin in pregnancy. *Anesthesia* 1985; 40: 655.
54 Hofmann H, Goerz G, Plewig G. Anaphylactic shock from chlorobutanol-preserved oxytocin. *Contact Derm* 1986; 15: 241.
55 Morriss WW, Lavies NG, Anderson SK, Southgate HJ. Acute respiratory distress during cesarean section under surgery from spina bifida. *Anesthesiology* 1990; 73: 556.
56 Kawarabayashi T, Narisawa Y, Nakamura K, Sugimori H, Oda M, Taniguchi Y. Anaphylactoid reaction to oxytocin during cesarean section. *Gynecol Obstet Invest* 1988; 25(4): 277.
57 Maycock EJ, Russell WC. Anaphylactoid reaction to syntocinon. *Anaesth Intens Care* 1993; 21: 211.
58 Cohn JR, Cohn JB, Fellin F, Cantor R. Systemic anaphylaxis from low dose methotrexate. *Ann Allergy* 1993; 70(5): 384.
59 Barbier P, Jonville AP, Autret E. Fetal risks with dextrans during delivery. *Drug Saf* 1992; 7: 71.
60 Ring J. Anaphylactoid reactions to intravenous solutions used for volume substitution. *Clin Rev Allergy* 1991; 9: 397.
61 Berg EM, Fasting S, Sellevoid OFM. Serious complications with dextran-70 despite hapten prophylaxis. Is it best avoided prior to delivery? *Anesthesia* 1991; 46: 1033.
62 Paull J. A prospective study of dextran-induced anaphylactoid reactions in 5475 patients. *Anaesth Intens Care* 1987; 15: 163.
63 Smith HS. Delivery as a cause of exercise-induced anaphylactoid reaction: case report. *Br J Obstet Gynaecol* 1985; 92; 1196.
64 Ahmed SM, Aw TC, Adisesh A. Toxicological and immunological aspects of occupational latex allergy. *Toxicol Rev* 2004; 23: 123.
65 Allmers H, Schmengler J, John SM. Decreasing incidence of occupational contact urticaria caused by natural rubber latex allergy in German health care workers. *J Allergy Clin Immunol* 2004; 114: 347.
66 Edde RR, Burtis BB. Lung injury in anaphylactoid shock. *Chest* 1973; 63: 637.
67 Fisher MM. Clinical observations on the pathophysiology and treatment of anaphylactic cardiovascular collapse. *Anaesth Intens Care* 1986; 14: 17.
68 Lehane L. Update on histamine fish poisoning. *Med J Aust* 2000; 173: 149.

43 Fetal Considerations in the Critically Ill Gravida

Jeffrey P. Phelan[1] & Shailen S. Shah[2]

[1]Department of Obstetrics and Gynecology, Citrus Valley Medical Center, West Covina *and* Clinical Research, Childbirth Injury Prevention Foundation, City of Industry, Pasadena, CA, USA

[2]Maternal-Fetal Medicine, Virtua Health, Voorhees, NJ *and* Thomas Jefferson University Hospital, Philadelphia, PA, USA

Introduction

Unlike any other medical or surgical specialty, obstetrics deals with the simultaneous management of two–and sometimes more–individuals. Under all circumstances, the obstetrician must delicately balance the impact of each treatment decision on the pregnant woman and her fetus, seeking, when possible, to minimize the risks of harm to each person. Throughout this text, the primary focus has been on the critically ill obstetric patient and, secondarily, her fetus. Although the fetal effects of those illnesses were reviewed in part, the goal of this chapter is to highlight, especially for the non-obstetric clinician, the important clinical fetal considerations encountered when caring for these complicated pregnancies. To achieve that objective, this chapter reviews: (i) current techniques for assessing fetal well-being; (ii) fetal assessment in the intensive care unit; (iii) fetal considerations in several maternal medical and surgical conditions; (iv) the contemporary management of the gravida who is brain-dead or in a persistent vegetative state; and (v) the role of perimortem cesarean delivery in modern obstetrics.

Detection of fetal distress in the critically ill obstetric patient

More than four decades ago, Hon and Quilligan [1] demonstrated the relationship between certain fetal heart rate (FHR) patterns and fetal condition by using continuous electronic FHR monitoring in laboring patients. Since then, continuous electronic FHR monitoring has become a universally accepted method of assessing fetal well-being during labor [2,3] with the goal of permitting the clinician to identify those fetuses at a greater likelihood of intrapartum fetal death [4] and to intervene when certain FHR abnormalities are present.

Critical Care Obstetrics, 5th edition. Edited by M. Belfort, G. Saade, M. Foley, J. Phelan and G. Dildy.

In addition to the intrapartum assessment of fetal well-being, the fetal monitor has been used to assess fetal health before labor [5] and attempt to identify those fetuses at risk for intrauterine death and convert those fetuses so identified from outpatient to inpatient care. Once in labor and delivery, continuous fetal monitoring is used to determine whether continued expectant management or delivery by induction of labor or cesarean is the next form of intervention. It is this area of fetal monitoring, antepartum rather than intrapartum fetal assessment that is used more frequently in the arena of the critically ill gravida. Regardless, the focus of this chapter will be on applications of fetal monitoring to assess fetal status both in the intensive care unit setting and intrapartum during labor.

Although the presence of a reassuring FHR tracing is virtually always associated with a well-perfused and oxygenated fetus [5,6], an "abnormal tracing" is not necessarily predictive of an adverse fetal outcome. While it was anticipated that the detection of abnormal FHR patterns during labor and expeditious delivery of such fetuses would impact the subsequent development of cerebral palsy, this expectation has not been realized because the number of fetuses injured during labor was highly overestimated and the number of fetuses injured before labor were highly underestimated [7]. However, with the ubiquitous use of electronic FHR monitoring during labor and a rise in the cesarean delivery rate for the past two decades from 5% to over 25%, a decline in the rate of asphyxia-induced cerebral palsy among singleton term infants has been observed [8,9]. For example, Smith and associates [9] documented a 56% decline over two decades in the incidence of hypoxic ischemic encephalopathy (HIE) among singleton term infants. During this time, the incidence of HIE dropped from 1 per 8000 to 1 per 12500 births.

While the specific entity of cerebral palsy is, in most cases, unrelated to the events associated with labor and delivery, it is more often related to prenatal developmental events, infection, or complications of prematurity. Nevertheless, the basic physiologic observations relating to specific FHR patterns remain, for the most part, valid. The critically ill mother will necessarily shunt blood from the splanchnic bed (including the uterus) in response to shock. Because of this and the fact that the fetus operates on the steep portion of the oxyhemoglobin dissociation curve, any degree of maternal hypoxia or hypoperfusion may first be manifested as an abnormality of the FHR. In this sense, the late second- and third-trimester fetus serves as a physiologic oximeter and cardiac output computer. Observation of FHR changes, thus, may assist or alert the clinician to subtle degrees of physiologic instability, which would be unimportant in a non-pregnant adult but may have potentially detrimental effects to the fetus [10].

The next few pages present an overview of FHR patterns pertinent to the critically ill gravida. Interpretations of FHR patterns, like all diagnostic tests, depend on the index population, and consequently, certain of these observations may not be applicable to the laboring but otherwise well mother. For a more detailed description of antepartum and intrapartum FHR tracings associated with fetal brain injury the reader is referred to the classic descriptions by Phelan and Ahn [11], Phelan and Kim [12], Phelan [13] and Phelan and associates [14].

Baseline fetal heart rate

The baseline FHR is the intrinsic heart rate of the fetus. A normal baseline FHR is between 110 beats per minute (bpm) and 160 bpm. A baseline FHR below 110 bpm is termed a bradycardia and 160 bpm or higher is considered a tachycardia.

Bradycardia

Bradycardia is defined as the intrinsic heart rate of the fetus of less than 110 bpm, as opposed to a sudden, rapid, and sustained deterioration of the FHR from a previously normal or tachycardic rate that lasts until delivery. As such, a FHR bradycardia may be associated with an underlying congenital fetal abnormality, such as a structural defect of the fetal heart. In addition, congenital bradyarrhythmias may involve fetal heart block secondary to a prior maternal infection, a structural defect of the fetal heart, or systemic lupus erythematosus with anti-Ro/SSA antibodies [15]. In these circumstances, the FHR bradycardia is not usually a threat to the fetus. But, alternative methods of fetal assessment, such as the fetal biophysical profile (FBP) [16], are necessary in this select group of patients to assure fetal well-being before and during labor. Given the inherent difficulties in providing continuous fetal monitoring and assuring fetal well-being in fetuses with a bradyarrhythmia, cesarean delivery may well represent the preferred route of delivery for these patients. Obviously, the decision to proceed directly to a cesarean will depend on the overall clinical circumstances and appropriate patient informed consent.

Prolonged fetal heart rate deceleration or a sudden, rapid and sustained deterioration of the fetal heart rate

Prolonged FHR deceleration is distinctly different from a bradycardia. In the former, the fetal monitor strip is typically reactive with a normal or tachycardic baseline rate; but, due to a sentinel hypoxic event, such as those depicted in Table 43.1, the FHR suddenly drops and remains at a lower level unresponsive to remedial measures and/or terbutaline therapy. In the critical care setting, a sudden, rapid, and sustained deterioration of the FHR or a prolonged FHR deceleration may arise from a partial or complete abruption in cases of markedly elevated maternal blood pressures or an aggressive lowering of maternal BP with antihypertensive agents [17]. This type of FHR pattern may also herald a sudden maternal hypoxic event, such as amniotic fluid embolus syndrome [18], acute respiratory insufficiency, or an eclamptic seizure [17,19]. Prolonged FHR decelerations have also been associated with maternal operative procedures such as cardiopulmonary bypass with inadequate maternal flow rates [20,21], and brain surgery during hypothermia [22].

Table 43.1 Sentinel hypoxic events associated with a sudden, rapid, and sustained deterioration of the fetal heart rate that was unresponsive to remedial measures and/or terbutaline lasting until delivery from a previously reactive fetal heart rate.

Umbilical cord prolapse
Uterine rupture
Placental abruption
Maternal arrest, e.g. AFE syndrome
Fetal exsanguination

AFE, amniotic fluid embolus.

In a patient with a prior normal baseline FHR, the abrupt occurrence and persistence of a fetal heart rate of less than 110 bpm for an extended period of time unresponsive to remedial measures and/or terbutaline therapy constitutes an obstetric emergency. Under these circumstances, and assuming the pregnant woman is hemodynamically and clinically stable and the fetus is potentially viable, these patients should be managed as if the fetus has had a cardiac arrest and be delivered as rapidly as it is technically feasible for the level of the institution.

Tachycardia

Fetal tachycardia is defined as a baseline FHR of 160 bpm or greater. Most commonly, this type of baseline FHR abnormality can be associated with prematurity, maternal pyrexia, or chorioamnionitis. In addition, betamimetic administration, hyperthyroidism, or fetal cardiac arrhythmias may also be responsible. The clinical observation of a FHR tachycardia, in and of itself, is probably not an ominous finding but probably reflects a normal physiologic adjustment to an underlying maternal or fetal condition. Although operative intervention is rarely required, a search for the underlying basis for the tachycardia and a reanalysis of the admission FHR pattern may be helpful.

For example, the patient with a previously reactive FHR pattern with a normal baseline rate (Figure 43.1) who develops the Hon pattern of intrapartum asphyxia or ischemia [11] which is characterized by a substantial rise in the baseline rate often to a level of tachycardia (Figures 43.2 & 43.3) in association with an inability to accelerate or non-reactivity, repetitive FHR decelerations,

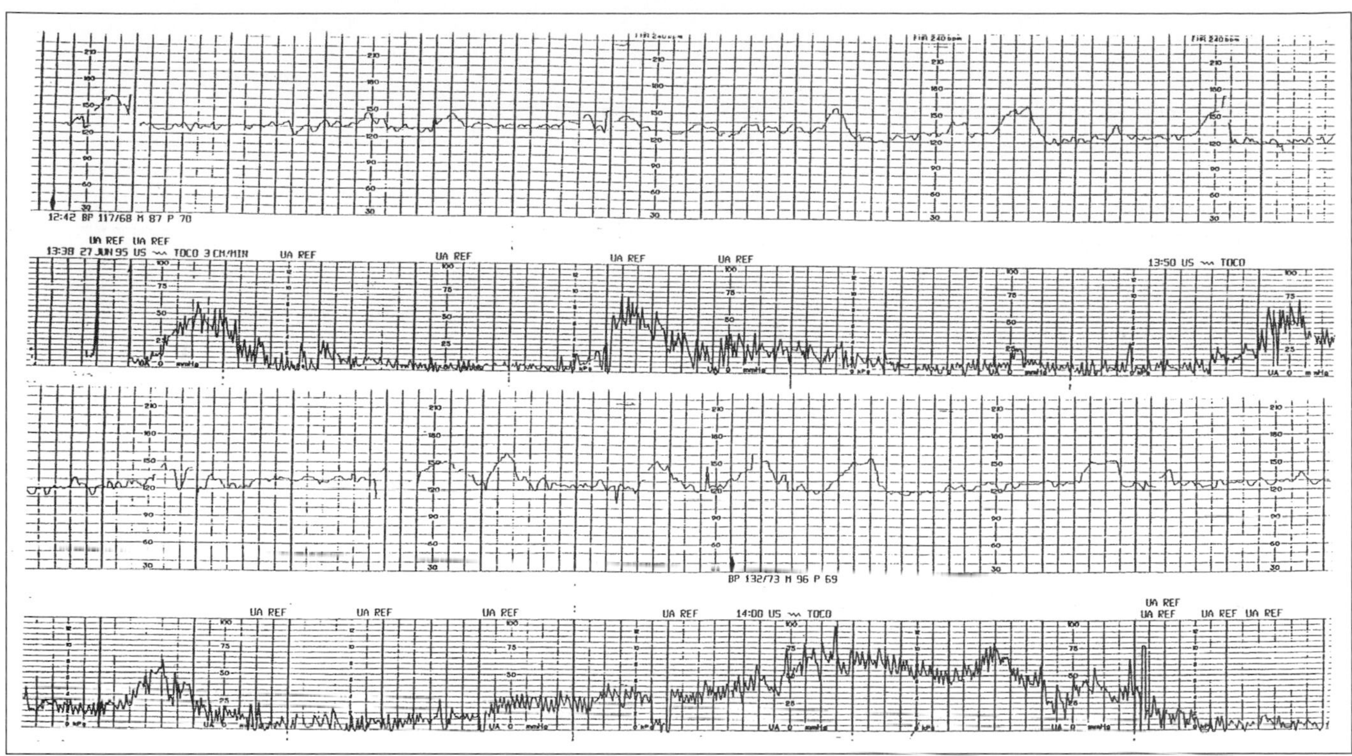

Figure 43.1 Admission FHR of this term pregnancy with spontaneously ruptured membranes exhibits a baseline rate around 120 bpm and numerous FHR accelerations or a reactive FHR pattern.

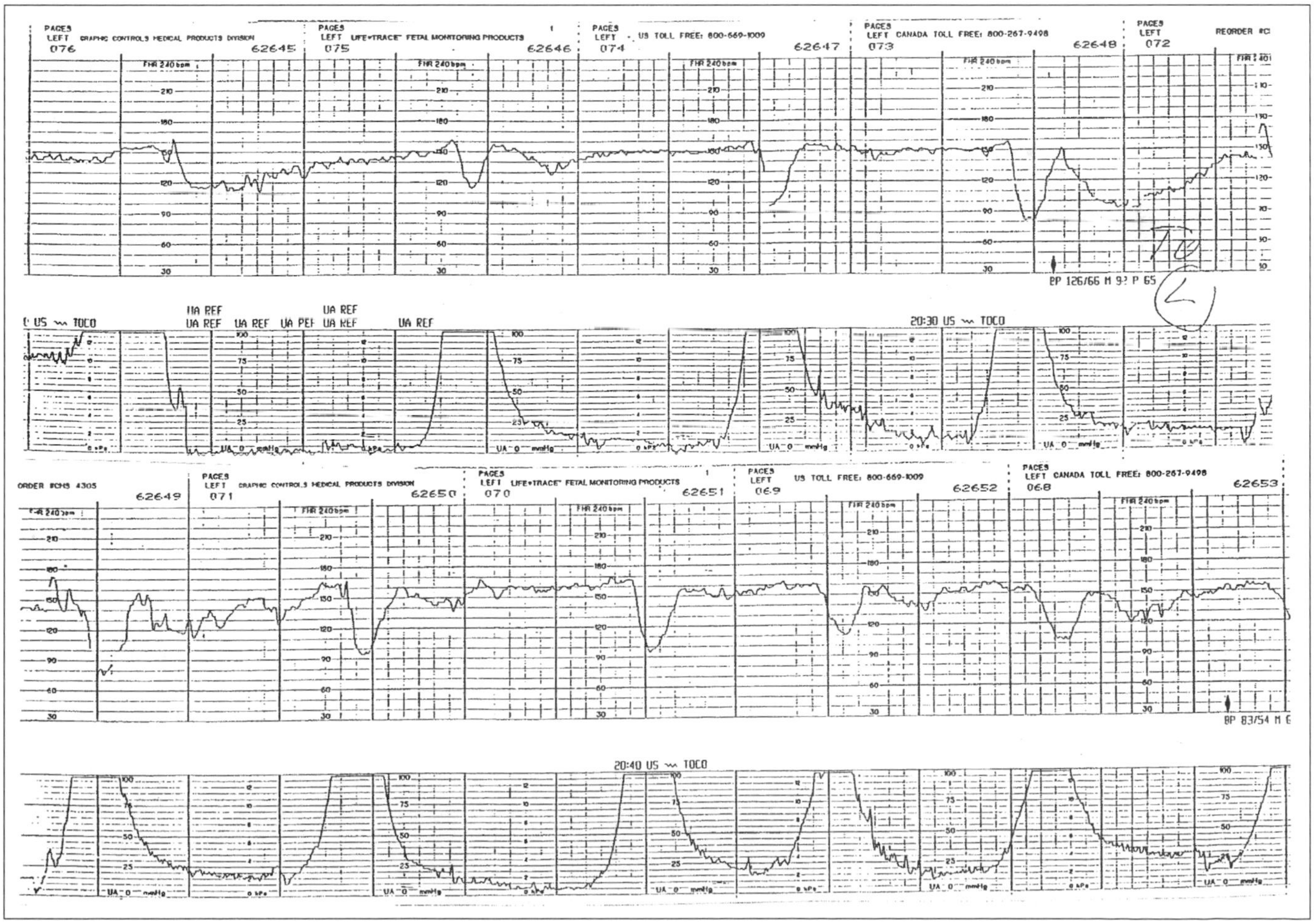

Figure 43.2 Some time later, the fetus exhibits an FHR tachycardia around 160 bpm, repetitive FHR decelerations and non-reactivity.

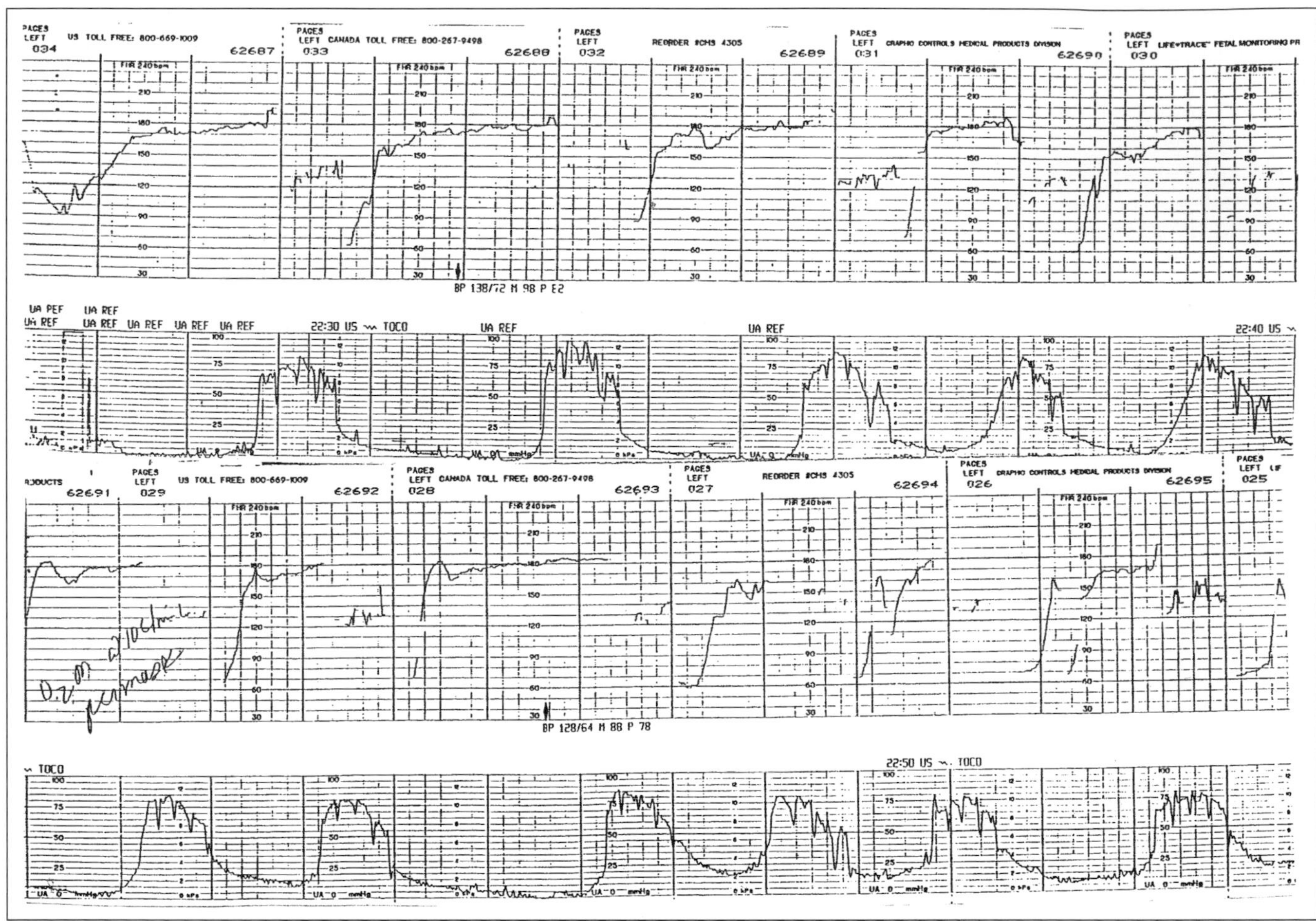

Figure 43.3 Later in the labor, the baseline FHR reaches 180 bpm and continues to exhibit repetitive FHR decelerations, non-reactivity, and diminished variability. The fetus was born with spastic quadriplegia due to hypoxic ischemic encephalopathy.

and usually a loss of FHR variability, flags fetal brain injury [23] and the fetus is at risk for hypoxic ischemic brain injury [11–13]. In this clinical setting, assessment of the usual causes of FHR tachycardia should be undertaken. If the mother does not have a fever to account for the change in fetal status, assessment of fetal acid–base status with scalp or acoustic stimulation [6,12] or delivery as soon as it is practical, in keeping with the capability of the hospital, should be considered. If the gravida has a fever, she should be cultured, and treated with antibiotics and anti-pyretics. If the FHR pattern does not return to normal (i.e. the same FHR pattern the fetus had on admission – normal baseline FHR and reactive) within approximately an hour of the initiation of medical therapy and regardless of whether the fetal heart rate variability is average [11–13,24], the patient should be delivered as expeditiously as possible.

Fetal heart rate variability

Fetal heart rate variability (FHRV) is defined as the beat-to-beat variation in the FHR resulting from the continuous interaction of the parasympathetic and sympathetic nervous systems on the fetal heart. For clinical purposes, normal FHRV may be viewed as a beat-to-beat variation of the FHR of 6 bpm or more above and below the baseline FHR.

Currently, two approaches, the National Institutes of Child Health and Human Development (NICHD) [25] and the Childbirth Injury Prevention Foundation (CIPF) [11,14] are available to classify FHRV. The NICHD and CIPF approaches subclassify FHRV into 4 and 2 categories, respectively. This means that the CIPF classification incorporates the NICHD criteria of undetectable (absent FHRV) and minimal (more than absent but ≤5 bpm) into one category known as diminished FHRV (<6 bpm). Similarly, the CIPF approach merges the NICHD criteria of moderate (6–25 bpm) and marked (>25 bpm) into their average FHRV classification. Regardless of the approach used, the more simplified approach of the CIPF or the more complicated one of the NICHD, a uniform approach for the classification of FHR variability should be used in your institution and established by the Department of Obstetrics and Gynecology.

Decreased FHRV (<6 bpm), in and of itself, is not an ominous observation. In most cases, the diminished FHRV represents normal fetal physiologic adjustments to a number of medications, illicit substances or simply behavioral state changes such as 1F to 4F [26]. For example, narcotic administration [27] or magnesium sulfate infusion [28] can alter FHRV by inducing a change in the behavioral state of the fetus to one of a sleep state or behavioral state 1F. Clinically, diminished FHRV appears to be clinically significant in cases of the Hon pattern of intrapartum asphyxia [11–13]. As observed herein (Figures 43.1–43.3), the FHR pattern was first reactive and exhibited a normal baseline rate. Subsequently, the FHR pattern changed. Then, the diminished FHRV was associated with a loss of FHR reactivity, a substantial rise in the baseline FHR, a FHR tachycardia, and repetitive FHR decelerations. Under these circumstances, the potential for fetal asphyxia is increased. Additionally, the presence of diminished FHRV [24] in the setting of the Hon pattern of intrapartum asphyxia is associated with significantly higher rates of neonatal cerebral edema.

Sinusoidal fetal heart rate pattern

A sinusoidal FHR pattern is defined as a persistent regular sine wave variation of the baseline FHR that has a frequency of 3–6 cycles per minute [29]. The degree of oscillation correlates with fetal outcome [30]. For instance, infants with oscillations of 25 bpm or more have a significantly greater perinatal mortality rate than do infants whose oscillations are less than 25 bpm (67% vs 1%). A favorable fetal outcome also is associated with the presence of FHR accelerations and/or non-persistent sinusoidal FHR pattern.

The key to the management of a persistent sinusoidal FHR pattern is recognition. Once a sinusoidal FHR pattern is recognized, a clinical evaluation of the patient and a search for the underlying cause should be considered. Non-persistent or an intermittent sinusoidal FHR pattern is commonly related to maternal narcotic administration [31]. In the absence of maternal narcotic administration, the sudden appearance of a persistent sinusoidal FHR pattern and a lack of FHR accelerations do suggest the potential for fetal anemia and fetomaternal hemorrhage.

Fetal anemia may be associated with a number of obstetric conditions such as placental abruption or previa, fetomaternal hemorrhage, vasa previa, Rh sensitization, and non-immune hydrops [31]. If, for example, a persistent sinusoidal FHR pattern is observed in a patient who recently has been involved in a motor vehicle accident, placental abruption is one consideration. Evidence of an abruption or other forms of fetal hemorrhage may also be suggested by a positive Kleihauer–Betke (K-B) test for fetal RBCs in the maternal circulation. Finally, as suggested by Katz and associates [30], a persistent sinusoidal FHR pattern in the absence of accelerations is a sign of potential fetal compromise. In this latter circumstance, a Kleihauer–Betke test with either delivery or some form of fetal acid–base assessment with scalp or acoustic stimulation should be considered [32,33]. Often, patients with a persistent sinusoidal FHR pattern will have a history of reduced fetal activity, usually a stair–step reduction over several days [34] and, occasionally, an abnormal Kleihauer–Betke test [33,35].

Periodic changes or FHR changes in response to uterine contractions

The focus of this section is on periodic FHR changes that occur in response to uterine contractions, such as FHR accelerations and variable and late decelerations. FHR decelerations, in and of themselves, are not associated with an increased risk of perinatal morbidity and mortality. To be associated with adverse fetal outcome, i.e. cerebral palsy due to hypoxic ischemic encephalopathy, FHR decelerations should be repetitive and in association with usually diminished FHR variability, a rising baseline rate to a level of FHR tachycardia, and a non-reactive FHR pattern [11,14]. To understand these periodic changes, the reader is encouraged to review the NICHD and CIPF approaches to the interpretation of periodic FHR decelerations. The CIPF approach is based on the criteria established in the 1960s and 1970s and published in the Corometric's Teaching Program around 1974 [36] for FHR interpretation. Each of these periodic changes will be discussed separately to assist the reader in their understanding of FHR patterns during labor.

Accelerations

A FHR acceleration is defined as an abrupt increase in the FHR above baseline, spontaneously or in relation to uterine activity, fetal body movement, or fetal breathing. Criteria for FHR accelerations (i.e. a "reactive" tracing) include a rise in the FHR of at least 15 bpm from baseline, lasting at least 15 seconds from the time it leaves baseline until it returns [5]. Since the acceleration does not need to remain at 15 bpm or higher for 15 seconds, acceptable FHR accelerations are in the form of a triangle rather than a rectangle. Whenever spontaneous or induced FHR accelerations are present, a healthy and non-acidotic fetus is probably present. This is true, regardless of whether otherwise "worrisome" features of the FHR tracing are present [5,6,37].

The presence of FHR accelerations is the basis to assess fetal well-being both before and during labor [5,6].

The presence of FHR accelerations is a sign of fetal well-being with a low probability of fetal compromise [5], brain damage [38], or death within several days to a week of fetal surveillance testing [5]. This observation persists irrespective of whether the acceleration is spontaneous or induced [5]. In contrast, the findings of a persistent non-reactive FHR pattern lasting longer than 120 minutes from admission to the hospital or the physician's office is a sign of pre-existing compromise due to a preadmission to the hospital or pre-NST fetal brain injury [14], structural [39] or chromosomal abnormality [40], fetal infection due to cytomegalovirus or toxoplasmosis [41], or maternal substance abuse.

Briefly, the clinical approach to assessing fetal health begins with monitoring the baseline FHR for a reasonable period to determine the presence of FHR accelerations or reactivity. In using an outpatient approach such as the NST, the goal is to identify the fetus at risk of death *in utero*. In this circumstance, a certain number of accelerations are required within a 10- or 20-min window to satisfy the criteria for a reactive NST. In contrast, in the patient in the hospital or ICU, the criteria for reactivity can be less because surgical intervention is readily available.

If the NST is considered non-reactive after a 40-minute monitoring period, several options are available to the clinician. These include, but are not limited to the following: to continue fetal monitoring, or, to perform a contraction stress test [41], fetal biophysical profile [42,43] or some form of fetal stimulation. If, after acoustic stimulation, the fetus has a persistent non-reactive pattern, a contraction stress test [41] or the FBP [16,43] can be used to evaluate fetal status.

In the critical care setting, the FBP (Table 43.2) is the easiest approach to use after fetal monitoring. Since the introduction of the FBP, this technique has been modified to include the amniotic fluid index to estimate the amniotic fluid volume [44,45]. Based on the work of Phelan and associates [5,44,45], an amniotic fluid index (AFI) of ≤5.0 cm is considered oligohydramnios. Consequently, if a patient has an AFI ≤5.0 cm, her FBP score for that component will be 0. Additional components of the FBP include fetal breathing movements, fetal limb movements, fetal tone, and reactivity on an NST. Based on the presence or absence of each component, the patient receives 0 or 2 points.

An FBP score of 8 or 10 is considered normal. In patients whose score is 6, the test is considered equivocal or suspicious. In such patients, a repeat FBP is recommended in 12–24 hours. If the patient is considered to be at term, she should be evaluated for delivery [43]. The patient with a biophysical profile score of 0, 2, or 4 is considered for delivery; but this FBP score does not mandate a cesarean. A trial of labor is reasonable whenever the cervix is favorable for induction, the amniotic fluid volume is normal (AFI >5.0 cm) and the fetus is not growth impaired. In the preterm fetus with a FBP score of 4 or less, the subsequent clinical management does not mandate delivery but does require an evaluation and a balancing of the risks of prematurity with those of continued intrauterine existence. If delivery is determined to be the best course of action under the circumstances, the options of induction of labor and cesarean are available.

Table 43.2 Fetal biophysical profile (FBP) components required over a 30-min period*.

Components	Normal result	Score
Non-stress test	Reactive	2
Fetal breathing	Duration ≥1 min	2
Fetal movement	≥3 movements	2
Fetal tone	Flexion and extension of limb	2
Amniotic fluid volume	Amniotic fluid index >5.0 cm	2
Maximum score		10

Components of the FBP, which includes the modification for determining the amniotic fluid volume using the amniotic fluid index [43,44,45].
*This represents one approach to the FBP.

Variable decelerations

Variable FHR decelerations have a variable or non-uniform shape and bear no consistent relationship to a uterine contraction. In general, the decline in rate is rapid and abrupt (onset of deceleration to beginning of nadir <30 seconds) and is followed by a quick recovery. Umbilical cord compression leading to an increased fetal BP and baroreceptor response is felt to be the most likely etiology. Umbilical cord compression is more likely to occur in circumstances of nuchal cords, knots, cord prolapse [46], or a diminished amniotic fluid volume [47,48].

To simplify intrapartum management, investigators such as Kubli et al. [49] and Krebs et al. [50] have attempted to classify variable decelerations. For example, Kubli and associates [49] have correlated fetal outcome with mild, moderate, or severe variable decelerations. Kubli's criteria, however, are cumbersome and do not lend themselves to easy clinical use. In contrast, Krebs et al.'s [50] criteria rely on the visual characteristics of the variable decelerations rather than on the degree or amplitude of the FHR deceleration. Krebs has shown that when repetitive, atypical variable decelerations are present over a prolonged period in a patient with a previously normal FHR tracing, the risk of low Apgars is increased. Atypical variables, in and of themselves, are clinically insignificant.

However, these atypical features in the circumstance of a Hon pattern of intrapartum asphyxia [11–13,51] can be associated with fetal brain injury. When persistent, atypical variable FHR decelerations arise in association with a substantial rise in the baseline FHR to a level of tachycardia, an absence of FHR accelerations or non-reactivity and with or without a loss of FHRV (Figures 43.1–43.3), expeditious delivery should be considered.

Late decelerations

Late decelerations are a uniform deceleration pattern with onset at the peak of the uterine contraction, the nadir in heart rate at the offset of the uterine contraction, and a delayed return to baseline after the contraction has ended [36]. The NICHD definition varies from the CIPF in the decelerations relationship to the contraction. With the NICHD definition, the onset of the deceleration can be at the beginning of the contraction, the nadir after the peak of the contraction, and recovery after the end of the contraction. The differences between these approaches will be reviewed after this section.

To be clinically significant, late decelerations must be repetitive (i.e. occur with each contraction of similar magnitude, and be associated with a substantial rise in baseline FHR, a loss of reactivity, with or without a loss of FHRV [11–14]. Non-persistent or intermittent late decelerations are probably variables, and consequently, appear to have no bearing on fetal outcome [52]. In fact, Nelson and associates [52] found that 99.7% of late decelerations observed on a fetal monitor strip were associated with favorable fetal outcome.

Whenever a patient with a reactive admission FHR pattern develops repetitive late decelerations in association with a fetal tachycardia and a loss of reactivity, traditional maneuvers of intrauterine resuscitation such as maternal repositioning, oxygen administration, and increased intravenous fluids are warranted. If this pattern persists, assessment of the fetal ability to accelerate its heart rate [5,6] or delivery should be considered.

In the critical care setting reversible, late decelerations can be seen in a number of clinical circumstances, such as diabetic ketoacidosis [53,54], sickle cell crisis [55], acute hypovolemia, or anaphylaxis [56–59]. With correction of the underlying maternal metabolic and hemodynamic abnormality, the FHR abnormality usually will resolve, and operative intervention is often unnecessary. Persistence of the FHR pattern after maternal metabolic recovery, however, may suggest an underlying fetal diabetic cardiomyopathy [60] or pre-existing fetal compromise [11–13,51] and should, when accompanied by the aforementioned additional signs of fetal compromise, lead to assessment for fetal reactivity or delivery.

Overview of periodic changes

The major distinctions between the NICHD [25] and CIPF [11–14] approaches are as follows.

1 The NICHD criteria broadened the definition of a late deceleration to include a deceleration with its onset at any time during the contraction as opposed to at the peak of the contraction. Additionally, the nadir or the lowest point of a late deceleration can occur after the peak of the contraction rather than at the offset of the contraction [25].

2 To determine whether a variable deceleration is present, the NICHD approach requires the practitioner to review successive contractions but does not appear to impose a similar requirement for late or early decelerations [25].

3 Recurrent FHR decelerations means persistent decelerations with more than 50% of contractions in any 20-minute segment [25]. This definition is broader than the previous requirement of "repetitive" FHR decelerations or decelerations which occur with each and every contraction.

4 The characterization of variable decelerations is patterned after those of Kubli [49] which is based on the depth and duration of the deceleration ("the big, the bad and the ugly"). This in contrast with the approach described by Krebs and associates [50]. With the latter approach, an atypical deceleration is defined as one that has lost its normal characteristics such as the loss of the primary and secondary accelerations associated with a typical or normal variable.

5 While both approaches focus on the FHR characteristics of the fetus becoming asphyxiated, the CIPF approach [13,14] focuses on the change of fetal status from admission to the hospital or the doctor's office followed by the changes previously discussed in this section pertaining to the Hon pattern of intrapartum asphyxia [13,14].

6 The other key difference is that the CIPF approach also focuses on the fetus at risk for asphyxia [13]. With the CIPF approach, the issue is whether there is any notice or warning of the potential for a sudden, rapid, or sustained deterioration of the fetal heart rate that could potentially last until delivery [13].

Fetal acid–base assessment

Fetal acid–base assessment continues to have minimal to no role in the contemporary practice of obstetrics. In the past, fetal acid–base status was thought to be a valuable adjunct for the assessment of fetal health during labor. This practice stemmed from the work of Saling [61]. In that work, Saling found that infants with a pH of less than 7.2 were more likely to be delivered physiologically depressed. Conversely, a normal fetal outcome was more likely to be associated with a non-acidotic fetus (pH ≥7.20) [62]. Even at the peak of its popularity, fetal scalp blood sampling was used in a limited number of pregnancies (~3%) [63]. Notwithstanding, Goodwin and associates [64] concluded in 1994 that fetal scalp blood sampling "... has been virtually eliminated without an increase in the cesarean rate for fetal distress or an increase in indicators of perinatal asphyxia. [Its continued role] in clinical practice is questioned."

A profound metabolic acidemia or mixed acidemia at birth, as reflected by an umbilical artery pH of less than 7.00 and a base deficit of 12 or greater, although often a direct result of a sentinel hypoxic event, usually reflects the impact of a slow heart rate (<100 bpm) at the time of birth [65] and seems to be a poor predictor of long-term neurologic impairment [66]. For example, Myers [67] demonstrated that animals whose blood pH was maintained at 7.1 showed no hypoxic brain injury, and that fetuses who had a pH of less than 7.00 could survive several hours before they died. Thus, the initial abnormal pH that surrounds a given birth may not be, in and of itself, indicative of an intrapartum injury [14].

If the clinical circumstances suggest the need for fetal acid–base assessment and the clinician is concerned about fetal status, the clinician should look alternatively for the presence of FHR accelerations. In key studies, Phelan [5] and Skupski and colleagues [6] have demonstrated with labor stimulation tests such as scalp or acoustic stimulation, that FHR accelerations were associated with a significantly greater likelihood of normal fetal acid–base status and a favorable fetal outcome. If the fetus fails to respond to the sound or scalp stimulation, delivery should be considered.

As with fetal scalp blood sampling, umbilical cord blood gas data do not appear to be useful in predicting long-term neurologic impairment. It is interesting to note that of 314 infants with severe umbilical artery acidosis identified in the world literature, 27 (8.6%) children were subsequently found to have permanent brain damage [66]. In the Fee study [68], for example, minor developmental delays or mild tone abnormalities were noted at the time of hospital discharge in 9 of 110 (8%) singleton term infants. When 108 of these infants were seen on long-term follow-up, all were considered neurologically normal, and none of these infants, which included a neonate with an umbilical artery pH of 6.57 at birth, demonstrated major motor or cognitive abnormality. In contrast, the neonatal outcomes for 113 infants in the Goodwin study [64] were known. Of these, 98 (87%) had normal outcomes. In the remaining 15 infants with known outcomes, five neonates died and 10 infants were brain damaged. Of interest, Dennis and colleagues [69] commented in their series of patients that "the very acidotic children did not perform worse than [the non-acidotic children]. Thus, the finding of severe fetal acidosis on an umbilical artery cord gas does not appear to be linked to subsequent neurologic deficits."

In contrast, the absence of severe acidosis does not ensure a favorable neurologic outcome. For example, Korst and associates [70,71] had previously shown that neonates with sufficient intrapartum asphyxia to produce persistent brain injury did not have to sustain severe acidosis (umbilical arterial pH ≤7.00). When her two studies are combined, 42 (60%) fetuses did not have severe acidosis, and all were neurologically impaired. Of 94 infants with reported permanent brain damage, Dennis and associates [69] also noted that children without acidosis appeared to fare worse than acidotic children. Thus, it appears that factors other than the presence of severe acidosis are probably responsible for fetal brain injury.

It is interesting to note that severe acidosis may not be a proper endpoint to study intrapartum asphyxia [72] nor to define whether a fetus has sustained intrapartum brain damage [73–75]. These findings suggest that the pathophysiologic mechanisms responsible for fetal brain damage appear to operate independently of central fetal acid–base status and to be more likely related to the adequacy of cerebral perfusion and the presence of neurocellular acidemia [14].

Severe acidosis, rather than fetal brain damage, continues to be used as an endpoint in the study of intrapartum asphyxia [75] and to define whether a fetus has sustained intrapartum brain damage [73–75]. This alleged clinical relationship remains a puzzlement when you consider that "there is no pH value that separates cleanly those babies who have experienced intrapartum injury from those who have not – no prognosis can be made or refuted on the basis of a single laboratory study" [76]. The lack of a consistent relationship between the presence or absence of fetal acidosis suggests that the pathophysiologic mechanisms that are responsible for fetal brain damage seem more likely to be related to the adequacy of cerebral perfusion [14] in that fetus rather than the mere presence of metabolic acidosis. Thus, as has happened with fetal scalp blood sampling, the use of umbilical cord blood gases to define or time fetal brain damage or the quality of care may not have a role in the contemporary or future practice of obstetrics.

FHR patterns in the brain-damaged infant

Term infants found to be brain damaged do not manifest a uniform FHR pattern [11–14,51]. However, these fetuses do manifest distinct FHR patterns intrapartum that can be easily categorized and identified based on the admission FHR pattern and subsequent changes in the baseline rate.

Reactive admission test and subsequent fetal brain damage

When a pregnant woman is admitted to hospital, the overwhelming number of obstetric patients will have a reactive FHR pattern. Of these, more than 98% will go through labor uneventfully and most will deliver vaginally. In the few patients (typically 1–2%) that develop intrapartum "fetal distress" [77,78], the characteristic "fetal distress" is usually, but not always, acute, usually precipitated by a sentinel hypoxic event, and manifested by a sudden, rapid, and sustained deterioration of the FHR unresponsive to remedial measures and/or terbutaline and lasts until delivery. Of these, an even smaller number of fetuses will ultimately experience a CNS injury. So, while unusual, fetal brain injury in the fetus with a reactive fetal admission test may arise, in the absence of trauma, as a result of a sudden, rapid, and sustained deterioration of the FHR or a Hon pattern of intrapartum asphyxia.

Acute fetal brain injury

In this group (Table 43.1) the FHR pattern is reactive on admission is followed by a sudden, rapid and sustained deterioration of the FHR that lasts until the time of delivery. In the circumstances of an abruption and/or a uterine rupture, this FHR deceleration is usually unresponsive to remedial measures and/or subcutaneous or intravenous terbutaline. For example, a fetus who has a sudden, rapid, and sustained deterioration of the FHR that is unresponsive to remedial measures and/or terbutaline and lasts for a prolonged period of time typically sustains in an injury

Table 43.3 Five factors useful in determining the susceptibility of a fetus to fetal brain injury under the circumstances of a sudden, rapid, and sustained deterioration of the fetal heart rate (FHR) from a previously reactive FHR [13].

Prior FHR pattern
Fetal growth pattern
Degree of intrafetal shunting
Duration of the FHR deceleration
Intactness of the placenta

to the basal ganglia or the deep gray matter. Injury to the deep gray matter gives rise to athetoid or dyskinetic cerebral palsy [14,79]. In this circumstance, the fetal brain injury is the result of a sudden reduction of fetal cardiac output and blood pressure or "cerebral hypotension due to an ineffective or non-functional cardiac pump" usually following a sentinel hypoxic event, such as a uterine rupture or a cord prolapse. That is not to say that the fetus cannot have injury to both the deep gray matter and the cerebral hemispheres with this specific FHR pattern. Whether both areas of the fetal brain are affected often depends on the five factors illustrated in Table 43.3. Fetal brain injuries that arise from this FHR pattern are associated with an array of hypoxic sentinel events (Table 43.1) such as uterine rupture, placental abruption, and cord prolapse. Given the acute nature of this FHR pattern, limited time is available to preserve normal CNS function.

Timing of fetal neurologic injury in this specific FHR group is a function of multiple factors (Table 43.3). Each variable plays a role in determining the length of time required to sustain fetal brain damage. For example, the admission FHR pattern provides an indicator of fetal status before the catastrophic event. If, for example, the FHR pattern is reactive with a normal baseline rate and a sudden prolonged FHR deceleration occurs, the window to fetal brain injury will be longer than in the patient with a tachycardic baseline [80]. As with the baseline rate, the other variables also play a role. But, it is not within the scope of this chapter to detail this information. The reader is referred to the work of Phelan and associates [14]. In general, our experience [11–14] would suggest an even shorter time to neurologic injury of less than 16 minutes whenever the placenta has completely separated. If the placenta remains intact, a longer period of time appears to be available before the onset of CNS injury. Thus, the intactness of the placenta plays an important role in determining long-term fetal outcome.

Hon pattern of asphyxia

The Hon pattern of intrapartum asphyxia (Figures 43.1–43.3) is uniquely different because the asphyxia evolves over a longer period of time [11–14,51]. This FHR pattern begins with a reactive FHR pattern on admission to the hospital. Subsequently during labor, the fetus develops a non-reactive FHR pattern or loses its ability to accelerate its heart rate [11–14,36]. As the labor continues, a substantial rise in baseline heart rate from admission (135 ± 10 bpm) to a mean maximum (186 ± 15 bpm) baseline heart rate is seen [11]. The maximum FHR ranged from 155 bpm to 220 bpm. This constituted a 39 ± 13% mean percentage rise in baseline heart rate from admission and ranged from 17% to 82% [11]. This rise in baseline FHR is usually not accompanied by maternal pyrexia. When a substantial rise in baseline FHR is encountered, the FHR pattern is also associated with repetitive FHR decelerations but not necessarily late decelerations and usually a loss of FHR variability [11–14,51]. "As labor progresses and the fetus nears death, the slopes become progressively less steep until the FHR does not return to its baseline rate and ultimately terminates in a profound bradycardia" [81] or a stairsteps-to-death pattern [11,12].

Once a FHR tachycardia begins in association with the fetal inability to accelerate its heart rate at least 15 bpm for 15 seconds from the time the FHR leaves baseline until it returns, repetitive FHR decelerations, and usually a loss of FHR variability, the subsequent FHR pattern [11] does one of the following: (i) the FHR pattern remains tachycardic and/or continues to rise until the fetus is delivered; (ii) the fetus develops a sudden, rapid, and sustained deterioration of the FHR that lasts until delivery; or (iii) the fetus initiates a stairsteps-to-death pattern or a progressive bradycardia is seen. Of particular clinical relevance is that all patients manifested a substantial rise in their baseline heart rates, lost their ability to generate FHR accelerations, became non-reactive and exhibited repetitive FHR decelerations. Of note, the repetitive FHR decelerations were not necessarily late decelerations and were frequently variable decelerations [11–13,75].

In the Hon FHR group, FHR variability appeared to be a predictor of neonatal cerebral edema [11]. For example, many brain-damaged fetuses exhibited average FHR variability at the time of their deliveries [11]. In the neonatal period, brain-damaged fetuses that had the Hon pattern of intrapartum asphyxia with average FHR variability had significantly less cerebral edema [24]. Kim's cerebral edema [24] findings suggest that the use of diminished FHR variability as an endpoint for the Hon pattern of intrapartum asphyxia to decide the timing of operative intervention is probably unreasonable. This means that the fetal brain may well be injured before the loss of FHR variability.

The Hon pattern characteristically results in damage to both cerebral hemispheres and gives rise to spastic quadriplegia [14,79]. Here, the mechanism for injury is not an ineffective pump, because these fetuses usually demonstrate tachycardic baseline heart rates. The brain damage in this situation relates more to cerebral ischemia (Figure 43.4). The triggering mechanism may be meconium [82,83] or infection [84,85] that may be bacterial, anerobic or aerobic, or viral [86,87], but is not related to uterine contractions [14]. The resultant fetal vasoconstriction or intrafetal shunting probably reflects the fetal efforts to maintain blood pressure and/or enhance fetal cerebral blood flow. Nevertheless, once the fetus develops ischemia or is unable to perfuse its brain cells, neurocellular hypoxia or injury occurs. Thus, the hypoxia encountered in the fetus is at the cellular level and not yet at the central or systemic level. By the time the fetus

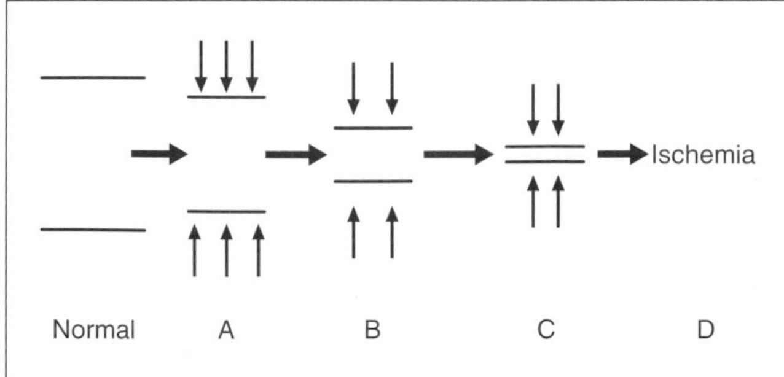

Figure 43.4 Persistent fetal vasoconstriction over time or intrafetal shunting leads to progressive narrowing of the fetal vascular tree leading ultimately to ischemia.

develops systemic or central hypoxia, the fetus, in our opinion, has already been brain injured and is probably near death [12,14]. Thus, cerebral perfusion deficits due to intrafetal and intracerebral shunting rather than fetal systemic hypoxia are most likely responsible for the fetal brain injury [88].

This means, for example, that a fetus that develops the Hon pattern of intrapartum asphyxia would appear to move to ischemia or from point C to point D (Figure 43.4). During this transition, a progressive and substantial rise in FHR is observed in an effort to preserve cerebral perfusion and neurocellular oxygenation. During this period, fetal systemic oxygenation and oxygen saturation is maintained. In our opinion [11], only after progressive and prolonged ischemia and brain injury do central fetal oxygen saturations begin to fall.

Additionally, it is important to emphasize that the pattern of fetal brain injury may change depending on the circumstances that gave rise to the delivery of the fetus. For example and as previously discussed, this FHR pattern characteristically results in cerebral palsy of the spastic quadriplegic type due to cerebral hemispheric injury. If, however, the FHR pattern moves from a Hon pattern followed by a sudden, rapid, and sustained deterioration of the FHR that lasts until delivery, the pattern of brain damage becomes more global and involves not only the cerebral hemispheres but also the deep gray matter. As such, the fetuses with this latter FHR pattern have a more severe injury and shorter life expectancies.

The persistent non-reactive FHR pattern

The persistent non-reactive FHR pattern from admission to the hospital or a non-stress test accounted for 45% of the FHR patterns observed in a population of 300 brain-damaged babies [11] and 33% of an updated population of 423 singleton term brain-damaged children [13,14]. This population is typically, but not always, characterized by the presence of reduced fetal activity before admission to the hospital, male fetuses, old meconium, meconium sequelae such as meconium aspiration syndrome and persistent pulmonary hypertension, and oligohydramnios [88]. Along with these observations, these fetuses usually but not always have elevated nucleated red blood cell counts [90,91], prolonged NRBC clearance times [90], low initial platelet counts [92], significant multiorgan system dysfunction [70,71,90], delayed onset of seizures from birth [93,94], and cortical or hemispheric brain injuries [13,14]. The typical FHR pattern is non-reactive with a fixed baseline rate that normally does not change from admission until delivery [13,14] in association with diminished or average variability.

When looking at the admission FHR pattern, the persistent non-reactive FHR pattern group can be divided into three phases. These three phases, in our opinion, represent a post-CNS insult compensatory response in the fetus. Moreover, this FHR pattern, in our opinion, does not represent ongoing asphyxia or worsening of the CNS injury [11–14,89]. For a fetus to have ongoing fetal asphyxia, a FHR pattern similar to the Hon pattern of intrapartum asphyxia would have to be seen. There, a progressive and substantial rise in baseline heart rate in association with repetitive FHR decelerations is observed in response to ongoing fetal asphyxia (Figures 43.1–43.3). In contrast, the FHR baseline in the non-reactive group usually but not always remains fixed. Infrequently, a FHR tachycardia is seen; however, the rise in baseline rate is usually insubstantial. Thus, the phase of recovery appears to equate with the length of time from the fetal CNS insult. Thus, phase I would appear to be closer to the time of the insult, and phase III would appear to be more distant in time from the injury-producing event [12].

The persistent non-reactive FHR pattern is not, in our opinion, a sign of ongoing fetal asphyxia but rather represents a static encephalopathy [11–14]. This means that earlier intervention in the form of a cesarean on admission to the hospital would not, in our opinion, substantially alter fetal outcome.

Fetal monitoring made simple during labor

In light of the lessons learned from the children damaged *in utero* before and during labor, current fetal monitoring interpretation will need to change to reflect and include the significance of the initial fetal monitoring period. When a patient presents to labor and delivery, the initial fetal assessment should include an initial fetal monitoring period to assess reactivity (the presence of FHR accelerations) and to ascertain from the patient the quality and quantity of fetal movement. In the patient with a reactive FHR pattern and normal fetal movement, the key to clinical management before and during labor is to follow the baseline fetal heart rate.

This means that the physician and nurse will need to watch for persistent elevations of the baseline rate to a level of tachycardia or higher or look for the potential for the baseline rate to fall suddenly. To assist with the identification of the Hon pattern, medical and nursing personnel should try to compare the current tracing with the one obtained on admission. If the characteristics of the Hon pattern of intrapartum asphyxia develop, subsequent clinical management will depend on whether the gravida is febrile and as outlined earlier in this chapter. In the non-reactive group, clinical management is to first evaluate the maternal and fetal status with respect to the etiology of the FHR pattern. These causes include, but are not limited to, the following: maternal substance abuse, fetal–maternal hemorrhage, fetal anomaly, and the potential for a fetal chromosomal abnormality. During this period of maternal and fetal evaluation, continuous fetal monitoring is used, if technically feasible, to assess fetal status. In addition, fetal stimulation tests, a contraction stress test, or a biophysical profile may be used to further determine fetal status. Once fetal status is clarified in the non-reactive group, the subsequent management with respect to the route of delivery in the term or near-term pregnancy will depend on the discussion with the family and the clinical findings.

Maternal and surgical conditions

Anaphylaxis

Anaphylaxis is an acute allergic reaction to food ingestion or drugs. It is generally associated with rapid onset of pruritus and urticaria and may result in respiratory distress, edema, vascular collapse, and shock. Medicines, primarily penicillins [58,95], food substances such as shellfish, exercise, contrast dyes, laminaria [96], and latex [97] are common causes of anaphylaxis [98,99].

Anaphylaxis may also arise during the use of allergen immunotherapy [100]. While allergen shots have been shown to be effective in improving asthma in patients with allergies and have not been associated with any adverse effects during pregnancy [101,102], anaphylaxis remains a risk early in pregnancy when the dose is being escalated. Thus, a risk/benefit analysis should be considered in such patients as to continuing or initiating allergen immunotherapy during pregnancy [100].

When an anaphylactic reaction occurs during pregnancy, the accompanying maternal physiologic changes may result in fetal distress. In a case described by Klein and associates [57], a woman at 29 weeks' gestation presented with an acute allergic reaction after eating shellfish. On admission, she had evidence of regular uterine contractions and repetitive, severe late decelerations. The "fetal distress" was believed to be the result of maternal hypotension and relative hypovolemia, which accompanied the allergic reaction. Prompt treatment of the patient with intravenous fluids and ephedrine corrected the FHR abnormality. Subsequently, the patient delivered a healthy male infant at term with normal Apgar scores.

As suggested by these investigators and by Witter and Niebyl [56], while acute maternal allergic reactions do pose a threat to the fetus, treatment directed at the underlying cause often remedies the accompanying fetal distress. To afford the fetus a wider margin of safety, efforts should be directed at maintaining maternal systolic BP above 90 mmHg. In addition, oxygen should be administered to correct maternal hypoxia; in the absence of maternal hypovolemia, a maternal P_aO_2 in excess of 60–70 mmHg will assure adequate fetal oxygenation [56,57]. A persistent fetal tachycardia, bradycardia [58], or other abnormal FHR patterns suggest the need for additional maternal hemodynamic support or oxygenation, even in the nominally "stable" mother.

Eclampsia

Maternal seizures are a well-known but infrequent sequel of pre-eclampsia [17]. Although the maternal hemodynamic findings in patients with eclampsia are similar to those with severe pre-eclampsia [103], maternal convulsions require prompt attention to potentially prevent harm to both mother and fetus [17]. During a seizure, the fetal response usually is manifested as an abrupt, prolonged FHR deceleration [19,104]. During the seizure, which generally lasts less than 1–2 minutes [19], transient maternal hypoxia and uterine artery vasospasm occur and combine to produce a decline in uterine blood flow. In addition, uterine activity increases secondary to the release of norepinephrine, resulting in additional reduction *in utero*placental perfusion. Ultimately, the reduction of uteroplacental perfusion causes the FHR deceleration. Such a deceleration may last up to 10 minutes after the termination of the convulsions and the correction of maternal hypoxemia [17,19]. Following the seizure and recovery from the FHR deceleration, a loss of FHRV and a compensatory rise in baseline FHR are characteristically seen. Transient late decelerations are not uncommon but usually resolve once maternal metabolic recovery is complete. During this recovery period, it is reasonably believed to be beneficial for the fetus to permit recovery *in utero* from convulsion induce hypoxia and hypercarbia [17]. During this time, the patient should not be rushed to an emergency cesarean based on the FHR changes associated with an eclamptic seizure [17]. This is especially true if the patient is unstable.

The cornerstone of patient management during an eclamptic seizure is to maintain adequate maternal oxygenation and to administer appropriate anticonvulsants. After a convulsion occurs, an adequate airway should be maintained and oxygen administered. To optimize uteroplacental perfusion, the mother is repositioned onto her side. Anticonvulsant therapy with intravenous magnesium sulfate [17,105–107] to prevent seizure recurrence is recommended. In spite of adequate magnesium sulfate therapy, adjunctive anticonvulsant therapy occasionally may be necessary in about 10% of patients [17,19,105].

In the event of persistent FHR decelerations, intrauterine resuscitation with a betamimetic [108] or additional magnesium sulfate [109] may be helpful in relieving eclampsia-induced uterine hypertonus. Continuous electronic fetal monitoring should be used to follow the fetal condition. After the mother has been stabilized, and if the fetus continues to show signs of a FHR bradycardia and/or repetitive late decelerations after a reasonable period of recovery, delivery should be considered.

Disseminated intravascular coagulopathy

Disseminated intravascular coagulopathy (DIC) occurs in a variety of obstetric conditions, such as abruptio placentae, amniotic fluid embolus syndrome, severe pre-eclampsia/

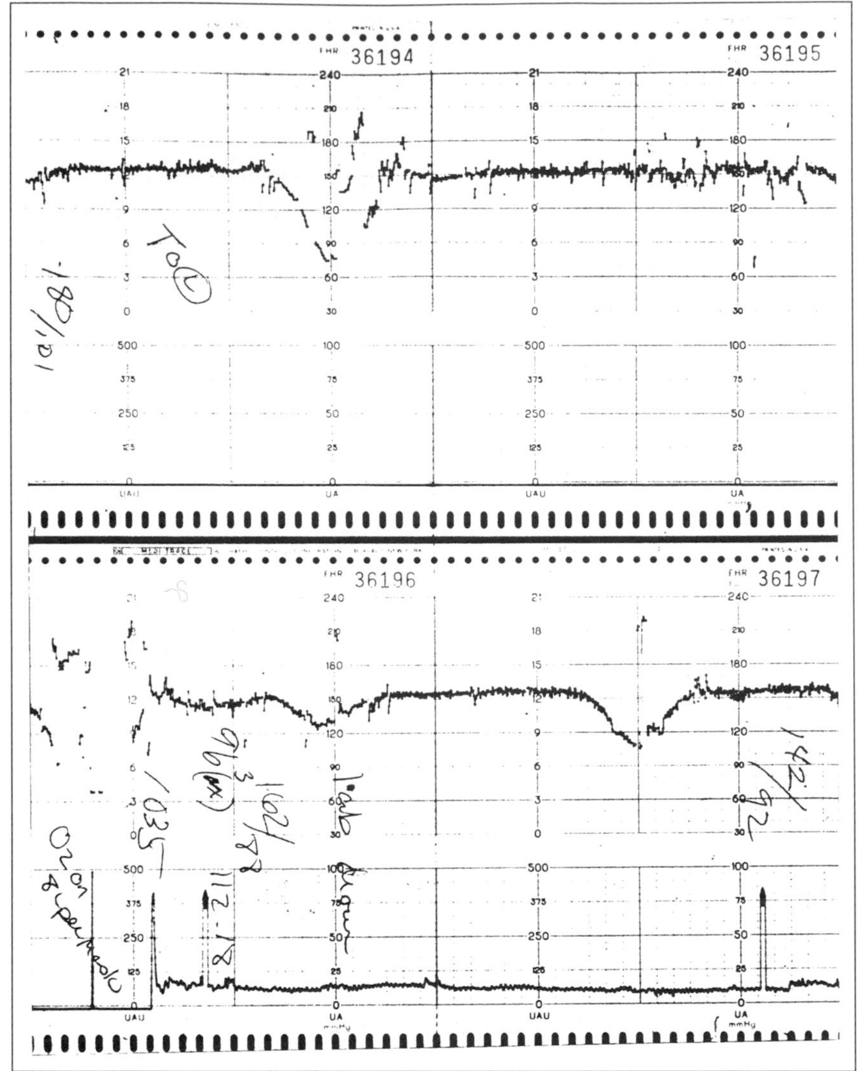

Figure 43.5 The FHR pattern from a 33-week fetus with asymmetric intrauterine growth impairment whose mother presented with clinical disseminated intravascular coagulation.

eclampsia and the dead fetus syndrome. The pathophysiology of this condition is discussed in greater detail in Chapter 31.

Infrequently, DIC may be advanced to a point of overt bleeding [110]. Under these circumstances, laboratory abnormalities accompany the clinical evidence of consumptive coagulopathy. In the rare circumstance of overt "fetal distress" and a clinically apparent maternal coagulopathy, obstetric management requires prompt replacement of deficient coagulation components before attempting to deliver the distressed fetus. This frequently requires balancing the interests of the pregnant woman with those of her unborn child.

For example, a 34-year-old woman presented to the hospital at 33 weeks gestation with the FHR tracing illustrated in Figure 43.5. Real-time sonography demonstrated asymmetric intrauterine growth retardation. Oxygen was administered, and the patient was repositioned on her left side. Appropriate laboratory studies were drawn, and informed consent for a cesarean was obtained. When a Foley catheter was inserted, grossly bloody urine was observed. The previously drawn blood did not clot, and she was observed to be bleeding from the site of her intravenous line. The abnormal FHR pattern persisted.

In this circumstance, the interests of the mother and fetus are at odds with one another, and a difficult clinical decision must now be made. Whose interest does the obstetrician protect in this instance? Immediate surgical intervention without blood products would have lessened the mother's chances of survival. On the other hand, if the clinician waits for fresh frozen plasma and platelet infusion before undertaking surgery, the fetus will be at significant risk of death or permanent neurologic impairment. Ideally, the mother and/or her family should participate in such decisions. In reality, because of the unpredictable nature of these dilemmas and the need for rapid decision-making, family involvement often is not always possible. Under such circumstances, it is axiomatic that maternal interests take precedence over those of the fetus.

Because blood products were not readily available, the decision was made to stabilize the mother and to move the patient to the operating room. Once in the operating room, the clinical management would include, but is not limited to, the following: to continue to oxygenate the mother; to maintain her in the left lateral recumbent position; to have an anesthesiologist, operating room personnel, and surgeons present; and to be prepared to operate. As soon as the blood products are available, and the fetus is alive, transfuse with fresh frozen plasma, platelets, and packed cells. Then, the clinician should begin the cesarean under general anesthesia. In this case, maternal and fetal outcomes were ultimately favorable.

In summary, the cornerstone of management of the patient with full-blown DIC and clinically apparent fetal distress is to stabilize the mother by correcting the maternal clotting abnormality before initiating surgery. While waiting for the blood products to be infused, the patient should be prepared and ready for immediate cesarean delivery. If the fetus dies in the interim, the cesarean should not be performed, and the patient should be afforded the opportunity to deliver vaginally, to reduce maternal hemorrhagic risks.

The burn victim

Although burn victims are uncommonly encountered in high-risk obstetric units, the pregnant burn patient is sufficiently complex to require a team approach to enhance maternal and perinatal survival [111,112]. In most cases, this will require maternal–fetal transfer to a facility skilled to handle burn patients. Transfer will depend primarily on the severity of the burn and the stability of the pregnant woman and her fetus. For greater detail and discussion on the clinical management of various types of thermal injuries, the reader is referred to Chapter 38.

The first step in the management of the pregnant burn patient is to determine the depth and size of the burn. The depth of a burn may be partial or full thickness. A full-thickness burn, formerly called a third-degree burn, is the most severe and involves total destruction of the skin. As a result, regeneration of the epithelial surface is not possible.

The second element of burn management is to determine the percentage of body surface area involved (Table 43.4). The percentage of maternal total body surface area covered by the burn is linked to maternal and perinatal outcome. The more severe the maternal burn, the higher is the maternal and perinatal mortality [111,112]. The risk of mortality becomes significant whenever 60% or more of the maternal total body surface area is burned [111].

Table 43.4 Classification of burn patients based on the percentage of body surface area involved.

Classification	Body surface area (%)
Minor	<10
Major	
Moderate	10–19
Severe	20–39
Critical	≥40

The subsequent clinical management of the pregnant burn patient will depend on the patient's burn phase (e.g. acute, convalescent, or remote) or burn period [113](e.g. resuscitation, postresuscitation, inflammation/infection, or rehabilitation). Each phase has unique problems. For example, the acute phase is characterized by premature labor, electrolyte and fluid disturbances, maternal cardiopulmonary instability, and the potential for fetal compromise. In contrast, the convalescent and remote periods are unique for their problems of sepsis and abdominal scarring, respectively. Because the potential for fetal compromise is greatest during the window of time immediately following the burn, the focus in this chapter is on acute-phase burn patients.

In the acute phase of a severe burn, the primary maternal focus centers on stabilization [112]. Here, electrolyte disturbances due to transudation of fluid and altered renal function mandate close attention to the maternal intravascular volume and prompt and aggressive fluid resuscitation. At the same time, these patients are also potentially compromised from airway injury and/or smoke inhalation, and ventilator support may be necessary to maintain cardiopulmonary stability. Additionally, a high index of suspicion for venous thrombosis and sepsis with early and aggressive treatment should be considered. Given the complexities of these patients, invasive hemodynamic monitoring may be necessary. Because most of these patients will be in an ICU, appropriate medical consultation and intensive nursing care for the mother and fetus are essential.

Assessing fetal well-being in the burn patient may be difficult. The ability to determine fetal status with ultrasound or fetal monitoring will depend on the size and location of the burn. If, for example, the burn involves the maternal abdominal wall, alternative methods of fetal assessment, such as fetal kick counts (alone or in response to acoustic stimulation) [26] or a modified FBP [16,42,43] using vaginal ultrasound, may be necessary. Whenever abdominal burns are present, a sterile transducer cover for the ultrasound device, fetal monitor, or doptone should be used to reduce the risk of infection. In the absence of a maternal abdominal burn, continuous electronic fetal monitoring can generally be used. Because of such monitoring difficulties and the direct relationship between the size of the maternal burn and perinatal outcome (see Figure 43.6), Matthews [114] and Polko and McMahon [111] have recommended immediate cesarean delivery (assuming maternal stability) in any pregnant burn patient with a potentially viable fetus and a burn that involves 50% or more of the maternal body surface area. In contrast, Guo [112] recommends early delivery if the pregnancy is in the third trimester. As a reminder, burn patients with electrolyte disturbances may exhibit alterations in fetal status similar to those of a patient in sickle cell crisis [55] or diabetic ketoacidosis [53,54].

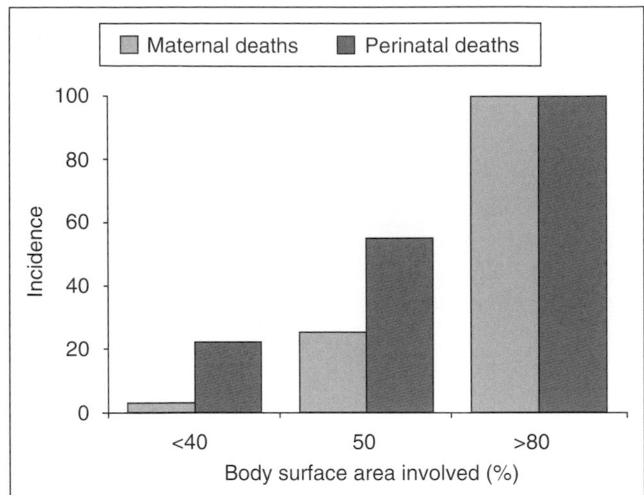

Figure 43.6 Estimated maternal and perinatal mortality rates following maternal burn injuries according to the amount of body surface area involved.

Once the maternal electrolyte disturbance is corrected, fetal status may return to normal and intervention often can be avoided.

Fetal considerations specific to cardiac bypass procedures and electrical shock are discussed in Chapters 14 and 38.

Maternal brain death or persistent vegetative state

With the advent of artificial life-support systems, prolonged viability of the brain-dead pregnant woman [115–126] or one in a persistent vegetative state (PVS) [127–141] is no longer unusual in a perinatal unit. As a consequence, an increasing number of obstetric patients on artificial life support will be encountered in the medical community. Maternal brain death or vegetative state poses an array of medical, legal, and ethical dilemmas for the obstetric healthcare provider [117,140,142–146].

In each case of maternal brain death or PVS, multiple questions need to be addressed depending on the role, if any, of continued somatic survival. When first confronted by the clinical circumstances of confirmed maternal brain death or PVS, the focus shifts to that of the fetus. If the fetus is alive, the question arises as to whether extraordinary care for the brain-dead patient should be initiated to preserve the life of her unborn child, and if so, at what gestational age? If artificial life support is elected to permit further maturation of the fetus, how should the pregnancy be managed, and, when and under what circumstances should the fetus be delivered? When should maternal life support be terminated? Is consent required to maintain the pregnancy? If so, from whom should consent be obtained? Such questions barely touch the surface of the complexities associated with these cases. But, it is clearly not within the scope of this chapter to deal with the ethical, moral, and legal issues related to the obstetric care of the brain-dead gravida or the gravida with PVS. Rather, the emphasis is on the clinical management of these patients when a decision has been made to maintain somatic support for the benefit of the unborn child.

The key distinction between brain death and PVS is that in PVS, the brainstem is usually but not always functioning normally. In the initial phases, it is arguably difficult to separate the two entities. With time, the distinction becomes clearer. For example, a PVS patient could appear to be awake, be capable of swallowing, and have normal respiratory control, but have no purposeful interactions. PVS patients are "truly unconscious because, although they are wakeful, they lack awareness" [140]. Nevertheless, the clinical management of the brain-dead or PVS gravida is similar initially.

To date, 13 cases of maternal brain death [115–126] and 17 cases of PVS [127–141] during pregnancy have been reported (Table 43.5 and 43.6). In general, PVS patients require less somatic support than do brain-dead pregnant women but can require a similar degree of medical management. The review by Bush and associates [140] illustrates the key differences between these two groups. When compared with the brain-dead group, the PVS population is more likely to demonstrate the following [140]:

1 longer time interval between maternal brain injury and delivery
2 heavier birth weights at delivery
3 delivery at a more advanced gestational age.

It is important to note that these differences may be more a reflection of the severity of the maternal condition in the brain-dead gravida [140]. Moreover, prolonged "maternal survival" is related to the ability to maintain euthermia, to have spontaneous respirations, and to have a functioning cardiovascular system [140].

Therefore it is easy to see that for optimal care of such patients and fetuses, a cooperative effort among various healthcare providers is essential. The goal is to maintain maternal somatic survival until the fetus is viable and reasonably mature. To achieve this goal, a number of maternal and fetal considerations must be addressed to enhance fetal outcome [117] (Table 43.7).

As demonstrated in Table 43.7, Field and associates [117] have tried to capture the complexities associated with the medical management of these patients. Maternal medical management involves the regulation of most, if not all, maternal bodily functions. For example, the loss of the pneumotaxic center in the pons, which is responsible for cyclic respirations, and the medullary center, which is responsible for spontaneous respirations, make mechanical ventilation mandatory. Ventilation, under these circumstances, is similar to that for the non-pregnant patient. In contrast to the non-pregnant patient, the desirable gas concentrations are stricter due to the presence of the fetus. As such, the maternal P_aCO_2 should be kept between 30 mmHg and 35 mmHg [142] and the maternal P_aO_2 greater than 60–70mmHg to avoid deleterious effects on uteroplacental perfusion.

Maternal hypotension occurs frequently in these patients and may be due to a combination of factors, including hypothermia, hypoxia, and panhypopituitarism. Maintenance of maternal BP can often be achieved with the infusion of low-dose dopamine, which elevates BP without affecting renal or splanchnic blood

Table 43.5 Perinatal outcome in 13 reported cases of maternal brain death during pregnancy [NA-Not Available; SVD- spontaneous vaginal delivery].

		Gestation age (weeks)					
Reference	Year	Brain death	Delivery	Indication for delivery	Mode of delivery	Apgar score at 5min	Birth Weight (grams)
Dillon 1 (115)	1982	25	26	Fetal distress	Cesarean	8	850
Dillon 2	1982	18	19	Life support Terminated	SVD	NA	NA
Heikkinen (116)	1985	21	31	Maternal hypotension	Cesarean	7	1,600
Field (117)	1988	22	31	Growth impaired Maternal Sepsis	Cesarean	8	1,440
Bernstein (118)	1989	15	32	Fetal distress	Cesarean	9	1,555
Wuermeling (119)	1994	14	NA	NA	SVD	NA	NA
Iriye (120)	1995	30	30	Maternal hypotension FHR decelerations	Cesarean	8	1,610
Vives (121)	1996	27	27	Fetal distress Maternal Hypotension	Cesarean	10	1,150
Catanzarite (122)	1997	25	29	Chorioamnionitis	Cesarean	7	1,315
Lewis (123)	1997	25	31	Fetal Lung Maturity	Cesarean	NA	NA
Spike (124)	1999	16	31	Maternal Hypotension	Cesarean	8	1,440
Souza (125)	2006	25	28	Oligohydramnios Growth Impaired	Cesarean	10	815
Hussein (126)	2006	26	28	Oligohydramnios	Cesarean	NA	1,285

flow. Along with vasopressors to support the maternal blood pressure and organ perfusion, the patient should be kept, when possible, in the lateral recumbent position to maintain uteroplacental blood flow. At the same time, care should be exercised to avoid decubitus ulcers.

With maternal brain death, the thermoregulatory center located in the ventromedian nucleus of the hypothalamus does not function, and maternal body temperature cannot be maintained normally. As a result, maternal hypothermia is the rule. Maintenance of maternal euthermia is important and usually can be accomplished through the use of warming blankets and the administration of warm, inspired, humidified air.

Maternal pyrexia suggests an infectious process and the need for a thorough septic work-up. Thus, infection surveillance for, and the treatment of, infectious complications is helpful to prolong maternal somatic survival [142]. If the maternal temperature remains elevated for a protracted period, cooling blankets may be necessary to avoid potentially deleterious effects on the fetus [146].

Nutritional support, usually in the form of enteral or parenteral hyperalimentation, is required for maternal maintenance and fetal growth and development (see Chapter 12). Because of poor maternal gastric motility, parenteral rather than enteral hyperalimentation is often preferred [117] to maintain a positive nitrogen balance. The use of hyperalimentation during pregnancy does not appear to have deleterious effects on the fetus [147]. As a rule, the amount of hyperalimentation should be in keeping with the caloric requirements for that gestational age of the pregnancy and be sufficient to avoid maternal hyperglycemia.

In such patients, panhypopituitarism frequently occurs. As a result, a variety of hypoendocrinopathies, such as diabetes insipidus, secondary adrenal insufficiency, and hypothyroidism, may develop, each mandating therapy to maintain the pregnancy. Treatment of these conditions requires the use of vasopressin, corticosteroids, and thyroid replacement, respectively.

Because of the hypercoagulable state of pregnancy and the immobility of the brain-dead gravida, these patients also are at

Table 43.6 Perinatal outcome in 17 reported cases of persistent vegetative state during pregnancy.

		Gestation age (weeks)					
Reference	Year	PVS	Delivery	Indication for delivery	Mode of delivery	Apgar score at 5min	Birth Weight (grams)
Lucas (127)	1976	6 mo	8 mo	NONE	SVD-Breech	NA	1,760
Sampson (128)	1979	6	34	Premature Labor	Forceps	5	1,640
BenAderet (129)	1984	17	35	Premature Rupture Of Membranes	Cesarean	9	2,450
Hill (130)	1985	14	34	Fetal Lung Maturity	Cesarean	9	1,600
Diamond (131)	1986	22	34	Contraction Stress Test	Cesarean	5	2,835
Landye (132)	1987	5 mo	37		Vacuum	9	2,530
Koh (133)	1993	13	37	Failed VBAC	Cesarean	9	3,680
Webb (134)	1996	14	31	Abruption	Cesarean	7	2,240
Wong (135)	1997	22	33	Chorioamnionitis	Cesarean	9	2,150
Finerty-1 (136)	1999	12	NA	NA	Cesarean	NA	NA
Finerty-2 (136)	1999	17	33	NA	SVD	NA	NA
Ayorinde (137)	2000	12	35	Premature Labor	SVD	10	2,200
Feldman (138)	2000	15	31	Seizures/hypertension	Cesarean	9	1,506
Sim (139)	2001	4	33	Premature Rupture Of Membranes	Cesarean	6	1,680
Bush (140)	2003	15	24	FHR Bradycardia	Cesarean	1	740
Chiossi-1 (141)	2006	10	34	Hypotension Fetal Lung Maturity	Cesarean	9	2,680
Chiossi-2 (141)	2006	19	31	Abnormal FHR Pattern Biophysical Profile 6/10	Cesarean	7	1,701

NA-Not Available; SVD- Spontaneous Vaginal Delivery; FHR – Fetal Heart Rate; mo- Months; PVS-Persistent Vegetative State.

an increased risk for thromboembolism. Therefore, to minimize the potential for deep venous thrombosis or pulmonary embolus, heparin prophylaxis (5000–7500 units twice or three times a day) and/or intermittent pneumatic calf compression are recommended [148].

By artificially supporting the maternal physiologic system, the intrauterine environment can be theoretically maintained to allow for adequate fetal growth and development (Table 43.7). Obstetric management should focus on monitoring fetal growth with frequent ultrasound evaluations, antepartum FHR assessment, and the administration of corticosteroids between 24 and 34 weeks gestation to enhance fetal lung maturation [117,149]. For stimulation of fetal lung maturity, betamethasone or dexamethasone is recommended. Repeat steroid injections in subsequent weeks are not recommended due to the concern over the effect of repeated steroid injections on fetal brain growth, and the absence of proven additive benefit [142].

Another obstetric concern is the development of premature labor. Here, tocolytic therapy has been used successfully [122,150]. Catanzarite et al. [122] described the use of a magnesium sulfate infusion and indomethacin to control uterine contractions, allowing prolongation of the pregnancy for 25 days. Other agents

Table 43.7 Medical and obstetric considerations in providing artificial life support to the brain-dead gravida.

Maternal considerations
Mechanical ventilation
Cardiovascular support
Temperature lability
Hyperalimentation
Panhypopituitarism
Infection surveillance
Prophylactic anticoagulation
Fetal considerations
Fetal surveillance
Ultrasonography
Steroids
Timing of delivery

Table 43.8 Perimortem cesarean delivery with the outcome of surviving infants from the time of maternal death until delivery [152,153].

Time interval (min)	Surviving infants (no.)	Intact neurologic status of survivors (%)
0–5	9	8 (89%)
6–15	5	2 (60%)
>15	7	4 (57%)

available for tocolysis include betamimetics, calcium-channel blockers, and oxytocin antagonists. The hemodynamic effects of betamimetics and calcium channel-blocking agents may make these drugs less than ideal choices in these settings, in which maternal hemodynamic instability is common [122].

The timing of delivery is based on the deterioration of maternal or fetal status or the presence of fetal lung maturity. Classical cesarean is the procedure of choice [117,142] and is the least traumatic procedure for the fetus. To assure immediate cesarean capability, a cesarean pack and neonatal resuscitation equipment should be immediately available in the intensive care unit.

Perimortem cesarean delivery

For centuries, perimortem cesarean delivery has been described as an attempt to preserve the life of the unborn child when the pregnant woman dies [151]. The first description of a perimortem cesarean was by Pliny the Elder in 237 AD. This delivery related to that of Scipio Africanus. Over a thousand years later in 1280, the Catholic Church at the Council of Cologne decreed that a perimortem cesarean delivery must be performed to permit the unborn child to be baptized and to undergo a proper burial. Failure to perform the delivery constituted a punishable offense. Moreover, perimortem cesarean was mandated specifically in those women whose pregnancies were advanced beyond 6 months. To date, there have been 307 cases of perimortem cesarean delivery reported in the English literature [152,153]. Of these cesareans, there have been 222 surviving infants [152,153].

Since Weber's monumental review of the subject in 1971, the causes of maternal death leading to a perimortem cesarean delivery have not changed substantially [152,153] but are more reflective of contemporary obstetric care [130,131]. These include traumatic events, pulmonary embolism from amniotic fluid, clot or air, acute respiratory or cardiac failure, and sepsis. In the case of a sudden, unanticipated maternal arrest, the timing of cesarean delivery becomes the quintessential element [152,153].

If a pregnant woman does sustain a cardiopulmonary arrest, cardiopulmonary resuscitation (CPR) should be initiated immediately (Chapter 7). Optimal performance of CPR in the non-pregnant patient results in a cardiac output less than a third of normal [153]. In the pregnant woman at term, CPR, under optimal circumstances, produces a cardiac output around 10% of normal. To optimize maternal cardiac output, the patient should be placed in the supine position. Dextrorotation of the uterus and compression of the major vessels of the uterus may impede venous return and may further compromise this effort. Lateral uterine displacement may help to remedy this problem; but CPR in this position is extremely awkward. Ultimately, a cesarean may be necessary to alleviate this impedance to CPR.

If maternal and fetal outcomes are to be optimized, the timing of the cesarean delivery is critical. According to Katz and associates [152] in 1986 and reaffirmed in 2005 [153], the theory behind a perimortem cesarean is that if CPR fails to produce a pulse within 4 minutes, a cesarean delivery should be begun and the baby delivered within 5 minutes of maternal cardiac arrest. Once the baby is delivered, maternal CPR should continue because many women will have "sudden and profound improvement" [153] after evacuation of the uterus. Hence, the "4-minute rule" came into effect and has been adopted by the American Heart Association when maternal CPR has been ineffective [153,154]. Thus, the standard ABCs of cardiopulmonary resuscitation (airway, breathing, circulation) should be expanded to include D (delivery).

As demonstrated in Table 43.8, fetal survival is linked consistently with the interval between maternal arrest and delivery. It is clear from the available data [152,153] that the longer the time interval from maternal death to the delivery of the fetus, the greater is the likelihood of permanent neurologic impairment of the fetus. Ideally, the fetus should be delivered within 5 minutes of maternal arrest. Within that 5-minute window rests the greatest likelihood of delivering a child who will be neurologically normal (Table 43.8). However, the potential exists for a favorable fetal outcome beyond 15 minutes of maternal cardiac arrest, and therefore, delivery should not be withheld even if beyond 5 minutes, if the fetus is still alive [152,153].

While the timing of cesarean delivery is a major determinant of subsequent fetal outcome, the gestational age of the fetus also is an important consideration. The probability of survival is related directly to the neonatal birth weight and gestational age

[155–158]. At what gestational age should a perimortem cesarean delivery be considered? Is there a lower limit? It becomes obvious immediately that there are no clear answers to these questions. As a general rule, intervention appears prudent whenever the fetus is potentially viable or is "capable of a meaningful existence outside the mother's womb" [159]. According to Gdansky and Schenker [143], the gray zone rests between 23 and 26 weeks' gestation. But, this threshold is continually pushed to earlier gestational ages in keeping with the advances in neonatal care. Ideally, criteria for intervention in such circumstances should be formulated with the aid of an institution's current neonatal survival statistics and guidance from its bioethics committee. In light of the continual technologic advances in neonatology, care must be taken to periodically review these criteria because the gestational age and weight criteria may be lowered in the future [155–159].

When maternal death is an anticipated event, is informed consent necessary? For instance, patients hospitalized with terminal cancer, class IV cardiac disease, pulmonary hypertension, or previous myocardial infarction are at an increased risk of death during pregnancy. Although these cases are infrequent, it seems reasonable to prepare for such an eventuality. Decisions regarding intervention should be made in advance with the patient and family. When intervention has been agreed to, one consideration is to have a cesarean delivery pack and neonatal resuscitation equipment immediately available in the ICU.

References

1 Hon EH, Quilligan EJ. Electronic evaluation of the fetal heart rate. *Clin Obstet Gynecol* 1968; 11: 145–155.

2 Paul RH, Gauthier RJ, Quilligan EJ. Clinical fetal monitoring: the usage and relationship to trends in cesarean delivery and perinatal mortality. *Acta Obstet Gynecol Scand* 1980; 59: 289–295.

3 Shenker L, Post RC, Seiler JS. Routine electronic monitoring of fetal heart rate and uterine activity during labor. *Obstet Gynecol* 1980; 46: 185–189.

4 Yeh SY, Diaz F, Paul RH. Ten year experience in fetal monitoring at Los Angeles County/University of Southern California Medical Center. *Am J Obstet Gynecol* 1982; 143: 496–500.

5 Phelan JP. Labor admission test. *Clin Perinatol* 1994; 21(4): 879–885.

6 Skupski DW, Rosenberg CR, Eglinton GS. Intrapartum fetal stimulation tests: a meta-analysis. *Obstet Gynecol* 2002; 99: 129–134.

7 Perkins, RP. Perspectives on perinatal brain damage. *Obstet Gynecol* 1987; 69: 807–819.

8 Rosen M, Dickinson MG. The incidence of cerebral palsy. *Am J Obstet Gynecol* 1992; 167: 417–423.

9 Smith J, Wells L, Dodd K. The continuing fall in incidence of hypoxic-ischemic encephalopathy in term infants. *Br J Obstet Gynecol* 2000; 107: 461–466.

10 Clark SL. Shock in the pregnant patient. *Semin Perinatol* 1990; 14: 52–58.

11 Phelan JP, Ahn MO. Fetal heart rate observations in 300 term brain-damaged infants. *J Matern Fetal Invest* 1998; 8: 1–5.

12 Phelan JP, Kim JO. Fetal heart rate observations in the brain-damaged infant. *Semin Perinatol* 2000; 24: 221–229.

13 Phelan JP. Perinatal risk management: obstetric methods to prevent birth asphyxia. *Clin Perinatol* 2005; 32: 1–17.

14 Phelan JP, Korst LM, Martin GI. Causation – fetal brain injury and uterine rupture. *Clin Perinatol* 2007; 34(3): 409–438.

15 Lockshin MD, Bonfa E, Elkon D, Druzin ML. Neonatal lupus risk to newborns of mother with systemic lupus erythematosus. *Arthritis Rheum* 1988; 31: 697–701.

16 Manning FA, Platt LD, Sipos L. Antepartum fetal evaluation: development of a fetal biophysical profile. *Am J Obstet Gynecol* 1980; 136: 787–795.

17 Sibai BM. Diagnosis, prevention, and management of eclampsia. *Obstet Gynecol* 2005; 105: 402–410.

18 Clark SL, Hankins GD, Dudley DA, et al. Amniotic fluid embolism: analysis of the National Registry. *Am J Obstet Gynecol* 1995; 172: 1158–1167.

19 Paul RH, Koh KS, Bernstein SG. Change in fetal heart rate: uterine contraction patterns associated with eclampsia. *Am J Obstet Gynecol* 1978; 130: 165–169.

20 Koh KD, Friesen RM, Livingstone RA, et al. Fetal monitoring during maternal cardiac surgery with cardiopulmonary bypass. *Can Med Assoc J* 1975; 112: 1102–1106.

21 Korsten HHM, van Zundert AAJ, Moou PNM, et al. Emergency aortic valve replacement in the 24th week of pregnancy. *Acta Anaestesiol Belg* 1989; 40: 201–205.

22 Strange K, Halldin M. Hypothermia in pregnancy. *Anesthesiology* 1983; 58: 460–465.

23 Bates B. Hon fetal heart rate pattern flags brain damage. *Ob Gyn News* 2005; 40(10): 1–2.

24 Kim JO, Martin G, Kirkendall C, Phelan JP. Intrapartum fetal heart rate variability and subsequent neonatal cerebral edema. *Obstet Gynecol* 2000; 95: 75S.

25 National Institute of Child Health and Human Development Research Planning Workshop. Electronic fetal heart rate monitoring: research guidelines for interpretation. *Am J Obstet Gynecol* 1997; 177: 1385–1390.

26 Smith CV. Vibroacoustic stimulation for risk assessment. *Clin Perinatol* 1994; 21: 797–808.

27 Petrie RH, Yeh SY, Maurata Y, et al. Effect of drugs on fetal heart rate variability. *Am J Obstet Gynecol* 1978; 130: 294–299.

28 Babakania A, Niebyl R. The effect of magnesium sulfate on fetal heart rate variability. *Obstet Gynecol* 1978; 51(Suppl): 2S–4S.

29 Clark SL, Miller FC. Sinusoidal fetal heart rate pattern associated with massive fetomaternal transfusion. *Am J Obstet Gynecol* 1984; 149: 97–99.

30 Katz M, Meizner I, Shani N, et al. Clinical significance of sinusoidal fetal heart rate pattern. *Br J Obstet Gynaecol* 1984; 149: 97–100.

31 Modanlou HD, Freeman RK. Sinusoidal fetal heart rate pattern: its definition and clinical significance. *Am J Obstet Gynecol* 1982; 142: 1033–1038.

32 Theard FC, Penny LL, Otterson WN. Sinusoidal fetal heart rate: ominous or benign? *J Reprod Med* 1984; 29: 265–268.

33 Kirkendall C, Romo M, Phelan JP. Fetomaternal hemorrhage in fetal brain injury. *Am J Obstet Gynecol* 2001; 185(6): S153.

34 Heise RH, van Winter JT, Ogburn PL Jr. Identification of acute transplacental hemorrhage in a low-risk patient as a result of daily counting of fetal movements. *Mayo Clin Proc* 1993; 68: 892–894.

35 Kosasa TS, Ebesugawa I, Nakayama RT, Hale R. Massive fetomaternal hemorrhage preceded by decreased fetal movement and a nonreactive fetal heart rate pattern. *Obstet Gynecol* 1993; 82: 711–714.
36 Corometrics Teaching Program, 1974. Corometrics Inc, Wallingford, CT, GE Medical Systems, Milwaukee, WI.
37 Shaw K, Clark SL. Reliability of intrapartum fetal heart rate monitoring in the postterm fetus with meconium passage. *Obstet Gynecol* 1988; 72: 886–889.
38 Ahn MO, Korst LM, Phelan JP. Normal fetal heart rate patterns in the brain-damaged infant: a failure of intrapartum fetal monitoring? *J Matern Fetal Invest* 1998; 8: 58–60.
39 Garite TJ, Linzey EM, Freeman RK, et al. Fetal heart rate patterns and fetal distress in fetuses with congenital anomalies. *Obstet Gynecol* 1979; 53: 716–720.
40 Slomka C, Phelan JP. Pregnancy outcome in the gravida with a nonreactive nonstress test and positive contraction stress test. *Am J Obstet Gynecol* 1981; 139: 11–15.
41 Phelan JP, Smith CV. Antepartum fetal assessment: the contraction stress test. In: Hill A, Volpe JJ, eds. *Fetal Neurology*. New York: Raven, 1989: 75–90.
42 Manning FA, Morrison I, Harman CR, Menticoglou SM. The abnormal fetal biophysical profile score V: predictive accuracy according to score composition. *Am J Obstet Gynecol* 1990; 162: 918–927.
43 Phelan JP. Antepartum fetal assessment: newer techniques. *Semin Perinatol* 1988; 12: 57–65.
44 Phelan JP, Smith CV, Broussard P, Small M. Amniotic fluid volume assessment using the four quadrant technique at 36–42 weeks' gestation. *J Reprod Med* 1987; 32: 540–543.
45 Phelan JP, Ahn MO, Smith CV, Rutherford SE, Anderson E. Amniotic fluid index measurements during pregnancy. *J Reprod Med* 1987; 32: 601–604.
46 Phelan JP, Lewis PE. Fetal heart rate decelerations during a nonstress test. *Obstet Gynecol* 1981; 57: 228–232.
47 Gabbe SG, Ettinger RB, Freeman RK, et al. Umbilical cord compression with amniotomy: laboratory observations. *Am J Obstet Gynecol* 1976; 126: 353–355.
48 Phelan JP. The postdate pregnancy: an overview. *Clin Obstet Gynecol* 1989; 32(2): 221–227.
49 Kubli FW, Hon EH, Hhazin AF, et al. Observations in heart rate and pH in the human fetus during labor. *Am J Obstet Gynecol* 1969; 104: 1190–1206.
50 Krebs HB, Petres RE, Dunn LH, et al. Intrapartum fetal heart rate monitoring: VII. Atypical variable decelerations. *Am J Obstet Gynecol* 1983; 145: 297–305.
51 Greenberg J, Economy K, Mark A, et al. In search of "true" birth asphyxia: labor characteristics associated with the asphyxiated term infant. *Am J Obstet Gynecol* 2001; 185: S94.
52 Nelson KB, Dambrosia JM, Ting TY, Grether JK. Uncertain value of electronic fetal monitoring in predicting cerebral palsy. *N Engl J Med* 1996; 334: 613–618.
53 LoBue C, Goodlin RC. Treatment of fetal distress during diabetic ketoacidosis. *J Reprod Med* 1978; 20: 101–104.
54 Rhodes RW, Ogburn PL. Treatment of severe diabetic ketoacidosis in the early third trimester in a patient with fetal distress. *J Reprod Med* 1984;29:621–625.
55 Cruz AC, Spellacy WN, Jarrell M. Fetal heart rate tracing during sickle cell crisis: a cause for transient late decelerations. *Obstet Gynecol* 1979; 54: 647–649.
56 Witter FR, Niebyl JR. Drug intoxication and anaphylactic shock in the obstetric patient. In: Berkowitz RL, ed. *Critical Care of the Obstetric Patient*. New York: Churchill Livingstone, 1983: 527–543.
57 Klein VR, Harris AP, Abraham RA, Niebyl JR. Fetal distress during a maternal systemic allergic reaction. *Obstet Gynecol* 1984; 64(Suppl): 15S–17S.
58 Dunn AB, Blomquist J, Khouzami V. Anaphylaxis in labor secondary to prophylaxis against group B Streptococcus: a case report. *J Reprod Med* 1999; 44: 381–384.
59 Stannard L, Bellis A. Maternal anaphylactic reaction to a general anesthetic at emergency cesarean section for fetal bradycardia. *Br J Obstet Gynecol* 2001; 108: 539–540.
60 Sheehan PQ, Rowland TW, Shah BL, et al. Maternal diabetic control and hypertrophic cardiomyopathy in infants of diabetic mothers. *Clin Pediatr* 1986; 25: 226–230.
61 Saling E. Technik der endoskopischen microbluentnahme am feten. *Geburtshilfe Frauenheikd* 1964; 24: 464–467.
62 Saling E, Schneider D. Biochemical supervision of the fetus during labor. *J Obstet Gynaecol Br Cwlth* 1967; 74: 799–803.
63 Clark SL, Paul RH. Intrapartum fetal surveillance: the role of fetal scalp sampling. *Am J Obstet Gynecol* 1985; 153: 717–720.
64 Goodwin TM, Milner-Masterson L, Paul RH. Elimination of fetal scalp blood sampling on a large clinical service. *Obstet Gynecol* 1994; 83: 971–974.
65 Phelan JP, Kirkendall C, Korst L, Martin G. In cases of fetal brain injury, a slow heart rate at birth is an indicator of severe acidosis. *Am J Obstet Gynecol* 2003; 189(6): S184.
66 Kirkendall C, Phelan JP. Severe acidosis at birth and normal neurological outcome. *Prenat Neonat Med* 2001; 6: 267–270.
67 Myers RE. Two patterns of perinatal brain damage and their conditions of occurrence. *Am J Obstet Gynecol* 1972; 112: 246–277.
68 Fee SC, Malee K, Deddish R, et al. Severe acidosis and subsequent neurologic status. *Am J Obstet Gynecol* 1990; 162: 802–806.
69 Dennis J, Johnson A, Mutch L, et al. Acid-base status at birth and neurodevelopmental outcome at four and one-half years. *Am J Obstet Gynecol* 1989; 161: 213–220.
70 Korst LM, Phelan JP, Ahn MO, Martin GI. Can persistent brain injury resulting from intrapartum asphyxia be predicted by current criteria? *Prenat Neonat Med* 1997; 2: 286–293.
71 Korst L, Phelan JP, Wang YM, Martin GI, Ahn MO. Acute fetal asphyxia and permanent brain injury: a retrospective analysis of current indicators. *J Matern Fetal Med* 1999; 8: 101–106.
72 Garite TJ, Dildy GA, McNamara H, et al. A multicenter controlled trial of fetal pulse oximetry in the intrapartum management of nonreassuring fetal heart rate patterns. *Am J Obstet Gynecol* 2000; 183: 1049–1058.
73 American College of Obstetricians and Gynecologists. *Fetal and Neonatal Injury*. Technical Bulletin No. 163. Washington, DC: American College of Obstetricians and Gynecologists, 1992.
74 MacLennan A. A template for defining a causal relation between acute intrapartum events and cerebral palsy: international consensus statement. *BMJ* 1999; 319: 1054–1059.
75 American College of Obstetricians and Gynecologists and American Academy of Pediatrics. Neonatal Encephalopathy Committee Opinion. Washington, DC: American College of Obstetricians and Gynecologists and American Academy of Pediatrics, 2003.
76 Schifrin B. The CTG and the timing and mechanism of fetal neurological injuries. *Best Pract Res Clin Obstet Gynaecol* 2004; 18: 437–456.

77 Krebs HB, Petres RE, Dunn LH, et al. Intrapartum fetal heart rate monitoring: VI. Prognostic significance of accelerations. *Am J Obstet Gynecol* 1982; 142: 297–305.
78 Ingemarsson I, Arulkumaran S, Paul RH, et al. Admission test: a screening test for fetal distress in labor. *Obstet Gynecol* 1986; 68: 800–806.
79 Pasternak JF, Gorey MT. The syndrome of acute near-total intrauterine asphyxia in the term infant. *Pediatr Neurol* 1998; 18: 391–398.
80 Leung A, Leung EK, Paul RH. Uterine rupture after previous cesarean delivery: maternal and fetal consequences. *Am J Obstet Gynecol* 1993; 169: 945–950.
81 Hon EH, Lee ST. Electronic evaluation of the fetal heart rate: VIII. Patterns preceding fetal death, further observations. *Am J Obstet Gynecol* 1963; 87: 814–826.
82 Altschuler G, Hyde S. Meconium induced vasoconstriction: a potential cause of cerebral and other fetal hypoperfusion and of poor pregnancy outcome. *J Child Neurol* 1989; 4: 1337–1342.
83 Altschuler G, Arizawa M, Molnar-Nadasy G. Meconium-induced umbilical cord vascular necrosis and ulceration: a potential link between the placenta and poor pregnancy outcome. *Obstet Gynecol* 1992; 79: 760–766.
84 Yoon BH, Kim CJ, Jun JK. Amniotic fluid interleukin 6: a sensitive test for antenatal diagnosis of acute inflammatory lesions of preterm placenta and prediction of perinatal morbidity. *Am J Obstet Gynecol* 1995; 172: 960–970.
85 Perlman JM, Risser R, Broyles RS. Bilateral cystic leukomalacia in the premature infant: associated risk factors. *Pediatrics* 1996; 97: 822–827.
86 Gibson CS, Maclennan AH, Goldwater PN, Haan E, Priest K, Dekker GA. Neurotropic viruses and cerebral palsy: population based case-control study. *BMJ* 2006; 332: 76–80.
87 Euscher E, Davis J, Holzman J, Nuovo GJ. Coxsackie virus infection of the placenta associated with neurodevelopmental delays in the newborn. *Obstet Gynecol* 2001; 98: 1019–1026.
88 Visser GHA, deVries LS, Groeneudaul F. How bad is a low pH at birth? *Prenat Neonat Med* 2001; 6: 265–266.
89 Phelan JP, Ahn MO. Perinatal observations in forty-eight neurologically impaired term infants. *Am J Obstet Gynecol* 1994; 171: 424–431.
90 Phelan JP, Martin GI, Korst LM. Birth asphyxia and cerebral palsy. *Clin Perinatol* 2005; 32: 61–76.
91 Blackwell SC, Refuerzo JS, Wolfe HM, et al. The relationship between nucleated red blood cell counts and early-onset neonatal seizures. *Am J Obstet Gynecol* 2000; 182: 1452–1457.
92 Korst LM, Phelan JP, Wang YM, Ahn MO. Neonatal platelet counts in fetal brain injury. *Am J Perinatol* 1999; 16: 79–83.
93 Ahn MO, Korst LM, Phelan JP, Martin GI. Does the onset of neonatal seizures correlate with the timing of fetal neurologic injury. *Clin Pediatr* 1998; 37: 673–676.
94 Kirkendall C, Ahn MO, Martin G, Korst L, Phelan JP. The brain injured baby, neonatal seizures, and the intrapartum fetal heart rate pattern: is there a relationship? *Am J Obstet Gynecol* 2000; 182: S184.
95 Gallagher JS. Anaphylaxis in pregnancy. *Obstet Gynecol* 1988; 71: 491–493.
96 Cole DS, Bruck LR. Anaphylaxis after laminaria insertion. *Obstet Gynecol* 2000; 95: 1025.
97 Deusch E, Reider N, Marth C. Anaphylactic reaction to latex during cesarean delivery. *Obstet Gynecol* 1996; 88: 727.
98 Van Arsdel PP. Drug allergy update. *Med Clin North Am* 1981; 65: 1089–1092.
99 Reisman RE. Responding to acute anaphylaxis. *Contemp Obstet Gynecol* 1989; 33: 45–57.
100 American College of Obstetricians and Gynecologists. *Asthma in Pregnancy*. ACOG Practice Bulletin No. 90. Washington, DC: American College of Obstetricians and Gynecologists, 2008.
101 Metzger WJ, Turner E, Patterson R. The safety of immunotherapy during pregnancy. *J Allergy Clin Immunol* 1978; 61: 268–272.
102 Shaikh WA. A retrospective study on the safety of immunotherapy in pregnancy. *Clin Exp Allergy* 1993; 23: 857–860.
103 Clark SL, Divon M, Phelan JP. Preeclampsia/eclampsia: hemodynamic and neurologic correlations. *Obstet Gynecol* 1985; 66: 337–340.
104 Boehm FH, Growdon JH. The effect of eclamptic convulsions of the fetal heart rate. *Am J Obstet Gynecol* 1974; 120: 851–853.
105 Pritchard JA, Cunningham FG, Pritchard SA. The Parkland Memorial Hospital protocol for treatment of eclampsia: evaluation of 245 cases. *Am J Obstet Gynecol* 1984; 148: 951–963.
106 Lucas MJ, Leveno KJ, Cunningham FG. A comparison of magnesium sulfate with phenytoin for the prevention of eclampsia. *N Engl J Med* 1995; 333: 201–205.
107 Naidu S, Payne AJ, Moodley J, et al. Randomised study assessing the effect of phenytoin and magnesium sulfate on maternal cerebral circulation in eclampsia using transcranial doppler ultrasound. *Br J Obstet Gynaecol* 1996; 103: 111–116.
108 Barrett JM. Fetal resuscitation with terbutaline during eclampsia-induced uterine hypertonus. *Am J Obstet Gynecol* 1984; 150: 895.
109 Reece E, Chervenak F, Romero R, Hobbins J. Magnesium sulfate in the management of acute intrapartum fetal distress. *Am J Obstet Gynecol* 1984; 148: 104–106.
110 Porter TF, Clark SL, Dildy GA, et al. Isolated disseminated intravascular coagulation and amniotic fluid embolism. *Am J Obstet Gynecol* 1996; 174: 486.
111 Polko LE, McMahon MJ. Burns in pregnancy. *Obstet Gynecol Surv* 1998; 53: 50–56.
112 Guo SS, Greenspoon JS, Kahn AM. Management of burn injuries during pregnancy. *Burns* 2001; 27: 394–397.
113 Demling RH. Management of the burn patient. In: Grenvik A, Holbrook PR, Shoemaker WC, eds. *Textbook of Critical Care*, 3rd edn. Philadelphia: WB Saunders, 1995: 1499.
114 Matthews RN. Obstetric implications of burns in pregnancy. *Br J Obstet Gynaecol* 1982; 89: 603–609.
115 Dillon WP, Lee RV, Tronolone MJ, et al. Life support and maternal brain death during pregnancy. *JAMA* 1982; 248: 1089–1091.
116 Heikkinen JE, Rinne RI, Alahuhta SM, et al. Life support of 10 weeks with successful fetal outcome after fatal maternal brain damage. *BMJ Clin Res Ed* 1985; 290: 1237–1238.
117 Field DR, Gates EA, Creasy RK, et al. Maternal brain death during pregnancy: medical and ethical issues. *JAMA* 1988; 260: 816–822.
118 Bernstein IM, Watson M, Simmons GM, Catalano PM, Davis G, Collings R. Maternal brain death and prolonged fetal survival. *Obstet Gynecol* 1989; 74: 434–437.
119 Wuermeling H. Brain-death and pregnancy. *Forens Sci Int* 1994; 68: 243–245.
120 Iriye BK, Asrat T, Adashek JA, Carr MH. Intraventricular hemorrhage and maternal brain death associated with antepartum cocaine abuse. *Br J Obstet Gynaecol* 1995; 102: 68–69.

121 Vives A, Carmona F, Zabala E, Fernandez C, Cararach V, Iglesia X. Maternal brain death during pregnancy. *Int J Gynecol Obstet* 1996; 52: 67–69.

122 Catanzarite VA, Willms DC, Holdy KE, et al. Brain death during pregnancy: tocolytic therapy and aggressive maternal support on behalf of the fetus. *Am J Perinatol* 1997; 14: 431–434.

123 Lewis DD, Vidovich RR. Organ recovery following childbirth in a brain-dead mother: a case report. *J Transpl Coord* 1997; 7: 103–105.

124 Spike J. Brain death, pregnancy, and posthumous motherhood. *J Clin Ethics* 1999; 10: 57–65.

125 Souza JP, Cecatta JG, Amaral E, et al. The prolongation of somatic support in a pregnant woman with brain death: a case report. *J Reprod Health* 2006; 3: 3.

126 Hussein IY, Govenden V, Grant JM, Said MR. Prolongation of pregnancy in a woman who sustained brain death at 26 weeks of gestation. *Br J Obstet Gynaecol* 2006; 113: 120–122.

127 Lucas B. Pregnant car crash victim. *Nurs Times* 1976; 72: 451–453.

128 Sampson MB, Peterson LP. Post-traumatic coma during pregnancy. *Obstet Gynecol* 1979; 53: 25–35.

129 BenAderet N, Cohen I, Abramowicz JS. Traumatic coma during pregnancy with persistent vegetative state. Case report. *Br J Obstet Gynecol* 1984; 91: 939–941.

130 Hill LM. Management of maternal vegetative state during pregnancy. *Mayo Clin Proc* 1985; 60: 469–472.

131 Diamond MP, Boehm FH, Allen G. Long term management of pregnancy in a comatose patient. *J Tenn Med Assoc* 1986; 79: 557–566.

132 Landye ST. Successful enteral nutrition support of a pregnant comatose patient: a case study. *J Am Diet Assoc* 1988; 88: 718–720.

133 Koh ML, Lipkin EW. Nutrition support of a pregnant comatose patient via percutaneous endoscopic gastrostomy. *J Parenter Enteral Nutr* 1993; 17: 384–387.

134 Webb GW, Huddleston JF. Management of the pregnant woman who sustains severe brain damage. *Clin Perinatol* 1996; 23: 453–464.

135 Wong M, Apodaca CC. Nutrition management in a pregnant comatose patient. *NCP Bull* 1997; 12: 63–67.

136 Finerty JJ, Chisolm CA, Chapple H, et al. Cerebral arterio-venous malformation in pregnancy: presentation and neurologic, obstetric, and ethical significance. *Am J Obstet Gynecol* 1999; 181: 296–303.

137 Ayorinde BT, Scudamore I, Buggy DJ. Anaesthetic management of a pregnant patient in a persistent vegetative state. *Br J Anaesth* 2000; 85: 478–491.

138 Feldman DM, Borgida AF, Rodis JF, Campbell WA. Irreversible maternal brain injury during pregnancy: a case report and review of the literature. *Obstet Gynecol Surv* 2000; 55: 708–714.

139 Sim KH. Maternal persistent vegetative state with successful fetal outcome. *J Korean Med* 2001; 16: 669–672.

140 Bush MC, Nagy S, Berkowitz RC, Gaddipati S. Pregnancy in a persistent vegetative state: case report, comparison to brain death, and review of literature. *Obstet Gynecol Surv* 2003; 50: 738–748.

141 Chiossi G, Novic K, Celebreeze JU, Thomas RL. Successful neonatal outcome in 2 cases of maternal persistent vegetative state treated in a labor and delivery suite. *Am J Obstet Gynecol* 2006; 195: 316–322.

142 Mallampalli A, Powner DJ, Gardner MO. Cardiopulmonary resuscitation and somatic support of the pregnant patient. *Crit Care Clin* 2004; 20: 747–761.

143 Gdanski E, Schenker G. Management of pregnancy in women with circulatory and brain death. *Prenat Neonat Med* 1998; 3: 327–333.

144 Black PM. Brain death. *N Engl J Med* 1978; 229(7): 338–344, and 299(8): 393–401.

145 Bernat JL, Culver CM, Gert B. On the definition and criterion of death. *Ann Intern Med* 1981; 94: 389–394.

146 Edwards MJ, Wanner RA. Extremes of temperature. In: Wilson JG, Graser FC, eds. *Handbook of Teratology, vol. 1.* New York: Plenum, 1977: 421.

147 Smith CV, Rufleth P, Phelan JP, et al. Longterm enteral hyperalimentation in the pregnant woman with insulin dependent diabetes. *Am J Obstet Gynecol* 1981; 141: 180–183.

148 Clark-Pearson DL, Synan IS, Dodge R, et al. A randomized trial of low-dose heparin and intermittent pneumatic calf compression for the prevention of deep venous thrombosis after gynecologic oncology surgery. *Am J Obstet Gynecol* 1993; 168: 1146–1154.

149 National Institutes of Health. Consensus Conference on Effect of Corticosteroids for Fetal Maturation on Perinatal Outcomes. *JAMA* 1995; 273: 413–418.

150 Powner DJ, Bernstein J. Extended somatic support for pregnant women after brain death. *Crit Care Med* 2003; 31: 1241–1249.

151 Weber CE. Postmortem cesarean section: review of the literature and case reports. *Am J Obstet Gynecol* 1971; 110: 158–165.

152 Katz VL, Dotters DJ, Droegemueller W. Perimortem cesarean delivery. *Obstet Gynecol* 1986; 68: 571–576.

153 Katz VL, Balderston K, DeFreest M. Perimortem cesarean delivery: were our assumptions correct? *Am J Obstet Gynecol* 2005; 192: 1916–1921.

154 American Heart Association, International Liaison Committee on Resuscitation. Guidelines 2000 for cardiopulmonary resuscitation and emergency cardiovascular care: international consensus on science, part 3: adult basic life support. *Circulation* 2000; 102(Suppl l): 22–59.

155 Copper RL, Goldenberg RL, Creasy RK, et al. A multicenter study of preterm birth weight and gestational age specific neonatal mortality. *Am J Obstet Gynecol* 1993; 168: 78–84.

156 Hussain N, Galal M, Ehrenkranz RA, Herson VC, Rowe JC. Predischarge outcomes of 22–27 weeks gestational age infants born at tertiary care centers in Connecticut: implications for perinatal management. *Conn Med* 1998; 62: 131–137.

157 Draper ES, Manktelow B, Field DJ, James D. Prediction of survival for preterm births by weight and gestational age: retrospective population based study. *BMJ* 1999; 319: 1093–1097.

158 Aschner JL, Walsh MC. Long-term outcomes: what should the focus be? *Clin Perinatol* 2007; 34: 205–217.

159 Roe v. Wade, 410 U.S. 113, 93 S. Ct. 705 (1973).

44 Fetal Effects of Drugs Commonly Used in Critical Care

Mark Santillan & Jerome Yankowitz

Department of Obstetrics and Gynecology, University of Iowa College of Medicine, Iowa City, IA, USA

Introduction

Rarely must a physician in an intensive care unit (ICU) consider the fetal effects of drugs commonly used in this setting. The incidence of ICU admissions during pregnancy is 0.17–1.1% [1]. This infrequent occurrence coupled with the lack of drug data in parturients complicates treatment of the pregnant ICU patient. A brief review of the physiologic changes in pregnancy that affect pharmacodynamics reveals some of this complexity.

The four aspects of pharmacokinetics affected by pregnancy are absorption, distribution, metabolism and excretion. Overall, absorption increases during pregnancy. Gastric pH, small bowel motility, and the rate of gastric emptying are decreased [2]. The increased cardiac output during pregnancy also helps increase the delivery of medications to tissues to increase absorption [3]. An increase in plasma volume, total body water, some plasma proteins, and body fat has been shown to increase the volume of distribution for some drugs. Increased cardiac output also contributes to increased distribution [4]. Various metabolic enzymes, such as cytochrome P-450, CYP1A2, and cholinesterase have different activity levels in the face of pregnancy. Cytochrome P-450 is upregulated. In contrast, CYP2C19 and cholinesterase are downregulated. These activities attenuate how drugs are metabolized in pregnancy. Ten to twenty per cent of the population has lower metabolic enzyme activity. This further causes variation in how pregnant women metabolize drugs [4]. An increase in drug elimination is driven by the increased glomerular filtration rate [5]. Of note, renal secretion and reabsorption of drugs increase in pregnancy. Drug processing also occurs through respiration. The changes in pulmonary function during pregnancy make respiration a more important factor in drug elimination [4]. These physiologic changes during pregnancy make predicting pharmacokinetics difficult.

Critical Care Obstetrics, 5th edition. Edited by M. Belfort, G. Saade, M. Foley, J. Phelan and G. Dildy.

The fetal effects of medications provide an additional challenge in treating the pregnant patient. Particularly in preterm fetuses, the poorly developed blood–brain barrier can lead to a higher concentration of drugs in the fetal CNS. The preterm fetus also has fewer protein binding sites. Consequently, more unbound drug is in the fetal circulation. In addition, preterm hyperbilirubinemia further increases the effects of drugs as bilirubin competes with drugs for protein binding sites [6]. Overall, preterm physiology increases the effects of most drugs. The challenge of treating two patients colors all therapeutic decisions of those caring for pregnant patients. A summary of the drugs that may commonly be encountered in the critical care unit are shown in Table 44.1.

Maternal analgesia and sedation

Analgesia and sedation are essential components of critical care medicine. Although there are many drugs to use for sedation, analgesia, and neuromuscular blockade, multiple practice surveys point to a pattern of commonly used medications in the ICU [7–9]. The most commonly used sedatives are midazolam, lorazepam, propofol, and haldol. The most common pain medications are morphine and fentanyl. The most frequently used neuromuscular blocking agents are pancuronium and vecuronium.

Midazolam

Midazolam is a water-soluble benzodiazepine. As a sedative/hypnotic, it is often used in combination with other anesthetic protocols. It has a rapid onset and a short duration of action. The elimination half-life is 1 hour in pregnant women [10], and 6.3 hours in neonates [11]. Placental transfer of the drug is very rapid. Rapid drug clearance makes midazolam a more acceptable sedative for use in pregnancy. Although cases of infant respiratory depression requiring resuscitation have occurred if midazolam is given before a cesarean section [12], there are no controlled trials investigating the embryotoxic effect of midazolam or cases of congenital anomalies in newborns of midazolam-exposed mothers.

Table 44.1 Summary of drugs.

Safe in pregnancy	Use in acute/limited situations	Contraindicated in pregnancy	Unknown effects
Midazolam	Propofol	Angiotensin converting enzyme inhibitors	Milrinone
Lorazepam	Pancuronium	Angiotensin II receptor blockers (ARBs)	Amrinone
Haloperidol	Vecuronium		
Morphine	Amiodarone		
Adenosine	Atropine		
Calcium channel blockers	Epinephrine		
Lidocaine	Ibutilide		
Digoxin	Procainamide		
Furosemide	Dopamine		
Hydralazine	Dobutamine		
Labetalol	Isoproterinol		
Heparins	Hydrochlorothiazide		
Insulin	Nitroglycerin		
Thyroxine	Nitroprusside		
Propylthiouracil	Warfarin		
	Thrombolytics		
	Corticosteroids		
	Methimazole		
	Mannitol		

In doses greater than 30 mg, diazepam, a similar benzodiazepine, has been linked to fetal hypothermia, hypotonia, poor feeding, and increased risk of jaundice [6]. Even though the manufacturer suggests caution in use of midazolam in pregnancy based on these adverse neonatal effects of diazepam at high doses, midazolam's rapid onset of action and rapid clearing coupled with medical needs in the ICU, makes use of midazolam in an ICU setting during pregnancy acceptable.

Midazolam is excreted in small amounts in breast milk and considered likely safe for breastfeeding [31].

Lorazepam

Lorazepam, like midazolam, is a water-soluble benzodiazepine with a longer duration of action. Lorazepam is more often used as an acute anxiolytic. It has a rapid onset and a short duration of action relative to diazepam. Its elimination half-life in adults is approximately 12 hours [13]. Lorazepam does cross the placenta, but fetal levels of the drug are uniformly lower than maternal levels [14]. In addition, neonatal rate of metabolism of the drug is less than maternal rates [13]. A "floppy infant syndrome" characterized by muscular hypotonia, hypothermia, low Apgar scores, and neurologic depression has been associated with this drug [14].

The question of embryotoxicity of lorazepam has not been adequately answered. Previous studies investigating this question showed no correlation with congenital malformations [15]. A large French retrospective review of 13 703 congenital malformations documented in the French Central East registry demonstrates that overall there is no increase of malformations with the use of first-trimester benzodiazepines. When the data were analyzed specifically for lorazepam there was a significant association of lorazepam with anal atresia (OR 6.2, 95% CI 2.4–15.7, $P = 0.01$) [16]. Of note, only 262 of the 13 703 infants were exposed to a benzodiazepine. Six cases of anal atresia were identified in this subgroup, 5 of which were exposed to lorazepam. Although there was a statistically significant correlation between lorazepam and anal atresia, the clinical significance of this finding is in question. Given the study design and the small number of cases of anal atresia, one should not use these data to restrict the use of lorazepam in pregnancy, particularly in the acute setting after the teratogenic period.

In terms of breastfeeding, only small amounts of lorazepam have been detected in breast milk [17] and it is considered likely safe for breastfeeding.

Propofol

Propofol is a widely used intravenous anesthetic. It is used in many general anesthesia protocols. Propofol has a rapid onset of action with a short duration of action. In pregnant women undergoing a cesarean section, onset of action is reported at 75 s after administration with a half-life of 4.7 min [18]. Placental transfer is also rapid, with rapid uptake by fetal tissues. In multiple studies, the fetal levels of the drug are lower than maternal levels. One case report describes a prolonged exposure to propofol greater than 48 hours in a pregnant woman with no adverse neonatal outcome except for prolonged neonatal sedation [19]. There is little written on adverse neonatal outcomes associated with propofol. One study suggests that there is a decrease in the Early

Neonatal Neurobehavioral Scale score at 1 hour of life in infants exposed to propofol *in utero* during a cesarean section. This change in the ENNS score resolved at the fourth hour of life [20]. This same study also states that these infants have satisfactory arterial pH and Apgar scores at delivery. There are multiple studies showing that fetuses exposed *in utero* to propofol show no significant neonatal depression as assessed by Apgar scores, arterial pH, and neurologic and adaptive capacity scores (NACS) [21–23]. No fetal structural abnormalities have been reported with propofol. Therefore, propofol is a safe induction agent in pregnancy.

Propofol is present only in very small amounts in breast milk. Breastfeeding is considered safe after propofol exposure [24].

Haloperidol

Haloperidol is often used as an acute tranquilizer, or in chronic disorders such as schizophrenia and Tourette's syndrome. Haloperidol has a relatively rapid onset of action with a time to peak plasma concentration of 20 min. The average half-life of haloperidol of both intravenous and intramuscular administrations is 20 min [25]. The lipophilic nature of haloperidol makes it available to the fetal circulation very rapidly [26]. The side-effect profile of haloperidol includes the side effects of other neuroleptic drugs including akathisia and tardive dyskinesia. There are some case reports discussing the occurrence of these side effects in the fetus post delivery. In particular, one case report describes a subtype of tardive dyskinesia in an infant exposed to 2–5 mg/day of haloperidol throughout pregnancy [27]. Human fetal structural abnormalities have not been conclusively linked to haloperidol. In a review of 100 pregnancies exposed to haloperidol, no association with structural anomalies was noted [28]. Consequently, the use of haloperidol is considered safe in pregnancy, particularly in the acute setting.

Haloperidol is excreted in the breast milk. It is estimated that the infant will ingest 3% of the maternal dose through breast milk [29]. This small exposure to haloperidol has not been linked to any adverse neonatal outcomes [30]. Despite these findings, given the case reports of infant side effects, the American Academy of Pediatrics has classified haloperidol as a drug "for which the effect on nursing infants is unknown but may be of concern" [31].

Morphine

Morphine was widely used for pain control during labor in the 1940s. It has long since been replaced by newer narcotics secondary to its delayed onset of action, prolonged duration of action, and adverse side effects to mother and fetus [6]. One of the most concerning of these side effects is maternal and fetal respiratory depression. Intrathecal morphine has proved to be safe analgesia without fetal toxicity [32]. The placental transfer of morphine is rapid. Morphine, like other opioids, has a corresponding fetal withdrawal syndrome in opioid-addicted mothers. There have been no conclusive studies linking congenital malformations to morphine [33]. As with most agents, the long-term effects of neurobehavior and development are unknown but the use of morphine is considered compatible with pregnancy.

The American Academy of Pediatrics noted that morphine is compatible with breastfeeding [34]. Even in a case of chronic maternal use of morphine for severe pain, the infant was estimated to receive 0.8–12% of the maternal dose with no adverse side effects observed in the infant [35].

Fentanyl

Fentanyl is a synthetic narcotic agonist. It is often used in transdermal form for chronic pain indications. In obstetrics, it is a common component of epidural analgesia. The half-life has been reported from 3 to 12 hours with an average of 7 hours [36]. Placental transfer of fentanyl is well documented in all three trimesters with a mean cord to maternal venous fentanyl concentration ratio of 0.94 [37]. There are no reports linking congenital defects conclusively to *in utero* fentanyl exposure [31]. As a labor analgesic, IV fentanyl demonstrated no statistical difference versus matched controls not requiring analgesia in terms of different neonatal outcomes including Apgar scores, incidence of respiratory depression, and use of naloxone [38]. The same study does link morphine with the loss of fetal heart rate variability with no evidence of fetal hypoxia. There is a case report of fentanyl-linked fetal respiratory muscle rigidity which made neonatal resuscitation more difficult [39]. This is noteworthy since respiratory muscle rigidity is a common adult side effect. The use of fentanyl is considered compatible with pregnancy given the overall favorable neonatal outcomes.

Fentanyl is transferred to human milk in small proportions. It has been reported that 0.033% of the maternal dose of fentanyl is transferred to breast milk. Fentanyl has also been found in low doses in colostrum. In this study, the colostrum concentrations were higher than serum concentrations. The authors state that given the low oral bioavailability of fentanyl that it is still safe in breastfeeding. Given the above data, the AAP agrees and considers it compatible with breastfeeding [31].

Pancuronium

Pancuronium is a non-depolarizing curaremimetic neuromuscular blockade agent. It is a competitive inhibitor of acetylcholine at the neuromuscular junction level. It is commonly used to aid ventilation and intubation for general anesthesia for surgical cases including cesarean sections. In obstetrics, it is also used for acute, *in utero* neuromuscular blockade of a fetus for fetal therapy procedures such as intrauterine blood transfusions [40,41]. In term pregnant women, the half-life of pancuronium is reported between 72 and 114 minutes [42]. Term placental transfer of pancuronium has been well documented. In comparison to other non-polarizing neuromuscular blockage agents, pancuronium has a higher mean cord to maternal venous concentration ratio at varying maternal doses [40]. This is supported by the finding that a 1-min Apgar score greater than 7 occurs as low as 20% of the time in term cesarean sections using pancuronium. To date, there have been no cases of human teratogenesis linked to pancuronium. In the fetal therapy literature, there is a well-documented short-term fetal response to the administration of pancuronium to the fetus. In addition to decreased movement, a decrease in heart rate variability and accelerations is observed [43]. It has been reported that fetal heart variability can be reduced by 60% [44]. These changes are temporary and revert to normal after the fetus has recovered from the drug. Although not statistically significant, pancuronium proves to have a more significant neonatal effect on 15-min Neurologic Adaptive Capacity Scores than vecuronium, with 29% of those neonates exposed to pancuronium having normal NACS versus 73% of those born exposed to vecuronium [45]. Pancuronium can be used during pregnancy.

There are no reports on pancuronium and human lactation.

Vecuronium

Like pancuronium, vecuronium is a non-depolarizing curaremimetic neuromuscular blockade agent. It has a similar mechanism of action and is used in general anesthesia protocols for surgeries including cesarean sections. Vecuronium is also used for fetal immobility during intrauterine blood transfusions. There is a report of *in utero* use of vecuronium for fetal MRI [46]. In term pregnant women, the half-life of vecuronium is an average of 36 minutes with an onset of action of 125–175 seconds [40]. Vecuronium has a lower mean cord to maternal venous concentration ratio than pancuronium with average ratios between 0.11 and 0.14 [40]. The decreased fetal uptake of vecuronium gives it an advantage over pancuronium in the treatment of parturients. In direct comparisons between pancuronium and vecuronium, retrospective data shows that vecuronium displayed no fetal heart rate changes [47]. As with pancuronium, there are no reports of human congenital malformations linked to vecuronium.

There are no studies evaluating vecuronium and human lactation.

Cardiovascular drugs

Acute or chronic cardiovascular disease poses a significant risk to the parturient. In the UK, heart disease is the leading indirect cause of maternal mortality, causing 16.5% of all maternal deaths during the period of 1997–1999 [48]. In the United States the maternal mortality rate is 13.1 per 100 000 live births as of 2004 [49]. A majority of those deaths were due to cardiovascular causes. It is important to emphasize that in the case of acute cardiovascular collapse of a pregnant woman, the potential fetal effects of drugs can become secondary to maternal health. To evaluate specific therapeutics related to this field, this section will divide the drugs by functional classes.

ACLS drugs

Adenosine

Adenosine is a ubiquitous nucleoside. It has been used in pregnancy for the therapy of supraventricular tachycardias including Wolff–Parkinson–White syndrome. Its mechanism of action is based on changing ion channels in order to suppress the AV node. It has a short half-life of 0.6–1.5 seconds. Given this short elimination half-life, there are no studies examining placental transfer. One survey suggests that a higher dose of adenosine is required in pregnant women, likely representing the effect of the increased volume of distribution [50]. Intravenous adenosine may produce flushing, chest pain, and dyspnea. These side effects are transient and resolve in 5–20 seconds [51]. Given this data, it is an ideal cardiovascular drug in pregnancy. Fetal effects of adenosine are transient. There are varied reports of the effect of adenosine on fetal heart tracings from no change to short episodes of fetal bradycardia [52,53]. Given these transient changes, it is suggested that adenosine should be administered in conjunction with fetal heart rate monitoring [48]. To date, there are no reports of human teratogenesis secondary to adenosine use.

There are no data specifically evaluating adenosine and lactation. Again, given the short elimination half-life and use in acute settings, it is likely present in negligible amounts in human breast milk.

Amiodarone

Amiodarone is a class III antiarrhythmic agent. It is commonly used in maternal or fetal ventricular tachycardia/fibrillation and atrial fibrillation. It works by prolonging phase III of the cardiac action potential. It also has β-blocker and calcium channel blocker-like activity at the level of the SA and AV nodes. Amiodarone and its major active metabolite, mono-N-desethylamiodarone, have long mean elimination half-lives of 53 and 61 days, respectively [54]. They also have large volumes of distribution. Studies have documented placental transfer of amiodarone with approximately 25% of active drug still found in cord blood [55]. These pharmacokinetic aspects of amiodarone predispose it to more maternal and fetal side effects. Maternal side effects include thyroid abnormalities, liver dysfunction, skin discoloration, and most importantly idiopathic pulmonary fibrosis. Despite the increased volume of distribution during pregnancy, it is not clear if the risk of the side effects is increased with pregnancy. In a study of 12 *in utero* exposed fetuses, six had first-trimester exposure. One of the six infants was born with congenital nystagmus. Another infant with amiodarone exposure at 20 weeks had developmental delay, hypotonia, hypertelorism and micrognathia. This infant was exposed to multiple drugs during pregnancy [56]. Yet, there are no conclusive studies linking amiodarone and human teratogenicity.

There are multiple reports of different fetal side effects linked to *in utero* amiodarone exposure. Amiodarone is 37% iodine by weight with a chemical structure that is similar to thyroxine [57]. Consequently, a common fetal side effect is congenital goiter with hypo- or hyperthyroidism. In a recent 2004 review of neonatal thyroid dysfunction and amiodarone exposure, the authors examined 69 reported cases of amiodarone use pregnancy. Duration of use ranged from 2 days to 40 weeks. Of all these cases, 23% of the infants developed hypothyroidism requiring varying durations of replacement (5 weeks–20 months). Only two infants developed hyperthyroidism [55]. Growth restriction has also been seen in multiple series. It is not clear if this finding is secondary to amiodarone, the cardiac polypharmacy to which these fetuses were exposed, or the underlying condition requiring treatment. Given these findings, it is recommended that amiodarone be used only in refractory cases [58].

Recommendations about the use of amiodarone during breastfeeding are controversial. The WHO Working Group on Drugs and Human Lactation discourage the use of amiodarone in breastfeeding patients given the clinically effective concentrations in human milk [59]. In contrast, the American Academy of Pediatrics states that amiodarone may be used as long as maternal doses are minimized and the infant is monitored for thyroid disturbances [60]. Clearly, amiodarone should be used cautiously during breastfeeding.

Atropine

Atropine is an anticholinergic agent that is frequently combined in a variety of pharmaceutical products. In the setting of advanced cardiac life support, atropine is used for the treatment of sinus bradycardia, pulseless electrical activity, and asystole. Atropine has a half-life of 2 hours. Atropine is known to cross the placenta [61]. Despite this, the connection of human congenital anomalies and atropine is not well established. The rate of congenital abnormalities with the use of atropine has been reported at 4.2% [62]. This data from the Collaborative Perinatal Project illustrates that this rate of abnormalities is not dependent on the trimester of exposure. More recent findings quote a small risk of skeletal malformations with exposure, yet it is not clear from the data if this is due to teratogenicity or maternal toxicity of atropine [63]. Atropine has been associated with changes in fetal heart rate and a decrease in fetal breathing [64]. Despite these findings, there are no studies conclusively linking poor fetal outcomes with the use of atropine. In settings of no alternative treatments and an acute life-threatening situation, one may consider the use of atropine in the parturient.

There are no studies linking atropine exposure through breast milk and neonatal toxicity. The American Academy of Pediatrics deems atropine compatible with breastfeeding [31].

Epinephrine

Epinephrine is a sympathomimetic drug with a wide variety of uses. In the critical care setting, it is used in anaphylaxis, bradycardia, and cardiac arrest. Epinephrine does cross the placenta. Early reports have associated epinephrine with human congenital abnormalities. More recent studies show that there is no increase in congenital abnormalies with epinephrine exposure in any trimester of pregnancy [65]. Inguinal hernia is the only abnormality that has been specifically linked to epinephrine exposure [66]. Animal studies have linked epinephrine to uterine hypoperfusion, cardiovascular malformations, and cleft palate [67–69]. There have been no studies to substantiate these findings in humans. In addition, there are no studies discussing neonatal outcomes with *in utero* exposure of epinephrine. In an acute life-threatening situation, one may consider the use of epinephine in the parturient.

There are also no studies showing epinephrine secretion in human milk.

Diltiazem and other calcium channel blockers

Diltiazem is a calcium channel blocker. In acute settings, it is used to control ventricular rate in atrial fibrillation. It is also used to terminate supraventricular or reentrant tachycardias. Placental transfer of diltiazem has not specifically been investigated in humans. There are no studies conclusively linking diltiazem with human congenital abnormalities. One study of 78 women exposed to calcium channel blockers cites a slightly higher risk of congenital malformations [70]. Limb malformations were seen in two of the neonates. The authors note that these findings were likely not due to the calcium channel exposure. Animal studies have shown more significant association with limb abnormalities and fetal loss [71,72]. These findings have not been substantiated in humans. The use of diltiazem is considered compatible with pregnancy.

Data concerning diltiazem and breastfeeding are based on one lactating woman [73]. The reported milk to plasma ratio was 1.0. The American Academy of Pediatrics considers diltiazem compatible with breastfeeding [58].

Verapamil is a calcium channel blocking agent and is an alternative drug to terminate paroxysmal supraventricular tachycardia. It is used to control the ventricular response in atrial fibrillation, atrial flutter, or multifocal atrial tachycardia. The fetal to maternal drug concentration ratio is reported at 0.1–0.2 [74]. In the aforementioned study, the 25 neonates exposed to verapamil had no associated congenital abnormalities [67]. One case of unexplained fetal death has been associated with verapamil in the transplacental treatment of fetal supraventricular tachycardia [75]. Thus, verapamil can be used in pregnancy.

There have been no reports of fetal effects secondary to the transfer of drug through human milk. It is considered safe for breastfeeding [31].

Ibutilide

Ibutilde has been used for the treatment of supraventricular tachycardias like atrial fibrillation and atrial flutter. It works by prolonging the cardiac action potential. Little is known about the use of ibutilide in pregnancy. One review suggests that class III antiarrhythmic drugs like ibutilide have similar teratogenic effects as phenytoin including distal digital defects and orofacial clefts [76]. These data and others show this effect in animal studies [77]. To date, there are no human studies on ibutilide concerning its potential effects on the human fetus and lactation. In an ICU setting with few alternative treatments, one may consider the use of ibutilide in the parturient.

Lidocaine

Lidocaine has multiple uses in medicine. In the cardiovascular realm, it is used to treat cardiac arrest secondary to ventricular fibrillation or flutter. It is a class I antiarrhythmic that blocks sodium channels. The placental transfer of lidocaine has been reported with fetal to maternal concentration ratios of 50% [78,79]. There are no human studies reporting specific congenital abnormalities connected with lidocaine. Data from the Collaborative Perinatal Project shows no increase of congenital abnormalities with *in utero* exposure to lidocaine [60].

Small amounts of lidocaine have been shown to be excreted in human breast milk. Therefore, lidocaine is unlikely to cause any untoward effects on the neonate and may be used during breastfeeding [80].

Procainamide

Procainamide is a class I antiarrhythmic drug which works by blocking sodium channels. It is used in a wide variety of arrhythmias including recurrent ventricular tachycardia and fibrillation. It is also used to treat fetal tachycardias *in utero* [81,82]. There are no studies reporting any human teratogenicity.

In addition, little procainamide is secreted in human milk, making it safe for breastfeeding [83].

Other cardiovascular drugs

Inotropes

Digoxin

Digoxin is a digitalis glycoside that is used to slow the ventricular response in atrial fibrillation and atrial flutter. It is used in a wide variety of maternal and fetal arrhythmias. The placental transfer of digoxin has been well documented [84]. Multiple studies have shown that there are no congenital malformations associated with digoxin exposure in any trimester [85,86]. Digoxin is transferred to human milk at 2–4% of the maternal dose [57].

There have been no adverse fetal effects published from digoxin through maternal milk. It is considered safe in breastfeeding [31].

Dopamine

Dopamine is a natural postganglionic sympathetic transmitter in renal vessels. As a catecholamine, it increases cardiac contractility for the treatment of congestive heart failure and increases arterial pressure in treatment of shock. There are no studies that link dopamine with human teratogenesis. There are cases of the treatment of acute renal failure during pregnancy using dopamine. There are no reported adverse effects on the fetus related to its use [87,88].

Dopaminergic agents have been used to suppress lactation. Yet, there are no studies investigating dopamine and its effects on breastfed babies.

Dobutamine

Dobutamine is a synthetic catecholamine that affects α_1- and β_1-receptors. It is commonly used to treat heart failure and shock to increase cardiac output with a decrease in ventricular filling pressure. There are no studies specifically investigating the use of dobutamine in pregnancy. There are no studies linking human teratogenesis with dobutamine. One report describes a parturient who underwent bypass surgery and was treated with dobutamine. No adverse fetal effects were noted [89].

There are no studies describing the effect of dobutamine during breastfeeding.

Isoproterinol

Isoproterinol is a β-receptor agonist. It has positive chronotropic and inotropic effects. It is a vasodilator and bronchodilator. Isoproterinol or isoprenaline is used in asthma and heart failure. It has also been investigated for the *in utero* treatment of fetal complete heart block [90]. There are no studies that link isoproterinol with human teratogenesis. Caution should be used in pre-eclamptic patients as it has a more pronounced chronotropic effect in this particular population [91].

There are no studies evaluating breastfeeding with isoproterinol.

Milrinone and amrinone

Milrinone and amrinone are newer inotropic phosphodiesterase III inhibitors used in acute heart failure and cardiogenic shock. There are no studies evaluating congenital malformations or breastfeeding in milrinone- or amrinone-exposed human fetuses.

Diuretics

Furosemide

Furosemide is a loop diuretic used in congestive heart failure during pregnancy. It has also been investigated as a diuretic in postpartum pre-eclamptic hypertension [92]. It also been shown to increase fetal urine production and has been used to evaluate fetal hydronephrosis [93]. The placental transfer of furosemide is well documented [94]. Furosemide does bind to fetal albumin and slightly increases free bilirubin thereby theoretically increasing the risk of kernicterus [95], although there have been no studies verifying an increased risk of kernicterus in furosemide-exposed fetuses. Neonatal sensorineural hearing loss has been associated with furosemide exposure in one study [96], but this association has not been substantiated in a more recent study [97]. These negative effects of furosemide were found in small studies. Also, there are no human studies correlating human congenital malformations to furosemide. Given this information, furosemide is considered safe for use in pregnancy.

It is excreted in human milk. No studies have reported untoward effects of furosemide transmitted through breastfeeding.

Hydrochlorothiazide

Hydrochlorothiazide (HCTZ) is a thiazide diuretic used to treat hypertension. It is known to cross the placenta [98]. HCTZ has been correlated with neonatal thrombocytopenia [99]. Yet there are no recent studies confirming this report. In addition, it has been shown to induce maternal hyperglycemia with resultant neonatal hypoglycemia [100]. Glucose levels should be checked in neonates exposed to hydrochlorothiazide. One study suggests that HCTZ decreases placental perfusion. Consequently, it is suggested that pregnant women chronically on HCTZ may continue its use, but HCTZ should not be initiated in the middle of pregnancy [101]. For the treatment of hypertension, there are other first-line agents that may be used instead of HCTZ. HCTZ may also be considered a second-line agent for fluid overload diuresis. There is no data showing that HCTZ should be contraindicated in pregnancy.

HCTZ is excreted in small amounts in human milk. No studies have reported untoward effects of HCTZ transmitted through breastfeeding. It has been associated with decreased milk production. Therefore, it has been suggested that it should be not be used in the first month of breastfeeding [102].

Vasodilators

Hydralazine

Hydralazine is a direct-acting vasodilator. It often used to control blood pressure in cases of gestational hypertension or pre-eclampsia. Hydralazine crosses the placenta with cord blood drug concentrations higher than maternal serum concentrations [103]. There are no studies linking human congenital abnormalities with *in utero* exposure. Case reports indicate that the use of hydralazine has been associated with abnormal heart tracings [104], fetal premature atrial contractions [105], and neonatal thrombocytopenia [106]. Yet, these case reports do cause sufficient concern to restrict the use of hydralazine in pregnancy.

Hydralazine is transferred to breast milk in small amounts [93]. No studies have reported untoward neonatal effects of hydralazine transmitted through breastfeeding.

Enalapril and other angiotensin converting enzyme inhibitors

Enalapril is an angiotensin-converting enzyme (ACE) inhibitor used for the treatment of hypertension and congestive heart failure. Enalapril and other ACE inhibitors are known to cross the placenta. When used in the second and third trimesters, ACE inhibitors are correlated with decreased fetal urine production, hypotension and fetal death [107,108]. There is a small risk of congenital malformations. There are multiple cases reporting the underdevelopment of skull bones and other skeletal abnormalities. In addition, IUGR and pulmonary hypoplasia have been associated with *in utero* exposure to ACE inhibitors [109]. Because of these findings, ACE inhibitor use in pregnancy is contraindicated. A study of 209 infants with first-trimester only exposure to ACE inhibitors showed an increased risk of major congenital malformations (RR = 2.71, 95% CI 1.72–4.27), primarily of the cardiovascular and central nervous systems, when compared to those infants with no exposure to antihypertensive agents [110].

Enalapril and other ACE inhibitors are secreted in small amounts in breast milk. They are considered compatible with breastfeeding by the American Academy of Pediatrics [31].

Losartan and other angiotensin receptor blockers

Losartan is an angiotensin receptor blocker also used in the treatment of heart failure and hypertension. Losartan and other ARBs have a similar fetal side-effect profile in the second and third trimester as ACE inhibitors. Because of skeletal abnormalities, effects on the fetal renal system and associated fetal death, ARBs are contraindicated in pregnancy [111]. There are no human studies evaluating ARBs and lactation.

Labetalol and other β-blockers

Labetalol has both α- and β-receptor blocking activity. During pregnancy, it is used for the treatment of mild to severe hypertension. Labetalol crosses the placenta. The pharmacokinetics of oral labetalol in hypertensive pregnant women have been studied. Labetalol has rapid absorption with peak concentrations at 20 minutes after ingestion. The half-life is 1.7 hours. It has also been found at 50% of the maternal concentration in cord blood [112]. There are no studies linking labetalol to human congenital malformations. The reports of adverse fetal or neonatal affects of labetalol have been controversial. There are reports that labetalol is associated with intrauterine growth restriction, bradycardia, or hypoglycemia; yet, there are other studies that refute these findings [113,114]. According to a recent Cochrane review, the effectiveness of β-blockers in general were evaluated in the treatment of mild to moderate hypertension during pregnancy. When compared to placebo, β-blockers decrease the risk of severe hypertension and the need for additional antihypertensives. When labetalol was analyzed for maternal and fetal outcomes, including cesarian section rates, Apgar scores, and fetal deaths, in comparison to hydralazine, labetalol faired better than or the same as hydralazine [103]. Given the data, labetalol is an acceptable first-line drug to use for blood pressure control during pregnancy.

Labetalol is transferred in human milk in small concentrations and is considered compatible with breastfeeding [31].

Nitroglycerin

Nitroglycerin is a smooth muscle relaxant and a potent vasodilator. It is used in the treatment of angina and severe hypertension. It has previously been used as a uterine relaxant for multiple indications including external version and preterm contractions [115,116]. The successful use of nitroglycerin treatment of myocardial infarction during pregnancy has also been reported [117]. There are no studies linking nitroglycerin to human teratogenesis. Fetal heart rate abnormalities including fetal heart decelerations have been reported with the use of nitroglycerin [118]. Yet these findings should not restrict the use of nitroglycerin in pregnancy. Given its short duration of action and its use in life-threatening conditions, a clinician should consider the use of nitroglycerin during these conditions in pregnancy safe.

There are no studies investigating the use of nitroglycerin during breastfeeding.

Nitroprusside

Nitroprusside is a powerful vasodilator used to treat hypertensive emergencies and heart failure. Its most important side effects are those caused by the accumulation of cyanide, namely metabolic acidosis, arrhythmias, hypotension, and death. There are no studies linking human teratogenesis with nitroprusside. The use of nitroprusside during pregnancy has been reported for aneurysm surgery and severe pre-eclampsia. Transient fetal bradycardia was the only side effect reported. In addition, cyanide levels in fetal cord blood have not shown toxic levels [119,120]. In a setting of no alternative treatments and an acute life-threatening situation, one may consider the use of nitroprusside in the parturient as long as cyanide levels are monitored appropriately.

There are no studies investigating the use of nitroprusside during breastfeeding.

Anticoagulation

Warfarin and coumarin derivatives

Warfarin and coumarin derivatives are used for oral anticoagulation. They inhibit the synthesis of vitamin K dependent clotting factors II, VII, IX, and X. Warfarin is a class D drug with known patterns of embryopathy. The clinical picture of fetal warfarin syndrome includes nasal hypoplasia, epiphyseal stippling, hypoplasia of nails and fingers, low birth weight, mental retardation, and seizures. The critical time for warfarin teratogenicity is between 6 and 9 weeks [121]. In a study evaluating the exposure of coumarin derivatives throughout pregnancy, the authors report an increased risk of spontaneous abortions and stillbirth [122]. Neurological delay related to intracranial hemorrhage has also been associated with *in utero* warfarin exposure. Only 70% of exposed pregnancies are expected to have a normal infant [31]. Warfarin *in utero* exposure should be avoided during pregnancy. In cases where maternal mortality is higher, such as parturients with mechanical heart valves, the use of warfarin may be considered. In a large literature review of anticoagulation for parturients with mechanical heart valves, the authors evaluated three main regimens: (i) warfarin only; (ii) heparin during the first trimester then warfarin; and (iii) heparin only. The data show that maternal death rates increase between regimens 1, 2, and 3 (1.8%, 4.2%, and 15.0%, respectively). In addition, the rate of embryopathy is halved if heparin is used in the first trimester (3.4%) and the rate is zero if no warfarin is used at all [123]. These data are based on the best available studies which lack prospective trials. Based on these data, the American College of Chest Physicians recommends heparin in the first trimester then warfarin or aggressive dose heparinoids throughout the pregnancy [124]. In the particular subgroup of women with high risk mechanical valves, the use of warfarin during pregnancy is very likely warranted.

The studies regarding breast milk transfer have not shown any transfer of the drug to human milk [125]. It is considered safe for breastfeeding.

Heparins

Heparin is a large, heterogenous sulfated glycosaminoglycan with a molecular weight ranging between 5000 and 30 000 Da. It activates antithrombin III to inhibit clotting factors most notably factor Xa. Because of its large molecular weight, heparin does not cross the placenta, nor is it transferred to breast milk [126]. The same has been found in low molecular weight heparins. Therefore, there is no potential for teratogenicity due to heparins alone. It considered safe for use in pregnancy during any gestational age [127]. There have been no studies linking heparin with congenital defects. Known side effects related to heparin are osteoporosis and heparin-induced thrombocytopenia. Heparin-induced thrombocytopenia is an immune mediated disorder that in high-risk populations has an incidence of 3–5%. The risk of HIT is 10 times higher with the use of unfractionated heparin versus low molecular weight heparin. With regard to use in pregnant patients, the incidence of HIT is 0.9%. [128] In general, routine platelet monitoring is not recommended in pregnant patients unless they are at high risk for HIT as defined by The Seventh ACCP Conference on Antithrombotic and Thrombolytic Therapy [129]. Thirty per cent of patients on long-term heparin therapy have decreased bone density leading to osteopenia [130]. Overall, the risk of osteopenia is low in pregnant patients because the majority of patients are on prophylactic doses of UFH or LMWH. There are data to show that this risk of osteoporosis may be lower with use of LMWH [112].

Thrombolytic therapy

Historically, the use of thrombolytic therapy has been considered relatively contraindicated during pregnancy. Risks include abruption, abortion, uterine bleeding, and postpartum hemorrhage. There are no large controlled trials evaluating the use of thrombolytics during pregnancy. There are only case series and case reports of their use with different indications. More than 200 pregnancies have been reported with an overall maternal mortality of 1%, fetal loss rate of 6%, and preterm delivery incidence of 6% [131]. Most reported cases have involved streptokinase and urokinase. The relative safety of those thrombolytics have led authors to consider tissue plasminogen activator safe in pregnancy. In a series of 172 pregnant patients exposed to thrombolytics, all infants were found to be normal on initial exams [132]. There are no studies evaluating tissue plasminogen activator for human teratogenesis and use during pregnancy. Streptokinase has been shown to cross the placenta in very small amounts [133]. There are no studies linking streptokinase with congenital malformations.

Use during breastfeeding has not been specifically evaluated with thrombolytics. It is not known if these agents cross into breast milk.

Endocrinologic emergencies

Endocrinologic emergencies are commonly seen in the ICU setting. Some of the important emergencies include diabetic ketoacidosis, Addisonian crisis, myxedema coma, and thyroid storm. Although altogether less common than cardiopulmonary reasons for admission to the ICU, they still represent significant patient morbidity and mortality [134]. This section will review some of the common drugs involved in the treatment of these emergencies.

Insulin

Insulin is pancreatic peptide that is used in the treatment of hyperglycemia and diabetes. It is a key element in the treatment of diabetic ketoacidosis. There are no studies linking the use of insulin specifically to human congenital malformations. Many studies are confounded by rate of malformations related to uncontrolled diabetes itself [135].

Insulin does not cross the placenta and is not transmitted in the milk. It is considered safe for pregnancy and breastfeeding [33].

Corticosteroids: hydrocortisone and dexamethasone

Stress doses of hydrocortisone are used to treat emergencies like Addisonian crisis and myxedema coma [127]. Corticosteroids like hydrocortisone and dexamethasone are known to cross the placenta and are used for fetal lung maturity induction [136]. Epidemiologic studies have shown a correlation between use of corticosteroids and oral clefting with odds ratios between 3 and 5 [137] . Repeat doses of corticosteroids for fetal lung maturity have been correlated with poor fetal growth [138]. These negative effects are seen in chronic administrations. Yet, the use of corticosteroids should not be restricted in pregnancy. The total amount of corticosteroids used for Addisonian crisis treatment has not been specifically studied for congenital malformations. An acute use of corticosteroids,does not require prolonged fetal evaluation. If corticosteroids are used chronically, one may consider an ultrasound to evaluate appropriate growth and anomalies.

Small of amounts of corticosteroids have been found in human milk, but they are considered compatible with breastfeeding [31].

Thyroxine

Intravenous thyroxine can be used to reverse hypothyroidism in myxedema coma. Thyroxine is known to cross the placenta and has been used to treat fetal hypothyroidism and goiter [139]. The Collaborative Perinatal Project has not demonstrated any significant birth defect association with the use of thyroxine during any trimester [140].

Thyroxine is known to be transmitted through human milk in small doses and is considered safe for breastfeeding [141].

Antithyroid medications: PTU and methimazole

Propylthiouracil is used to treat hyperthyroidism with thyroid storm. It is considered the drug of choice for the treatment of hyperthyroidism in pregnancy in the USA [142]. It is known to cross the placenta and can cause transient neonatal hypothyroidism or fetal goiter [143]. There are no studies correlating PTU to congenital malformations. Long-term follow-up on children who had been exposed to PTU *in utero* has shown no decrease in motor or intellectual function [144]. For the treatment of thyroid storm and hyperthyroism, PTU is considered safe in pregnancy [31].

PTU is excreted in the human milk in small amounts with no known neonatal effects [145]. It is considered safe for breastfeeding.

Methimazole is another antithyroid medication that is used in the treatment of thyroid storm. Three times more methimazole is known to cross the placenta than PTU [146]. The correlation of congenital malformations and methimazole exposure is controversial. There are some studies that suggest that exposure is correlated with aplasia cutis. Other studies do not show any increase in specific defects [147].

Methimazole is excreted in human milk in small amounts and is safe for breastfeeding [31].

Mannitol

Mannitol is an alcohol derived from glucose that is used to treat different manifestations of cerebral edema. There are no studies evaluating human congenital malformations and mannitol. In addition, there are no studies evaluating mannitol and breastfeeding.

Conclusion

As with any treatment in medicine, a consideration of therapeutic risks and benefits to the patient is important. This consideration is further complicated in pregnant patients by altered physiology. In addition, those caring for pregnant patients also must invariably care for another patient, the fetus. Due to the paucity of data of therapeutics in pregnancy, there are few medications such as ACE inhibitors and angiotensin receptor blockers that are clearly contraindicated in pregnancy. This therapeutic dilemma forces the clinician to rely on judgement of the clinical situation with an evaluation of the best possible data. In the realm of the ICU where life-threatening conditions are commonplace, it is important to remember that when a mother is not optimally treated for an acute life-threatening condition, the fetus will be placed at increased risk, as well. In cases where acuity is less of an issue, then consideration of fetal morbidities should become of paramount importance.

References

1 Martin SR, Foley MR. Intensive care in obstetrics: qn evidence-based review. *Am J Obstet Gynecol* 2006; 195: 673–689.
2 Baron TH, Ramirez B, Richter JE. Gastrointestinal motility disorders during pregnancy. *Ann Intern Med* 1993; 118: 366–375.
3 Mattison DR. Physiologic variations in pharmacokinetics during pregnancy. In: *Drug and Chemical Action in Pregnancy: Pharmacologic and Toxicologic Principles*. New York: Thieme-Stratton, 1984: 74–86.
4 Little BB. Pharmacokinetics during pregnancy: evidence-based maternal dose formulation. *Obstet Gynecol* 1999; 93: 858–868.
5 Dunlop W. Serial changes in renal haemodynamic during pregnancy. *Br J Obstet Gynaecol* 1981; 8: 1–9.
6 Mattingly JE, Alessio JD, Ramanathan J. Effects of obstetric analgesic and anesthetics on the neonate. *Pediatr Drugs* 2003; 5: 615–627.

7 Rhoney DH, Murry KR. National survey of the use of sedating drugs, neuromuscular blocking agents, and reversal agents in the intensive care unit. *J Intensive Care Med* 2003; 18: 139–145.

8 Mehta S, Burry L, Fischer S, et al., for the Canadian Critical Care Trials Group. Canadian survey of the use of sedatives, analgesics, and neuromuscular blocking agents in critically ill patients. *Crit Care Med* 2006; 34: 374–380.

9 Soliman HM, Melot C, Vincent JL. Sedative and analgesic practice in the intensive care unit: the results of a European survey. *Br J Anaesth* 2001; 87: 186–192.

10 Kanto J, Aaltonen L, Erkkola R, Aarimaa L. Pharmacokinetics and sedative effect of midazolam in connection with cesarean section performed under epidural analgesia. *Acta Anaesthesiol Scand* 1984; 28: 116–118.

11 Bach V, Carl P, Ravlo O, et al. A randomized comparison between midazolam and thiopental for elective cesarean section anesthesia. III. Placental transfer and elimination in neonates. *Anesth Analg* 1989; 68: 238–242.

12 Wilson CM, Dundee JW, Moore J, et al. A comparison of the early pharmacokinetics of midazolam in pregnant and nonpregnant women. *Anaesthesia* 1987; 42: 1057–1062.

13 Whitelaw AGL, Cummings AJ, McFadyen IR. Effect of maternal lorazepam on the neonate. *Br J Anaesth* 1979; 51: 971–978.

14 McBride RJ, Dundee JW, Moore J, Toner W, Howard PJ. A study of the plasma concentrations of lorazepam in mother and neonate. *Br J Anaesth* 1979; 51: 971–978.

15 Ornoy A, Arnon J, Shechtman S, Moerman, L, Lukashova I. Is benzodiazepine use during pregnancy really teratogenic? *Reprod Toxicol* 1998; 12: 511–515.

16 Bonnot O, Vollset SE, Godet PF, d'Amato T, Dalery J, Robert E. In utero exposure to benzodiazepine. Is there a risk of anal atresia with lorazepam? *Encephale* 2003; 29: 553–559.

17 Summerfield RJ, Nielsen MS. Excretion of lorazepam into breast milk. *Br J Anaesth* 1985; 57: 1042–1043.

18 Sanchez-Alcaraz A, Quintana MB, Laguarda M. Placental transfer and neonatal effects of propofol in caesarean section. *J Clin Pharm Ther* 1998; 23: 19–23.

19 Bacon RC, Razis PA The effect of propofol sedation in pregnancy on neonatal condition. *Anaesthesia* 1994; 49: 1058–1060.

20 Celleno D, Capogna G, Tomassetti M, Costantino P, di Feo G, Nisini R. Neurobehavioural effects of propofol on the neonate following elective caesarean section. *Br J Anaesth* 1989; 62: 649–654.

21 Aaltonen M, Kanto J, Rosenberg P. Comparison of propofol and thiopentone for induction of anaesthesia for elective caesarian section. *Anaesthesia* 1989; 44: 758–762.

22 Abboud TK, Zhu J, Richardson M, Peres da Silva E, Donovan M. Intravenous propofol vs thiamylal-isoflurane for caesarean section, comparative maternal and neonatal effects. *Acta Anaesthesiol Scand* 1995; 39: 205–209.

23 Siafaka I, Vadalouca A, Gatziou B, Petropoulos G, Salamalekis E. Comparative study of propofol and thiopental as induction agents for elective caesarean section. *Exp Obstet Gynecol* 1992; 19: 93–96.

24 Dailland P, Cockshott ID, Lirzin JD. Intravenous propofol during cesarean section: placental transfer, concentrations in breast milk, and neonatal effects. *Anesthesiology* 1989; 71: 827–834.

25 Kudo S, Ishizaki T. Pharmacokinetics of haloperidol: an update. *Clin Pharmacokinet* 1999; 37: 435–456.

26 Baldessarini RJ. Drugs and the treatment of psychiatric disorders In: Gilman AG et al., eds. *Goodman and Gilman's The Pharmacological Basis of Therapeutics*, 8th edn. New York: Macmillan, 1990: 384.

27 Sexson WR, Barak Y. Withdrawal emergent syndrome in an infant associated with maternal haloperidol therapy. *J Perinatol* 1989; 9: 170–172.

28 Van Waes A, van de Velde E. Safety evaluation of haloperidol in the treatment of hyperemesis gravidarum. *J Clin Pharmacol* 1969; 9: 224–227.

29 Yoshida K, Smith B, Craggs M, Kumar R. Neuroleptic drugs in breast-milk: a study of pharmacokinetics and of possible adverse effects in breast-fed infants. *Psychol Med* 1998; 28: 81–91.

30 Whalley LJ, Blain PG, Prime JK. Haloperidol secreted in breast milk. *BMJ* 1981; 282: 1746–1747.

31 Committee on Drugs, American Academy of Pediatrics. The transfer of drugs and other chemicals into human breast milk. *Pediatrics* 2001; 108: 776–789.

32 Baraka A, Noueihid R, Hajj S. Intrathecal injection of morphine for obstetric analgesia. *Anesthesiology* 1981; 54: 136–140.

33 Briggs GG, Freeman RK, Yaffe SJ. *Drugs in Pregnancy and Lactation*, 6th edn. Philadelphia: Lippincott Williams and Wilkins, 2002.

34 Committee on Drugs, American Academy of Pediatrics. The transfer of drugs and other chemicals into human milk. *Pediatrics* 1994; 93: 137–150.

35 Robieux I, Koren G, Vandenbergh H, Schneiderman J. Morphine excretion in breast milk and resultant exposure of a nursing infant. *J Toxicol Clin Toxicol* 1990; 28: 365–370.

36 Nitsun M, Szokol JW, Saleh J, et al. Pharmacokinetics of midazolam, propofol, and fentanyl transfer to human breast milk. *Clin Pharmacol Ther* 1980; 28: 106–114.

37 Bader AM, Fragneto R, Terui K, Arthur GR, Loferski B, Datta S. Maternal and neonatal fentanyl and bupivacaine concentrations after eipdural infusion during labor. *Anesth Analg* 1995; 81: 829–832.

38 Rayburn W, Rathke A, Leuschen MP, Chleborad J, Weidner W. Fentanyl citrate analgesia during labor. *Am J Obstet Gynecol* 1989; 161: 202–206.

39 Lindemann R. Respiratory muscle rigidity in a preterm infant after use of fentanyl during Caesarian section. *Eur J Pediatr* 1998; 157: 1012–1013.

40 Seeds JW, Corke BC, Spielman FJ. Prevention of fetal movement during invasive procedures with pancuronium bromide. *Am J Obstet Gynecol* 1986; 15: 818–819.

41 Moise KJ Jr, Deter RL, Kirshon B, Adam K, Patton DE, Carpenter RJ Jr. Intravenous pancuronium bromide for fetal neuromuscular blockade during intrauterine transfusion for red-cell alloimmunization. *Obstet Gynecol* 1989; 74: 905–908.

42 Guay J, Grenier Y, Varin F. Clinical pharmacokinetics of neuromuscular relaxants in pregnancy. *Clin Pharmacokinet* 1998; 34: 483–496.

43 Pielet BW, Socol ML, MacGregor SN, Dooley SL, Minogue J. Fetal heart rate changes after fetal intravascular treatment with pancuronium bromide. *Am J Obstet Gynecol* 1988; 159: 640–643.

44 Spencer JA, Ryan G, Ronderos-Dumit D, Nicolini U, Rodeck CH. The effect of neuromuscular blockade on human fetal heart rate and its variation. *Br J Obstet Gynaecol* 1994; 101: 121–124.

45 Daily PA, Fisher DM, Shnider SM. Pharmacokinetics, placental transfer, and neonatal effects of vecuronium and pancuronium

administered during cesarean section. *Anesthesiology* 1984; 60: 569–574.

46 Daffos F, Forestier F, MacAleese J, et al. Fetal curarization for prenatal magnetic resonance imaging. *Prenat Diagn* 1988; 8: 312–314.

47 Watson WJ, Atchison SR, Harlass FE. Comparison of pancuronium and vecuronium for fetal neuromuscular blockade during invasive procedures. *J Matern Fetal Med* 1996; 5: 151–154.

48 De Sweit M. Cardiac disease In: Lewis G, Drife J, eds. *Why Mothers Die, 1997–1999. The Confidential Enquiries into Maternal Deaths in the United Kingdom.* London: Royal College of Obstetricians and Gynaecologists, 2001: 153–164.

49 National Center for Health Statistics. *Deaths: Final Data for 2004.* Available at: www.cdc.gov/nchs/products/pubs/pubd/hestats/finaldeaths04/finaldeaths04.htm.

50 Elkayam U, Goodwin TM. Adenosine therapy for supraventricular tachycardia during pregnancy. *Am J Cardiol* 1995; 75: 521–523.

51 Afridi I, Moise KJ Jr, Rokey R. Termination of supraventricular tachycardia with intravenous adenosine in a pregnant woman with Wolff-Parkinson-White syndrome. *Obstet Gynecol* 1992; 80: 481–483.

52 Leffler S, Johnson DR. Adenosine use in pregnancy: lack of effect on fetal heart rate. *Am J Emerg Med* 1992; 10: 548–549.

53 Dunn JS Jr, Brost BC. Fetal bradycardia after IV adenosine for maternal PSVT. *Am J Emerg Med* 2000; 18: 234–235.

54 Freedman MD, Somberg JC. Pharmacology and pharmacokinetics of amiodarone. *J Clin Pharmacol* 1991; 31: 1061–1069.

55 Plomp TA, Vulsma T, de Vijlder JJM. Use of amiodarone during pregnancy. *Eur J Obstet Gynecol Reprod Biol* 1992; 43: 201–207.

56 Magee LA, Downar E, Sermer M, et al. Pregnancy outcome after gestational exposure to amiodarone in Canada. *Am J Obstet Gynecol* 1995; 172: 1307–1311.

57 Lomenick JP, Jackson WA, Backeljauw PF. Amiodarone-induced neonatal hypothyroidism: a unique form of transient early-onset hypothyroidism. *J Perinatol* 2004; 24: 397–399.

58 Strasburger JF, Cuneo BF, Michon MM, et al. Amiodarone therapy for drug-refractory fetal tachycardia. *Circulation* 2004; 109(3): 375–379.

59 WHO Working Group, Bennet PN, ed. *Drugs and Human Lactation.* Amsterdam: Elsevier, 1988.

60 Committee on Drugs, American Academy of Pediatrics. The transfer of drugs and other chemicals into human breast milk. *Pediatrics* 2001; 108: 776–789.

61 Kanto J, Virtanen R, Iisalo E, Maenpaa K, Liukko P. Placental transfer and pharmacokinetics of atropine after a single maternal intravenous and intramuscular administration. *Acta Anaesthesiol Scand* 1981; 25: 85–88.

62 Heinonen OP, Slone D, Shapiro S, eds. *Birth Defects and Drugs in Pregnancy.* Littleton, MA: Publishing Sciences Group, 1977: 346–347.

63 Rosa F. Personal communication, 1993. Cited in: Briggs GG, Freeman RK, Yaffe SJ. *Drugs in Pregnancy and Lactation: A Reference Guide to Fetal and Neonatal Risk*, 6th edn. Philadelphia: Lippincott Williams and Wilkins, 2002: 111.

64 Roodenburg PJ, Wladimiroff JW, van Weering HK. Effect of maternal intravenous administration of atropine (0.5mg) on fetal breathing and heart pattern. *Contrib Gynecol Obstet* 1979; 6: 92–97.

65 Czeizel AE, Toth M. Birth weight, gestational age and medications during pregnancy. *Int J Gynaecol Obstet* 1998; 60: 245–249.

66 Heinonen OP, Slone D, Shapiro S, eds. *Birth Defects and Drugs in Pregnancy.* Littleton, MA: Publishing Sciences Group, 1977: 439.

67 Adamsons K, Mueller-Heubach E, Myers RE. Production of fetal asphyxia in the rhesus monkey by administration of catecholamines to the mother. *Am J Obstet Gynecol* 1971; 109: 248–262.

68 Hodach RJ, Gilbert EF, Fallon JF. Aortic arch anomalies associated with administration of epinephrine in chick embryos. *Teratology* 1974; 9: 203–210.

69 Loevy H, Roth BF. Induced cleft palate development in mice: comparison between the effect of epinephrine and cortisone. *Anat Rec* 1968; 160: 386.

70 Magee LA, Schick B, Donnenfeld AE, et al. The safety of calcium channel blockers in human pregnancy: a prospective, multicenter cohort study. *Am J Obstet Gynecol* 1996; 174: 823–828.

71 Scott WJ Jr, Resnick E, Hummler H. Cardiovascular alterations in rat fetuses exposed to calcium channel blockers. *Reprod Toxicol* 1997; 11(2/3): 207–214.

72 Ariyuki F. Effects of diltiazem hydrochloride on embryonic development: species differences in the susceptibility and stage specificity in mice, rats, and rabbits. *Okajimas Folia Anat Jpn* 1975; 52: 103–117.

73 Okada M, Inoue H, Nakamura Y, Kishimoto M. Excretion of diltiazem in human milk. *N Engl J Med* 1985; 312: 992–993.

74 Ito S. Transplacental treatment of fetal tachycardia: implications of drug transporting proteins in placenta. *Semin Perinatol* 2001; 25: 196–201.

75 Owen J, Colvin EV, Davis RO. Fetal death after successful conversion of fetal supraventricular tachycardia with digoxin and verapamil. *Am J Obstet Gynecol* 1988; 158: 1169–1170.

76 Danielsson BR, Skold AC, Azarbayjani F. Class III antiarrhythmics and phenytoin: teratogenicity due to embryonic cardiac dysrhythmia and reoxygenation damage. *Curr Pharm Des* 2001; 7: 787–802.

77 Marks TA, Terry R. Developmental toxicity of ibutilide fumarate in rats after oral administration. *Teratology* 1996; 54: 157–164.

78 Cavalli R, Lanchote VL, Duarte G, et al. Pharmacokinetics and transplacental transfer of lidocaine and its metabolite for perineal analgesic assistance to pregnant women. *Eur J Clin Pharmacol* 2004; 60: 569–574.

79 Johnson RF, Herman N, Arney TL, et al. Transfer of lidocaine across the dual perfused human placental cotyledon. *Int J Obstet Anesth* 1999; 8: 17–23.

80 Ortega D, Viviand X, Lorec AM, Gamerre M, Martin C, Bruguerolle B. Excretion of lidocaine and bupivacaine in breast milk following epidural anesthesia for cesarean delivery. *Acta Anaesthesiol Scand* 1999; 43: 394–397.

81 Hallak M, Neerhof MG, Perry R, Nazir M, Huhta JC. Fetal supraventricular tachycardia and hydrops fetalis: combined intensive, direct, and transplacental therapy. *Obstet Gynecol* 1991; 78: 523–525.

82 Dumesic DA, Silverman NH, Tobias S, Golbus MS. Transplacental cardioversion of fetal supraventricular tachycardia with procainamide. *N Engl J Med* 1982; 307: 1128–1131.

83 Prittard III WB, Glazier H. Procainamide excretion in human milk. *J Pediatr* 1983; 102: 631–633.

84 Padeletti L, Porciani MC, Scimone G. Placental transfer of digoxin (beta-methyl-digoxin) in man. *Int J Clin Pharmacol Biopharm* 1979; 17: 82–83.

85 Jick H, Holmes LB, Hunter JR, Madsen S, Stergachis A. First-trimester drug use and congenital disorders *JAMA* 1981; 246: 343–346.

86 Laros RK. Pregnancy and heart valve prostheses. *Obstet Gynecol* 1970; 35: 241–247.

87 Nasu K, Yoshimatsu J, Anai T, Miyakawa I. Low-dose dopamine in treating acute renal failure caused by preeclampsia. *Gynecol Obstet Invest* 1996; 42: 140–141.

88 Mantel GD, Makin JD. Low dose dopamine in postpartum pre-eclamptic women with oliguria: a double-blind, placebo controlled, randomised trial. *Br J Obstet Gynaecol* 1997; 104: 1180–1183.

89 Strickland RA, Oliver WC Jr, Chantigian RC, Ney JA, Danielson GK. Anesthesia, cardiopulmonary bypass, and the pregnant patient. *Mayo Clin Proc* 1991; 66: 411–429.

90 Groves AM, Allan LD, Rosenthal E. Therapeutic trial of sympathomimetics in three cases of complete heart block in the fetus. *Circulation* 1995; 92: 3394–3396.

91 Leighton BL, Norris MC, DeSimone CA, Darby MJ, Menduke H. Pre-eclamptic and healthy term pregnant patients have different chronotropic responses to isoproterenol. *Anesthesiology* 1990; 72: 392–393.

92 Ascarelli MH, Johnson V, McCreary H, Cushman J, May WL, Martin JN Jr. Postpartum preeclampsia management with furosemide: a randomized clinical trial. *Obstet Gynecol* 2005; 105: 29–33.

93 Barrett RJ, Rayburn WF, Barr M Jr. Furosemide (Lasix) challenge test in assessing bilateral fetal hydronephrosis. *Am J Obstet Gynecol* 1983; 147: 846–847.

94 Beermann B, Groschinsky-Grind M, Fahraeus L, Lindstrom B. Placental transfer of furosemide. *Clin Pharmacol Ther* 1978; 24: 560–562.

95 Turmen T, Thom P, Louridas AT, LeMorvan P, Aranda JV. Protein binding and bilirubin displacing properties of bumetanide and furosemide. *J Clin Pharmacol* 1982; 22: 551–556.

96 Brown DR, Watchko JF, Sabo D. Neonatal sensorineural hearing loss associated with furosemide: a case-control study. *Dev Med Child Neurol* 1991; 33: 816–823.

97 Rais-Bahrami K, Majd M, Veszelovszky E, Short BL. Use of furosemide and hearing loss in neonatal intensive care survivors. *Am J Perinatol* 2004; 2: 329–332.

98 Garnet J. Placental transfer of hydrochlorothiazide. *Obstet Gynecol* 1963; 21: 123–125.

99 Rodriguez SU, Leikin SL, Hiller MC. Neonatal thrombocytopenia associated with ante-partum administration of thiazide drugs. *N Engl J Med* 1964; 270: 881–884.

100 Christianson R, Page EW. Diuretic drugs and pregnancy. *Obstet Gynecol* 1976; 48: 647–652.

101 Shoemaker ES, Gant NF, Madden JD, MacDonald PC. The effect of thiazide diuretics on placental function. *Tex Med* 1973; 69: 109–115.

102 Miller ME, Cohn RD, Burghart PH. Hydrochlorothiazide disposition in a mother and her breast-fed infant. *J Pediatr* 1982; 101: 789–791.

103 Liedholm H, Wahlin-Boll E, Hanson A, Ingemarsson I, Melander A. Transplacental passage and breast milk concentrations of hydralazine. *Eur J Clin Pharmacol* 1982; 21: 417–419.

104 Kirshon B, Wasserstrum N, Cotton DB. Should continuous hydralazine infusions be utilized in severe pregnancy-induced hypertension? *Am J Perinatol* 1991; 8: 206–208.

105 Lodeiro JG, Feinstein SJ, Lodeiro SB. Fetal premature atrial contractions associated with hydralazine. *Am J Obstet Gynecol* 1989; 160: 105–107.

106 Widerlov E, Karlman I, Storsater J. Hydralazine-induced neonatal thrombocytopenia. *N Engl J Med* 1980; 303: 1235–1238.

107 Tabacova S, Vega A, McCloskey C, Kimmel CA. Enalapril exposure during pregnancy: adverse developmental outcomes reported to FDA. *Teratology* 2000; 61: 520.

108 Burrows RF, Burrows EA. Assessing the teratogenic potential of angiotensin-converting enzyme inhibitors in pregnancy. *Aust NZ J Obstet Gynaecol* 1998; 38: 306–311.

109 Piper JM, Ray WA, Rosa FW. Pregnancy outcome following exposure to angiotensin-converting enzyme inhibitors. *Obstet Gynecol* 1992; 80: 429–432.

110 Cooper WO, Hernandez-Diaz S, Arbogast PG, et al. Major congenital malformations after first-trimester exposure to ACE inhibitors. *N Engl J Med* 2006; 354(23): 2443–2451.

111 Alwan S, Polifka JE, Friedman JM. Angiotensin II receptor antagonist treatment during pregnancy. *Birth Defects Res A Clin Mol Teratol* 2005; 73: 123–130.

112 Rogers RC, Sibai BM, Whybrew WD. Labetalol pharmacokinetics in pregnancy-induced hypertension. *Am J Obstet Gynecol* 1990; 162: 362–366.

113 Stevens TP, Guillet R. Use of glucagon to treat neonatal low-output congestive heart failure after maternal labetalol therapy. *J Pediatr* 1995; 127(1): 151–153.

114 Magee LA, Duley L. Oral beta-blockers for mild to moderate hypertension during pregnancy. *Cochrane Database Syst Rev* 2003; 3: CD002863.

115 Dufour P, Vinatier D, Puech F. The use of intravenous nitroglycerin for cervico-uterine relaxation: a review of the literature. *Arch Gynecol Obstet* 1997; 261: 1–7.

116 Lees C, Campbell S, Jauniaux E, et al. Arrest of preterm labour and prolongation of gestation with glyceryl trinitrate, a nitric oxide donor. *Lancet* 1994; 343: 1325–1326.

117 Sheikh AU, Harper MA. Myocardial infarction during pregnancy: management and outcome of two pregnancies. *Am J Obstet Gynecol* 1993; 169: 279–284.

118 Cotton DB, Longmire S, Jones MM, Dorman KF, Tessem J, Joyce TH 3rd. Cardiovascular alterations in severe pregnancy-induced hypertension: effects of intravenous nitroglycerin coupled with blood volume expansion. *Am J Obstet Gynecol* 1986; 154: 1053–1059.

119 Donchin Y, Amirav B, Sahar A, Yarkoni S. Sodium nitroprusside for aneurysm surgery in pregnancy. *Br J Anaesth* 1978; 50: 849–851.

120 Paull J. Clinical report on the use of sodium nitroprusside in severe pre-eclampsia. *Anaesth Intensive Care* 1975; 3: 72.

121 Jones KL, ed. *Smith's Recognizable Patterns of Human Malformation*, 5th edn. Philadelphia: WB Saunders, 1997: 568.

122 Salazar E, Zajarias A, Gutierrez N, Iturbe I. The problem of cardiac valve prosthesis, anticoagulants, and pregnancy. *Br J Obstet Gynaecol* 1984; 91: 1070–1073.

123 Chan WS, Anand S, Ginsberg JS. Anticoagulation of pregnant women with mechanical heart valves: a systematic review of the literature. *Arch Intern Med* 2000; 160: 191–196.

124 Salem DN, Stein PD, Al-Ahmad A, et al. Antithrombotic therapy in valvular heart disease – native and prosthetic: the Seventh ACCP Conference on Antithrombotic and Thrombolytic Therapy. *Chest* 2004; 126: 457S–482S.

125 De Swiet M, Lewis PJ. Excretion of anticoagulants in human milk. *N Engl J Med* 1997; 297: 1471.

126 Uszynski M. Heparin neutralization by an extract of the human placenta: measurements and the concept of placental barrier to heparin. *Gynecol Obstet Invest* 1992; 33: 205–208.

127 Bates SM, Greer IA, Hirsh J, Ginsberg JS. Use of antithrombotic agents during pregnancy: the Seventh ACCP Conference on Antithrombotic and Thrombolytic Therapy. *Chest* 2004; 126(3 Suppl): 627S–644S.

128 Arepally GM, Ortel TL. Clinical practice. Heparin-induced thrombocytopenia. *N Engl J Med* 2006; 355: 809–817.

129 Warkentin TE, Greinacher A. Heparin-induced thrombocytopenia: recognition, treatment, and prevention: the Seventh ACCP Conference on Antithrombotic and Thrombolytic Therapy. *Chest* 2004; 126: 311S–337S.

130 Hawkins D, Evans J. Minimising the risk of heparin-induced osteoporosis during pregnancy. *Expert Opin Drug Saf* 2005; 4: 583–590.

131 Ahern GS, Hadjiliadis D, Govert JA, Tapson VF. Massive pulmonary embolism during pregnancy successfully treated with recombinant tissue plasminogen activator. *Arch Intern Med* 2002; 162: 1221–1227.

132 Turrentine MA, Braems G, Ramirez MM. Use of thrombolytic for the treatment of thromboembolic disease during pregnancy. *Obstet Gynecol Surv* 1995; 50: 534–541.

133 Pfeifer GW. Distribution and placental transfer of 131-I streptokinase. *Aust Ann Med* 1970; 19: 17–18.

134 Goldberg PA, Inzucchi SE. Critical issues in endocrinology. *Clin Chest Med* 2003; 24: 583–606.

135 Khoury MJ. Clinical-epidemiologic assessment of pattern of birth defects associated with human teratogens: application to diabetic embryopathy. *Pediatrics* 1989; 84: 658–665.

136 Creasy RK, Resnik R, eds. *Maternal Fetal Medicine: Principles and Practice*, 5th edn. Philidelphia: Saunders, 2004.

137 Park-Wyllie L, Mazzotta P, Pastuszak A, et al. Birth defects after maternal exposure to corticosteroids: prospective cohort study and meta-analysis of epidemiological studies. *Teratology* 2000; 62: 385–392.

138 Wapner RJ, Sorokin Y, Thom EA, et al., National Institute of Child Health and Human Development Maternal Fetal Medicine Units Network. Single versus weekly courses of antenatal corticosteroids: evaluation of safety and efficacy. *Am J Obstet Gynecol* 2006; 195: 633–642.

139 Bruner JP, Dellinger EH. Antenatal diagnosis and treatment of fetal hypothyroidism. *Fetal Diagn Ther* 1997; 12: 200–204.

140 Heinonen OP, Slone D, Shapiro S, eds. *Birth Defects and Drugs in Pregnancy*. Littleton, MA: Publishing Sciences Group, 1977: 388–400.

141 Varma SK, Collins M, Row A, Haller WS, Varma K. Thyroxine, tri-iodothyronine, and reverse tri-iodothyronine concentrations in human milk. *J Pediatr* 1978; 93: 803–806.

142 American College of Obstetricians and Gynecologists. Thyroid disease in pregnancy. ACOG Technical Bulletin No. 181. *Obstet Gynecol* 1993; 43: 82–88.

143 Masiukiewicz US, Burrow GN. Hyperthyroidism in pregnancy: diagnosis and treatment. *Thyroid* 1999; 9: 647–652.

144 Burrow GN. Children exposed in utero to propylthiouracil. Subsequent intellectual and physical development. *Am J Dis Child* 1968; 116: 161–166.

145 Kampmann JP, Johansen K, Hansen JM, Helweg J. Propylthiouracil in human milk. *Lancet* 1980; 1: 736–738.

146 Marchant B, Brownlie BE, Hart DM, Horton PW, Alexander WD. The placental transfer of propylthiouracil, methimazole and carbimazole. *J Clin Endocrinol Metab* 1977; 45: 1187–1193.

147 Di Gianantonio E, Schaefer C, Mastroiacovo PP, et al. Adverse effects of prenatal methimazole exposure. *Teratology* 2001; 64: 262–266.

45 Anesthesia Considerations for the Critically Ill Parturient with Cardiac Disease

Shobana Chandrasekhar & Maya S. Suresh
Department of Anesthesiology, Baylor College of Medicine, Houston, TX, USA

Introduction and epidemiology

Cardiac disease, a leading cause of non-obstetric mortality in pregnancy, occurs in 1–3% of pregnancies and accounts for 10–15% of maternal mortality [1,2]. Even though the incidence of rheumatic heart disease is declining in developing countries, it still accounts for a majority of mortality in obstetric cases. The incidence of congenital heart disease in pregnant women is increasing in developed countries because of advances in the diagnosis and treatment of congenital heart defects in childhood.

Cardiovascular maternal morbidity and mortality during pregnancy correlate strongly with maternal functional status [1–3]. Women with NYHA class I and II (no or minor symptoms) tolerate pregnancy without major deterioration, whereas those with NYHA class III and IV during pregnancy are at risk for major morbidity resulting in mortality upwards of 50% [4]. Because of the physiologic changes in pregnancy, further deterioration in functional status in the range of 15–55% of symptomatic patients can be expected during pregnancy [2]. When a pregnant woman presents with onset of cardiorespiratory deterioration the main differential diagnoses include thromboembolism, cardiomyopathy, dysrhythmia, pre-eclampsia, hemorrhage, and sepsis. A less commonly considered differential is underlying heart disease, and this is something that should be excluded in all of these cases. Therefore the diagnosis of cardiac disease by history, physical exam, ECG, CXR, and echocardiogram is essential to obstetric and anesthetic management.

In the United Kingdom Report of the Confidential Enquiries into Maternal and Child Health (CEMACH; formerly Confidential Enquiries into Maternal Deaths (CEMD)), cardiac disease was the second commonest cause of maternal mortality. Significant and increasing numbers of deaths occur in women without previously known disease, either in those with risk factors or in those who develop conditions in the absence of risk factors [5].

Labor analgesic techniques and anesthetic management in the critically ill parturient are determined largely by the nature of the presenting illness. Issues dictating choice of anesthetic technique are the patient's ability to maintain her airway, coagulation status, intravascular volume, and requirements for ventilatory support and intensive care. Fetal well-being is an important issue in the antepartum period. Uteroplacental blood flow should be maintained and hypotension should be avoided. Maternal survival clearly takes priority. Anesthesia itself is associated with known hazards, and the risks of each technique must be balanced against the possible benefits to both mother and baby in the context of the presenting illness.

Physiologic changes of pregnancy relevant to the cardiorespiratory system

Pregnancy-induced alterations of the cardiovascular and respiratory systems are the result of both anatomic and functional changes. The cardiovascular changes that occur during pregnancy improve oxygenation and flow of nutrition to the fetus. Cardiac output increases up to 50% in the first half of pregnancy due to increased stroke volume, and later in the pregnancy due to increased heart rate. Hypotension and decreased cardiac output can occur due to inferior vena cava compression by the enlarged uterus. Peripheral vascular resistance is decreased due to smooth muscle relaxation caused by increased circulating progesterone levels. Systolic murmurs are a normal occurrence due to increased blood flow. However, a diastolic murmur is not a normal finding during pregnancy. During labor, cardiac output increases an additional 45% above that found in late pregnancy. Mean arterial pressure increases 10 mmHg during each contraction. Immediately after delivery, cardiac output increases by as much as 80% due to autotransfusion. The autotransfusion results from an increase in preload secondary to release of vena caval obstruction by the enlarged uterus, and from autotransfusion of the blood during

Critical Care Obstetrics, 5th edition. Edited by M. Belfort, G. Saade, M. Foley, J. Phelan and G. Dildy.

contraction and involution of the uterus. Simultaneously, systemic vascular resistance increases dramatically in the immediate postpartum period (Table 45.1 & Figure 45.1).

Pulmonary anatomic and physiologic changes during pregnancy place the pregnant patient at increased risk for hypoxemia. The anatomic changes occur to compensate for an enlarging uterus. The increased subcostal angle increases the chest circumference. There is increased diaphragmatic excursion and the diaphragm is elevated 4 cm in late pregnancy. Pulmonary function is also altered in pregnancy. A 30% increase in tidal volume occurs, with a corresponding 30–40% increase in minute ventilation. The expiratory reserve volume and functional residual capacity decrease by 20%. Respiratory rate, vital capacity, and inspiratory reserve volume do not change. P_aO_2 is increased while P_aCO_2 and HCO_3 are decreased. $PaCO_2$ decreases to 27–32 mmHg in the second half of pregnancy as a result of the increased minute ventilation. Oxygen consumption increases progressively during pregnancy and is maximum during the stress of labor.

Table 45.1 Comparison of hemodynamic parameters in pregnant and non-pregnant patients.

	Non-pregnant	Pregnant
Central venous pressure (mmHg)	1–10	Unchanged
Pulmonary artery pressure (mean) (mmHg)	9–16	Unchanged
Pulmonary capillary wedge pressure (mmHg)	3–10	Unchanged
Cardiac output (L/min)	4–7	↑ 30–45%
Systemic vascular resistance (dyne-sec cm^{-5})	770–1500	↓ 25%
Pulmonary vascular resistance (dyne-sec cm^{-5})	20–120	↓ 25%
Heart rate	65–72/min	↑10–20%

Congenital heart disease (CHD)

Congenital heart diseases with small left to right intracardiac shunts account for 60–80% of cardiac disease in pregnant patients in the United States [2]. Women with significant uncorrected congenital heart lesions, significantly dilated aortic root in Marfan's disease, congestive heart failure (NYHA class III and IV) despite optimized medical treatment and palliative surgery, and those with increased pulmonary vascular resistance, are at increased risk for major morbidity and mortality and should be advised against pregnancy (Table 45.2) [6]. The risks to mother and fetus of congenital heart disease during pregnancy are shown in Table 45.3. The two most important predictors of fetal mor-

Table 45.2 Absolute contraindications to pregnancy.

Severe primary and secondary pulmonary hypertension
Marfan's syndrome with aortopathy and ascending aorta diameter >40 mmHg
Eisenmenger syndrome (cyanosis due to R to L intracardiac shunt)

Table 45.3 Risks of congenital heart disease to mother and fetus during pregnancy.

Risk to the mother	Risk to the fetus
Pulmonary edema	Intrauterine growth restriction
Arrhythmias	Prematurity
Heart failure	Congenital heart disease (inherited)
Hemorrhage from anticoagulation	Teratogenic effect of drugs administered to the mother
Death	Intracranial hemorrhage
	Fetal loss

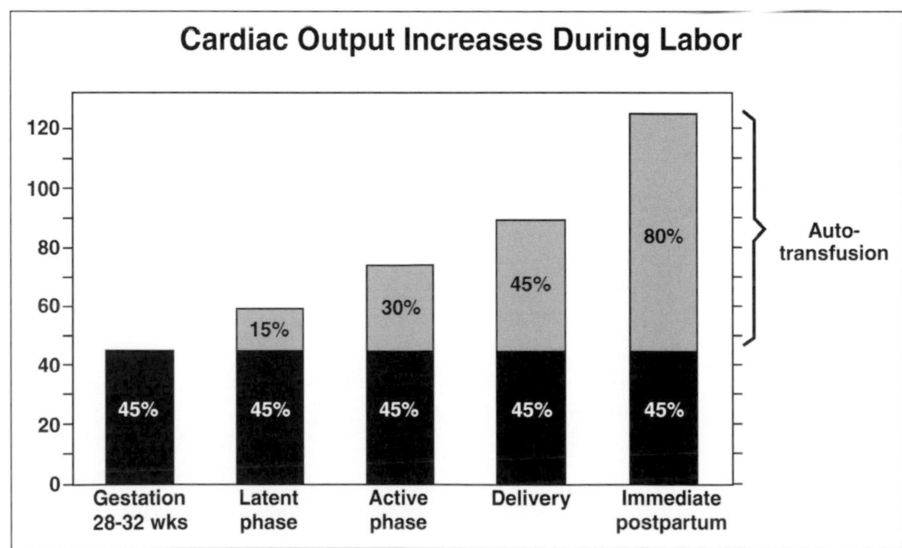

Figure 45.1 Cardiac output increases during labor.

bidity in these parturients are the presence of congestive heart failure and persistent cyanosis in the mother.

Left to right shunts

Pathophysiology

The hemodynamic alterations depend on the size of the defect. Patients with atrial shunts, such as atrial septal defect (ASD) are at low risk of hemodynamic deterioration or onset of arrhythmias. In the rare case of a marked clinical deterioration, catheter-based closing of the shunt is the first-line treatment. Ventricular septal defect (VSD), and persistent patent ductus arteriosus (PDA) are also usually well tolerated during pregnancy although arrhythmias should be anticipated in these conditions. The hemodynamic alterations, complications and prognosis are summarized in Table 45.4.

Anesthetic management considerations in left to right intracardiac shunts

With small shunts right ventricular (RV) and pulmonary artery (PA) pressures are unchanged and there is not much change in pulmonary blood flow. Risk of bacterial endocarditis is increased. With larger shunts, there is progressively increased pulmonary blood flow with resultant increase in RV and PA pressures. Ultimately RV and left ventricular (LV) pressures equalize, leading to pulmonary vasoconstriction and irreversible vascular changes resulting in pulmonary hypertension and Eisenmenger's syndrome.

One of the primary goals in the anesthetic management of these women is to avoid pain thus mitigating the hemodynamic increases in pulmonary and systemic vascular resistance. Avoidance of sudden decrease in systemic vascular resistance is also of paramount importance because it increases the L to R shunt thus increasing the incidence of hypoxemia.

Because of hemodynamic responses secondary to increased stress hormones and catecholamines seen during labor and delivery, parturients with NYHA class III and IV may require invasive monitoring to note the beat to beat changes. In such cases continuous arterial blood pressure monitoring with an arterial line, continuous ECG and central venous pressure (CVP) monitoring may be useful during both labor and cesarean section.

Antibiotic prophylaxis for prevention of bacterial endocarditis, particularly in patients with ASD for uncomplicated delivery, is not advocated by the American Heart Association [4]. (See Table 45.5.)

Table 45.4 Left to right shunts.

Size of defect	Hemodynamic alterations	Pregnancy complications	Prognosis
Small	RV and PA are unchanged	Increased risk of endocarditis	Usually uncomplicated course
Moderate	RV and PA pressures are increased but remain below systemic pressures Increased pulmonary blood flow Pulmonary vascular disease unlikely	LV volume overload and failure	CHF and arrhythmias are likely High chance of cardiac decompensation during pregnancy
Large	RV and LV pressures equalize Eisenmenger's syndrome Pulmonary vascular disease likely	Heart failure, fetal hypoxemia	Mortality can reach as high as 50% Pregnancy is contraindicated

RV, right ventricle; PA, pulmonary artery; LV, left ventricle; CHF, congestive heart failure.

Table 45.5 Antibiotic Prophylaxis for Genitourinary/Gastrointestinal Procedures.

	Standard Regimen
Ampicillin, gentamicin, and amoxicillin	Intravenous or intramuscular administration of ampicillin, 2 g plus gentamicin 1.5 mg/kg (not to exceed 80 mg), 30 min before procedure; followed by amoxicillin, 1.5 g orally 6 h after initial dose; alternatively the parenteral regimen may be repeated once 8 h after initial dose
	Ampicillin/Amoxicillin/Penicillin Allergic Patient Region
Vancomycin and gentamicin	Intravenous administration of vancomycin, 1 g over 1 hr plus intravenous or intramuscular administration of gentamicin 1.5 mg/kg (not to exceed 80 mg), 1 hr before procedure; may be repeated once 8 hr after initial dose
	Alternative Low-risk Patient Regimen
Amoxicillin	3 g orally 1 hr before procedure; then 1.5 g 6 hr after initial dose

Table 45.6 Anesthetic management principles in left to right intracardiac shunts.

Management principles	Rationale
Supplemental oxygen	Increases oxygen reserves, especially in second stage of labor
Loss of resistance to saline technique for epidural anesthesia	Decreases risk of venous air embolism and paradoxic air embolism
Early combined spinal epidural technique with intrathecal narcotics and ultra-low concentration of epidural infusion analgesia for good pain control throughout labor	Avoid increases in maternal catecholamines
Cut short second stage of labor with forceps/vacuum assist	Avoids Valsalva and hemodynamic changes associated with pushing

In parturients with left to right shunts, the primary considerations are alleviation of pain during labor and therefore the use of a combined spinal/epidural (CSE) technique in early labor is particularly advantageous. Intrathecal lipophilic narcotics such as fentanyl can be used to alleviate pain without causing any changes in the hemodynamics (specifically the SVR). Furthermore, this can be followed with ultra-low dose epidural infusion which provides continuous labor analgesia without any adverse effects on the hemodynamics or progress of labor [7].

The technique of loss of resistance to saline should be used during epidural placement in order to prevent air entry into an epidural vein which can lead to paradoxical air embolism [8]. In addition, in those patients with potential intracardiac shunts air filters should be used on all venous and arterial lines.

Decompensation in the cardiac status is most likely immediately after delivery due to the autotransfusion that occurs from the uteroplacental unit. Close monitoring of the hemodynamics are important. Prevention of the Vasalva maneuver in the second stage is important and decreasing the duration of the second stage of labor by operative vaginal delivery and provision of adequate analgesia is important. Supplemental oxygen is helpful to increase oxygen reserves and to enhance oxygen delivery to both mother and fetus (Table 45.6).

Cyanotic heart disease

Tetralogy of Fallot

Pathophysiology

Tetralogy of Fallot (TOF) is the commonest congenital heart disease associated with the following conditions: right to left shunt, VSD, right ventricular hypertrophy, pulmonary stenosis with right ventricular outflow tract obstruction, and an overriding aorta. Most women have correction in childhood but some may present with residual defects. The degree of intracardiac shunting, severity of right ventricular outflow obstruction, and right ventricular function are primary determinants of outcome.

Anesthetic management

Goals of anesthetic management include:

- avoiding decreases in systemic vascular resistance, thus minimizing the magnitude of the right to left shunt
- maintaining adequate intravascular volume and venous return.

Amongst the neuraxial anesthesia labor analgesic techniques the combined spinal/epidural (CSE) technique is most preferable. Early establishment of CSE in labor with the use of intrathecal narcotics followed by epidural infusion of ultra low concentrations of local anesthetics can provide excellent analgesia without decreasing the systemic vascular resistance. Phenylephrine is the drug of choice for managing hypotension in these patients. The advantage of a CSE technique for labor analgesia is the ability to provide surgical anesthesia if a cesarean section is needed. In the event that general anesthesia becomes necessary (due to lack of time to establish a regional block or if there are contraindications to regional anesthesia), it is important to avoid decreases in SVR with intravenous induction and inhalational agents, and increases in pulmonary vascular pressures. Following acid aspiration prophylaxis, controlled induction with ketamine, or short-acting narcotics such as remifental is preferable in order to prevent large hemodynamic perturbations, and to minimize adverse effects on the fetus.

Consultation with the neonatologist and plans for neonatal resuscitation are also important.

Eisenmenger's syndrome

Pathophysiology

Eisenmenger's complex is described as pulmonary hypertension with a reversible or bidirectional shunt through a large VSD. The systemic and pulmonary circulations are in open communication. When the pulmonary vascular resistance rises or systemic vascular resistance falls, severe hypoxemia ensues due to blood bypassing the lungs.

When flow through the pulmonary vascular bed is increased, as in patients with congenital intracardiac (left to right) shunts, the vasculature is initially able to compensate for the increased volume. However, over a prolonged period, there is thickening of the vessel walls, resulting in an increase in pulmonary vascular resistance. Eventually, as a result of the increased pulmonary vascular resistance, right-sided cardiac pressures become elevated leading to reversal in the intracardiac shunt. The conversion or reversal to a right to left shunt with longstanding atrial or ventricular septal defect or a patent ductus arteriosus results in Eisenmenger's syndrome. A retrospective analysis (1978–1996) [9], showed an increase in pulmonary artery pressure and pulmonary vascular resistance during gestation in some patients with moderate pulmonary hypertension at the beginning of the pregnancy. The maternal death rate was 36% in a series of 73 patients with Eisenmenger syndrome. Three women died during pregnancy and 23 died at the time of delivery or within 1 month postpartum. Mortality was strongly associated with late diagnosis and late hospital admission, while severity of pulmonary hypertension was also found to be a contributing factor. Neither the mode and timing of delivery, nor the type of anesthesia and monitoring correlated with maternal outcome. Most fatalities were described as sudden death or therapy-resistant heart failure.

Because maternal and fetal mortality can be as high as 50% in parturients with Eisenmenger's syndrome, this condition is considered an absolute contraindication to pregnancy. If the patient decides to continue pregnancy despite counseling then the following modalities should be implemented: bed rest, hospital admission by second trimester, continuous pulse oximetry, supplemental oxygenation, and prophylactic antithrombotic prophylaxis with heparin.

Anesthetic management

The important considerations in patients with large VSD and severe symptoms are:

- avoidance of decrease in SVR and increase in PVR
- prevention of hypercarbia, hypoxemia, acidosis and high airway pressures.

Invasive monitoring should include continuous invasive blood pressure measurement. Assessment of central venous pressure (CVP) is equally important to monitor the trends in right ventricular filling pressures and the intravascular volume status. Continuous supplemental oxygen must be used throughout labor.

Perioperative risk in Eisenmenger's syndrome is high for patients undergoing non-cardiac surgery, and regional anesthesia should be avoided because of the potential deleterious hemodynamic effects. Spinal or epidural anesthesia could decrease the afterload, causing an increase in the magnitude of the right to left shunt. A review of 57 articles describing 103 anesthetic procedures in patients with Eisenmenger's syndrome showed the overall perioperative mortality based on anesthetic management to be 14%. Patients receiving regional anesthesia had a mortality of 5%, whereas those receiving general anesthesia had a mortality of 18%. This trend favored the use of regional anesthesia but was not statistically significant [10].

Since the primary objectives involve maintaining cardiac output, preserving systemic vascular resistance and lowering pulmonary vascular resistance, general anesthesia is the preferred technique for parturients with Eisenmenger's syndrome who are undergoing cesarean section delivery. However there are anecdotal case reports of the use of regional anesthesia for both operative and vaginal delivery.

As mentioned earlier, combined/spinal epidural is the preferred technique for labor analgesia in these high-risk patients. A combination of 10–15 μg of fentanyl and bupivacaine 2.5 mg intrathecally provides excellent analgesia with minimal hemodynamic perturbation. This is followed by a low-dose epidural infusion of bupivacaine 0.0625 mg/mL and fentanyl 2 μg/mL at 10–15 mL/hour.

If cesarean section is needed the authors recommend general anesthesia with ketamine as an induction agent and the use of short-acting narcotics such as remifental. Close monitoring in the intensive care unit is recommended post operatively for at least 48 hours after delivery due to the increased risk of thromboembolism in these patients.

Stenotic lesions

Pathophysiology

Congenital aortic stenosis

Congenital aortic stenosis is usually associated with a bicuspid aortic valve [11]. Patients with aortic stenotic lesions, functional class NYHA >2, cyanosis, severe left ventricular outflow obstruction (aortic valve area <1.5 cm^2) resulting in decreased cardiac output and uteroplacental blood flow, or impaired left ventricular function are considered at high risk for morbidity and mortality during pregnancy.

Severe aortic stenosis (a peak transvalvular gradient greater than 50 mmHg) must be corrected before pregnancy. Severe aortic stenosis carries a high risk of mortality during pregnancy. Siu et al. reported a maternal mortality rate of 11% and a perinatal mortality rate of 4% [3]. A Canadian study described 49 cases with a 10% risk of complications in patients with severe stenosis [12].

Conservative medical management is acceptable for mild to moderate aortic stenosis. However, once surgical valve replacement for severe aortic stenosis is required during pregnancy, there is an increased (30%) fetal mortality [13]. Intrapartum balloon valvuloplasty has been reported, but it is not widely available and needs to be done in centers with the necessary experience [14].

Pulmonary stenosis

Pulmonic valve stenosis is rare as an isolated condition. Untreated severe/symptomatic pulmonary stenosis causes arrhythmias and right heart failure leading to high maternal and fetal morbidity and mortality. The right ventricular failure is a result of an inability to compensate for the increases in heart rate, right ventricular preload, and oxygen delivery and consumption associated with pregnancy.

Management of isolated pulmonic stenosis by percutaneous balloon valvuloplasty has been shown to improve the outcome of pregnancy and has been used in some institutions with success [14;15]. Beta-blockade and diuretics, as well as close hemodynamic monitoring, should be continued throughout the pregnancy.

Pain control during labor is often inadequate with the systemic analgesics that have been recommended by some authors, and fetal cardiorespiratory depression is an unwanted side effect when high-dose narcotic analgesia is used.

Anesthetic management

Epidural/spinal local anesthetics should be avoided due to the risk of hypotension and the risk of decreasing preload which may not be well tolerated in patients with mild to moderate aortic and pulmonary stenosis. However, epidural and intrathecal narcotics using fentanyl or sufentanil are very effective for pain control with minimal hemodynamic consequences. The disadvantage of this technique is the short duration of action of the neuraxial narcotics, necessitating repeated lumbar punctures with the single-shot technique. A successful case using continuous spinal anesthesia with narcotics (sufentanil) has been reported and other lipid-soluble narcotics like fentanyl may also be used [16].

Left ventricular outflow tract obstruction

Aortic coarctation

Pathophysiology

Aortic coarctation is a fixed left ventricular outflow obstruction, causing elevated blood pressure proximal to the lesion and hypoperfusion distally. The decreased left ventricular outflow causes decreased uteroplacental perfusion with a fetal mortality that can approach 20% [12]. Parturients with uncorrected coarctation are usually unable to meet the increased hemodynamic demands of pregnancy. Complications include left ventricular failure, aortic rupture, aortic dissection and endocarditis due to associated bicuspid aortic valve [11]. These patients are also prone to cerebrovascular accidents due to an association with aneurysms in the circle of Willis.

Uncomplicated uncorrected coarctation carries a maternal mortality risk of less than 3%. Severe complications include aortic dissection and rupture (particularly in the third trimester), congestive heart failure secondary to the increased pressure load on the left ventricle, and bacterial endocarditis. The increased demands of pregnancy predispose to aortic dissection. Coarctation of aorta is also associated with a high incidence of bicuspid aortic valve, aneurysms of the circle of Willis, ventricular septal defects, and Turner syndrome. An MRI of the brain in such patients is not unreasonable to exclude berry aneurysms.

Recent data on the outcome of pregnancy in patients with this rare condition is limited. A Mayo clinic review included a comparison of 50 women who underwent repair of aortic coarctation before pregnancy and parturients who had unrepaired lesions. In 118 pregnancies the miscarriage rate was 9% and the preterm delivery rate was 3%. One third of the women who had uncorrected coarctation had significant hypertension during pregnancy. There was one maternal death and a very low incidence of cardiovascular complications [17].

Anesthetic management

Patients with corrected coarctation and no arm/leg blood pressure discrepancy; and those with an arm to leg residual gradient of less than 20 mmHg, usually can expect a good pregnancy outcome. In these patients, both vaginal delivery with neuraxial labor analgesia, and cesarean section with neuraxial anesthesia, have been conducted with minimal morbidity [18].

Pregnant patients with uncorrected coarctation are, however, at much greater risk, and anesthetic goals should focus on maintaining a normal or high cardiac preload, SVR and heart rate. In most situations, abdominal delivery by cesarean section under general anesthesia is recommended. This includes pre- and post-ductal arterial catheters in the upper and lower extremities and PA catheter monitoring with intravenous β-blockade. A high-dose narcotic induction offers good hemodynamic stability and invasive monitors should be used to guide fluid management. The mild chronotropic effect of vasopressors like ephedrine and dopamine is helpful in managing decreases in blood pressure. In general neuraxial blockade (particularly spinal anesthesia) for cesarean section is not recommended. There have been some case reports showing success using titrated epidural analgesia for vaginal delivery [19].

Vaginal delivery has been reported in uncomplicated coarctation [17]. When cesarean section is needed for obstetric indications, or in patients with poorly controlled blood pressure, general anesthesia is administered with invasive hemodynamic monitoring, intravenous antihypertensive drugs, including β-blockade, and postoperative intensive care management.

Aortic dissection

Pathophysiology

Patients with Marfan syndrome or bicuspid aortic valve may proceed to aortic root dilatation and dissection, secondary to the hyperdynamic and hypervolemic condition associated with pregnancy. There is an increased chance of acute Type A dissection in parturients with Marfan syndrome, particularly when aortic root dilatation is greater than 4 cm, or if an increase in aortic size is detected during pregnancy [20].

Numerous case series have been reported with favorable outcomes in the mother, but fetal outcome, in majority of the cases (especially when acute aortic dissection occurred necessitating emergency surgery), is relatively poor [21,22].

It is hard to draw conclusions from so few patients, but it seems logical that emergent delivery of a viable fetus is preferable before emergent repair of aortic dissection. In situations where, based on gestational age, fetal viability is not assured, the mother's condition takes priority and emergent repair of the dissection should be performed with the knowledge that the fetus will be unlikely to tolerate cardiopulmonary bypass and deep hypothermic circulatory arrest. Fetal protection can be attempted with pulsatile perfusion and minimizing the circulatory arrest time.

Anesthetic management

The considerations are similar to those in non-pregnant patients who undergo emergent cardiac surgery and cardiopulmonary bypass.

Acquired heart disease

Rheumatic mitral stenosis

Pathophysiology (Figure 45.2 & Table 45.7)

Rheumatic mitral valve stenosis is the most frequent rheumatic heart disease (RHD) encountered in the pregnant population worldwide. Mitral stenosis is the lesion that most frequently requires therapeutic intervention during pregnancy.

In severe mitral stenosis the valve area reduction decreases left ventricular filling and causes a fixed cardiac output state, elevated

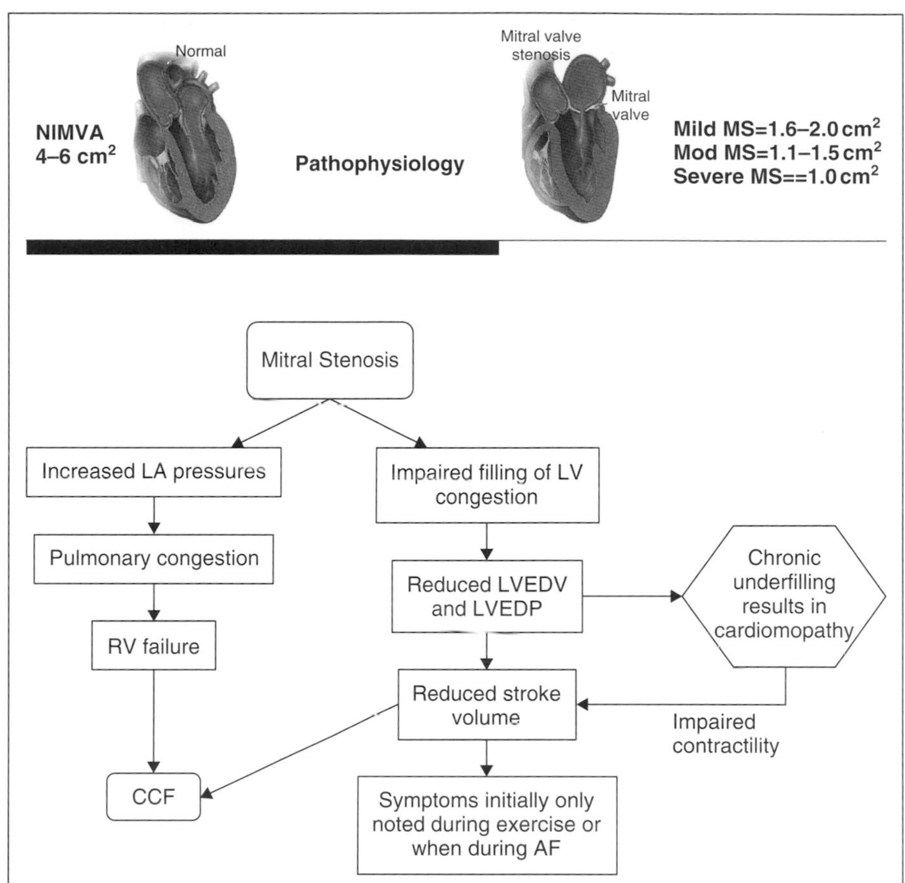

Figure 45.2 Pathophysiology of mitral stenosis. MS, mitral stenosis; Nl MVA, normal mitral valve area; LV, left ventricle; LVEDV, left ventricle end-diastolic volume; LVEDP, left ventricle end-diastolic pressure; RV, right ventricle; CCF, congestive cardiac failure; AF, atrial fibrillation.

Table 45.7 Interaction of Hemodynamic Changes on Pregnancy and Mitral Stenosis.

- Mitral stenosis limits ability to increase CO during pregnancy
- The increase in HR during pregnancy limits the time available for filling of the LV & results in LAP & PAP pulmonary edema
- With the increase in HR, blood volume, and demands for increase in CO(late trimester and L&D) causes the pressure gradient across the valve to quadruple – thus increasing the functional cardiac status (NYHAC)
- Approximately 80% off cases of systemic emboli occur in patients with atrial fibrillation

CO, cardiac output; HR, heart rate; LV, left ventricle; LAP, left atrial pressure; PAP, pulmonary artery pressure; L&D, labor and delivery; NYHAC, New York Heart Association classification.

left atrial and pulmonary arterial pressures, and eventually pulmonary edema. Compensatory RV hypertrophy leads to right heart failure. During gestation and labor, the increased cardiac output and demands, plus the increased heart rate and decreased left ventricular filling, increase the risk for pulmonary edema. The time of highest risk for pulmonary edema is immediately after delivery due to the auto transfusion from uterine contraction, with resultant augmentation in cardiac output.

Mitral stenosis with chronic left ventricular failure can result in pulmonary hypertension by causing back-pressure distal to the pulmonary vasculature in either the left atrium or left ventricle. This condition eventually causes structural changes in the vasculature and an increase in pulmonary vascular resistance. Tolerance of pregnancy when a woman has mitral disease depends upon the severity of the valve disease, the heart rate and rhythm, atrial compliance, circulating blood volume, and pulmonary vascular response.

Patients with a mitral orifice area >1.5 cm^2 can usually be treated medically, whereas parturients with more advanced mitral stenosis often require percutaneous mitral balloon valvotomy, a procedure with a very low complication rate in experienced hands. Closed and open mitral commissurotomy has been performed with low maternal risk and a fetal survival of greater than 90% [23]. Closed or open mitral commissurotomy, balloon valvuloplasty, and valve replacement, are usually considered in patients with a valve area <1.2 cm^2, a poor response to medical therapy, and the absence of valve calcification [25]. Percutaneous balloon valvuloplasty of the mitral valve is the preferred method when intervention is needed during pregnancy [24]. Kasb et al. [25] have shown that pregnant patients with symptomatic mitral stenosis can be safely treated with β-blockade which significantly reduces the incidence of pulmonary edema. It has also been shown that patients with severe symptoms who undergo valvuloplasty or valve surgery before pregnancy have fewer complications than those treated medically. Early preconceptional counseling regarding management and risk of adverse cardiac outcomes is important, especially in patients with severe mitral stenosis (Tables 45.8 & 45.9).

Anesthetic management (Tables 45.10 & 45.11)

Principles of anesthetic management include:

- prevention of pain and avoidance of increased sympathetic stimulation which can result in tachycardia and augmentation of cardiac output
- judicious preload with crystalloids
- invasive hemodynamic monitoring with a pulmonary artery pressure catheter.

In laboring parturients an early epidural can be placed and boluses of medication can be given slowly. Combined spinal/epidural labor analgesia with a lipophilic narcotic and ultralow concentration of bupivacaine as described above and in Tables 45.12 and 45.13 is the preferred technique. Figure 45.3 shows a technique of combining a lipophilic narcotic (fentanyl), given intrathecally, with a hydrophilic narcotic like morphine, which provides longer-lasting labor analgesia than a single narcotic. This technique also offers hemodynamic stability with reasonable

Table 45.8 Impact of Pregnancy-Induced Hemodynamic Changes and Complications with Mitral Stenosis.

An anatomically moderate stenosis become functionally severe

- ↑ NYHAC during pregnancy
- ↑ Pulmonary congestion
- ↑ Atrial fibrillation
  - Systemic emboli
- ↑ Paroxysmal tachycardia

NYHAC, New York Heart Association Classification.

Table 45.9 Preanesthetic evaluation.

Clinical	Physical examination

• Fatigue
• Dyspnea on exertion, paroxysmal nocturnal dyspnea
• Orthopnea
• Dyspnea
• Hemoptysis
  ○ Rupture of bronchopulmonary varices
• Arrhythmias (atrial fibrillation)
• Pulmonary embolism
• Congestive heart failure
	Murmur
	• Presystolic accentuation or mid-diastolic murmur
	  ○ Opening snap
	Signs of failure
	  ○ Pulmonary edema
	  ○ Jugular venous distension
	  ○ Liver enlargement
	  ○ Ascites

Table 45.10 Maternal Monitoring.

- EKG
  - Maintain NSR
  - Detect arrhythmias
- Arterial catheterization
  - Beat-to-Beat monitoring(Labor & Delivery a dynamic state)
  - ABGs
  - Laboratory studies
- Swan Ganz catheter
  - Following trends
  - PAP & PCWP
  - Calculate parameters PVR, (R/O Pulmonary HTN), SVR, Assess CO, CI,

EKG, electrocardiogram; ABGs, arterial blood gases; NSR, normal sinus rhythm; PAP, pulmonary artery pressure; PCWP, pulmonary capillary wedge pressure; PVR, pulmonary vascular resistance; HTN, hypertension; SVR, systemic vascular resistance; CO, cardiac output; CI, Cardiac Index.

Table 45.11 Anesthetic Considerations and Challenges in Mitral Stenosis.

- Prevent rapid ventricular rates
- Maintain sinus rhythm
- Minimize decreases in systemic vascular resistance
- Minimize or prevent increases in central blood volume
- Prevent increases in pulmonary artery pressure
  - Immediate postpartum
  - Avoid hypoxemia/hypoventilation

Table 45.12 Selection of Anesthetic Technique-Pros & Cons.

- Combined Spinal – Epidural technique
  - Optimal technique
  - Intrathecal opioids during stage I (excellent analgesia without sympathetic block)
    - 15–25ugs fentanyl+0.25–0.5mgs morphine (preservative-free)
  - Dilute local anesthetics for late 1st stage and second stage of labor
    - 0.625–0.125% bupivacaine + fentanyl 2–2.5ugs/ml
- Epidural with dilute local anesthetics
  - 0.625–0.125% bupivacaine + fentanyl 2–2.5ugs/ml

ugs/ml: micrograms per milliliter.

Table 45.13 Advantages of anesthetic techniques.

Intraspinal Narcotic	Epidural Local Anesthetics

• Quick onset
• Selective analgesia
• No sympathetic block
• No motor block
	Titratability of block
	• Unlimited duration analgesia (catheter)
	• Relative hemodynamic stability
	• Ability to use different Local Anesthetics/ different situation
	  – 1st stage labor
	  – 2nd stage labor
	  – c/section
	  – post op

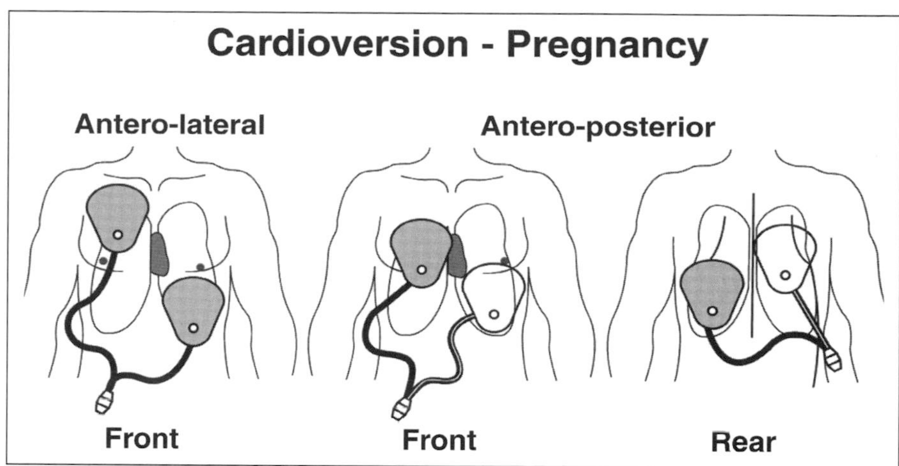

Figure 45.3 Cardioversion in pregnancy.

pain control in this high-risk group of parturients (personal experience of senior author). Clark et al. have previously suggested preloading with 5% albumin, but this is no longer routinely advocated [26]. Phenylephrine is the vasopressor of choice to manage hypotension rather than ephedrine which causes tachycardia and decreases the ventricular filling time, resulting in decreased cardiac output. Epinephrine-containing epidural solutions must be avoided because of the potential for accidental epidural intravascular injection and the associated adverse maternal hemodynamic and uteroplacental blood flow effects. Avoidance of the Valsalva maneuver, and shortening the second stage of labor with forceps or vacuum, are strategies that have been used successfully in these patients. Another advantage of an epidural analgesia for delivery is the increased venous capacitance caused by the sympathetic blockade. This is analogous to the effect of nitroglycerine, and helps to accommodate the autotranfused fluid from the uterus, mitigating the increased preload and preventing the development of pulmonary edema.

In our institution, when cesarean section is needed, gradual titration of an epidural block with continuous monitoring of blood pressure, pulmonary artery pressure and cardiac output is performed. A general anesthesia with a balanced anesthetic that includes a high-dose narcotic and β-blocker has been used successfully with intense invasive and/or transesophageal echocardiography hemodynamic monitoring.

Aortic stenosis

Pathophysiology

Amongst the acquired cardiac lesions, advanced aortic stenosis is rare in patients of childbearing age. If the aortic valve orifice area is >1.5 cm^2, the hemodynamic changes of pregnancy are usually well tolerated. In those cases of more advanced aortic stenosis, there is considerable risk of myocardial decompensation. The development of symptoms such as dyspnea, chest pain, syncope, and arrhythmias are indicators of a complicated course. Patients with severe stenosis of <0.5 cm^2 and a flow gradient greater than 60 mmHg are at high risk for left ventricular failure [27]. Balloon valvuloplasty, which carries the risk of severe regurgitation, has been attempted in some centers as a temporizing procedure. Aortic valve replacement performed antenatally has a maternal mortality of up to 11% [28].

Anesthetic management

The goals of anesthetic management include maintenance of a slow heart rate, preservation of adequate preload and circulating blood volume, and control of systemic vascular resistance. Oxygen supplementation, hemodynamic monitoring (continuous ECG, arterial catheter, central venous catheter/PA catheter), careful preloading and fluid management strategies, left uterine displacement and cesarean delivery under general anesthesia, have all been recommended in patients with severe disease. Phenylephrine is the vasopressor of choice to restore coronary perfusion pressure in patients with severe aortic stenosis when under general anesthesia [29].

In patients with milder aortic stenosis who are undergoing cesarean section single-shot spinal anesthesia is contraindicated. However epidural anesthesia with incremental and careful titration of local anesthetic has been administered with good maternal and fetal outcomes [30,31]. In a case of mitral stenosis with pulmonary hypertension undergoing general anesthesia for urgent cesarean section, Batson and Longmire [32] demonstrated that alfentanil provided cardiovascular stability and allowed immediate postoperative extubation, and that subsequent epidural morphine provided excellent postoperative analgesia. Currently, ultra short-acting remifentanil is also used for induction of anesthesia in pregnant patients with cardiac disease. The combination of general anesthesia followed by postoperative epidural morphine allows early ambulation and helps with the prevention of thromboembolism. Any neonatal respiratory depression that occurs as a result of this technique can usually be reversed with naloxone.

Management of atrial fibrillation in parturients with mitral stenosis

New-onset atrial fibrillation must be treated aggressively in pregnant patients with mitral stenosis because of the increased reliance on the atrial component for cardiac output during pregnancy.

Parturients with moderate mitral stenosis have an increased incidence of atrial fibrillation and an associated increased maternal mortality [33](Table 45.14). Pharmacologic therapy includes β-blockers, calcium channel blockers and digoxin for heart rate control. Procainamide and quinidine are the preferred drugs for suppressive antiarrhythmic therapy because of their safety profile in pregnancy [34]. Although the safety of other antiarrhythmic drugs such as sotalol and flecainide has not been established in pregnancy they have been used in the management of fetal tachycardia and no obvious maternal or fetal morbidity has been recognized. Amiodarone, on the other hand, has been associated with neonatal hypothyroidism, congenital anomalies and teratogenicity.

Direct cardioversion should be considered if the patient is hemodynamically unstable and this has been safely performed in pregnancy [35]. Cardioversion , if needed, should be undertaken in the operating room with simultaneous preparation for cesarean section. Recommendations for cardioversion are described in Table 45.14 and Figure 45.1.

Anticoagulation therapy in a parturient

Mechanical heart valves, new-onset atrial fibrillation, dilated cardiomyopathy, and cardiopulmonary bypass surgery are some of the indications for anticoagulation in a pregnant cardiac patient.

Table 45.14 Cardioversion in Pregnancy.

- Recommendations
  - Prepare for Emergency C-section
  - Monitoring – FHR monitoring
  - MAC Low energy levels biphasic
  - Anterior Posterior Gel Pad Placement
  - GETA for High energy levels

MAC, monitored anesthesia care; GETA, general endotracheal anesthesia; FHR, fetal heart rate.

Oral anticoagulation with warfarin has been associated with the lowest maternal mortality and rate of thromboembolism during pregnancy. However, it is well known that warfarin use in the first trimester can cause fetal growth restriction, spontaneous abortion, embryopathy and premature birth, and fetal and placental hemorrhage in the third trimester [36].

Any decision to use warfarin or its derivatives in pregnancy should be accompanied by an in-depth informed consent discussion with the patient and her family, in which the relative fetal and maternal risks are outlined.

Unfractionated heparin and low molecular weight heparin do not cross the placenta, and are thought to have no fetal teratogenic effects. These drugs may not be as effective as warfarin in preventing thrombosis. One accepted strategy is to use heparin in the first trimester of pregnancy, switch to warfarin or enoxaparin until 35–36 weeks, and then restart heparin until delivery.

A special concern in the anesthetic management of anticoagulated patients is the risk of epidural or spinal hematoma development during neuraxial anesthesia. The American Society for Regional Anesthesia Consensus on anticoagulation and neuraxial anesthesia has stated that the decision to administer a neuraxial anesthetic in a patient receiving anticoagulants, particularly LMWH, should be based on an individual assessment of the risks and benefits for each patient. Table 45.15 discusses some of these recommendations [37].

Ischemic heart disease

Pathophysiology

Ischemic heart disease occurs in 1 in 10,000 pregnancies. Risk factors in pregnancy include older age, smoking, hypercholesterolemia, hypertension, class H diabetes, intravenous administration of ergometrine, pheochromocytoma, cocaine and other drug

Table 45.15 Recommendations based on American Society of Regional Anesthesia Guidelines for neuraxial block placement in parturients receiving anticoagulation.

Anticoagulant	Timing of needle insertion	Timing of epidural catheter removal
NSAIDs/aspirin	No specific concerns	No specific timing
Warfarin (Coumadin)	Stop drug for at least 48 hours PT/INR checked subsequently should be within normal limits before neuraxial attempts	PT/INR checked and confirmed to be within normal limits before removal
Low molecular weight heparin	Stop LMWH 12 hours before placing epidural catheter If larger doses of LMWH have been used (e.g. enoxaparin 1 mg/kg), a 24-hour interval is needed before attempting neuraxial technique	At least 2 hours should elapse after removal of catheter before redosing LMWH to reinstitute anticoagulation

Monitoring anti-Xa levels is not recommended for LMWH activity.
Thromboelastogram is used in some centers to determine coagulation status but cannot be recommended.
NSAID, non-steroidal anti-inflammatory drugs; PT, prothrombin time; INR, International Normalized Ratio (normal value is 1.2); LMWH, low molecular weight heparin.

abuse, and severe hemorrhage. The mortality rate is as high as 50% in the event of a myocardial infarction [38]. Delivery should be avoided for 2 weeks postinfarction if at all possible since the mortality rate is extremely high. Early diagnosis, consultation with a cardiologist, and aggressive therapy are the keys to reducing morbidity and mortality. One study showed that patients with severe postpartum hemorrhage admitted to the ICU had elevated troponin levels and myocardial injury, and that tachycardia and hypotension were independent predictors of myocardial ischemia [39]. Spontaneous coronary dissection can occur in the immediate postpartum period and usually involves the left anterior descending coronary artery. Interventions such as coronary stenting and angioplasty have been successful in pregnant patients. Tissue plasminogen activator has been administered for thrombolysis; it has a short half-life of about 5 minutes and does not cross the placenta.

Anesthetic management

Hemodynamic monitoring, oxygen supplementation, heart rate control with β-blockade, assisted vaginal delivery and effective pain control with epidural analgesia are all effective strategies to reduce the myocardial work and oxygen consumption. Epidural anesthesia has been used successfully for labor and delivery in these patients as it reduces the pain and consequent tachycardia. Successful pregnancy outcomes have been reported after myocardial infarction with close monitoring and multidisciplinary management [40].

Pulmonary hypertension

Pathophysiology

Pulmonary hypertension is a condition characterized by chronic elevation of mean pulmonary artery pressure >25 mmHg at rest, or >30 mmHg with exercise, and it is associated with a pulmonary capillary wedge pressure lower than 12 mmHg diagnosed by right heart catheterization (Table 45.16). The World Health Organization has also recently defined pulmonary hypertension to be present when a systolic pulmonary artery pressure is >40 mmHg. This level of pulmonary hypertension can be estimated non-invasively by using the velocity of the tricuspid jet seen when assessing tricuspid regurgitation, and corresponds to a velocity of 3–3.5 m/s. Pulmonary hypertension is self-perpetuating, and causes structural changes in the pulmonary vasculature, including intimal proliferation, smooth muscle hypertrophy, atheromatous changes, narrowing of the arterial bed, and in situ thrombosis.

Table 45.16 Criteria for pulmonary hypertension.

1. Chronic elevation of mean PAP >25 mmHg at rest
2. Mean PAP >30 mmHg with exercise
3. PCWP <12 mmHg

PAP, pulmonary artery pressure; PCWP, pulmonary capillary wedge pressure.

Diagnosis of pulmonary hypertension is confirmed by various diagnostic modalities (Table 45.17).

A word of caution is needed when relying on non-invasive measurements of pulmonary artery pressure in pregnancy. A recent study has revealed that echocardiography significantly overestimates pulmonary artery pressures compared with catheterization in pregnant patients with suspected pulmonary hypertension. Thirty-two per cent of pregnant patients with normal pulmonary artery pressures may be misclassified as having pulmonary artery hypertension when measured by echocardiography alone [41]. For this reason we suggest right heart catheterization in such women before making the diagnosis of pulmonary hypertension.

Maternal mortality in the setting of severe pulmonary hypertension is over 50% [42,43] and primary pulmonary hypertension is a contraindication to pregnancy. Most fatalities occur during labor and the early postpartum period. Management of these patients is challenging, and invasive hemodynamic monitoring during labor and delivery is recommended [44].

Despite improvements in medical, obstetric, anesthetic, and intensive care, mortality rates have remained stable over the past decades.

Pharmacologic therapies

Pharmacologic therapies include calcium channel blockers, angiotensin-converting enzyme (ACE) inhibitors, adenosine, cardiac glycosides, anticoagulants, diuretics, and supplemental oxygen, but no combination has resulted in increased survivability or a long-term response. Diuretics are frequently used to treat excessive edema that compromises the patient's current condition, and must be used with caution to avoid significant

Table 45.17 Diagnosis of pulmonary hypertension.

Diagnostic modalities	Changes seen in pulmonary hypertension
Electrocardiogram	Right axis deviation, right ventricular hypertrophy, right ventricular strain or right atrial enlargement
Chest X-ray	May show enlargement of the central pulmonary arteries with peripheral tapering
Transthoracic echocardiography	May show evidence of tricuspid regurgitation, right ventricular and right atrial enlargement, paradoxic motion of the interventricular septum, and a reduction in left ventricular size
Right heart catheterization	Reveals elevated pulmonary artery pressures and normal pulmonary capillary wedge pressure

reductions in preload and electrolyte abnormalities. Long-term oral therapy with calcium channel blockers has produced sustained improvement in approximately 25–30% of patients. In patients whose condition responds to calcium channel blockers, the 5-year survival rate approximates 95% [9].

Vasodilators are the most important new development in the treatment of primary pulmonary hypertension. Continuous epoprostenol (prostacyclin 12, PG12) infusion lowered pulmonary vascular resistance and improved right ventricular function in several series of primary pulmonary hypertension and secondary vascular pulmonary hypertension patients [44]. Short-term application of aerosolized PG12 or its analogue iloprost more effectively reduced pulmonary artery pressure as compared to intravenous PG12 and inhaled nitric oxide in patients. Oral or long-acting transdermally delivered prostacyclin analogues, endothelin receptor antagonists and converting enzyme inhibitors, thromboxane inhibitors and antagonists, or new angiotensin-converting enzyme inhibitors with specific affinity for the pulmonary vasculature might be expected to further improve the efficacy of treatment and life expectancy in patients with pulmonary vascular disease. These therapies, however, remain experimental.

Sildenafil is a new class of medication being utilized in the treatment of acute and chronic pulmonary hypertension. It is at least as effective as inhaled nitric oxide in relaxing the pulmonary vasculature, and may have fewer side effects Coadministration of sildenafil with nitric oxide also leads to less rebound pulmonary hypertension.

An atrial balloon septostomy is an optional postpartum intervention for cases that are resistant to treatment. Congenital or iatrogenic intra-atrial communication may postpone the occurrence of right heart failure or acutely decompress the right heart at the expense, of course, of the right-to-left shunt blood flow.

Surgical pulmonary thrombendarterectomy is indicated in patients with chronic thromboembolic disease involving the proximal pulmonary arteries. Excellent results have been reported after surgery, including moderate morbidity rates, survival of small for gestational age neonates, and excellent maternal survival rates [9].

Perioperative management

While the literature on the management of the non-pregnant patient with primary pulmonary hypertension is extensive, information on pregnant patients is very limited.

In a recent study, the authors reviewed the charts of all pregnant women with severe pulmonary hypertension who were followed up at their institution during the past 10 years, to assess the multidisciplinary treatment and outcome of these patients. They concluded that despite the most modern treatment efforts, the maternal mortality was 36% [44].

Pain, anxiety, stress, hypercarbia, hypoxia, and acidosis during labor and delivery further complicate the management of a patient with pulmonary hypertension by increasing pulmonary vascular resistance. These avoidable factors should be minimized. The degree of pulmonary hypertension and right ventricular failure must be assessed before proceeding with anesthesia. The reactivity of the pulmonary vasculature should also be examined to determine if pharmacologic pulmonary vasodilatation is feasible. Preoperatively, drugs likely to produce depression of ventilation should be avoided. Excessive doses of systemic analgesics can cause respiratory depression resulting in hypercarbia and acidosis, which further exacerbates the pulmonary hypertension.

ECG, pulse oximetry, and invasive arterial blood pressure monitoring is advocated at the time of delivery. Transesophageal echocardiography has been used intraoperatively during cesarean section. Continuous invasive monitoring for instrumental or surgical delivery allows frequent determinations of arterial blood gases and subsequent adjustments in inspired oxygen concentrations and minute ventilation. A right atrial catheter can give important information such as abrupt increases in right atrial pressure, which may signal right ventricular dysfunction and increased pulmonary vascular resistance.

The optimum mode of delivery and anesthetic management remain unclear. Methods of delivery should be discussed with the delivery team and the patient because of the deleterious effects of anesthesia. The literature reports a mortality rate of 37% for vaginal delivery and almost 63% for cesarean section [45], which should be reserved for accepted obstetric indications.

The most serious anesthetic complication in women with pulmonary hypertension is right ventricular dysfunction. Monitoring the central venous pressure can warn of early dysfunction. If the central venous pressure gradually increases, hypercarbia, acidosis, hypoxia, and light anesthesia should be excluded as causal and if present should be immediately corrected. Inotropic therapy or pulmonary vasodilator therapy intraoperatively usually requires intraoperative consultation with a cardiologist.

Intravenous opioids, inhalational analgesia, intrathecal morphine, and paracervical and pudendal nerve blocks are recommended for labor and vaginal delivery. Vaginal delivery using segmental epidural analgesia with local anesthetics (low-dose bupivacaine and fentanyl) [46] has been reported. Low-dose epidural analgesia alone does not have any significant deleterious hemodynamic effect, and it considerably decreases the adverse hemodynamic consequences of labor. If a continuous epidural technique with local anesthetic agents is used, a very cautious and slow titration of local anesthetics is recommended with careful attention to venous capacitance and resistance. Continuous intravenous fluid titration is necessary and only marked decreases in systemic vascular resistance should be corrected using careful ephedrine titration.

Breen and Janzen [47] have described the successful use of epidural anesthesia as a safe alternative to general anesthesia for cesarean section in a patient with pulmonary hypertension, cardiomyopathy, and a patent foramen ovale. Duggan and Katz [45] described the successful use of a combined spinal/epidural technique, using both intrathecal morphine and fentanyl, followed by epidural local anesthetic for the cesarean section, in a patient with primary pulmonary hypertension who failed to respond to nitric oxide.

Some authors have described the use of general anesthesia for cesarean section with good maternal outcome. However, others have reported increased pulmonary arterial pressure during laryngoscopy and tracheal intubation, and that positive-pressure ventilation may reduce venous return and ultimately lead to cardiac failure. Low tidal volumes of 5–10 mL/kg are recommended. Intermittent positive pressure breathing is most often selected for the intraoperative management of ventilation in patients with cor pulmonale. Marked decreases in venous return caused by lung inflation, aortocaval compression, or by conduction anesthesia must be minimized. Excessive reductions in the P_aCO_2 during controlled ventilation should be avoided because metabolic alkalosis causes hypokalemia; this is particularly important in patients on digitalis therapy.

There are now an increasing number of case reports highlighting the use of regional anesthesia with good outcome. However, a single-shot spinal anesthesthetic is contraindicated in these patients. Therefore, epidural anesthesia with incremental doses is currently regarded as the best regional technique. Nonetheless, the dense and extended block needed to prevent pain during cesarean delivery may have significant hemodynamic consequences.

The postpartum period is critical in women with primary pulmonary hypertension because dramatic increases in pulmonary vascular resistance generally precede irreversible right ventricular failure and death. After placental extraction, oxytocin must be infused slowly, because direct intravenous boluses of large doses can be fatal in patients with an unstable hemodynamic status [48].

Symptomatic therapy during the postpartum period includes inhaled nitric oxide and epoprostenol infusion or inhaled iloprost. Many advocate long-term anticoagulation as part of the postpartum therapy. Postoperative management in an intensive care unit is critical and close observation in a high-dependency unit should continue for at least 1 week postpartum because of the high incidence of sudden death during this period.

Peripartum cardiomyopathy

The primary criteria for peripartum cardiomyopathy are listed in Table 45.18. Secondary criteria include multiparity, black race, older maternal age, multiple gestation, tocolytic therapy with β-agonists, and viral myocarditis. A notable feature is its tendency to recur in subsequent pregnancies. Signs and symptoms include dyspnea, extensive lower extremity edema, fatigue, nocturnal cough, paroxysmal nocturnal dyspnea, pulmonary edema, elevated jugular venous pressure, hepatomegaly and new regurgitant murmurs, all of which are indicative of congestive heart failure. Chest X-ray needs to be done to determine the presence of cardiomegaly. The ECG findings usually include tachycardia, dysrhythmias, left ventricular hypertrophy, and/or ST segment changes. Echocardiography confirms the diagnosis by revealing new left ventricular systolic dysfunction. Endomyocardial biopsy demonstrates myocarditis in up to 76% of patients. Persistent cardiomegaly results in a poor prognosis [49].

Table 45.18 Criteria for peripartum cardiomyopathy.

Criteria
Heart failure in the last month of pregnancy or within 5 months post partum
Absence of identifiable cause
Absence of prior heart disease
Echocardiography shows left ventricle dysfunction with ejection fraction <45% and/or fractional shortening <30% and end-diastolic dimension >2.7 cm/sq m body surface area

Perioperative management

The treatment of peripartum cardiomyopathy, particularly in patients with severe systolic dysfunction, involves the use of diuretics, salt restriction, and afterload reduction with vasodilators. Hydralazine, nitrates or calcium channel blockers like amlodipine are some of the drugs that have been recommended for afterload reduction.

ACE inhibitors are generally contraindicated in the antepartum period due to the risk of teratogenicity, neonatal anuric renal failure and neonatal death [50]. However, these drugs may be used under specific circumstances where maternal condition mandates them. This clearly involves a clear informed consent discussion. ACE inhibitors are used effectively postpartum even if the mother is breastfeeding. Newer therapy includes pooled polyclonal antibodies [45] which have been shown to improve overall survival in pregnant patients with dilated cardiomyopathy.

Atrial arrhythmias can be treated with digoxin and other indicated anti-arrhythmia drugs as required. Drug choice in such patients is best made in consultation with a cardiologist.

Anticoagulation with unfractionated or low molecular weight heparin should be considered in patients with very low ejection fraction due to the risk of thromboembolism. Oral anticoagulation with warfarin is useful in the postpartum period.

The mode of delivery in patients with peripartum cardiomyopathy is usually determined by obstetric indications and the maternal functional status. A multidisciplinary approach helps with delivery planning and in most cases vaginal delivery is appropriate in a well compensated and medically optimized mother [51]. The advantages of vaginal delivery are greater hemodynamic stability, decreased blood loss, minimal surgical stress and lower risk of postoperative infection. Epidural analgesia with slow titration of low concentrations of local anesthetic has the advantages of decreasing preload and afterload, and helps in accommodating volume from uterine autotransfusion after delivery. It also provides excellent pain control and minimizes the effect of sympathetic responses on the heart as a consequence of pain. Combined spinal/epidural anesthesia with very low dose infusion of bupivacaine (0.0625–0.04%) as a continuous epidural has also been used with success. Contraindications to regional anesthesia include the presence of an anticoagulated state.

Cesarean delivery may be performed under general anesthesia or neuraxial anesthesia. The principles of anesthetic management in patients undergoing general anesthesia include maintenance of a low to normal heart rate and avoidance of large changes in blood pressure. An opioid-based technique for induction is helpful. This avoids the myocardial depression and vasodilatation caused by large doses of agents such as thiopental and propofol.

There should be adequate preparation for neonatal resuscitation following high-dose narcotic induction in mothers undergoing general anesthesia. Use of sufentanil and low-dose thiopental for induction in a diabetic obese parturient with peripartum cardiomyopathy has been described [52]. In patients with severe cardiac dysfunction inotropic support can be provided along with general anesthesia. A recent review by the National Heart, Lung and Blood institute suggests that patients with EF <35% benefit from anticoagulation therapy [49].

Monitoring usually includes an arterial line and a pulmonary artery catheter. Transesophageal echocardiography is a very useful tool to assess ventricular function and wall motion when general anesthesia is used. Regional anesthesia for cesarean delivery has been performed with a combined spinal/epidural technique, but such a choice should be made on a case-by-case basis.

Arrhythmias during pregnancy and management

Significant supraventricular and ventricular arrhythmias are very uncommon in healthy parturients. The additional circulatory burden of pregnancy, and enhanced adrenergic receptor excitability mediated by progesterone and estrogen can promote mild arrhythmias (PACs and PVCs) but these are usually self-limited and not hemodynamically significant. In clinically relevant arrhythmias the usual causes are structural cardiac defects or residual defects after repair, and most of these arrhythmias are supraventricular in origin.

Management of arrhythmias includes the following.

- Avoidance of stimuli including smoking, caffeine, and substance abuse including amphetamines, ephedrine and cocaine.
- Correction of electrolyte abnormalities if present.
- Vagal maneuvers for paroxysmal supraventricular arrhythmias can be attempted.

Echocardiography for structural cardiac defects and 24-hour monitoring should be considered. Drug therapy should be avoided in the first trimester unless arrhythmias result in severe symptoms or in patients with severe ventricular hypertrophy or dysfunction.

Electrical cardioversion is generally safe during pregnancy. Firm application of paddles, adequate sedation, and aspiration prophylaxis are all important considerations. Fetal ventricular arrhythmias have been reported after cardioversion. The energy needed for defibrillation is unchanged in pregnancy.

In maternal paroxysmal supraventricular tachycardia, adenosine can be administered if vagal maneuvers are unsuccessful. Cardioselective β-blockers may also be useful. Esmolol is associated with a higher incidence of fetal bradycardia and may cause fetal acidosis. It should be avoided unless clearly indicated. Amiodarone should also be avoided as a first line of therapy and reserved for resistant cases. Ventricular arrhythmias can be treated with intravenous lidocaine, procainamide or cardioversion. In patients with long QT syndrome and torsades de pointes, β-blockade should be continued into the postpartum period.

Pregnancy in patients with an implantable cardioversion defibrillator (ICDs) has had favorable maternal and fetal outcomes.

Pregnancy and the transplanted heart

Pathophysiology

Pregnancy in heart transplant recipients is generally tolerated provided the transplanted heart was functioning well before the onset of the pregnancy [53]. A transplanted heart is denervated and the response to the hemodynamic demands of pregnancy is atypical because of the adaptive mechanisms. The increased circulating blood volume leads to an increased preload and an increased stroke volume response as defined by the Frank Starling relationship. There is also a delayed increase in cardiac output in response to increased demands because it is only mediated by the release of catecholamines from the adrenal medulla and not via the sympathetic nerves [54].

Anesthetic considerations

Spontaneous labor and vaginal delivery is well tolerated and cesarean section is reserved for obstetric indications. In a case series of pregnancies after heart transplantation, 16 out of 22 pregnancies resulted in live births, and 10 out of the 22 pregnancies delivered vaginally. Five patients had cesarean section for labor complications and one was for pre-eclampsia. Neuraxial anesthesia was used in five cesarean deliveries and four vaginal deliveries without any adverse maternal or fetal outcomes [55].

Complications seen in these pregnancies include gestational hypertension, pre-eclampsia, renal insufficiency, and infections. Most infections are consequent to immunosuppressive therapy [56]. Episodes of acute rejection can occur. Fetal/neonatal morbidity is generally the result of spontaneous abortion, premature-birth and low birth weight, and intrauterine growth restriction. Cesarean sections are associated with a higher risk of infection in these patients due to use of immunosuppressive therapy [57].

Ventricular assist devices are usually used as a bridge to transplantation in patients with cardiogenic shock. They are designed to provide full hemodynamic support to patients with severe heart decompensation but their limitations include operative risks, infections and other device-related morbidity such as thromboembolism [58,59]. Even though the ventricular assist devices are used mostly as a bridge to heart transplantation, several successful cases of their use for bridge to recovery have been reported [60].

Cardiac transplantation should be considered in patients with severe end-stage failure, especially in women with postpartum cadiomyopathy. The survival rates are similar to those with idiopathic dilated cardiomyopathy. However patients with postpartum cardiomyopathy have higher rates of early rejection and infection.

Intra-aortic balloon pumps have also been used during cardiopulmonary bypass (CPB) in pregnancy (see Chapter 14). The authors claimed that the balloon pump provided an effective pulsatile flow pattern throughout CPB, and they postulated that the balloon pump may benefit maternal circulation and secondarily help fetal hemodynamics [61].

Cardiopulmonary resuscitation in pregnancy

Cardiopulmonary resuscitation has been dealt with in detail in Chapter 7 and will not be dealt with further here .There are a number of excellent reference articles for those interested in this subject [62–67].

Cardiovascular surgery during pregnancy

Cardiac surgery during pregnancy, particularly with cardiopulmonary bypass, is associated with very high fetal and maternal mortality [68,69]. Medical therapy remains the treatment of choice. Interventional cardiology procedures and cardiac surgery should be reserved as an option only for the extremely critically ill parturients who are not candidates for medical or palliative therapy. Recent studies have suggested maternal mortality as high as 8–10%, especially in pregnant patients with NYHA class III or IV disease undergoing emergency cardiac surgery [70]. Hospitalization in late pregnancy, and surgery performed immediately postpartum, significantly worsened the outcome. Cardiovascular surgery is better tolerated in early pregnancy [71]. A prolonged interval between surgery and pregnancy, and delivery before reaching term seem to improve maternal outcome. A systematic review of the outcome of cardiovascular surgery and pregnancy in the period 1984–1996 showed maternal morbidity and mortality of 24% and 6% respectively. Fetal/neonatal risks of maternal surgery during pregnancy can be high and unpredictable. Fetal morbidity is around 9% and fetal mortality is as high as 30%. Hospitalization after 27 weeks of pregnancy and emergency surgery contributed to poor maternal outcome. In contrast fetal outcome was better when the gestational age was higher. The duration of the surgery and CPB, and the temperature of CPB blood did not affect outcomes [28].

Cardiopulmonary bypass in pregnancy

This has been dealt with in Chapter 14 and will not be covered here except to say that the pros and cons of intraoperative fetal monitoring must be assessed on a case-by-case basis [72]. Fetal bradycardia, sinusoidal patterns, and late decelerations may occur during CPB soon after initiation or emergence from CPB [73]. The reasons include reduced systemic vascular resistance, low uteroplacental blood flow, hemodilution, particulate or air embolism, obstruction of venous drainage during inferior vena caval cannulation, prolonged bypass, or maternal administration of high-dose narcotics. Fetal protection strategies in such conditions include hyperoxygenation, maintenance of the hematocrit above 28%, high CPB perfusion pressures, high pump flow, normothermic CPB, minimization of aortic cross-clamp, and CPB duration, and tocolytic therapy. Pulsatile perfusion seems to offer theoretical benefit but still controversial [74].

References

1 Bitsch M, Johansen C, Wennevold A, Osler M. Maternal heart disease. A survey of a decade in a Danish university hospital. *Acta Obstet Gynecol Scand* 1989; 68(2): 119–124.

2 Shime J, Mocarski EJ, Hastings D, Webb GD, McLaughlin PR. Congenital heart disease in pregnancy: short- and long-term implications. *Am J Obstet Gynecol* 1987; 156(2): 313–322.

3 Siu SC, Sermer M, Harrison DA, Grigoriadis E, Liu G, Sorensen S, et al. Risk and predictors for pregnancy-related complications in women with heart disease. *Circulation* 1997; 96(9): 2789–2794.

4 American College of Obstetricians and Gynecologists. ACOG Practice Bulletin No. 47. Prophylactic antibiotics in labor and delivery. *Obstet Gynecol* 2003; 102(4): 875–882.

5 Malhotra S, Yentis SM. Reports on Confidential Enquiries into Maternal Deaths: management strategies based on trends in maternal cardiac deaths over 30 years. *Int J Obstet Anesth* 2006; 15(3): 223–226.

6 Elkayam U, Ostrzega E, Shotan A, Mehra A. Cardiovascular problems in pregnant women with the Marfan syndrome. *Ann Intern Med* 1995; 123(2): 117–122.

7 Wong CA, Scavone BM, Peaceman AM, McCarthy RJ, Sullivan JT, Diaz NT, et al. The risk of cesarean delivery with neuraxial analgesia given early versus late in labor. *N Engl J Med* 2005; 352(7): 655–665.

8 Saberski LR, Kondamuri S, Osinubi OY. Identification of the epidural space: is loss of resistance to air a safe technique? A review of the complications related to the use of air. *Reg Anesth* 1997; 22(1): 3–15.

9 Weiss BM, Zemp L, Seifert B, Hess OM. Outcome of pulmonary vascular disease in pregnancy: a systematic overview from 1978 through 1996. *J Am Coll Cardiol* 1998; 31(7): 1650–1657.

10 Martin JT, Tautz TJ, Antognini JF. Safety of regional anesthesia in Eisenmenger's syndrome. *Reg Anesth Pain Med* 2002; 27(5): 509–513.

11 Reimold SC, Rutherford JD. Clinical practice. Valvular heart disease in pregnancy. *N Engl J Med* 2003; 349(1): 52–59.

12 Silversides CK, Colman JM, Sermer M, Farine D, Siu SC. Early and intermediate-term outcomes of pregnancy with congenital aortic stenosis. *Am J Cardiol* 2003; 91(11): 1386–1389.
13 Chambers CE, Clark SL. Cardiac surgery during pregnancy. *Clin Obstet Gynecol* 1994; 37(2): 316–323.
14 Kan JS, White RI Jr, Mitchell SE, Gardner TJ. Percutaneous balloon valvuloplasty: a new method for treating congenital pulmonary-valve stenosis. *N Engl J Med* 1982; 307(9): 540–542.
15 Loya YS, Desai DM, Sharma S. Mitral and pulmonary balloon valvotomy in pregnant patients. *Indian Heart J* 1993; 45(1): 57–59.
16 Ransom DM, Leicht CH. Continuous spinal analgesia with sufentanil for labor and delivery in a parturient with severe pulmonary stenosis. *Anesth Analg* 1995; 80(2): 418–421.
17 Beauchesne LM, Connolly HM, Ammash NM, Warnes CA. Coarctation of the aorta: outcome of pregnancy. *J Am Coll Cardiol* 2001; 38(6): 1728–1733.
18 Vriend JW, Drenthen W, Pieper PG, Roos-Hesselink JW, Zwinderman AH, van Veldhuisen DJ, et al. Outcome of pregnancy in patients after repair of aortic coarctation. *Eur Heart J* 2005; 26(20): 2173–2178.
19 Zwiers WJ, Blodgett TM, Vallejo MC, Finegold H. Successful vaginal delivery for a parturient with complete aortic coarctation. *J Clin Anesth* 2006; 18(4): 300–303.
20 Rossiter JP, Repke JT, Morales AJ, Murphy EA, Pyeritz RE. A prospective longitudinal evaluation of pregnancy in the Marfan syndrome. *Am J Obstet Gynecol* 1995; 173(5): 1599–1606.
21 Sakaguchi M, Kitahara H, Seto T, Furusawa T, Fukui D, Yanagiya N, et al. Surgery for acute type A aortic dissection in pregnant patients with Marfan syndrome. *Eur J Cardiothorac Surg* 2005; 28(2): 280–283.
22 Wakiyama H, Nasu M, Fujiwara H. Two surgical cases of acute aortic dissection n pregnancy with marfan syndrome. *Asian Cardiovasc Thorac Ann* 2007; 5: 63–65.
23 Rahimtoola SH. The year in valvular heart disease. *J Am Coll Cardiol* 2006; 47(2): 427–439.
24 Avila WS, Rossi EG, Ramires JA, Grinberg M, Bortolotto MR, Zugaib M, et al. Pregnancy in patients with heart disease: experience with 1,000 cases. *Clin Cardiol* 2003; 26(3): 135–142.
25 al Kasab SM, Sabag T, al Zaibag M, Awaad M, al Bitar I, Halim MA, et al. Beta-adrenergic receptor blockade in the management of pregnant women with mitral stenosis. *Am J Obstet Gynecol* 1990; 163(1 Pt 1): 37–40.
26 Clark SL, Phelan JP, Greenspoon J, Aldahl D, Horenstein J. Labor and delivery in the presence of mitral stenosis: central hemodynamic observations. *Am J Obstet Gynecol* 1985; 152(8): 984–988.
27 Naidoo DP, Moodley J. Management of the critically ill cardiac patient. *Best Pract Res Clin Obstet Gynaecol* 2001; 15(4): 523–544.
28 Weiss BM, von Segesser LK, Alon E, Seifert B, Turina MI. Outcome of cardiovascular surgery and pregnancy: a systematic review of the period 1984–1996. *Am J Obstet Gynecol* 1998; 179(6 Pt 1): 1643–1653.
29 Goertz AW, Lindner KH, Schutz W, Schirmer U, Beyer M, Georgieff M. Influence of phenylephrine bolus administration on left ventricular filling dynamics in patients with coronary artery disease and patients with valvular aortic stenosis. *Anesthesiology* 1994; 81(1): 49–58.
30 Patharkar M, Cohen S, Wang M, Solina A. Epidural anesthesia for cesarean section in a parturient with subaortic stenosis. *Int J Obstet Anesth* 2007; 16(3): 294.
31 Xia VW, Messerlian AK, Mackley J, Calmes SH, Matevosian R. Successful epidural anesthesia for cesarean section in a parturient with severe aortic stenosis and a recent history of pulmonary edema – a case report. *J Clin Anesth* 2006; 18(2): 142–144.
32 Batson MA, Longmire S, Csontos E. Alfentanil for urgent caesarean section in a patient with severe mitral stenosis and pulmonary hypertension. *Can J Anaesth* 1990; 37(6): 685–688.
33 Walsh CA, Manias T, Patient C. Atrial fibrillation in pregnancy. *Eur J Obstet Gynecol Reprod Biol* 2008; 138(1): 119–120.
34 Qasqas SA, McPherson C, Frishman WH, Elkayam U. Cardiovascular pharmacotherapeutic considerations during pregnancy and lactation. *Cardiol Rev* 2004; 12(5): 240–261.
35 Slavik Z. Treatment of cardiac arrhythmias during pregnancy. *Amiodarone Pharmacother* 2004; 24: 792–798.
36 Chan WS, Anand S, Ginsberg JS. Anticoagulation of pregnant women with mechanical heart valves: a systematic review of the literature. *Arch Intern Med* 2000; 160(2): 191–196.
37 Horlocker TT, Wedel DJ, Benzon H, Brown DL, Enneking FK, Heit JA, et al. Regional anesthesia in the anticoagulated patient: defining the risks (the second ASRA Consensus Conference on Neuraxial Anesthesia and Anticoagulation). *Reg Anesth Pain Med* 2003; 28(3): 172–197.
38 Hankins GD, Wendel GD Jr, Leveno KJ, Stoneham J. Myocardial infarction during pregnancy: a review. *Obstet Gynecol* 1985; 65(1): 139–146.
39 Karpati PC, Rossignol M, Pirot M, Cholley B, Vicaut E, Henry P, et al. High incidence of myocardial ischemia during postpartum hemorrhage. *Anesthesiology* 2004; 100(1): 30–36.
40 Vinatier D, Virelizier S, Depret-Mosser S, Dufour P, Prolongeau JF, Monnier JC, et al. Pregnancy after myocardial infarction. *Eur J Obstet Gynecol Reprod Biol* 1994; 56(2): 89–93.
41 Penning S, Robinson KD, Major CA, Garite TJ. A comparison of echocardiography and pulmonary artery catheterization for evaluation of pulmonary artery pressures in pregnant patients with suspected pulmonary hypertension. *Am J Obstet Gynecol* 2001; 184(7): 1568–1570.
42 Abboud TK, Raya J, Noueihed R, Daniel J. Intrathecal morphine for relief of labor pain in a parturient with severe pulmonary hypertension. *Anesthesiology* 1983; 59(5): 477–479.
43 Easterling TR, Ralph DD, Schmucker BC. Pulmonary hypertension in pregnancy: treatment with pulmonary vasodilators. *Obstet Gynecol* 1999; 93(4): 494–498.
44 Bonnin M, Mercier FJ, Sitbon O, Roger-Christoph S, Jais X, Humbert M, et al. Severe pulmonary hypertension during pregnancy: mode of delivery and anesthetic management of 15 consecutive cases. *Anesthesiology* 2005; 102(6): 1133–1137.
45 Duggan AB, Katz SG. Combined spinal and epidural anaesthesia for caesarean section in a parturient with severe primary pulmonary hypertension. *Anaesth Intens Care* 2003; 31(5): 565–569.
46 Slomka F, Salmeron S, Zetlaoui P, Cohen H, Simonneau G, Samii K. Primary pulmonary hypertension and pregnancy: anesthetic management for delivery. *Anesthesiology* 1988; 69(6): 959–961.
47 Breen TW, Janzen JA. Pulmonary hypertension and cardiomyopathy: anaesthetic management for caesarean section. *Can J Anaesth* 1991; 38(7): 895–899.
48 Thomas JS, Koh SH, Cooper GM. Haemodynamic effects of oxytocin given as i.v. bolus or infusion on women undergoing Caesarean section. *Br J Anaesth* 2007; 98(1): 116–119.

49 Pearson GD, Veille JC, Rahimtoola S, Hsia J, Oakley CM, Hosenpud JD, et al. Peripartum cardiomyopathy: National Heart, Lung, and Blood Institute and Office of Rare Diseases (National Institutes of Health) workshop recommendations and review. *JAMA* 2000; 283(9): 1183–1188.

50 Mastrobattista JM. Angiotensin converting enzyme inhibitors in pregnancy. *Semin Perinatol* 1997; 21(2): 124–134.

51 George LM, Gatt SP, Lowe S. Peripartum cardiomyopathy: four case histories and a commentary on anaesthetic management. *Anaesth Intens Care* 1997; 25(3): 292–296.

52 Kaufman I, Bondy R, Benjamin A. Peripartum cardiomyopathy and thromboembolism: anesthetic management and clinical course of an obese, diabetic patient. *Can J Anaesth* 2003; 50(2): 161–165.

53 Armenti VT, Radomski JS, Moritz MJ, Philips LZ, McGrory CH, Coscia LA. Report from the National Transplantation Pregnancy Registry (NTPR): outcomes of pregnancy after transplantation. *Clin Transpl* 2000; 123–134.

54 Abukhalil IE, Govind A. Pregnancy in heart transplant recipients. Case report and review. *Clin Exp Obstet Gynecol* 1995; 22(2): 111–114.

55 Morini A, Spina V, Aleandri V, Cantonetti G, Lambiasi A, Papalia U. Pregnancy after heart transplant: update and case report. *Hum Reprod* 1998; 13(3): 749–757.

56 Scott JR, Wagoner LE, Olsen SL, Taylor DO, Renlund DG. Pregnancy in heart transplant recipients: management and outcome. *Obstet Gynecol* 1993; 82(3): 324–327.

57 Baxi LV, Rho RB. Pregnancy after cardiac transplantation. *Am J Obstet Gynecol* 1993; 169(1): 33–34.

58 Lewis R, Mabie WC, Burlew B, Sibai BM. Biventricular assist device as a bridge to cardiac transplantation in the treatment of peripartum cardiomyopathy. *South Med J* 1997; 90(9): 955–958.

59 Monta O, Matsumiya G, Fukushima N, Miyamoto Y, Sawa Y, Koseki M, et al. Mechanical ventricular assist system required for sustained severe cardiac dysfunction secondary to peripartum cardiomyopathy. *Circ J* 2005; 69(3): 362–364.

60 Frazier OH, Myers TJ. Left ventricular assist system as a bridge to myocardial recovery. *Ann Thorac Surg* 1999; 68(2): 734–741.

61 Willcox TW, Stone P, Milsom FP, Connell H. Cardiopulmonary bypass in pregnancy: possible new role for the intra-aortic balloon pump. *J Extra Corpor Technol* 2005; 37(2): 189–191.

62 Syverson CJ, Chavkin W, Atrash HK, Rochat RW, Sharp ES, King GE. Pregnancy-related mortality in New York City, 1980 to 1984: causes of death and associated risk factors. *Am J Obstet Gynecol* 1991; 164(2): 603–608.

63 Rees GA, Willis BA. Resuscitation in late pregnancy. *Anaesthesia* 1988; 43(5): 347–349.

64 Lindsay SL, Hanson GC. Cardiac arrest in near-term pregnancy. *Anaesthesia* 1987; 42(10): 1074–1077.

65 Sanders AB, Kern KB, Ewy GA. Time limitations for open-chest cardiopulmonary resuscitation from cardiac arrest. *Crit Care Med* 1985; 13(11): 897–898.

66 Greiss FC Jr. Uterine vascular response to hemorrhage during pregnancy, with observations on therapy. *Obstet Gynecol* 1966; 27(4): 549–554.

67 European Resuscitation Council. Part 8: advanced challenges in resuscitation. Section 3: special challenges in ECC. 3F: cardiac arrest associated with pregnancy. *Resuscitation* 2000; 46(1–3): 293–295.

68 Kole SD, Jain SM, Walia A, Sharma M. Cardiopulmonary bypass in pregnancy. *Ann Thorac Surg* 1997; 63(3): 915–916.

69 Parry AJ, Westaby S. Cardiopulmonary bypass during pregnancy. *Ann Thorac Surg* 1996; 61(6): 1865–1869.

70 Arnoni RT, Arnoni AS, Bonini RC, de Almeida AF, Neto CA, Dinkhuysen JJ, et al. Risk factors associated with cardiac surgery during pregnancy. *Ann Thorac Surg* 2003; 76(5): 1605–1608.

71 Pomini F, Mercogliano D, Cavalletti C, Caruso A, Pomini P. Cardiopulmonary bypass in pregnancy. *Ann Thorac Surg* 1996; 61(1): 259–268.

72 Lamb MP, Ross K, Johnstone AM, Manners JM. Fetal heart monitoring during open heart surgery. Two case reports. *Br J Obstet Gynaecol* 1981; 88(6): 669–674.

73 Karahan N, Ozturk T, Yetkin U, Yilik L, Baloglu A, Gurbuz A. Managing severe heart failure in a pregnant patient undergoing cardiopulmonary bypass: case report and review of the literature. *J Cardiothorac Vasc Anesth* 2004; 18(3): 339–343.

74 Tripp HF, Stiegel RM, Coyle JP. The use of pulsatile perfusion during aortic valve replacement in pregnancy. *Ann Thorac Surg* 1999; 67(4): 1169–1171.

46 The Organ Transplant Patient in the Obstetric Critical Care Setting

Calla Holmgren & James Scott
Department of Obstetrics and Gynecology, University of Utah Medical Center, Salt Lake City, UT, USA

Background

Successful pregnancies have been reported in women with virtually all types of organ and tissue allografts now used clinically. However, all transplant patients have significant underlying medical disorders that can adversely affect the outcome. Problems may occur unpredictably, and each group of organ recipients has its own array of specific issues. Pregnancy in transplant patients also represents a natural experiment in immunologic aspects of gestation. The implanted conceptus is itself a graft of living tissue, and it is still not clear how the developing semiallogeneic placenta and fetus survive the normal immunocompetent maternal environment. Pregnancy in allograft recipients takes place in a relative state of generalized immune deficiency because of the immunosuppressive agents these women must take. This combination of factors presents unique management challenges to the physician.

Organ and tissue transplantation have evolved from a clinical experiment into a contemporary treatment which restores many patients to near-normal life styles. The first reported post-transplant pregnancy was in a woman who had received a kidney from her identical twin sister in 1958 [1]. Since then, the number of young women with allografts has dramatically increased and thousands have become pregnant (Table 46.1). There are no randomized trials that have investigated pregnancy management options for transplant patients, but a great deal has been learned through experience. The largest experience is with patients receiving living donor or cadaver kidney transplants, but many recipients of liver, heart, lung and pancreas allografts and bone marrow transplants have also become pregnant. Potential problems in these women include adverse effects of immunosuppressive drugs, medical and obstetric complications, and the psychological stress of being both transplant recipient and an expectant mother. Although the prognosis for a live birth is usually good, it is clear that these are high-risk pregnancies that require expert obstetric care.

Critical Care Obstetrics, 5th edition. Edited by M. Belfort, G. Saade, M. Foley, J. Phelan and G. Dildy.

Prepregnancy evaluation

Preconception counseling is desirable for all transplant patients, but it is often difficult to decide how to advise these couples [2–4]. Any woman contemplating pregnancy after transplantation should be in good health with no evidence of graft rejection (Table 46.2). Medical problems, such as diabetes mellitus, recurrent infections, and serious side effects from the immunosuppressive drugs make pregnancy inadvisable. Most transplantation centers advise that it is safe to attempt pregnancy after the second post-transplantation year. This is with the condition that the graft is performing well [5]. An assessment of the patient's family support as well as a tactful but honest discussion of the potential pregnancy problems is important. Those who have followed many of these patients are aware that the literature can be overly optimistic about pregnancy and long-term prognosis. It needs to be appreciated that the long-term organ allograft survival rates are not 100%, and many transplant recipients will not live to raise their children to adulthood [6].

Prenatal care

Much of the information regarding pregnancy and transplantation is from experience with renal transplant patients. However, antepartum care is similar with essentially all other organ allografts. Early diagnosis of pregnancy is important, and a first-trimester ultrasound examination is valuable to establish an accurate date of delivery. Antenatal management should be meticulous and includes serial assessment of maternal allograft function, detection of graft rejection episodes, and prompt diagnosis and treatment of infections, anemia, hypertension, and pre-eclampsia. Close fetal surveillance is also necessary, and the

Table 46.1 Pregnancies in female transplant recipients reported to the National Transplantation Pregnancy Registry (NTPR).[37]

Kidney	1097
Liver	187
Heart	54
Pancreas-kidney	56
Lung	15
Heart-lung	3

Table 46.2 Important prognostic factors for optimum pregnancy outcome in transplant patients.

Two years since transplant
Good general health and prognosis
Satisfactory graft function with no evidence of rejection
No or minimal hypertension and proteinuria
Family support
Stable immunosuppressive regimen
No or minimal hypertension and proteinuria

known risk for fetal growth restriction is monitored by serial ultrasound examinations.

Dysplastic cervical lesions can occur in up to 9% of renal transplant recipients and the risk of cervical carcinoma has been estimated to be 3–16 times higher for renal transplant recipients than for the general population [7]. This is related to the increased risk for human papillomavirus in the immunosuppressed population. At present, it is recommended that all women greater than age 18 and girls less than 18 who are sexually active undergo pelvic examinations, with pap smears, annually. The effect of HPV vaccination on this rate has yet to be assessed but there may be a reduction in women previously vaccinated. Urinary tract infections are particularly common in kidney transplant patients, with up to a twofold increase in the incidence of pyelonephritis. Asymptomatic bacteriuria should be treated for 2 weeks with follow-up urine cultures, and suppressive doses of antibiotics may be needed for the rest of the pregnancy. Other bacterial and fungal infections may be associated with immunosuppression including endometritis, wound infections, skin abscesses, and pneumonia often with unusual organisms such as *Aspergillus*, *Pneumocystis*, *Mycobacterium tuberculosis*, and *Listeria*.

Some patients have become Rh-sensitized from the allograft, and commonly acquired viral infections such as cytomegalovirus (CMV), herpes genitalis (HSV), human papillovirus (HPV), human immunodeficiency virus (HIV) and hepatitis B (HBV) and C (HCV) pose a risk for both the mother and her fetus. The transplanted graft is a source of CMV, and patients typically receive prophylaxis against CMV for 1–3 months postoperatively when the risk for infection is highest. The greatest risk of congenital infection in the fetus is with primary CMV infection during pregnancy, but recurrent CMV infection in immunosuppressed women has also caused congenital CMV in the infant [8]. HBV and HCV are usually acquired through dialysis and blood transfusions prior to transplantation. Hepatitis B immune globulin (HBIG) and HBV vaccine should be given to the newborn and are 90% effective in preventing chronic hepatitis. Acyclovir as prophylaxis or treatment of HSV can be used safely during pregnancy.

The management of antepartum obstetric complications is similar to that for non-transplant patients. However, the risk of infection warrants a more aggressive approach and avoidance of invasive procedures when possible.

Immunosuppression during pregnancy

This is a class of drugs that not all obstetricians are familiar with, but it is crucial that they become aware of the impact on pregnancy and potential side effects when caring for these women. Most maintenance immunosuppressive regimens in transplant patients include combinations of daily corticosteroids, azathioprine, cyclosporine, tacrolimus (FK 506) and mycophenolate mofetil. Multiple drug regimens are common, and both the dose and timing of drug administration require close monitoring during pregnancy. The potential fetal risks for each drug categorized by the US Food and Drug Administration are shown in Table 46.3.

Corticosteroids have been used by physicians for immunosuppression in renal transplant patients since the 1950s [9]. Prednisone is the corticosteroid used in most transplant patients, and intravenous glucocorticoids are used to treat acute rejection reactions. These anti-inflammatory medications inhibit both humoral and cell-mediated immune responses. Maternal adverse effects include glucose intolerance, hirsutism, acne, weight gain, cushingoid appearance, striae formation, osteonecrosis, osteoporosis, fluid retention, hypertension, severe infections, impaired wound healing, and mood changes. Since prednisone is largely metabolized by placental 11-hydroxygenase to the relatively inactive 11 keto form, the fetus is exposed to only 10% of the maternal dose of the active drug. [10] Most patients are maintained on moderate doses of prednisone (10–30 mg/day) that are relatively safe with few fetal effects. However, it is uncertain whether the increased incidence of premature rupture of membranes, preterm birth, pre-eclampsia and fetal growth restriction are due exclusively to the underlying condition or whether prednisone might contribute to these complications [11,12]. There is also evidence that *prolonged* exposure to other glucocorticoids, such as betamethasone used to accelerate fetal lung maturation, may lead to decreased fetal and neonatal somatic brain growth, adrenal suppression, neonatal sepsis, chronic lung disease, psychomotor delay and behavioral problems [12–17]. Two doses of 12 mg 24 h apart have been shown to improve fetal outcomes without exposure of the fetus to the complications listed above [12,13].

Azathioprine and its more toxic metabolite 6-mercaptopurine is a purine analogue whose principal action is to decrease delayed

Table 46.3 Classification and fetal risks for immunosuppressive drugs used in transplantation.

Medication	Pregnancy category	Associated fetal risks
Corticosteroids	B	Premature rupture of membranes, preterm birth, fetal growth restriction, adrenal suppression, neonatal sepsis, chronic lung disease, psychomotor delay, behavioral problems
Azathioprine (Imuran)	D	Fatal neonatal anemia, thrombocytopenia, leukopenia, acquired chromosome breaks
Cyclosporine	C	Unknown
Tacrolimus (Prograf)	C	Unknown
Sirolimus, rapamycin	C	Unknown
Mycophenolate mofetil (CellCept)	D	Possible problems with organogenesis; no structural malformations have been noted in offspring exposed to this drug
Antithymocyte globulin (ATGAM, ATG, thymoglobulin)	C	Unknown
Muromonab-CD3 (Othroclone OKT3)	C	Unknown
Basilizimab (Simulect)	B	None
Daclizumab (Zenapax)	C	Unknown

A, controlled studies, no risk; B, no evidence of risk in humans; C, risks cannot be ruled out; D, positive evidence of risk; X, contraindicated.

hypersensitivity and cellular cytotoxicity. The primary maternal hazards of azathioprine administration are an increased risk of infection and neoplasia. Maternal liver toxicity and bone marrow depression with anemia, leucopenia and thrombocytopenia have occurred but usually resolve with a decrease in dose. Between 64% and 90% of azathioprine crosses the placenta in human pregnancies, but the majority is the inactive form, thiouric acid [18]. Classification of azathioprine as Category D is based largely on two early series that reported an incidence of congenital anomalies of 9% and 6.4% [19,20]. No specific pattern has emerged, and further experience has shown that azathoiprine is not associated with more congenital malformations than seen in the normal population. [21,22]. Other fetal effects that have occasionally occurred include fatal neonatal anemia, thrombocytopenia, leucopenia, and acquired chromosome breaks. One approach suggested recently to minimize neonatal effects is to adjust doses to keep the maternal leukocyte count within normal limits for pregnancy [23].

Cyclosporine is a fungal metabolite whose major inhibitory effect is on T cell-mediated responses by preventing formation of interleukin-2 (IL-2). Cyclosporine has improved survival in transplant recipients and is a standard component of many immunosuppressant regimens. Bone marrow depression is infrequent, but the drug has a propensity for nephrotoxicity and hypertension. Other side effects include hirsutism, tremor, gingival hyperplasia, viral infections, hepatotoxicity and an increased risk of neoplasia such as lymphomas. Cyclosporine levels drop during pregnancy, but graft function has remained stable in most patients despite decreases in trough levels [24]. Cyclosporine readily crosses the placenta, but there is no evidence of teratogenicity of cyclosporine in the human.

Tacrolimus (FK 506) is a macrolide obtained from streptomyces. The incidence of post-transplant diabetes mellitus with tacrolimus is 11–20%; the median time to onset is 68 days, but it is reversible in up to 50% of patients after 2 years [25,26]. Nephrotoxicity and hyperkalemia develop in at least one-third of patients, and neurotoxicities such as headache, tremor, change in motor function, mental status or sensory function have also been described. Cord blood concentrations are approximately 50% of maternal levels [27], but there is no proven association with congenital malformations to date.

Mycophenolate mofetil is another medication more recently utilized to prevent organ rejection, and approximately 79.6% of patients receiving renal transplantation in the United States are placed on this medication. In animal studies, fetal developmental abnormalities have been noted, but there are limited data regarding human teratogenicity. One case report demonstrated major congenital malformation while on mycophenolate mofetil during the organogenesis period of pregnancy. The anomalies were similar to those described in animal models [28]. In 2002, the US National Transplantion Pregnancy Registry reported a total of 14 pregnancies in 10 women with mycophenolate mofetil exposure during pregnancy. Of these, there were six spontaneous abortions. Of the eight live births, there were two newborns with congenital anomalies [29]. Given concerning animal studies and the lack of human data, the use of this medication in pregnancy should be approached with caution. In general, it is recommended that treatment with mycophenolate mofetil should be stopped 6 weeks prior to conception [28].

It is apparent that all immunosuppressive drugs cross the placental barrier and diffuse into the fetus during the development of its own immune system. Yet, there is no convincing evidence that prednisone, azathioprine, cyclosporine or tacrolimus produce congenital abnormalities in the human fetus, and they remain the drugs of choice during pregnancy. Other than fetal growth restriction and preterm birth, the majority of offspring born to immunosuppressed mothers have had relatively uncomplicated courses. Respiratory distress syndrome (RDS), increased susceptibility to infection, hypoglycemia, hypocalcemia, adrenal insufficiency, thymic atrophy, bone marrow hypoplasia, transient leucopenia, reduced levels of IgM and IgG, and transiently elevated serum creatinine levels have all been reported, but these conditions are also commonly present in premature infants not exposed to these drugs. Most neonates have also progressed normally through infancy and childhood, [30] but as they reach adulthood there are concerns about the possibility of delayed adverse effects [31]. Fetal exposure to immunosuppressive agents could be associated with later development of fertility problems, autoimmune disease, and neoplasia [32–34]. With newer agents, it may be even more difficult to accurately identity a cause and effect. It is hoped that lower dosages now possible with drug combinations resulting in less exposure to each specific drug will decrease the potential for teratogenesis. However, potentiating effects among drugs as well as unknown interactions in multiple drug regimens could also result in as yet unrecognized adverse fetal effects. Thus, it is important that all offspring exposed to these agents have long-term follow-up.

Renal transplantation

Approximately 1 in 20 women of childbearing age with a functioning renal allograft become pregnant [2], and it is estimated that more than 10 000 pregnancies have now occurred. Many women have now had more than one pregnancy, and some have successfully delivered twins and triplets. One patient has had five live births and one spontaneous abortion with no evident deleterious effect on the kidney evident 25 years after transplantation [34] (Figure 46.1).

If preconception graft function is adequate as evidenced by a plasma creatinine <1.5 mg/dL and a rate of urinary protein excretion less than 500 mg per day, the pregnancy can be expected to progress normally until near term. Although the transplanted kidney usually functions satisfactorily during gestation, most patients do not have an increased glomerular filtration rate (GFR) seen in normal pregnant women. GFR, instead, characteristically decreased during the third trimester, although this has been reversible after delivery except in a few cases. Proteinuria also occurs in 40% of renal transplant patients in the third trimester, but this characteristically resolves postpartum. If there are no signs of pre-eclampsia, this proteinuria requires no specific treatment [35].

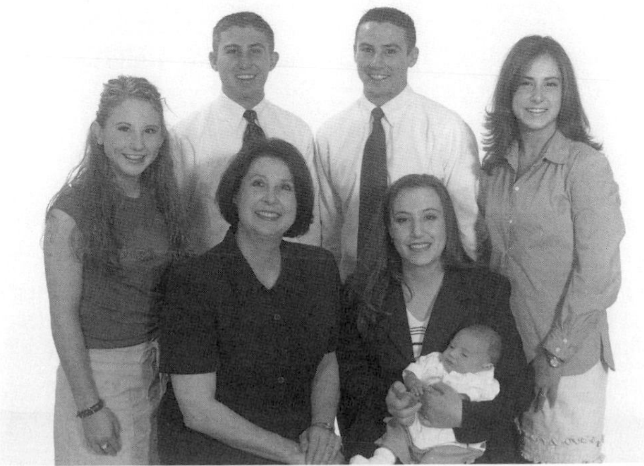

Figure 46.1 Two generations following renal transplantation. The patient is pictured with her five children and recently born granddaughter.

Pregnancy is almost always more complicated in patients with elevated creatinine levels and those with chronic rejection episodes. Deterioration of renal function, rejection and even maternal death has occurred. There is no evidence that pregnancy has a deleterious effect on the transplanted kidney. Rejection of the renal graft with irreversible impairment of renal function during pregnancy or postpartum occurs in 10–20% of women, a risk similar to non-pregnant patients [36]. The clinical hallmarks of rejection include fever, oliguria, deteriorating renal fuction, enlargement of the kidney and tenderness to palpation. The diagnosis can be difficult because the findings overlap with other disorders, such as pyelonephritis, recurrent glomerulopathy, pre-eclampsia and nephrotoxicity from immunosuppressant drugs. It is crucial to establish the diagnosis of rejection before initating additional antirejection therapy, and the clinical situation of failing renal function demands prompt hospitalization. Imaging studies, such as ultrasound, are useful to detect changes in the renal parenchyma and an indistinct corticomedullary boundary indicative of rejection. If the diagnosis is still unclear, renal biopsy is sometimes necessary.

Chronic hypertension and pre-eclampsia are the most prominent complications in these pregnancies and contribute to the increase in preterm births, fetal growth restriction and occasional fetal death (Table 46.2). Hypertension has been reported in anywhere from 47 to 73 percent of patients with a kidney transplant [37]. Pre-eclampsia rates vary, but it is described that one-third of patients with a kidney or kidney/pancreas transplant will develop the syndrome. In women with a renal transplant, blood pressure greater than 140/90 mmHg should usually be managed pharmacologically. Most commonly used antihypertensive agents can be continued during pregnancy with little risk to the fetus, but ACE inhibitors and angiotensin receptor blockers should not be used because of adverse effects on the fetus such as oligohydramnios, pulmonary hypoplasia, long-lasting neonatal anuria and possible fetal cardiac defects [7]. Calcium channel blockers are the preferred agents, and they appear to be beneficial in countering the vasoconstrictive effect of cyclosporine. Pre-eclampsia should be anticipated, and the management is the same as that in the non-transplant patient.

Patients with systemic disease require even closer surveillance, but successful pregnancies have occurred in recipients who received their renal allografts for diabetes, type I oxalosis, previous urinary diversion, Favry's disease, systemic lupus erythematosus, cystinosis, sickle cell disease, and Wegener's and Goodpasture's syndrome [24]. Although renal transplantation allows diabetic women to become pregnant, immunosuppression adds to the complexity of management because of the risk of infection and potentially poor diabetic control. Maternal complications in diabetic transplant patients have included weight-bearing foot fractures, diabetic neuropathy, and vascular complications leading to maternal and fetal death. Neonatal hypocalcemia and hypoglycemia have also been reported in the offspring of these mothers [24].

The data regarding allograft survival following pregnancy are conflicting. However, in general, women with poor prepregnancy renal function (defined as a serum creatinine level greater than 1.5 mg/dL), the risk of irreversible loss of renal allograft function is increased. In addition, this increased risk is present during and after pregnancy. The risk is lower if there is good renal function prior to conception. The risk of allograft rejection with pregnancy is less in patients with renal transplant than those with lung or heart transplant.

Other organ transplantation

Pancreas

The first pancreas transplants were performed in humans in 1966 [38]. Whole or segmental pancreas transplantation is now a treatment option for certain patients with insulin-dependent diabetes mellitus. Based on the international pancreas transplant registry from 1998 to 2000, 1-year survival rate is greater than 95%. Graft survival rates vary depending on treatment and were 95% when pancreas and kidney were transplanted simultaneously, 74% when pancreas was transplanted after kidney transplantation, and 76% when pancreas alone was transplanted. The 10-year probability of insulin independence is about 90% if the patient has a functioning graft at 5 years [39]. Findings of pancreatic rejection are pain at the graft site, elevated serum amylase, hyperglycemia, and histologic evidence. Most cases of pancreas transplantation are performed in patients who already have or will receive a kidney allograft at the same time as they receive the pancreas. Since many issues are the same, antepartum and intrapartum management is similar to kidney transplant patients. However, the diabetogenic effects of pregnancy, corticosteroids, cyclosporine and other immunosuppressive drugs can all aggravate hyperglycemia, macrosomia and other sequelae in pancreas transplant patients. Euglycemia should be achieved preconception, and glucose tolerance testing (GTT) is warranted prior to 20 weeks, particularly in patients who receive a segmental graft. If hypoglycemia is present, diet and insulin therapy should be instituted at that time. If the GTT screen is normal, it should be repeated at 24–28 weeks as with any pregnant patient. In reality, most pancreas transplant patients will maintain euglycemia throughout pregnancy and labor [40]. Nevertheless, complications characteristic of diabetes have occurred in these patients including osteoporosis, fractures, diabetic neuropathy, chronic vascular insufficiency, maternal death, stillbirth, neonatal hypocalcemia and hypoglycemia [24].

Liver

Improvements in immunosuppressant drug therapy and surgical techniques have resulted in longer life expectancy and many pregnancies in women with liver allografts. Currently, 11% of all patients receiving liver transplants are women of reproductive age, and an additional 15% are younger patients who will survive to and beyond the childbearing age [41]. As in renal transplant patients, conception can be attempted approximately 2 years following liver allograft placement if the patient has a stable immunosuppressive regimen and no signs of liver rejection [42]. Clinical signs suggesting liver rejection are fever, right upper quadrant pain, leukocytosis, elevated serum bilirubin and amniotransferase levels. Because these tests are non-specific, suspected graft rejection requires biopsy confirmation. Most rejection episodes can be managed by adjustments in the drug regimen. Maternal complications have included elevated liver function tests, rejection, recurrent hepatitis, decreased renal function, urinary tract infection, adrenal insufficiency, and endometritis [22,41,43]. There are also increased rates of fetal growth restriction, pre-eclampsia, premature rupture of membranes, preterm birth, cesarean delivery, and neonatal infection (Table 46.4). These complications are in part dependent on maternal health before pregnancy and the immunosuppressive regimen employed. Management of these pregnancy complications is similar to those in renal transplant patients.

Table 46.4 Representative pregnancy outcome in organ allograft recipients reported to the NTPR.[37]

	Graft rejection	Graft loss	Pre-eclampsia	Live born	Mean GA (weeks)	Mean BW (grams)	Newborn complications	Neonatal deaths
Kidney	2–4%	4–13%	30%	75%	36	2439	48%	<1%
Liver	8%	7%	35%	73%	37	2705	29%	0%
Heart	21%	0%	10%	69%	37	2717	22%	0%
Pancreas	6%	16%	34%	79%	34	2096	57%	2%
Lung	27%	21%	13%	53%	35	2285	75%	0%

It is also important to note that, although pregnancy does not increase the risk of maternal mortality in liver transplant recipients, there are implications for these patients related to long-term survival and ability to care for children. In one reported series of women undergoing liver transplantation from 1992 to 2002, five of 29 patients died between 10 and 54 months postpartum [42].

Heart

The first successful pregnancy in a cardiac transplant patient was reported in 1988 [44]. Since then, more than 5000 women in North America have undergone heart transplants at a current rate of more than 500 per year. In the past, patients with a history of cardiac transplantation have been dissuaded from pregnancy by physicians. This is, in part, related to the risks to the prospective mother. In addition, one must consider long-term survival and implications for child rearing. However, many pregnancies have been managed successfully following cardiac transplantation.

There are many cardiovascular changes that occur during pregnancy and the transplanted denervated heart must adapt to the physiologic changes. Arrhythmias may be present and the deneravated heart may not respond to some vasopressors in a predictable way. Only direct-acting vasoactive drugs will have an effect, and the transplanted heart may be more sensitive to β-adrenergic agonists due to an increase in β-receptors [45]. One-third of patients have tricuspid regurgitation 1 year post transplant, and it may worsen with the increased blood volume associated with pregnancy. Almost one-third of cardiac transplant patients have atherosclerotic coronary vessel stenosis by 3 years after the transplant and up to 50% have atherosclerosis at 5 years [46]. Chest pain from myocardial ischemia will not be present since there is no afferent innervation, and paroxysmal dyspnea may be the only presenting symptom.

Many signs and symptoms observed in normal pregnancies, including fatigue, dyspnea, and peripheral edema, may be confusing in heart transplant recipients. However, many women have had heart transplants for peripartum cardiomyopathy which has not recurred with subsequent pregnancies [47]. The incidence of acute graft rejection is not increased during pregnancy. Maternal graft rejections episodes occur in 20–30% of pregnancies, but most are not clinically evident and are diagnosed by routine surveillance biopsies. Surveillance endomyocardial biopsies are performed most frequently in the first 3–6 months after transplantation. Endomyocardial biopsies are generally performed in a specialized facility, with access obtained through the right internal jugular vein or, less commonly, through a femoral vein. A specialized cardiac bioptome is then guided into the superior vena cava and through the right atrium and tricuspid valve into the right ventricle using fluoroscopy or occasionally echocardiography [48]. Biopsy specimens are taken from the right ventricle. Rejection episodes are usually successfully managed by increasing the immunosuppression regimen.

The increased incidence of hypertension, pre-eclampsia, prematurity and low birth weights are similar to that for other transplant patients [24,49,50]. It is well to utilize a multidisciplinary approach for care of these patients. Particular attention should address the involvement of an anesthesiologist during late second trimester to formulate a well-organized plan for labor and delivery. An important intrapartum consideration is the denervated heart's increased sensitivity to hypovolemia and catecholamines. Cesarean delivery in these patients should be performed for usual obstetric indications. Antibiotic prophylaxis for subacute bacterial endocarditis is recommended [51]. Opiates can be used to relieve pain and anxiety. Lumbar epidural anesthesia, for either vaginal or cesarean delivery, is effective in controlling pain and lowering pain-induced elevations of sympathetic activity [52]. It is also important to remember that these patients remain at significant risk postpartum secondary to increases in maternal blood volume. Careful attention to cardiac function and maternal immunosuppressive blood levels is crucial to good care [53].

Lung

In North America, there are approximately 30 female heart–lung transplant procedures annually. The most frequent indications are congenital heart disease with Eisenmenger's syndrome, primary pulmonary hypertension and less commonly, cystic fibrosis and emphysema. The 1-year survival rate for heart–lung recipients is 63% and this decreases to approximately 40% at 5 years [50]. There are few cases of pregnancy following heart–lung transplantation in the literature [24,54–56]. In addition to the management issues related to heart transplant patients, there are specific issues to be considered in the heart–lung transplant recipient. Diagnosing chronic rejection of the lung allograft may be challenging, but one of the first symptoms can be a mild cough with subsequent deterioration in pulmonary function. Very little is known about the changes that occur in the gravid heart–lung recipient. During the transplant, there is a loss of pulmonary innervation, bronchial arterial supply and pulmonary lymphatics. The denervation leads to compromise of the cough reflex and difficulty protecting the airway. Decreased lung compliance may result in a persistent alveolar–arterial oxygen gradient. Pulmonary edema is a definite possibility in these patients, and excess intravenous hydration should be avoided. Two patients have died postpartum from complications of obliterative bronchiolitis [56].

Bone marrow

The use of stem cell transplantation for women of childbearing age with leukemia and other malignant and non-malignant hematologic disorders has increased steadily for the past 20 years. Pretransplant conditioning protocols include alkylating agents and irradiation which can cause germ cell injury, ovarian failure and infertility, but many normal children have been born to women after bone marrow transplantation (BMT).

Clinically significant acute graft-versus-host disease (GVHD) occurs in 9–50% of patients who receive an allogenic stem cell transplant. Immunosuppressive agents, such as methotrexate, cyclosporine, tacrolimus, corticosteroids, or antithymocyte globulin are used for prophylaxis in an attempt to prevent GVHD. The skin, liver, gastrointestinal tract, and the hematopoietic system are the organs typically targeted. Diagnosis of acute GVHD can be established clinically in a patient presenting with a classic rash, abdominal cramps with diarrhea, and a rising serum bilirubin concentration [59]. Histologic confirmation, by biopsy of skin or GI tract, can also be useful. In a patient with acute GVHD, the first and most effective treatment option is the use of corticosteroids with the most commonly used corticosteroid being methylprednisolone [60].

As with solid organ transplant recipients, infection is a potentially important contributor to maternal morbidity and mortality. Immediately following engraftment (3 weeks to 3 months after transplant), risks include bacterial (listeria and legionella), fungal and viral (CMV, human herpetic viruses and enteric and respiratory viruses) infections. Parasitic infections and mycobacteria are also a concern. Following this time period, infectious complications can be present as well. Encapsulated bacteria (*Streptococcus pneumoniae*, *Haemophilus influenzae*, *Neisseria meningitidis*) [61,62], staphylococci and Gram-negative bacteria, such as *Pseudomonas* pose the greatest risk to these patients as do viral infections resulting from varicella zoster and Epstein–Barr [63]. In addition, there is concern for loss of immunity acquired early in life to diseases such as measles and environmental exposures. Because of the concern for infectious risk, all pregnant patients with a history of BMT with a fever should be treated empirically with broad-spectrum antibiotics and evaluated carefully for source of infection.

Miscarriage, pre-eclampsia, IUGR, and preterm birth are the most frequent complications in patients with a history of BMT and pregnancy, but most have had relatively uncomplicated pregnancies and deliveries [57,58,64]. One study evaluated pregnancy outcome among 113 women after stem cell transplant and found that 85% of pregnancies resulted in live births. Less than 1% of the pregnancies had an anomalous fetus; a rate similar to that of the general population. There was an increased risk for cesarean delivery, preterm delivery and low birth weight infant in those patients with a history of stem cell transplant [58,64].

Labor and delivery

The timing of delivery is often dictated by events such as premature labor, premature ruptured membranes, or severe pre-eclampsia. The extraperitoneal location of the transplanted kidney in the iliac fossa usually does not interfere with vaginal delivery. Obstructed labor from soft tissue dystocia due to the graft or pelvic osteodystrophy is very rare. If the fetal head is not engaged in the pelvis during labor, dystocia can be assessed by ultrasound and CT scan of the pelvis. There are no particular contraindications to induction, labor or vaginal delivery in organ graft recipients. Because of an increased susceptibility to infection, vaginal examinations should be kept to a minimum and artificial rupture of membranes and internal monitoring performed only when specifically indicated. Cultures and antibiotics are warranted with the earliest sign of infection.

Delivery by cesarean is based on accepted obstetric indications. Operative deliveries in these patients are managed with prophylactic antibiotics and additional glucocorticoids, and require strict asepsis, careful attention to hemostasis and good surgical technique. A lower midline vertical incision provides the greatest exposure and avoids the region of the transplanted kidney. A low transverse uterine incision is almost always possible, but the obstetrician should be aware of the anatomic alterations associated with the transplanted kidney to avoid inadvertent damage to the blood supply or urinary drainage.

Obstetric emergencies

Acute emergencies may arise in transplant patients during pregnancy with severe consequences that require aggressive management and intensive care. These patients are best managed in a tertiary setting where the transplant surgeon, obstetrician, nephrologists and other subspecialists and intensivists can work together. Most difficult is severe and chronic rejection or allograft vasculopathy with loss of graft function which threatens the life of the mother and fetus. In some cases, patients have deliberately stopped their immunosuppression drugs resulting in acute rejection episodes and even death [47,65]. Renal allograft patients with deteriorating function may have to be placed back on dialysis therapy for the remainder of the pregnancy, and other organ recipients need a variety of supportive measures or including re-transplantation. Sepsis and overwhelming infections are also a constant threat in these women, and patients have died of meningitis, pneumonia, gastroenteritis, hepatitis C and B and AIDS [24,47]. With the high incidence of hypertension and pre-eclampsia, it is not surprising the HELLP syndrome, stroke and eclampsia have occurred [3,24]. Other causes of morbidity that have required emergent surgery include rupture of renal vessel anastomosis, mechanical obstruction of the ureter, antepartum bleeding, uterine rupture, small bowel injury at cesarean delivery, severe postpartum hemorrhage, abdominal wound dehiscence, and pelvic abscess [3,24].

The baby

All immunosuppressive drugs cross the placental barrier and diffuse into the fetal circulation. Again, because there is no convincing evidence that prednisone, azathioprine, cyclosporine or tacrolimus produce congenital abnormalities in the human fetus, they are the drugs of choice during pregnancy. Other than fetal growth restriction and preterm birth, most offspring born to these mothers have had relatively uncomplicated neonatal courses. Mothers are usually empirically advised against breastfeeding since the immunosuppressive drugs are detected in breast milk [3]. However, the dosage delivered to the infant is generally small. If a woman decides to breastfeed, she should understand there is limited information available to make this decision.

Most neonates have progressed normally through childhood [46,47]. Concerns have recently been raised about the possibility of delayed adverse effects in adulthood such as the later development of fertility problems, autoimmune disease and neoplasia [47–49]. Thus, it is important that all offspring exposed to these agents have long-term follow-up.

References

1 Murray JE, Reid DE, Harrison JH, Merrill JP. Successful pregnancies after human renal transplantation. *N Engl J Med* 1963; 269: 341–343.

2 Alston PK, Kuller JA, McMahon MJ. Pregnancy in transplant recipients. *Obstet Gynecol Surv* 2001; 56(5): 289–295.

3 Norton PA, Scott JR. Gynecologic and obstetric problems in renal allograft recipients. In: Buchsbaum H, Schmidt J, eds. *Gynecologic and Obstetric Urology*, 3rd edn. Philadelphia: WB Saunders, 1993: 657–674.

4 Scott JR. Pregnancy in transplant recipients. In: Coulam CB, Faulk WP, McIntyre JA, eds. *Immunology and Obstetrics*. New York: WW Norton, 1992: 640–644.

5 McKay DB, Josephson MA. Pregnancy in recipients of solid organs – effects on mother and child. *N Engl J Med* 2006; 354(12): 1281–1293.

6 Davison JM. Towards long-term graft survival in renal transplantation: pregnancy. *Nephrol Dial Transplant* 1995; 10(Suppl 1): 85–89.

7 Kasiske BL, Vazquez MA, Harmon WE, et al. Recommendations for the outpatient surveillance of renal transplant recipients. American Society of Transplantation. *J Am Soc Nephrol* 2000; 11(Suppl 15): S1–86.

8 American College of Obstetricians and Gynecologists. Perinatal viral and parasitic infections. ACOG Practice Bulletin No. 20. *Int J Gynaecol Obstet* 2002; 76(1): 95–107.

9 Brent L. The discovery of immunologic tolerance. *Hum Immunol* 1997; 52(2): 75–81.

10 Levitz M, Jansen V, Dancis J. The transfer and metabolism of corticosteroids in the perfused human placenta. *Am J Obstet Gynecol* 1978; 132(4): 363–366.

11 Scott JR. Fetal growth retardation associated with maternal administration of immunosuppressive drugs. *Am J Obstet Gynecol* 1977; 128(6): 668–676.

12 Baud O, Zupan V, Lacaze-Masmonteil T, Dehan M. Neurological adverse effects of early postnatal dexamethasone in very preterm infants. *Arch Dis Child Fetal Neonatal Ed* 1999; 80(2): F159.

13 Ballard PL, Ballard RA. Scientific basis and therapeutic regimens for use of antenatal glucocorticoids. *Am J Obstet Gynecol* 1995; 173(1): 254–262.

14 Cowchock FS, Reece EA, Balaban D, Branch DW, Plouffe L. Repeated fetal losses associated with antiphospholipid antibodies: a collaborative randomized trial comparing prednisone with low-dose heparin treatment. *Am J Obstet Gynecol* 1992; 166(5): 1318–1323.

15 Abbasi S, Hirsch D, Davis J, et al. Effect of single versus multiple courses of antenatal corticosteroids on maternal and neonatal outcome. *Am J Obstet Gynecol* 2000; 182(5): 1243–1249.

16 Esplin MS, Fausett M, Smith S. Multiple courses of antenatal steroids are associated with a delay in long term psychomotor development in children with birth weights <1500 grams. *Am J Obstet Gynecol* 2000; 182: 524.

17 National Institutes of Health. *Antenatal Corticosteroids Revisited: Repeat Courses*. NIH Consensus Statement. Bethesda, MD: National Institutes of Health, 2000; 17: 1–18.

18 Saarikoski S, Seppala M. Immunosuppression during pregnancy: transmission of azathioprine and its metabolites from the mother to the fetus. *Am J Obstet Gynecol* 1973; 115(8): 1100–1106.

19 Penn I, Makowski EL, Harris P. Parenthood following renal transplantation. *Kidney Int* 1980; 18(2): 221–233.

20 Registration Committee of the European Dialysis and Transplant Association. Successful pregnancies in women treated by dialysis and kidney transplantation. *Br J Obstet Gynaecol* 1980; 87: 839–845.

21 Rizzoni G, Ehrich JH, Broyer M, et al. Successful pregnancies in women on renal replacement therapy: report from the EDTA Registry. *Nephrol Dial Transplant* 1992; 7(4): 279–287.

22 Armenti VT, Moritz MJ, Radomski JS, et al. Pregnancy and transplantation. *Graft* 2000; 3: 59–63.

23 Davison JM, Dellagrammatikas H, Parkin JM. Maternal azathioprine therapy and depressed haemopoiesis in the babies of renal allograft patients. *Br J Obstet Gynaecol* 1985; 92(3): 233–239.

24 Bumgardner GL, Matas AJ. Transplantation and pregnancy. *Transplant Rev* 1992; 6: 139–162.

25 Miller J, Mendez R, Pirsch JD, Jensik SC. Safety and efficacy of tacrolimus in combination with mycophenolate mofetil (MMF) in cadaveric renal transplant recipients. FK506/MMF dose ranging kidney transplant study group. *Transplantation* 2000; 69: 875–880.

26 Pirsch JD, Miller J, Deierhoi MH, Vincenti F, Filo RS. A comparison of tacrolimus (FK506) and cyclosporine for immunosuppression after cadaveric renal transplantation. FK506 Kidney Transplant Study Group. *Transplantation* 1997; 63(7): 977–983.

27 Winkler ME, Niesert S, Ringe B, Pichlmayr R. Successful pregnancy in a patient after liver transplantation maintained on FK 506. *Transplantation* 1993; 56(6): 1589–1590.

28 Le Ray C, Coulomb A, Elefant E, Frydman R, Audibert F. Mycophenolate mofetil in pregnancy after renal transplantation: a case of major fetal malformations. *Obstet Gynecol* 2004; 103(5 Pt 2): 1091–1094.

29 Armenti VT, Radomski JS, Moritz MJ, et al. Report from the National Transplantation Pregnancy Registry (NTPR): outcomes of pregnancy after transplantation. *Clin Transpl* 2002; 121–130.

30 Lau RJ, Scott JR. Pregnancy following renal transplantation. *Clin Obstet Gynecol* 1985; 28(2): 339–350.

31 Scott JR. Development of children born to mothers with connective tissue diseases. *Lupus* 2002; 11(10): 655–660.

32 32Classen BJ, Shevach EM. Evidence that cyclosporine treatment during pregnancy predisposes offspring to develop autoantibodies. *Transplantation* 1991; 51: 1052–1057.

33 Willis FR, Findlay CA, Gorrie MJ, Watson MA, Wilkinson AG, Beattie TJ. Children of renal transplant recipient mothers. *J Paediatr Child Health* 2000; 36(3): 230–235.

34 Scott JR, Branch DW, Holman J. Autoimmune and pregnancy complications in the daughter of a kidney transplant patient. *Transplantation* 2002; 73(5): 815–816.

35 Scott JR, Branch DW, Kochenour NK, Larkin RM. The effect of repeated pregnancies on renal allograft function. *Transplantation* 1986; 42: 694–695.

36 First MR, Combs CA, Weiskittel P, Miodovnik M. Lack of effect of pregnancy on renal allograft survival or function. *Transplantation* 1995; 59(4): 472–476.

37 Armenti VT, Radomski JS, Moritz MJ, et al. Report from the National Transplantation Pregnancy Registry (NTPR): outcomes of pregnancy after transplantation. *Clin Transpl* 2004; 103–114.
38 Kelly WD, Lillehei RC, Merkel FK, Idezuki Y, Goetz FC. Allotransplantation of the pancreas and duodenum along with the kidney in diabetic nephropathy. *Surgery* 1967; 61(6): 827–837.
39 Sutherland DE, Gruessner A. Long-term function (>5 years) of pancreas grafts from the International Pancreas Transplant Registry database. *Transplant Proc* 1995; 27(6): 2977–2980.
40 Barrou BM, Gruessner AC, Sutherland DE, Gruessner RW. Pregnancy after pancreas transplantation in the cyclosporine era: report from the International Pancreas Transplant Registry. *Transplantation* 1998; 65(4): 524–527.
41 Casele HL, Laifer SA. Pregnancy after liver transplantation. *Semin Perinatol* 1998; 22(2): 149–155.
42 Nagy S, Bush MC, Berkowitz R, Fishbein TM, Gomez-Lobo V. Pregnancy outcome in liver transplant recipients. *Obstet Gynecol* 2003; 102(1): 121–128.
43 Armenti VT, Radomski JS, Moritz MJ, Philips LZ, McGrory CH, Coscia LA. Report from the National Transplantation Pregnancy Registry (NTPR): outcomes of pregnancy after transplantation. *Clin Transpl* 2000; 123–134.
44 Lowenstein BR, Vain NW, Perrone SV, Wright DR, Boullon FJ, Favaloro RG. Successful pregnancy and vaginal delivery after heart transplantation. *Am J Obstet Gynecol* 1988; 158(3 Pt 1): 589–590.
45 Camann WR, Goldman GA, Johnson MD, Moore J, Greene M. Cesarean delivery in a patient with a transplanted heart. *Anesthesiology* 1989; 71(4): 618–620.
46 Uretsky BF, Murali S, Reddy PS, et al. Development of coronary artery disease in cardiac transplant patients receiving immunosuppressive therapy with cyclosporine and prednisone. *Circulation* 1987; 76(4): 827–834.
47 Scott JR, Wagoner LE, Olsen SL, Taylor DO, Renlund DG. Pregnancy in heart transplant recipients: management and outcome. *Obstet Gynecol* 1993; 82(3): 324–327.
48 Kim KM, Sukhani R, Slogoff S, Tomich PG. Central hemodynamic changes associated with pregnancy in a long-term cardiac transplant recipient. *Am J Obstet Gynecol* 1996; 174(5): 1651–1653.
49 Wagoner LE, Taylor DO, Olsen SL, et al. Immunosuppressive therapy, management, and outcome of heart transplant recipients during pregnancy. *J Heart Lung Transplant* 1993; 12(6 Pt 1): 993–999; discussion 1000.
50 Branch KR, Wagoner LE, McGrory CH, et al. Risks of subsequent pregnancies on mother and newborn in female heart transplant recipients. *J Heart Lung Transplant* 1998; 17(7): 698–702.
51 Durack DT. Prevention of infective endocarditis. *N Engl J Med* 1995; 332: 38.
52 Kim KM, Sukhani R, Slogoff S, Tomich PG. Central hemodynamic changes associated with pregnancy in a long-term cardiac transplant recipient. *Am J Obstet Gynecol* 1996; 174(5): 1651–1653.
53 Mendelson MA. Pregnancy after cardiac transplantation. In: Gleicher N, ed. *Principles and Practice of Medical Therapy in Pregnancy*, 2nd edn. Norwalk, CT: Appleton and Lange, 1992: 841.
54 Parry D, Hextall A, Banner N, Robinson V, Yacoub M. Pregnancy following lung transplantation. *Transplant Proc* 1997; 29(1–2): 629.
55 Troche V, Ville Y, Fernandez H. Pregnancy after heart or heart-lung transplantation: a series of 10 pregnancies. *Br J Obstet Gynaecol* 1998; 105(4): 454–458.
56 Rigg CD, Bythell VE, Bryson MR, Halshaw J, Davidson JM. Caesarean section in patients with heart-lung transplants: a report of three cases and review. *Int J Obstet Anesth* 2000; 9(2): 125–132.
57 Sanders JE, Hawley J, Levy W, et al. Pregnancies following high-dose cyclophosphamide with or without high-dose busulfan or total-body irradiation and bone marrow transplantation. *Blood* 1996; 87(7): 3045–3052.
58 Salooja N, Szydlo RM, Socie G, et al. Pregnancy outcomes after peripheral blood or bone marrow transplantation: a retrospective survey. *Lancet* 2001; 358(9278): 271–276.
59 Firoz BF, Lee SJ, Nghiem P, Qureshi AA. Role of skin biopsy to confirm suspected acute graft-vs-host disease: results of decision analysis. *Arch Dermatol* 2006; 142(2): 175–182.
60 Bacigalupo A, van Lint MT, Frassoni F, et al. High dose bolus methylprednisolone for the treatment of acute graft versus host disease. *Blut* 1983; 46(3): 125–132.
61 Wessels, M, Nevill, T, Ford, K, et al. Late bacteremia after stem cell transplantation: incidence and risk factors analysis. Proceedings of the 25th Annual Meeting of the European Group or Blood and Marrow Transplantation and 15th Meeting of the Nurses Group, March 21–25 1999, Hamburg, Germany.
62 Sheridan JF, Tutschka PJ, Sedmak DD, Copelan EA. Immunoglobulin G subclass deficiency and pneumococcal infection after allogeneic bone marrow transplantation. *Blood* 1990; 75(7): 1583–1586.
63 Kawasaki H, Takayama J, Ohira M. Herpes zoster infection after bone marrow transplantation in children. *J Pediatr* 1996; 128(3): 353–356.
64 Carter A, Robison LL, Francisco L, et al. Prevalence of conception and pregnancy outcomes after hematopoietic cell transplantation: report from the Bone Marrow Transplant Survivor Study. *Bone Marrow Transplant* 2006; 37(11): 1023–1029.
65 Sims CJ. Organ transplantation and immunosuppressive drugs in pregnancy. *Clin Obstet Gynecol* 1991; 34(1): 100–111.

47 Ethics in the Obstetric Critical Care Setting

Fidelma B. Rigby
Department of Obstetrics and Gynecology, MFM Division, MCV Campus of Virginia Commonwealth University, Richmond, VA, USA

Introduction

Ethical issues remain a relevant topic in the obstetric setting. This is especially true when one considers that obstetrics often deal with the care of two or more individuals at any one moment. In essence, ethics is "the determination of what ought to be done, all things considered" [1]. This definition, a form of ethics in action, requires differentiating "what could be done" from "what ought to be done" and calls for special thought regarding nonprofessional factors [1]. Chervenak and McCullough [2] describe medical ethics as the "disciplined study of morality in medicine regarding obligations of physicians and institutions to patients and the obligations of patients." They note that medical ethics calls for examining concrete and clinically applicable accounts of how physicians ought to conduct themselves with patients. Tools for answering ethical dilemmas derive from ethical principles that assist practitioners in interpreting and implementing their general moral obligations to protect and promote the interest of the patient [2].

This chapter first introduces four ethical principles that form the framework for ethical decision-making, i.e. autonomy, nonmaleficence, beneficence, and justice. Boxes 47.1 and 47.2 provide a glossary of ethical terms and review of important legal cases. The doctrine of informed consent and the relative status of the fetus are then examined in relation to the mother. Applications to the critical care setting are then made. Issues involving competency, critically ill patients, and maternal–fetal conflict are addressed. Specific concerns regarding Jehovah's Witness cases are reviewed, and finally letters of condolence are discussed. With the aid of this chapter the reader should have an understanding of how to apply ethical principles to the care of the critically ill obstetric patient.

Critical Care Obstetrics, 5th edition. Edited by M. Belfort, G. Saade, M. Foley, J. Phelan and G. Dildy.

Ethical principles

Four principles frame the values of the underlying common morality in the community formed by the patient–physician relationship: beneficence, non-malficence, patient autonomy and justice. These principles should guide the approach to the patient in medical ethics [3]. Until the 1960s, the Hippocratic tradition served as the basis for medical ethics discussion in the United States [1]. Physicians were expected to be beneficent, thereby promoting patient well-being. Beneficence obligates the physician to act in a manner that produces the greater good for the patient. The coinciding ethical principle of non-maleficence obligated the physician to do no harm [1,3]. The technological advances and cultural change that accompanied the 1960s expanded the framework to include respect for autonomy. This principle emphasizes the decision-making capacity of the competent person [3]. The prior assumption that the physician is the main decision maker came to be shunned as paternalism. The emphasis shifted from the physician making decisions "in the patient's best interests" to the patient's right to self-determination. Patient autonomy rose to the foremost of the ethical principles and tended to overpower other ethical considerations [1]. More recently, limitations on a patient's absolute autonomy have been raised in light of affirmation of the physician's autonomy, consideration for the physician's character, and efforts to protect physicians from compromising their own principles. The final ethical principle which should be considered is justice. Justice is the principle which involves weighing the obligation to the patient with the physician's obligation to society as a whole. Justice obligates the physician to consider the allocation of limited resources in the community [4]. These varied emphases merged into a model of shared decision-making.

Informed consent

The legal right to informed consent is well summarized in Justice Benjamin Cardozo's ruling in the 1914 case of Schloendorff vs Society of New York Hospital: "Every being of adult years and

Box 47.1 Glossary of ethical and legal terminology

Battery Harmful or offensive touching of another person: physicians may commit battery if they operate without patient's consent.
Beneficence The physician's obligation to act in the patient's best interest.
Competence Capacity to understand and appreciate the nature and consequences of one's actions.
Dependent moral status A moral status which is dependent on someone else's actions.
Ethical principles Guidelines for ethical behavior (i.e. beneficence, autonomy, non-maleficence).
Independent moral status Having a moral status in and of one's self.
Justice Consideration of risks and benefits to society as a whole.
Negligence Breach of duty to the patient from which the patient suffers harm.
Non-maleficence The physician's obligation to do no harm.
Paternalism Overriding the patient's wishes to act in a way the physician feels would most benefit the patient.
Respect for autonomy Respect for the patient's wishes and right to self-determination.
Substituted judgment When a surrogate decision makes attempts to determine what a patient would have decided.

Adapted from Chervenak & McCullough [63], Annas & Densberger [10], Pinkerton [44], ACOG Patient Choice, 2004 [62].

sound mind has a right to determine what shall be done with his body, and a surgeon who performs an operation without his patient's consent commits an assault for which he is liable in damages" [5]. The original concept of informed consent centered on the legal doctrine regarding battery: the harmful or offensive touching of another person [6]. This concept of battery for unauthorized surgery applies even if the surgery is appropriately and skillfully done [6]. This point was underscored in the classic case of Mohr vs Williams in which the consent was obtained for surgery on the patient's right ear (Mohr vs Williams, 1905 [87]). However, increased disease was noted in the patient's left ear at the time of surgery. Although appropriate surgery was done on the more severely affected left ear, the courts ruled that the patient had not consented to the surgery and held the physician liable (Mohr vs Williams, as presented in Beauchamp & Childress, 2001 [3]).

The breach of informed consent in today's legal setting is more commonly interpreted as a form of negligence [6]. Negligence involves a breach of duty to the patient from which the patient suffers harm. In the case of informed consent, negligence occurs when the physician has not disclosed a risk of the surgery and this risk occurs, causing harm to the patient. The patient could then claim that she would not have consented to the surgery if the risk had been disclosed.

Exceptions to this concept of informed consent do occur. In an emergency setting, where the patient is incapable of providing informed consent and there is not time to find a proxy decision maker, doctors may provide lifesaving procedures (as long as they do not go against any known beliefs of the patient) [6]. In the case of minors, parental consent is usually needed except when state laws provide for emancipation of minors. Pregnancy is generally one of the conditions that allows minors to consent to procedures on their own behalf. The essence and interpretation of these laws can vary from state to state.

Other exceptions to informed consent occur. One of these rare exceptions may include a waiver of informed consent [7]. In this case, a patient with a serious illness specifically requests that the physician make decisions regarding treatment options the patient does not feel capable of making (such as surgery vs radiation treatment). As Lo points out, self-determination is undermined when reluctant patients are forced to engage in decision-making against their wishes. Shared decision-making is a goal but not an absolute requirement in this particular setting [6]. In fact, accepting the patient's decision to waive her right to decide can be seen as respect for her autonomy to make such decisions [7]. Physicians should be aware that such patients can change their minds and choose to actively participate in a later phase of their therapy [6].

The American College of Obstetrics and Gynecology was among the first specialty societies to establish an ethics committee [1]. The concept of informed consent evolved in the 1970s when the central concern for the medical well-being of the patient evolved to include increasing concern for the autonomy of the patient in making medical decisions [8]. In the 1980s, the concept of shared decision-making evolved [8]. The issue of informed consent is addressed by ACOG in its 2004 document *Informed Consent*. In this document, two main aspects of informed consent are addressed: free consent and comprehension. Free consent is defined as an act that is intentional and voluntary by which the individual is authorized to act in certain ways. For medicine, free consent means the patient freely authorizes a medical intervention [7]. "Consent" implies that no coercion is present. "Free" implies that the person is choosing among alternatives.

The document also emphasizes the element of comprehension, i.e. an awareness and understanding of the information regarding one's care and the possibilities that surround it [7]. The ideal of informed consent works best in a relationship of mutual respect and is best seen as a process, as opposed to a task of getting the patient to sign the consent form. In the critical care setting, decisions are often made under periods of stress with limited time. Special effort must be made to allow the patient (or the designated surrogate) to help in the decision process as much as possible.

Competency

Informed consent presupposes the patient's competency. Competency questions lead to ethical dilemmas when the patient refuses life-sustaining interventions. In Lane vs Candura, a

Box 47.2 Summaries of important medical–legal cases

Informed Consent	
Mohr v. Williams (1904) [87]	Physician was held accountable for operating on opposite ear without consent.
Schloendorff v. Society of New York Hospital (1914) [5]	Judge Cardozo's classic case where patient was not properly informed re nature of surgery.
In the Matter of Karen Quinlan (1976) [12]	Court permitted withdrawal of respirator in first "right to die" case, introduced "substituted judgment" stand and spurred development of ethics committees.
Lane v. Candura (1987) [9]	Case affirmed competency of woman who declined amputation of her gangrenous leg.
Superintendent of Belchertown v. Bouvia (1983) [88]	Court granted right of patient with cerebral palsy to refuse nutrition.
Cruzan v. Missouri Department of Health (1990) [13]	Courts permitted parents to withdraw feeding tube from patient with persistent vegetative state: spurred development of living wills.
Maternal–Fetal Conflict	
Smith v. Brennan (1960) [47]	Court permitted neonate to sue for damages inflicted during gestation.
Jefferson v. Griffer Spalding Hospital Authority (1981) [46]	Court ordered cesarean section for patient with complete previa at term.
Re: Maydun (1986) [49]	Court ordered cesarean after 60 hours of ruptured membranes.
Re: A.C. (1990) [39]	Patient with terminal cancer underwent court-ordered cesarean with subsequent demise of mother and neonate. Appeals Court overturned decision.
Baby Doe v. Mother Doe (1999) [43]	Court declined to order cesarean section for placental insufficiency, citing re: A.C. as precedent Supreme Court Case.
Rowland Case (2004) [55]	Pregnant woman charged in stillborn birth of one twin. She accepted plea bargain for child endangerment charge.
Supreme Court Cases	
Roe v. Wade (1973) [38]	Landmark decision permitting abortion in first trimester with regulation in second and third trimesters.
Calauttiv v. Franklin (1979) [45]	Supreme Court invalidated statute that required post- viability termination using least destructive techniques.
Webster v. Reproductive Health Services (1989) [50]	Court permitted ultrasounds of fetus above 20 weeks undergoing termination.
Planned Parenthood v. Casey (1992) [51]	Court permitted restrictions on abortions after viability.
Jehovah's Witness	
Raleigh-Fitkin (1964) [77]	Court gave permission for forced transfusion of pregnant woman but she left hospital before transfusion.
Georgetown Hospital Case (1964) [80]	Court ordered transfusion to prevent abandonment of young child.
Application of Jamaica Hospital (1985) [79]	Court ordered transfusion at 18 weeks gestation in pregnant women with esophageal varices.

77-year-old widow with diabetes refused amputation of a gangrenous lower leg [9]. She was considered competent when she consented to the earlier amputations of her toe and then a portion of her foot. When she initially vacillated and then firmly and repeatedly declined the further amputation, her competency was called into question. Although the lower court ruled against her, the appeals court ruled in her favor, stating, "Mrs. Candura's decision may be regarded by most as unfortunate but … it is not the uninformed decision of a person incapable of appreciating the nature and consequence of her act." (Lane vs Candura in Annas, 1984 [10]). Thus the mere fact that she was declining a life-saving operation did not in itself make her incompetent.

Ethical guidelines must allow for decision-making to proceed when the patient is judged to be incompetent. The Karen Quinlan case in 1976 was pivotal in the evolution of the substituted judgment standard in these cases. Karen Quinlan was a 22-year-old woman in a persistent vegetative state. She was initially intubated and placed on a respirator using consent to treatment implied by the emergency doctrine [11]. As the vegetative state continued without hope of recovery, her father petitioned to be named her legal guardian so that he could ask that she be taken off the respirator. The court ruling discussed the right to privacy, which includes a right to decline treatment. The court decided the father could exercise this right on his daughter's behalf. The question that needed to be addressed was, "What would the patient decide if the patient were able to decide?" [12]. Decision-makers for the patient were expected to "render their best judgment" [6]. This expectation became known as the "substituted judgment standard" [6]. The complications surrounding this case spurred the development of ethics committees [6]. This case in particular made clear the limitations of medicine in predicting the outcome of critically ill patients, as Karen Quinlan lived for years after being removed from the respirator [6].

Further evolutions in the ethical and legal response to critically ill patients occurred in the Cruzan, Brophy, and Bouvia cases. Cruzan was a young woman in a persistent vegetative state following a 1983 motor vehicle accident. In 1986, her parents asked that her gastrostomy feeding tube be discontinued because she had previously stated that she "didn't want to live" as a "vegetable" (Cruzan vs Missouri Dept of Health, 1990 [13] as presented in Lo, 2000 [6]). In 1990, the Supreme Court affirmed the Missouri court ruling that states may require life-sustaining interventions in cases where there is no clear convincing evidence that the incompetent patient would refuse such. Many states allow the family to make decisions on the patient's behalf, but the Supreme Court ruled that states could intervene on the patient's behalf to continue life-sustaining measures if there were no clear indications of the patient's preferences [6]. Ironically, the court was repetitioned after more evidence of Cruzan's wishes was discovered. In this phase of the proceedings, the State of Missouri withdrew from the proceedings and Cruzan's attending physician no longer challenged the removal of the feeding tube. The Court then ruled that the tube could be removed (Cruzan vs Missouri Dept of Health adapted from Lo, 2000 [6]). This case was a landmark case involving the refusal of treatment and spurred the development of living wills and advance directive statutes.

The Brophy case in 1986 also confirmed the right for patients' families to allow the removal of feeding tubes in patients in persistent vegetative states [14]. Brophy was a firefighter who fell into a persistent vegetative state following a ruptured aneurysm in 1983. In 1985 his wife petitioned the court to remove his feeding tube, and in 1986 a four to three decision by the Supreme Judicial Court of Massachusetts affirmed that the tube could be removed ([14] adapted from Beauchamp, 2001 [3]).

The Bouvia case presented the judicial system with the issue of removing a feeding tube from a competent patient who was not terminally ill [15]. Elizabeth Bouvia was a 26-year-old woman with cerebral palsy. Her disease left her with only limited use of her right hand such that she could operate an electric wheelchair but could only eat when fed by another person. In 1983 the courts originally upheld the hospital's right to feed her due to the onerous effect her refusal to eat would have had on the staff and other patients [10]. She went to court again 2 years later and lost again. However, this decision was overturned by the appeals court which held "a person of adult years and in sound mind has the right, in the exercise of control over his own body, to determine whether or not to submit to lawful medical treatment … It follows that such a patient has the right to refuse any medical treatment, even that which may save or prolong her life" [15]. Thus the Bouvia case permitted withdrawal of nutrition from a competent patient with a non-terminal illness.

We will consider how these cases and ethical principles should influence our approach to critically ill obstetric patients after first addressing the status of the fetus.

Status of the fetus

One of the special aspects of obstetric medical ethics is that there are two patients involved: the mother and fetus. The status of the fetus can significantly influence the approach to ethical issues surrounding the pregnancy. The debate regarding the moral/legal/political status of the fetus as a person has been going on since antiquity [1]. Many authors have addressed this issue during the last two decades [16–29]). Three main views can be distinguished in much of today's debate regarding fetal status: the fetus never has moral status, has independent moral status, or has dependent moral status.

One view is that the fetus never has moral status. Annas argues that there is no justification for considering forced treatment of pregnant women because the fetus has no independent moral status and maternal autonomy concerns should therefore prevail in any situation [30,31].

Problems with this view have become more evident as knowledge of fetal status and beneficial prenatal fetal interventions have become more common. The expanding ability to treat the fetus has encouraged viewing the issue of the fetus as a patient. The idea of a graded moral status for the fetus has been introduced as a way to relieve this dilemma. Brown and Elkins credit Fletcher with introducing the concept of the fetus as a patient [1,18]. In this 1981 editorial in JAMA, he identified several important ethical dilemmas in the emerging field of fetal therapy. Central to his analysis was the pressure to consider the fetus as a separate entity in that specific interventions were becoming possible on its behalf. Many authors have addressed this issue of fetal status [17–29]).

McCullough and Chervenak have developed a framework to discuss the issue of fetal status by presenting the concepts of independent and dependent moral status of the fetus [32]. They argue that the fetus is a being who can be reliably linked to later "achieving" independent moral status as its development progresses. Knowing when to confer "independent moral status" is the problematic issue. They hold that the fetus does not have subjective interests *per se* due to the immaturity of its central nervous system. Therefore, there can be no autonomy-based obligations to the fetus [32]. They conclude that there are, therefore, no fetal rights in the sense that the fetus itself can "generate" these rights.

This conclusion leads McCullough and Chervenak to propose a dependent moral status for the viable fetus in that viability is the first important step the fetus achieves in progressing towards an independent moral status [32]. The age at which the fetus achieves independent moral status could vary in different countries but in the US it is approximately 24–25 weeks. Viability means that the fetus can begin to have "interests" that deserve to be protected/promoted by obstetric interventions [32]. The potential protection of the fetus, however, can only occur when the pregnant woman presents the fetus to the healthcare team when she seeks prenatal care. To McCullough and Chervenak's viewpoint, the dependent moral status of the fetus obligates the pregnant woman to take reasonable risks to protect the fetus. She is not obligated to take unreasonable risks [32].

According to this view of fetal moral status, the previable fetus has no claim on the pregnant woman or her physician to remain *in utero* because the fetus requires the use of the pregnant woman's body to achieve viability. The fetus needs the pregnant woman to make an autonomous decision in order for the "patient" status to be conferred during the previable period [32]. The pregnant woman has no ethical obligation to present her previable fetus to her physician. If and only if she presents her fetus to the physician for treatment, is the physician then obligated to protect and promote fetal interests. Thus the previable fetus in this view has only dependent moral status [32]. If the mother is undecided regarding her views toward the fetus, McCullough and Chervenak recommend using Pascal's wager (if you are unsure regarding the existence of God then it would make more sense to act as if God exists) and proceeding in ways that promote full fetal benefit (until the mother withholds the status from her fetus). This view of the fetus as having dependent moral status provides a useful framework to look at the issues which confront the physician during dilemmas in critical care obstetric settings.

Practical applications of ethical principles to high-risk obstetrics

Maternal–fetal conflict

Advocates of strong maternal autonomy

One's approach to the issue of maternal–fetal conflict is largely defined by how one approaches the status of the fetus. Strong maternal autonomy advocates such as Annas argue that it is an assumption in Anglo-American law that every competent adult is at liberty to consent or to refuse any proposed medical treatment. This legal right to refuse treatment is viewed by Annas as part of the common law right to self-determination and associated with the constitutional right to privacy [10]. He notes that forcing compliance with medical advice would give the fetus status as a patient which is not correct as the fetus can only be treated (without the mother's consent) by drastically curtailing the mother's liberties [31]. He warns against using an "outcome" approach to judge competency in cases of maternal–fetal conflict wherein the mother's competency comes into question only when her wishes go against the beliefs of her doctors [10]. Annas outlines questions he considers helpful in assessing patient competency.

Can the patient describe:

1 her current medical problem
2 the therapy suggested for the problem
3 the risks associated with the recommended therapy
4 the risks associated with foregoing this therapy
5 the other available therapies and their risks/benefits?

(Adapted from [10])

Annas notes that if the patient is not decisive and treatment is immediately needed to save her life or prevent severe damage, then reasonable treatment can be done as this promotes society's general interest in health. However, if a question persists and non-emergent treatment is indicated, then evaluation of the patient for competency is called for. If the patient is determined incompetent, then a proxy decision-maker must be identified. When psychiatric assistance is needed, it is important to note that psychiatry determines whether the patient is competent to make treatment decisions. The psychiatric evaluation should not play a direct role in determining which treatment to use, but should only be used to determine whether the patient is competent to decide among the different treatment options [10]. Annas argues that the unusual case of a pregnant woman's refusal to consent to an intervention that would benefit her fetus should always be honored. He notes that this may seem callous to the rights of fetuses, but this is the price society should be prepared to pay in order to protect the rights of all competent adults [30].

Other authors also argue for full maternal autonomy for resolving ethical conflicts that arise during pregnancy. Mahowald bases her arguments on four issues: the right to informed consent, the right of bodily integrity, the questionable personhood of the fetus, and the maternal risks in undergoing forced treatments such as cesarean section. Mahowald agrees with Annas that forcing women to undergo any treatment for the sake of the fetus marks women as "unequal citizens" equivalent to "fetal containers" [33]. Rhoden also advocates strong maternal autonomy, noting that there is a "quantum leap in logic" when using the oft-cited Roe vs Wade decision where prohibitions on abortions were allowed when the fetus reached viability. Rhoden notes that there is a marked difference between prohibiting destruction and requiring surgical preservation [34]).

Harris supports strong maternal autonomy and proposes that fetal needs exist only as a projection by a third party (i.e. the physician). This projection can become problematic. It has been estimated that up to one-third of court-ordered interventions use wrong medical judgment [35].

Advocates of fetal rights

In contrast to those who believe the fetus never has moral status, there are advocates of fetal rights. Strong is supportive of fetal rights in maternal–fetal conflict cases. He proposes intervention with treatments that pose insignificant or no health risks to the mother or treatments that would promote her interests in life/health. He advocates interventions that protect fetal life or prevent serious harm to the fetus. He surpasses some other authors in finding supportive compelling reasons to override maternal autonomy. These other reasons include preventing abandonment of dependent children, preserving the ethical integrity of physicians, and promoting the well-being of the community. For instance, he sanctions the transfusion of blood in a Jehovah's Witness at term if the pregnant woman has multiple dependent children and there are no other people to assume care of the children [36,37].

Review of prominent court cases

Background: Roe vs Wade

The groundwork for maternal and fetal rights cases was in many ways laid by the Supreme Court's 1973 decision in Roe v. Wade [38]. Roe vs Wade changes the status assigned to the fetus as the fetus progresses through the three trimesters. In the first trimester, a woman's right to privacy is emphasized. The first-trimester fetus is noted to lack personhood (as defined by the 14th Amendment) and no societal obligations to the fetus are granted. This landmark decision establishes that during the first trimester, no states can interfere with the right of the pregnant woman to have an abortion. In the second trimester, increasing regulation of pregnancy termination is permitted to safeguard the mother's health. In the third trimester, stricter restrictions by the states are permitted to protect the rights of the viable fetus. It is this protective language regarding the third-trimester fetus that has been increasingly used by fetal advocates to justify interventions for the fetus at this stage [34]. The Supreme Court has revisited this issue in several cases since Roe vs Wade.

Cases affirming maternal autonomy

Several cases have settled in favor of maternal autonomy. One of the more celebrated of these cases is the Angela Carder case in 1990 [39]. Angela Carder had developed bone cancer at age 13 but was felt to be in remission when she married at the age of 27 and subsequently became pregnant. When she reached 25 weeks' gestational age, Angela was discovered to have metastases to her lungs and was admitted to the hospital for further work-up. At 26 weeks gestational age, Angela's condition began to deteriorate and she decided that she would undergo chemotherapy with the goal of reaching 28 weeks before delivery might be indicated. However, her condition degenerated rapidly and 1 day later the question of whether the fetus should be delivered earlier was raised (re: AC [39] as noted in Mohaupt & Sharma, 1998 [40]). Her feelings about the pregnancy were noted to be equivocal and the hospital sought a declaratory judgment regarding a caesarean delivery for the fetus. A hearing was convened at the bedside but Angela was not coherent at the time and the judge ruled in favor of proceeding with the cesarean section. A short time later Angela and her attending obstetrician had communications that strongly suggested she did not want the surgery performed (re: AC as noted in Brown, 2001 [41]).

A session was reconvened at the bedside. The attending obstetrician and Angela's family were opposed to the cesarean section. The counsel for the District of Columbia suggested that Angela's current refusal did not change the situation because the court would not have been called in the first place had she consented for the surgery. The judge agreed and reaffirmed his order that the cesarean section be performed. Less than 1 hour later, a three-judge panel heard arguments for a stay of the procedure. Angela's lawyer argued that the surgery would likely end his client's life and that it should not be done without her consent. The lawyer for the fetus argued that fetal concerns should outweigh maternal concerns because the mother was clearly going to die soon, but the fetus had a chance for life. It was argued that the fetus had a better chance of survival than the mother. The three-judge panel denied the request for a stay but reserved the right to file an opinion at a later date. The fetus was delivered via cesarean section and lived just a few hours. Angela died 2 days later without awakening from the surgery. The D.C. Court of Appeals reviewed the case (although the outcome was long decided) and vacated the lower court's decision, arguing that substituted judgment by one of the family members should have been used if Angela's competency was in question. They ruled against the court-ordered cesarean section (re: AC as noted in Brown, 2001 [41] and Adams, 2003 [42]).

A more recent case has also favored maternal autonomy: Baby Doe vs Mother Doe [43]. This case involved a woman at 36 weeks of gestation who was thought to have placental insufficiency so severe that the fetus would die *in utero* or be severely damaged unless it was delivered via cesarean section immediately. The mother expressed her faith in God's healing powers and declined the cesarean section. The attending physician and hospital took the case to the Cook County State Attorney who brought it to court. The Court of Appeal's decision strongly reaffirmed the right of a competent pregnant woman to decline invasive medical treatments. They could find no other case in which any person has an obligation to undergo invasive surgery for the sake of another. The Carder case was cited as a precedent (re: Baby Doe as presented in Pinkerton & Finnerty, 1996 [44]).

The Supreme Court has addressed the maternal versus fetal rights issue several times. In 1979, in Colautti vs Franklin, the Court ruled in favor of maternal rights and invalidated a state statute that had protected the fetus by requiring that post-viability abortions be done in a manner least destructive to the fetus [45]. The statute had required that a more destructive abortion technique was permitted only if it were indispensable to the life of the mother. The Supreme Court ruled that this language was too restrictive (Colautti vs Franklin as reported in Rhoden, 1987 [34]).

Cases affirming fetal rights

Several court cases have granted the fetus or neonate certain rights relative to that of the mother. One of the frequently cited cases is Jefferson vs Griffen [46]). This case involved a woman diagnosed with a complete placenta previa at term. The hospital asked the court for permission to perform a cesarean section and give blood if necessary should the patient present to the hospital. The trial court gave permission for all medical procedures deemed necessary to preserve the life of the unborn child, but the order was only valid if the mother sought admission to Griffen Hospital. The Georgia Department of Human Resources then petitioned the juvenile court for temporary custody of the child. The petition was granted with a ruling that the Georgia Department of Human Resources could give permission for the cesarean section. The Supreme Court of Georgia then ordered Jefferson to undergo a cesarean section due to the state's compelling interest in preserving life after viability. Most accounts of this case note that the patient left the hospital but subsequently delivered successfully via a vaginal delivery [40,44].

The Smith vs Brennan case involved a neonate, but applied to injuries sustained during the gestational period [47]. This case recognized the right of a child after birth to sue for damages for injuries wrongfully inflicted by a third party prior to birth [48]. Some have interpreted this case as a basis for the fetus' legal right to develop without injury. The pertinent section said, "justice requires that the principle be recognized that a child has a legal right to begin life with a sound mind and body." (Smith vs Brennan as noted in Nelson & Milliken, 1988 [48]). Nelson disagrees with this view, noting that the case refers to a child *after* birth who has a right to sue for damages but who had no such rights as a fetus. The wording of the case does explicitly state that this decision applied to an injured, live-born child. The decision makes explicit that it was "immaterial whether before birth the child is considered a person in being" that could have definite legal rights (Smith vs Brennan, 1960 [47] as referenced in Nelson, 1988 [48]).

In the Maydun case, a 19-year-old primagravida at term was transferred to Georgetown University Hospital from an outlying hospital following 48 hours of labor with ruptured membranes and failure to progress [49]. She insisted upon a vaginal delivery. She was observed until the duration of ruptured membranes reached 60 hours, at which time a cesarean section was again recommended. The patient and her husband declined the procedure, noting that they understood the infection risk to the fetus and that as a Muslim woman she had the right to determine if a risk to her fetus warranted the risk to her own health from the cesarean section. The hospital then requested from the courts a sanction to allow delivery by cesarean section. The court ruled that, while a competent adult does have the right to refuse treatment on religious grounds, the state has a compelling interest to ensure the health of the viable fetus. The court ruled that parents do not have the right to make a martyr of the unborn child and ordered the hospital to take medically necessary steps, including a cesarean if needed (in re: Maydun as presented in Pinkerton & Finnerty, 1996 [44]).

The Supreme Court has also had several post-Roe-vs-Wade rulings that have supported fetal rights. In 1989, the Court decided in Webster vs Reproductive Health Services that a Missouri statute was constitutional [50]. This law required ultrasound, prior to termination, for gestations of at least 20 weeks. The statute was deemed constitutional because the Roe vs Wade decision affirmed the state's interest in protecting potential human life after a certain gestational age. To justify this interpretation, the Court had to modify the first-, second-, and third-trimester framework of Roe vs Wade in order to permit testing as early as 20 weeks [40]. In 1992 the Court again took up the abortion issue in Planned Parenthood v. Casey ([51] as reported in Lo, 2000 [6]). In this case, the court affirmed that states may ban abortions after viability has been reached as long as there are exceptions to protect the life and health of the mother and there are not excessive restrictions placed prior to viability. For example, if the state has parental notification laws, then judicial reviews for juveniles must be made available ([51] as reported in Lo, 2000 [6]). Thus the Supreme Court has both affirmed maternal autonomy, particularly in clearly previable fetuses, and has granted restrictions on the practice of abortion, especially as the fetus nears viability.

More recently there have been several court cases which appear to curtail a pregnant woman's right to complete autonomy. Most notable among these is the case of Melissa Rowland. Ms. Rowland was a 28-year-old woman who was reportedly mentally ill and had been brought to Utah by a Florida adoption agency. She was pregnant with twins and was to give the babies up for adoption [52]. She had six previous children and had had two previous caesarean sections [53]. She was advised to undergo a caesarean section due to concerns regarding the twins' well-being. She initially declined the surgery for several days. When she finally consented to the surgery, one twin was stillborn and the other tested positive for cocaine and alcohol [53,54]. She was charged with homicide but pleaded guilty to the lesser charge of child endangerment. Multiple observers view this case as a dangerous precedent constricting maternal autonomy [52,54,55]. Others view the case as not abrogating her autonomy rights, but holding her responsible for her actions regarding the manner in which she chose to assert her autonomy [56,57].

The most recent ACOG Committee Opinion mentions several other recent cases concerning maternal autonomy. These include the January 2004 case of a woman (with pelvis proven to 11 pounds) who declined a caesarean section for macrosomia. Although the Pennsylvania hospital obtained a court order for a cesarean delivery, she and her husband went to another hospital where a successful vaginal birth occurred [52]. There was also the September 2003 case of a 22-year-old woman who was convicted in Glen Falls, NY after her newborn infant tested positive for alcohol. This was overturned on appeal. Finally, there is the May 1999 case of a South Carolina woman who gave birth to a stillborn infant while using cocaine. She was convicted of homicide and sentenced to 12 years. The South Carolina Supreme Court upheld the conviction, and the US Supreme Court declined to hear it. [52].

Special considerations following case reviews

There are drawbacks to placing an emphasis too strongly on either maternal or fetal rights. This section discusses problems with maternal autonomy and fetal rights viewpoints. A case is then presented in which a seemingly bad outcome (forcibly restraining a woman for cesarean section) ended with a good outcome for both mother and fetus.

Problems with emphasizing maternal autonomy viewpoint

One of the strongest arguments for giving priority to maternal autonomy is the seemingly discriminatory nature of the application of court-ordered interventions for minority women. However, a closer review of the situation highlights concerns about this viewpoint.

Many strong maternal autonomy advocates refer to Kolder's study of the practice of court-ordered interventions [58]. This study of court-ordered cesarean sections noted that 81% of the cases studied involved African American, Hispanic, or Asian women. Of this study population 44% were not married and 24% did not speak English as their first language [58]. Harris suggests that the consideration of forced treatment of pregnant women can be regarded as racism masked as fetal protection [35]. Kolder's study is to be commended as it is the most complete review of the demographics of women in the situation of court-ordered interventions. However, a closer look at the study population also reveals the difficulty in adequately addressing this issue. As Nelson makes clear, Kolder's study only questioned maternal–fetal medicine fellowship heads (preferably in University settings) or (in their absence) residency directors [48]. Although there was an 83% response rate, significant selection bias can be introduced by studying the population in this manner. For instance, there were five states (Alaska, Idaho, Montana, North Dakota, and Wyoming) that were not represented. The patient population of the hospitals studied (preferably university centers or at least those with residency programs) would also have a disproportionate number of minority or non-English-speaking patients. It would be helpful to know if the proportion of patients for whom court-ordered interventions were contemplated differed in general from the patient population in these medical centers. The study is a good first step in quantifying a difficult demographic situation, but the use of its demographics to condemn the practice of seeking court interventions does not take into account the biases that may have been introduced by the types of programs surveyed for this study.

One must also be cautious regarding the "reported" outcomes of the maternal autonomy cases. The Jefferson case is often cited as ending with the safe vaginal delivery of the child. What is not usually presented in this scenario is that the patient voluntarily returned to her original hospital where another ultrasound was obtained several days later. This ultrasound showed the previa was no longer present, and she labored under the care of the original hospital, which had earlier sought a cesarean delivery [59].

When courts decline to intervene, the outcome can sometimes be poor. Elkins reports another case in 1975 where a 27-year-old primagravida was seen by Planned Parenthood and requested pregnancy termination [60]. She was noted to be 30–34 weeks with blood pressures of 180/110 mmHg and was transferred to a tertiary care center. A decision was made the following morning to induce labor. Internal monitoring found no variability with late decelerations. The scalp pH was noted to be 7.09. The patient was advised that her baby needed to be delivered abdominally, but she declined, stating that she did not want the baby. The hospital attorney was unsuccessful in getting any of the three judges he contacted to hear the case. Oxytocin was begun and the fetal heart tracing continued to worsen with severe late decelerations and longer periods of bradycardia. A sister of the patient was summoned to the hospital but was unable to convince the patient to undergo a cesarean section. A second scalp pH was noted to be 6.71. Labor continued and finally a stillborn female infant weighing 2140 g was delivered [60]. Strict adherence to maternal autonomy thus resulted in the death of a viable fetus.

Problems with advocating fetal rights

In contrast, there have been cases where court orders have affected the opposite of their intention. Strong (1991) cites the case of Barbara Jefferies, a 33-year-old Michigan woman with a placenta previa who declined cesarean delivery on religious grounds. The court ordered the police to escort the patient to the hospital but the patient had fled to another state, thereby increasing risks to the mother and fetus. Thus the court order had the opposite of its intended effect.

Forcible restraint with good outcome

There are also cases where severe fetal harm may be avoided with timely court interventions and this outcome was subsequently appreciated by the mother. Elkins reports a case involving a 24-year-old primagravida who presented at 34 weeks with thick meconium [60]. She had recently left another hospital against medical advice because a cesarean section had been recommended. She presented with severe hypertension (160/110 mmHg) and 3 proteinuria. The fetal heart tracing showed no variability, with recurrent late decelerations and episodic severe bradycardia. The patient repeatedly declined all recommendations for cesarean delivery. She was noted to have a flat affect and did not wish to discuss her decision. Her mother noted that her daughter had been in a similar state for several weeks during which she would not communicate with her either. Serial fetal scalp blood sampling was performed which noted progressive acidemia (pH drop from 7.1 to 6.96). After 4 hours, a juvenile court judge was contacted on behalf of the fetus and a court order obtained to proceed with cesarean section. The patient needed to be restrained while general anesthesia was given. A 4-pound male infant was delivered with Apgars of 2, 5, and 7 at 1, 5, and 10 minutes. The postoperative course was uneventful, and the infant did well after an initial period of seizures. After the surgery the patient said she now understood why the surgery was necessary. At 1 year follow-up the patient and her child appeared to be doing well [60].

As the cases above have illustrated, there can be problems with either a strict maternal autonomy or fetal rights viewpoint. Maternal advocates may rely on minority bias and ultimately good outcomes for mother and fetus to help justify their position, but with a closer examination, these factors may be misleading. The maternal advocate's approach can also result in the unnecessary death of a fetus that is viable. On the other hand, a strict adherence to fetal rights can result in unintended consequences such as maternal flight to avoid a court order. The next section critiques viewpoints that address both issues.

Compromise views regarding maternal–fetal conflict

Fortunately, the vast majority of maternal–fetal interactions in the context of a viable fetus do not result in maternal–fetal conflict. However, the potential for scenarios such as those mentioned above does exist, especially in the high-risk setting, and the obstetrician must be prepared to deal with complex ethical situations. Three more balanced responses to maternal–fetal conflict situations should be considered: the ACOG, the American Academy of Pediatrics (AAP), and Chervenak and McCullough. These views are examined in regard to risks to pregnant women, risks to the fetus without the procedure, effect of the procedure on the fetus, and special considerations. The different viewpoints are summarized in Table 47.1.

The APP revised its statement on maternal–fetal conflict in 1999. The new statement requires that the proposed treatment of the mother against her will should be of negligible risk to the health and well-being of the pregnant woman. The treatment should prevent irrevocable and substantial fetal harm and be effective therapy [61].

The most discussion on maternal fetal conflict by ACOG is reflected in its 2005 Committee Opinion "Maternal Decision Making, Ethics and the Law" and its document "Patient Choice in the Maternal-Fetal Relationship" [52,62]. The Committee Opinion asserts that there needs to be high probability the treatment will help or cause minimal harm to the mother. It also requires that there be a high probability of serious harm to the fetus and a high probability that treatment will significantly decrease fetal harm. The statement strongly recommends that an ethics committee be consulted before appealing to a court case. In fact, The Committee on Ethics states "in the absence of extraordinary circumstances, circumstances that, in fact, the Committee on Ethics cannot currently imagine, judicial authority should not be used to implement treatment regimens aimed at protecting the fetus" [52].

The Committee on Ethics also strongly opposes the criminal prosecution of pregnant women whose activities cause harm to their fetuses. It notes three relatively recent cases where pregnant women were (at least initially) successfully prosecuted for using illicit substances which were associated with adverse pregnancy outcomes [52].

Chervenak and McCullough are two authors who deal extensively with maternal–fetal conflict. They present a thorough approach to maternal–fetal conflict that complements the guidelines proposed by ACOG and AAP. Chervenak and McCullough require that: (i) the mortality risk and the risk of disease, injury, or disability to the pregnant woman be reliably low or manageable in order to consider coercing the intervention; and (ii) there be a high probability that the procedure will be life-saving or will prevent serious or irreversible damage to a viable fetus. They expect that the treatment will also reliably have a low mortality or have a manageable risk of serious injury to the fetus [63].

Chervenak and McCullough address the issue of the possible use of court orders in the case of a woman with a well-documented complete placenta previa at term who is demanding to be delivered via the vaginal route. They address the argument that

Table 47.1 Considerations for treatment of fetus without maternal consent.

Reference	Risk to pregnant woman	Risk to fetus without procedure	Effects of procedure on fetus	Special considerations
ACOG, 1999 [85] Committee Opinion	High probability that treatment helps or has very little risk for pregnant woman	High probability of serious harm to fetus	High probability that treatment will significantly decrease fetal harm	Always consult ethics committee before considering legal approach
AAP, 1999 [61] Statement	Negligible risk to health/well-being of pregnant woman	Serious harm	Effective treatment that prevents irrevocable and substantial fetal harm	No less invasive way to help the fetus
Chervenak & McCullough, 1985 [86]	Mortality risk and risk of disease/injury/disability to pregnant woman reliably low or manageable	High probability of saving life or preventing serious and irreversible disease/injury/disability for viable fetus	Treatment reliably has low mortality and low or manageable risk of serious disease/injury/disability to fetus	Do not force pregnant woman but use court order to help persuade
Strong, 1991 [37]	Insignificant or no health risk *or* would promote her health	Serious fetal harm/death	Prevent serious fetal harm	Promote well-being of community. Prevent abandonment of dependent children. Preserve ethical integrity of physician

court-ordered cesarean sections can never be ethically justified. They state that no physician should be justified in accepting a patient's refusal of cesarean section in the case of a complete previa at term because of the unreliability of the patient's clinical judgement. They note that physicians are justified in resisting a patient's exercise of her positive right if the fulfilling of her positive right would contradict the physician's best clinical judgment and negate all beneficence-based interests of the woman and her fetus. A woman does not have a right to make her physician practice medicine that is against the physician's best clinical judgment. They argue that a court-ordered cesarean in this instance does not treat a woman as a "mere instrument" to benefit her fetus, one of Rhoden's claims [34], because in this case the cesarean benefits the woman as well. There is no violation of her autonomy without justification because a pregnant woman who has taken a pregnancy to term has an ethical obligation to accept reasonable risks on behalf of her fetus. An exercise of someone's positive and negative rights can be limited when the exercise of those rights brings certain serious harm to others. They argue that the woman's fear of surgery cannot be used to justify her claim because her claim is an irrational fear and irrational beliefs disable the exercise of autonomy. Even objections on religious grounds can be overcome in that courts have ordered the treatment of pediatric patients over the religious objections of their parents.

Chervenak and McCullough then turn to arguments to justify court intervention in the case of complete previa at term. They note that the use of a state's power to enforce a pregnant woman's beneficence-based obligations to her fetus at term is justified when the net risk to her is non-existent. Maternal autonomy rights are not absolute in this case and can be constrained by the probability of severe, preventable harm to third parties. Judge Belson stated this obligation succinctly in his commentary in the Angela Carder case:

> A woman who carries a child to viability is in fact a member of a unique category of persons. Her circumstances differ fundamentally from those of other potential patients for medical procedures that will aid another person, for example, a potential donor of bone marrow for transplant. This is so because she has undertaken to bear another human being, and has carried an unborn child to viability. Another unique feature of the situation we address arises from the singular nature of the dependence of the unborn child upon the mother ... The expectant mother has placed herself in a special category of person who is bringing another person into existence, and upon whom that other person's life is totally dependent. Also, uniquely, the viable unborn child is literally captive within the mother's body. No other potential beneficiary of a surgical procedure on another person is in that position.
>
> (In re: AC as reported in McCullough & Chervenak, 1994 [32])

As Chervenak and McCullough state, the primary moral relationship of a pregnant woman and her viable fetus is one of obligation as opposed to unrestrained freedom. The analogous relationship is that of a parent to a child rather than a potential organ donor and recipient. Legal issues can also be framed in terms of the legal obligations of parents to their children in terms of child neglect and abuse cases. They conclude that, in cases similar to that of a placenta previa at term, there are cases when ethical and legal court sanctions can be sought for cesarean delivery. Whether physical force can be used to perform the surgery is not clearly defined. They oppose the use of force in this situation if there is no time to obtain a court order, but do not address the issue if the court order is obtained. They also stop short of condoning court orders for cesarean delivery in cases where there is no clear benefit for the mother (i.e. fetal distress cases). Their criteria for intervention include that the mortality risk to the pregnant woman be very low and the risk of injury or handicap be low or manageable. They acknowledge that any attempt to go beyond these criteria faces a "considerable, perhaps daunting, burden of proof" [32].

Suggestions for managing maternal–fetal conflict

The above sections have dealt with court cases and theories regarding how to deal with maternal–fetal conflicts. In their 1996 article, Pinkerton and Finnerty present a logical outline for preparing for and dealing with issues of maternal–fetal conflict by using a proactive team approach that attempts to deal with these issues across departmental lines [44]. This has become the model at the University of Virginia Health Sciences Center. They developed a subcommittee of the hospital ethics committee consisting of representatives of the departments of obstetrics and gynecology, pediatrics, anesthesiology, family medicine, ethics committee, and hospital counsel. All subcommittee members reviewed relevant literature on maternal–fetal conflict, and guidelines were then developed. The guidelines were discussed in the individual departments and finally discussed with the full ethics committee. Many diverse opinions were noted and many revisions occurred over the course of 1 year. The guidelines evolved from being a staunch advocate of full maternal autonomy to including references to some instances where court-mandated interventions could be considered. Separate guidelines were developed for incompetent women. The final consensus was that the courts should be used very rarely and maternal autonomy should prevail in almost all instances [44]. The purpose of the guidelines was to provide a framework to foster communication between the patient and the healthcare team members. Unresolved conflicts could then be mediated by the ethics consultation service. If the conflict remained unresolved then the ethics committee and departmental representatives were available for assistance. Only after these avenues had failed was turning to the courts considered [44].

Although the process of developing these guidelines was long and difficult, the end result was a greater appreciation for the nuances of cases and the judicial decisions surrounding them. This increased awareness should decrease the likelihood of resorting to the courts for assistance. Should a court order a direct intervention, the policy stated that physical force should not be used in its implementation. The court order should rather be used to help persuade the patient to agree to the intervention [44].

A common theme among many authors is the responsibility of ethics committees to help mediate in difficult situations. To do so in a viable manner for high-risk obstetric cases, the ethics committee needs to have members available on an emergency basis. At Louisiana State University Health Sciences Center (LSUHSC) in New Orleans, one member carries a beeper so that response can be immediate if necessary. Also important in this process is an awareness and appreciation for the role of the ethics committee. The more the ethics committee is involved in service to the hospital community (e.g. by sponsoring workshops and lectures), the more people will feel comfortable approaching the committee. It is also important to let patients and their family members know that the committee is available and to allow, if possible, their direct access to its services as well [41].

Moral differences between the healthcare team and the patient do not have to end up in court. Ethics consultations can sometimes have unexpected results. Gill et al. refer to the case of a couple requesting late termination of a Down's pregnancy. The patient underwent amniocentesis at 25 weeks due to a finding of fetal duodenal atresia. The results indicated a trisomy 21 (Down's syndrome) fetus and the parents requested termination. The physician requested an acute clinical ethics service (ACES) consultation. The ACES team met with the obstetrician, social worker and labor ward midwife (the parents supported the process but did not want direct involvement). The ACES team supported the termination of the pregnancy, citing maternal autonomy. However, the ACES team felt this would only work if the mother received further counseling and the labor ward staff agreed to carry out the procedure. The team also recommended involving the hospital's CEO. The CEO recommended a formal psychiatric consultation; that evaluation found that the pregnancy was not a risk to maternal mental health. The CEO further requested that the full Institutional Clinical Ethics Committee meet. No consensus was reached (despite lengthy debate) at the full committee meeting. After input from several sources, the CEO declined to authorize termination of the pregnancy. The couple was advised of this decision which was reached 2 weeks after the initial consultation. The family actually accepted the result and was appreciative of the manner in which their case was handled. In fact, they chose to continue obstetric care and deliver at the same hospital [64].

Issues regarding brain death

Background

Cesarean sections were first used to deliver the living fetus from dead mothers [65,66]. In Greek mythology, Asklepios (the famous Greek physician and Apollo's son) was said to be delivered from his dead mother in this manner [66]. In the fourth century BC Susruta's Samhita recommended cesarean delivery when the woman's life was in great danger or where she had died. Pliny the Elder was said to have been delivered by postmortem cesarean in 23 AD. The Babylonian Talmud recommended opening the abdomen immediately to deliver the child of a mother who died in childbirth. Postmortem cesarean section was practiced in Hellenistic times by Roman authorities and in 17th century Venice [66]. In approximately 700 BC Numa Popilus forbade burial of a pregnant woman before the child was removed. This edict, which may have been used to rescue a live child or allow separate burial of the child, became part of the Roman's King's Law (Lex Regia) which in turn became the Emperor's Law or Lex Caesare, which may be the origin of the term *cesarean*. It is unlikely that Julius Caesar was delivered in this manner because there are references to his mother being alive 40 years later. In 1280 the Council of Cologne required postmortem cesareans to allow for baptism and proper burial of children from mothers who had died [65,66]. Not until approximately 1500 were cesareans performed successfully to save a mother and child. Jacob Nufer, a Swiss sow gelder, accomplished such a delivery [66].

Only in the past century have cesarean sections been used regularly to save both mother and child [65]. Ironically, improvements in the care of critically ill obstetric patients have brought us full circle, making it now possible to contemplate postmortem sections in which the mother has been brain dead for prolonged periods of time. With intensive care, it is possible to prolong fetal maturation in a mother who would otherwise have been declared dead and taken off life support. Rapid evacuation of the uterus (especially after 5 minutes of a full code with no significant response from the mother) is still recommended in mothers with a fetus of significant size impeding blood flow during a code situation.

This section deals with cases of fatally ill women who can be stabilized with life support techniques. In some of these cases, care of the mother with monitoring of the fetus allows for fetal growth. The means for providing a rapid abdominal delivery at the bedside is reviewed (Table 47.2).

There is a significant moral distinction between a rapid postmortem cesarean section and maintaining viability solely for the sake of the fetus. Some would have concerns about using brain-dead mothers as incubators, merely as a means to justify an end. However, the moral value of brain-dead pregnant women can also be viewed as secondary moral status [66]. The brain-dead mother's worth is secondary in that she has symbolic worth and value for others but cannot have actual or potential harm or benefit directly herself [66]. On the other hand, the fetus has real and symbolic value. Its real moral value is based on its potential for being harmed or benefited. The symbolic value can be derived from its role as a symbol of renewal or continuity of life. The concept of "flesh of her flesh" underscores the continuity of her life and could justify the prolonged use of brain-dead mothers to continue fetal life [66]. The embryo can be viewed as having inherent interests, with the discussion focusing on where those interests lie relative to those of the mother. With a brain-dead mother, her interests still exist, but in a secondary status [66]. With technological advances, there comes an increasing probabil-

Table 47.2 Suggested equipment for emergency cesarean in ICU setting.

Maternal equipment	Infant equipment
Surgical drapes	Warmer
Cesarean section instrument tray	Blankets
Suction	Infant identification kit (i.e. ID bands, footprint sheet)
Bovie with grounding pad (optional)	
Gloves/gowns/masks	Blood tubes for cord blood
Sutures	Cord blood gas kit
Laps	Suction/laryngoscope/endotracheal tube
Cord clamps/bulb suction	Neonatal resuscitation medications

ity of success defined as a viable infant who is not severely damaged. However, such cases must still be considered experimental, and therefore the risks and benefits cannot be clearly outlined. Informed consent from the patient's surrogate decision-maker is critical in deciding courses of action [66]. The job of the high-risk pregnancy team is to coordinate the response and give this decision-maker the information required to proceed.

Outcomes regarding brain-damaged pregnant women

In 1982, Dillon and colleagues presented two cases involving brain-dead pregnant women. From these, he concluded that at less than 24 weeks no continued life support be offered; between 24 and 27 weeks intensive support be considered and by 28 weeks delivery be accomplished [65].

Since that time Bush and colleagues have presented a review of the literature involving 11 cases of brain-dead pregnant women and 15 cases of pregnancies in a vegetative state where the decision to continue support was made [67]. In the eleven cases associated with brain death, 46 days on average was gained with an average EGA of 29.7 weeks achieved. In the 15 cases involving vegetative state pregnancies, 124 days on average was obtained. These authors conclude that it is very possible to obtain good outcomes with intensive management, but families need to be aware of the difficult course that can ensue [67].

Decision to maintain support in vegetative state with complicated family dynamics

Webb presented the case of a 24-year-old G1 P 0, who at 12 weeks of gestation in 1995 declared her desire to have an elective termination [68]. At 14 weeks of gestation, she took an overdose of her mother's insulin. The father of the child was unknown. After several days of care there was no significant recovery of brain function. Some family members inquired about the feasibility of an abortion in this setting. They were interested in pursuing this course even if it would not improve the clinical outcome of the patient. The ethics committee was consulted, prompting the patient's mother to have further discussions with other family members. The patient's mother decided not to terminate the pregnancy because she then felt that, had the patient not been depressed, she would not have desired termination. At 16 weeks cerebral imaging showed "toxic injury" and the EEG was "severely abnormal" [68]. She was diagnosed to be in a chronic vegetative state with little chance of recovery. It was decided to withdraw all treatment (except nutrition) and give her DNR status. At 23 weeks, pneumonia was diagnosed and ultrasound showed a normal-size fetus. The ethics committee was reconsulted and met with the obstetric and medical teams and with family members. It was determined that care could be given that would help the fetus as long as there was a chance of a normal outcome. Antibiotics and other medications could be provided. Fetal monitoring was to start at 28 weeks. At 31 weeks late decelerations and vaginal bleeding were noted. An abruption was diagnosed and cesarean section was performed with delivery of a 2240g fetus with Apgars of 4 and 7. The mother died on postoperative day 3. The baby developed bronchopulmonary dysplasia and was discharged from the hospital at 2 months of age. At 5 months the child was noted to be "otherwise apparently well" [68].

Guidelines for management in the severely brain damaged pregnant woman

For any pregnant patient with severe neurological involvement, an attempt to support the fetus while aggressively pursuing maternal diagnosis and prognosis should be done. As noted earlier, the exception to this management is acute anoxia due to maternal cardiac arrest that is unresponsive to immediate resuscitative efforts. In these cases, rapid delivery of the fetus can significantly improve maternal survival [68].

The etiology and extent of the injury as well as its prognosis are necessary before making decisions regarding fetal status [68]. This assessment may take time, as the improvement (or lack thereof) over time may be crucial in determining the extent of injury as well as the prognosis. A team approach is critical in managing these complex medical and ethical cases. It is important for the obstetric team to discuss and agree on plans and options with the consultants before talking with the family. Frequent discussions are needed to keep the family updated. It is also important to keep the nurses and residents updated on changes in the patient's status [68].

When the patient is deemed incapable of consent, a neurologist should be consulted to assess mental status and to determine the patient's state of chronic brain damage (coma, stupor, or chronic vegetative state) (Table 47.3). A commonly used diagnosis of brain death is often the one adopted in 1981 by the President's Commission for the Study of Ethical Problems in Medicine and Biomedical and Behavioral Research [69]. These criteria called for the irreversible cessation of circulatory or respiratory function or the irreversible cessation of all functioning of the brain (including the brain stem). Table 47.4 describes some of the tests used for this determination. Studies that can be useful for documentation of clinical findings include EEG, brainstem evoked potentials, and cerebral blood flow studies [70].

When a patient is deemed incompetent, identify who speaks for the patient. If there is no advance directive, the person who is the next of kin should provide guidance for what decisions the

Table 47.3 States of brain damage.

Stupor	Coma	Chronic vegetative state	Brain death
Patient can be aroused *only* by vigorous or continuous circulatory/respiratory stimulation function	Patient cannot be aroused by any stimulus	Intermediate state Can be initial presentation or can evolve Patient has brain stem function without cerebral function. Has sleep–wake cycles, opens eyes to verbal stimuli, normal respiratory control but no apparent understanding or discrete localizing motor responses	Irreversible cessation of circulatory/respiratory function *or* irreversible cessation of *all* functions of brain, including brain stem (President's Commission for the Study of Ethical Problems in Medicine and Biomedical and Behavioral Research, 1981) [69]

From Webb G, Huddleston J. Management of the pregnant woman who sustains severe brain damage. *Clin Perinatol* 1996; 23: 453–464.

Table 47.4 Brain death criteria and tests.

Need to exclude reversible causes of coma (i.e. drug toxicity, hypothermia)
Allow time for brain to recover function
Cerebral criteria: no clinical response to stimuli
Brain stem criteria:
No response to cranial nerve testing. Absence of reflexes: papillary/corneal/oculocephalic/oculovestibular/oropharyngeal
Apnea test for respiratory function
Studies to help document lack of brain function:
EEG
Brain stem evoked potential study

From Halevy A, Brody B. Brain death: reconciling definitions, criteria and test. Ann Intern Med 1993; 119: 519–525.

patient would have made. The medical team needs to be updated by legal counsel regarding the right-to-die and living will statutes applicable in their state [68]. Many such statutes have pregnancy clauses that change their interpretation during pregnancy [71]. There may also be hospital bylaws addressing these situations. Requesting input from an ethics committee can also be helpful [68].

Assessment of fetal status is also important. Establishment of estimated gestational age by ultrasound and electronic fetal heart rate monitoring should be performed as soon as feasible. Fetal brain function in the older fetus can be indirectly assessed by beat-to-beat variability, accelerations, or biophysical profile. Serial sonography may reveal more regarding developmental brain injury. Intrauterine growth restriction (IUGR) can be a sign of early first- or second-trimester injury. Microcephaly can be due to anoxia and decreased cortical growth can cause enlarged cerebral ventricles. Periventricular leukoencephalopathy can sometimes be seen and MRI can be used to assess the fetal brain [68].

The effort spent in keeping the pregnant woman alive for fetal growth must also be assessed in terms of fetal status. If there is no evidence of fetal harm, then directive counseling for fetal benefit may be appropriate. If evidence of significant fetal injury develops (such as microcephaly or IUGR), then aggressive versus non-aggressive interventions may be recommended [68].

The mother's autonomy, beneficence, and non-maleficence should be balanced. In the brain-dead patient, maternal autonomy concerns remain important (as expressed through maternal proxy) but can be seen as secondary moral claims compared to those of the fetus. One would not wish to violate the tenet of non-maleficence by prolonging maternal death but should also consider beneficence-based claims for the fetus. In the case of first-trimester fetuses or mid-to-late second-trimester fetuses with hard to control maternal conditions, the issue of non-maleficence toward the fetus must be considered. If there is little chance of the fetus reaching viability in a relatively intact state, then the claim of non-maleficence for the fetus may favor withdrawing maternal life support so as to avoid simply postponing fetal death [68]. As the cases above illustrate, it can be relatively easy to manage a fetus in a patient in a chronic vegetative state but much more challenging when more extensive brain damage has occurred. Counseling for the patient's proxy must then take into account the fetal status just after the injury. Subsequent evaluations of the fetus must be conducted. The gestational timing of the injury is important. Informed consent for the patient's proxy is key to any endeavors involving prolonged maternal support as this must still be considered an experimental procedure in many regards [68].

If it is decided to prolong the pregnancy in a mother with significant brain damage, many obstacles lie ahead. Mallampalli et al. outline these challenges well with suggestions for dealing with them. One must be prepared to provide extensive cardiovascular, endocrine, respiratory, temperature regulation, nutritional and infectious disease treatment to allow for a potentially successful outcome [72].

In summary, the first ethical tasks in these cases are to clarify maternal diagnosis and to assess the prognosis for both the mother and the chances for relatively intact survival for the fetus. An appropriate proxy decision-maker must be identified and provided with appropriate information to guide informed consent. Extensive efforts must be made to educate this person and to empathize with the family [68]. Consultation with the ethics committee and legal guidance as to the applicability of living will statutes in pregnancy can also be helpful.

Management of the Jehovah's Witness

Patient

This last section will address treatment of the Jehovah's Witness pregnant patient. The history of this religious faith and the origins of its tenets regarding blood transfusions are reviewed. Important legal cases regarding Jehovah's Witnesses are introduced. Finally, general guidelines for the management of these patients are given.

Background

To properly address the ethical issues which accompany the care of Jehovah's Witness patients, the background of their religion and its tenets regarding blood product transfusion should be understood. Jehovah's Witnesses are a fundamentalist Christian sect founded in Philadelphia in 1884 that emphasizes a literal reading of the Bible [73,74]. There are currently about 2 million worldwide members with half of these in the United States [75]. This religious faith concentrates on prophecies regarding the end of this world and the coming reign of Jehovah. Converts tend to come from the working class and have limited educational background [73]. They are characteristically deeply devout with a great commitment to the tenets of their faith. One of these tenets causing controversy is the refusal to acknowledge the authority of any earthly establishment. Therefore, controversies have arisen in the past regarding not pledging allegiance to the flag or taking oaths of loyalty. They are also conscientious objectors to military service [73].

Prior to 5 July, 1945 there were no explicit prohibitions regarding blood product transfusion. It was on this date that an article in *The Watchtower*, the official journal for Jehovah's Witnesses, forbade the taking of blood into the body. The penalty for doing so would be loss of eternal life in God's Kingdom [74]. The basis for this proclamation was the reviewed interpretations of several Biblical passages (Genesis 9: 3–4, Leviticus 17: 13–14, Acts 15: 19–21). The Christian writing Acts of the Apostles restated the Hebrew scripture's prohibition against eating blood or flesh with blood in it [76]: "And whatsoever man there be among you, that eateth any manner of blood: I will even set my face against that would that eateth blood and will cut him off from amongst his people" (Leviticus 17: 10–14). The first leaders of the newly founded Christian faith meeting in Jerusalem appealed to this prohibition when they instructed non-Jewish converts to observe Jewish law insofar as it required abstinence "from things polluted by idols, from fornication and from what is strangled and from blood" (Acts 15: 19–21 as noted in Jonsen, 1986 [73]). The article in *The Watchtower* forbids the taking of blood into the body by any route: "the issue for Jehovah's Witnesses involves the most fundamental principle on which they as Christians base their lives. Their relationship with their creator and God is at stake" [73]. The Jehovah's Witness who violates this tenet not only jeopardizes his or her eternal future but more immediately risks being "disfellowshipped", excommunication and shunning by family and friends. This risk may be influenced by how vigorously the member resists the transfusion [74]. It is clear that this tenet of faith is definite, absolute, and important to practitioners of this religion [73].

However, several points remain unclear. Why was this tenet expanded to include the routes of intake that were not oral? Why was the proclamation done at this particular time? Who was in charge of the decision for this proclamation? Was it a governing board or an individual? Is it just blood that is forbidden or are certain blood components and organ transplants also forbidden? [73,74]. Can this sin be forgiven? Are they still guilty if they are unconscious and/or it is given against their will? [76]. These issues are not addressed in the tract that Jehovah's Witnesses give to their physicians. Some have even addressed these questions to Church authorities and been given different answers [76].

What constitutes a forbidden product is not entirely clear. Whole blood, packed red blood cells, plasma, and platelets seemed to be banned but the transfusion of albumin, immune serum globulin and antihemophilic preparations, and organ transplants appear to be left to the conscience of the individual member [74]. Even within these guidelines, there appears to be individual variations. For instance, a confidential questionnaire of one Witness congregation noted that some would accept plasma and one person would accept autotransfusion [74].

Despite their reluctance to accept blood component therapy, Jehovah's Witnesses actively seek medical care and have been in the forefront of developing artificial blood components and other pharmacological methods of helping the body increase its blood count (e.g. erythropoietin). There are alternatives that many Witnesses will accept which can lessen the risk of surgeries where a large blood loss is expected. For example, open heart surgery has been successfully performed on Witnesses who underwent extracorporeal dilution of their blood. This technique can be acceptable as long as the blood is always in physical continuity with their circulatory systems. It involves removing a portion of their blood and diluting it with an intravenous solution, then returning it back to their circulatory system. The blood lost at surgery will be more dilute and, volume for volume, the patient will be able to tolerate larger losses of volume during the surgery [74].

Legal cases regarding treatment of Jehovah's Witnesses

The issue of court-ordered transfusions in cases of pregnant Jehovah's Witnesses has been addressed. In Raleigh Fitkin-Paul Morgan Hospital vs Anderson, a woman at 32 weeks' gestation was thought to be at high risk for hemorrhage prior to birth and a transfusion was recommended [77]. She declined on religious grounds because she was a Jehovah's Witness. The issue went to court and the initial trial court upheld her refusal. The hospital then appealed to the New Jersey Supreme Court. By this time, the woman had left the hospital against medical advice. However, the New Jersey Supreme Court determined that the unborn child was "entitled to the law's protection" and that blood could be given "if necessary to save her life or the life of her child, as the physician in charge at the time may determine" ([78], Raleigh Fitkin-Paul Morgan Hospital vs Anderson [77] as described in [75]). This case determined that the First Amendment embodied two freedoms: the freedom to believe and the freedom to act on those beliefs. The court held that only the first of these two concepts is absolute. The second concept in this case is limited by the child's right to live [75]. This case has been criticized for the shortness of the opinion and the fact that the judgment was not enacted because the patient left the hospital [78].

In re: Jamaica Hospital in 1985, the New York Supreme Court addressed the issue of a Jehovah's Witness who was 18 weeks pregnant and bleeding extensively from esophageal varices [79]. The mother refused blood. She was noted to be the single mother of 10 children with her only relative being a sister who was unavailable at the time. The court allowed the transfusion to protect the fetus [37]. It decided that a person does have the right to refuse medical treatment but that the state is permitted (under Roe vs Wade) to interfere with reproductive choices when it has a compelling interest. The court acknowledged that, in the case of a non-viable fetus, the interest is not compelling but rather "significant." This interest was felt to outweigh the patient's right to refuse a blood transfusion and she was ordered to receive blood (re: Jamaica Hospital, 1985 [79] as presented in Mohaupt & Sharma, 1998 [40]).

In the Georgetown Hospital case, the court also ordered a transfusion for a non-pregnant woman who was the sole provider for a 7-month-old child. This decision aimed to prevent child abuse and abandonment (Application of the President and Directors of Georgetown College Hospital [80], as presented in Elkins, 1994 [75]). There have been inconsistent decisions involving patients without dependents or those who are not the sole providers for their children [75]. There have been frequent rulings in favor of intervention for transfusions for the children of Jehovah's Witness against their parents' wishes [75]. The courts have ruled that parents cannot make martyrs of their children [81]. It is now commonplace for court orders for transfusion to be given in the case of children.

There have also been cases of successful lawsuits against physicians who have knowingly transfused Witness patients in emergency settings. In a Canadian case, a 57-year-old woman was brought unconscious to the emergency room with multiple injuries from a motor vehicle accident. In searching her belongings, a nurse located a note in her wallet that stated she was a Jehovah's Witness and never wished to receive blood products. It was signed but not dated or witnessed. The treating physician decided to proceed with the blood transfusion despite this note. The patient recovered and sued, alleging battery. The court noted that the transfusion was necessary to save the patient's life but the physician knowingly did so against her wishes. The court could not absolve the physician from respecting the patient's wishes on the basis that the wishes were unreasonable. The patient was awarded $20 000 (Malette vs Shulman [82] as presented in Sanbar, 2001 [11]). Not many successful lawsuits of this nature have been reported. This may be due to pretrial settlements or to feelings on the part of the Witness that the injuries inflicted cannot be compensated by monetary awards [74].

Guidelines for approaching Jehovah's Witness patients

One of the more important aspects in dealing with adult or emancipated Witness patients is for the physician to be honest regarding whether he or she can respect their wishes regarding transfusion of blood products. If it would be impossible for the physician to allow the patient to die without a transfusion then he or she needs to be honest at the first patient encounter and if possible find an alternative physician to assume care. It is important to determine the exact wishes of the Witness patient regarding which blood products are acceptable. There are local and individual variations in Witness' interpretation of the prohibition, and it is important to ascertain what products would be acceptable in individual cases. Maximizing acceptable alternatives to blood product therapy, such as erthypoietin treatments and hemodilution of blood prior to major surgeries, should be emphasized. Remember that Jehovah's Witnesses are in general very active and compliant in seeking alternatives to replacement therapy. This conversation should occur as early as possible in the care of the patient. In the critical care setting, this may not always be possible to do in early gestation. The conversation should occur in private because the presence of family or church members may unduly influence the patient in a potential life or death situation where the decision should belong to the patient. There are also Jehovah Witness patients who will allow transfusion if they do not sign a consent form putting their wishes in writing. This obviously would put the physician in a very awkward position later if the patient were transfused and then stated that a previous conversation with the physician never occurred. Whether to transfuse in this situation would be up to the individual physician. Other Witness patients may accept transfusions and consent in writing but not wish any family or church members to know they have done so. All conversations of this nature should be clearly documented in the patient chart so that anyone who assumes care of the patient is aware of the patient's wishes.

The physician should acquire support of other members of the healthcare team. The anesthesiology team needs to be aware of the patient's wishes and be willing to honor them. Some hospitals have detailed written protocols regarding care of pregnant Jehovah's Witnesses [83].

Other issues can develop after this initial conversation. It is important to affirm that the patient's wishes remain the same when faced with imminent loss of life during a critical bleeding episode. If the patient's wishes have previously been clearly documented, efforts to confirm these wishes should not come across as attempts to change the patient's mind, but rather as offers to reassess the beliefs when facing a life-threatening hemorrhage. It is important to keep in mind that most of the Witness population are dealing with much more than a life or death situation. They feel the use of blood products can prevent them from reaching eternal salvation. There is also the very real concern regarding being isolated from their community.

A more difficult situation occurs when there is no time for conversation during a life-threatening hemorrhage (i.e. the patient is unconscious). This is especially difficult when dealing with a Witness who is unknown to the medical team and is only identified by a card in the wallet. In these cases, patient autonomy should probably prevail and the patient's wishes against transfusion be honored. As noted above, doctors have been successfully sued in these cases, but the amounts awarded have been relatively small, probably indicative of the court's recognition that the physicians were trying to save the lives of the involved patients. Prior documentation regarding alternatives such as autotransfusion devices may be helpful in these situations. Considerations such as leaving the patient intubated significantly longer after surgery can also be effective in minimizing the workload on the patient's metabolism (personal communication, Gary Dildy III, November 2001).

Jehovah's Witness patients who are minors represent another special category. In general, the courts have been quick to allow transfusions of minors against parental wishes. However, most states consider pregnancy to place minors in an emancipated category, which would give them the same decision-making capacities as adults. Even in non-emancipated minor cases, there has been a trend to allow more autonomy as the patient approaches the age of emancipation and is clearly able to articulate her beliefs [81].

Some physicians and courts have placed the pregnant Jehovah's Witness in a special category, especially when the fetus is viable. The presence of the fetus is used to justify transfusions in these settings, with the feeling that the transfusion is not as much an assault as a cesarean delivery on the patient's autonomy. By comparison, a transfusion is a more minor procedure. This author finds such reasoning troubling. To the Witness, the blood transfusion is much more of an assault than is cesarean delivery. In the case of a viable fetus with a hemorrhaging mother, delivery of the baby would seem to be a more ethical alternative than a blood transfusion.

Thus, care of the Jehovah's Witness in the critical care setting entails many ethical issues. It is important to respect the patient's autonomy and to exercise beneficence by understanding the alternative treatments the patient may allow consideration. If one has trouble caring for the patient within these limitations, it is imperative to inform the patient and assist in obtaining alternative care.

Letter of condolence

It is fitting to conclude a chapter on ethics in high-risk obstetrics with a reminder that a physician's duty to his patient does not end with the death of the patient. There remains one final responsibility: to assist the family members who are left behind. The idea of writing a letter of condolence was recently presented by Bedell, Cadenhead, and Graboys in the *New England Journal of Medicine* [84]. This responsibility was an accepted part of a physician's practice in 19th century America. Bedell et al. illustrate with this letter from Dr James Jackson to Mrs. Louisa Higgonson in 1892 [84]:

> My Dear Friend,
>
> I need not tell you how much I have sympathized with you. I think I realize in some measure how much you will miss Dear Aunt Nancy for a long time – for the rest of your life. I know that she has been a part of you ... mind as well as body was duly exercised, and she always had stock from which she poured out stores for the delight of her friends, – stores of wit and wisdom, affording pleasure with profit to all around her.
>
> How constantly will the events of life recall her to our minds – realizing what she said or did under interesting and important circumstances – or perhaps suggesting imperfectly what she would have said under new and unexpected occurrences.
>
> For you my dear friend I implore God's blessing.
>
> Your old friend,
>
> J. Jackson

A letter of condolence can be a great help to the family during their grieving process. This is particularly true when the death is unexpected or comes after complications that occurred during hospitalization [84]. The loss of a fetus, and even more so of a mother, could fall into this category. This letter can be of great assistance to the family in dealing with the anger that naturally accompanies such a loss [84]. This letter can be much more comforting than expressions of sympathy given in person or via telephone in that it can be referenced over and over. The absence of a visible sign of sympathy can be quite distressing to the family. Bedell mentions a family member who felt strongly about this: "After my mom died, the doctor never even wrote me. He ran and hid" [84]. Bedell, Cadenhead, and Graboys encourage all physicians, house staff, and fellows who have had personal contact with their deceased patients to write condolence letters.

Suggestions for writing condolence letters

Phrases to avoid

Expressions that de-emphasize the loss or suffering: "it was meant to be"; "I know how you must feel"; "it is better that she died".

Avoid revisiting the medical details of the death (also helps to avoid legal liability issues).

Suggestions for inclusion

Begin with a direct expression of sorrow for the loss, such as "I would like to send you our condolences on the death of your wife."

Include a personal memory of the patient and/or a reference to her family or work. References to the patient's achievements, devotion to family, character, or strength during the hospitalization are also helpful.

Mention the strength the patient received from the family's love.

Tell the family that it was a privilege to participate in the care of their loved one.

Let the family know your thoughts are with them in their hour of need [84].

The above suggestions are meant simply as guidelines for helping start a letter of condolence. The letter may be a few short sentences or a more detailed description of the physician–patient relationship. The physician should write the type of letter with which he or she is most comfortable. As Bedell, Cadenhead, and Graboys point out, "the letter of condolence is a professional responsibility of the past that is worth reviving" [84]. Such a letter provides a sense of comfort to the patient's family and affects positively the family's interactions with physicians in the future. On the other hand, a failure to communicate our sadness at the loss can be seen as a lack of interest or concern.

Conclusion

This book has detailed how to technologically deal with many of the high-risk situations that confront us in the care of our critically ill obstetric patients. This chapter helps the physician take a step back from the technology and look at the patient and her family as individuals who need to be dealt with at more levels than just the technological ones. Doing so is not always an easy process, especially when balancing the physician's ethical responsibility of beneficence with the patient's right to autonomy. Identifying possible ethical conflicts early in the decision process and clarifying these issues through communication can often help resolve them. Ethics committees can be helpful when communication between the physician, the patient, and her family is at an impasse. Rarely, if ever, should the courts be called upon to help in this decision process. The old French proverb to "cure sometimes, help often and comfort always" is especially applicable to the ethical dilemmas that face the high-risk obstetrician. When the best medical technologies do not result in the best outcome, it is also important to remember that a thoughtful letter of condolence can further the healing process.

Acknowledgments

The author wishes to thank Doug Brown PhD, Thomas Nolan MD, Cliona Robb Esq., Ginger Vehaskari PhD, and Ms Betty Rowe for their invaluable assistance in preparation of the manuscript.

References

1 Brown D, Elkins T. Ethical issues in obstetrics cases involving prematurity. *Clin Perinatol* 1992; 19: 469–481.

2 Chervenak F, McCullough L. Ethical and LEGAL ISSUES. In: *Danforth's Obstetrics and Gynecology*, 8th edn. Philadelphia: Lippincott, Williams and Wilkins, 1999: 939–953.

3 Beauchamp T, Childress J. *Principles of Biomedical Ethics*, 5th edn. New York: Oxford University Press, 2001: 57–164.

4 American College of Obstetricians and Gynecologists. Ethical decision making in obstetrics and gynecology. In: *Ethics in OB/GYN*, 2nd edn. Washington, DC: American College of Obstetricians and Gynecologists, 2004: 3–8.

5 Schloendorff v. Society of New York Hospitals. 211 N.Y. 125, at 129, 105 N.E. 92, at 93 (1914).

6 Lo B. *Resolving Ethical Dilemmas: A Guide for Clinicians*, 2nd edn. Philadelphia: Lippincott, Williams and Wilkins, 2000: 19–29, 181–188.

7 American College of Obstetricians and Gynecologists. Informed consent. In: *Ethics in OB/GYN*, 2nd edn. Washington, DC: American College of Obstetricians and Gynecologists, 2004: 9–17.

8 American College of Obstetricians and Gynecologists, Committee on Ethihcs Opinion 108. Ethicak Dimensions of Informed Consent. Washington, DC: ACOG, 1992: No.108.

9 Lane v. Candura 6 Mass. App. Ct 377, 376 N.E. 2d 1232 (1978).

10 Annas GJ, Densberger JE. Competence to refuse medical treatment: autonomy vs paternalism. *Toledo Law Rev* 1984; 15: 561 592.

11 Sanbar S, Firestone M, Gibofsky A. *Legal Medicine*, 5th edn. St Louis: Mosby, 2001; 292, 341.

12 In the Matter of Karen Quinlan 70 N.J. 10, 335A, 2d 647, cert. Denied U.S. 922 (1976).

13 Cruzan v. Missouri Department of Health, 497 U.S. 261 110 S. Ct. 2842 (1990).

14 Brophy v. New England Sinai Hospital, Inc. 497 N.E. 2d 626 (Mass. 1986).

15 Bouvia v. Superior Court, 179 Cal. App. 3d 1127, 225 Cal Rpt. 297 (Ct. App. 1986).

16 Leiberman J, Mazor M, Chaim W, Cohen A. The fetal right to live. *Obstet Gynecol* 1979; 53: 515–517.

17 Fost N, Chudwin D, Wikler D. The limited moral significance of "fetal viability". *Hastings Cent Rep* 1980; 10–13.

18 Fletcher J. The fetus as patient: ethical issues. *JAMA* 1981; 24: 772–773.

19 Chervenak F, Farley A, Walters L, Hobbins JC, Mahoney MJ. When is termination of pregnancy during the third trimester morally justifiable? *N Engl J Med* 1984; 310: 501–504.

20 Gillon R. Pregnancy, obstetrics and the moral status of the fetus. *J Med Ethics* 1988; 14: 3–4.

21 Abrams F. Polarity within beneficence: additional thoughts on nonaggressive obstetric management. *JAMA* 1989; 261: 3454–3455.

22 Chervenak F, McCullough L. Nonaggressive obstetric management: an option for some fetal anomalies during the third trimester. *JAMA* 1989; 261: 3439–3440.

23 Chervenak F, McCullough L. The limits of viability. *J Prenat Med* 1997; 25: 418–420.

24 Mahoney M. The fetus as patient. *West J Med* 1989; 150: 459–460.

25 Newton E. The fetus as a patient. *Med Clin North Am* 1989; 73: 517–540.
26 Strong C, Garland A. The moral status of the near-term fetus. *J Med Ethics* 1989; 15: 25–27.
27 Beller F, Zlatnik G. The beginning of human life: medical observations and ethical reflections. *Clin Obstet Gynecol* 1992; 35: 720–727.
28 Mattingly S. The maternal fetal dyad: exploring the two-patient obstetric model. *Hastings Cent Rep* 1992; 13–18.
29 Botkin J. Fetal privacy and confidentiality. *Hastings Cent Rep* 1995; 32–39.
30 Annas G. Forced cesareans: the most unkindest cut of all. *Hastings Cent Rep* 1982; 16–17, 45.
31 Annas G. Protecting the Liberty of Pregnant Patients. *N Engl J Med* 1987; 316: 1213–1214.
32 McCullough L, Chervenak F. *Ethics in Obstetrics and Gynecology*. New York: Oxford University Press, 1994: 96–129, 241–265.
33 Mahowald M. Beyond abortion: refusal of caesarean section. *Bioethics* 1989; 3: 106–121.
34 Rhoden N. Cesareans and Samaritans. *Law Med Healthcare* 1987; 15: 118–125.
35 Harris L. Rethinking maternal–fetal conflict: gender and equality in perinatal ethics. *Obstet Gynecol* 2000; 96: 786–791.
36 Strong C. Ethical conflicts between mothers and fetus in obstetrics. *Clin Perinatol* 1987; 14: 313–328.
37 Strong C. Court ordered treatment in obstetrics: the ethical views and legal framework. *Obstet Gynecol* 1991; 78: 861–868.
38 Roe v. Wade: United States Supreme Court: 35 LED 2d 147 (1973).
39 Re: AC, District of Columbia, 573 A. 2d 1235 (D.C. App. 1990).
40 Mohaupt S, Sharma K. Forensic implications and medical-legal dilemmas of maternal versus fetal rights. *J Forensic Sci* 1998; 43(5): 985–992.
41 Brown D. Maternal Fetal Topic II. Presented at AC Clinical Ethics for Practitioners Symposium, Hard Choices at the Beginning of Life, November 16 2001, Nashville, TN.
42 Adams F, Mahowald MB, Gallagher J. Refusal of treatment during pregnancy. *Clin Perinatol* 2003; 30: 127–140.
43 Baby Doe v. Mother Doe, 632 NF2d 326 (III App 1 Dist 1994).
44 Pinkerton J, Finnerty J. Resolving the clinical and ethical dilemma involved in fetal-maternal conflicts. *Am J Obstet Gynecol* 1996; 175: 289–295.
45 Colautti v. Franklin 439 U.S. 379 (1979).
46 Jefferson v. Griffen Spalding Hospital Authority, Ga., 274 S.F. 2d 457 (1981).
47 Smith v. Brennan 157 A 2d 497 (NJ 1960).
48 Nelson L, Milliken N. Compelled medical treatment of pregnant women: life, liberty and law in conflict. *JAMA* 1988; 259: 1060–1068.
49 Re: Maydun, 114 Daily Wash L. Rptr 2233 (DC Super Ct 1986).
50 Webster v. Reproductive Health Services, Daily Appellate Report, July 6, 1989;8724.
51 Planned Parenthood of Southeastern Pennsylvania v. Casey 112 U.S. 674 (1992).
52 American College of Obstetricians and Gynecologists, Committee on Ethics. *Opinion 321. Maternal Decision Making, Ethics and the Law*. Washington, DC: American College of Obstetricians and Gynecologists, 2005.
53 Dalton K. Refusal of interventions to protect the life of the viable fetus – a case-based transatlantic overview. *Medico-Legal J* 2006; 74(1): 16–24.
54 Berdowitz RL. Should refusal to undergo a cesarean delivery be a criminal offense? *Obstet Gynecol* 2004; 104(6): 1220–1221.
55 Minkoff H, Paltrow LM. Melissa Rowland and the rights of pregnant women. *Obstet Gynecol* 2004; 104(6): 1234–1236.
56 Haack S. Letter to the Editor. *Obstet Gynecol* 2005: 105(5): 1147.
57 Habiba M. Letter to the Editor. *Obstet Gynecol* 2005; 105(5): 1147–1148.
58 Kolder V, Gallagher J, Parson M. Court ordered obstetrical interventions. *N Engl J Med* 1987; 316: 1192–1196.
59 Berg RN. Georgia Supreme Court orders caesarean section – mother nature reverses on appeal. *J Med Assoc Ga* 1981; 70: 451–543.
60 Elkins T, Andersen H, Barclay M, et al. Court-ordered cesarean section: an analysis of ethical concerns in compelling cases. *Am J Obstet Gynecol* 1989; 161: 150–154.
61 American Academy of Pediatrics, Committee on Bioethics. Fetal therapy – ethical considerations. *Pediatrics* 1999; 103: 1061–1063.
62 American College of Obstetricians and Gynecologists. Patient choice in the maternal-fetal relationship. In: *Ethics in OB/GYN*, 2nd edn. Washington, DC: American College of Obstetricians and Gynecologists, 2004: 34–36.
63 McCullough LA, Chervenak F. Ethics IN Obstetrics and Gynecology. New York, NY. Oxford University Press, 1994: 196–237.
64 Gill AW, Saul P, McPhee J, Kerridge I. Acute clinical ethics consultation: the practicalities. *Med J Aust* 2004; 181(4): 204–206.
65 Dillon W, Lee R, Tronolone MJ, et al. Life support and maternal brain death during pregnancy. *JAMA* 1982; 248: 1089–1091.
66 Loewy E. The pregnant brain dead and the fetus: must we always try to wrest life from death? *Am J Obstet Gynecol* 1987; 157: 1097–1101.
67 Bush MC, Nagy S, Berkowitz R, Gaddipati S. Pregnancy in a persistent vegetative state: case report, comparision to brain death, and review of the literature. *Obstet Gynecol Surv* 2003; 58(11): 738–748.
68 Webb G, Huddleston J. Management of the pregnant woman who sustains severe brain damage. *Clin Perinatol* 1996; 23: 453–464.
69 President's Commission for the Study of Ethical Problems in Medicine and Biomedical and Behavorial Research. Guidelines for the determination of death. Report of the Medical Consultants on the Diagnosis of Death to the President's Commission. *JAMA* 1981; 246(19): 2184–2186.
70 Halevy A, Brody B. Brain death: reconciling definitions, criteria and test. *Ann Intern Med* 1993; 119: 519–525.
71 Burch TJ. Incubator or individual: the legal and policy deficiencies of pregnancy clauses in living wills and advance healthcare directive statutes. *Maryland Law Rev* 1995; 54: 528–570.
72 Mallampalli A, Powner DJ, Gardner MO. Cardiopulmonary resuscitation and somatic support of the pregnant patient. *Crit Care Clin* 2004; 20: 747–761.
73 Jonsen A. Blood transfusions and Jehovah's Witnesses: the impact of the patient's unusual beliefs in critical care. *Crit Care Clin* 1986; 2(1): 91–99.
74 Sacks DH, Koppes RH. Caring for the female Jehovah's Witness: balancing medicine, ethics, and the First Amendment. *Am J Obstet Gynecol* 1994; 170(2): 452–455.
75 Elkins T. *Exploring Medical-Legal Issues in Obstetrics and Gynecology*. Washington, DC: Association of Professors of OB/GYN, 1994: 35–38.
76 Macklin R. The inner workings of an ethics committee: latest battle over Jehovah's Witnesses. *Hastings Cent Rep* 1988; 15–20.
77 Raleigh Fitkin-Paul Morgan Hospital v. Anderson 42. NJ421, 201 A2d, 537 cert. Denied 377 U.S. 985 (1964).

78 Elias S, Annas G. *Reproductive Genetics and the Law*. Chicago: Yearbook Medical Publishers, 1987: 83–120, 143–271.
79 Re: Jamaica Hospital, 491 NYS 2d 898 (1985).
80 Application of the President and Directors of Georgetown College Hospital, F2d 1000 (1964).
81 Cain J. Refusal of blood transfusion. In: Elkins T. *Exploring Medical-Legal Issues in Obstetrics and Gynecology*. Washington, DC: Association of Professors of OB/GYN, 1994: 62–64.
82 Malette v. Shulman 630 R. 2d, 243, 720R. 2d, 417 (O.C.A.).
83 Gyamfi C, Gyamfi M, Berkowitz R. Ethical and medicolegal considerations in the obstetric care of a Jehovah's Witness. *Obstet Gynecol* 2003; 102(1): 173–180.
84 Bedell SE, Cadenhead K, Graboys TB. The doctor's letter of condolence. *N Engl J Med* 2001; 344(15): 1162–1164.
85 American College of Obstetricians and Gynecologists, Committee on Ethics. *Opinion 214. Patient Choice and the Maternal-Fetal Relationship*. Washington, DC: American College of Obstetricians and Gynecologists, 1999.
86 Chervenak FA, McCullough FB. Perinatal ethics: a practical method of analysis of obligations to mother and fetus. *Obstet Gynecol* 1985; 66: 442–446.
87 Mohr v. Williams, Minn, 261,265;104 N.W. 12, 15 (1905).
88 Superintendent of Belchertown v. Bouvia (1983).

48 Acute Psychiatric Conditions in Pregnancy

Ellen Flynn, Carmen Monzon & Teri Pearlstein

Alpert Medical School of Brown University, Women and Infants Hospital, Providence, RI, USA

Introduction

Visits to emergency departments (EDs) that involve psychiatric issues have substantially increased in the past 15 years, particularly among persons covered by Medicaid and the uninsured [1]. The decreased rates of inpatient hospitalization and decreased availability of psychiatric and substance abuse outpatient care have contributed to this increase in ED visits. Patients presenting to EDs have an increased prevalence of psychiatric diagnoses compared to community prevalence figures, and the psychiatric diagnoses are often missed or not included in the treatment plan [2]. Substance use disorders, which can present as depression or psychosis, are also suboptimally evaluated and treated [3]. A recent survey reported that ED clinicians were less likely to administer psychotropic medications to patients with active suicidal ideation or substance abuse, and there was no indication that receiving a prescription for a psychotropic medication at discharge from the ED improves the likelihood of follow-up with outpatient care [4]. This chapter will focus on some of the acute behavioral health problems that commonly present in an ED or other medical setting: depression, suicidality, and agitation/psychosis. These topics will be discussed in terms of general adult populations followed by specific issues that arise in the perinatal woman.

Assessment of depression

Major depressive disorder (MDD) is more common in women than in men, and the peak prevalence of MDD occurs in women during the reproductive years [5]. MDD is characterized by depressed mood, hopelessness, guilt, decreased motivation, low energy, poor concentration, change in sleep, change in appetite, decreased libido and decreased enjoyment of relationships and activities [5]. MDD can also include recurrent suicidal ideation, suicide attempt, and completed suicide. MDD is a serious disorder associated with behavioral and functional impairments. MDD is currently one of the world's leading causes of disability [6]. MDD is underdiagnosed and undertreated in medical settings and can negatively influence the course of comorbid medical illnesses [7]. Studies have suggested that two screening questions: "Over the last two weeks, how often have you been bothered by little interest or pleasure in doing things?" or "how often have you been feeling down, depressed or hopeless?" can reliably screen for depression in medical settings [8].

Depression during pregnancy

Perinatal depression is also under-recognized and undertreated [9–12]. Even with obstetrician encouragement and on-site availability of mental health treatment, pregnant women are unlikely to pursue treatment for depression [13]. A recent systematic review reported that the point prevalence of MDD ranged from 1.0 to 5.6% through pregnancy, while the point prevalence of major and minor depression was 11.0% in the first trimester and 8.5% in the second and third trimesters [14]. The Edinburgh Postnatal Depression Scale (EPDS) [15] is commonly used to screen for depression during pregnancy and the postpartum period. An EPDS score of 15 or higher has been suggested as a threshold that warrants further evaluation [16]. The evaluation of depression in pregnancy is complicated since the symptoms of sleep change, appetite change, fatigue and decreased libido are common in both normal pregnancy and MDD. Symptoms that are more specific to MDD include feelings of worthlessness, hopelessness, helplessness, guilt, and ruminations about death, dying and/or suicide. Risk factors for increased depressive symptoms or MDD during pregnancy include being adolescent, unmarried, financially disadvantaged, African American or Hispanic, having had a prior MDD, lack of social support and a recent negative life event [17].

Pregnancy has long been thought to be a time of enhanced well-being and quiescence of mental illness. A recent large cohort

Critical Care Obstetrics, 5th edition. Edited by M. Belfort, G. Saade, M. Foley, J. Phelan and G. Dildy.

study conducted in Denmark confirmed that pregnancy was a time of decreased risk of new-onset psychiatric disorders in primigravid women [18]. However, recent studies have suggested that women with previous psychiatric diagnoses are not protected against relapse during pregnancy, particularly if they discontinue their maintenance psychotropic medication. One study reported that 68% of women with treated depression who discontinued their antidepressant medication had a recurrence of depression compared to 26% of women who maintained their antidepressant [19]. Abrupt discontinuation of medication during pregnancy also significantly increases the risk of relapse, psychiatric decompensation and suicide in pregnant women with bipolar disorder [20,21]. Since both untreated psychiatric disease and psychotropic medications have potential adverse risks on the developing fetus, how pre-existing psychiatric illness is managed during pregnancy poses significant treatment dilemmas.

Untreated depression in pregnancy has deleterious consequences for both the mother and the developing infant. Obstetric complications reported with untreated prenatal stress and depression include pre-eclampsia, preterm delivery, low birth weight, miscarriage, growth restricted babies, low Apgar scores and neontatal complications [22]. Untreated prenatal anxiety and depression have also been correlated with language and cognitive impairment, impulsivity, and psychopathology in children [23,24]. Depression in pregnancy is associated with poor attention to maternal health, nutrition, and prenatal care, as well as an increased risk of impulsive and potentially dangerous activities, substance abuse, and tobacco use. In addition, undertreated depression in pregnancy places women at risk for completed suicide and for attempted suicide with its sequelae.

Depression during the postpartum period

When women present with depression during the postpartum period, the differential diagnosis includes postpartum blues, postpartum depression (PPD), and postpartum psychosis (PPP). Postpartum blues occur in 15–85% of women, depressive symptoms peak at postdelivery day 5, and symptoms are usually resolved by day 10 [25]. Postpartum blues may include mood swings, irritability, tearfulness, confusion, fatigue and mild elation. Postpartum blues are so common that they can be considered normal. Postpartum blues are not accompanied by significant functional impairment and the symptoms rarely require treatment. However, postpartum blues are a risk factor for subsequent PPD [26].

The prevalence of PPD is similar to non-puerperal prevalence rates of MDD in women. The systematic review by Gavin and colleagues reported that the point prevalence of MDD ranged from 1.0 to 5.7% through the first 6 postpartum months, peaking at 3 months post delivery, and most episodes were with postpartum onset of depressive symptoms [14]. The point prevalence of major and minor depression ranged from 6.5 to 12.9% through the first 6 postpartum months. Depression in pregnancy is the leading risk factor in the development of PPD. Other risk factors include anxiety during pregnancy, lack of social support and a stressful life event [27]. The EPDS is the most widely used and validated screening measure for PPD. A score of 13 or higher suggests probable PPD, and a full diagnostic evaluation should ensue [16]. Restlessness, agitation and decreased concentration may be more common in PPD compared to MDD occurring outside of the postpartum period [28].

The recent large cohort study conducted in Denmark reported that the first 90 days postpartum represented a time of increased risk of new-onset psychiatric disorder, inpatient admission and outpatient treatment in new mothers, but not in new fathers [18]. Primiparity was a significant risk factor, and PPD was the most common new-onset psychiatric disorder. In women with pre-existing MDD or bipolar disorder, the postpartum period is a time of increased risk of relapse [20,29]. There is a large body of literature describing the long-term negative consequences of untreated PPD on infant development. Children of mothers with untreated maternal depression are more likely to have slowed motor and cognitive development, behavioral difficulties, poor affect tolerance, poor social development, and increased risk of psychiatric and medical disorders [30,31]. Thus, the need to effectively screen for and treat the psychiatric disorders that appear *de novo* or as a relapse during the early postpartum period is of paramount public health significance [32,33].

Additional perinatal risk factors for depression

When evaluating the pregnant woman for depression, it is important to note that other pregnancy-related circumstances may contribute to an increased risk of depression. A literature review of emotional symptoms associated with induced abortion for unwanted pregnancy reported that prior to abortion 40–45% of women have significant levels of anxiety and 20% have significant levels of depression [34]. One month following elective abortion, mood and anxiety symptoms decrease in most women. Women with previous or current depressive and anxiety disorders are at risk for post-abortion depression [35] and a proportion of women who undergo an induced abortion will be at risk for later development of MDD, anxiety disorder, suicidal ideation and alcohol dependence [36]. Some studies have suggested increased risk of suicide following induced abortion [37,38].

Miscarriage, defined as an involuntary pregnancy loss before 20 weeks gestation, is associated with depressive symptoms and an increased risk of MDD [39,40]. Miscarriage is also associated with anxiety symptoms for at least 4 months, and an increased risk for acute stress disorder, post-traumatic stress disorder and obsessive–compulsive disorder [41,42]. Stillbirth is likewise associated with subsequent depression, anxiety and post-traumatic stress disorder [43,44]. The benefit of holding the stillborn or the promotion of a quick next conception is debated [44–46]. Women who have had a previous reproductive loss may experience depression, anxiety and unresolved grief in a subsequent pregnancy [41,47,48].

Pregnant women experiencing intimate partner violence (IPV) during pregnancy are more likely to have depressive symptoms than non-abused women [49]. IPV has been estimated to occur in 1–20% of pregnant women [49,50]. Homocide, often the result of IPV, occurs in 12–63% of pregnancy-associated deaths [37]. A recent large population-based study reported that IPV during pregnancy was associated with preterm labor, vaginal bleeding, nausea and vomiting, urinary tract infections, increased ED visits and hospitalizations, preterm delivery and low birth weight [51]. A systematic review identified similar adverse pregnancy outcomes as well as increased rates of maternal and fetal deaths with IPV during pregnancy [52]. Several national health organizations promote universal screening for domestic violence, and screening is acceptable to the majority of pregnant women although reporting mandates may decrease disclosure [53,54]. Healthcare providers' concern and recommendations for safe options often need to be repeated several times, and pregnant women may wait to act until after the infant is born [53].

The American College of Obstetricians and Gynecologists (ACOG) recommends screening perinatal women for psychosocial risk factors such as barriers to care, unstable housing, unintended or unwanted pregnancy, communication barriers, nutrition, tobacco use, substance use, psychiatric symptoms, safety, IPV and stress [54]. Psychosocial stressors can also include employment instability, economic burdens, and lack of social support. At the time of delivery, a premature infant and neonatal medical complications may be unexpected stressors. Pediatricians and other medical clinicians are also encouraged to screen for maternal depression and know of available resources [33]. Referral to appropriate intervention, social support, and counseling should ideally improve maternal, fetal and infant outcomes.

Treatment of depression during pregnancy and postpartum

Pregnant patients presenting with depression need to be informed of the potential risks to the fetus associated with not treating their symptoms as well as the risks with fetal exposure to antidepressant medications. If the depressive symptoms are not severe and are not jeopardizing the well-being of the woman, her fetus, and her family, non-pharmacologic treatments may be recommended initially. These would include supportive psychotherapy, interpersonal psychotherapy (IPT), and cognitive behavioral psychotherapy (CBT). IPT is a short-term treatment that addresses role transitions and promotes the increase of social support which has been demonstrated to improve depression during pregnancy [55]. Preliminary controlled trials with light therapy [56], massage [57], and acupuncture [58], and a preliminary open trial with fish oil [59] suggest alternative options for pregnant depressed women that deserve further study.

Antidepressant medications during pregnancy should be considered if the depressive symptoms are severe and disabling, the symptoms do not respond to non-pharmacologic treatments, or a woman is already on an antidepressant and her tapering the medication would pose a risk of recurrence. It is imperative that severely depressed women be referred to a clinician with expertise in psychotropic prescription during pregnancy and lactation so that she and her family can make the best informed decision for her treatment. Factors that govern the selection of treatment options include her previous psychiatric history, response to treatment, plans for breastfeeding, the clinician's presentation of treatment choices with their risks and benefits, the patient's perception of the treatment choices with their risks and benefits, and cultural expectations [60].

Recent published studies regarding the safety of antidepressant medication during pregnancy have led to worrying and often contradictory conclusions, widespread public concern in lay and media venues, and the introduction of warnings by regulatory authorities. Meta-analytic reviews have reported a small increased risk of spontaneous miscarriages with first-trimester selective serotonin reuptake inhibitor (SSRI) use [61,62]. Although several prospective studies have failed to identify increased congenital malformations with first-trimester antidepressant exposure [61,63], a recent study reported a 1.34 increased relative risk [64]. A retrospective unpublished study reported a 2.2 increased relative risk of congenital malformations with paroxetine which led to an FDA and Health Canada Advisory in 2005 and the revision of paroxetine's safety category from "C" to "D" [65]. A recent study reported that first-trimester exposure to paroxetine doses in excess of 25 mg/day, but not lower daily paroxetine doses, was associated with increased risk of congenital cardiac and other malformations [66].

Recent studies have characterized symptoms that appear in about one-third of neonates exposed to SSRIs in the third trimester that include jitteriness, poor muscle tone, respiratory distress, hypoglycemia and possible seizures [67]. These symptoms are usually mild and transient, and may be due to excess serotonin, SSRI discontinuation or cholinergic overdrive [67–69]. An FDA Alert about neonatal symptoms with third-trimester antidepressant use was issued in 2004. A compelling study that controlled for the level of maternal depression, comparing depressed women treated with SSRIs, depressed mothers not treated with SSRIs, and non-exposed control mothers, reported that infants of depressed mothers exposed to SSRIs were more likely to have lower birth weight, prematurity, and increased respiratory distress than control mothers [70]. An FDA Alert was issued in 2006 about an increased risk of persistent pulmonary hypertension of the newborn in women exposed to SSRIs after week 20 of gestation [71].

Untreated depression, anxiety and stress have known adverse effects on the fetus and infant as outlined above. Discontinuation of an antidepressant in a euthymic pregnant woman carries a risk of relapse with its attendant potential adverse effects. The risks to the fetus with SSRI exposure summarized above, and the paucity of studies of the effects of fetal SSRI exposure on long-term cognitive, behavioral and motor development, pose difficult treatment dilemmas for the pregnant woman with depression. A position paper by ACOG advised that paroxetine not be used during pregnancy and that the use of SSRIs should be individualized [72].

As with depression in pregnancy, there are no FDA-approved antidepressants for PPD. It is generally assumed that antidepressants would work for PPD as well as for non-puerperal MDD, although this has not been tested. Three published randomized controlled trials in PPD have reported equal efficacy of sertraline and nortriptyline [73], superiority of fluoxetine to placebo [74], and equal efficacy of paroxetine and combined paroxetine/CBT in women with comorbid PPD and anxiety [75]. It should be noted that most open and controlled pharmacotherapy trials of PPD have excluded breastfeeding women.

Although double-blind placebo-controlled studies of antidepressant medication for PPD in breastfeeding mothers do not exist, there is a growing observational database. A pooled analysis of antidepressant levels in mother–infant dyads concluded that sertraline, paroxetine and nortriptyline usually yield undetectable infant serum levels and that elevated serum levels are more likely with fluoxetine and citalopram [76]. There has also been an absence of adverse effects reported with sertraline, paroxetine and nortriptyline. Adverse reports in breastfeeding infants have been reported with fluoxetine, citalopram, bupropion and doxepin [77–80]. Breast milk and infant serum antidepressant levels are not routinely monitored. Breastfeeding mothers should monitor the infant for new-onset somnolence, irritability, poor feeding, colic, or change in temperament. Adverse effects in the infant should be reported to the prescribing clinician and pediatrician, and a change of antidepressant or lowering of dose may be necessary.

Breastfeeding mothers with PPD often prefer non-pharmacologic treatments rather than antidepressant medication. IPT has been demonstrated to be superior to a waitlist control [81]. Positive results have also been reported with CBT, lay peer support, health visitors in the home, and group therapy [82–84]. Initial positive reports with light therapy, maternal sleep deprivation, massage, exercise, infant sleep intervention, herbs and fish oil deserve further study [85]. The adverse effects on infant and child development of untreated maternal depression are substantial and well characterized. However, many barriers to seeking care exist including perceived negative stigmata, availability of highly trained IPT or CBT psychotherapists, childcare and time commitment issues, cost, and sensitivity of the therapist to cultural sociodemographic variables [77,86]. Discussions of treatment options for PPD need to include the risks of not treating, psychotherapy options, available data about the safety of medications with breastfeeding, the woman's previous psychiatric history and responses to treatment, and her individual treatment preferences and expectations [60].

Suicidality

The annual suicide rate in the general population is 10.7 per 100 000 persons [87] and men commit suicide at a 4 times greater rate than women [88]. The general population suicide rate for women in the United States aged 20–45 was 3.2–6.4 per 100 000 in 2000 [88] and 3.5–7.7 per 100 000 in 2002 [89]. The single most significant risk factor for suicide is psychiatric illness and elevated rates are found with MDD (14.6%), bipolar disorder (15.5%) and mixed drug abuse (14.7%) [87]. Besides the presence of psychiatric illness, prior suicide attempts represent a major risk factor for suicide, particularly in women (see Table 48.1) [90]. In a systematic review of risk factors for suicide in bipolar disorder, previous suicide attempt and hopelessness were the strongest risk factors [91]. Methods of suicide in women include in decreasing frequency firearms, overdose and hanging, followed by all other forms [88]. For every completed suicide, there have usually been 18–20 attempts [92] and women account for most of the attempts [88]. Suicide attempts substantially increase the risk of subsequent suicide, and need to be taken seriously [93,94].

The suicidal patient represents one of the most significant challenges to the healthcare professional. Failed suicide attempts account for 1–2% of ED visits, 5% of ICU admissions and 10% of admissions to general medical services [92]. The assessment of suicidality includes the evaluation of current suicidal thoughts

Table 48.1 Risk factors for suicide in women.

Increased suicide risk
Psychiatric illness
Depression
Anhedonia*
Hopelessness*
Insomnia*
Anxiety*
Persistent symptoms*
Psychotic symptoms (delusions)*
Cigarette smoking
Substance use or abuse
Psychiatric history
Psychiatric hospitalization
Postpartum psychiatric hospitalization
History of suicide attempts
Personality characteristics*
Impulsive*
Aggressive
History of violence
Family history of suicide*
Abortion
Child has died
Child has psychiatric illness
Demographic characteristics
Single or unmarried
Higher levels of education
Middle-aged
Firearm access
Decreased suicide risk
Pregnancy
Postpartum
Young children (under 18 years old) in the home

Adapted from [88] and [90].
* Risk factors identified in mixed gender groups, not specific to women.

and plans, inquiry about past suicidal behavior, and inquiry about risk factors. It is common lore that asking a patient about suicidal thoughts or plans for suicide will "give them ideas". In fact, the exploration of suicidal thoughts and plans often allows the patient to feel less isolated and it may lead to further discussion of the patient's thoughts and feelings because the topic has been normalized to some degree by the healthcare provider's inquiry. There are multiple self-report and clinician-rated suicide assessment tools that can be helpful to the psychiatric evaluation [87]. Screening for suicidal ideation and plan is a critical part of the evaluation of a patient presenting with depression and other psychiatric disorders.

Self-injurious behavior

Often in medical settings, when patients present with self-injurious behaviors such as cutting, scarring, or burning oneself, it is assumed that this represents a suicide attempt. The single most important question is the intent, i.e. does the patient intend to die? The self-injurious behaviors may be coping mechanisms that patients employ to modulate difficult emotional states. However, careful examination for suicidal intent and plan is always prudent and necessary. A recent study reported that self-injury or suicide gesture in women tended to represent a means to communicate with others while self-injury in men tended to represent an intent to die [93]. The authors caution that even though an intent to die is associated with medical lethality and completed suicide, self-injury and suicidal gestures without an intent to die are dangerous and warrant clinical attention [93].

Assessment and management of the suicidal patient

The most important goal with a suicidal patient is to assure the patient's safety. The safest means of transfer from home or from an outpatient setting is by ambulance, or police if necessary, to the nearest ED for further evaluation and management. A suicidal patient should be immediately admitted to the ED due to the patient's high risk status. It should be ascertained at admission if the patient possesses means for suicide, e.g. firearms, knives, or pills. A suicidal patient should not be isolated in the ED. The suicidal patient requires maximal supervision via nursing staff as well as constant observation with a one-to-one sitter, including trips to the bathroom. This is recommended even if a family member is present. As with an agitated patient, items in the room that could be used as self-inflicting weapons should be removed. Suicidal patients should not be permitted to leave the ED even to smoke, due to the risks of imminent self-harm and elopement. Hospital security should be involved, if needed, to hold the patient until a thorough risk and safety assessment can be accomplished by psychiatric staff. Securing the suicidal patient's safety may involve the use of physical and or chemical restraints.

Once the patient is in a safe and secure environment, a thorough medical and psychiatric work-up should be initiated. Toxicology screens should be obtained. Psychiatry and social work should be contacted immediately upon arrival of a suicidal patient to the ED. The pregnant patient should receive a focused medical and obstetric examination to address any acute medical or obstetric problems that may be life-threatening or contributing to the patient's presentation. Attention should be paid to maximizing the patient's comfort, addressing such symptoms such as nausea, hunger, cramping, pain, etc. Anxiety can be managed with a low-dose benzodiazepine. It is important, however, not to overly sedate the patient, as this can interfere with psychiatric and medical assessment.

The essential feature of the management of suicidal patients is risk assessment with particular attention to modifiable risk factors. Risk factors that need to be inquired about include the lethality of previous suicide attempts, depression, panic disorder, unremitting anxiety, psychosis, borderline personality disorder, antisocial personality disorder, alcohol or substance abuse, medical illness including delirium, childhood sexual or physical abuse, family history of suicide, hopelessness, impulsiveness, aggression, and a recent psychosocial stressor such as IPV, loss of employment, or loss of a close relationship [87]. In evaluating the lethality of a previous suicide attempt, several features should be noted such as number of prior suicide attempts, the means, availability of firearms, was medical admission or ICU level of care necessary, likelihood of discovery, communication with others, disappointment about survival and intention to die.

If the patient has a specific current suicidal plan, the intent to die and lethality must be evaluated. It is important to ascertain whether there are contributing life stressors that are impacting the current situation. It is critical to assess how and why suicide appears to be a reasonable alternative to their current situation. Feelings of worthlessness, hopelessness and ruminations about death, dying and suicide are characteristic of severe depression. When these thoughts increase or are associated with changes in behavior, this may represent an increased likelihood or imminence of acting on suicidal ideation. The following could signify concerning behavioral alterations: becoming more isolative, giving objects away, writing a suicide note, disconnecting from family and community, poor self-care, increasing impulsive and risky behaviors, and obtaining firearms. Corollary information from family members can provide critical information that the patient might be unwilling to disclose or is minimizing. Collaboration with family is also important in the treatment planning process. The exception to this is involvement of the domestically violent partner or abusive family member. While it is helpful to obtain consent from the patient to contact family, because of the risk of death, patients do not need to provide consent for such contact to take place.

Patients in imminent danger of suicide usually warrant psychiatric admission. If the patient is deemed not to be at imminent danger of suicide, collaboration with outpatient healthcare providers, as well as the mobilization of family and community resources with attention to current psychosocial stressors, is critical. Social work can be extremely helpful in identifying community and support services that can assist the patient and family in addressing specific psychosocial concerns, such as shelter programs for IPV victims, rent and housing assistance, and food assistance. In addition, besides inpatient psychiatric hospitalization, other treatment options may offer psychiatric stabilization such as partial hospital programs, intensive outpatient programs, substance abuse treatment, individual or family therapy and psychotropic medications. A multimodality treatment plan is best achieved through collaboration between psychiatry, social work, obstetrics and gynecology, and medicine services.

Although there is not definite evidence that antidepressant medication specifically reduces suicidality in MDD, antidepressants are the mainstay treatment for reducing depressive symptoms. There is also not compelling evidence that mood stabilizers, antipsychotics or benzodiazepines acutely reduce suicidality in psychiatric disorders, whereas lithium has been demonstrated to reduce suicide and suicide attempts in bipolar disorder [87].

Suicidality during pregnancy and postpartum

Completed suicides are less prevalent in pregnancy [95,96] and the postpartum period [38,96] compared to non-puerperal times in a woman's life. Adolescents may not have lower suicide rates than older postpartum women [38]. Results from a Danish cohort reported that suicide risk increased 70-fold in the first year after giving birth in the presence of a psychiatric disorder [97]. An examination of perinatal maternal deaths in the United Kingdom in 1997–99 suggested that suicide was the leading cause of maternal death, was increased in women with psychiatric and substance abuse disorders, and was more likely to be a violent death compared to the suicides of men and non-childbearing women [98]. Other studies confirm that although suicide rates may be lower during pregnancy and the postpartum period, perinatal women complete suicide by more violent and lethal means than when not perinatal [94]. Lindahl and colleagues have suggested that when assessing suicidality in the pregnant or postpartum woman, specific inquiry should be made about reasons for dying, reasons for living, prior suicide attempts, prior psychiatric illness, previous trauma, and current marital violence [94].

Pregnant and postpartum women also have lower rates of self-injury and suicide attempts than non-puerperal women, ranging from one-half to two-thirds the expected rates [94]. Suicidal ideation occurs in up to 14% of perinatal women [94]. Suicide attempts (mostly poisoning) have been associated with unwanted pregnancy [99]. A recent study of a United States population sample reported that fetal demise and infant death in the first year after delivery increased the risk of a suicide attempt threefold (mostly poisonings) and increased inpatient psychiatric admissions [100]. In this study, labor and delivery complications, cesarean section, preterm delivery, low birth weight and congenital malformations were not associated with increased risk of suicide attempts.

Another recent study examined the characteristics of 2132 women who delivered and had attempted suicide during their pregnancy compared to women who did not attempt suicide [101]. Again, the majority of the women (86%) attempted suicide by ingestion of a drug overdose or poisoning. Suicide attempts were correlated with psychiatric illness, substance abuse, younger age, being single, less education, poor prenatal care, being multiparous, and being African-American. The consequences of attempted suicide on the neonate included preterm labor, low birth weight, respiratory distress syndrome, and cesarean delivery. The women who delivered during the hospitalization for attempted suicide had an increased risk of neonatal and infant death. The authors stress the importance of prenatal treatment of an underlying psychiatric and/or substance abuse disorder, and the need to counsel women about potential adverse neonatal outcomes if suicide is attempted [101].

Agitation and psychosis

Acute agitation or violence is a symptom present in a wide range of psychiatric illnesses such as bipolar disorder, schizophrenia, substance abuse or personality disorders with impulsivity (such as borderline or antisocial) [102,103]. Agitation in psychosis can be from confusion, akathisia, fearfulness, paranoia, delusions or command hallucinations. Alcohol and substance abuse increase agitation and violence in patients with depression, bipolar disorder and schizophrenia [104]. Agitation can also occur in medical conditions such as brain trauma, meningitis, encephalitis, dementia, thyrotoxicosis, infection or fever in the elderly and delirium [102]. Agitation has been defined as excessive motor activity associated with a feeling of inner tension [5] and motor restlessness, heightened responsivity to external or internal stimuli, irritability, inappropriate and/or purposeless verbal or motor activity, decreased sleep, and fluctuation of symptoms over time [105].

The neuroanatomy and neurochemical basis of agitation are not well understood [104,106]. In patients with psychosis, the proposed pathophysiologic mechanisms include reduction of inhibitory γ-aminobutyric acid (GABA) action, hyperdopaminergia in the basal ganglia, altered serotonin function and increased norepinephrine tone. Frontal lobe dysfunction has been implicated by neuroimaging and other studies [107] and a mutation in the catechol O-methyltransferase (COMT) gene has been identified [104].

Even though men exhibit a higher rate of aggression than women, the gender gap disappears among psychiatric inpatients and patients evaluated in an ED [108]. Violence is common in the medical ED, and surveys indicate frequent occurrence of assaults of staff members and use of restraints [109]. The incidence of agitation and violence is higher in psychiatric EDs [104]. Determinants of violence in the ED include patient factors, such as psychiatric disorder, medical disorder, drug intoxication or withdrawal, transport to the hospital involuntarily, negative perception of hospital staff, and possession of a weapon at presentation; staff factors, such as impoliteness, insensitivity, and inadequate training; environmental factors, such as high noise levels, overcrowding and uncomfortable waiting rooms; and system factors such as high patient volumes, prolonged waiting and evaluation times, inadequate security staff, and absent or inadequate formal training in the management of hostile and aggressive patients [109].

Cultural issues can influence patient, staff and system factors involved in a clinical emergency [110]. Specific psychiatric symptoms and behaviors can present from a culturally determined response to a specific event rather than from a clinical disorder. An acute psychotic episode may be related to a religious trance or misleading somatic symptoms may be part of a depressive crisis in certain ethnic groups. Reactions to a trauma may look very different in Hispanic compared to Asian patients [110]. Clinicians evaluating patients need to achieve cultural competence which requires the understanding of cultural beliefs, assumptions and expectations, the acceptance of alternative perspectives and the expression of compassion and empathy.

Management of agitation and psychosis

The immediate goal is the rapid reduction of agitation or psychosis while maintaining the safety of the patient and staff. The long-term goal is the treatment of the underlying condition and reduction of future agitation. One of the first tasks is to try to discern the etiology of the agitation. A quick medical evaluation should be done to determine if there are any life-threatening medical conditions. Much of the time, staff must start with presumptive diagnoses. Precautions must be taken to modify or manipulate the environment to maximize the safety of all individuals present [111]. These may include assuring that the patient is physically comfortable, minimizing wait time, removing potentially dangerous objects, decreasing external stimuli through use of a quiet and private examination room, and communicating a respectful, safe and caring attitude [112].

Personnel should be educated to maintain calmness, keep a safe distance, identify cues for violence, respect the patient's personal space, avoid direct confrontation, refrain from prolonged or intense eye contact, and avoid any body language that might be interpreted as threatening or confrontational [111]. The first treatment approach generally involves verbal de-escalation or "defusing" or "talking down". The staff should be seen as calm and in control while at the same time conveying empathy, professional concern for the patient's well-being, and continuous reassurance that the patient is safe. At least one staff member should form a therapeutic alliance that could be used later if the patient's agitation escalates. This staff member should not be involved with the use of physical or chemical restraints since he or she may be helpful later for the patient to re-establish normal interpersonal relationships. If, despite initial interventions, the patient's agitation is so severe that the threat of harm to self or others is a paramount concern, the immediate goal of treatment is safety.

Restraints may need to be employed when other methods of de-escalation and attempts to calm the patient have failed [113]. There are two types of restraints used in emergency situations: physical and chemical restraints. Physical restraints, e.g. four-point leather restraints (both arms, both legs), are important adjuncts to the emergency treatment of agitated patients. Advantages include minimal side effects when used correctly, immediate reversibility, and no change to the mental state of the patient that might hinder further assessment. Leather restraints are preferred because they are more reliable and cause less injury than other types of physical restraints. One of the disadvantages of physical restraints is that they require significant training: how to take the patient down, how to apply them and how to monitor their use. Poor training or incorrect use can result in injury to the patient or others. Chemical restraints require that the patient agrees to take medications or medications may be administered to a patient involuntarily, which involves holding a patient down until the medication starts exerting its calming effect. An advantage of chemical restraints is that the administered medication may also constitute initiation of treatment for the underlying cause of the agitation. Restraints should be used for the least amount of time as clinically indicated, in the least restrictive manner possible, and staff must adhere to hospital policies about training, monitoring and documentation [112,113].

The Expert Consensus Panel for Behavioral Emergencies 2005 recommends specific chemical restraints (see Figure 48.1) [114]. Benzodiazepines are the recommended choice when the cause of agitation is not known, when there is no specific treatment (e.g. personality disorders), or when there might be specific benefits (e.g. intoxication with certain substances). The first-line recommended benzodiazepine is lorazepam due to its complete and rapid intramuscular absorption, an elimination half life of 12–15 hours, and a duration of action of 8–10 hours [102]. The goal is to calm the patient without excessive sedation. Lorazapam 2 mg IM may be sufficient to calm the patient and allow the clinician to further assess the patient. Benzodiazepines have the potential to cause respiratory depression, ataxia, excessive sedation and paradoxical disinhibition [102].

Combination treatment with both an antipsychotic and a benzodiazepine is often necessary to control agitation. Several studies have reported benefit with haloperidol (5 mg IM) combined with lorazepam (2 mg IM), and this regimen is preferred in pregnant agitated women due to the existence of a fair amount of safety data with exposure to haloperidol in pregnancy [114]. Haloperidol 5 mg IM or IV will have an onset of action of 30–60 minutes, an elimination half-life of 12–36 hours, and a duration of effect of up to 24 hours [102]. Droperidol is also effective but is now used infrequently due to concerns about a risk of fatal cardiac arrhythmias caused by possible prolongation of the QTc interval [115]. Possible adverse effects with typical antipsychotics include extrapyramidal symptoms (EPS), cardiac arrhythmias, and neuroleptic malignant syndrome (NMS). EPS include dystonia, akathisia and parkinsonian-like effects and are unwelcome due to their potential to increase patient distress and medication refusal. Dystonic reactions can be managed with diphenhydramine, which is not contraindicated during pregnancy. It should be noted that diphenhydramine may be eliminated before a dose of haloperidol is completely eliminated, creating the potential for a return of EPS. Akathisia from neuroleptics is difficult to assess in a patient who is already agitated. Akathisia may partially respond to lorazepam. NMS is a rare complication of typical antipsychotic

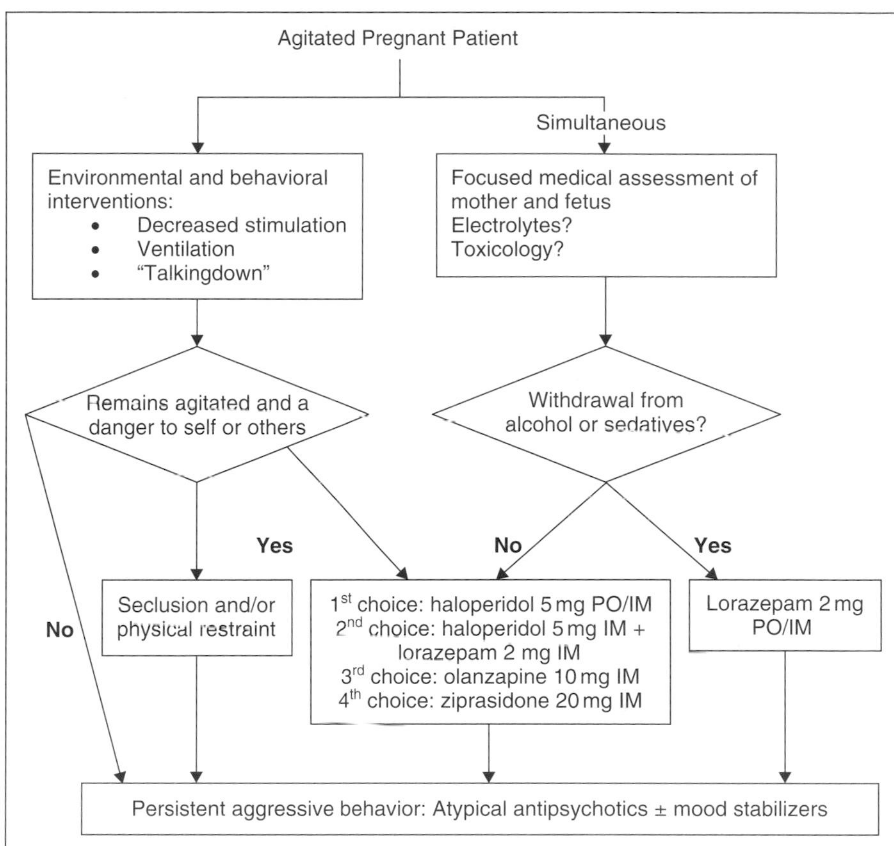

Figure 48.1 Management of the agitated pregnant patient. Adapted from [103].

use, but the risk increases in highly agitated patients who are poorly hydrated, restrained, and kept in poorly ventilated holding areas. It is imperative that periodic monitoring of vital signs and muscular rigidity are performed in the patient receiving typical antipsychotics [112].

The newer second-generation atypical antipsychotics (SGAs) include clozapine, olanzapine, risperidone, quetiapine, aripiprazole and ziprasidone. SGAs are alternatives to haloperidol that offer some advantages, e.g. absence of risk of EPS and a smoother transition to long-term oral pharmacotherapy. However, fewer safety data are available about risks with fetal exposure. Ziprasidone and olanzapine are available PO and IM, and olanzapine and risperidone are available as dissolvable oral tablets. Ziprasidone 10 mg and 20 mg IM and olanzapine 5 mg and 10 mg IM have been reported to effectively decrease agitation in several studies [112,114,116]. However, olanzapine has been associated with hypotension and some fatalities, and concern exists with the potential prolongation of the QTc interval with ziprasidone [114–116].

Once the patient is stable enough to undergo a medical evaluation, a physical examination should be performed and laboratory tests and toxicology screens should be obtained. Medical illnesses that can present as psychiatric emergencies should be ruled out. These include hypothyroidism, hyperthyroidism, diabetic ketoacidosis, hypoglycemia, urinary tract infection, pneumonia, myocardial infarction, alcohol intoxication, alcohol withdrawal, other substance withdrawal, acute liver disease and chronic obstructive pulmonary disease [105]. Less common medical illnesses that can present with psychiatric symptoms include pulmonary embolism, subarachnoid hemorrhage, epidural hemorrhage, encephalitis, malignant hypertension, hypokalemia, hypocalcemia, splenic rupture, subacute bacterial endocarditis, cocaine intoxication, amphetamine intoxication, steroid-induced psychosis and phencyclidine psychosis [105].

After potentially life-threatening medical conditions have been ruled out, a full psychiatric assessment should be conducted to determine if there is a new-onset psychiatric disorder or an ongoing psychiatric disorder. An emergency psychiatric evaluation in an agitated patient should focus on specific questions: "What is the problem?" "Why now?" "What are the patient's expectations?" Determining what is wrong may be difficult to ascertain. The patient may feel that nothing is wrong; and the collection of collateral information from significant others may be crucial. Are chronic symptoms suddenly exacerbated? Clarifying the precipitating factor is crucial for determining further treatment. Is there a psychosocial stressor? Is the patient trying to communicate something to a significant other or provider? Has there been a change in the pattern or amount of substance use? The patient's expectations are also important. Patients that come in willingly to a medical service are expecting something such as a cure, alleviation of a particular symptom, avoidance of incarceration, hospitalization to avoid a situation at home or on the streets, a prescription, or a note to be out of work for a few days. Sometimes the expectation is overtly displayed. For example, a pregnant patient may become acutely agitated and complain of contractions to be hospitalized in order to avoid arrest or incarceration. Sometimes the expectations are covert and the patient expects the clinician to infer what the patient's desires are.

Every emergency evaluation of agitation requires identification of any underlying conditions and the circumstances that led to the agitation. A new-onset psychiatric disorder involves education of the patient and family about the disorder and treatment options. For chronic psychiatric disorders, adjustment of medication may be necessary. It is necessary to ascertain whether or not treatment can be administered in an outpatient setting, or if admission to a medical or psychiatric hospital is necessary. Contact with existing outpatient clinicians is important for continuity of care. If alcohol or substance abuse is present, the patient should be referred to a detoxification or rehabilitation program.

Management of agitation in the pregnant and postpartum patient

The management of agitation in the pregnant patient represents additional challenges. Specific precipitants that can arise with a pregnant woman include an unwanted pregnancy or discontinuation of psychotropic medications due to fears of harming the fetus. Since the well-being of the fetus is important, the physical assessment becomes a primary concern. The risks to the fetus with medication or physical restraints need to be considered. One of the concerns in the use of physical restraints is harm to the fetus during takedown, particularly during the second or third trimester when the gravid abdomen is prominent. However, if leather restraints are necessary the fetus is already likely to be at physical risk due to the mother's level of agitation. An agitated pregnant patient elicits concern in family members, ED staff and police. A psychiatric ED is more equipped to deal with agitation, violence and psychosis than a medical ED, but is less experienced in the physical assessment treatment of a pregnant woman and her fetus.

If an agitated pregnant woman is being evaluated in a medical or obstetrics and gynecology facility, the setting in which the assessment and management of the agitation is taking place presents challenges. In the ED, how the patient presents is important. Was she brought in unwillingly or did the patient request an evaluation? A patient that is brought involuntarily may be belligerent and agitated from the start. The noise in an ED may lead to further escalation. Effort should be made to locate a room away from the most active areas of the ED and away from patients in active labor or requiring much care. Equipment commonly found in an obstetrics ED triage area or on a unit can quickly become a weapon in the hands of an agitated and hostile patient. Potentially dangerous articles should be removed from the proximity of an agitated patient. An agitated patient can break off bathroom parts when utilizing a toilet or shower unit that can be used to inflict injury to self or others. It is usually easier to work with an agitated patient who presents voluntarily. In this case, the woman is likely to want help for herself and her fetus, and it may be possible to de-escalate her agitation by reminding her of her initial purposes in seeking help. Sometimes patients are very close to their "breaking point" when they finally decide to come to an ED, and a noisy environment or perceived disrespect can quickly escalate a situation that otherwise could have been managed. The labor and delivery units present similar issues as the obstetric ED, i.e. noise and equipment that can be dangerous. The antepartum units have visitors and children that need to be protected from a risk of injury from an agitated and violent patient. A private and quiet room on the antepartum or postpartum floor can be helpful in secluding an agitated pregnant or postpartum woman.

Obstetrics and gynecology attendings, residents and nurses often feel uncomfortable managing acutely agitated pregnant and postpartum patients. Unfortunately, the patient may perceive rising levels of anxiety in the staff. If the staff–patient relation is fragile this can lead to escalation in an agitated patient. Staff should honestly assess their feelings and reactions and use those reactions to help manage their interactions. If they feel fear, staff should maintain a safe distance. If they feel anger, it is important to remember that the patient and fetus need help and the patient may not know how to ask for help. If they feel hostility, forming an alliance with another staff member that feels sympathy for the patient can be helpful. In an emergency situation it may be tempting to allow a belligerent and agitated patient to leave (or hope that they will leave) without an evaluation. However, a belligerent patient that is demanding to leave may have a life-threatening condition and deserves a full medical and psychiatric evaluation. Having the involvement of a psychiatry consultation service familiar with the management of psychiatric illness in the context of pregnancy can make the management of acute agitation easier for obstetrics and gynecology clinicians.

Psychosis and mania during pregnancy and postpartum

Schizophrenia is characterized by delusions, hallucinations, disorganized speech, disorganized behavior, and flattened emotions [5]. Women with schizophrenia have a high risk of unplanned and unwanted pregnancies and they tend to have poorer prenatal care, poorer nutrition, more alcohol, drug and tobacco use, and a higher risk of suicide and injury to others than women without schizophrenia [117]. Psychosis itself is associated with low birth weight, small for gestational age babies, stillbirth, prematurity and infant death [118–120]. Women with schizophrenia and schizoaffective disorder have an increased risk of relapse in the first 3 months after delivery, possibly due to the decrease in antidopaminergic activity with the fall of estrogen following delivery [121]. Mothers with active psychosis have severely impaired functioning and adverse effects on child development. Because of the negative effects of active psychosis on fetal and infant development, women with psychotic disorders should strongly consider continuation of their psychotropic medication through pregnancy and the postpartum period. If they do wish to discontinue their medication, a slow taper over 2 months reduces the risk of relapse, compared to a taper in less than 2 weeks [122]. The woman's competence to make decisions and her treatment preferences must be taken into account [123].

Bipolar disorder is a chronic psychiatric disorder characterized by recurrent mania, hypomania, depression, mixed states and euthymic mood. Mania involves elevated, expansive or irritable mood and may be accompanied by inflated self-esteem or grandiosity, pressured speech, racing thoughts, decreased need for sleep, increased goal-directed activity, psychomotor agitation, and risky behaviors [5]. Pregnancy is neither protective nor a time of increased risk for bipolar episodes if medication is maintained. However, decreasing a mood stabilizer during pregnancy (or at any time), especially a rapid decrease, leads to a high risk of relapse [20]. The postpartum risk of recurrence of bipolar disorder is 20–50% [117]. A woman with active mania is severely impaired in her functioning, as is an actively psychotic woman. There is an elevated risk of risk-taking behaviors, poor self-care and nutrition, substance abuse and risk of suicide. Again, due to the deleterious effects of active psychosis on fetal and infant development, women with bipolar disorder should strongly consider continuation of their psychotropic medication through pregnancy and the postpartum period.

Postpartum psychosis (PPP) occurs in 1 in 500 mothers, with rapid onset in the first 2–4 weeks after delivery. PPP includes delusions, paranoid thinking, confused thinking, mood swings, disorganized behavior, poor judgement and impaired functioning [124]. It is considered a psychiatric emergency and usually results in inpatient psychiatric hospitalization. Risk factors include a previous episode of PPP, obstetric complications, primiparity, sleep deprivation, environmental stressors, family history, and recent discontinuation of mood stabilizers [124–126]. Having a family member with previous PPP was associated with an increased risk of PPP in women with bipolar disorder compared to not having a relative with previous PPP [127]. Longitudinal studies suggest that the majority of PPP cases are related to bipolar disorder, not schizophrenia [124]. Overall, the prognosis for recovery from PPP is good with adequate treatment [124].

One of the most serious risks of PPP is infanticide. The rate of homicide of infants up to 1 year of age is 8 per 100 000 in the United States [128], but it is unknown how many women with PPP commit infanticide. Symptom exacerbation, command hallucinations and the stressor of being postpartum can increase the risk of infanticide in a postpartum mother with psychosis [129]. However, not all infanticide is committed by psychotic mothers. Infanticide also occurs in the context of severe depression, due to neglect and abuse, due to the child being unwanted, or as revenge against the infant's father [129]. Between 16 and 29% of mothers who kill their children also kill themselves [128]. Neonaticide is defined as killing of a newborn within 24 hours of birth. It is associated with denial of pregnancy, relative lack of prenatal care, dissociative hallucinations, depersonalization, and intermittent amnesia of delivery [128,130]. Infanticidal thoughts can occur in mothers with PPD and who have babies with colic, but most women do not act on infanticidal thoughts. More study is needed of specific risk factors for neonaticide and infanticide [128].

Treatment of mania and psychosis during pregnancy and postpartum

The treatment of mania, psychosis and agitated behavior in the pregnant woman is likely to involve mood stabilizers, antipsychotics and, on occasion, benzodiazepines. It is assumed that the response rates to these medications approximate the response rates with non-puerperal use, but this assumption has not been studied. As with antidepressant medications, exposure of the fetus to mood stabilizers and antipsychotic medications is associated with potential risks that need to be discussed with the mother. The goal of treatment of the pregnant or breastfeeding woman with mania or psychosis is to maintain emotional and physical stability for the mother, fetus and infant. Psychosocial support and psychotherapy can be useful adjuncts to pharmacotherapy.

Women with a postpartum manic episode or PPP should be stabilized with a mood stabilizer [126]. Antipsychotic medication and electroconvulsive therapy (ECT) should also be considered, as well as an antidepressant if a woman with PPP has had previous psychotic depression [124]. Postpartum administration of estrogen has demonstrated mixed efficacy for PPP and is currently considered investigational [131]. In one study, 12 days of transdermal estradiol did not reduce PPP in 29 women with previous mania or psychosis [132]. Divalproex was reported not to be superior to no drug in preventing PPP in women with bipolar disorder [133]. Olanzapine was recently reported to be superior to no drug in preventing PPP and mood episodes in women with bipolar disorder [134]. PPP may preferentially respond to ECT compared to non-puerperal psychosis [135].

Studies of congenital malformations with first-trimester benzodiazepine exposure have suggested both no teratogenic risk [136] and a small increased risk of oral cleft [137]. Neonatal concerns with third-trimester benzodiazepine use include floppy infant syndrome and benzodiazepine withdrawal [138]. Benzodiazepines have been safely administered during lactation, but excessive sedation is a risk [138].

First-trimester exposure to lithium confers an increased risk of Ebstein's cardiac anomaly from 1 in 2000 to 1 in 1000 [139]. The appearance of this anomaly can be evaluated by ultrasound at 16–18 weeks gestation. Neonatal concerns with third-trimester lithium use include floppy infant syndrome, hypotonicity, cyanosis, hypothyroidism, and neonatal diabetes insipidus [140,141]. It has been suggested to discontinue lithium prior to delivery to avoid toxicity with the sudden decrease in vascular volume at delivery and immediately restarting lithium after delivery, with serum monitoring, to prevent postpartum relapse [142]. Lithium is generally not recommended during breastfeeding due to its elevated levels in breast milk [124,141].

First-trimester exposure to carbamazepine increases the risk of neural tube defects, craniofacial abnormalities, fingernail hypoplasia and growth retardation [143]. The teratogenic risks with first-trimester exposure with valproate are more profound, particularly with doses above 800–1000 mg/day. Valproate has been associated with neural tube defects, craniofacial abnormalities, cardiac abnormalities and developmental delay. With third-trimester exposure, neonatal symptoms of jitteriness, difficulty feeding, abnormal tone, bradycardia, hypoglycemia and liver toxicity have been reported [141]. Supplemental folic acid (3–5 mg/day) is recommended with carbamazepine and valproate, ideally started prior to conception. Vitamin K 20 mg/day is recommended in the last month of pregnancy to decrease the risk of a bleeding diathesis [144]. Less information is available about the teratogenicity of lamotrigine, topiramate, gabapentin and newer antiepileptic drugs. Monotherapy confers less teratogenic risk than the use of multiple antiepileptic mediations [145]. Carbamazepine and valproate are considered relatively safe with breastfeeding, and minimal safety data are available for the newer antiepileptic medications with breastfeeding [141,143,146].

As mentioned above, antipsychotic medications may be needed during pregnancy for the treatment of agitation, bipolar disorder or chronic schizophrenia. Reviews of studies of haloperidol use in pregnancy have suggested both no increased risk of congenital malformations [147] and a possible increase in limb defects [148]. First-trimester exposure to phenothiazines confers a small increase in risk of congenital malformations compared to the general population rate [149]. It is important to note that untreated psychosis itself is associated with adverse birth outcomes [117,119]. Third-trimester use of traditional antipsychotics has been associated with neonatal dyskinesias, hypertonicity, tremor, motor restlessness, poor feeding and cholestatic jaundice [147]. The newer SGAs are currently used more frequently in psychosis and bipolar disorder than traditional antipsychotics due to their easier tolerability and decreased risk of EPS. Studies have reported both an absence of congenital malformations [150,151] and a small increase in congenital malformations with olanzapine and clozapine [121,152]. Neonatal concerns with third trimester exposure to SGAs have not been reported, except with clozapine (seizures and theoretical risk of agranulocytosis) [121,150]. Concerns with SGA use during pregnancy include the potential weight gain with hyperinsulinemia and hypertension and their adverse effects on birth outcomes [121]. Few data have been published on the safety of SGAs with breastfeeding but low infant serum levels and absence of adverse effects have been reported [124]. Clozapine is not recommended with breastfeeding due to reports of high concentrations in breast milk and infant serum, agranulocytosis, excess sedation and seizures [121,153].

Conclusions

The recommendations for the assessment and treatment of depression, suicidality and agitation during pregnancy and the postpartum period are similar to those for adults in general. Abortion may be a specific risk factor for suicide, and this should be taken into account. Although pregnancy and the postpartum period are associated with fewer suicide attempts and completed suicides, perinatal women should be asked about unwanted pregnancy, hopelessness, IPV, social support, preparations for the infant, attention to self-care and prenatal care, and alcohol and substance abuse. Women may have discontinued psychotropic medication that had been working due to fears of harming the fetus. The treatment of depression, bipolar disorder, psychosis and agitation should involve medications with the best-known safety profile in pregnancy and lactation. Women and their families need to make informed decisions about the risks and benefits of both treating and not treating psychiatric disorders. The goal is maternal–fetal and maternal–infant well-being.

References

1 Hazlett S, McCarthy M, Londner M, et al. Epidemiology of adult psychiatric visits to US emergency departments. *Acad Emerg Med* 2004; 11: 193–195.

2 Boudreaux E, Cagande C, Kilgannon H, et al. A prospective study of depression among adult patients in an urban emergency department. *Prim Care Companion J Clin Psychiatry* 2006; 8: 66–70.

3 Schanzer B, First M, Dominguez B, et al. Diagnosing psychotic disorders in the emergency department in the context of substance use. *Psychiatr Serv* 2006; 57: 1468–1473.

4 Ernst C, Bird S, Goldberg J, et al. The prescription of psychotropic medications for patients discharged from a psychiatric emergency service. *J Clin Psychiatry* 2006; 67: 720–726.

5 American Psychiatric Association. *Diagnostic and Statistical Manual of Mental Disorders*, 4th edn, rev. Washington, DC: American Psychiatric Press, 2000.

6 Lopez A, Mathers C, Ezzati M, et al. Global and regional burden of disease and risk factors, 2001: systematic analysis of population health data. *Lancet* 2006; 367: 1747–1757.

7 Cassano P, Fava M. Depression and public health: an overview. *J Psychosom Res* 2002; 53: 849–857.

8 Kroenke K, Spitzer R, Williams J. The Patient Health Questionnaire-2: validity of a two-item depression screener. *Med Care* 2003; 41: 1284–1292.

9 Flynn H, Blow F, Marcus S. Rates and predictors of depression treatment among pregnant women in hospital-affiliated obstetrics practices. *Gen Hosp Psychiatry* 2006; 28: 289–295.

10 Smith M, Rosenheck R, Cavaleri M, et al. Screening for and detection of depression, panic disorder, and PTSD in public-sector obstetric clinics. *Psychiatr Serv* 2004; 55: 407–414.

11 Sundstrom I, Bixo M, Bjorn I, et al. Prevalence of psychiatric disorders in gynecologic outpatients. *Am J Obstet Gynecol* 2001; 184: 8–13.

12 Miranda J, Azocar F, Komaromy M, et al. Unmet mental health needs of women in public-sector gynecologic clinics. *Am J Obstet Gynecol* 1998; 178: 212–217.

13 Flynn H, O'Mahen H, Massey L, et al. The impact of a brief obstetrics clinic-based intervention on treatment use for perinatal depression. *J Womens Health* 2006; 15: 1195–1204.

14 Gavin N, Gaynes B, Lohr K, et al. Perinatal depression: a systematic review of prevalence and incidence. *Obstet Gynecol* 2005; 106: 1071–1083.

15 Cox J, Holden J, Sagovsky R. Detection of postnatal depression. Development of the 10-item Edinburgh Postnatal Depression Scale. *Br J Psychiatry* 1987; 150: 782–786.

16 Matthey S, Henshaw C, Elliott S, et al. Variability in use of cut-off scores and formats on the Edinburgh Postnatal Depression Scale – implications for clinical and research practice. *Arch Womens Ment Health* 2006; 9: 309–315.

17 Halbreich U. Prevalence of mood symptoms and depressions during pregnancy: implications for clinical practice and research. *CNS Spectr* 2004; 9: 177–184.

18 Munk-Olsen T, Laursen T, Pedersen C, et al. New parents and mental disorders: a population-based register study. *JAMA* 2006; 296: 2582–2589.

19 Cohen L, Altshuler L, Harlow B, et al. Relapse of major depression during pregnancy in women who maintain or discontinue antidepressant treatment. *JAMA* 2006; 295: 499–507.

20 Viguera A, Nonacs R, Cohen L, et al. Risk of recurrence of bipolar disorder in pregnant and nonpregnant women after discontinuing lithium maintenance. *Am J Psychiatry* 2000; 157: 179–184.

21 Dell D, O'Brien BW. Suicide in pregnancy. *Obstet Gynecol* 2003; 102: 1306–1309.

22 Halbreich U. The association between pregnancy processes, preterm deliv ery, low birth weight, and postpartum depressions – the need for interdisciplinary integration. *Am J Obstet Gynecol* 2005; 193: 1312–1322.

23 Van den Bergh B, Mulder E, Mennes M, et al. Antenatal maternal anxiety and stress and the neurobehavioural development of the fetus and child: links and possible mechanisms. A review. *Neurosci Biobehav Rev* 2005; 29: 237–258.

24 Wadhwa PD. Psychoneuroendocrine processes in human pregnancy influence fetal development and health. *Psychoneuroendocrinology* 2005; 30: 724–743.

25 Henshaw C. Mood disturbance in the early puerperium: a review. *Arch Womens Ment Health* 2003; 6: S33-S42.

26 Henshaw C, Foreman D, Cox J. Postnatal blues: a risk factor for postnatal depression. *J Psychosom Obstet Gynaecol* 2004; 25: 267–272.

27 Robertson E, Grace S, Wallington T, et al. Antenatal risk factors for postpartum depression: a synthesis of recent literature. *Gen Hosp Psychiatry* 2004; 26: 289–295.

28 Bernstein I, Rush A, Yonkers K, et al. Symptom features of postpartum depression: are they distinct? *Depress Anxiety* 2008; 25: 20–26.

29 Kendell R, Wainwright S, Hailey A, et al. The influence of childbirth on psychiatric morbidity. *Psychol Med* 1976; 6: 297–302.

30 Grace S, Evindar A, Stewart DE. The effect of postpartum depression on child cognitive development and behavior: a review and critical analysis of the literature. *Arch Womens Ment Health* 2003; 6: 263–274.

31 Weissman M, Wickramaratne P, Nomura Y, et al. Offspring of depressed parents: 20 years later. *Am J Psychiatry* 2006; 163: 1001–1008.

32 Wisner K, Chambers C, Sit D. Postpartum depression: a major public health problem. *JAMA* 2006; 296: 2616–2618.

33 Chaudron L, Szilagyi P, Campbell A, et al. Legal and ethical considerations: risks and benefits of postpartum depression screening at well-child visits. *Pediatrics* 2007; 119: 123–128.

34 Bradshaw Z, Slade P. The effects of induced abortion on emotional experiences and relationships: a critical review of the literature. *Clin Psychol Rev* 2003; 23: 929–958.

35 Sit D, Rothschild A, Creinin M, et al. Psychiatric outcomes following medical and surgical abortion. *Hum Reprod* 2007; 22: 878–884.

36 Fergusson D, Horwood L, Ridder E. Abortion in young women and subsequent mental health. *J Child Psychol Psychiatry* 2006; 47: 16–24.

37 Shadigian E, Bauer S. Pregnancy-associated death: a qualitative systematic review of homicide and suicide. *Obstet Gynecol Surv* 2005; 60: 183–190.

38 Gissler M, Hemminki E, Lonnqvist J. Suicides after pregnancy in Finland, 1987–94; register linkage study. *BMJ* 1996; 313: 1431–1434.

39 Klier C, Geller P, Ritsher J. Affective disorders in the aftermath of miscarriage: a comprehensive review. *Arch Womens Ment Health* 2002; 5: 129–149.

40 Neugebauer R, Kline J, Shrout P, et al. Major depressive disorder in the 6 months after miscarriage. *JAMA* 1997; 277: 383–388.

41 Geller P, Kerns D, Klier C. Anxiety following miscarriage and the subsequent pregnancy: a review of the literature and future directions. *J Psychosom Res* 2004; 56: 35–45.

42 Brier N. Anxiety after miscarriage: a review of the empirical literature and implications for clinical practice. *Birth* 2004; 31: 138–142.

43 Turton P, Hughes P, Evans C, et al. Incidence, correlates and predictors of post-traumatic stress disorder in the pregnancy after stillbirth. *Br J Psychiatry* 2001; 178: 556–560.

44 Hughes P, Turton P, Evans C. Stillbirth as risk factor for depression and anxiety in the subsequent pregnancy: cohort study. *BMJ* 1999; 318: 1721–1724.

45 Badenhorst W, Hughes P. Psychological aspects of perinatal loss. *Best Pract Res Clin Obstet Gynaecol* 2007; 21: 249–259.

46 Hughes P, Turton P, Hopper E, et al. Assessment of guidelines for good practice in psychosocial care of mothers after stillbirth: a cohort study. *Lancet* 2002; 360: 114–118.

47 O'Leary J. Grief and its impact on prenatal attachment in the subsequent pregnancy. *Arch Womens Ment Health* 2004; 7: 7–18.

48 Chaudron L. Critical issues in perinatal psychiatric emergency care. *Psychiatr Issues Emerg Care Sett* 2005; 4: 11–18.

49 Martin S, Li Y, Casanueva C, et al. Intimate partner violence and women's depression before and during pregnancy. *Violence Against Women* 2006; 12: 221–239.

50 Gazmararian J, Lazorick S, Spitz A, et al. Prevalence of violence against pregnant women. *JAMA* 1996; 275: 1915–1920.

51 Silverman J, Decker M, Reed E, et al. Intimate partner violence victimization prior to and during pregnancy among women residing in 26 U.S. states: associations with maternal and neonatal health. *Am J Obstet Gynecol* 2006; 195: 140–148.

52 Boy A, Salihu H. Intimate partner violence and birth outcomes: a systematic review. *Int J Fertil Womens Med* 2004; 49: 159–164.

53 Renker P, Tonkin P. Women's views of prenatal violence screening: acceptability and confidentiality issues. *Obstet Gynecol* 2006; 107: 348–354.

54 American College of Obstetricians and Gynecologists, Committee on Healthcare for Underserved Women ACOG Committee Opinion

No. 343: psychosocial risk factors: perinatal screening and intervention. *Obstet Gynecol* 2006; 108: 469–477.
55 Spinelli M, Endicott J. Controlled clinical trial of interpersonal psychotherapy versus parenting education program for depressed pregnant women. *Am J Psychiatry* 2003; 160: 555–562.
56 Epperson C, Terman M, Terman J, et al. Randomized clinical trial of bright light therapy for antepartum depression: preliminary findings. *J Clin Psychiatry* 2004; 65: 421–425.
57 Field T, Diego M, Hernandez-Reif M, et al. Massage therapy effects on depressed pregnant women. *J Psychosom Obstet Gynaecol* 2004; 25: 115–122.
58 Manber R, Schnyer R, Allen J, et al. Acupuncture: a promising treatment for depression during pregnancy. *J Affect Disord* 2004; 83: 89–95.
59 Freeman M, Hibbeln J, Wisner K, et al. An open trial of omega-3 fatty acids for depression in pregnancy. *Acta Neuropsychiatr* 2006; 18: 21–24.
60 Sit D, Wisner K. Decision making for postpartum depression treatment. *Psychiatr Ann* 2005; 35: 577–585.
61 Rahimi R, Nikfar S, Abdollahi M. Pregnancy outcomes following exposure to serotonin reuptake inhibitors: a meta-analysis of clinical trials. *Reprod Toxicol* 2006; 22: 571–575.
62 Hemels M, Einarson A, Koren G, et al. Antidepressant use during pregnancy and the rates of spontaneous abortions: a meta-analysis. *Ann Pharmacother* 2005; 39: 803–809.
63 Einarson T, Einarson A. Newer antidepressants in pregnancy and rates of major malformations: a meta-analysis of prospective comparative studies. *Pharmacoepidemiol Drug Saf* 2005; 14: 823–827.
64 Wogelius P, Norgaard M, Gislum M, et al. Maternal use of selective serotonin reuptake inhibitors and risk of congenital malformations. *Epidemiology* 2006; 17: 701–704.
65 Williams M, Wooltorton E. Paroxetine (Paxil) and congenital malformations. *Can Med Assoc J* 2005; 173: 1320–1321.
66 Berard A, Ramos E, Rey E, et al. First trimester exposure to paroxetine and risk of cardiac malformations in infants: the importance of dosage. *Birth Defects Res B Dev Reprod Toxicol* 2007; 80: 18–27.
67 Moses-Kolko E, Bogen D, Perel J, et al. Neonatal signs after late in utero exposure to serotonin reuptake inhibitors: literature review and implications for clinical applications. *JAMA* 2005; 293: 2372–2383.
68 Nordeng H, Spigset O. Treatment with selective serotonin reuptake inhibitors in the third trimester of pregnancy: effects on the infant. *Drug Saf* 2005; 28: 565–581.
69 Sanz E, De-las-Cuevas C, Kiuru A, et al. Selective serotonin reuptake inhibitors in pregnant women and neonatal withdrawal syndrome: a database analysis. *Lancet* 2005; 365: 482–487.
70 Oberlander T, Warburton W, Misri S, et al. Neonatal outcomes after prenatal exposure to selective serotonin reuptake inhibitor antidepressants and maternal depression using population-based linked health data. *Arch Gen Psychiatry* 2006; 63, 898–906.
71 Chambers C, Hernandez-Diaz S, van Marter L, et al. Selective serotonin-reuptake inhibitors and risk of persistent pulmonary hypertension of the newborn. *N Engl J Med* 2006; 354: 579–587.
72 American College of Obstetricians and Gynecologists, Committee on Obstetric Practice. Committee Opinion No. 354: treatment with selective serotonin reuptake inhibitors during pregnancy. *Obstet Gynecol* 2006; 108: 1601–1603.
73 Wisner K, Hanusa B, Perel J, et al. Postpartum depression: a randomized trial of sertraline versus nortriptyline. *J Clin Psychopharmacol* 2006; 26: 353–360.
74 Appleby L, Warner R, Whitton A, et al. A controlled study of fluoxetine and cognitive-behavioural counselling in the treatment of postnatal depression. *BMJ* 1997; 314: 932–936.
75 Misri S, Reebye P, Corral M, et al. The use of paroxetine and cognitive-behavioral therapy in postpartum depression and anxiety: a randomized controlled trial. *J Clin Psychiatry* 2004; 65: 1236–1241.
76 Weissman A, Levy B, Hartz A, et al. Pooled analysis of antidepressant levels in lactating mothers, breast milk, and nursing infants. *Am J Psychiatry* 2004; 161: 1066–1078.
77 Abreu A, Stuart S. Pharmacologic and hormonal treatments for postpartum depression. *Psychiatr Ann* 2005; 35: 568–576.
78 Eberhard-Gran M, Eskild A, Opjordsmoen S. Use of psychotropic medications in treating mood disorders during lactation: practical recommendations. *CNS Drugs* 2006; 20: 187–198.
79 Gentile S. The safety of newer antidepressants in pregnancy and breastfeeding. *Drug Saf* 2005; 28: 137–152.
80 Hallberg P, Sjoblom V. The use of selective serotonin reuptake inhibitors during pregnancy and breast-feeding: a review and clinical aspects. *J Clin Psychopharmacol* 2005; 25: 59–73.
81 O'Hara M, Stuart S, Gorman L, et al. Efficacy of interpersonal psychotherapy for postpartum depression. *Arch Gen Psychiatry* 2000; 57: 1039–1045.
82 Dennis C. Treatment of postpartum depression, part 2: a critical review of nonbiological interventions. *J Clin Psychiatry* 2004; 65: 1252–1265.
83 Kopelman R, Stuart S. Psychological treatments for postpartum depression. *Psychiatr Ann* 2005; 35: 556–566.
84 Bledsoe S, Grote N. Treating depression during pregnancy and the postpartum: a preliminary meta-analysis. *Res Soc Work Pract* 2006; 16: 109–120.
85 Pearlstein T. Perinatal depression: treatment options and dilemmas. *J Psychiatry Neurosci* 2008; 33: 302–318.
86 Dennis C, Chung-Lee L. Postpartum depression help-seeking barriers and maternal treatment preferences: a qualitative systematic review. *Birth* 2006; 33: 323–331.
87 Practice guideline for the assessment and treatment of patients with suicidal behaviors. *Am J Psychiatry* 2003; 160: 1–60.
88 Chaudron L, Caine E. Suicide among women: a critical review. *J Am Med Womens Assoc* 2004; 59: 125–134.
89 Knox K, Caine E. Establishing priorities for reducing suicide and its antecedents in the United States. *Am J Public Health* 2005; 95: 1898–1903.
90 Oquendo M, Bongiovi-Garcia M, Galfalvy H, et al. Sex differences in clinical predictors of suicidal acts after major depression: a prospective study. *Am J Psychiatry* 2007; 164: 134–141.
91 Hawton K, Sutton L, Haw C, et al. Suicide and attempted suicide in bipolar disorder: a systematic review of risk factors. *J Clin Psychiatry* 2005; 66: 693–704.
92 Stern T, Perlis R, Lagomasino I. Suicidal patients. In: Stern T, Fricchione G, Cassem N, et al., eds. *Massachusetts General Hospital Handbook of General Hospital Psychiatry*, 5th edn. Philadelphia: Mosby, 2004: 93–104.
93 Nock M, Kessler R. Prevalence of and risk factors for suicide attempts versus suicide gestures: analysis of the National Comorbidity Survey. *J Abnorm Psychol* 2006; 115: 616–623.

94 Lindahl V, Pearson J, Colpe L. Prevalence of suicidality during pregnancy and the postpartum. *Arch Womens Ment Health* 2005; 8: 77–87.

95 Marzuk P, Tardiff K, Leon A, et al. Lower risk of suicide during pregnancy. *Am J Psychiatry* 1997; 154: 122–123.

96 Appleby L. Suicide during pregnancy and in the first postnatal year. *BMJ* 1991; 302: 137–140.

97 Appleby L, Mortensen P, Faragher E. Suicide and other causes of mortality after post-partum psychiatric admission. *Br J Psychiatry* 1998; 173: 209–211.

98 Oates M. Suicide: the leading cause of maternal death. *Br J Psychiatry* 2003; 183: 279–281.

99 Czeizel A, Timar L, Susanszky E. Timing of suicide attempts by self-poisoning during pregnancy and pregnancy outcomes. *Int J Gynaecol Obstet* 1999; 65: 39–45.

100 Schiff M, Grossman D. Adverse perinatal outcomes and risk for postpartum suicide attempt in Washington state, 1987–2001 *Pediatrics* 2006; 118: e669–e675.

101 Gandhi S, Gilbert W, McElvy S, et al. Maternal and neonatal outcomes after attempted suicide. *Obstet Gynecol* 2006; 107: 984–990.

102 Battaglia J. Pharmacological management of acute agitation. *Drugs* 2005; 65: 1207–1222.

103 Citrome L, Volavka J. Treatment of violent behavior. In: Tasman A, Kay J, Lieberman J, eds. *Psychiatry*, 2nd edn. Chichester: John Wiley, 2003: 2136–2146.

104 Sachs G. A review of agitation in mental illness: burden of illness and underlying pathology. *J Clin Psychiatry* 2006; 67: 5–12.

105 Fauman B. Other psychiatric emergencies. In: Kaplan H, Sadock B, eds. *Comprehensive Textbook of Psychiatry, VI*. Baltimore, MD: Williams and Wilkins, 1995: 1752–1765.

106 Lindenmayer J. The pathophysiology of agitation. *J Clin Psychiatry* 2000; 61: 5–10.

107 Brower M, Price B. Neuropsychiatry of frontal lobe dysfunction in violent and criminal behaviour: a critical review. *J Neurol Neurosurg Psychiatry* 2001; 71: 720–726.

108 Lam J, McNiel D, Binder R. The relationship between patients' gender and violence leading to staff injuries. *Psychiatr Serv* 2000; 51: 1167–1170.

109 Onyike C, Lyketsos C. Aggression and violence. In: Levenson J, ed. *Textbook of Psychosomatic Medicine*. Arlington, VA: American Psychiatric Publishing, 2005: 171–191.

110 Alarcon R, Hart D. The influence of culture in emergency psychiatry. *Psychiatr Issues Emerg Care Sett* 2006; 5: 13–22.

111 Petit J. Management of the acutely violent patient. *Psychiatr Clin North Am* 2005; 28: 701–711.

112 Marder S. A review of agitation in mental illness: treatment guidelines and current therapies. *J Clin Psychiatry* 2006; 67: 13–21.

113 Nelstrop L, Chandler-Oatts J, Bingley W, et al. A systematic review of the safety and effectiveness of restraint and seclusion as interventions for the short-term management of violence in adult psychiatric inpatient settings and emergency departments. *Worldviews Evid Based Nurs* 2006; 3: 8–18.

114 Allen M, Currier G, Carpenter D, et al. Treatment of behavioral emergencies 2005. *J Psychiatr Pract* 2005; 11: 5–108.

115 Lukens T, Wolf S, Edlow J, et al. Clinical policy: critical issues in the diagnosis and management of the adult psychiatric patient in the emergency department. *Ann Emerg Med* 2006; 47: 79–99.

116 Rund D, Ewing J, Mitzel K, et al. The use of intramuscular benzodiazepines and antipsychotic agents in the treatment of acute agitation or violence in the emergency department. *J Emerg Med* 2006; 31: 317–324.

117 Howard L. Fertility and pregnancy in women with psychotic disorders. *Eur J Obstet Gynecol Reprod Biol* 2005; 119: 3–10.

118 Jablensky A, Morgan V, Zubrick S, et al. Pregnancy, delivery, and neonatal complications in a population cohort of women with schizophrenia and major affective disorders. *Am J Psychiatry* 2005; 162: 79–91.

119 Nilsson E, Lichtenstein P, Cnattingius S, et al. Women with schizophrenia: pregnancy outcome and infant death among their offspring. *Schizophr Res* 2002; 58: 221–229.

120 Bennedsen B, Mortensen P, Olesen A, et al. Congenital malformations, stillbirths, and infant deaths among children of women with schizophrenia. *Arch Gen Psychiatry* 2001; 58: 674–679.

121 Yaeger D, Smith H, Altshuler L. Atypical antipsychotics in the treatment of schizophrenia during pregnancy and the postpartum. *Am J Psychiatry* 2006; 163: 2064–2070.

122 Gilbert P, Harris J, McAdams L, et al. Neuroleptic withdrawal in schizophrenic patients. A review of the literature. *Arch Gen Psychiatry* 1995; 52: 173–188.

123 Seeman M. Relational ethics: when mothers suffer from psychosis. *Arch Womens Ment Health* 2004; 7: 201–210.

124 Sit D, Rothschild A, Wisner K. A review of postpartum psychosis. *J Womens Health* 2006; 15: 352–368.

125 Blackmore E, Jones I, Doshi M, et al. Obstetric variables associated with bipolar affective puerperal psychosis. *Br J Psychiatry* 2006; 188: 32–36.

126 Sharma V. Pharmacotherapy of postpartum psychosis. *Expert Opin Pharmacother* 2003; 4: 1651–1658.

127 Jones I, Craddock N. Familiality of the puerperal trigger in bipolar disorder: results of a family study. *Am J Psychiatry* 2001; 158: 913–917.

128 Friedman S, Horwitz S, Resnick P. Child murder by mothers: a critical analysis of the current state of knowledge and a research agenda. *Am J Psychiatry* 2005; 162: 1578–1587.

129 Spinelli M. Maternal infanticide associated with mental illness: prevention and the promise of saved lives. *Am J Psychiatry* 2004; 161: 1548–1557.

130 Spinelli M. A systematic investigation of 16 cases of neonaticide. *Am J Psychiatry* 2001; 158: 811–813.

131 Gentile S. The role of estrogen therapy in postpartum psychiatric disorders: an update. *CNS Spectr* 2005; 10: 944–952.

132 Kumar C, McIvor R, Davies T, et al. Estrogen administration does not reduce the rate of recurrence of affective psychosis after childbirth. *J Clin Psychiatry* 2003; 64: 112–118.

133 Wisner K, Perel J, Peindl K, et al. Prevention of postpartum episodes in women with bipolar disorder. *Biol Psychiatry* 2004; 56: 592–596.

134 Sharma V, Smith A, Mazmanian D. Olanzapine in the prevention of postpartum psychosis and mood episodes in bipolar disorder. *Bipolar Disord* 2006; 8: 400–404.

135 Reed P, Sermin N, Appleby L, et al. A comparison of clinical response to electroconvulsive therapy in puerperal and non-puerperal psychoses. *J Affect Disord* 1999; 54: 255–260.

136 Eros E, Czeizel A, Rockenbauer M, et al. A population-based case-control teratologic study of nitrazepam, medazepam, tofisopam, alprazolum and clonazepam treatment during pregnancy. *Eur J Obstet Gynecol Reprod Biol* 2002; 101: 147–154.

137 Dolovich L, Addis A, Vaillancourt J, et al. Benzodiazepine use in pregnancy and major malformations or oral cleft: meta-analysis of cohort and case-control studies. *BMJ* 1998; 317: 839–843.

138 Iqbal M, Sobhan T, Ryals T. Effects of commonly used benzodiazepines on the fetus, the neonate, and the nursing infant. *Psychiatr Serv* 2002; 53: 39–49.

139 Cohen L, Friedman J, Jefferson J, et al. A reevaluation of risk of in utero exposure to lithium. *JAMA* 1994; 271: 146–150.

140 Viguera A, Cohen L, Baldessarini R, et al. Managing bipolar disorder during pregnancy: weighing the risks and benefits. *Can J Psychiatry* 2002; 47: 426–436.

141 Yonkers K, Wisner K, Stowe Z, et al. Management of bipolar disorder during pregnancy and the postpartum period. *Am J Psychiatry* 2004; 161: 608–620.

142 Newport D, Viguera A, Beach A, et al. Lithium placental passage and obstetrical outcome: implications for clinical management during late pregnancy. *Am J Psychiatry* 2005; 162: 2162–2170.

143 Pennell P. 2005 AES annual course: evidence used to treat women with epilepsy. *Epilepsia* 2006; 47: 46–53.

144 Crawford P. Best practice guidelines for the management of women with epilepsy. *Epilepsia* 2005; 46(Suppl 9): 117–124.

145 Tatum W. Use of antiepileptic drugs in pregnancy. *Expert Rev Neurother* 2006; 6: 1077–1086.

146 Gentile S. Prophylactic treatment of bipolar disorder in pregnancy and breastfeeding: focus on emerging mood stabilizers. *Bipolar Disord* 2006; 8: 207–220.

147 Trixler M, Gati A, Fekete S, et al. Use of antipsychotics in the management of schizophrenia during pregnancy. *Drugs* 2005; 65: 1193–1206.

148 Diav-Citrin O, Shechtman S, Ornoy S, et al. Safety of haloperidol and penfluridol in pregnancy: a multicenter, prospective, controlled study. *J Clin Psychiatry* 2005; 66: 317–322.

149 Altshuler L, Cohen L, Szuba M, et al. Pharmacologic management of psychiatric illness during pregnancy: dilemmas and guidelines. *Am J Psychiatry* 1996; 153: 592–606.

150 Gentile S. Clinical utilization of atypical antipsychotics in pregnancy and lactation. *Ann Pharmacother* 2004; 38: 1265–1271.

151 McKenna K, Koren G, Tetelbaum M, et al. Pregnancy outcome of women using atypical antipsychotic drugs: a prospective comparative study. *J Clin Psychiatry* 2005; 66: 444–449.

152 Howard L, Webb R, Abel K. Safety of antipsychotic drugs for pregnant and breastfeeding women with non-affective psychosis. *BMJ* 2004; 329: 933–934.

153 Aichhorn W, Whitworth A, Weiss E, et al. Second-generation antipsychotics: is there evidence for sex differences in pharmacokinetic and adverse effect profiles? *Drug Saf* 2006; 29: 587–598.

49 Fetal Surgery Procedures and Associated Maternal Complications

Robert H. Ball[1] & Michael A. Belfort[2]

[1]HCA Fetal Therapy Initiative, St Mark's Hospital, Salt Lake City *and* Division of Perinatal Medicine and Genetics, Departments of Obstetrics, Gynecology and Reproductive Sciences, UCSF Fetal Treatment Center, University of California, San Francisco, CA, USA

[2]Department of Obstetrics and Gynecology, Division of Maternal-Fetal Medicine, University of Utah, Salt Lake City, UT *and* HCA Healthcare, Nashville, TN, USA

Introduction

A discussion of the potential maternal complications of fetal surgery is pertinent given the fact that such complications are in theory absolutely avoidable. As the term suggests, fetal surgery is performed for the sole physical benefit of the fetus, and any risk to which the mother is exposed is for a purely altruistic purpose. There is no direct health benefit to the mother.

Many of the first fetal surgical procedures depended on maternal laparotomy to expose the uterus and hysterotomy to expose the fetus. This approach then evolved into laparotomy with uterine endoscopy rather than hysterotomy to preserve the integrity of the uterus. With further experience laparotomy has been for the most part been replaced with percutaneous procedures using telescopic devices with a diameter of 3 mm or less. The progression to microinvasive fetoscopic approaches has reduced the potential for morbidity, but not eliminated it [1] (Table 49.1.). Each one of these approaches and associated complications will be discussed in more detail below.

Hysterotomy

Hysterotomy, while less frequently used now, is still employed in some cases where endoscopic techniques are not possible. These include repair of neural tube defects, and the removal of sacrococcygeal teratomas and other masses. Hysterotomy-based procedures are usually dependent on intraoperative ultrasound guidance (both before and after abdominal wall incision). Once the patient has had anesthesia (general endotracteal) and the sterile field has been established, ultrasound is used to determine the fetal lie. If the lie is unsuitable for the proposed surgery, external version and transabdominal manipulation is employed under ultrasound guidance to position the fetus such that the fetal surgical site is near the fundus. Depending on the maternal body habitus and fetal size and position this may be quite challenging. Laparotomy is then performed and the ultrasound transducer, covered in a sterile sleeve, is placed directly on the surface of the uterus. The placental edge is identified, a critical step in making the decision on where to perform the uterine entry. Ideally the uterine incision is best centered as far from the placental edge as possible because once amniotic fluid escapes the uterus deflates. Despite taking this precaution the uterine incision will almost always still be in relatively close proximity to the placental edge – which increases the risk of bleeding and abruption. If significant bleeding cannot be readily controlled immediate delivery will be required for maternal safety.

Generally the incision in the uterus will have been made such as to have optimal access to the fetal part to be surgically addressed. Ultrasound is used for transuterine monitoring of the fetal heart during the procedure.

Following completion of the fetal intervention, the membranes and myometrium are closed with several layers of suture. A catheter is left in the uterine cavity to allow lactated Ringer's solution to be infused together with antibiotics. Ultrasound is used to determine the volume of "amniotic" fluid, which generally is left at a low normal level to minimize stress on the suture line.

Postoperative management usually involves tocolytic therapy of some sort. The regimen in San Francisco included 24 hours of intravenous magnesium sulfate and oral indomethacin for a total of 48 hours. Long-term tocolytic maintenance with nifedipine is then substituted and continued until delivery. Prophylactic antibiotics are continued for 24 hours. Ultrasound monitoring is used daily to evaluate fetal health (biophysical profile and ductus arteriosus patency), amniotic fluid volume, and cervical length. Hospital discharge generally occurs 4–5 days after surgery. If all goes well long-term monitoring with ultrasound continues at a weekly frequency.

Critical Care Obstetrics, 5th edition. Edited by M. Belfort, G. Saade, M. Foley, J. Phelan and G. Dildy.

Table 49.1 Maternal morbidity and mortality for 178 interventions at UCSF with postoperative continuing pregnancy and divided into operative subgroups.

Operative technique	Open hysterotomy	Endoscopy FETENDO/Lap-FETENDO	Percutaneous FIGS/Lap-FIGS	All interventions
Patients with postoperative continuing pregnancy	79	68	31	178
Gestational age at surgery [wks]	25.1	24.5	21.1	24.2
Range [wks]	17.6–30.4	17.9–32.1	17.0–26.6	17.0–32.1
Gestational age at delivery [wks]	30.1	30.4	32.7	30.7
Range [wks]	21.6–36.7	19.6–39.3	21.7–40.4	19.6–40.4
Interval surgery to delivery [wks]	4.9	6.0	11.6	6.5
Range [wks]	0–16	0–19	0.3–21.4	0–21.4
Pulmonary edema	22/79 (27.8%)	17/68 (25.0%)	0/31 (0.0%)	39/178 (21.9%)
Bleeding requiring blood transfusion	11/87 (12.6%)	2/69 (2.9%)	0/31 (0.0%)	13/187 (7.0%)
PTL leading to delivery	26/79 (32.9%)	18/68 (26.5%)	4/31 (12.9%)	48/178 (27.0%)
Preterm premature rupture of membranes (PPROM)	41/79 (51.9%)	30/68 (44.1%)	8/31 (25.8%)	79/178 (44.4%)
Chorioamnionitis	7/79 (8.9%)	1/68 (1.5%)	0/31 (0.0%)	8/178 (4.5%)

FETENDO, fetal endoscopic procedure; Lap-FETENDO, laparotomy and fetal endoscopic procedure; FIGS, fetal image-guided surgery; Lap-FIGS, laparotomy and fetal image-guided surgery.

We have recently reviewed our experience at UCSF with maternal hysterotomy [1] (Table 49.1). Eighty-seven hysterotomies were performed between 1989 and 2003. There were significant immediate postoperative complications. In the early experience, pulmonary edema was common and is believed to be related to the use of multiple tocolytic agents (particularly nitroglycerin and beta stimulants) combined with steroid use and aggressive fluid management [2]. Thirteen per cent of women having a hysterotomy required transfusion for intraoperative blood loss. Fifty two per cent of these patients suffered postoperative preterm premature rupture of the membranes (PPROM) and 33% developed preterm contractions refractory to maximal therapy and delivered preterm. The mean time from hysterotomy to delivery was 4.9 weeks (range 0–16 weeks). The mean gestational age at the time of delivery was 30.1 weeks (range 21.6–36.7 weeks). Others [3,4] have had similar experience with preterm delivery following hysterotomy. With experience much of the morbidity associated with hysterotomy has decreased and clinically significant pulmonary edema and blood loss are now less common. The mean gestational age at the time of delivery following repair of meningomyelocele (MMC) is now approximately 34 weeks [5].

Discussion of the risks, benefits and alternatives of the procedure are important, and must include a clear disclosure of the experimental nature of the surgery. The risks to the mother are similar to those seen in any major abdominal surgery, although in this case as mentioned above, there is no direct physical benefit to her. She should understand the risks associated with aggressive tocolytic therapy and those resulting from bed rest in a hypercoagulable state (venous thromboembolism). The risks to the fetus are primarily the result of intraoperative vascular instability and hypoperfusion (leading to injury or death) and the pathology of preterm delivery. The risks to the pregnancy are primarily preterm labor, premature rupture of the membranes, and preterm delivery. Infectious complications are rare, except when premature rupture of the membranes leads to prolonged latency. An important additional discussion point is that all subsequent deliveries, including the index pregnancy, must be by cesarean section. Data regarding future fertility are reassuring, with no increased incidence of infertility in the UCSF experience in those patients attempting pregnancy [6]. Experience from the Children's Hospital of Phildelphia (CHOP) suggests a concerning risk for uterine rupture/dehiscence in subsequent pregnancies that may be as high as 6–12% [7], which would be considerably higher than the risk after previous low transverse cesarean section (1% or less) [8] or classical cesarean section (5–10%) [9]. Another theoretical risk in subsequent pregnancies is placenta accreta. This is because the hysterotomy performed in the second trimester is never in the transverse lower uterine segment and therefore the patient is exposed to two uterine incisions during the pregnancy. The risk of accreta increases when implantation is in an area of uterine scarring and multiple incisions will increase the likelihood of implantation in such an area. To our knowledge there has not been a single case of placenta accreta in a fetal surgical patient from UCSF in a subsequent pregnancy.

Fetoscopy

The growing popularity of videoendoscopic surgery in the 1990s, combined with the earlier experience with fetoscopy, paved the way for endoscopic fetal surgery. The belief was that a smaller disruption of the amniotic membranes would ameliorate some of the limiting steps in fetal surgery, viz. (i) preterm labor, which was believed to be triggered by the large uterine incision required for open fetal surgery, and (ii) significant maternal morbidity associated with a large laparotomy. The ultimate hope was that fetoscopic interventions would be possible by a percutaneous approach.

Patients are given a preoperative tocolytic agent, often indomethacin, and also receive prophylactic IV antibiotics. The procedures are performed under local or regional anesthesia. Depending on the gestational age and the tradition of the center, the surgery may be performed in the surgical operating rooms, the labor and delivery operating room, or the ultrasound suite. The endoscopes and fetoscopic instruments have undergone tremendous development and improvement over the last decade. Operative fetoscopy has now evolved into a combined sono-endoscopic procedure in which the fetal surgical team use both the ultrasound and fetoscopic images simultaneously to perform the operations. Purpose-designed embryo- or fetoscopes typically have remote eyepieces, to reduce weight and facilitate precise movements. Nearly all are bendable fibre-endoscopes rather than conventional rod lens scopes, and as the number of pixels increases over time, image quality improves. Typical diameters are between 1.0 and 2.0 mm. Thin-walled semi-flexible plastic cannulas (7–10 French diameter) are used to provide access to the amniotic sac and this allows different instruments to be inserted into the uterus without multiple puncture wounds.

Ultrasound is used to identify an appropriate entry point and is then used to direct the trochar into the amniotic cavity, avoiding the placenta, fetus, and maternal organs such as bowel and bladder. One group has documented the safety, in their hands, of a transplacental approach [10] but most operators still avoid deliberate transplacental passage of instruments if at all possible.

Ultrasound is initially used to direct and position the fetoscope within the uterus, since its field and depth of view can be relatively limited. These procedures are truly "sono-endoscopic".

One of the most commonly performed fetoscopic procedures is laser ablation of placental blood vessels in twin–twin transfusion syndrome (TTTS). In these cases the endoscope is placed into the sac of the recipient twin, which is the sac with polyhydramnios. The insertion point of the fetoscope is determined by placental location, the lie of the donor baby, the umbilical cord insertion sites and the presumed membrane and vascular equators between the twins. Once the fetoscope is positioned and the placental surface is being visualized, the whole vascular equator is then explored. Unpaired vessels consistent with abnormal communications are ablated using a laser fiber that is advanced through the operating channel of the endoscope sleeve. After ablation of the abnormal communications the endoscope is withdrawn and the polyhydramnios is then drained through the cannula under ultrasound guidance. Once the fluid has reached a normal level (deepest vertical pocket of around 5–6 cm) the cannula is removed. This amnioreduction reduces the risk of port-site leaking and amniotic fluid irritation of the peritoneal cavity. It may also improve placental perfusion and makes the patient more comfortable. In many cases little or no tocolytic medication is needed and patients are generally discharged within 24 hours or less of the procedure.

The risks of fetoscopy are related to uterine puncture as well as to the specific procedure that is being treated. In some cases adverse outcomes may be inherent in the disease state itself such as mirror syndrome (Ballantyne syndrome) in TTTS [11].

Preoperative measurement of the cervix can be used to assess the risk for premature delivery after fetoscopy [12]. When the cervix is less than 30 mm the data suggest a 74% risk for delivery prior to 34 weeks. If the cervix is shorter than 20 mm the vast majority of patients miscarry. After fetoscopy the risk for preterm premature rupture of membranes (PPROM) is estimated to be approximately 10 % or less and the risk for abruption is 1–2%. The rate of abruption is believed to be related more to the amnioreduction than the use of the fetscope. Less common complications are chorioamnionitis and hemorrhage.

Shunts and radiofrequency ablation

Shunts are used for chronic drainage of fluid-filled fetal cavities, organs and cysts. The first shunt was developed by Harrison at UCSF in the early 1980s [13]. This was essentially a double pigtail shunt introduced through a 14G introducer (Cook Medical, USA). The Rodeck shunt, developed during the same time period in the UK, is also a double pigtail shunt, but is longer and has a greater diameter (Rocket Medical, UK) than the Harrison shunt, and it uses a larger diameter introducer [14]. These shunts are placed in fetuses with an obstructed bladder, pleural effusion(s) and large type I congenital cystic adenomatoid malformations (CCAMs). With most shunt procedures, a small incision is made in the maternal skin, and the introducer with the trochar in place is advanced into the amniotic cavity. Care is taken to evaluate the myometrium that will be traversed with a high-frequency transducer (to improve the resolution of the tissue) and with color flow Doppler with low flow settings, to avoid damaging large veins. We generally avoid a transplacental approach but if no other approach is available shunts can be placed transplacentally. The trochar and introducer are then advanced into the area to be drained. Once in position the trochar is removed and care is taken to not allow sudden decompression of the fluid-filled cavity by placing a finger over the end of the introducer. The shunt is then loaded into the introducer and advanced using a pusher until the internal coils exit the introducer. It is critical to continuously image this process with ultrasound. Once the inner coils are appropriately positioned, the introducer is carefully withdrawn, while at the same time advancing the shunt so that the outer coil is positioned on the skin of the fetus, within the amniotic cavity. Care must be taken to have sufficient amniotic fluid between the fetus and the wall of the uterus during this procedure to prevent the outer end of the shunt from being left in the myometrium or maternal abdominal wall. In the case of the shunt penetrating the uterus there is the risk of an amnioperitoneal shunt. Shunt placement procedures may be the most frequently performed fetal surgical intervention.

Complications from shunt placement include maternal and fetal bleeding, placental abruption, amniotic–peritoneal shunt, and infection.

Radiofrequency ablation (RFA) is most commonly used for destruction of tumor tissue in solid organs such as the liver. This technique was first used for localized cautery of fetal vascular communications. Additionally it has been used for ablating the feeding vessels to the anomalous fetus in twin reversed arterial perfusion (TRAP) sequence [15,16]. Further applications include selective reduction in monochorionic twin gestations discordant for severe anomalies, and in severe twin–twin transfusion without hope for salvage of one of the twins.

The RFA device that we currently use is a 17G needle device (Rita Medical, USA). The perioperative management is identical to that discussed above with shunts except that local anesthesia alone is usually sufficient. In the case of TRAP, the instrument is guided into the tissue of the acardiac twin at the level of the cord insertion. The prongs are deployed and energy transmission to the device initiated. Because of the heat generation there is outgassing that is readily visible with ultrasound. The procedure is considered completed when there is no evidence of flow in the acardiac twin (or in the cord leading to it) as evidenced by color and pulse Doppler ultrasound. The prongs are then retracted and the device withdrawn. Postoperative monitoring is similar to that used in shunt placement cases and further tocolytic management is rarely necessary. The patients can generally be discharged within hours of the procedure.

The risks of complications following shunt placement and RFA are lower than for the more invasive fetal surgical interventions requiring hysterotomy. Obviously, by definition, all invasive procedures involve a risk of hemorrhage and infection (Table 49.1) [1]. The triggering of preterm delivery by these procedures is also quite unusual, although the risk of PPROM remains. There is also the risk of fetal injury, which in cases of monochorionic twins generally is related to hypotension from acute hypovolemia in the normal cotwin secondary to exsanguination into the placental vascular bed and the other fetus.

Over time, as teams have become more comfortable with fetoscopic procedures, the length of hospitalization, complexity of perioperative management and type of anesthesia have changed. In many cases these operations can be performed under ultrasound guidance as an outpatient procedure (23-hour admission) with a single dose of indomethacin for tocolysis. Routine preoperative antibiotic prophylaxis is given. For most procedures spinal or local anesthesia is sufficient.

Postoperative management involves maternal and fetal monitoring (in cases of fetal viability). Further tocolytic management is based on contraction activity. Frequently no further medication is necessary. Maternal vital signs should be followed carefully as direct observation of the uterine puncture is not possible to determine hemostasis, because of the percutaneous approach. One benefit of not needing tocolysis is that the hemostatic mechanism of the uterus in response to a puncture is a localized contraction.

In summary, the fact that many fetal and particularly placental procedures can now be performed using microendoscopes and that hysterotomy is infrequently needed except for a few rare indications, has improved the rate and severity of maternal complications. Nevertheless none of these procedures are risk free. There have been intraoperative maternal deaths reported and this must be discussed with a patient and her family in balancing the risks and benefits of a prospective intervention.

References

1 Golombeck K, Ball RH, Lee H, et al. Maternal morbidity after maternal-fetal surgery. *Am J Obstet Gynecol* 2006; 194(3): 834–839

2 DiFederico EM, Burlingame JM, Kilpatrick SJ, Harrison MR, Matthay MA. Pulmonary edema in obstetric patients is rapidly resolved except in the presence of infection or of nitroglycerin tocolysis after open fetal surgery. *Am J Obstet Gynecol* 1998; 179: 925–933

3 Wilson RD, Johnson MP, Crombleholme TM, et al. Chorioamniotic membrane separation following open fetal surgery: pregnancy outcome. *Fetal Diagn Ther* 2003; 18(5): 314–320.

4 Bruner JP, Tulipan NB, Richards WO, Walsh WF, Boehm FH, Vrabcak EK. In utero repair of myelomeningocele: a comparison of endoscopy and hysterotomy. *Fetal Diagn Ther* 2000; 15(2): 83–88.

5 Johnson MP, Gerdes M, Rintoul N, et al. Maternal-fetal surgery for myelomeningocele: neurodevelopmental outcomes at 2 years of age. *Am J Obstet Gynecol* 2006; 194(4): 1145–1150.

6 Farrell JA, Albanese CT, Jennings RW, Kilpatrick SJ, Bratton BJ, Harrison MR. Maternal fertility is not affected by fetal surgery. *Fetal Diagn Ther* 1999; 14: 190–192.

7 Wilson RD, Johnson MP, Flake AW, et al. Reproductive outcomes after pregnancy complicated by maternal-fetal surgery. *Am J Obstet Gynecol* 2004; 191(4): 1430–1436.

8 Macones GA, Peipert J, Nelson DB, et al. Maternal complications with vaginal birth after cesarean delivery: a multicenter study. *Am J Obstet Gynecol* 2005; 193(5): 1656–1662.

9 McMahon MJ. Vaginal birth after cesarean. *Clin Obstet Gynecol* 1998; 41(2): 369–381.

10 Yamamoto M, El Murr L, Robyr R, et al. Incidence and impact of perioperative complications in 175 fetoscopy-guided laser coagulations of chorionic plate anastomoses in fetofetal transfusion syndrome before 26 weeks of gestation. *Am J Obstet Gynecol* 2005; 193(3 Pt 2): 1110–1116

11 Gratacos E, Deprest J. Current experience with fetoscopy and the Eurofoetus registry for fetoscopic procedures. *Eur J Obstet Gynecol Reprod Biol* 2000; 92: 151–160.

12 Robyr R, Boulvain M, Lewi L, et al. Cervical length as a prognostic factor for preterm delivery in twin-to-twin transfusion syndrome

treated by fetoscopic laser coagulation of chorionic plate anastomoses. *Ultrasound Obstet Gynecol* 2005; 25: 37–41.

13 Harrison MR, Golbus MS, Filly RA, et al. Management of the fetus with congenital hydronephrosis. *J Pediatr Surg* 1982; 17(6):728–742.

14 Nicolini U, Rodeck CH, Fisk NM. Shunt treatment for fetal obstructive uropathy. *Lancet* 1987; 2(8571): 1338–1339.

15 Tsao K, Feldstein VA, Albanese CT, et al. Selective reduction of acardiac twin by radiofrequency ablation. *Am J Obstet Gynecol* 2002; 187(3): 635–640.

16 Lee H, Wagner AJ, Sy E, et al. Efficacy of radiofrequency ablation for twin-reversed arterial perfusion sequence. *Am J Obstet Gynecol* 2007; 196(5): 459.

50 Cancer in the Pregnant Patient

Kenneth H. Kim, David M. O'Malley & Jeffrey M. Fowler

Division of Gynecologic Oncology, Department of Obstetrics and Gynecology, James Cancer Hospital and Solove Research Institute, The Ohio State University, Columbus, OH, USA

Introduction

The diagnosis of cancer in pregnancy complicates anywhere between 1 in 1000 and 1 in 2000 live births. According to the 2004 Annual National Vitals Statistics Report Provisional Data, malignancy is the second most common cause of mortality in reproductive-age women aged 25–44 years; however, it is a rare cause of maternal death in pregnancy [1,2]. As the trend continues toward delaying childbearing, the incidence of malignancy occurring in pregnancy is expected to increase. The most common type of cancer diagnosed during pregnancy is melanoma (complicating approximately 1 in 350 pregnancies), followed by cervical cancer (1 in 2250), Hodgkin's lymphoma (1 in 3000), breast cancer (1 in 7500), ovarian cancer (1 in 18 000), and leukemia (1 in 75 000) [3].

Cancer in pregnancy can be categorized into those discovered during the antenatal period, those discovered at the time of delivery, and those discovered up to 1 year postpartum. In over 50% of cases, cancers complicating pregnancy are found in the postpartum period, within 1 year of delivery. At least one-quarter of cancers are found in the antenatal period, and a small minority are found at the time of delivery [4].

When the diagnosis of a malignant neoplasm is made in pregnancy, particular care must be taken to balance both maternal and fetal well-being. This often leads to an extremely challenging therapeutic dilemma. In the antenatal period, the clinical picture is simplified if the fetus is mature and can be delivered prior to any treatment initiation, or if the pregnancy is unwanted and the fetus is not viable. When cancer is diagnosed in a desired pregnancy, and the fetus has not achieved maturity, the clinical situation is more complex. If prognosis is such that delaying treatment will not affect or worsen maternal outcome, treatment may be deferred until the fetus has achieved maturity. However, if the prognosis will deteriorate with a delay in treatment, the risks and benefits of more immediate treatment must be weighed against the risks to the pregnancy and the fetus.

Certainly, a patient should not be penalized for being pregnant and the necessary steps required to assure appropriate management and therapy should be taken. Treatment should be individualized with emphasis on the parents' participation in the decision-making process. In addition, a multidisciplinary team must be utilized to ensure that the patient, the physicians, and all else who are involved are well informed of the risks, benefits, and alternatives to the treatment choices. It is important to not only consider the medical aspects of the condition but also to consider ethical, moral, spiritual, and cultural issues of the patients. Physicians may be faced with unique psychosocial challenges in addition to the clinical diagnosis of cancer, or findings that are suspicious for cancer in pregnancy. Examples of this may include those patients who are carrying their first, and potentially only pregnancy, or those who have had difficulties with conception and have undergone assisted reproductive technologies to achieve pregnancy, both cases in which the pregnancy is truly desired. There are also patients that may be opposed to terminating the pregnancy regardless of gestational age for various personal, religious or ethical reasons. The patient's goal may not necessarily be to undergo curative therapy for their malignancy, but to give birth to a healthy infant, no matter what the risk. Some patients may not believe in cesarean delivery for cultural or other reasons and choose to defer any surgery until after delivering vaginally. A small subset may also refuse not only cesarean delivery, but any labor-inducing agents as well, preferring to go into "natural labor." There may be those who refuse blood products of any sort on the basis of religion or culture and may also choose to deliver vaginally, deferring surgery to the postpartum period to reduce the risk of blood loss. In these cases, the patient must be thoroughly informed of the risks, benefits, and alternatives of therapy for their specific clinical scenario while heeding their cultural, ethical, religious, and moral beliefs.

Critical Care Obstetrics, 5th edition. Edited by M. Belfort, G. Saade, M. Foley, J. Phelan and G. Dildy.

Surgical principles during pregnancy

While every pregnancy comes with inherent risk such as stillbirth or preterm labor, patients generally never expect to require surgery during this time. It is clear that pregnant patients are not immune to processes that require surgical intervention, whether it be gallbladder disease, appendicitis or invasive cancer. Pregnant patients generally tolerate surgical procedures well, depending on the nature and complexity of the surgery performed. Moreover, the risks of adverse pregnancy outcomes appear to be small when uncomplicated, non-emergent surgical procedures are performed. Nevertheless, the ramifications can be grave if the surgery becomes complicated secondary to the clinical scenario (e.g. ruptured viscera) or the procedure itself (e.g. postoperative bleeding, infection or anesthetic complications).

Various non-obstetric surgical procedures have been performed and reported in the literature. The largest study involves 5405 patients undergoing a large variety of procedures throughout pregnancy, with the majority occurring in the second trimester [5]. This study, which employed the Swedish Birth Registry, observed that the difference in rate of stillbirth and congenital anomalies was insignificant, although an increase in the rate of low birth weight and preterm delivery was noted. Factors associated with an increased risk of pregnancy loss include first-trimester surgery, peritonitis, and longer procedure times [6]. Thus if the surgery is needed, recommendations for timing of surgery have generally been to electively defer procedures until the second trimester under controlled circumstances. The use of prophylactic tocolytics at the time of surgery in the second trimester has not been shown to decrease the risk of preterm labor or preterm delivery in these patients, but may be beneficial in the third trimester [7]. However, there are no randomized or prospective trials to address this specific issue. Clearly, these decisions must be individualized for each patient. If the patient is unstable, or requires emergent surgery, this should be carried out in an efficient, timely manner. When counseling patients it is important to note that intra-abdominal surgery, as opposed to extra-abdominal sites, is associated with a higher risk of pregnancy-related complications.

With advancing technology, the use of minimally invasive laparoscopic and robotic techniques have entered the surgeon's armamentarium. The complexity of the decision to proceed with surgery during the gestation is therefore further layered with what surgical approach to employ. Abundant case reports and studies are present in the literature regarding the well-tolerated nature of laparoscopic surgery during pregnancy [8–12]. Benefits of the minimally invasive approach include less pain in the postoperative period, less use of analgesics, less use of tocolytics, and overall shorter length of bedrest and hospitalization as compared to laparotomy. The most common indications for laparoscopic surgery during pregnancy are cholecystectomy, evaluation of an adnexal mass, and appendectomy [13,14].

Surgical risks inherent to minimally invasive surgery do not appear to be increased in pregnancy. Laparoscopic techniques in pregnant patients should not differ greatly from that of open procedures. As with open procedures, fetal heart tones should be obtained before and after the procedure. In those cases where the fetus is viable continuous monitoring of the fetal heart rate is advised so that intervention can be undertaken in the event of fetal decompensation. Naso/orogastric decompression should be utilized, and the patient should be placed in a leftward tilt to minimize aortocaval compression. The primary port should be inserted via the open technique or the left upper quadrant direct technique to decrease the risk of uterine perforation or laceration. There has been one reported case of incorrect placement of the Verres needle, leading to pneumoamnion that contributed to fetal loss [15]. Ancillary ports should be placed under direct visualization in the cephalad direction, and then rotated carefully. Due to an intra-abdominal space that is progressively compromised, laparoscopy should generally not be attempted after 26–28 weeks gestation [14]; however, this should be evaluated on a case-by-case basis. Promising reports of robotic gynecologic surgery are now appearing in the literature but there is no information yet on the use of this novel technique in a pregnant patient to date.

Another theoretical risk of laparoscopy is that the developing fetus could potentially be susceptible to acidosis caused by maternal absorption of the carbon dioxide gas with subsequent hypercarbia and serum conversion to carbonic acid. There have been two studies performed in pregnant ewes to evaluate the response in fetal sheep to the use of CO_2 insufflation. In the first study [16], one fetus that was compromised prior to the study succumbed during the pneumoperitoneum. The second study [17] had no such complications. There have been no subsequent reports of fetal loss attributable to acidosis secondary to pneumoperitoneum, and this risk appears to be theoretical. Notwithstanding, if the duration of the case is anticipated to be rather lengthy, it may be prudent to employ traditional open methods of surgery. Until randomized trials are available, the decision of surgical approach should be individualized and made in consultation with the perinatologist and the surgeon, ensuring that the risks, benefits, and alternatives are discussed at great length with the patient.

Cervix

In 2007 there will be approximately 11 000 new cases of cervical cancer in the United States with an estimated 3600 deaths from the disease according to the National Cancer Institute. The incidence of invasive cervical cancer in pregnancy is low, comprising only approximately 1% of total cervical cancers diagnosed; however, preinvasive cervical neoplasia is quite common in reproductive age women, occurring in 5–50 cases per 1000 pregnancies [18–20]. The recent downward trend in the incidence of cervical neoplasia in pregnancy coincides with the general decreasing incidence of cervical cancer. Therefore the practicing obstetrician/gynecologist is more likely to encounter the issue of evaluation and management of an abnormal pap smear rather than management of a pregnant woman with invasive cervical cancer. While Pap smears and routine screening are readily available in developed countries, most patients diagnosed with cervical cancer have not had appropriate screening. Pregnancy and prenatal care affords an opportunity to screen and appropriately treat many patients who would otherwise not seek healthcare. Thus, at the antenatal visit, it is important to stress the importance of cervical neoplasia screening and appropriate follow-up of any abnormal Pap results with colposcopic evaluation, in addition to routine obstetric care.

Intraepithelial neoplasia

As many as 5% of pregnancies are complicated by an abnormal Pap smear [20]. Cervical cytology and physical examination, complemented with colposcopy, are the mainstay for cervical cancer screening during pregnancy. Studies have shown that use of either spatula- or liquid-based smear methods result in similar detection rates. While an endocervical curettage should be avoided during pregnancy, an endocervical cytology brush should be employed as it improves the adequacy of the smear. Use of the brush may increase the incidence of post-collection spotting, but appears to have no effect on increasing the risk of serious adverse outcomes related to the pregnancy [21]. During pregnancy the emphasis is on evaluation and diagnosis of the extent of neoplasia while definitive therapeutic management is usually delayed until after delivery. This evaluation of an abnormal Pap smear in the pregnant patient mirrors the management in the non-pregnant state.

The Bethesda system remains the standard for classification and management of abnormal cervical cytology. Atypical squamous cells of uncertain significance (ASCUS) should be managed in the same manner as in the non-pregnant state with high-risk human papilloma virus (HPV) type testing and colposcopy when indicated, immediate colposcopy, or colposcopy after a repeated abnormal Pap result. Pap smears revealing atypical glandular cells (AGC) of any variety, however rare in pregnancy, warrant further evaluation with colposcopic examination. In the case of AGC, pregnancy complicates the cytologic interpretation with sloughed decidual cells, endocervical gland hyperplasia, and/or cells demonstrating an Arias–Stella reaction, all of which are benign changes occurring in normal pregnancy. Compared to non-pregnant counterparts, AGC found in pregnancy may have decreased probability of being associated with malignancy, but should still be followed closely [22–25]. Patients who are found to have low- or high-grade intraepithelial lesions, or any other results that cannot exclude high-grade disease, must also undergo colposcopic evaluation.

Colposcopic evaluation, which is facilitated in pregnancy by the fact that the transformation zone is everted, should be performed when indicated by the Pap cytology. Colposcopy should be performed by clinicians who are familiar with the cervical cytological and colposcopic changes associated with pregnancy. Biopsies should be taken of the most suspicious lesions seen at the time of colposcopic evaluation. Multiple biopsies at one examination and use of the endocervical curettage should be avoided [26]. Colposcopic diagnostic accuracy, with or without biopsy, is 95–99% and complications rarely arise [27]. The most common complication associated with colposcopically directed biopsy is hemorrhage secondary to the hyperemic state of the cervix during pregnancy. Should this problem present itself, a number of methods can stop the bleeding including direct pressure to the site, Monsel solution, silver nitrate, vaginal packing, and/or rarely suture.

When the possibility of invasive disease has been excluded, conservative management with close observation of cervical intraepithelial neoplasia is reasonable and acceptable [27–32]. While an inadequate colposcopic evaluation is indication for loop electrical excisional procedure (LEEP) or cone biopsy in the non-pregnant patient, this approach can be modified during pregnancy. Pregnant patients with unsatisfactory colposcopic evaluation may undergo repeat colposcopic examination 6–12 weeks from the initial colposcopy. As the transformation zone undergoes further eversion through the gestation, a repeated colposcopy may subsequently yield a satisfactory examination. In pregnancy, the biopsy-proven progression rate from lower-grade to higher-grade dysplasia was found to be approximately 7%, and there was no progression to invasive disease [31]. However, it has also been demonstrated that regression rates of moderate and even severe dysplasia 6 months after delivery appear higher than regression rates in the non-pregnant population [31,33]. Regression rates in these studies were found to be 68% in patients with CIN 2, and 70% in CIN 3 [31]. Therefore, biopsy-proven dysplasia may be followed with serial colposcopic examinations during pregnancy. The patient may be allowed to have a vaginal delivery, and then followed up 6–8 weeks postpartum for definitive management.

In the pregnant state, LEEP and cone biopsy should be reserved for excluding invasive disease. Risks of these procedures in pregnancy include cramping, bleeding, infection, preterm premature rupture of membranes, spontaneous abortion and/or preterm labor, and subsequent loss of the pregnancy. Comparatively, the rates of complication with LEEP and cone biopsy are similar [34]. Cold knife cone biopsy may be favored over LEEP to allow for adequate assessment of the margins. If a LEEP or cone biopsy is indicated, this can be performed any time during the first trimester and up to 20 weeks gestational age. If fetal maturity is attainable in a reasonable amount of time, these procedures can also be deferred until after delivery. Alternatively, cone cerclage, where a McDonald cerclage is placed at the time of conization, has been proposed to try and prevent hemorrhage, preterm labor, and pregnancy loss. While there were no complications in the study, it was quite underpowered, involving only 17 patients [35].

Cervical carcinoma

The occurrence of cervical carcinoma in pregnancy is rare, comprising only 1% of all cervical cancers diagnosed per year. Presentation will usually be postcoital bleeding or persistent bleeding during pregnancy, but many patients will be asymptomatic. The vast majority of patients with cervical cancer found in pregnancy will be diagnosed with stage I disease. In the past it was thought that pregnancy altered the course of cervical cancer compared with non-pregnant cohorts. However, it has been demonstrated that there is no difference in survival outcomes when matched cohorts were studied [33,36,37]. When compared with non-pregnant counterparts, pregnant patients with cervical cancer are over three times more likely to be stage I, the majority having stage IB disease [36,38–41]. Because of the physiologic and anatomic changes that develop with pregnancy, indurations or nodularities at the base of the broad ligament will be less prominent during pregnancy, thus risking underestimation of the degree of involvement during staging of the tumor. Regardless, studies have shown that pregnancy does not affect overall survival rate when compared to non-pregnant women, with survival rates of 80% in pregnant subjects compared with 82% in non-pregnant control cohorts [42].

Cervical cancer is primarily staged by physical examination, but disease extent may be difficult to determine in the pregnant state. Ancillary studies that may aid in the evaluation of the extent of tumor involvement include limited CT scans of the lower abdomen and pelvis. Sigmoidoscopy and cystoscopy are safe in pregnancy for the evaluation of mucosal involvement, and, in some cases, MRI has been utilized to help determine the extent of urinary tract involvement [43,44].

Once staging has been determined, management must be individualized for each patient. A multidisciplinary team, which includes perinatologist, neonatologist, and gynecologic oncologist, should be recruited to extensively counsel the patient on all of the treatment options available to her. These should take into account the tumor stage, her prognosis with immediate treatment versus delayed treatment, and the fetal issues including timing of delivery. The patient's desire to continue or terminate the pregnancy may impact treatment decisions. In most instances of invasive cancer, relatively prompt treatment is expected and ideal. During pregnancy, effecting definitive treatment will depend on the stage of disease and the gestational age of the fetus.

Microinvasive disease may be suspected after colposcopy; however, the diagnosis is formally made only after cervical conization. If it is determined the patients has International Federation of Gynecology and Obstetrics (FIGO) stage Ia1 disease, she can be followed closely and delivered as obstetrically indicated with definitive management deferred to the postpartum period. However, if there is evidence of frank invasion (FIGO stage Ia2 or higher), further options must be discussed with the patient regarding definitive management, particularly if the patient desires to continue the pregnancy. Standard management for the non-pregnant patient would be prompt definitive therapy. However, with informed consent, the pregnant patient can be followed with close observation with definitive therapy deferred until after delivery once fetal maturity is attained.

Fortunately, most pregnant patients diagnosed with cervical cancer have early stage disease. Case reports and small series have demonstrated relative success with delivery once fetal maturity is obtained and delaying cancer therapy until that time or until the postpartum period, even if the cancer is diagnosed at an early gestational age [40,45,46]. Although the risk of recurrence is low in these relatively small case series, the recurrence rate of cervical cancer after intentional delay of treatment to optimize fetal maturity cannot be quantified. Thus, if the pregnancy is desired, the patient must be thoroughly counseled on this unquantifiable but likely low risk of recurrence if therapy were to be delayed. If the malignancy is diagnosed in the latter half of the pregnancy, treatment can likely be delayed with only slight risk of progression and worsened outcome. With advancing neonatal intensive care technology, the threshold for fetal maturity will continue to decrease, and patients who present at less than 20 weeks will likely have improved risk/benefit ratio with delay of treatment. In those patients who are diagnosed in the first half of the gestation, and wish to terminate the pregnancy and future fertility, immediate treatment may be offered and recommended. The majority of patients diagnosed with invasive disease in pregnancy will be stage Ia2 to Ib1; in these patients, and those with up to stage IIA disease, standard treatment is usually radical hysterectomy with pelvic lymphadenectomy. Care must be taken in evaluating pelvic lymph nodes as they may contain decidual reaction from the pregnancy which can be confused with metastatic cells. Depending on the size of the uterus at the time of surgery, hysterectomy can be performed with the fetus *in utero*, or a hysterotomy may be performed immediately preceding hysterectomy. Definitive radiation therapy offers similar cure rates in these stages of disease; however, this has been avoided mainly secondary to the potential adverse effects of therapeutic radiation. Definitive surgical management is associated with baseline perioperative morbidity but offers the advantage of surgical staging and preservation of ovarian function. Use of definitive radiation therapy exposes the ovaries, vagina, gastrointestinal and urinary tracts to high doses of radiation, leading to loss of ovarian function and risk of long-term chronic toxicity [47].

Mode of delivery with concomitant cervical cancer remains a controversial topic. There appears to be a slight trend toward worsening prognosis in vaginal deliveries through a cancerous cervix yet this is not well established [36,37,48]. A bulky, friable cervix is at risk for significant complications with life-threatening intrapartum and/or postpartum hemorrhage that may lead to emergent hysterectomy in a less than ideal, uncontrolled and acute situation. In addition, case reports describe recurrence at the episiotomy site, most of which occurred within 6 months of delivery [49,50]. Thus close follow-up with careful palpation and inspection of any laceration or episiotomy site is recommended; if recurrence at this site is noted, management should entail excision followed by radiation therapy. Vaginal delivery should likely be reserved for intraepithelial lesions and potentially early stage I candidates who wish to preserve pregnancy and fertility. Consequently, most clinicians favor abdominal delivery, especially if radical hysterectomy with lymphadenectomy is indicated and can be performed at the time of cesarean delivery.

For the subset of patients with early-stage tumors who wish to defer definitive treatment until the postpartum period and who wish to conserve fertility, radical trachelectomy performed vaginally or abdominally may be a viable option [51]. A total of 212 patients collected from six studies were evaluated for survival, fertility and pregnancy outcomes after radical trachelectomy. Of these 212 patients, 2% developed recurrence, and 56% delivered a viable pregnancy with 28% being full term, and 28% being preterm [52,53].

Advanced-stage cervical cancer is rare in pregnancy and there is a paucity of data in the literature regarding management. For higher-stage disease and those few patients who are medically unfit for surgery, radiation therapy with concurrent chemotherapy is indicated. If this occurs in the third trimester, delay of therapy until after delivery is reasonable [46]. If the patient chooses not to continue the pregnancy, external-beam radiation with concomitant chemotherapy can be given in the first trimester, and if spontaneous miscarriage does not occur, dilation and curettage or extraction can be performed. In the middle trimester, abortion may be induced or delayed, depending on spiritual/religious, moral, and ethical considerations. If delayed, teletherapy may be administered; however, hysterotomy may be required for up to one-fourth of cases [45]. One week post-abortion, after uterine involution, external radiation can be administered, followed by brachytherapy. In general, the anatomic distortion that occurs in pregnancy must be taken into consideration to ensure that the radiation field includes all targeted regions. The use of neoadjuvant chemotherapy without radiation may be helpful in the pregnant patient [54]. The most important factor in administration of the chemotherapy during pregnancy is the gestational age of the fetus. If the fetus is exposed to chemotherapeutic agents within 2 weeks postconception, it will either spontaneously abort or develop normally. Organogenesis occurs in the first trimester; thus, chemotherapy should be avoided during this period, as this is the most likely time that the fetus will develop a malformation. Though limited, reports have shown relative success with administration of chemotherapy during the second and third trimesters, with very low risk of fetal malformations; however, there has been increased tendency toward interuterine growth restriction, low birth weight, spontaneous abortion, and/or preterm labor. Timing of chemotherapy administration with relation to the planned delivery date is also important. Chemotherapy given within 3 weeks of delivery may lead to maternal myelosuppression with resultant neutropenia, thrombocytopenia, and/or anemia. Furthermore, the neonate may be incapable of handling such high levels of chemotherapeutic agents and metabolites because of its immature hepatorenal excretion mechanisms [55].

Management of adnexal masses occurring in pregnancy

The finding of an adnexal mass during pregnancy has increased as ultrasound has become commonplace in the practice of obstetrics. Prior to routine ultrasonography, these masses were usually found at the time of abdominal delivery, during the postpartum period, or during the gestation when associated symptoms prompted a physical exam. Currently, many asymptomatic masses that would otherwise be unrecognized are incidentally found at the time of first-trimester sonogram. The actual incidence is not well documented since many masses that are incidentally discovered in pregnancy undergo regression, are not reported, or may not require/receive any intervention. It has been estimated that 0.2–2% of pregnancies are complicated by an adnexal mass, and that approximately 1–3% of these are malignant [56–63]. While a significant portion of these masses are benign corpus luteum and other cysts that will undergo spontaneous regression by the second trimester, a proportion of these masses will be neoplastic and persist through the second trimester and beyond, potentially causing major complications during the pregnancy. Some of these will need extensive surgical intervention.

It has been demonstrated that approximately three-quarters of adnexal masses found in pregnancy are simple-appearing cysts measuring less than 5 cm in diameter. The remaining one-quarter of adnexal masses discovered in pregnancy are either simple or complex, and measure greater than 5 cm in diameter. Of all adnexal masses found in pregnancy, 70% will spontaneously resolve by the early middle trimester, becoming undetectable by 14–15 weeks gestational age [59,64]. Functional cysts, including theca lutein cysts, are the most common masses detected, while dermoid cysts are the most common neoplasm encountered in pregnancy. Other common benign findings are cystadenomas, paraovarian cysts, endometriomas, and leiomyomas [64–66].

Adnexal masses measuring greater than 8 cm are at risk of complications, including pain, torsion, rupture, and hemorrhage. A minority of pregnant women with an adnexal mass will have an acute presentation where surgery is clearly indicated [67–69]. Rarely a mass can be associated with preterm labor, preterm premature rupture of membranes, pregnancy loss, obstruction of labor, and/or fetal/neonatal death [66,68,69]. The risk of torsion peaks in two periods during the pregnancy: the first trimester or early second trimester, when the uterus is growing out of the true pelvis; and the puerperium, when the uterus undergoes rapid involution. If a patient develops clinical signs or symptoms consistent with torsion, emergent surgery is indicated and should not be delayed, regardless of gestational age.

In the non-emergent setting, ultrasound, occasionally supplemented with other imaging modalities, has been traditionally used to guide management decisions. Generally, if the mass appears benign on ultrasonographic evaluation, it is extremely unlikely to be malignant. Tumor markers including AFP, LDH, hCG, and CA-125 levels may be elevated with pregnancy and are generally not reliable or useful. If the origin of the mass is not clear, occasionally, magnetic resonance imaging can be employed to differentiate between ovarian versus other possible sources. Masses that are simple and cystic in nature and which measure less than 6 cm have a low risk of malignancy (less than 1%) and can be closely observed [64,66,70]. Masses that persist into the second trimester, particularly those that are rapidly enlarging, larger than 8 cm, and/or appear complex and multiseptated, most often require surgical exploration [64].

It has generally been advised that surgical exploration be undertaken at approximately 16–20 weeks gestation. This is a time when physiological cysts have regressed and the placenta is hormonally functional and the fetus is supported independent of the corpus luteum. If an oophorectomy which removes a functional corpus luteum is required during the first trimester, the pregnancy should be supported with supplemental progesterone to prevent spontaneous abortion. If the mass is discovered in the third trimester, definitive work-up, management, and surgical exploration can usually be deferred until after vaginal delivery or during cesarean section.

The various options available for the surgical approach must also be considered. Traditionally, patients in these clinical situations have undergone open laparotomy. More recently with technologic advances more surgical options are now available for use in the pregnant patient. The use of minimally invasive techniques (including robotic surgery) has been shown to be generally safe and effective. In any surgical approach, the gravid uterus should be manipulated as little as possible to minimize any potential risk of spontaneous preterm labor, rupture of membranes or any other potential complication that may lead to fetal loss. If the mass is benign, unilateral cystectomy is performed whenever possible and the contralateral ovary should then be inspected to ensure normal appearance. While most masses in pregnancy are confined to a single ovary, it is not uncommon to find bilateral involvement.

There are currently insufficient data to determine the optimal management of patients who require surgery during pregnancy. These decisions should be made on a case-by-case basis in consultation with the patient and all involved medical personnel. The general emphasis in surgical management should be removal of the mass, and confirmation of the diagnosis with minimal impact on the pregnancy.

Ovarian cancer

One in 20 000 pregnancies is complicated by an ovarian malignancy [56,57,71]. Approximately 1 in 1000 pregnant women undergo some sort of exploratory surgery to evaluate an adnexal mass, and 1–5% of these masses are found to be malignant [72,73]. This percentage is lower than found in non-pregnant women, likely owing to that fact that pregnancy occurs in younger women and that most masses found in pregnancy are corpus luteum cysts or some other benign simple cyst. The majority of ovarian neoplasms found in pregnancy are teratomas or cystadenomas [63,65,70]. Most malignancies found in pregnancy are classically germ cell tumors; however, with the increasing trend of delaying childbearing, there has more recently been an increase in epithelial ovarian malignancies.

The management of ovarian cancer in pregnancy does not greatly differ from that of the non-pregnant patient. Many pregnant women who are diagnosed with an invasive neoplasm are young and have not completed childbearing. Fortunately, as most masses are asymptomatic and found incidentally, they are often early stage. Fertility-sparing treatment is an appropriate option for that subset of patients whose disease is found to be of low malignant potential (LMP), such as stage IA tumors or germ cell tumors (any stage). While complete surgical staging (peritoneal washings, biopsies of the parietal and pelvic peritoneal surfaces and diaphragm, omentectomy, and pelvic and aortic lymph node dissections) is necessary to document correct staging, it is not always practical in the gravid patient, especially as gestational age advances. The surgeon should attempt to biopsy any area suspicious for extraovarian disease if feasible. If the patient requires adjuvant chemotherapy, there is a risk of subsequent ovarian failure of varying severity; however, most patients will not suffer from persistent premature ovarian failure, and will be able to conceive with the remaining ovary and uterus after completion of chemotherapy.

Rarely, a patient will have more advanced disease, and more extensive surgery may be required. Management is individualized for patients with advanced disease depending on fertility desires, gestational age and extent of disease. If the malignancy is diagnosed when the fetus is mature treatment may be initiated after delivery. If the patient does not wish to continue the pregnancy, appropriate cytoreduction and subsequent treatment may be undertaken, and termination of the pregnancy. If the pregnancy is desired, and the fetus is not mature, management becomes more complex. In selected patients, if clinically indicated, both ovaries may be removed, the pregnancy continued and subsequent treatment delayed. One option is to offer neoadjuvant chemotherapy until fetal maturity is achieved followed by interval cytoreductive surgery at the time of delivery or shortly thereafter. If the patient chooses to delay therapy after adequate counseling, continuing advances in neonatal intensive care capability allows for much shorter delay in treatment as the threshold for fetal viability decreases. Active coordination between the gynecologic oncologist and perinatologist is critical and individualized consideration must be given to gestational age, maternal condition, and prognosis.

Germ cell tumors are the most common ovarian malignancy found in pregnancy; up to 30% of malignancies in pregnancy are dysgerminomas. They are often discovered when a patient presents with torsion or incarceration of a massive ovary. This can occur in the late first or early second trimester when the uterus is rapidly growing out of the pelvis. Of note, LDH levels are not affected in pregnancy, and may be employed as a useful tumor marker. Alpha fetoprotein levels do change in pregnancy; however, an extremely elevated AFP level may be associated with an endodermal sinus tumor. Standard treatment in these cases is unilateral oophorectomy with pelvic and para-aortic lymph node dissection. Fifteen per cent of dysgerminomas can be bilateral, but blind wedge resection or biopsy of a normal-appearing contralateral ovary is generally no longer accepted procedure. For those with advanced disease beyond stage IA, adjuvant chemotherapy is indicated, usually with first-line therapy comprising bleomycin, etoposide, and cisplatin (BEP). The recurrence rate of stage IA disease is approximately 10%, but the majority of these cases are cured with chemotherapy or radiation therapy [74].

The sex-cord stromal tumors are uncommon in pregnancy. When they occur in pregnancy, they are less frequently associated with hormonal manifestations and more frequently associated with hemorrhagic rupture leading to hemoperitoneum than in non-pregnant cohorts. These patients tend to do well and can usually be managed with conservative measures. This most commonly involves unilateral salpingo-oophorectomy, though some patients have undergone postoperative chemotherapy and/or radiation therapy, as well as complete surgical staging.

Chemotherapy is necessary for most patients diagnosed with epithelial ovarian cancer. Attention must be given to the drug's mechanism of action and side-effect profile, especially in the pregnant patient. Various other factors must also be taken into account including nutritional status (which can alter protein-binding and serum free-drug concentration), maternal habitus (which can affect fat sequestration of the agent), and the expanded plasma volume found in the pregnant state (which can affect an agent's pharmacokinetics) [75–77]. The potential for transplacental passage must also be considered since chemotherapeutic agents tend to non-selectively kill rapidly dividing cells found in both carcinomas and fetal tissues [78]. The most susceptible period for the fetus is the first trimester when organogenesis occurs [79]. The risk of malformation and spontaneous abortion can be minimized by deferring administration of chemotherapy until after this critical time. Folate antagonists can increase the risk of malformations [75] and supplemental folic acid should be administered in such cases in an effort to reduce the risk of an anomaly. If chemotherapy must be given during the first trimester, the issue of potential teratogenicity must be fully understood by the patient when deciding whether to continue or abort the pregnancy.

Chemotherapy administered during second and third trimester has been associated with low birth weight, intrauterine growth restriction, and premature delivery [75,80]. These pregnancies should be closely followed, with antenatal monitoring of fetal growth and functional well-being. Administration of chemotherapy near the time of delivery should be avoided if possible. A 3-week buffer period prior to a planned delivery date may prevent potential complications close to term. Long-term follow-up studies of children who were exposed to antineoplastic agents *in utero* demonstrate normal birth weights, educational performance, and reproductive capacity [81–84].

Non-gynecologic cancers in pregnancy

Breast

Cancer of the breast is the most common malignancy in women of all ages and, according to American Cancer Society and the National Cancer Institute, will afflict over 178 000 women in 2008. It is one of the most common causes of cancer death in women, second only to lung cancer. It is apparent that the incidence of breast cancer during pregnancy is increasing, likely secondary to recent trends toward delaying childbearing into the third and fourth decade of life. As many as 3 in 10 000 gravid women will have a pregnancy complicated by carcinoma of the breast [3,85,86].

The evaluation of a breast mass during pregnancy should not differ from that of a non-pregnant patient and therefore should not be delayed. Mammography may be of use but is associated with a higher rate of a false-positive test when compared with non-pregnant women because of the increased density of breast tissue in pregnancy. Because of this an ultrasound may be a useful first step in the diagnostic process. Magnetic resonance imaging (MRI) of the breast may also be useful in prenatal diagnosis of breast cancer; data are currently limited on its use in pregnancy, but it appears to be a safe modality [87–90].

If a mass appears suspicious for malignancy on radiographic evaluation, a biopsy is indicated. Ideally, this is acquired through a core biopsy. A fine needle aspiration may also yield the diagnosis but requires a pathologist with experience in pregnancy-associated breast cancer [91].

If a malignancy is discovered further evaluation is mandatory. In non-pregnant patients, this has been achieved through careful history and physical exam, serologic tests and chest X-ray; bone scans and CT are also performed in patients at high risk or who have suspected metastases. Traditionally, CT has been avoided in pregnancy because of concerns about exposure of the fetus especially during the first trimester. MRI may be selectively used in patients where metastasis is suspected.

When matched for stage and other prognostic factors, pregnancy does not appear to worsen the prognosis [92–94]. In those women who have no evidence of metastasis, surgical management may be definitive [91]. For smaller tumors, breast-conserving surgery can be performed; if the tumor is larger, the patient may require more substantial surgical management with modified radical or total mastectomy with axillary node staging [95]. While radiation therapy is employed in non-pregnant women with breast-conserving surgery [96,97], this is avoided in pregnancy, because of the potential radiation exposure to the fetus. In node-positive or advanced cases, chemotherapy is recommended; current recommendations include cyclophosphamide, doxorubicin, and 5-fluorouracil. Methotrexate can also be used beyond the first trimester [98].

Individualization of care and good communication amongst a multidisciplinary care team including the obstetrician/perinatologist, neonatologist, and surgical and medical oncologists is extremely important. Traditionally, women have been counseled to abort pregnancy; however, therapeutic abortion has not been shown to alter disease course or improve survival rates in pregnant women with breast cancer [92]. In addition, with advancing neonatal intensive care technology, the threshold for fetal maturity has decreased, and patients who present at earlier gestations will likely have an improved risk/benefit ratio with delay of treatment.

As previously discussed, if the patient requires adjuvant chemotherapy, there is a risk of varying degrees of ovarian failure, although most patients will not suffer from persistent premature ovarian failure and will be able to conceive after completion of chemotherapy. Subsequent pregnancy after treatment of breast cancer does not appear to worsen the prognosis of breast cancer when compared to patients, matched for age and stage, who did not become pregnant [99]. Studies have also shown that the number of subsequent pregnancies, the interval between treatment and subsequent pregnancy, and termination of pregnancy versus continuing pregnancy to delivery does not affect maternal outcome [100]. Notwithstanding, patients are counseled to delay subsequent pregnancy for at least 2–3 years, as risk of recurrence is greatest during this interval after treatment.

Melanoma

Melanoma is one of the most common cancers diagnosed during pregnancy, although the exact incidence during this period is unknown [101,102]. The median age for patients diagnosed with melanoma is 45 years; 30–40% of patients are reproductive age, and up to 8% of these women are pregnant at the time of diagnosis. With the increasing trend toward delaying childbearing among other reasons, the incidence of melanoma found in pregnancy has increased drastically in the past 5 decades [103,104]. The estimated incidence is approximately 0.14–2.8 cases per 1000 births [105]. However, according to Salopek and colleagues [106], cases of melanoma are greatly underreported, with a large proportion of patients being treated on an outpatient basis, and thus never entering a tumor registry.

The vast majority of melanomas arise from the pigment-producing melanocytes, usually from a pre-existing nevus. Therefore, any nevus that appears suspicious in appearance should be biopsied. Characteristics that have classically been described as associated with invasive disease include, but may not be limited to, irregular lesions or changes in shape or contour, surface elevation or increase in thickness, itching, bleeding or ulceration, or discolorations.

Once diagnosed, these cancers are clinically staged. Fortunately, the majority, between 50 and 85%, of pregnant patients with melanoma have stage I disease [105,107,108]. Prognosis in stage I disease is dictated by tumor thickness (epidermis, dermis, subcutaneous fat) as measured with the Clark classification or the Breslow scale.

While melanomas are generally not considered to be hormonally dependent or responsive, there has been concern for various endocrinologic factors that occur during pregnancy which could potentially influence the course and prognosis of the tumor. There is a well-known association with increased pigmentation of nipples, vulva, linea nigra, and/or pre-existing nevi in pregnancy that begins in the first trimester, and typically disappears shortly after the birth [109]. This increase in pigmentation is likely secondary to the pregnancy-associated increase in production of adrenocorticotropic hormone (ACTH) and melanocyte-stimulating hormone (MSH); however, a clear association between increased MSH in pregnancy and melanoma has not been established [110]. With regard to the effects of estrogen on melanocytes, previous animal studies have shown an increase in melanocyte activity; this has not been the case with pregnancy, oral contraceptive use, and hormone replacement therapy, none of which have shown a direct association with melanoma [105,111].

Until recently, melanoma occurring in pregnancy was thought to carry a poorer prognosis compared with non-pregnant controls. Earlier anecdotal reports suggesting this association have been countered by more recent studies showing no major differences in tumor location, presentation or prognosis in pregnancy [103,105,112,113]. There does, however, seem to be an increased tumor thickness associated with pregnancy [114,115]. With respect to overall survival rates, there is no significant difference between pregnant patients and their non-pregnant counterparts [104,112,116]. The current standard of care in non-pregnant patients has now changed from routine lymph node dissection towards sentinel node mapping and sampling, with formal lymphadenectomy if the sentinel node contains evidence of metastasis [104,117,118]. In pregnant patients, this can be undertaken with a ^{99m}Tc-sulfur colloid which has a fetal dose of less than 100 mGy [119,120].

Surgical treatment of melanoma is dictated by tumor stage. Since many pregnant patients have stage I disease, most undergo wide local resection with or without regional lymph node dissection. Prophylactic chemotherapy or immunotherapy is generally avoided during pregnancy, although this is dependent on tumor stage and maternal prognosis. If the tumor is noted to have distant metastases, palliation may be the goal of therapy. Notably, the only adjuvant agent proven to be effective in improving survival, though modest, in non-pregnant cohorts is high-dose interferon-α2b; there are no reports involving the use of immunotherapy in melanoma in the pregnant state [104].

The standard chemotherapy agent used to treat melanoma is dacarbazine. Several studies are currently investigating the use of combination chemotherapy and radiation therapy in malignant melanoma [121]. Therapeutic abortion has not been shown to improve survival. There is at least one case report of a pregnant patient with progressive metastatic disease who was treated with combination chemotherapy during pregnancy and who died due to systemic complications after giving birth to an unaffected infant that developed normally [76].

While transplacental tumor metastasis is exceedingly rare, melanoma is the most commonly cited tumor to have placental and fetal metastases [122–125]. Up to a third of placental metastases are attributed to melanoma; according to Alexander [126], 27 of 87 cases of metastatic placental disease were attributed to malignant melanoma with five of six affected infants dying of metastatic melanoma. Reports of spontaneous regression in the infant are exceedingly rare [127]. Other reported cancers to have metastasized to the products of conception include breast, lung, maxilla, vulvar, neuroendocrine and pancreatic cancer, lymphoma, leukemia, and one case of vaginal sarcoma.

Other non-gynecologic cancers

Hodgkin's lymphoma is the most common hematologic malignancy found in women of reproductive age. The median age of presentation is 30 years, and it been reported to occur in 1 in 1000 to 1 in 6000 pregnancies [128–130]. Non-Hodgkin's lymphoma is rarer than Hodgkin's disease in this age group as this disease typically presents after the childbearing years. Nevertheless a recent increase in the incidence of Hodgkin's lymphoma in pregnancy can be attributed to trends toward delaying childbearing and the increased incidence of human immunodeficiency syndrome (HIV). The condition frequently presents as painless enlargement of the supradiaphragmatic lymph nodes, particularly supraclavicular, along with various "B" symptoms such as fever, night sweats, malaise, weight loss, and pruritus. In pregnancy, radiologic work-up may be limited by a desire to avoid exposing the fetus to ionizing radiation. The protocol may be modified to include chest radiograph, bone marrow biopsies, and abdominal imaging. Computed tomography (CT) can be adjusted to reduce the amount of radiation exposure to the fetus, and magnetic resonance imaging (MRI) may provide an alternative to CT which avoids ionizing radiation exposure of the fetus. Treatment usually involves radiation and/or chemotherapy. Once the diagnosis of lymphoma is made, consultation and coordination with a hematologic oncologist are important.

Colorectal cancers are common in women overall, but are relatively rare in age groups less than 40 years. One report cites fewer than 250 cases of colon cancer occurring with concomitant pregnancy, and of these, approximately 80% occur in the rectum [131–133]. Presentation may include abdominal pain, nausea, vomiting, constipation, or bloody stool; diagnosis can be difficult as most of these symptoms can also be found in normal pregnancy. Work-up may involve digital rectal exam, occult blood testing, and flexible sigmoidoscopy or colonoscopy. Carcinoembryonic antigen (CEA) can be elevated in normal pregnancy, and may not provide useful insight into cases of colorectal cancer. Once diagnosed, treatment does not differ from non-pregnant patients. Surgical intervention can be timed with respect to the gestational age and the mother's desire to keep or abort the fetus. Vaginal delivery may be possible, however this is usually not recommended with larger rectal lesions in which labor dystocia or hemorrhage may occur, necessitating urgent or emergent surgical intervention [134]. Other gastrointestinal cancers, such as gastric cancer [135–137], hepatocellular carcinoma [138–141], and pancreatic cancer [142,143] are exceedingly rare during the childbearing years. Few case reports exist in the literature regarding these rare malignancies. Other tumors reported in pregnancies include renal [144–146], thyroid [147–149], bone and soft tissue [150], carcinoid [151], and brain tumors [152–154].

Conclusion

The treatment of any cancer occurring in pregnancy must be individualized. A multidisciplinary team consisting of a perinatologist, neonatologist, and gynecologic, surgical and/or medical oncologist should be assembled to extensively counsel the patient on all treatment options based on tumor stage and the prognosis based on immediate treatment versus delayed treatment. Each case should be evaluated on a case-by-case basis, and each patient should be counseled and managed with respect to their desires for the current pregnancy and future fertility.

References

1 Landis SH, Murray T, Bolden S, Wingo PA. Cancer statistics, 1998. *CA Cancer J Clin* 1998; 48: 6–29.

2 Landis SH, Murray T, Bolden S, Wingo PA. Cancer statistics, 1999. *CA Cancer J Clin* 1999; 49: 1,8–31.

3 Dinh TA, Warshal DP. The epidemiology of cancer in pregnancy. In: Barnea ER, Jauniaux E, Schwartz PE, eds. *Cancer and Pregnancy*. London: Springer, 2001: 1–5.

4 Smith LH, Danielsen B, Allen ME, et al. Cancer associated with obstetric delivery: results of linkage with the California cancer registry. *Am J Obstet Gynecol* 2003; 189: 1128–1135.

5 Mazze RI, Kallen B. Reproductive outcome after anesthesia and operation during pregnancy: a registry study of 5405 cases. *Am J Obstet Gynecol* 1989; 161: 1178–1185.

6 Stepp KJ, Sauchak KA, O'Malley DM, et al. Risk factors for adverse outcomes after intraabdominal surgery during pregnancy. *Obstet Gynecol* 2002; 99: 23S.

7 Kort B, Katz VL, Watson WJ. The effect of nonobstetric operation during pregnancy. *Surg Gynecol Obstet* 1993; 177: 371–376.

8 Soriano D, Yefet Y, Seidman DS, et al. Laparoscopy versus laparotomy in the management of adnexal masses during pregnancy. *Fertil Steril* 1999; 71: 955–960.

9 Akira S, Yamanaka A, Ishihara T, et al. Gasless laparoscopic ovarian cystectomy during pregnancy: comparison with laparotomy. *Am J Obstet Gynecol* 1999; 180: 554–557.

10 Al-Fozan H, Tulandi T. Safety and risks of laparoscopy in pregnancy. *Curr Opin Obstet Gynecol* 2002; 14: 375–379.

11 Mathevet P, Nessah K, Dargent D, Mellier G. Laparoscopic management of adnexal masses in pregnancy: a case series. *Eur J Obstet Gynecol Reprod Biol* 2003; 108: 217–222.

12 Stepp K, Falcone T. Laparoscopy in the second trimester of pregnancy. *Obstet Gynecol Clin North Am* 2004; 31: 485–496, review vii.

13 Lachman E, Schienfeld A, Voss E, et al. Pregnancy and laparoscopic surgery. *J Am Assoc Gynecol Laparosc* 1999; 6: 347–351.

14 Fatum M, Rojansky N. Laparoscopic surgery during pregnancy. *Obstet Gynecol Surv* 2001; 56: 50–59.

15 Friedman JD, Ramsey PS, Ramin KD, Berry C. Pneumoamnion and pregnancy loss after second-trimester laparoscopic surgery. *Obstet Gynecol* 2002; 99: 512–513.

16 Hunter JG, Swanstrom L, Thornburg K. Carbon dioxide pneumoperitoneum induces fetal acidosis in a pregnant ewe model. *Surg Endosc* 1995; 9: 272–279.

17 Barnard JM, Chaffin D, Droste S, et al. Fetal response to carbon dioxide pneumoperitoneum in the pregnant ewe. *Obstet Gynecol* 1995; 85: 669–674.
18 Jolles CJ. Gynecologic cancer associated with pregnancy. *Semin Oncol* 1989; 16: 417–424.
19 Hacker NF, Berek JS, Lagasse LD, et al. Carcinoma of the cervix associated with pregnancy. *Obstet Gynecol* 1982; 59: 735–746.
20 Campion MJ, Sedlacek TV. Colposcopy in pregnancy. *Obstet Gynecol Clin North Am* 1993; 20: 153–163.
21 Paraiso MF, Brady K, Helmchen R, Roat TW. Evaluation of the endocervical Cytobrush and Cervex-Brush in pregnant women. *Obstet Gynecol* 1994; 84: 539–543.
22 Michael CW, Esfahani FM. Pregnancy-related changes: a retrospective review of 278 cervical smears. *Diagn Cytopathol* 1997; 17: 99–107.
23 Kim TJ, Kim HS, Park CT, et al. Clinical evaluation of follow-up methods and results of atypical glandular cells of undetermined significance (AGUS) detected on cervicovaginal Pap smears. *Gynecol Oncol* 1999; 73: 292–298.
24 Chieng DC, Elgert P, Cangiarella JF, Cohen JM. Significance of AGUS Pap smears in pregnant and postpartum women. *Acta Cytol* 2001; 45: 294–299.
25 Boardman LA, Goldman DL, Cooper AS, Heber WW, Weitzen S. CIN in pregnancy: antepartum and postpartum cytology and histology. *J Reprod Med* 2005; 50: 13–18.26.
26 Wright TC Jr, Cox JT, Massad LS, et al. 2001 Consensus guidelines for the management of women with cervical cytological abnormalities. *JAMA* 2002; 287: 2120–2129.
27 Economos K, Perez-Veridiano N, Delke I, et al. Abnormal cervical cytology in pregnancy: a 17-year experience. *Obstet Gynecol* 1993; 81: 915–918.
28 Benedet JL, Boyes DA, Nichols TM, Millner A. Colposcopic evaluation of pregnant patients with abnormal cervical smears. *Br J Obstet Gynaecol* 1977; 84: 517–521.
29 Depetrillo AD, Townsend DE, Morrow CP, et al. Colposcopic evaluation of the abnormal Papanicolaou test in pregnancy. *Am J Obstet Gynecol* 1975; 121: 441–445.
30 Woodrow N, Permezel M, Butterfield L, et al. Abnormal cervical cytology in pregnancy: experience of 811 cases. *Aust N Z J Obstet Gynaecol* 1998; 38: 161–165.
31 Yost NP, Santoso JT, McIntire DD, et al. Postpartum regression rates of antepartum cervical intraepithelial neoplasia II and III lesions. *Obstet Gynecol* 1999; 93: 359–362.
32 Palle C, Bangsboll S, Andreasson B. Cervical intraepithelial neoplasia in pregnancy. *Acta Obstet Gynecol Scand* 2000; 79: 306–310.
33 Kiguchi K, Bibbo M, Hasegawa T, et al. Dysplasia during pregnancy: a cytologic follow-up study. *J Reprod Med* 1981; 26: 66–72.
34 Robinson WR, Webb S, Tirpak J, et al. Management of cervical intraepithelial neoplasia during pregnancy with LOOP excision. *Gynecol Oncol* 1997; 64: 153–155.
35 Goldberg GL, Altaras MM, Block B. Cone cerclage in pregnancy. *Obstet Gynecol* 1991; 77: 315–317.
36 Hopkins MP, Morley GW. The prognosis and management of cervical cancer associated with pregnancy. *Obstet Gynecol* 1992; 80: 9–13.
37 Zemlickis D, Lishner M, Degendorfer P, et al. Maternal and fetal outcome after invasive cervical cancer in pregnancy. *J Clin Oncol* 1991; 9: 1956–1961.
38 Senekjian EK, Hubby M, Bell DA, et al. Clear cell adenocarcinoma (CCA) of the vagina and cervix in association with pregnancy. *Gynecol Oncol* 1986; 24: 207–219.
39 Greer BE, Easterling TR, McLennan DA, et al. Fetal and maternal considerations in the management of stage I-B cervical cancer during pregnancy. *Gynecol Oncol* 1989; 34: 61–65.
40 Duggan B, Muderspach LI, Roman LD, et al. Cervical cancer in pregnancy: reporting on planned delay in therapy. *Obstet Gynecol* 1993; 82: 598–602.
41 Monk BJ, Montz FJ. Invasive cervical cancer complicating intrauterine pregnancy: treatment with radical hysterectomy. *Obstet Gynecol* 1992; 80: 199–203.
42 Van der Vange N, Weverling GJ, Ketting BW, et al. The prognosis of cervical cancer associated with pregnancy: a matched cohort study. *Obstet Gynecol* 1995; 85: 1022–1026.
43 Hannigan EV. Cervical cancer in pregnancy. *Clin Obstet Gynecol* 1990; 33: 837–845.
44 Gilstrap LG, van Dorsten PV, Cunningham FG, eds. Cancer in pregnancy. In: *Operative Obstetrics*, 2nd edn. New York: McGraw-Hill, 2001: 421–442.
45 Sood AK, Sorosky JI, Krogman S, et al. Surgical management of cervical cancer complicating pregnancy: a case-control study. *Gynecol Oncol* 1996; 63: 294–298.
46 Takushi M, Moromizato H, Sakumoto K, Kanazawa K. Management of invasive carcinoma of the uterine cervix associated with pregnancy: outcome of intentional delay in treatment. *Gynecol Oncol* 2002; 87: 185–189.
47 Nisker JA, Shubat M. Stage IB cervical carcinoma and pregnancy: report of 49 cases. *Am J Obstet Gynecol* 1983; 145: 203–206.
48 Nevin J, Soeters R, Dehaeck K, et al. Cervical carcinoma associated with pregnancy. *Obstet Gynecol Surv* 1995; 50: 228–239.
49 Cliby WA, Dodson MK, Podratz KC. Cervical cancer complicated by pregnancy: episiotomy site recurrences following vaginal delivery. *Obstet Gynecol* 1994; 84: 179–182.
50 Goldman NA, Goldberg GL. Late recurrences of squamous cell cervical cancer in an episiotomy site after vaginal delivery. *Obstet Gynecol* 2003; 101: 1127–1129.
51 Gershenson DM. Fertility-sparing surgery for malignancies in women. *J Natl Cancer Inst Monogr* 2005; 34: 43–47.
52 Plante M, Roy M. Fertility-preserving options for cervical cancer. *Oncology* 2006; 20: 479–488; discussion 491–493.
53 Carter J, Sonoda Y, Abu-Rustum NR. Reproductive concerns of women treated with radical trachelectomy for cervical cancer. *Gynecol Oncol* 2007; 105(1): 13–16.
54 Bader AA, Petru E, Winter R. Long-term follow-up after neoadjuvant chemotherapy for high-risk cervical cancer during pregnancy. *Gynecol Oncol* 2007; 105(1): 269–272.
55 Goff BA, Paley PJ, Koh WJ, et al. Cancer in the pregnant patient. In: Hoskins WJ, Perez CA, Young RC, eds. *Principles and Practice of Gynecologic Oncology*. Philadelphia: Lippincott Williams and Wilkins, 2000.
56 Creasman WT, Rutledge F, Smith JP. Carcinoma of the ovary associated with pregnancy. *Obstet Gynecol* 1971; 38: 111–116.
57 Roberts JA. Management of gynecologic tumors during pregnancy. *Clin Perinatol* 1983; 10: 369–382.
58 Ueda M, Ueki M. Ovarian tumors associated with pregnancy. *Int J Gynaecol Obstet* 1996; 55: 59–65.

59 Bernhard LM, Klebba PK, Gray DL, Mutch DG. Predictors of persistence of adnexal masses in pregnancy. *Obstet Gynecol* 1999; 93: 585–589.

60 Marino T, Craigo SD. Managing adnexal masses in pregnancy. *Contemp Ob/Gyn* 2000; 45: 130–143.

61 Hermans RH, Fischer DC, van der Putten HW, van de Putte G, et al. Adnexal masses in pregnancy. *Onkologie* 2003; 26: 167–172.

62 Agarwal N, Parul, Kriplani A, Bhatla N, Gupta A. Management and outcome of pregnancies complicated with adnexal masses. *Arch Gynecol Obstet* 2003; 267: 148–152.

63 Leiserowitz GS, Xing G, Cress R, et al. Adnexal masses in pregnancy: how often are they malignant? *Gynecol Oncol* 2006; 101: 315–321.

64 Leiserowitz GS. Managing ovarian masses during pregnancy. *Obstet Gynecol Surv* 2006; 61: 463–470.

65 Thornton JG, Wells M. Ovarian cysts in pregnancy: does ultrasound make traditional management inappropriate? *Obstet Gynecol* 1987; 69: 717–721.

66 Bromley B, Benacerraf B. Adnexal masses during pregnancy: accuracy of sonographic diagnosis and outcome. *J Ultrasound Med* 1997; 16: 447–452.

67 Beischer NA, Buttery BW, Fortune DW, Macafee CA. Growth and malignancy of ovarian tumours in pregnancy. *Aust N Z J Obstet Gynaecol* 1971; 11: 208–220.

68 Struyk AP, Treffers PE. Ovarian tumors in pregnancy. *Acta Obstet Gynecol Scand* 1984; 63: 421–424.

69 Hess LW, Peaceman A, O'Brien WF, et al. Adnexal masses occurring with intrauterine pregnancy: report of fifty-four patients requiring laparotomy for definitive management. *Am J Obstet Gynecol* 1988; 158: 1029–1034.

70 Hogston P, Lilford RJ. Ultrasound study of ovarian cysts in pregnancy: prevalence and significance. *Br J Obstet Gynaecol* 1986; 93: 625–628.

71 Rahman MS, Al-Sibai MH, Rahman J, et al. Ovarian carcinoma associated with pregnancy: a review of 9 cases. *Acta Obstet Gynecol Scand* 2002; 81: 260.

72 Jacob JH, Stringer CA. Diagnosis and management of cancer during pregnancy. *Semin Perinatol* 1990; 14: 79–87.

73 Whitecar MP, Turner S, Higby MK. Adnexal masses in pregnancy: a review of 130 cases undergoing surgical management. *Am J Obstet Gynecol* 1999; 181: 19–24.

74 De Palo G, Pilotti S, Kenda R, et al. Natural history of dysgerminoma. *Am J Obstet Gynecol* 1982; 143: 799–807.

75 Doll DC, Ringenberg QS, Yarbro JW. Antineoplastic agents and pregnancy. *Semin Oncol* 1989; 16: 337–346.

76 Dipaola RS, Goodin S, Ratzell M, et al. Chemotherapy for metastatic melanoma during pregnancy. *Gynecol Oncol* 1997; 66: 526–530.

77 Buekers TE, Lallas TA. Chemotherapy in pregnancy. *Obstet Gynecol Clin North Am* 1998; 25(2): 323–329.

78 Williams SF, Schilsky RL. Antineoplastic drugs administered during pregnancy. *Semin Oncol* 2000; 27: 618–622.

79 Beeley L. Adverse effects of drugs in the first trimester of pregnancy. *Clin Obstet Gynaecol* 1986; 13: 177–195.

80 Sutcliffe SB. Treatment of neoplastic disease during pregnancy: maternal and fetal effects. *Clin Invest Med* 1985; 8: 333–338.

81 Aviles A, Neri N. Hematological malignancies and pregnancy: a final report of 84 children who received chemotherapy in utero. *Clin Lymphoma* 2001; 2: 173–177.

82 Partridge AH, Garber JE. Long-term outcomes of children exposed to antineplastic agents in utero. *Semin Oncol* 2000; 27: 712–726.

83 Zemlickis D, Lishner M, Degendorfer P, et al. Fetal outcome after in utero exposure to cancer chemotherapy. *Arch Intern Med* 1992; 152: 573–576.

84 Garber JE. Long-term follow-up of children exposed in utero to antineoplastic agents. *Semin Oncol* 1989; 16: 437–444.

85 Moore HC, Foster RS Jr. Breast cancer and pregnancy. *Semin Oncol* 2000; 27: 646–653.

86 Gallenberg MM, Loprinzi CL. Breast cancer and pregnancy. *Semin Oncol* 1989; 16: 369–376.

87 American College of Radiology. MR safety and sedation. In: *American College of Radiology Standards*. Reston, Va: American College of Radiology, 1998: 457.

88 Levine D. The role of computed tomography and magnetic resonance imaging in obstetrics. In: Callen PW, ed. *Ultrasonography in Obstetrics and Gynecology*, 4th edn. Philadelphia: WB Saunders, 2000: 725.

89 Chew S, Ahmadi A, Goh PS, et al. The effects of 1.5T magnetic resonance imaging on early murine in-vitro embryo development. *J Magn Reson Imaging* 2001; 13: 417–420.

90 Chung SM. Safety issues in magnetic resonance imaging. *J Neuroophthalmol* 2002; 22: 35–39.

91 Woo JC, Yu T, Hurd TC. Breast cancer in pregnancy. *Arch Surg* 2003; 138: 91–98, discussion 99.

92 King RM, Welch JS, Martin JK Jr, Coulam CB. Carcinoma of the breast associated with pregnancy. *Surg Gynecol Obstet* 1985; 160: 228–232.

93 Nugent P, O'Connell TX. Breast cancer and pregnancy. *Arch Surg* 1985; 120: 1221–1224.

94 Zemlickis D, Lishner M, Degendorfer P, et al. Maternal and fetal outcome after breast cancer in pregnancy. *Am J Obstet Gynecol* 1992; 166: 781–787.

95 Isaacs JH. Cancer of the breast in pregnancy. *Surg Clin North Am* 1995; 75: 47–51.

96 Fisher B, Anderson S, Bryant J, et al. Twenty-year follow-up of a randomized trial comparing total mastectomy, lumpectomy, and lumpectomy plus irradiation for the treatment of invasive breast cancer. *N Engl J Med* 2002; 347: 1233–1241.

97 Veronesi U, Cascinelli N, Mariani L, et al. Twenty-year follow-up of a randomized study comparing breast conserving surgery with radical mastectomy for early breast cancer. *N Engl J Med* 2002; 347: 1227–1232.

98 Sorosky JI, Scott-Conner CE. Breast disease complicating pregnancy. *Obstet Gynecol Clin North Am* 1998; 25: 353–363.

99 Bunker ML, Peters MV. Breast cancer associated with pregnancy or lactation. *Am J Obstet Gynecol* 1963; 85: 312–321.

100 Danforth DN Jr. How subsequent pregnancy affects outcome in women with a prior breast cancer. *Oncology (Williston Park)* 1991; 11: 23–30; discussion 30–31, 35.

101 Mackie RM, Bray CA, Hole DJ, et al. Incidence of and survival from malignant melanoma in Scotland: an epidemiological study. *Lancet* 2002; 360: 587–591.

102 Katz VL, Farmer RM, Dotters D. Focus on primary care: from nevus to neoplasm. Myths of melanoma in pregnancy. *Obstet Gynecol Surv* 2002; 57: 112–119.

103 Kjems E, Krag C. Melanoma and pregnancy. A review. *Acta Oncol* 1993; 32: 371–378.

104 Lang PG Jr. Malignant melanoma. *Med Clin North Am* 1998; 82: 1325–1358.

105 Wong DJ, Strassner HT. Melanoma in pregnancy: a literature review. *Clin Obstet Gynecol* 1990; 33: 782–791.

106 Salopek TG, Marghoob AA, Slade JM, et al. An estimate of the incidence of malignant melanoma in the United States: based on a survey of members of the American Academy of Dermatology. *Dermatol Surg* 1995; 21: 301–305.

107 Daryanani D, Plukker JT, de Hullu JA, et al. Pregnancy and early stage melanoma. *Cancer* 2003; 97: 2248–2253.

108 Squatrito RC, Harlow SP. Melanoma complicating pregnancy. *Obstet Gynecol Clin North Am* 1998; 25: 407–416.

109 Zanetti R, Franceschi S, Rosso S, et al. Cutaneous malignant melanoma in females: the role of hormonal and reproductive factors. *Int J Epidemiol* 1990; 19: 522–526.

110 Shiu MH, Schottenfield D, Maclean B, Fortner JG. Adverse effect of pregnancy on melanoma: a reappraisal. *Cancer* 1976; 37: 181–187.

111 Smith MA, Fine JA, Barnhill RL, Berwick M. Hormonal and reproductive influences and risk of melanoma in women. *Int J Epidemiol* 1998; 27: 751–757.

112 Slingluff CL Jr, Reintgen DS, Vollmer RT, Seigler HF. Malignant melanoma arising during pregnancy. A study of 100 patients. *Ann Surg* 1990; 211: 552–559.

113 Wong JH, Sterns EE, Kopald KH, et al. Prognostic significance of pregnancy in stage I melanoma. *Arch Surg* 1989; 124: 1227–1231.

114 Travers RL, Sober AJ, Berwick M, et al. Increased thickness of pregnancy-associated melanoma. *Br J Dermatol* 1995; 33: 40–46.

115 Mackie RM. Pregnancy and exogenous hormones in patients with cutaneous malignant melanoma. *Curr Opin Oncol* 1999; 11: 129–131.

116 Reintgen DS, McCarty KS Jr,Vollmer R, et al. Malignant melanoma and pregnancy. *Cancer* 1985; 55: 1340–1344.

117 Morton DL, Thompson JF, Cochran AJ, et al. Sentinel-node biopsy or nodal observation in melanoma. *N Engl J Med* 2006; 355: 1307–1317. Erratum in *N Engl J Med* 2006; 355: 1944.

118 Gannon CJ, Rousseau DL Jr, Ross MI, et al. Accuracy of lymphatic mapping and sentinel lymph node biopsy after previous wide local excision in patients with primary melanoma. *Cancer* 2006; 107: 2647–2652.

119 Schwartz JL, Morzurkewich EL, Johnson TM. Current management of patients with melanoma who are pregnant, want to get pregnant, or do not want to get pregnant. *Cancer* 2003; 97: 2130–2133.

120 Mondi MM, Cuenca RE, Ollila DW, et al. Sentinel lymph node biopsy during pregnancy: initial clinical experience. *Ann Surg Oncol* 2007; 14: 218–221.

121 Atallah E, Flaherty L. Treatment of metastatic malignant melanoma. *Curr Treat Options Oncol* 2005; 6: 185–193.

122 Ferreira CM, Maceira JM, Coelho JM. Melanoma and pregnancy with placental metastases. Report of a case. *Am J Dermatopathol* 1998; 20: 403–407.

123 Baergen RN, Johnson D, Moore T, Benirschke K. Maternal melanoma metastatic to the placenta: a case report and review of the literature. *Arch Pathol Lab Med* 1997; 121: 508–511.

124 Marsh RD, Chu NM. Placental metastasis from primary ocular melanoma: a case report. *Am J Obstet Gynecol* 1996; 174: 1654–1655.

125 Dildy GA 3rd, Moise KJ, Carpenter RJ Jr, Klima T. Maternal malignancy metastatic to the products of conception: a review. *Obstet Gynecol Surv* 1989; 44: 535–540.

126 Alexander A, Samlowski WE, Grossman D, et al. Metastatic melanoma in pregnancy: risk of transplacental metastases in the infant. *J Clin Oncol* 2003; 21: 2179–2186.

127 Rothman LA, Cohen CJ, Astarloa J. Placental and fetal involvement by maternal malignancy: a report or rectal carcinoma and review of the literature. *Am J Obstet Gynecol* 1973; 116: 1023–1034.

128 Jacobs C, Donaldson SS, Rosenberg SA, Kaplan HS. Management of the pregnant patient with Hodgkin's disease. *Ann Intern Med* 1981; 95: 669–675.

129 Lishner M, Zemlickis D, Degendorfer P, Panzarella T, Sutcliffe SB, Koren G. Maternal and foetal outcome following Hodgkin's disease in pregnancy. *Br J Cancer* 1992; 65: 114–117.

130 Pereg D, Koren G, Lishner M. The treatment of Hodgkin's and Non-Hodgkin's lymphoma in pregnancy. *Haematologica* 2007; 92: 1230–1237.

131 Walsh C, Fazio VW. Cancer of the colon, rectum, and anus during pregnancy. The surgeon's perspective. *Gastroenterol Clin North Am* 1998; 27: 257–267.

132 Skilling JS. Colorectal cancer complicating pregnancy. *Obstet Gynecol Clin North Am* 1998; 25: 417–421.

133 Chan YM, Ngai SW, Lao TT. Colon cancer in pregnancy: a case report. *J Reprod Med* 1999; 44: 733–736.

134 Donegan WL. Cancer and pregnancy. *CA Cancer J Clin* 1983; 33: 194–214.

135 Hirabayashi M, Ueo H, Okudaira Y, et al. Early gastric cancer and a concomitant pregnancy. *Am Surg* 1987; 53: 730–732.

136 Davis JL, Chen MD. Gastric carcinoma presenting as a exacerbation of ulcers during pregnancy: a case report. *J Reprod Med* 1991; 36: 450–452.

137 Chan YM, Ngai SW, Lao TT. Gastric adenacarcinoma presenting with persistent, mild gastrointestinal symptoms in pregnancy: a case report. *J Reprod Med* 1999; 44: 986–988.

138 Gisi P, Floyd R. Hepatocellular carcinoma in pregnancy: a case report. *J Reprod Med* 1999; 44: 65–67.

139 Hsieh TT, Hou HC, Hsu JJ, et al. Term delivery after hepatocellular carcinoma resection in previous pregnancy. *Acta Obstet Gynecol Scand* 1996; 75: 77–78.

140 Balderston KD, Tewari K, Azizi F, Yu JK. Intrahepatic cholangiocarcinoma masquerading as the HELLP syndrome (hemolysis, elevated liver enzymes, and low platelet count) in pregnancy: case report. *Am J Obstet Gynecol* 1998; 179: 823–824.

141 Hsu KL, Ko SF, Cheng YF, et al. Spontaneous rupture of hepatocellular carcinoma during pregnancy. *Obstet Gynecol* 2001; 98: 913.

142 Gamberdella FR. Pancreatic carcinoma in pregnancy: a case report. *Am J Obstet Gynecol* 1984; 148: 15–17.

143 Levy C, Pereira L, Dardarian T, et al. Solid pseudopapillary pancreatic tumor in pregnancy. A case report. *J Reprod Med* 2004; 49: 61–64.

144 Walker JL, Knight EL. Renal cell carcinoma in pregnancy. *Cancer* 1986; 58: 2343–2347.

145 Smith DP, Goldman SM, Beggs DS, et al. Renal cell carcinoma in pregnancy: report of three cases and review of the literature. *Obstet Gynecol* 1994; 83: 818–820.

146 Fazeli-Matin S, Goldfarb DA, Novick AC. Renal and adrenal surgery during pregnancy. *Urology* 1998; 52: 510–511.

147 Morris PC. Thyroid cancer complicating pregnancy. *Obstet Gynecol Clin North Am* 1998; 25: 401–405.

148 Tewari K, Balderston KD, Carpenter SE, et al. Papillary thyroid carcinoma manifesting as thyroid storm of pregnancy: case report. *Am J Obstet Gynecol* 1998; 179: 818–819.

149 Rossing MA, Voigt LF, Wicklund KG, et al. Reproductive factors and risk of papillary thyroid cancer in women. *Am J Epidemiol* 2000; 151: 765–772.

150 Maxwell C, Barzilay B, Shah V, et al. Maternal and neonatal outcomes in pregnancies complicated by bone and soft-tissue tumors. *Obstet Gynecol* 2004; 104: 344–348. Comment in *Obstet Gynecol* 2005; 105: 447; author reply 447–448.

151 Durkin JW Jr. Carcinoid tumor and pregnancy. *Am J Obstet Gynecol* 1983; 145: 757–761.

152 Isla A, Alvarez F, Gonzalez A, et al. Brain tumor and pregnancy. *Obstet Gynecol* 1997; 89: 19–23.

153 Finfer SR. Management of labour and delivery in patients with intracranial neoplasms. *Br J Anaesth* 1991; 67: 784–787.

154 Tewari KS, Cappuccini F, Asrat T, et al. Obstetric emergencies precipitated by malignant brain tumors. *Am J Obstet Gynecol* 2000; 182: 1215–1221.

51 Pregnancy in Women with Complicated Diabetes Mellitus

Martin N. Montoro

Departments of Medicine and Obstetrics and Gynecology, Keck School of Medicine, University of Southern California, Los Angeles, CA, USA

Introduction

The outcome of pregnancy in women with diabetes mellitus has steadily improved over the last several decades. However, women with pregestational diabetic complications still have elevated fetal, neonatal and maternal morbidity and mortality. At the highest risk are those with severe retinal, renal, or ischemic heart disease. Advances in the medical treatment of diabetes and in obstetric and neonatal care have improved the outcome of pregnancy in women with complicated diabetes. Until recently, many women with complicated diabetes mellitus were advised to avoid pregnancy or have a therapeutic abortion if they became pregnant. At present, absolute recommendations against pregnancy are few and limited to women with unusually severe complications, particularly ischemic heart disease.

Obtaining optimal diabetic control before pregnancy is of paramount importance because at present, perinatal mortality due to congenital anomalies accounts for over 50% of perinatal losses. Emphasis should be placed on preconceptual diabetic control since organogenesis may be complete by the time the pregnancy is recognized.

Diabetic retinopathy

Course of retinopathy during pregnancy

Publications on the prevalence and risk factors affecting the progression of diabetic retinopathy during pregnancy still vary widely. One study reports a rate of progression as high as 78% in women with pre-existing retinopathy [1] while another reports a much lower rate of 5% [2]. Still others report that sight-threatening deterioration during pregnancy is not more common than in non-pregnant, age- and duration-matched type 1 diabetic women controls [3]. The findings of the Diabetes Control and Complications Trial (DCCT) [4] are considered to be very important since conducting future similar studies will be difficult to accomplish (180 women with 270 pregnancies compared to 500 women who did not become pregnant and followed for an average of 6.5 years, all with type 1 diabetes). These investigators reported a 1.63-fold greater risk of worsening retinopathy in the intensive treatment group versus a 2.48-fold increase in the conventionally treated group. The increased risk peaked during the second trimester but persisted for as long as 1 year postpartum. The risk of progression was attributed to "a pregnancy effect" as well as an additional effect resulting from establishing rapid diabetic control. The worsening that occurred during pregnancy did not result in long-term morbidity. Of the 270 pregnancies, 183 were in women who had absent or minimal changes (only microaneurysms) just before pregnancy. The progression to severe retinopathy in this group was extremely low (1.6%). Patients who progressed to severe retinopathy commonly had lesions before pregnancy [5]. Other studies have shown a higher (up to 33%) rate of background retinopathy developing during pregnancy in women without detectable lesions before pregnancy. However, those lesions were considered mild, did not require treatment and regressed after delivery [3,6–9].

The sudden institution of tight diabetic control may also be a factor in the worsening of retinopathy [4]. However, not all studies confirm these findings. Lauszus et al. report that tight diabetic control may actually prevent the progression of retinopathy rather than contribute to its worsening [10].

Is there a "pregnancy factor"?

Several publications have reported on the levels of vasoactive hormones in pregnant women with and without diabetes followed with serial retinal photographs before, during and up to 6–12 months postpartum. Levels of plasma atrial natriuretic peptide (ANP) and angiotensin II were not statistically significantly different in type 1 diabetic women compared with healthy controls. Both groups showed retinal arteriolar constriction during pregnancy and in the diabetic women the change in

Critical Care Obstetrics, 5th edition. Edited by M. Belfort, G. Saade, M. Foley, J. Phelan and G. Dildy.

arteriolar diameter did not correlate with retinopathy, arterial blood pressure or HbA1c levels. One interesting finding was that diabetic women who smoked did not show retinal vasoconstriction during pregnancy [11], although smoking is an independent risk factor for worsening retinopathy.

Other studies have reported on the possible role of vasoactive mediators and retinopathy during pregnancy. In one study, plasma renin activity (RAS) and ANP were significantly lower in diabetic compared with non-diabetic women throughout pregnancy and postpartum. The authors speculate that the lower levels of RAS and ANP may contribute to hyperdynamic blood flow and progression of retinopathy in diabetic pregnancies. However, no significant differences were found in the levels of other natriuretic peptides (BNP and CNP), angiotensin II, aldosterone or adrenomedullin [12].

The insulin-like growth factor system has also been studied in pregnant diabetic women and higher levels of insulin-like growth factor-1 (IGF-1) were found to be significantly associated with worsening retinopathy (as well as with higher birth weight) [13]. Levels of IGF-1, IGF binding protein-1, highly phosphorylated IGF binding protein-1, and IGF binding protein-3 were not associated with progression of retinopathy [14].

Is there an insulin effect?

After the first rapid-acting insulin analog, Lispro was introduced, there were concerns, based on case reports, about its potential for worsening retinopathy during pregnancy [15]. However, subsequent publications involving larger series have shown that it is both safe and effective during pregnancy [16,17]. Insulin Aspart, another rapid-acting insulin analog, has also been reported to be safe and effective during pregnancy [18,19]. These two insulin analogs are preferred over regular insulin because they are much more effective than regular insulin in controlling postprandial serum glucose levels. A newer rapid-acting analog, insulin Glulisine has been recently released but reports of its safety during pregnancy are absent. There are also two long-acting insulin analogs available for use, insulin Glargine and insulin Detemir. The limited data on Glargine indicates that it is probably safe in animals [20] as well as in humans [21]. There is no information at present about the use of insulin Detemir in pregnancy. The main concern about the use of insulin analogs in pregnancy has been their higher binding affinity for the IGF-1 receptor and thus the potential for generating higher IGF-1 levels. However, at least with insulin Lispro, those concerns have not been found to be clinically relevant [16–17,22]. Therefore, insulin does not appear to be a factor affecting the progression or development of retinopathy during pregnancy.

Other important factors

Most studies reporting on diabetic retinopathy and pregnancy agree that the duration of diabetes is a strong independent variable associated with worsening retinopathy during pregnancy. The longer the duration of diabetes mellitus the higher the risk of worsening retinopathy [1–3,12], particularly after 5–10 years' duration. Another independent variable is the degree of metabolic control, with the highest risk involving women poorly controlled before pregnancy and who are brought rapidly under tight control [3,4]. Elevated blood pressure (acute or chronic) is also associated with worsening retinopathy, and pre-eclampsia seems to be a potent risk factor for exacerbation of retinal disease [1,3] (Table 51.1).

Table 51.1 Highest risk for retinopathy during pregnancy.

Diabetes of long duration (>5 years, particularly >10 years)
Rapid glucose normalization after prolonged poor control
Coexisting hypertension of any type (chronic hypertension, pre-eclampsia, eclampsia)
Treat pre-existing retinopathy before conception!

Management

The management of severe retinopathy during pregnancy remains controversial because there are no studies that have included photocoagulation as an independent variable. In addition, since retinopathy may regress after delivery it has been argued that treatment during pregnancy might not be needed [23]. Even though some regression may occur postpartum, most centers recommend treatment during pregnancy if significant neovascularization occurs, the same advice as for non-pregnant patients [24]. Ideally, treatment should be completed before conception in order to prevent or minimize progression during pregnancy. If proliferative retinopathy worsens during pregnancy, treatment may prevent further progression and preserve vision.

Proliferative retinopathy is no longer considered to be an absolute contraindication for pregnancy, given current treatment possibilities. However, these patients remain at high risk, and have to be monitored closely. They should be advised of their risk on an individual basis and before pregnancy if at all possible. General guidelines are as follows.

1 The highest risk for worsening retinopathy involves women (i) with diabetes for 5–10 years or longer, (ii) with diabetes which is poorly controlled and brought under tight control very rapidly, (iii) with chronic hypertension and (iv) developing pre-eclampsia/eclampsia.

2 An ophthalmologist should examine any patient with diabetes of longer than 5 years' duration before pregnancy, each trimester, and within 3 months after delivery. If the diabetes has been present for fewer than 5 years, the treating physician should perform periodic ophthalmoscopic exams. If any changes are noted, or if any visual symptoms develop, referral to an ophthalmologist is warranted. However, since early lesions may be easily missed by non-ophthalmologists it could be argued that all patients should have at least one examination by an ophthalmologist before or in early pregnancy. All diabetic women with documented retinopathy should be followed in conjunction with an ophthalmologist during pregnancy and postpartum.

3 Active proliferative retinopathy should, ideally, be treated before pregnancy. If it develops in early gestation (first trimester), and there is no response to treatment, pregnancy termination might have to be offered as an alternative.

4 Vaginal delivery may be allowed for those patients with background or successfully treated proliferative retinopathy. The optimal route of delivery for those patients with active proliferative retinopathy has not been determined, since in non-pregnant patients vitreous hemorrhages may occur even during periods of inactivity. Vitreous hemorrhages have been observed during both cesarean sections and vaginal deliveries, but there is concern that they may occur more readily during the active expulsion phase of vaginal birth. In patients with active proliferative retinopathy, it is recommended that the mode of delivery be determined on an individual basis and in consultation with both the obstetrician and ophthalmologist.

Nephropathy

Until fairly recently, women with diabetic nephropathy were strongly discouraged from attempting pregnancy, and therapeutic abortion was frequently recommended if pregnancy occurred. These recommendations are not supported by more recent reports, which show significantly improved perinatal outcome when good metabolic and blood pressure control is achieved along with current "state of the art" obstetric and neonatal care. Better outcomes are consistently obtained in centers offering a multidisciplinary team approach.

Perinatal complications may include congenital anomalies, fetal growth restriction, fetal death, stillbirth, and preterm delivery with its associated neonatal morbidity from prematurity. Maternal complications include worsening of renal function during or after pregnancy, anemia, superimposed pre-eclampsia or eclampsia, and worsening of other diabetic complications frequently coexisting with nephropathy, mainly retinopathy (see previous section). These women should also be aware that they may face future significant morbidity (e.g. dialysis, renal transplantation, etc.) and even shortened life spans due to macrovascular disease.

Diabetic nephropathy usually occurs in uncontrolled type 1 diabetes after 5–15 years' duration or longer, but it may also be seen with shorter duration of diabetes as well as in patients with type 2 diabetes. In the United Kingdom Prospective Diabetes Study (UKPDS) [25], 17% of newly diagnosed type 2 diabetics had pre-existing microalbuminuria, 3.8% had macroalbuminuria and 37% were hypertensive, most likely because many type 2 diabetics have had the disease for several years before the diagnosis.

It should be widely recognized that all reproductive-age women with diabetes could become pregnant. They should be thoroughly informed about the risks of pregnancy when the diabetes is poorly controlled and the additional risks of hypertension and overt diabetic nephropathy. These women should be strongly urged to use effective contraceptive measures while waiting to attempt pregnancy until a time when the diabetes and hypertension have been optimally controlled.

Prepregnancy evaluation

Women with diabetes should, ideally, be evaluated for the presence or absence of nephropathy before pregnancy. A 24-hour urine collection for protein excretion and creatinine clearance (CrCl) is recommended. A renal biopsy is no longer considered to be absolutely necessary for diagnosis.

Many diabetic women are currently prescribed angiotensin-converting enzyme (ACE) inhibitors or angiotensin receptor blockers (ARBs) in an effort to prevent or delay the onset of diabetic nephropathy. It has been suggested that using these compounds in the preconception period, until the pregnancy is diagnosed, might decrease complications during pregnancy [26,27]. However, more recent studies show that these compounds are not safe at any time during pregnancy and should be stopped before conception [28]. Therefore, prepregnancy counseling must include the discontinuation of ACE inhibitors and ARBs before conception. Counseling should also include the discontinuation of statin and fibrate medications before pregnancy. Omega-3 fatty acids may be continued or started during pregnancy because of potential benefits, particularly with diabetes [29].

Further evaluation should include an ophthalmologic exam and an ECG, as well as additional cardiovascular testing including an echocardiogram and/or stress test if clinically appropriate. All women with type 1 diabetes should have an evaluation of their thyroid function [30] including a TSH level and a thyroid peroxidase antibody titer along with the pertinent routine laboratory studies. Further dietary counseling should include the additional changes that are required when significant renal impairment is present.

It should be emphasized that excellent glycemic control before pregnancy may not only prevent or minimize the risk of congenital anomalies but also result in more stable renal function and lower complication rates later in the pregnancy as well [31].

Course during pregnancy

The expected increase in CrCl during pregnancy, in the presence of diabetic nephropathy, is seen in only about a third of these women; in another third the renal function remains stable. In the remainder, a decrease occurs which may reflect the natural progression of diabetic nephropathy and/or a pregnancy effect from glomerular hyperfiltration, heavy proteinuria, along with worsening hypertension and pre-eclampsia [32–35].

Microalbuminuria and blood pressure levels

The presence of microalbuminuria before or in early pregnancy is associated with a 35–60% risk for the development of pre-eclampsia, much higher than the 6–14% risk observed in diabetic women without microalbuminuria before conception [36–39]. Blood pressure levels alone in early pregnancy have been found to have a low sensitivity and specificity as sole predictors of hypertensive complications in the third trimester, while urinary microalbumin excretion was a better predictor of pre-eclampsia ([36]. The subset of women with both microalbuminuria and chronic hypertension is reported to have the highest rate of superimposed pre-eclampsia [40]. The highest pregnancy complication rate is seen in women with a serum creatinine level of ≥2.0 mg/dL or a CrCl <50 mL/min before or in early pregnancy [31–32,41–42]. Given the high rate of maternal and fetal complications in women with this advanced degree of diabetic nephropathy some experts recommend discouraging pregnancy.

Anemia

Anemia due to erythropoietin deficiency is a common complication of diabetic nephropathy and may further compromise fetal oxygenation. Erythropoietin has been used during pregnancy to treat anemia in diabetic nephropathy [43–45]. Recently, concerns have been raised about the long-term use of this medication. However, the short-term, judicious use of erythropoietin, during pregnancy is unlikely to be a cause of serious long-term morbidity and may be very beneficial for the developing fetus.

Asymptomatic bacteriuria and pyelonephritis

Screening for and treating asymptomatic bacteriuria seems justified in pregnant women with diabetic nephropathy because it occurs more frequently in these women. Pyelonephritis is a particularly serious, but preventable, consequence of untreated bacteriuria [46,47].

Cigarette smoking

Cigarette smoking should be strongly discouraged in all pregnant women and in diabetic women in particular. Smoking impairs fetal oxygenation and, as in the case of retinopathy, it is an independent risk factor for worsening nephropathy [48–50].

Worsening renal function

It is unusual for diabetic nephropathy to progress to end-stage renal disease during the course of pregnancy [31–33,41–43,51,52]. Nevertheless, pregnancy may have a deleterious effect and accelerate deterioration in those with more impaired renal function (Cr ≥1.2 mg/dL) in early pregnancy [32–35,41–43,51,52]. Overall, parity alone does not appear to be associated with more rapid deterioration of renal function according to data from long-term follow-up of diabetic women with similar degrees of nephropathy who do not have pregnancies [4,53–56].

Management

Strict diabetic control (HbA_1C <7%) should be achieved before conception and maintained at all times throughout pregnancy. Adequate rest at night (e.g. ≥8 hours, but it is not necessary to be asleep all those hours) and rest periods lasting 1–2 h each during the day (e.g. late moring and mid- to late afternoon) will be greatly beneficial for those with the more advanced nephropathy. These women should be made aware that a readjustment of their lifestyle and even their work schedule would likely be recommended later in the pregnancy.

Hypertension should be appropriately treated. There is evidence that blood pressure levels (e.g. ≤130/80 mmHg), lower than the ≤140/90 mmHg currently recommended, might provide additional benefits including a reduction in premature deliveries [57]. Antihypertensive agents that are considered safer during pregnancy, even during organogenesis, include α-methyldopa, clonidine and the β-adrenergic antagonists with low lipid solubility [58–61]. The non-dehydropyridine calcium channel blockers (e.g. diltiazem) are reportedly beneficial for glomerular function [62,63]. Calcium channel blockers during the first trimester were associated with the possibility of limb defects in one study [64] but not found to be teratogenic in a larger prospective study [65].

Frequent visits for close monitoring and liberal hospitalizations are recommended for worsening hypertension, deteriorating renal function, or fetal compromise. Periodic ultrasound examinations are useful for dating (first trimester), detection of congenital anomalies (later in second trimester), and assessment of fetal growth (monthly in third trimester). Intrauterine growth restriction, rather than macrosomia, is more likely in patients with vascular compromise even if the diabetes is not optimally controlled. Fetal surveillance should be instituted as soon as there is willingness to intervene for fetal distress. The mother should be carefully informed of the situation and her wishes taken into consideration. A consultation with a neonatologist is strongly recommended to make sure the mother is aware of the prematurity risks.

Outpatient therapy is acceptable as long as the diabetes and hypertension are well controlled and the renal function is at an acceptable level (determined at least every month in stable patients and more often if unstable); otherwise hospitalization, even prolonged, is strongly advised.

Delivery before term may be indicated due to maternal deterioration or fetal distress. For elective delivery before term, fetal lung maturation should be documented. The route of delivery should be considered on an individual basis. Many of these women (68–74%) will require cesarean section delivery secondary to prematurity, malpresentation, and fetal distress. Obviously, these decisions should be made in conjunction with the obstetrician/perinatologist and neonatal consultant.

Neonatal survival has steadily improved during the last 20–25 years. However, perinatal mortality is still reported to be 5–7% mainly due to congenital anomalies or severe fetal growth restriction. Respiratory distress syndrome is reported in 24–25% of cases. The improved outcome is most likely multifactorial and includes better control of diabetes and hypertension, improved fetal surveillance, as well as improved neonatal care. Predictors of poor outcome are outlined in Table 51.2.

Table 51.2 Diabetic nephropathy: predictors of poor outcome.

Proteinuria of ≥3g in the first trimester
Serum creatinine ≥1.2 mg/dL
Chronic hypertension, pre-eclampsia, eclampsia
Anemia (hematocrit <25%)
Poor compliance

Pregnancy in women on dialysis and after renal transplantation

Dialysis

The number of cases of hemodialysis and, less commonly, continuous ambulatory peritoneal dialysis during pregnancy, is increasing. This information comes primarily from observational studies of women with all varieties of kidney diseases, including diabetes mellitus. Most reported cases were women on the verge of requiring dialysis when they conceived (usually unplanned pregnancies) or women who experienced a rapid decline in renal function while pregnant [66]. Although it might be tempting to recommend termination of pregnancy under these circumstances, it rarely results in substantial improvement in renal function [67]. Interestingly, no increase risk of maternal death has been reported although severe hypertension, preterm delivery and oligohydramnios result in a perinatal mortality of 22–40% [68]. The judicious management of anemia (erythropoietin and/or transfusions) and of preterm labor may help to improve outcomes [69].

Renal transplantation

As a result of an overall increased number of renal transplantations coupled with a strong desire for motherhood, more pregnant patients with renal transplants will be seen in the future. About one-fourth of all patients on chronic dialysis or after renal transplantation have diabetes. Current recommendations emphasize the importance of waiting a minimum of 2 years before attempting pregnancy. Stable graft function including a serum creatinine <1.5 mg/dL, proteinuria <500 mg/day and optimal blood pressure and glucose control are also prudent requirements [70]. Data reported from pregnancies in women with kidney transplants secondary to conditions other than diabetes reveal an improved survival when serum creatinine levels are <1.5 mg/dL, 98% vs 75% [71]. The course during pregnancy is dependent on baseline glomerular function at the time of conception, control of hypertension and prompt diagnosis and treatment of urinary tract infections [72]. The outcome of pregnancy in women with combined pancreas/kidney transplants is similar to those with kidney transplant alone [73].

There appears to be a low rate of graft dysfunction during pregnancy; however, hypertension, pre-eclampsia and preterm delivery are frequent complications [74]. A surprising low rate of complications has been reported with the use of immunosuppressant agents. Azathioprine and cyclosporine cross the placenta but do not appear to be teratogenic or cause fetal growth restriction [75]. There is less experience with the newer immunosuppressants although tacrolimus has been reported to be associated with fetal/neonatal hyperkalemia [70,76,77].

Diabetic ketoacidosis

Diabetic ketoacidosis (DKA) is an acute and potentially life-threatening emergency with very serious consequences for both mother and fetus. Until recently, perinatal mortality, after an episode of maternal DKA, was reported to be as high as 90%. In the last 15–20 years however, it has been reduced to 10–35%, [78–82]. Maternal mortality was reported to be 4–15% [83], considerably higher than in the non-pregnant general diabetic population [84], but no maternal deaths have been reported in the most recent publications [78–82]. The frequency of DKA during pregnancy is 1.7–3% [78–82] and will likely decrease because of the widespread use of self-glucose monitoring.

The occurrence of DKA has, traditionally, been considered to be solely a complication of type 1 diabetes. However, the line differentiating type 1 from type 2 diabetes is becoming increasingly blurred and DKA is now reported in children, adolescents and adults with the apparent phenotype of type 2 diabetes [85,86]. Consequently, an amendment to the current classification of diabetes has been recently proposed [87,88]. DKA during pregnancy has been reported in gestational diabetes as well [89–91], which may represent new cases of ketosis-prone type 2 diabetes presenting as DKA during pregnancy [92].

There are no data about the long-term outcome of fetuses surviving maternal DKA. There is, however, information about the long-term intellectual development of fetuses exposed to ketosis *in utero*. Ketosis alone is unlikely to have serious long-term consequences except when there is a concomitant elevation of plasma β-hydroxybutyrate and/or free fatty acids. The offspring of those women had lower behavioral and intellectual development testing [93].

Pathophysiology

DKA occurs when there is an absolute or relative lack of insulin with excessive production of counter-regulatory hormones including glucagon, catecholamines, cortisol and growth hormone. This combination leads to increased lipolysis in insulin-sensitive tissues including adipose tissue, skeletal muscle and liver resulting in a massive release of free fatty acids (FFAs). In the liver, FFAs undergo β-oxidation with unrestrained ketoacid (β-hydroxybutyrate and acetoacetate) production, as well as gluconeogenesis which precipitates DKA. These conditions also favor proteolysis leading to elevated plasma aminoacids. Aminoacids serve as precursors for gluconeogenesis, which results in exacerbation of the hyperglycemia. Several glucose transporters (GLUT) are involved as well. Both GLUT 2 and GLUT 4 are reduced in insulin deficiency. GLUT 2 transports glucose in and out of liver cells and GLUT 4 regulates glucose uptake by muscle cells and adipopcytes [94]. Excess ketones cause acidosis and hyperglycemia leading to osmotic diuresis with resultant volume depletion, dehydration and electrolyte loss. Decreased cardiac output, hypotension and shock may occur. If there is inadequate tissue perfusion, lactic acid will accumulate resulting in worsening acidosis. In an effort to compensate for acidosis, hydrogen ions enter into cells causing exit of intracellular potassium. The serum (extracellular) potassium levels will be elevated initially but total body (intracellular) potassium depletion may be severe. With insulin therapy, the potassium quickly re-enters the cells resulting in low serum potassium. Serum potassium levels therefore, must be monitored closely and replaced accordingly.

Pregnant, diabetic women may develop DKA more rapidly than their non-pregnant counterparts due to accelerated lipolysis, ketosis and protein catabolism associated with pregnancy. In addition, buffering capacity is diminished because of higher minute alveolar ventilation (progesterone effect), which in turn results in a compensatory elevated renal bicarbonate excretion. Further potential contributing factors include the increased levels of hormones that cause insulin resistance during pregnancy, such as human placental lactogen. Persistent nausea and vomiting in early pregnancy is another potential contributing factor [81].

Precipitating factors

The common precipitating factors seen outside of pregnancy are also reported during pregnancy including infection, insulin omission, insulin pump failure, non-compliance, alcohol and drug use and medications including corticosteroids and adrenergic agonists which are frequently used in pregnancy. Failure to recognize new-onset diabetes presenting as DKA has been reported to be the main cause of fetal demise in several recent publications [80,92,95]. Given the increasing reports of ketosis-prone type 2 diabetes, more cases of DKA during pregnancy should be expected [87,88,92].

Clinical presentation

In general, DKA develops over a period of 3–7 days but it may develop more precipitously when alcohol ingestion is a contributing factor. The usual initial symptoms of uncontrolled diabetes are present, including polyuria, polydipsia, blurred vision, anorexia, nausea, vomiting, abdominal pain, and unintentional weight loss. The abdominal symptoms are caused by elevated ketones. With severe hypokalemia, gastroparesis and even ileus may occur or be greatly worsened if pre-existing. Without treatment, mental changes will develop, ranging from drowsiness to deep coma. Other signs include deep, rapid respirations (Kussmaul) with a fruity odor (caused by ketones), and signs of intravascular volume depletion (dry mucous membranes, poor skin turgor and warm dry skin). Sinus tachycardia and orthostatic hypotension are other signs of inadequate intravascular volume. The body temperature is usually normal or below normal. If fever is present, an infection should be suspected. A normal temperature, however, may not exclude infection. Symptoms and signs of shock will ensue if aggressive treatment is not rapidly instituted.

Table 51.3 Diagnosis of diabetic ketoacidosis in pregnancy.

Serum pH <7.30
Serum bicarbonate <15
Serum ketones >1:2 dilution
Any glucose level (can be <200 mg/dL and even <150 mg/dL

Laboratory diagnosis

DKA is defined as an arterial pH of ≤7.30, a serum bicarbonate of ≤15 mmol/L, ketosis (serum acetone present at 1:2 dilution), and hyperglycemia of ≥300 mg/dL. In pregnancy, however, DKA may occur with relatively low blood sugar levels, and it is very important not to dismiss the diagnosis because the blood sugar is "too low". There are reports of profound DKA in diabetic pregnant women with blood sugars of less than 200 mg/dL. This relative "euglycemia" may lead to misdiagnosis and inappropriate therapy [78,83,90,96,97] (Table 51.3).

Leukocytosis is almost always present and it does not indicate infection. A left shift in the differential is more suggestive of an active infection.

Calculating the anion gap $[Na - (Cl + HCO_3) = 8\text{–}12]$ is useful. In DKA it usually is ≥15 although it may also be elevated in lactic acidosis, chronic renal insufficiency and rhabdomyolysis, or after ingestion of acid substances such as salicylates, ethylene glycol, methanol, formaldehyde, sulfur, toluene and paraldehyde.

The serum osmolality $[2(Na + K) + \text{serum glucose}/18]$ is another useful calculation because the mental status correlates better with this than with any other metabolic derangement. A value of 320 mOsm/L or higher is significant with coma occurring with values of ≥340 mOsm/L.

It is very important to determine the corrected serum sodium (Na), which is very helpful to estimate water deficit:

$$(\text{measured Na} + 1.6 \times \text{plasma glucose} - 100)/100$$

Hyperglycemia dilutes plasma Na by 1.6 mEq/L for every 100 mg/dL of increased glucose and therefore the measured plasma Na should be lower than normal in the presence of significant hyperglycemia. A plasma Na that is normal or high at presentation is indicative of massive water deficit.

In pure metabolic acidosis the arterial PCO_2 level should be approximately equal to the last 2 numbers of the arterial pH. A lower than predicted PCO_2 value is indicative of respiratory alkalosis and sepsis should be suspected; if higher, respiratory acidosis should be suspected. When hypoxemia is also present, pneumonia or low-pressure pulmonary edema is most often the cause.

Differential diagnosis

It is the same as for the non-pregnant patient including alcohol and/or drug overdose, encephalopathy of any cause, hyperosmo-

Table 51.4 Management of diabetic ketoacidosis during pregnancy.

Must be in the intensive care unit!
Fetal monitoring (if viable)
Detailed flow chart (vital signs, I&O, electrolytes, glucose, insulin used and serum ketones)
Fluids: NS 500–1000 mL/h x 3 h, ½ NS thereafter
Change to D_5 when glucose ≤250 mg/dL
Start with D_5 if initial glucose ≤250 mg/dL
Insulin: 0.10 units/kg IV push
0.10 units/kg/h (5–10 units/h) IV drip
Readjust if glucose not decreasing by ≥60 mg/h
Potassium: None for the first 2–4 h
None if serum K >5 mEq/L
20 mEq/h if serum K 4–5, 30 mEq/h if 3–4 and 40 mEq/h if <3
Partial replacement may be given as potassium phosphate
Bicarbonate: None if pH >7.10
But if hypotensive, replace when pH ≤7.20

lar state, hypoglycemia, uremic coma, trauma, infection, psychosis, syncope and seizures.

Treatment

All patients with DKA must be managed in an intensive care setting and the fetus continuously monitored if at a viable gestational age (Table 51.4). A flow sheet detailing all aspects of management is extremely important and should include the following: dates/times, serial glucose measurements, serum ketones, electrolytes, arterial blood gases, anion gap, insulin administration, and intake and output (I & O).

Fluid and electrolytes

Restoring the extracellular volume with adequate fluids and electrolytes is the first priority of therapy. One of the most common mistakes made in the treatment of DKA is not giving adequate fluids. The average deficit is 5–7 L (about 100 mL/kg of body weight) but can be more severe. At least 75% of the fluid deficit must be replaced during the initial 24 hours. A rate of 500–1000 mL/h for the initial 4 hours and 250–500 mL/h for the following 4 hours is recommended. The replacement must take into account the urine output as well as insensible losses. Isotonic fluids (0.9% normal saline) are generally regarded as the optimal initial replacement (first 1–3 L). If the reported Na level is "normal" or high (here is when the corrected serum Na and osmolality are very helpful to guide treatment) the fluid deficit is massive and the patient very hyperosmolar. Under these severe hyperosmolar conditions using hypotonic fluids (0.45% saline) from the outset might be considered. Concerns about the development of cerebral edema following rapid fluid replacement in the treatment of DKA are important but it appears that cerebral edema may be more the result of reduced blood volume and elevated carbon dioxide leading to cerebral vasoconstriction, ischemia and hypoxia related to the severity and duration of the DKA [98,99]. Hyperchloremia almost always develops in the course of DKA treatment and the use of lactated Ringer's instead of saline has been proposed as prevention. However, in uncontrolled diabetes, lactate infusions might not be well tolerated.

When the serum glucose decreases to less than or equal to 250 mg/dL dextrose solutions should be administered (D5 0.9% saline or D5 0.45% saline). Since many pregnant women with DKA may have initial glucose levels well below 250 mg/dL, dextrose-containing solutions may be started from the outset.

Insulin

Insulin should be administered as soon as fluid replacement has been started because fluids alone will not reverse DKA. Treatment should be administered by continuous intravenous infusion using only regular insulin. Many experts initiate therapy with a primary bolus of intravenous regular insulin utilizing 0.1 units/kg ideal body weight. The general insulin requirements are also 0.1 units per kilogram of body weight per hour but this rate must be adjusted as often as necessary to maintain a steady glucose diminution. The rate of glucose fall should be greater than 10% every 1–2 hours, generally 60 mg/dL per hour. There is no benefit of a more rapid normalization of the serum glucose. If, however, desired glucose control is not achieved, the insulin infusion should be readjusted accordingly.

Potassium

The potassium deficit is usually greater than or equal to 3–5 mmol/kg. Potassium will start re-entering the cells quickly after the initiation of insulin and a fall in serum levels should be anticipated. No potassium is given during the first 2–4 hours except when the initial level is already critically low. The rate of administration has to be readjusted according to the serum levels and urinary output. Extreme caution is recommended if there is oliguria or anuria. General guidelines are: (i) 40 mEq/h when the serum K level is below 3; (ii) 30 mEq/h if between 3 and 4; (iii) 20 mEq/h if between 4 and 5 and (iv) none if the level is over 5 mEq/L. Administering potassium phosphate, instead of only potassium chloride, is advocated but not universally recommended.

Bicarbonate

There is almost universal agreement that bicarbonate should be administered when there is severe lactic acidosis in addition to DKA, and also in the presence of life-threatening hyperkalemia with electrocardiographic changes. Otherwise, bicarbonate administration is not recommended unless the arterial pH is below 7.10. However, if there is hypotension many experts advice bicarbonate administration when the pH is 7.20 or less in an effort to increase the left ventricular ejection fraction and vascular responsiveness. Under the above conditions the benefits are thought to outweigh the risks of the paradoxical lowering of intracerebral pH by CO_2 diffusion, impaired oxygenation from a shift in the oxygen dissociation curve, hyperosmolality, hypernatremia, hypokalemia, late alkalosis and cerebral dysfunction [98,99]. Nevertheless, if bicarbonate replacement is deemed necessary the use of dilute therapy (i.e. putting the bicarbonate in a liter of fluid) is preferable to direct concentrated administration.

Other DKA complications

If hypotension persists after adequate volume replacement, sepsis should be suspected. Another possibility could be a silent myocardial infarction, which would be unusual in a childbearing-age woman but possible in long-standing diabetes with nephropathy and hypertension. Pulmonary edema has been reported in pregnant women receiving large amounts of fluids, ß-adrenergic agonists for premature labor and steroids for lung maturation. These agents have been reported to cause DKA even in gestational diabetes [100]. Cerebral edema has been reported more frequently in children and young adults but may be seen at any age. This condition should be suspected when neurologic deficits reappear after initial improvement or if there is no improvement despite adequate biochemical normalization [98,99]. Other reported complications include pancreatitis, hyperlipidemia, hypocalcemia, renal failure and vascular thrombosis.

It is extremely important that the process of switching from intravenous to subcutaneous insulin, once DKA resolves and the patient is ready to resume oral intake, be done properly because worsening of or even a relapse back into DKA may occur. Intravenous insulin disappears from the plasma in a few minutes. This must be anticipated and subcutaneous insulin injected 1–2 hours before stopping intravenous insulin so that the patient is not left without adequate insulin coverage. In addition, gastrointestinal dysfunction is common while the CO_2 level is 20 mEq/L or less, even in the absence of other gastrointestinal conditions such as gastroparesis or gastritis. Therefore, feeding the patient prematurely may lead to nausea and vomiting.

Other considerations

The reports of the autopsies performed after fetal demise have not shown an obvious pathology and therefore a metabolic derangement is thought to be the most probable cause of fetal death. Contributing factors include:

1 reduced uterine blood flow (from maternal hypovolemia and excess catecholamines) and indeed transient abnormal blood flow has been reported by Doppler ultrasonography [101]

2 decreased myocardial contractility from hyperglycemia (shown in experimental animals) and

3 acidosis since ketoacids cross the placenta freely.

Examples of fetal stress that subsided after the maternal DKA was successfully treated have been published [80,102]. These reports form the basis for recommending rapid and aggressive treatment of maternal DKA, in an effort to correct the maternal condition, before emergently intervening for non-reassuring fetal heart rate tracing.

A review of published papers suggests that the women with DKA who had a fetal demise were at a more advanced gestational age, had higher glucose, BUN and osmolality levels, required more insulin and had a prolonged duration of recovery.

Coronary artery disease

There is little information regarding pregnancy and ischemic heart disease in diabetic women. Two recent papers have reported on the incidence, mortality and risk factors for pregnancy-related acute myocardial infarction in the United States. During the 10-year period from 1991 to 2000 [103], 151 women had an acute myocardial infarction for an incidence of 1 in 35 700 deliveries; 4% were women with diabetes mellitus but not identified as gestational or pre-gestational diabetes. The maternal mortality rate was 7.1% but fatalities occurred only in women with an acute myocardial infarction taking place before or at the time of delivery. The relative risk of the various factors identified by multivariate analysis using logistic regression were:

1 age, particularly 40 years or older: odds ratio (OR) 4.5 and confidence interval (CI) 2.0–9.8

2 diabetes mellitus: OR 4.3 (CI 2.3–7.9)

3 chronic hypertension: OR 24.5 (CI 14.8–40.3

4 severe pre-eclampsia: OR 6.9 (CI 3.7–13.1) and

5 eclampsia: OR 15.3 (CI 5.3–44.1).

In this report, hypertensive disorders greatly increased the risk of acute myocardial infarction and were a stronger risk factor than diabetes mellitus. The incidence of myocardial infarction during pregnancy, reporting data from the years 2000 to 2002 [104], was 6.2 cases per 100 000 deliveries and a mortality rate of 5.1%. Single independent variables associated with increased risk were, again, age over 40 years OR 30.2 (CI 17.2–43.2), hypertension OR 21.7 (CI 6.8–69.1), thrombophilia OR 25.6 (CI 9.1–71.2), smoking OR 8.4 (CI 5.4–12.9), need for blood transfusion OR 5.1 (CI 2.0–12.7), and diabetes mellitus OR 3.6 (CI 1.5–8.3).

The maternal mortality was much higher (73%), in the few cases reported before 1980 either because treatment was less effective at that time or because of a tendency toward reporting fatal cases. The prognosis is better if the myocardial infarction occurs before pregnancy or early in the first trimester than when it takes place later in the pregnancy or during labor. The few cases reported after angioplasty or coronary artery revascularization before conception tolerated pregnancy better and had less neonatal morbidity from prematurity [105,106].

Women with coronary artery disease tend to be older and have longstanding diabetes. A detailed history, physical examination, ECG, echocardiogram, a stress test and, if indicated, a coronary angiogram should be performed before conception in any woman contemplating pregnancy if coronary artery disease is suspected. Every effort should be made to treat coronary insufficiency before pregnancy. Because of the possibility of maternal mortality, pregnancy is usually discouraged in this group of patients. However, if pregnancy occurs before treatment and termination is not an option, the treatment should be the same as in non-pregnant patients with coronary insufficiency. Diabetes should be controlled but with care to avoid hypoglycemia in order to prevent catecholamine release and tachycardia, which will increase myocardial demands [105]. The route of delivery should be individualized and in consultation with the obstetrician/perinatologist. Shortening the duration of the second stage of labor, to decrease the Valsalva maneuver, has been suggested [107]. The route of delivery in the reported cases has been 60% cesarean section and 40% vaginal deliveries. Continuous cardiac monitoring is routinely advised but the placement of central line catheters is not universally endorsed and should be individualized. Continuous epidural anesthesia is recommended for patients in labor to avoid pain-related stress and tachycardia, which also increases myocardial demands and the risk of an acute cardiac event.

Diabetic neuropathy

The distal peripheral neuropathy commonly seen in many diabetic patients is seldom of any consequence during pregnancy. Several studies have concluded that pregnancy does not adversely affect neuropathy [108–110], and even improvement of nerve conduction has been observed towards the third trimester. This phenomenon was attributed to tight glucose control achieved during pregnancy [110]. It has been concluded that pregnancy is not a significant risk factor for neuropathy and improved glycemic control may actually ameliorate abnormalities with nerve conduction.

Diabetic autonomic neuropathy, however, may pose serious difficulties for pregnant women. It may be asymptomatic in the early stages and found only by specific examination. Diagnosing autonomic neuropathy for the first time during pregnancy may not be easy [111] because pregnancy affects the heart rate response during respiration, as well as the role of the autonomic nervous system in the cardiovascular adaptation to pregnancy. Symptoms may include loss of sweating in the feet, urinary bladder dysfunction (and higher risk of urinary tract infections), abnormal cardiovascular reflexes (e.g. loss of beat to beat variability, postural hypotension etc.), and in the more advanced states, sweat disturbances of the upper body, gastroparesis, diarrhea, and bladder atony.

Pregnancy may exacerbate gastroparesis and postural hypotension. Vomiting usually starts early in gestation and may not subside until after delivery. The women with asymptomatic autonomic neuropathy before pregnancy have a better prognosis for postpartum resolution of symptoms and a more benign course during pregnancy. Vomiting interferes with diabetic control and impairs the nutritional status of the mother (weight loss, ketone production, etc.) and the fetus (growth restriction). Autonomic neuropathy may block the early "alarm" symptoms of the catecholamine phase of hypoglycemia, thus making these women vulnerable to neuroglycopenia; this is particularly true when tight control of the diabetes is attempted, such as is commonly the case during pregnancy. Therefore, autonomic neuropathy may affect pregnancy in a variety of ways: (i) prevent adjustment to the hemodynamic demands of pregnancy; (ii) make it difficult, or impossible, to achieve the tight diabetes control usually recommended during pregnancy due to hypoglycemia unawareness and slow gastric emptying; (iii) maternal and fetal malnutrition; and (iv) increased fetal loss, intrauterine growth restriction and preterm labor [110,111].

The therapeutic possibilities are limited for this condition in general, and particularly during pregnancy. Antiemetics are seldom of value. Metoclopramide may provide symptomatic relief in some patients. Intravenous erythromycin (not as effective when given orally) has a motilin-like effect and has been reported to be useful in non-pregnant patients [112]. Erythromycin is safe for the fetus. We have used this form of therapy in several pregnant women after all other measures failed, with temporary improvement for days to weeks. Parenteral nutrition may become necessary despite its potential risks when used long term. It should be initiated before the mother becomes severely malnourished and when it becomes obvious that all other available measures have proven ineffective.

References

1 Axer-Siegel R, Hod M, Fink-Cohen S, et al. Diabetic retinopathy during pregnancy. *Ophthalmology* 1996; 103(11): 1815–1819.

2 Temple RC, Aldridge VA, Sampson MJ, et al. Impact of pregnancy on the progression of diabetic retinopathy in Type 1 diabetes. *Diabet Med* 2001; 18(7): 573–577.

3 Lovestam-Adrian M, Agardh CD, Aberg A, Agardh E. Pre-eclampsia is a potent risk factor for deterioration of retinopathy during pregnancy in Type 1 diabetic patients. *Diabet Med* 1997; 14(12): 1059–1065.

4 Diabetes Control and Complications Trial Research Group. Effect of pregnancy on microvascular complications in the Diabetes Control and Complications Trial. *Diabet Care* 2000; 23: 1084–1091.

5 Nathan DM, Davis M, Cleary P, Lachin J. Letter: Response to "Do all women require intensive retinal surveillance during pregnancy?" *Diabet Care* 2001; 24(4): 795–796.

6 Moloney JB, Drury MI. The effect of pregnancy on the natural course of diabetic retinopathy. *Am J Ophthalmol* 1986; 93: 745–756.

7 Serup L. The influence of pregnancy on diabetic retinopathy. *Acta Endocrinol* 1986; 277(Suppl): 122–124.

8 Phelps RL, Sakol P, Metzger BE, et al. Changes in diabetic retinopathy during pregnancy: correlation with regulation of hyperglycemia. *Arch Ophthalmol* 1986; 104: 1806–1810.

9 Klein BEK, Moss SE, Klein R. Effect of pregnancy on progression of diabetic retinopathy. *Diabet Care* 1990; 13: 34–40.

10 Lauszus F, Klebe JB, Bek T. Diabetic retinopathy in pregnancy during tight metabolic control. *Acta Obstet Gynecol Scand* 2000; 79(5): 367–370.

11 Larsen M, Colmorn LB, Bonnelycke M, et al. Retinal artery and vein diameters during pregnancy in diabetic women. *Invest Ophthalmol Vis Sci* 2005; 42(2): 709–713.

12 Loukovaara S, Immonen IJ, Yandie TG, et al. Vasoactive mediators and retinopathy during type 1 diabetic pregnancy. *Acta Ophthalmol Scand* 2005; 83(1): 57–62.
13 Lauszus FF, Klebe JG, Bek T, Flyvbjerg A. Increased serum IGF-I during pregnancy is associated with progression of diabetic retinopathy. *Diabetes* 2003; 52(3): 852–856.
14 Loukovaraa S, Immonen IJ, Koistinen R, et al. The insulin-like growth factor system and Type 1 diabetic retinopathy during pregnancy. *J Diabet Complications* 2005; 19(5): 297–304.
15 Kitzmiller J, Main E, Ward B, et al. Insulin lispro and the development of proliferative diabetic retinopathy during pregnancy. *Diabet Care* 1999; 22: 874.
16 Loukovaara S, Immonen I, Teramo KA, Kaaja R. Progression of retinopathy during pregnancy in type1 diabetic women treated with insulin lispro. *Diabet Care* 2003; 26(4): 1193–1198.
17 Garg SK, Frias JP, Anil S, et al. Insulin lispro therapy in pregnancies complicated by type 1 diabetes: glycemic control and maternal and fetal outcomes. *Endocr Pract* 2003; 9(3): 187–193.
18 Pettitt DJ, Ospina P, Kolaczynski JW, et al. Comparison of an insulin analog, insulin aspart, and regular human insulin with no insulin in gestational diabetes mellitus. *Diabet Care* 2003; 26: 183–186.
19 Mathiesen ER, Kinsley B, Amiel SA, et al. Maternal glycemic control and hypoglycemia in Type 1 diabetic pregnancy: a randomized trial of insulin aspart versus human insulin in 322 pregnant women. *Diabet Care* 2007; 30(4): 771–776.
20 Hofmann T, Horstmann G, Stammberger I. Evaluation of the reproductive toxicity and embryotoxicity of insulin glargine in rats and rabbits. *Int J Toxicol* 2002; 21: 181–189.
21 Price N, Bartlett C, Gillmer M. Use of insulin glargine during pregnancy: a case-control pilot study. *Br J Obstet Gynaecol* 2007; 114(4): 453–457.
22 Gluckman PD. The endocrine regulation of fetal growth in the late gestation: the role of insulin-like growth factors. *J Clin Endocrinol Metab* 1995; 80: 1047–1050.
23 Mein BEK, Moss SE, Klein R. Effect of pregnancy on progression of diabetic retinopathy. *Diabet Care* 1990; 13: 34.
24 Early Treatment Diabetic Retinopathy Study Research Group. Grading diabetic retinopathy from stereoscopic color fundus photographs: an extension of the modified Airlie House classification. ETDRS report number 10. *Ophthalmology* 1991; 98: 786.
25 UK Prospective Diabetes Study Group (UKPDS). X. Urinary albumin excretion over 3 years in diet-treated type 2 (non-insulin-dependent) patients, and association with hypertension, hyperglycemia and hypertriglyceridemia. *Diabetologia* 1993; 36: 1021.
26 Hod M, van Dijk DJ, Karp M, et al. Diabetic nephropathy and pregnancy: the effect of ACE inhibitors prior to pregnancy on maternal outcome. *Nephrol Dial Transplant* 1995; 10: 2328–2333.
27 Bar JB, Schoenfeld A, Orvieto R, et al. Pregnancy outcome in patients with insulin dependent diabetes mellitus and diabetic nephropathy treated with ACE inhibitors before pregnancy. *J Pediatr Endocrinol Metab* 1999; 12: 659.
28 Cooper WO, Hernandez-Diaz S, Arbogast PG, et al. Major congenital malformations after first-trimester exposure to ACE inhibitors. *N Engl J Med* 2006; 354: 2443–2451.
29 Norris JM, Yin X, Lamb MM, et al. Omega-3 polyunsaturated fatty acid intake and islet autoimmunity in children at increased risk for type1 diabetes. *JAMA* 2007; 298(12): 1420–1428.
30 Surks MI, Ortiz E, Daniels GH, et al. Subclinical thyroid diseases: scientific review and guidelines for diagnosis and management. *JAMA* 2004; 291: 228–238.
31 Jovanovic R, Jovanovic L. Obstetric management when normoglycemia is maintained in diabetic pregnant women with vascular compromise. *Am J Obstet Gynecol* 1984; 149: 617–623.
32 Mackie ADR, Doddridge MC, Gamsu HR, et al. Outcome of pregnancy in patients with insulin-dependent diabetes mellitus and nephropathy with moderate renal impairment. *Diabet Med* 1996; 13: 90.
33 Dunne FP, Chowdhury TA, Hartland A, et al. Pregnancy outcome in women with insulin-dependent diabetes mellitus complicated by nephropathy. *Q J Med* 1999; 92: 451.
34 Carr D, Binney G, Brown Z, et al. Relationship between hemodynamics, renal function, and pregnancy outcome in class F diabetes. *Am J Obstet Gynecol* 2002; 187(suppl): 152.
35 Biesenbach G, Grafinger P, Stoger H, et al. How pregnancy influences renal function in nephropathic type 1 diabetic women depends on their pre-conception creatinine clearance. *J Nephrol* 1999; 12: 41.
36 Ekbom P, Damm P, Norgaard K, et al. Urinary albumin excretion and 24-hour blood pressure as predictors of preeclampsia in type 1 diabetes. *Diabetologia* 2000; 43: 927.
37 Schroder W, Heyl W, Hill-Grasshof B, et al. Clinical value of detecting microalbuminuria as a risk factor for pregnancy-induced hypertension in insulin-treated diabetic pregnancies. *Eur J Obstet Gynecol Reprod Biol* 2000; 94: 155.
38 Ekbom P, Damm P, Feldt-Rasmussen O, et al. Pregnancy outcome in type 1 diabetic women with microalbuminuria. *Diabet Care* 2001; 24: 1739.
39 Lauszus FF, Rasmussen OW, Lousen T, et al. Ambulatory blood pressure as predictor of preeclampsia in diabetic pregnancies with respect to urinary albumin excretion rate and glycemic regulation. *Acta Obstet Gynecol Scand* 2001; 80: 1096.
40 Combs CA, Rosenn B, Kiztmiller JL, et al. Early-pregnancy proteinuria in diabetes related to preeclampsia. *Obstet Gynecol* 1993; 82: 802.
41 Kimmerle R, Zas RP, Cupisti S, et al. Pregnancies in women with diabetic nephropathy: long-term outcome for mothers and child. *Diabetologia* 1995; 38: 227.
42 Miodovnik M, Rosenn BM, Khoury JC, et al. Does pregnancy increase the risk for development and progression of diabetic nephropathy? *Am J Obstet Gynecol* 1996; 174: 1180.
43 McGregor E, Stewart G, Junor BJ, et al. Successful use of recombinant human erythropoietin in pregnancy. *Nephrol Dial Transplant* 1991; 6: 292.
44 Yankowitz J, Piraino B, Laifer A, et al. Use of erythropoietin in pregnancies complicated by severe anemia of renal failure. *Obstet Gynecol* 1992; 80: 485.
45 Braga J, Marques R, Branco A, et al. Maternal and perinatal implications of the use of human recombinant erythropoietin. *Acta Obstet Gynecol Scand* 1996; 75: 449.
46 Geerlings SE, Stolk RP, Camps MJL, et al. Risk factors for asymptomatic urinary tract infection in women with diabetes. *Diabet Care* 2000; 23: 1737.
47 Geerlings SE, Stolk RP, Camps MJL, et al. Consequences of asymptomatic bacteriuria in women with diabetes mellitus. *Arch Intern Med* 2001; 161: 1421.

48 Muhlhauser I, Bender R, Bott U, et al. Cigarette smoking and progression of retinopathy and nephropathy in type 1 diabetes. *Diabet Med* 1996; 13: 536.

49 Baggio B, Budakovic A, Dalla Vestra M, et al. Effect of cigarette smoking on glomerular structure and function in type 2 diabetic patients. *J Am Soc Nephrol* 2002; 13: 2730.

50 Chuahiran T, Wesson DE. Cigarette smoking predicts faster progression of type 2 established diabetic nephropathy despite ACE inhibition. *Am J Kidney Dis* 2002; 39: 376.

51 Purdy LP, Hantsch CE, Molitsch ME, et al. Effect of pregnancy on renal function in patients with moderate-to-severe diabetic renal insufficiency. *Diabet Care* 1996; 19: 1067.

52 Gordon M, Landon MB, Samuels P, et al. Perinatal outcome and long-term follow-up associated with modern management of diabetic nephropathy. *Obstet Gynecol* 1996; 87: 401.

53 Rossing K, Jacobsen P, Hommel E, et al. Pregnancy and the progression of diabetic nephropathy. *Diabetologia* 2002; 45: 36–41.

54 Chatuvedi N, Stephenson JM, Fuller JH, et al. The relationship between pregnancy and long-term maternal complications in the EURODIAB IDDM complications study. *Diabet Med* 1995; 12: 494.

55 Hemachandra A, Ellis D, Lloyd CE, et al. The influence of pregnancy on IDDM complications. *Diabet Care* 1995; 18: 950.

56 Kaaja R, Sjoberg L, Hellstedt T, et al. Long-term effects of pregnancy on diabetic complications. *Diabet Med* 1996; 13: 165.

57 Nielsen LR, Muller C, Damm P, Mathiesen ER. Reduced prevalence of early preterm delivery in women with Type 1 diabetes and microalbuminuria – possible effect of early antihypertensive treatment during pregnancy. *Diabet Med* 2006; 23(4): 426–431.

58 Conway, DL, Langer O. Selecting antihypertensive therapy in the pregnant woman with diabetes mellitus. *J Matern Fetal Med* 2000; 9: 66.

59 Magee LA. Treating hypertension in women of childbearing age and during pregnancy. *Drug Saf* 2001; 24: 457.

60 Rosenthal T, Oparil S. The effect of antihypertensive drugs on the fetus. *J Human Hypertens* 2002; 16: 293.

61 Sibai BM. Diagnosis and management of gestational hypertension and preeclampsia. *Obstet Gynecol* 2003; 102: 181.

62 Griffin KA, Picken M, Bakris GL, et al. Comparative effects of selective T-and L-type calcium channel blockers in the remnant kidney model. *Hypertension* 2001; 37: 1268.

63 Hayashi K, Ozawa Y, Fujiwara K, et al. Role of actions of calcium antagonists on efferent arterioles with special references to glomerular hypertension. *Am J Nephrol* 2003; 23: 229.

64 Danielsson BR, Reiland S, Rundqvist E, et al. Digital defects induced by vasodilating agents: relationships to reduction in uteroplacental blood flow. *Teratology* 1989; 40: 351.

65 Magee LA, Conover B, Schick B, et al. Exposure to calcium channel blockers in human pregnancy: a prospective, controlled, multicentre cohort study. *Teratology* 1994; 49: 372.

66 Okundaye I, Abrinko P, Hou S. Registry of pregnancy in dialysis patients. *Am J Kidney Dis* 1998; 31: 766.

67 Jones DC, Hayslett JP. Outcome of pregnancy in women with moderate or severe renal insufficiency. *N Engl J Med* 1996; 335: 226–232.

68 Chao AS, Huang JY, Lien R, et al. Pregnancy in women who undergo long-term dialysis. *Am J Obstet Gynecol* 2002; 187: 152–156.

69 Hou S. Pregnancy in women on dialysis. In: Nissenson AR, Fine RN, eds. *Dialysis Therapy*, 3rd edn. Philadelphia: Hanley and Belfus, 2002: 519–522.

70 Hou S. Pregnancy in renal transplant recipients. *Adv Ren Replace Ther* 2003; 10: 40–47.

71 Davidson JM. Pregnancy in renal allograft recipients: prognosis and management. *Bailliere's Clin Obstet Gynecol* 1994; 8:501–525.

72 Armenti VT, Ahlswede KM, Ahlswede BA, et al. National Transplantation Pregnancy Registry: outcomes of 154 pregnancies in cyclosporine-treated female kidney transplant recipients. *Transplantation* 1994; 57: 502–508.

73 McGrory CH, Groshek MA, Sollinger HW, et al. Pregnancy outcomes in female pancreas-kidney transplants. *Transplant Proc* 1999; 31: 652–656.

74 First MR, Combs CA, Weiskittel P, et al. Lack of effect of pregnancy on renal allograft survival or function. *Transplantation* 1995; 59: 472–476.

75 Oz B, Hackman R, Einarson T, et al. Pregnancy outcome after cyclosporine therapy during pregnancy: a meta-analysis. *Transplantation* 2001; 71: 1051–1060.

76 Kainz A, Harabicz I, Cowlrick IS, et al. Review of the course and outcome of 100 pregnancies in 84 women treated with tacrolimus. *Transplantation* 2000; 70: 1718–1725.

77 Pergola PE, Kancharia A, Riley DJ. Kidney transplantation during the first trimester of pregnancy: immunosuppression with mycophenolate mofetil, tacrolimus and prednisone. *Transplantation* 2001; 71: 994–999.

78 Cullen MT, Reece EA, Homko CJ, et al. The changing presentations of diabetic ketoacidosis during pregnancy. *Am J Perinatol* 1996; 13: 449–451.

79 Chauhan SP, Perry KG Jr, McLaughlin BN, et al. Diabetic ketoacidosis complicating pregnancy. *J Perinatol* 1996; 16: 173–175.

80 Montoro MN, Myers VP, Mestman JH, et al. Outcome of pregnancy in diabetic ketoacidosis. *Am J Perinatol* 1993; 10: 17–20.

81 Rodgers BD, Rodgers DE. Clinical variables associated with diabetic ketoacidosis during pregnancy. *J Reprod Med* 1991; 36: 797–800.

82 Kilvert JA, Nicholson HO, Wright AD. Ketoacidosis in diabetic pregnancy. *Diabet Med* 1993; 10: 278–281.

83 Gabbe SG, Mestman JH, Hibbard LT. Maternal mortality in diabetes mellitus: an 18-year survey. *Obstet Gynecol* 1976; 48: 549–551.

84 Wetterhal SF, Olson DR, de Stafano F, et al. Trends in diabetes and diabetic complications. *Diabet Care* 1992; 15: 960–967.

85 American Diabetes Association. Type 2 diabetes in children and adolescents. *Pediatrics* 2000; 105: 671–680.

86 Umpierrez GE, Smiley D, Kitabchi AE. Narrative review: ketosis-prone type 2 diabetes mellitus. *Ann Intern Med* 2006; 144: 350–357.

87 Balasubramanyan A, Garza G, Rodriguez L, et al. Accuracy and predictive value of classification schemes for ketosis-prone diabetes. *Diabet Care* 2006; 29: 2575–2579.

88 Umpierrez GE. Ketosis-preone type 2 diabetes. Time to revise the classification of diabetes. *Diabet Care* 2006; 29: 2755–2757.

89 Maislos M, Harman-Bohem I, Weizman S. Diabetic ketoacidosis: rare complication of gestational diabetes. *Diabet Care* 1992; 15: 968–970.

90 Clark JDA, McConnell A, Hartog M. Normoglycemic ketoacidosis in a woman with gestational diabetes. *Diabet Med* 1991; 8: 388–389.

91 Pitteloud N, Binz K, Caufield A, et al. Ketoacidosis during gestational diabetes. Case report. *Diabet Care* 1998; 21: 1031–1032.

92 Schneider MB, Umpierrez GE, Ramsey RD, et al. Pregnancy complicated by diabetic ketoacidosis. *Diabet Care* 2003; 26: 958–959.

93 Rizzo T, Metzger BE, Burns WJ, et al. Correlation between antepartum maternal metabolism and intelligence of the offspring. *N Engl J Med* 1991; 325: 911–916.

94 Fleckman AM. Diabetic ketoacidosis. *Endocrinol Metab Clin North Am* 1993; 22: 181–207.

95 Sills IN, Rapaport R. New onset IDDM presenting with diabetic ketoacidosis in a pregnant adolescent. *Diabet Care* 1994; 17: 904–905.

96 Franke B, Carr D, Hatem MH. A case of euglycemic diabetic ketoacidosis in pregnancy. *Diabet Med* 2001; 18: 858–859.

97 Oliver R, Jagadeesan P, Howard RJ, et al. Euglycemic diabetic ketoacidosis in pregnancy: an unusual presentation. *J Obstet Gynaecol* 2007; 27: 308.

98 Glaser N, Barnett P, Mc Caslin I, et al. Risk factors for cerebral edema in children with diabetic ketoacidosis. *N Engl J Med* 2001; 344: 264–269.

99 Dunger DB, Edge JA. Predicting cerebral edema during diabetic ketoacidosis. *N Engl J Med* 2001; 344: 302–303.

100 Bedalov A, Balasubramanyan A. Glucocorticoid-induced ketoacidosis in gestational diabetes. Sequela of acute treatment of preterm labor. *Diabet Care* 1997; 20: 922–924.

101 Takahashi Y, Kawabata I, Shinohara A, et al. Transient fetal blood flow redistribution induced by maternal ketoacidosis diagnosed by Doppler ultrasonography. *Prenat Diagn* 2000; 20: 524–525.

102 O'Shaughnessy MJ, Beingesser KR, Khieu WU. Diabetic ketoacidosis in pregnancy with a recent normal screening test. *West J Med* 1999; 170: 115–118.

103 Ladner HE, Danielsen B, Gilbert WM. Acute myocardial infarction in pregnancy and the puerperium: a population-based study. *Obstet Gynecol* 2005; 105(3): 480–484.

104 James AH, Jamison MG, Biswas MS, et al. Acute myocardial infarction in pregnancy: a United States population-based study. *Circulation* 2006; 113(12): 1564–1571.

105 Hankins GD, Wendel GD Jr, Leveno KJ, et al. Myocardial infarction during pregnancy: a review. *Obstet Gynecol* 1985; 65: 139–146.

106 Roth A, Elkayam U. Acute myocardial infarction associated with pregnancy. *Ann Intern Med* 1996; 125: 751–762.

107 Sheikh AU, Harper MA. Myocardial infarction during pregnancy: management and outcome of two pregnancies. *Am J Obstet Gynecol* 1993; 169: 179–184.

108 Chaturvedi N, Stephenson JM, Fuller JH, et al. The relationship between pregnancy and long-term maternal complications in the EURODIAB IDDM complications study. *Diabet Med* 1995; 12: 494–499.

109 Airaksinen KEJ, Salmela PI, Markku J, et al. Effect of pregnancy on autonomic nervous function and heart rate in diabetic and nondiabetic women. *Diabet Care* 1987; 10: 748–751.

110 Airaksinen KEJ, Anttila LM, Linnaluoto MK, et al. Autonomic influence on pregnancy outcome in IDDM. *Diabet Care* 1990; 13: 756.

111 Hagay Z, Weissman A. Management of diabetic pregnancy complicated by coronary artery disease and neuropathy. *Obstet Gynecol Clin North Am* 1996; 23: 205–220.

112 Richards RD, Davenport K, McCallum RW. The treatment of idiopathic and diabetic gastroparesis with acute intravenous and chronic oral erythromycin. *Am J Gastroenterol* 1993; 88: 203–207.

52 Biological, Chemical, and Radiological Attacks in Pregnancy

Shawn P. Stallings & C. David Adair

Division of Maternal-Fetal Medicine, Department of Obstetrics and Gynecology, University of Tennessee College of Medicine, Chattanooga, TN, USA

Introduction

It is an unfortunate reality that in many parts of the world there is an ongoing threat of terrorism against target groups that frequently include pregnant women. In addition to the concerns about injuries due to conventional weapons and explosions, there is now the potential for attacks using chemical and/or biological agents, as exemplified by the the release of Sarin gas in a Tokyo subway system in 1995, and the anthrax-contaminated letters mailed in 2001.

Pregnant women represent a unique population that differs from the populace at large both in terms of susceptibility to certain agents and in the management of any exposures. Transport and triage of the patient, and her long-term management in the face of continued pregnancy must be anticipated and planned for in advance to optimize outcomes. This chapter aims to address some of the special concerns of mass casualty management for pregnant women and to review some of the potential biological, chemical, or radioactive agents that might be involved in an intentional event.

Clinical vignette

"A 22 year-old primigravida at 30 weeks of gestation presented to her local hospital for evaluation due to fever, chills, cough, and malaise. The initial work-up revealed a temperature of 39.6°C, but at the time she had stable respiratory status. Her chest radiograph revealed a prominent pattern of diffuse infiltration without evidence of consolidation. After evaluation by the patient's midwife and obstetrician, she was placed on antibiotics for suspected community-acquired pneumonia or viral pneumonia and admitted to the antepartum-postpartum floor. Fetal testing was reassuring.

On the second day following admission she complained of severe headache and backache, and she developed frequent emesis. The following day her condition worsened, ultimately requiring oxygen supplementation to maintain her arterial oxygen saturation (S_pO_2) above 93%. At this time a maculopapular rash was noticed over most of her body and this was thought to be pregnancy related. Due to her headache and change in status, laboratory blood tests were repeated and showed an elevation in her liver enzymes, along with a falling platelet count. Despite meticulous intravenous hydration in response to the emesis, her urine output began to decline. The patient began to report uterine contractions, and was found to be 3 cm dilated with significant effacement. The fetal status, via electronic monitoring showed a change at this point, with a decrease in heart rate variability and intermittent decelerations.

Because of the fetal heart rate tracing, the patient was deemed too unstable for immediate transport to a tertiary center and preparations were made for cesarean delivery with a tentative diagnosis of severe pre-eclampsia. At the time of the surgical skin preparation, the patient's maculopapular rash was noted to have progressed to a vesicular form. The infant was delivered, failed to respond adequately to resuscitation and was pronounced dead in the delivery room. By this time, the medical team suspected a contagious infection, possibly varicella, and isolation measures were instituted. The patient was later transferred to a tertiary care facility for intensive care support."

In the above anecdote, a young, previously unvaccinated patient presented with an unknown exposure to what was later proven to be smallpox. At most community hospitals and birthing centers, the initial care providers are generally not emergency medicine or infectious disease personnel and recognition of contagious conditions may be delayed. The admission of such a patient to the antepartum/postpartum wing may inadvertently expose a large number of susceptible patients and staff. Under most circumstances, the personnel are not to be faulted. The presentation of a biological threat may be subtle and unexpected,

Critical Care Obstetrics, 5th edition. Edited by M. Belfort, G. Saade, M. Foley, J. Phelan and G. Dildy.

and thus the necessary isolation precautions and treatment may be delayed. It is clear that, as in so many other situations, a high index of suspicion, adequate training, and general preparedness are the only protection against uncommon occurrences.

General preparation

The specific needs of the pregnant patient are often lost among the basic humanitarian concerns of such disasters as the Indian Ocean Tsunami in 2004 and the flooding of the Gulf Coast after Hurricanes Katrina and Rita in 2005. While it is clearly impractical to focus on a specific subgroup of people in a disaster it is worthwhile having the issues faced by pregnant survivors in mind when preparing for dealing with evacuation and treatment on a massive scale. Some of these specific needs will be discussed below.

One of the major differences between a chemical and/or biological intentional attack and a natural disaster is that in the former, there is a pressing need to contain the spread of potent contaminants and highly contagious and lethal organisms. A second major difference relates to the temporal relationship between the injury and the time of the event. With a natural disaster, traumatic and other immediate injury is generally limited to the time around the event, whereas with chemical and biological agents, some of the worst effects may only become apparent days to weeks after the inciting event.

A major legislative step was taken by the United States government in 1996 with the "Defense Against Weapons of Mass Destruction Act" [1]. The bill highlighted the contemporary lack of preparedness of emergency medical systems for large-scale intentional destructive events, and included a mandate for funding and training first-responders to serve the general population in such events. While most patients will likely be encountered first by emergency services personnel and physicians, obstetric providers should be ready to participate or advise in the care of pregnant patients. In cases of natural disaster or industrial accident, management of resources will be run by a state or local law enforcement head, fire chief, or the person in charge of emergency services. Within the USA, in the the event of a terrorist attack, the Federal Bureau of Investigation (FBI) will take control of the disaster site from a security and investigation standpoint and the Federal Emergency Management Agency (FEMA) will be charged with the mobilization of federal resources to deal with the aftermath [2]. Most other countries have similar federal or national structures in place to cope with such events.

Problems that may be anticipated include difficulties in communication, differences in command structure and coordination, and the logistics of allocation of both personnel and physical resources [1]. Coordination between emergency first responders and hospital-based medical personnel is important, and back-up communication systems are vital. Reliable information from the scene of the event is critical for planning for the disposition of patients who are en route [1]. For example, knowledge of the approximate gestational age of any pregnant women involved will allow the providers to transport women with viable fetuses to hospitals where fetal monitoring is available and to triage those first and early second trimester patients to hospitals or facilities where there may not be fetal monitoring equipment.

In a major bioterrorism event, it is important to have protocols that help in the rapid identification of victims who have been exposed and who are showing symptoms, versus those who are exposed but as yet asymptomatic. Asymptomatic patients may require different interventions, such as prophylaxis, and quarantine, rather than active therapy. Pregnant women represent a unique population because of their predisposition to go into labor in times of stress. For this reason the treatment of preterm labor and a plan to deal with large numbers of potentially infected or affected preterm babies should be kept in mind when designing any master plan for population dense areas.

Local hospitals, along with regional tertiary care centers, will need to have a plan in place for the triage of victims near the site of contact with the harmful substance, or for containment of persons who may have been contaminated and are at risk of spreading the agent to others. In the case of pregnant women, those requiring intensive care and those with preterm fetuses will likely need to be transferred to a tertiary care center. The master plan should always include a back-up plan to deal with the possibility of failed communication lines or transportation modes.

Labor and delivery unit managers should be prepared to provide fetal monitoring to multiple patients in isolated or intensive care unit settings. Such monitoring, of course, must be accompanied by preparation of equipment and personnel to take care of any emergent deliveries that may become necessary. While some patients may require only evaluation, others will require a longer stay, which may strain both the physical resources at the hospital and the personnel involved in their care. Back-up plans for relief personnel may involve rotating duty for regular staff, part-time staff, or even volunteer personnel with known labor and delivery experience. Identifying such individuals in advance facilitates the rapid response to an acute event. Finally, it should always be borne in mind that attacks frequently do not occur in isolation, and coordinated second or third attacks might occur in rapid succession, generating new waves of victims.

Review of selected agents

The following review deals with a selcted group of agents which could be encountered in the setting of an intentional attack. This list is, of course, not exhaustive. Injuries from conventional weapons that involve blast injury or penetrating trauma from bullets or shrapnel are managed as described in the chapter on trauma in pregnancy, and are not covered here. The agents for intentional attack may be separated into three basic categories: biological, chemical, and radiological.

Biological agents

Biological agents have received the most attention from the news media as potential weapons of terrorism. In describing some of the concerning agents, Dr Gregory Moran has noted: "The ideal agent for biological terrorism (BT) would be capable of producing illness in a large percentage of those exposed, would be disseminated easily to expose many people (e.g. by way of aerosol), would remain stable and infectious despite environmental exposure, and would be available to terrorists for production in adequate amounts. Fortunately, few agents have all of these characteristics" [3]. The Centers for Disease Control and Prevention (CDC) have designated three different categories for agents that are potential threats for bioterrorism.

Category A agents include those that are easily disseminated and which have high morbidity and mortality rates or, alternatively, have great potential to cause widespread panic or disruption. These agents include anthrax, smallpox, plague, botulism, and viral hemorrhagic fevers [4,5].

Category B agents include those considered easy to disseminate but which do not cause such widespread injury. These agents include ricin, threats to food safety such as *E. coli* O157:H7, typhus and Q fever.

Category C agents include pathogens that have not historically been used for acts of terrorism or mass destruction, but whose high morbidity and mortality rate make them potential targets for deliberate engineering to allow widespread dissemination. Such agents could include various tick-borne hemorrhagic viruses and tick-borne encephalitides (see Table 52.1) [3–5].

Anthrax

Anthrax arises from infection with the Gram-positive, spore-forming bacterium *Bacillus anthracis*. Humans acquire naturally occurring disease from contact with infected animals or contaminated animal products. The disease more commonly infects herbivores which ingest the spores from the soil. Animal vaccination is a common practice and has decreased animal mortality from the disease [6]. There are three manifestations of the illnesses in humans depending on the route of contact: cutaneous, inhalational, and gastrointestinal. The cutaneous form is the most common naturally occurring disease, although outbreaks of gastrointestinal anthrax are occasionally reported due to consumption of undercooked, contaminated meat. Inhalational anthrax is rare, but has been raised as a concern for bioterrorism because of its high mortality rate and ease of dissemination [6].

Table 52.1 Examples of CDC category A, B, and C biological agents [3–5].

Category A	Category B	Category C
Inhalational anthrax	*Coxiella burnetti* (Q fever)	Hantavirus
Smallpox	Ricin toxin	Tickborne hemorrhagic fever
Pneumonic plague	*Salmonella* species	Tickborne encephalitis viruses
Viral hemorrhagic fevers	*E. coli* O157:H7	Yellow fever
Botulism		

The spores of *B. anthracis* are stable for many years, are resistant to sunlight, heat and disinfectants, and can be dispersed as a dry or moist aerosol cloud. It is reported that weaponized spores may be disseminated throughout an entire building even after delivery within a sealed envelope [4]. As an example of the deadly nature of the spores, it was reported from the former Soviet Union that an outbreak near one of their weapons facilities in 1979 resulted in 77 cases of inhalational anthrax with 66 deaths (85% mortality) [4]. In the fall of 2001, 22 cases of anthrax infection occurred following delivery of spores through the United States Postal Service. Eleven of the cases were inhalational, with five deaths occurring in that group, while the rest of the cases were cutaneous [4,6]. The knowledge that strains of *B. anthracis* have been modified and may potentially be released creates a whole new outlook in public health policies. It is estimated that more than 30 000 potentially exposed persons were placed on postexposure prophylaxis during the US outbreak of 2001 [4]. The direct and indirect costs of handling even as limited a contamination as the 2001 mailed attacks are undoubtedly high.

The spores germinate in an environment rich in amino acids, nucleic acids and glucose, such as in mammalian tissues or blood. The bacteria then multiply rapidly and will only form spores again when the nutrients are depleted, such as when contaminated body fluids are discharged and encounter ambient air. The vegetative bacteria do not survive long in ambient conditions, but the spores may remain stable for many years.

Inhalational anthrax begins when inhaled spore particles 1–5 microns in size enter alveolar spaces and are ingested by macrophages. Spores that survive and are not lysed may travel to the mediastinal lymphatic tissue where they germinate and multiply. The incubation period varies. Most often incubation occurs during 1–7 days, but can be delayed as many as 43 days [4–6]. The replicating *B. anthracis* produces toxins that will continue to cause cell damage even after living bacteria are eradicated with antibiotics [6]. This ongoing damage results in hemorrhagic lymphadenitis, hemorrhagic mediastinitis, necrosis, and pleural effusions. The patient may present initially with fever, cough, dyspnea, and malaise. An initial chest radiograph may be abnormal with widened mediastinum, infiltrates, and effusion. The more fulminant cases progress rapidly with a continued rise in fever, worsening dyspnea, chest pain, and respiratory failure. Blood culture will usually show the characteristic colony formation, but communication with the laboratory is important when *B. anthracis* is suspected since colonies may be mistaken for contaminant normal flora [5,6]. Hemorrhagic meningitis is also a frequent occurrence in such patients and the organism may be identified readily in the cerebrospinal fluid.

Cutaneous anthrax occurs following deposition of the spores in cuts or abrasion of the skin. Following germination in the skin, toxin production will cause local edema and necrosis. A vesicle typically forms which then dries to form a black eschar. Antibiotic therapy will not alter the course of skin destruction and eschar resolution. Systemic spread may be possible, and if untreated the mortality is reported to be as high as 20% [4,6]. Gastrointestinal anthrax may be contracted from ingestion of contaminated meat. Spores may germinate in either the upper or lower intestinal tract. Ulcer formation in the mouth or esophagus may lead to regional lymphadenitis. In the lower tract, infection of the terminal ileum or cecum may lead to nausea, vomiting, abdominal pain, and bloody diarrhea. In both cases, death may occur due to systemic illness, and mortality as high as 25–60% has been reported. [4–6]. There is little specific information available on anthrax infection during pregnancy [7].

It is important to remember that casual contact or respiratory droplets from coughing or sneezing do not spread anthrax. While person-to-person respiratory transmission does not occur, care should be exercised when caring for patients with non-intact skin from cutaneous anthrax [5]. Treatment of anthrax is by combination therapy that usually includes ciprofloxacin and doxycycline, and may also include clindamycin, rifampin, vancomycin, or chloramphenicol [6]. The recommendations for appropriate antibiotic therapy are the same for pregnant women or children as for non-pregnant adults. One should check with an infectious disease consultant or the CDC website for the latest recommended drug combination. Supportive therapy is also usually required for severe cases.

Prophylactic antimicrobial therapy is not needed unless law enforcement and public health officials document an actual exposure. It is recommended that the primary care women's health providers do not initiate therapy unless directed to do so by the appropriate public health officials [8]. Screening may be performed by way of nasal swab, but due to potential error, postexposure prophylaxis is recommended only after a confirmed exposure or high-risk encounter [8].

Adult exposure prophylaxis is typically given with ciprofloxacin 500 mg orally every 12 hours for 60 days or doxycycline 100 mg orally every 12 hours for 60 days [4–6,8]. The recommendation is the same for pregnant and lactating women. The potential morbidity and mortality from anthrax are felt to outweigh the historical concerns regarding these medications [8]. If the anthrax isolate in a current case is found to be sensitive to penicillin, the pregnant or lactating patient should be switched to amoxicillin 500 mg orally three times a day for the remainder of the prophylaxis period [8].

Vaccination against anthrax is available. The vaccine, called anthrax vaccine adsorbed (AVA), is a cell-free product given in a 6-dose series over 18 months [6]. While there has been significant media coverage of concerns over side effects of the vaccine following the US military's mandated vaccination of active-duty and reserve-duty personnel, AVA is thought to be acceptably safe [6]. Due to the potential for spores to remain dormant in tissues for prolonged periods despite antibiotic prophylaxis, there has been interest in the use of AVA for postexposure prophylaxis in conjunction with antibiotics [6,7]. The vaccine should theoretically be safe for use during pregnancy due to a lack of active organism. No published experience is available on the use of the vaccine during pregnancy, but the potential benefits may outweigh the risk associated with systemic disease in the event of a large-scale exposure. Experience from the military vaccination program suggests no adverse effect on pregnancy outcomes for women vaccinated prior to becoming pregnant [9].

Smallpox

Younger generations know very little of the devastation of smallpox infection, as a result of widespread vaccination and aggressive disease control measures. Ironically, this extraordinary medical accomplishment has left the vast majority of the world's population susceptible to the potential reintroduction of this disease. Initial dissemination may be difficult, but the number of secondary contacts and ease of transmission to secondary victims make this agent attractive to groups seeking to induce massive societal disruption.

Smallpox is caused by the DNA virus variola. It is easily transmitted from person to person by respiratory droplets. In addition, the virus may remain stable on fomites for up to 1 week [4]. The virus replicates in respiratory epithelium and then migrates to regional lymph nodes. An initial viremia, accompanied by mild fever and malaise, will lead to introduction of the virions into a variety of tissues, resulting in localized infection of the kidneys, lungs, intestines, skin, and lymphoid tissues. After an incubation period of 7–17 days, a second viremia occurs with high fever, headache, backache, rigors, and vomiting. A rash is usually apparent within 48 hours of this new phase. The rash is initially maculopapular, but changes soon to a vesicular eruption. The characteristic smallpox appearance is reached when the vesicles become pustules. Viral shedding may occur from the time of the rash until the lesions have crusted and separated. Death may occur in this phase due to overwhelming viremia and organ failure [4].

From historical series of pregnant women affected by smallpox it is known that there may be very high rates of prematurity and fetal loss [10]. In addition, pregnant women appear more susceptible to the disease, with historical case-fatality rates as high as 61% among unvaccinated individuals, and mortality rates of 27% even among vaccinated pregnant women. This compares with commonly reported mortality rates in non-pregnant adults of 3% when vaccinated and 30% among unvaccinated patients [5,10]. Pregnant women more commonly develop the hemorrhagic form of the disease in comparison with non-pregnant women and men [7,10]. The hemorrhagic form of smallpox is characterized by fever, backache, abdominal pain, and a diffuse red rash. Historically, spontaneous epistaxis, ecchymoses, and bleeding into various organs led to rapid death in such patients. The case-fatality rate among women with hemorrhagic smallpox was 100% in one series. Congenital smallpox among liveborn infants has been described in as many as 9–60%, with a very high mortality rate [7,10].

An infected patient should be isolated in a negative-pressure room. In the setting of large numbers of infected individuals, quarantine and separate physical facilities may be needed. Airborne and contact precautions must be used. All discarded laundry or waste should be placed in biohazard bags and autoclaved prior to disposal [4]. A certain number of hospital personnel may need to be vaccinated in advance in order to provide care in the event of a deliberate infection. The United States government made an attempt at vaccinating a core group of staff at hospitals all over the country in 2002, but the program met with limited success due to concerns about adverse reactions to the vaccine. Again, for obstetric units, planning to care for multiple pregnant, infectious victims will be challenging. Hospitals with maternity services should anticipate the need to designate obstetric and neonatal physicians and nurses for a team response.

Although Cidofovir has been tried with success against other pox viruses and has been reported to have *in vitro* activity against variola, it cannot yet be recommended as treatment for smallpox [5]. The principles of managing an outbreak of smallpox will be isolation and supportive care of infected patients and postexposure vaccination for contacts. Vaccination against smallpox is by inoculation of the related orthopoxvirus, vaccinia. Vaccination is moderately effective at aborting or attenuating the disease if given within 4 days of an exposure [5]. Complications from widespread vaccination with vaccinia in the past included localized dermal reactions, vaccinia gangrenosa (with local extensive skin necrosis at the site of inoculation), eczema vaccinatum (a superinfection of eczema with the vaccinia virus), progressive vaccinia, and post-vaccinial encephalitis [10]. While pregnant mothers may be vaccinated, there is a low risk of a potentially fatal fetal infection from the vaccinia virus. Therefore, routine vaccination of pregnant women in non-emergent settings is not recommended. In the event of an actual bioterrorism event, a pregnant woman at risk for exposure must weigh the relatively small risk of an adverse effect from the vaccine, against the devastating outcome associated with smallpox infection in pregnancy [10].

Plague

Plague has held a special place in world history with multiple pandemics leading to the deaths of millions of people. The bacillus, *Yersinia pestis*, is generally transmitted to humans from a rodent host by way of a flea vector. However, direct host-to-host transmission may occur by way of an infectious aerosol from affected individuals. This makes the disease extremely contagious. The disease is rapidly fatal in the absence of appropriate antibiotic treatment [4]. There have been attempts in the past to weaponize plague; however, most such attempts have met with limited success. Still, it is thought that plague represents a bioterrorism threat by way of an aerosol or inhalational route.

Typical bubonic plague is acquired from the bite of a flea, which regurgitates the *Y. pestis* from its foregut. The organisms rapidly multiply and spread to regional lymph nodes within 1–8 days. The infection of lymph nodes creates a characteristic bubo, which is a large tender area of inflammation within the regional lymph node. Once this occurs, the patient may become septic within several days. Some patients will develop pneumonia and begin to shed the *Yersinia* organisms in their cough droplets. Victims will typically develop a productive cough with blood-tinged sputum within 24 hours of the onset of symptoms [4]. The organism can also be ingested from a contaminated food source. The gastrointestinal form of the disease also follows a rapid course, with the buboes developing in mesenteric drainage sites. Persons infected by the inhalational route may not develop the typical buboes but may progress rapidly to septicemia.

The diagnosis is made by a sputum Gram stain showing Gram-negative coccobacilli with bipolar "safety pin" staining. Chest X-ray may show consolidating lobar pneumonia. Further tests include an IgM enzyme immunoassay, antigen detection, and PCR [5]. These tests are available typically through state health departments and CDC. This approach requires a high index of suspicion and the ordering of the requisite tests early enough to involve state organizations in containment. Patients with suspected bubonic plague should be separated from other patients, preferably under negative-pressure conditions, and body fluid precautions should be followed until at least 3 days of appropriate antibiotics have been completed [4]. Patients who are suspected of being septic, or having respiratory symptoms, or are diagnosed with pneumonic plague should be maintained under respiratory droplet precautions including negative pressure isolation until the completion of 4 days of antibiotic therapy [4].

Standard therapy is 10 days of intravenous antibiotic, which may be switched to oral therapy when there are positive signs of improved condition. For non-pregnant adults the recommended treatment is streptomycin 1 mg intramuscularly twice a day or gentamicin 5 mg/kg IM or IV every 24 hours. Other choices include chloramphenicol or fluoroquinolones. For patients with suspected meningitis, chloramphenicol (50–75 mg/kg per day) is considered mandatory because of its superior penetration of the CNS [4,5].

It is thought that the major determinant of the outcome of mother and child is the timing of antibiotic administration [6]. Historically, plague acquired during pregnancy led to nearly universal fetal loss and could be especially severe in pregnant women [7]. Gentamicin should be substituted for streptomycin in the case of pregnancy. Chloramphenicol should be used with caution in pregnant women due to potential adverse effects on fetus and newborn. Doxycycline and ciprofloxacin have also been considered as alternative regimens and use in this situation should represent the choice between the benefit of treating the infection versus any potential risks of the medication to the fetus [7]. Empiric treatment of the newborn following delivery of an infected mother should also be considered. In the event of a bioterrorist attack, it is thought that postexposure prophylaxis is necessary to prevent rapid spread of the disease. A decision regarding whether or not to place pregnant patients on the recommended prophylaxis of doxycycline 100 mg twice a day would need to be made based on the risk of exposure and the anticipated spread of the disease [7]. Timely treatment with the appropriate antibiotics is very important in affecting the outcome in pregnancy. Untreated, the mortality from plague is estimated to be close to 100%. Even in treated cases, pneumonic plague is highly lethal with up to 50–60% mortality despite appropriate antibiotic therapy. Given the small risk to the fetus of doxycycline use in pregnancy and the very high morbidity and mortality of the disease itself, most would agree that, if indicated, the prophylactic antibiotics should be given.

Viral hemorrhagic fevers

Extremely infectious body fluids also raise the potential for widespread transmission of some of the most feared tropical hemorrhagic viruses, such as Ebola or Marburg. These viruses could conceivably mutate to spread by inhalational routes that would allow wider dissemination. One documented outbreak of Ebola Zaire virus killed 9 out of 10 infected victims [11]. With no known cure or vaccine, intensive support and isolation are the only available responses, and any widespread infection would likely overload our current medical system. One has only to read an account of these viruses [11] to appreciate that advance preparation and containment may be our best approach.

Q fever

Q fever is caused by an intracellular bacterium, *Coxiella burnetii.* This agent may be considered for use in bioterrorism because of the ease with which it causes infection [5]. Most immunocompetent persons have a self-limited infection without serious long-term complications, although chronic infection and endocarditis may occur in a small proportion of infected individuals and this can be debilitating. An intentional release of Q fever would most likely cause social disruption and psychological effects rather than mass casualties. The organism has long been known for its association with infection leading to abortion in animals. More recent information suggests that there is a similar effect on fetal loss in humans as well.

Q fever is generally obtained through inhalation of *Coxiella* organisms. The organisms are carried in body fluids such as the amniotic fluid of farm animals. The incubation period is between 2 and 14 days. The clinical manifestations are similar to other non-specific viral illnesses with fever, chills and headache. The patient may also experience malaise, anorexia and weight loss. More serious complications include neurologic symptoms in at least 23% of acute cases [5].

The diagnosis is generally made on the basis of the clinical complaints along with the presence of patchy infiltrates seen on chest X-ray and a history consistent with exposure. Serology for *Coxiella* IgG and IgM may be useful, with antibodies appearing during the second week of the illness. The typical treatment for a non-pregnant adult is doxycycline twice a day for 5–7 days. Fluoroquinolones can also be used. The disease is not thought to be contagious from person to person [5].

While Q fever has long been known to cause low birth weight and abortion in farm animals, more recent data from France suggest that there is also a significant effect on human pregnancy [12]. Acute infection during the first trimester leads to a very high rate of abortion in untreated patients. Acute infection in the second or third trimester is less commonly associated with fetal loss but can be associated with low birth weight and premature delivery [12]. The recommended treatment is trimethoprim 320 mg with sulfamethoxazole 1600 mg daily for the duration of the pregnancy. Chronic infection is more common in women who develop the acute infection during pregnancy. This is thought to be related to the relatively immunocompromized state of pregnancy. The use of the trimethoprim/sulfamethoxazole during pregnancy reduces the frequency of abortion, and decreases the number of women with identifiable *Coxiella* in the placenta at birth [12]. Such treated patients are still at risk for preterm delivery and low birth weight. Prolonged therapy should be instituted after delivery, and the recommended postpartum regimen is doxycycline 100 mg twice daily and hydroxychloroquine 600 mg daily for 1 year following the pregnancy. For women who are appropriately treated, future pregnancies seem to be unaffected. Similarly, women who acquire and resolve the acute infection prior to becoming pregnant do not show any adverse pregnancy effects [12]. Breastfeeding is not recommended for women with acute Q fever.

Ricin

Ricin is a potent toxin easily derived from the beans of the castor plant (*Ricinus communis*). The history of ricin's use as a lethal agent goes back several years and crosses many political lines. Recently, this toxin received extensive media attention as an agent of terrorism following the arrest of six persons in Manchester, England, in December of 2002, who allegedly produced the toxin in an apartment for use in a potential attack. The discovery of powdered ricin in the mailroom serving US Senate Majority Leader Bill Frist's office in February 2004 resulted in renewed fears regarding vulnerability to an attack with this toxin. The potential for ricin to be a weapon of mass destruction rests in the ease with which it can be produced, its stability, and its relatively easy route of dissemination with low risk of detection. The amount of ricin necessary to produce effects is also very small.

The protein is derived in the processing of castor beans, the oil from which is used in a number of diverse industrial settings, including the manufacture of brake and hydraulic fluid [13]. The waste mash, or aqueous phase of the oil production, contains 5–10% ricin, which can then be isolated using chromatography. The toxins RCL III and RCL IV are relatively small dimeric proteins consisting of an "A" and "B" chain. After entry into the cell by binding to the cell surface glycoproteins, the toxin inhibits the 60S ribosomal subunit preventing continued protein synthesis. The interruption of protein synthesis eventually leads to cell death [13].

In the event of inhalational exposure, symptoms are related to irritation of the lungs. Respiratory symptoms will begin usually 4–8 hours after the exposure. Early symptoms can include fever, chest tightness, cough and dyspnea. Within 1–2 days, severe inflammation of the respiratory tract, cell death, and the development of acute respiratory distress syndrome may be expected. The only treatment is respiratory support with mechanical ventilation. [3,5]. There has been concern that ricin may be used to contaminate the water or food supply. In the event of a gastrointestinal exposure, necrosis of the gastrointestinal epithelium as well as damage to spleen, liver and kidneys may occur. Symptoms might manifest as abdominal cramps and nausea, as well as high-output gastrointestinal fluid loss. Ricin is thought to be much less toxic when ingested rather than inhaled, although a large gastrointestinal exposure could lead to enough necrotic multiorgan damage to produce hemorrhage and hypovolemic shock [3,5].

The diagnosis can be confirmed by ELISA testing. Patients should be treated with decontamination including removal of garments and cleansing of the body with soap and water. Outside of contact with residual, undetected toxin remaining on the victim, there is thought to be little secondary risk to emergency department personnel; however, universal contact precautions should be observed. There is no direct antidote to the toxin, although gastric decontamination with charcoal may be beneficial in some cases [3,5]. Supportive care is the main approach to management. In the case of exposure during pregnancy, the molecular weight of the toxin makes it unlikely to cross the placental barrier. The outcome for the baby will depend on maternal response to supportive care.

Toxins or chemicals

There are several compounds that may represent mass risk either as the result of a deliberate act (e.g. release of a nerve gas in the Tokyo subway system in 1995), or as a result of an industrial accident. Chemical weapons may be classified either by their lethality or by their ability to persist in the environment [14]. Lethal agents are classified into four categories: nerve agents or anticholinesterases, vesicants or blistering agents, choking or pulmonary agents, and cyanogens or "blood" agents [15]. For the most part, care of the pregnant patient will differ little from that in the non-pregnant patient, especially prior to fetal viability. As in trauma situations, the health and survival of the fetus depend most upon the mother's condition, as a result of both the immediate and the prolonged supportive care.

Whenever a chemical threat is suspected, the medical team should wear protective equipment including rubber boots and impermeable suits. Decontamination of the victims is a high priority, and patients should be moved to a well-ventilated setting for safe disposal of clothing and decontamination of the skin [14]. Dilute sodium hypochlorite solution is preferred to water, and the eyes should be irrigated with large amounts of water or normal saline [14].

Nerve agents – acetylcholinesterase inhibitors

Organophosphorus compounds such as tabun, sarin, soman, and VX primarily act through the inhibition of acetylcholinesterase at synapses and neuromuscular junctions [14,15]. Tyrylcholinesterase in plasma, and acetylcholinesterase in the red blood cell, are also inhibited by these agents. The result is an excess of acetylcholine leading to bronchial hypersecretion and bronchoconstriction, mental status changes, nausea, vomiting, and muscle fasciculations and weakness [15]. A large exposure may be rapidly fatal with loss of consciousness, seizures, and apnea from respiratory muscle paralysis and central nervous system depression. The agents are usually clear and colorless and may be disseminated as either a vapor or liquid. Exposure may occur through skin absorption, inhalation, or gastrointestinal ingestion.

Patients who have had significant exposure or who are presenting with obvious symptoms should be treated with atropine and pralidoxime (2-PAM) [14,15]. Atropine is commonly given as a 1-mg intramuscular or intravenous dose and is sometimes available for self-administration via an auto-injector. The patient should be reevaluated every 3–5 minutes, and repeat doses may be given (up to 6 mg total) until secretions decrease and ventilation improves. Pralidoxime, which reactivates the acetylcholinesterase at the nicotinic receptor, can also be given as a 600–1000 mg intramuscular injection or as a slow intravenous infusion [14,15]. In the event of severe respiratory compromise, intubation and mechanical ventilation may be required. Severely affected victims should be given a benzodiazepine (diazepam, lorazepam, or midazolam) to raise the seizure threshold and help prevent secondary anoxic brain injury [15]. Successfully treated patients will begin to recover within a few hours, but neurological symptoms may last for weeks.

There is little information on the fetal effects of such an exposure. The fetus will be particularly susceptible to any respiratory depression or anoxia in the mother. Theoretically, these compounds may be able to reach the fetal brain with resultant behavioral depression likely, and this may alter fetal biophysical and non-stress testing. Ultimately, fetal survival will depend on expeditious care of the mother.

Vesicants and pulmonary agents

Vesicants, such as mustard gas and Lewisite, are easily absorbed through the skin and mucous membranes [15]. The damage may not be evident until hours after the exposure. Damage is caused by cross-linking and methylation of DNA. Blisters may form on the skin in the early stages. Skin sloughing will later place the patient at risk for secondary infection. Similarly, damage to lung tissues results in a chemical pneumonia that may also lead to secondary infection. Mortality is generally low from an acute attack, but the number of people affected may be high, and because of the high morbidity associated with these agents caring for these victims, will consume significant medical resources [14,15].

In a similar vein, pulmonary agents, such as phosgene and chlorine, lead to respiratory tract injury within hours, with damage to the alveolar–capillary membrane and subsequent pulmonary edema. Victims of phosgene usually require mechanical ventilation and careful management of fluid balance, but survival beyond 48 hours suggests that recovery is likely [14,15].

Radiation

Public concern over radiation exposure has been elevated by worries about the safety of nuclear power facilities, the transport and disposal of nuclear waste, and the threatened use of radiation contaminated weapons – so-called "dirty bombs". Much is known about the consequences of inadvertent exposure. Damage can range from skin reddening to cancer induction and death. Particularly relevant to pregnancy is the fact that fetuses and children (in whom there is ongoing rapid cell division) are more susceptible to the subtle effects of radiation exposure than are adults [16,17]. Damage is also cumulative, with increasing or repetitive exposures resulting in more severe damage [16].

"Dirty bombs" are typically intended to spread radiation in such a way as to make large areas uninhabitable. Depending on the source, the amount of radiation released from such a weapon is unlikely to cause severe forms of acute radiation syndrome [16]. According to the United Nations' report of Iraq's testing of dirty bombs in 1987, the Iraqis deemed that radiation levels achieved were too low to cause significant damage and the project was abandoned. In a modern context, such weapons would likely be used to disrupt routines and generate fear in the general public.

Management of the initial exposure to radiation revolves around limiting the amount of time near the source, increasing the distance from the source, and use of physical barriers, such as glass or concrete to shield an individual from exposure [16]. In the event of an exposure, it is recommended that exposed individuals leave the area on foot (as opposed to using cars or public transportation that may harbor contaminated dusts), and to make use of barriers by entering buildings. Clothes should be removed and bagged for later disposal. A shower may remove contaminated dust or debris from the skin [16]. These principles of contamination must also be considered for the patient presenting to the hospital or clinic for evaluation.

Radiation exposure can result in significant dysfunction to many organs. Depending on the dose and duration of exposure, as well as the mechanism of exposure, injuries may range from local (such as a burn) to more widespread injury such as acute radiation syndrome (ARS) [18]. A local injury often involves exposed contact areas like the hands. Patients may present with erythema, blistering, desquamation, and ulceration of the skin. The patient may or may not know when the exposure occurred. For example, handling an unknown metallic object might be the source of exposure. Such injuries generally evolve slowly and the full extent of injury may not be known for several weeks. Conventional wound management may be ineffective [18].

The acute radiation syndrome (ARS) is a quickly developing illness caused by a total body exposure to radiation. It is characterized by simultaneous damage to several organ systems from ionizing radiation that caused deficiency in cell numbers or cell function. Radioactive sources provoking ARS might consist of machines that emit gamma rays, X-rays, or neutrons. There are three phases of ARS [18]. The first is a prodromal phase in which a patient might experience nausea, vomiting and loss of appetite. Generally these symptoms disappear within a day or two and a symptom-free latent period may follow. The length of the latent period may vary depending on the radiation dose. A period of fully expressed illness may then follow with electrolyte imbalances, diarrhea, hematologic abnormalities, and even CNS changes. The overt illness results either in death or in slow, eventual recovery [18]. Severe organ dysfunction may be present, including low white blood cell counts leading to immunodeficiency. A gastrointestinal syndrome also may occur with loss of the cells lining the small and large intestines, leading to water and electrolyte loss through vomiting, diarrhea and impaired absorption. The patient may also demonstrate confusion and disorientation resulting from the dramatic changes of dehydration and electrolyte imbalance. Such mental status changes, including periods of unconsciousness, are a poor prognostic sign [18]. Full recovery is possible and may occur over a prolonged period of time, from several weeks to 2 years.

The initial management of a large radiation exposure includes treating traumatic injuries (fractures, lacerations) as they would normally be managed. In addition, care should be taken to remove external contaminants. The history should focus on the details of the source of exposure including the type of radiation, the proximity to the source, and the duration of the exposure [18]. A careful medical history should be obtained and, in pregnant women, an estimate of the gestational age and a summary of the pregnancy history should be included. Diagnosis of ARS may be aided by following the complete blood count every 4–6 hours. A significant drop in the absolute lymphocyte count and platelet count may aid in timing the exposure. Suspected exposures less than 2 Gy may not require hospitalization. Prospective evaluation of the white blood cell count and the cell differential count over the course of the next few days may be appropriate. Nausea and vomiting might not be present in the early phase for someone with less than 7.5 Gy of exposure (see Table 52.2) [16,18].

For more severe ARS with a known higher exposed dose, supportive care should be the rule. Careful history and physical examination is imperative. Nausea and vomiting can be initially managed with selective serotonin $5HT_3$ receptor antagonists [18]. Admission to hospital will be necessary. The anticipated drop in blood cell counts merits prophylactic use of antiviral prophylaxis and possibly neutropenic precautions. Management should be performed in conjunction with a hematologist or others knowledgeable in radiation illness.

Potassium iodide has been considered as a means of protecting thyroid function in the event of an acute population exposure to radiation [19]. This becomes useful primarily in the event of

Table 52.2 Biological effects of total body irradiation [16].

Amount of exposure	Effect
50 mGy (5 rads)	No detectable injury
1 Gy (100 rads)	Nausea and vomiting for 1–2 days, temporary drop in new blood cell production
3.5 Gy (350 rads)	Nausea and vomiting initially, followed by periods of apparent wellness. At 3–4 weeks, may see deficiencies of white blood cells and platelets
>3.5 Gy	May be fatal

exposure to radioactive iodine, which is typically present early in a nuclear explosion and decays rapidly. Radioactive iodine is potentially taken up by the thyroid gland and leads to destruction of the normal glandular tissue. Potassium iodide salt taken within the first 3–4 hours of an event saturates the thyroid gland's iodine uptake mechanism, blocking uptake of the radioactive form. Due to the quick decay of radioactive iodine, only a single dose is usually needed [19].

Because of the relatively greater activity of the thyroid gland in children, potassium iodide is recommended for children as well. Adults should receive one tablet or 130 mg. Children aged 3–18 are to receive one half-tablet (65 mg). Children aged 1–3 years receive 32 mg, and under 1 year of age, 16 mg is the recommended dose. The adult dose therapy is recommended for pregnant women, as the fetus is also susceptible. Women who are breast-feeding should also be given the usual adult dose, and the child should receive the appropriate dose based on age [19].

Unfortunately, high-dose radiation exposure can have severe effects on the developing fetus. Estimates of the risk of injury from ionizing radiation are based in part on reports from Hiroshima and Nagasaki following the atomic explosions there. Along with other data, a linear relationship has been used to estimate risks to the fetus from smaller exposures. While no direct evidence links exposure to diagnostic medical imaging tests with childhood cancers or birth defects [17,20], exposures from an intentional event could pose significant fetal risk due to a much higher dose of ionizing radiation.

In the case of the pre-implantation embryo, the most likely outcomes are either no detectable effect or complete loss of the embryo [17,20]. For example, an exposure of 10,000 millirads (mrads) is associated with a 2% risk of death for the pre-implantation embryo [20]. In the first trimester, the threshold for detecting an increased risk of birth defects, such as brain malformation or injury to the mid-face, teeth or genitalia, is 5000–25 000 mrad. Microcephaly, developmental delay, and cognitive impairment can occur with large exposures, (greater than 12 000–20 000 mrad) particularly between 8 and 15 weeks [17,20]. Developmental delay and impairment may occur later in the gestation, but at doses that would induce ARS in the mother. The expected risk of mental impairment in the fetus exposed to 100 rad (1 Gy) is approximately 40%, while the risk climbs to 60% with 150 rad of ionizing radiation [17].

Summary

Most new information on these described agents will likely come in the form of case reports from isolated exposures or events. Basic science research must continue to discover the complex microbiology of some of these agents, particularly as it is altered by pregnancy. The most critical immediate need is for systems preparation. A written, well-instructed triage and management plan, including back-up plans for communication and personnel, is a necessary first step. Collaboration between obstetricians and members of other relevant hospital departments, such as emergency medicine, critical care, and the first-response and transport teams, is essential. Helpful resources and training centers exist, including the Department of Energy-sponsored Radiation Emergency Assistance Center/Training Site (REAC/TS) program in Oak Ridge, Tennessee, and the Department of Homeland Security's Center for Domestic Preparedness in Anniston, Alabama.

References

1 Disaster management. In: Holleran RS, ed. *Air and Surface Patient Transport: Principles and Practice*, 3rd edn. St. Louis: Mosby, 2003.

2 Bleck TP. Fundamentals of disaster management. In: Farmer JC, Jimenez EJ, Talmor DS, Zimmerman JL, eds. *Fundamentals of Disaster Management*. Des Plaines, IL: Society of Critical Care Medicine, 2003: 1–8.

3 Moran GJ. Threats in bioterrorism II: CDC category B and C agents. *Emerg Med Clin N Am* 2002; 20: 311–330.

4 Darling RG, Catlett CL, Huebner KD, Jarrett DG. Threats in bioterrorism I: CDC category A agents. *Emerg Med Clin N Am* 2002; 20: 273–309.

5 Agrawal AG, O'Grady NP. Biologic agents and syndromes. In: Farmer JC, Jimenez EJ, Talmor DS, Zimmerman JL, eds. *Fundamentals of Disaster Management*. Des Plaines, IL: Society of Critical Care Medicine, 2003: 71–93.

6 Inglesby TV, O'Toole T, Henderson DA, Bartlett JG, Ascher MS, Eitzen E, et al. Anthrax as a biological weapon, 2002; updated recommendations for management. *JAMA* 2002; 287(17): 2236–2252.

7 White SR, Henretig FM, Dukes RG. Medical management of vulnerable populations and co-morbid conditions of victims of bioterrorism. *Emerg Med Clin N Am* 2002; 20: 365–392.

8 American College of Obstetricians and Gynecologists. Management of asymptomatic pregnant or lactating women exposed to anthrax. ACOG Committee Opinion No. 268. *Obstet Gynecol* 2002; 99: 366–368.

9 Wiesen AR, Littell CT. Relationship between prepregnancy anthrax vaccination and pregnancy and birth outcomes among US army women. *JAMA* 2002; 287(12): 1556–1560.

10 Suarez VR, Hankins GDV. Smallpox and pregnancy: from eradicated disease to bioterrorist threat. *Obstet Gynecol* 2002; 100: 87–93.

11 Preston R. *The Hot Zone*. New York: Random House, 1994.

12 Raoult D, Fenollar F, Stein A. Q fever during pregnancy. *Arch Intern Med* 2002; 162: 701–704.

13 Mirarchi FL. CBRNE – Ricin. Available at www.emedicine.com/emerg/topic889.htm.

14 Evison D, Hinsley D, Rice P. Chemical weapons. *BMJ* 2002; 324: 332–335.

15 Lantz G, Talmor DS. Chemical agents and syndromes. In: Farmer JC, Jimenez EJ, Talmor DS, Zimmerman JL, eds. *Fundamentals of Disaster Management*. Des Plaines, IL: Society of Critical Care Medicine, 2003: 57–70.

16 Oak Ridge Institute for Science and Education, Radiation Emergency Assistance Center/Training Site. Guidance for Radiation Accident Management. Types of radiation exposure. Available at http://orise.orau.gov/reacts/guide/injury.htm. Retrieved January 7, 2007.

17 American College of Obstetricians and Gynecologists. Guidelines for diagnostic imaging during pregnancy. ACOG Committee Opinion No. 158, 1995. Available at www.acog.com/publications/committee_opinions/bco158.htm. Retrieved January 1, 2001.
18 Oak Ridge Institute for Science and Education, Radiation Emergency Assistance Center/Training Site. Guidance for Radiation Accident Management. Managing radiation emergencies: acute radiation syndrome. Available at http://orise.orau.gov/reacts/guide/syndrome.htm. Retrieved January 7, 2007.
19 Centers for Disease Control. Emergency Preparedness and Response. Radiation emergencies: potassium iodide. Available at www.bt.cdc.gov/radiation/ki.asp.
20 Miller JC. Risks from ionizing radiation in pregnancy. *Radiology Rounds* 2004; 2(2).

Index

Page numbers in *italics* represent figures, those in **bold** represent tables.